Transactions on Computational Science and Computational Intelligence

Computational Science (CS) and Computational Intelligence (CI) both share the same objective: finding solutions to difficult problems. However, the methods to the solutions are different. The main objective of this book series, "Transactions on Computational Science and Computational Intelligence", is to facilitate increased opportunities for cross-fertilization across CS and CI. This book series will publish monographs, professional books, contributed volumes, and textbooks in Computational Science and Computational Intelligence. Book proposals are solicited for consideration in all topics in CS and CI including, but not limited to, Pattern recognition applications; Machine vision; Brain-machine interface; Embodied robotics; Biometrics; Computational biology; Bioinformatics; Image and signal processing; Information mining and forecasting; Sensor networks; Information processing; Internet and multimedia; DNA computing; Machine learning applications; Multi-agent systems applications; Telecommunications; Transportation systems; Intrusion detection and fault diagnosis; Game technologies; Material sciences; Space, weather, climate systems, and global changes; Computational ocean and earth sciences; Combustion system simulation; Computational chemistry and biochemistry; Computational physics; Medical applications; Transportation systems and simulations; Structural engineering; Computational electro-magnetic; Computer graphics and multimedia; Face recognition; Semiconductor technology, electronic circuits, and system design; Dynamic systems; Computational finance; Information mining and applications; Astrophysics; Biometric modeling; Geology and geophysics; Nuclear physics; Computational journalism; Geographical Information Systems (GIS) and remote sensing; Military and defense related applications; Ubiquitous computing; Virtual reality; Agent-based modeling; Computational psychometrics; Affective computing; Computational economics; Computational statistics; and Emerging applications. For further information, please contact Mary James, Senior Editor, Springer, mary.james@springer.com.

More information about this series at http://www.springer.com/series/11769

Hamid R. Arabnia • Leonidas Deligiannidis
Hayaru Shouno • Fernando G. Tinetti
Quoc-Nam Tran
Editors

Advances in Computer Vision and Computational Biology

Proceedings from IPCV'20, HIMS'20, BIOCOMP'20, and BIOENG'20

Springer

Editors
Hamid R. Arabnia
Department of Computer Science
University of Georgia
Athens, GA, USA

Leonidas Deligiannidis
School of Computing and Data Sciences
Wentworth Institute of Technology
Boston, MA, USA

Hayaru Shouno
Graduate School of Information Science & Engineering
University of Electro-Communications
Chofu, Japan

Fernando G. Tinetti
Facultad de Informática - CIC PBA
Universidad Nacional de La Plata
La Plata, Argentina

Quoc-Nam Tran
Department of Computer Science
Southeastern Louisiana University
Hammond, LA, USA

ISSN 2569-7072 ISSN 2569-7080 (electronic)
Transactions on Computational Science and Computational Intelligence
ISBN 978-3-030-71050-7 ISBN 978-3-030-71051-4 (eBook)
https://doi.org/10.1007/978-3-030-71051-4

This Springer imprint is published by the registered company Springer Nature Switzerland AG
The registered company address is: Gewerbestrasse 11, 6330 Cham, Switzerland

Preface

It gives us great pleasure to introduce this collection of papers that were presented at the following international conferences: Image Processing, Computer Vision, and Pattern Recognition (IPCV 2020); Health Informatics and Medical Systems (HIMS 2020); Bioinformatics and Computational Biology (BIOCOMP 2020); and Biomedical Engineering and Sciences (BIOENG 2020). These four conferences were held simultaneously (same location and dates) at Luxor Hotel (MGM Resorts International), Las Vegas, USA, July 27–30, 2020. This international event was held using a hybrid approach, that is, "in-person" and "virtual/online" presentations and discussions.

This book is composed of seven parts. Parts I through III (composed of 21 chapters) include articles that address various challenges in the areas of Image Processing, Computer Vision, and Pattern Recognition (IPCV). Parts IV and V (composed of 29 chapters) present topics in the areas of Health Informatics and Medical Systems (HIMS). Part VI (composed of 14 chapters) includes articles in the areas of Bioinformatics and Computational Biology (BIOCOMP). Lastly, Part VII (composed of 4 chapters) discusses research topics in the areas of Biomedical Engineering and Sciences (BIOENG).

An important mission of the World Congress in Computer Science, Computer Engineering, and Applied Computing, CSCE (a federated congress to which this event is affiliated with) includes *"Providing a unique platform for a diverse community of constituents composed of scholars, researchers, developers, educators, and practitioners. The Congress makes concerted effort to reach out to participants affiliated with diverse entities (such as: universities, institutions, corporations, government agencies, and research centers/labs) from all over the world. The congress also attempts to connect participants from institutions that have* ***teaching*** *as their main mission with those who are affiliated with institutions that have* ***research*** *as their main mission. The congress uses a quota system to achieve its institution and geography diversity objectives."* By any definition of diversity, this congress is among the most diverse scientific meetings in the USA. We are proud to report that this federated congress had authors and participants from 54 different nations representing variety of personal and scientific experiences that arise from differences in culture and values.

The program committees (refer to subsequent pages for the list of the members of committees) would like to thank all those who submitted papers for consideration. About 47% of the submissions were from outside the USA. Each submitted paper was peer-reviewed by two experts in the field for originality, significance, clarity, impact, and soundness. In cases of contradictory recommendations, a member of the conference program committee was charged to make the final decision; often, this involved seeking help from additional referees. In addition, papers whose authors included a member of the conference program committee were evaluated using the double-blind review process. One exception to the above evaluation process was for papers that were submitted directly to chairs/organizers of pre-approved sessions/workshops; in these cases, the chairs/organizers were responsible for the evaluation of such submissions. The overall paper acceptance rate for regular papers was 17%; 12% of the remaining papers were accepted as short and/or poster papers.

We are grateful to the many colleagues who offered their services in preparing this book. In particular, we would like to thank the members of the Program Committees of individual research tracks as well as the members of the Steering Committees of IPCV 2020, HIMS 2020, BIOCOMP 2020, and BIOENG 2020; their names appear in the subsequent pages. We would also like to extend our appreciation to over 500 referees.

As Sponsors-at-large, partners, and/or organizers, each of the following (separated by semicolons) provided help for at least one research track: Computer Science Research, Education, and Applications (CSREA); US Chapter of World Academy of Science; American Council on Science and Education & Federated Research Council; and Colorado Engineering Inc. In addition, a number of university faculty members and their staff, several publishers of computer science and computer engineering books and journals, chapters and/or task forces of computer science associations/organizations from 3 regions, and developers of high-performance machines and systems provided significant help in organizing the event as well as providing some resources. We are grateful to them all.

We express our gratitude to all authors of the articles published in this book and the speakers who delivered their research results at the congress. We would also like to thank the following: UCMSS (Universal Conference Management Systems & Support, California, USA) for managing all aspects of the conference; Dr. Tim Field of APC for coordinating and managing the printing of the programs; the staff of Luxor Hotel (MGM Convention) for the professional service they provided; and Ashu M. G. Solo for his help in publicizing the congress. Last but not least, we would like to thank Ms. Mary James (Springer Senior Editor in New York) and Arun Pandian KJ (Springer Production Editor) for the excellent professional service they provided for this book project.

Athens, USA — Hamid R. Arabnia
Boston USA — Leonidas Deligiannidis
Chofu Japan — Hayaru Shouno
La Plata Argentina — Fernando G. Tinetti
Hammond USA — Quoc-Nam Tran
Savannah, Georgia, USA — Ray Hashemi
Savannah, Georgia, USA — Azita Bahrami

Image Processing, Computer Vision, and Pattern Recognition

IPCV 2020 – Program Committee

- *Prof. Emeritus Nizar Al-Holou (Congress Steering Committee); ECE Department; Vice Chair, IEEE/SEM-Computer Chapter; University of Detroit Mercy, Detroit, Michigan, USA*
- *Dr. Mahmood Al-khassaweneh; University of Detroit Mercy, Detroit, Michigan, USA*
- *Prof. Emeritus Hamid R. Arabnia (Congress Steering Committee); Department of Computer Science, The University of Georgia, USA; Editor-in-Chief, Journal of Supercomputing (Springer); Fellow, Center of Excellence in Terrorism, Resilience, Intelligence & Organized Crime Research (CENTRIC)*
- *Dr. Azita Bahrami (Vice-Chair); President, IT Consult, USA*
- *Prof. Dr. Juan-Vicente Capella-Hernandez; Universitat Politecnica de Valencia (UPV), Department of Computer Engineering (DISCA), Valencia, Spain*
- *Prof. Juan Jose Martinez Castillo; Director, The Acantelys Alan Turing Nikola Tesla Research Group and GIPEB, Universidad Nacional Abierta, Venezuela*
- *Prof. Emeritus Kevin Daimi (Congress Steering Committee); Department of Mathematics, Computer Science and Software Engineering, University of Detroit Mercy, Detroit, Michigan, USA*
- *Prof. Zhangisina Gulnur Davletzhanovna; Vice-rector of the Science, Central-Asian University, Kazakhstan, Almaty, Republic of Kazakhstan; Vice President of International Academy of Informatization, Kazskhstan, Almaty, Republic of Kazakhstan*
- *Prof. Leonidas Deligiannidis (Congress Steering Committee); Department of Computer Information Systems, Wentworth Institute of Technology, Boston, Massachusetts, USA*
- *Dr. Trung Duong; Research Faculty at Center for Advanced Infrastructure and Transportation (CAIT), Rutgers University, the State University of New Jersey, New Jersey, USA*

- *Prof. Fernando G. Tinetti (Congress Steering Committee); School of CS, Universidad Nacional de La Plata, La Plata, Argentina; also at Comision Investigaciones Cientificas de la Prov. de Bs. As., Argentina*
- *Prof. Hahanov Vladimir (Congress Steering Committee); Vice Rector, and Dean of the Computer Engineering Faculty, Kharkov National University of Radio Electronics, Ukraine and Professor of Design Automation Department, Computer Engineering Faculty, Kharkov; IEEE Computer Society Golden Core Member; National University of Radio Electronics, Ukraine*
- *Dr. Haoxiang Harry Wang (CSCE); Cornell University, Ithaca, New York, USA; Founder and Director, GoPerception Laboratory, New York, USA*
- *Prof. Shiuh-Jeng Wang (Congress Steering Committee); Director of Information Cryptology and Construction Laboratory (ICCL) and Director of Chinese Cryptology and Information Security Association (CCISA); Department of Information Management, Central Police University, Taoyuan, Taiwan; Guest Ed., IEEE Journal on Selected Areas in Communications.*
- *Prof. Layne T. Watson (Congress Steering Committee); Fellow of IEEE; Fellow of The National Institute of Aerospace; Professor of Computer Science, Mathematics, and Aerospace and Ocean Engineering, Virginia Polytechnic Institute & State University, Blacksburg, Virginia, USA*
- *Prof. Jane You (Congress Steering Committee); Associate Head, Department of Computing, The Hong Kong Polytechnic University, Kowloon, Hong Kong*

Health Informatics & Medical Systems

HIMS 2020 – Program Committee

- *Prof. Abbas M. Al-Bakry (Congress Steering Committee); University President, University of IT and Communications, Baghdad, Iraq*
- *Prof. Emeritus Nizar Al-Holou (Congress Steering Committee); Electrical & Computer Engineering Department; Vice Chair, IEEE/SEM-Computer Chapter; University of Detroit Mercy, Michigan, USA*
- *Prof. Emeritus Hamid R. Arabnia (Congress Steering Committee); Department of Computer Science, The University of Georgia, USA; Editor-in-Chief, Journal of Supercomputing (Springer); Fellow, Center of Excellence in Terrorism, Resilience, Intelligence & Organized Crime Research (CENTRIC)*
- *Prof. Dr. Juan-Vicente Capella-Hernandez; Universitat Politecnica de Valencia (UPV), Department of Computer Engineering (DISCA), Valencia, Spain*
- *Prof. Juan Jose Martinez Castillo; Director, The Acantelys Alan Turing Nikola Tesla Research Group and GIPEB, Universidad Nacional Abierta, Venezuela*
- *Prof. Emeritus Kevin Daimi (Congress Steering Committee); Department of Mathematics, Computer Science and Software Engineering, University of Detroit Mercy, Detroit, Michigan, USA*
- *Prof. Zhangisina Gulnur Davletzhanovna; Vice-rector of the Science, Central-Asian University, Kazakhstan, Almaty, Republic of Kazakhstan; Vice President of International Academy of Informatization, Kazskhstan, Almaty, Republic of Kazakhstan*
- *Prof. Leonidas Deligiannidis (Congress Steering Committee); Department of Computer Information Systems, Wentworth Institute of Technology, Boston, Massachusetts, USA*
- *Prof. Mary Mehrnoosh Eshaghian-Wilner (Congress Steering Committee); Professor of Engineering Practice, University of Southern California, California, USA; Adjunct Professor, Electrical Engineering, University of California Los Angeles, Los Angeles (UCLA), California, USA*

- *Prof. Fernando G. Tinetti (Congress Steering Committee); School of Computer Science, Universidad Nacional de La Plata, La Plata, Argentina; also at Comision Investigaciones Cientificas de la Prov. de Bs. As., Argentina*
- *Prof. Quoc-Nam Tran (Congress Steering Committee); Department of Computer Science, Southeastern Louisiana University, Hammond, Louisiana, USA*
- *Prof. Hahanov Vladimir (Congress Steering Committee); Vice Rector, and Dean of the Computer Engineering Faculty, Kharkov National University of Radio Electronics, Ukraine and Professor of Design Automation Department, Computer Engineering Faculty, Kharkov; IEEE Computer Society Golden Core Member; National University of Radio Electronics, Ukraine*
- *Prof. Shiuh-Jeng Wang (Congress Steering Committee); Director of Information Cryptology and Construction Laboratory (ICCL) and Director of Chinese Cryptology and Information Security Association (CCISA); Department of Information Management, Central Police University, Taoyuan, Taiwan; Guest Ed., IEEE Journal on Selected Areas in Communications.*
- *Dr. Yunlong Wang; Advanced Analytics at QuintilesIMS, Pennsylvania, USA*
- *Prof. Layne T. Watson (Congress Steering Committee); Fellow of IEEE; Fellow of The National Institute of Aerospace; Professor of Computer Science, Mathematics, and Aerospace and Ocean Engineering, Virginia Polytechnic Institute & State University, Blacksburg, Virginia, USA*
- *Prof. Jane You (Congress Steering Committee); Associate Head, Department of Computing, The Hong Kong Polytechnic University, Kowloon, Hong Kong*
- *Dr. Farhana H. Zulkernine; Coordinator of the Cognitive Science Program, School of Computing, Queen's University, Kingston, ON, Canada*

Bioinformatics and Computational Biology

BIOCOMP 2020 – Program Committee

- *Prof. Abbas M. Al-Bakry (Congress Steering Committee); University President, University of IT and Communications, Baghdad, Iraq*
- *Prof. Emeritus Nizar Al-Holou (Congress Steering Committee); Electrical and Computer Engineering Department; Vice Chair, IEEE/SEM-Computer Chapter; University of Detroit Mercy, Michigan, USA*
- *Prof. Emeritus Hamid R. Arabnia (Congress Steering Committee); Department of Computer Science, The University of Georgia, USA; Editor-in-Chief, Journal of Supercomputing (Springer); Fellow, Center of Excellence in Terrorism, Resilience, Intelligence & Organized Crime Research (CENTRIC)*
- *Prof. Hikmet Budak; Professor and Winifred-Asbjornson Plant Science Chair Department of Plant Sciences and Plant Pathology Genomics Lab, Montana State University, Bozeman, Montana, USA; Editor-in-Chief, Functional and Integrative Genomics; Associate Editor of BMC Genomics; Academic Editor of PLosONE*
- *Prof. Emeritus Kevin Daimi (Congress Steering Committee); Department of Mathematics, Computer Science and Software Engineering, University of Detroit Mercy, Detroit, Michigan, USA*
- *Prof. Leonidas Deligiannidis (Congress Steering Committee); Department of Computer Information Systems, Wentworth Institute of Technology, Boston, Massachusetts, USA*
- *Prof. Youping Deng (Congress Steering Committee); Professor & Director of Bioinformatics Core, Department of Complementary & Integrative Medicine; Co-Director, Genomics Shared Resource, University of Hawaii Cancer Center, University of Hawaii John A. Burns School of Medicine, Honolulu, Hawaii, USA*
- *Dr. Lamia Atma Djoudi (Chair, Doctoral Colloquium & Demos Sessions); France*
- *Prof. Mary Mehrnoosh Eshaghian-Wilner (Congress Steering Committee); Professor of Engineering Practice, University of Southern California, California,*

- *Prof. Shiuh-Jeng Wang (Congress Steering Committee); Director of Information Cryptology and Construction Laboratory (ICCL) and Director of Chinese Cryptology and Information Security Association (CCISA); Department of Information Management, Central Police University, Taoyuan, Taiwan; Guest Ed., IEEE Journal on Selected Areas in Communications.*
- *Prof. Layne T. Watson (Congress Steering Committee); Fellow of IEEE; Fellow of The National Institute of Aerospace; Professor of Computer Science, Mathematics, and Aerospace and Ocean Engineering, Virginia Polytechnic Institute & State University, Blacksburg, Virginia, USA*
- *Prof. Mary Yang (Steering Committee, BIOCOMP); Director, Mid-South Bioinformatics Center and Joint Bioinformatics Ph.D. Program, Medical Sciences and George W. Donaghey College of Engineering and Information Technology, University of Arkansas, USA*
- *Prof. Jane You (Congress Steering Committee); Associate Head, Department of Computing, The Hong Kong Polytechnic University, Kowloon, Hong Kong*
- *Dr. Wen Zhang; Icahn School of Medicine at Mount Sinai, New York City, Manhattan, New York, USA; Board member, Journal of Bioinformatics and Genomics; Board member, Science Research Association*
- *Dr. Hao Zheng; Novo Vivo, VP of Bioinformatics, California, USA*

Biomedical Engineering and Sciences

BIOENG 2020 – Program Committee

- *Prof. Emeritus Nizar Al-Holou (Congress Steering Committee); ECE Department; Vice Chair, IEEE/SEM-Computer Chapter; University of Detroit Mercy, Detroit, Michigan, USA*
- *Prof. Emeritus Hamid R. Arabnia (Congress Steering Committee); Department of Computer Science, The University of Georgia, USA; Editor-in-Chief, Journal of Supercomputing (Springer); Fellow, Center of Excellence in Terrorism, Resilience, Intelligence & Organized Crime Research (CENTRIC)*
- *Prof. Emeritus Kevin Daimi (Congress Steering Committee); Department of Mathematics, Computer Science and Software Engineering, University of Detroit Mercy, Detroit, Michigan, USA*
- *Prof. Leonidas Deligiannidis (Congress Steering Committee); Department of Computer Information Systems, Wentworth Institute of Technology, Boston, Massachusetts, USA*
- *Prof. Mary Mehrnoosh Eshaghian-Wilner (Congress Steering Committee); Professor of Engineering Practice, University of Southern California, California, USA; Adjunct Professor, Electrical Engineering, University of California Los Angeles, Los Angeles (UCLA), California, USA*
- *Prof. Ray Hashemi (Vice-Chair); College of Engineering and Computing, Georgia Southern University, Georgia, USA*
- *Prof. Byung-Gyu Kim (Congress Steering Committee); Multimedia Processing Communications Lab.(MPCL), Department of Computer Science and Engineering, College of Engineering, SunMoon University, South Korea*
- *Prof. Tai-hoon Kim; School of Information and Computing Science, University of Tasmania, Australia*
- *Prof. Dr. Guoming Lai; Computer Science and Technology, Sun Yat-Sen University, Guangzhou, P. R. China*
- *Dr. Muhammad Naufal Bin Mansor; Faculty of Engineering Technology, Department of Electrical, Universiti Malaysia Perlis (UniMAP), Perlis, Malaysia*

Contents

Part II Imaging Science – Detection, Recognition, and Tracking Methods

Part III Image Processing and Computer Vision – Novel Algorithms and Applications

Part I
Imaging Science and Applications of Deep Learning and Convolutional Neural Network

Evolution of Convolutional Neural Networks for Lymphoma Classification

Christopher D. Walsh and Nicholas K. Taylor

1 Introduction

Lymphoma is a haematological disease that is the tenth most common cause of death in the United Kingdom, with an overall incidence rate of approximately 18.3 cases per 100,000 people [1, p.3]. There are several subgroups of the disease. The two most common are Hodgkin's Lymphoma, which has approximately four known subtypes and Non-Hodgkin's Lymphoma, which has many more. The World Health Organisation revised its report on the classification of Lymphomas in 2016. They currently recognise over 60 subtypes of Non-Hodgkin's Lymphoma [2, p.2376]. Treatment usually involves immunotherapy, chemotherapy or radiotherapy either individually or in combination. Over recent decades, the survival rate of Lymphoma patients has improved dramatically. This improvement has taken place due to a better scientific understanding of the biology of the disease that researchers are rapidly transforming into type-specific and individualised therapies [1, p.4].

However, lymphoma does not easily fit into the standards developed for diagnosing solid cancers and requires a different approach to diagnose and classify. Haematoxylin and Eosin (H&E) stained biopsies are the only starting point for the histological diagnosis of suspected lymphoma [2]. Because of the difficulty in diagnosis and typing of these biopsies, the National Institute for Health and Care Excellence (NICE) and the National Cancer Action Team (NCAT) have laid down strict parameters for the classification of a tissue sample. They specify that sample typing should only be carried out by specialists in haematopathology. They require that a team of these specialists are assembled to serve each geographical region and cross-validation performed to ensure an accurate diagnosis. NICE and NCAT also

C. D. Walsh (✉) · N. K. Taylor
School of Mathematical and Computer Sciences, Heriot-Watt University, Edinburgh, UK
e-mail: c.walsh.1@research.gla.ac.uk; N.K.Taylor@hw.ac.uk

H. R. Arabnia et al. (eds.), *Advances in Computer Vision and Computational Biology*, Transactions on Computational Science and Computational Intelligence,
https://doi.org/10.1007/978-3-030-71051-4_1

specify that no more than 62 days must elapse between the patient presenting with symptoms and the commencement of treatment. Per the standards set by the Royal College of Pathologists, this means that the classification of these biopsies can take no more than 10–14 days from the time the sample taken from the patient.

The original guidance specified that each specialist pathology team covered a region with a population of 500,000. In 2012 due to NHS restructuring, NCAT issued an update that increased the population covered by each group to two million [1, p.5]. Due to the specialist knowledge required, tight deadlines for classification and increasing pressure on the NHS, it is recognised that, at present, not every region can meet the guidelines. Fewer can offer specialist diagnostics for all diseases within the lymphoma spectrum. Therefore, an automated and reproducible methodology could help to meet these standards.

In recent years, artificial neural networks (ANNs) have met and in some cases surpassed human-level accuracy at image recognition tasks. Several new network architectures have emerged that brought about this revolution; in particular, Convolutional Neural Networks. This improvement in accuracy indicates that ANNs have become increasingly relevant for medical image classification. There have already been encouraging successes in diagnosing solid cancer biopsies which merited the investigation into the application of ANNs to Lymphoma diagnosis and inspired this work.

2 Related Work

2.1 Artificial Neural Networks in Medical Diagnosis

Recent developments in deep neural networks along with a general increase in available computing power have presented a significant opportunity for the development of automated medical diagnosis. The following is a brief review of some of the relevant material to this work.

We found no prior work that expressly set out to investigate the effectiveness of lymphoma classification based on histopathological diagnosis using ANNs optimised with evolutionary algorithms. One of the closest pieces of work was a paper titled "Bioimage Classification with Handcrafted and Learned Features" published in March 2018 by L. Nanni et al. [3]. The paper investigated the effectiveness of a general-purpose bioimage classification system. They used and compared several methods of classification, mainly support vector machines, a hybrid convolutional network and support vector machine and purely convolutional approach. The networks were pre-trained on prior image data and repurposed to biological image classification. It is particularly relevant as one of the datasets used to test the classifier is the same as in this work. This allowed us to compare the test accuracy of our work with a human pathologist and another system with a similar goal. L. Nanni et al. tested their bioimage classification system on image data from source datasets ranging from 120×120 to 1600×1200 pixels. They pre-processed their data to reduce and standardise the dimensions to 128×128 pixels. The purely convolutional approach resulted in a validation accuracy of 71.20% on the lymphoma biopsy dataset [3, p.8].

Artificial Neural Networks have also been used in many other medical imaging tasks recently, one of the papers we reviewed was titled "Combining Convolutional Neural Network With Recursive Neural Network for Blood Cell Image Classification" by Liang et al. published in July 2018. Their work investigated the possibility of using recurrent neural networks to model the long-term dependence between key image features and classification. They combined a convolutional neural network and recurrent neural network to deepen the understanding of image content in sizeable medical image datasets. They pre-processed the data by rotating some of the images to increase the number of training instances. This approach achieved a validation accuracy of 90.79% [4, p.36194].

Another application of ANNs to medical diagnosis was "Applying Artificial Neural Networks to the Classification of Breast Cancer Using Infrared Thermographic Images" by Lessa et al. [5], published in 2016. They used multilayer feedforward networks with a FLIR thermal imaging camera to investigate the possibility of employing ANNs to identify breast cancer from the thermal data alone without using penetrating scans. Image masks were applied to the data to pick out specific regions of interest and remove unnecessary data and also converted the images to grey-scale. This approach achieved an 85% validation accuracy [5, p.1].

The success of Convolutional Networks in the reviewed work warranted further investigation into their application to Lymphoma classification, and to what extent Evolutionary Algorithms could optimise them for that task.

3 Approach

We aimed to test the feasibility of automatic classification of lymphomas using ANNs. Given the necessity for accuracy in classification, we also proposed to use Evolutionary Algorithms to optimise the Neural Networks. Therefore the research questions we sought to answer in this work were:

1. Can Artificial Neural Networks classify the subtype of a non-Hodgkin's lymphoma biopsy at a validation accuracy similar to experienced human pathologists?
2. Can Evolutionary Algorithms improve the network metrics of ANNs designed to classify non-Hodgkin's lymphoma?

3.1 Hypotheses

Given our aims and research questions, the following were our hypotheses:

- $H1_0$ **Null**: Artificial Neural Networks can classify the subtype of a non-Hodgkin's lymphoma biopsy at a validation accuracy similar to experienced human pathologists.
- $H1_1$ **Alternative**: Artificial Neural Networks can classify the subtype of a non-Hodgkin's lymphoma biopsy at a validation accuracy less than or greater than experienced human pathologists.
- $H2_0$ **Null**: Evolutionary Algorithms cannot alter the test accuracy of ANNs designed to classify non-Hodgkin's lymphoma.
- $H2_1$ **Alternative**: Evolutionary Algorithms can improve or worsen the test accuracy of ANNs designed to classify non-Hodgkin's lymphoma.

3.2 Overview

To test these hypotheses, we built a set of experiments to test the network accuracy and runtime as well as gather other quantitative metrics. We constructed two separate ANNs for comparison: a Feedforward Neural Network and a Convolutional Neural Network.

Before training and testing, the dataset was randomised and stratified. This process ensured that the networks received a representative sample of all classes within the dataset. The same prepared dataset was used across network types and variations in architecture configuration to ensure consistency. We iterated over the network design for many training runs of the two network types and evaluated how well each performed on the dataset based on the network metrics, mainly test accuracy and fitness.

We finally took the best architectures for the Convolutional and Feedforward networks and applied Evolutionary Algorithms to evolve an optimum set of weights to process this type of data and evaluated the results.

3.3 Network Evaluation Strategy

To evaluate each ANN prototype, we used k-fold Cross-validation to test the network accuracy and its ability to generalise to new data. This data was recorded for each network type and later used to answer the research questions and hypotheses. The details for how we applied k-fold Cross-Validation and the network metrics it generated is given below.

4 Materials and Methods

4.1 Dataset

The dataset chosen for this work was part of an image repository assembled by the US National Institute on Aging. Its purpose is to provide a benchmark when testing and analysing the performance of image analysis algorithms for biological imaging [6]. The dataset is composed of 374 images of Haematoxylin and Eosin stained tumour biopsies. Each instance of the dataset has been pre-labelled with the preparing pathologists classification of CLL, FL or MCL lymphoma. A randomly selected image from each class can be seen below in Fig. 1.

The samples were prepared across a variety of sites. Therefore the staining varies substantially across the dataset. The complete dataset is 1.5 Gb in size. Each image is 1388 by 1040 pixels, and there are 113 CLL, 139 FL and 122 MCL instances. The dataset classification benchmark was set at 85% test accuracy using the Wndchrm utility.

The dataset was made available by Elaine Jaffe and Nikita Orlov and was retrieved from and is available in full on the NIA website. More information about the dataset is available at https://ome.grc.nia.nih.gov/iicbu2008/lymphoma/index.html.

Several works used this dataset for classification research. The best-reported test accuracy using it *without* k-fold cross-validation was 97.33% [7]. The paper was titled "Towards Designing an Automated Classification of Lymphoma subtypes using Deep Neural Networks" and published in January of 2019. It used an Inception network rather than a purely convolutional one. These networks use convolutional layers with varying kernel sizes as well as connections between layers that allow some layers to be skipped depending on the input. Therefore 97.33% was the target benchmark for a single training run of the convolutional neural network augmented with evolutionary algorithms implemented in this work.

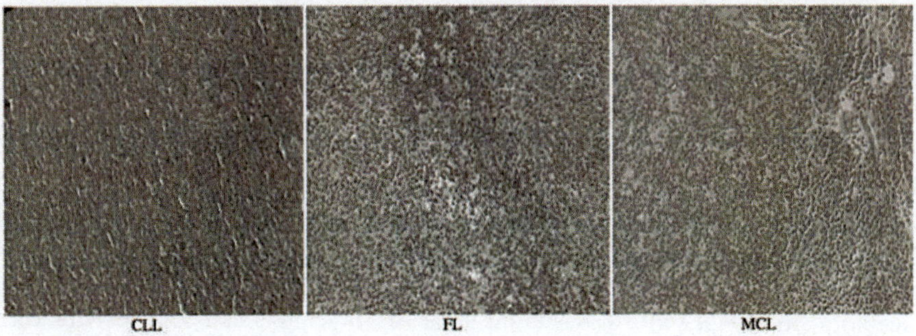

Fig. 1 Example dataset instances of FL, CLL, MCL

4.2 *Dataset Pre-processing*

This dataset contained a small number of samples. This is a common problem faced when training on medical image datasets. The generally accepted solution is to perform data augmentation. This technique increases the variation and number of training samples by rotating, mirroring and flipping the original images. This process has been shown to reduce overfitting due to a small sample set [8, p.41]. Therefore this was the first step in our pre-processing workflow.

As explained in the dataset description, the biopsy samples were prepared across a variety of sites by many pathologists. This variation resulted in a diverse range of stain colours. To account for this, we randomised the data so that any subset contained a representative variety of the possible variations in staining. We also stratified the dataset to ensure each of the three classes was presented to the networks in turn.

RGB images are encoded with pixel values in the range 0–255; therefore, normalisation was another step in our pre-processing workflow. We also split the dataset into training, validation and test sets.

4.3 *Artificial Neural Networks*

Feedforward Network

We began to design the network by reviewing research into medical image classification using Feedforward Networks; to identify the properties of successful architectures. Our first network was just the necessary three neurons in the output layer with a softmax activation function. This network had 12,991,683 trainable parameters due to the size of the images. This first design had a sizeable training loss which got larger as training continued indicating the network was not capable of learning the necessary features for classification. Y. Zhou et al. have shown that deeper networks with more significant numbers of neurons are better function approximators up to the point where overfitting happens [9, 1012]. Given this information, we decided to expand the network in breadth and depth.

Given the vast number of weights of even the most straightforward architecture, overfitting was going to be the most significant problem with this network type. Therefore we set out on a systematic search over the hyperparameters; learning rate, number of neurons, number of layers, batch size, normalisation, oversampling and image dimensionality, all while trying to minimise overfitting. The results and evaluation of this search are given below. The best network design achieved was a feedforward network with 128 neurons in the first layer, 64 in the second, with ReLu activation functions and three neurons in the output layer with a softmax activation function. One novel approach that we took to combat overfitting was to introduce a max-pooling layer after the input and hidden layers that reduced the dimensionality of the output of the previous layer by half.

Convolutional Network

We began to design the network architecture by reviewing current and past research into convolutional neural networks for image recognition; there had been a vast amount of work done in this area, including some for biopsy classification. However only a few papers had published work on lymphoma biopsy classification, and those that had were not merely a convolutional approach, some used hybrid convolutional and support vector machines, others used a residual convolutional network. We wanted to investigate the effectiveness of a purely convolutional network. Therefore we looked at the typical architecture of the best performing image classifiers based on these. We started our design based on Alex-Net [10]. This design was an eight-layer network with max-pooling layers after every second layer. The bottom three layers consisted of fully connected neurons. Given the dimensionality of the images in the dataset, the graphics card in use could not model the 2048 neurons present in each of them. After some initial testing, we decided to replace them with convolutional layers. The resulting network learned effectively; therefore, that was the design of our first base network.

We used this design for the search over the architecture choices and hyperparameters. The best performing network design was an eight-layer network, with 32 filters in the first two layers, 64 in the second two, 96 in the third pair and 128 in the final two layers with max-pooling layers after each layer pair. We used half-resolution images and ReLu activation functions. A diagram representing this architecture is available in Fig. 2.

4.4 Evolutionary Algorithms

Algorithm Design

We started our algorithm design by reviewing conventional methods of EA implementation. Tensorflow or Keras did not provide any evolutionary functionality;

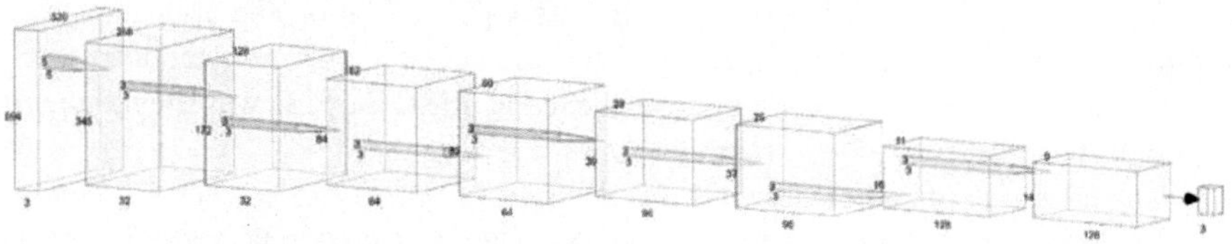

Fig. 2 Convolutional network architecture

consequently, we had to create it. From a review of the current literature, we decided to use a population-based algorithm. Specifically, we decided on a genetic algorithm. A genetic algorithm creates new generations by selecting a few parents at a time based on the ones with the best fitness and then creates new children using selection and crossover. Selection is made with replacement, so a few of the best performing parents can be used with multiple other favourable ones to produce better offspring. Other population methods use the whole population to create children. Therefore the best solutions are often diluted [11]. The pseudo-code for our chosen algorithm was provided by the book titled "the Essentials of Meta-heuristics" by Sean Luke. This was the basis for our evolutionary algorithm. It had to be adapted to work with the weights of a Convolutional Neural network by representing the weights as a vector for it to mutate.

5 Results

5.1 Feedforward Network

The first design choice investigated was the effect of data *normalisation*. Initially, a network with two layers was created, with two neurons in each layer. The Normalised dataset resulted in a maximum test accuracy of **45.83%** while the original images produced a maximum test accuracy of **33.33%**. This result revealed that the feedforward network could not learn without normalisation. Therefore the normalised dataset was used for the rest of this work.

The next design aspect studied was an *undersampled* dataset versus an *oversampled* one. The undersampled data reached a test accuracy of **44.72%** while the oversampled data reached a test accuracy of **46.03%**. The networks trained faster on the oversampled set and then seemed to generalise better. Given this result, the oversampled balanced dataset was used for the rest of the experiments.

We then varied the *number of neurons per layer*. Two hidden layers were used with an equal number of neurons in each layer. We began at one neuron per layer, then kept doubling the number of neurons until the memory required to run the training session exceeded the GPU memory. This occurred after only 128 neurons per layer. A graph of this search can be seen in Fig. 3. Test accuracy increased up until around 16 neurons per layers, then started to plateau and decreased around the 128 neuron mark. We reasoned that this was due to overfitting, therefore in order to reduce the number of trainable parameters while retaining the ability to learn, 128 neurons were left in the first layer and the second layer was reduced to 64. This resulted in the best test accuracy achieved at **73.02%**. This was the number of neurons used for subsequent training.

The next hyperparameter altered was the *number of layers*. We kept 128 neurons in the first layer and 64 in any further ones. We started from two layers and searched in increments up to twelve, again the limit of our machines graphics memory. A

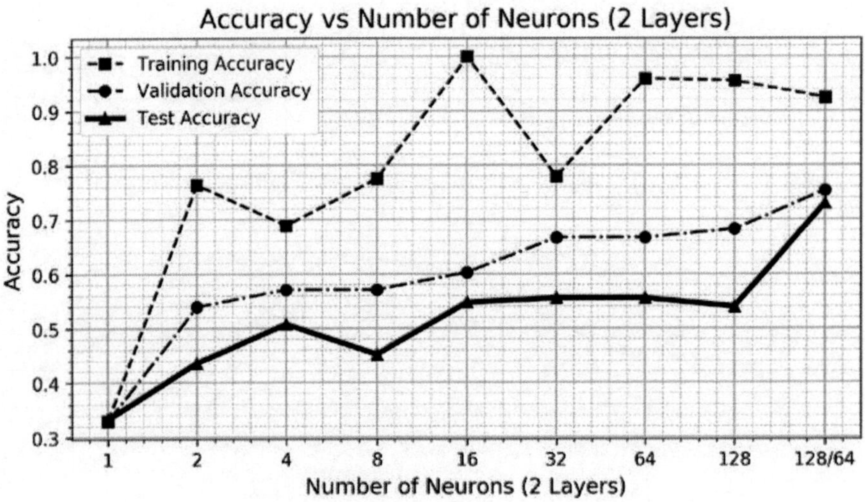

Fig. 3 Accuracy vs. number of neurons

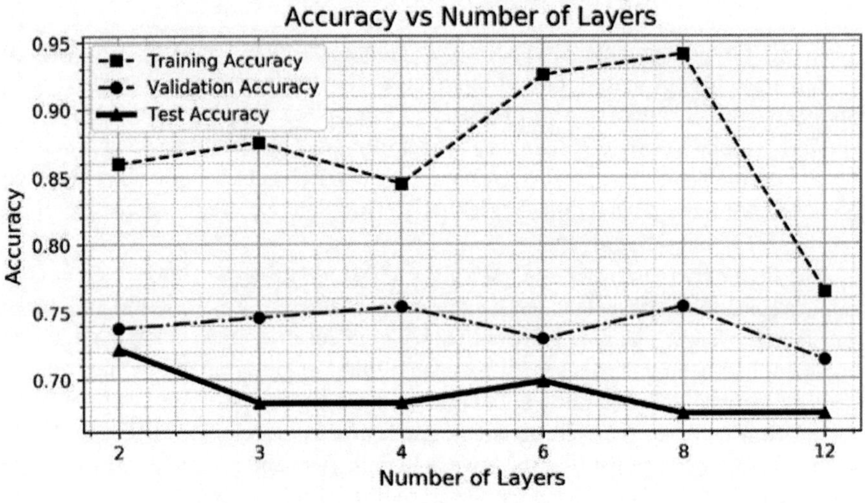

Fig. 4 Accuracy vs. number of layers

graph of this search is available in Fig. 4. In this case, it can be seen that all accuracy measures consistently decrease with an increasing number of layers. We attribute this result to overfitting, due to the much larger number of trainable parameters allowing the network to learn features too specific to each image and therefore poorly affecting generalisation and the ability to classify the test data correctly. Hence we continued the rest of the training with only two hidden layers before the output layer.

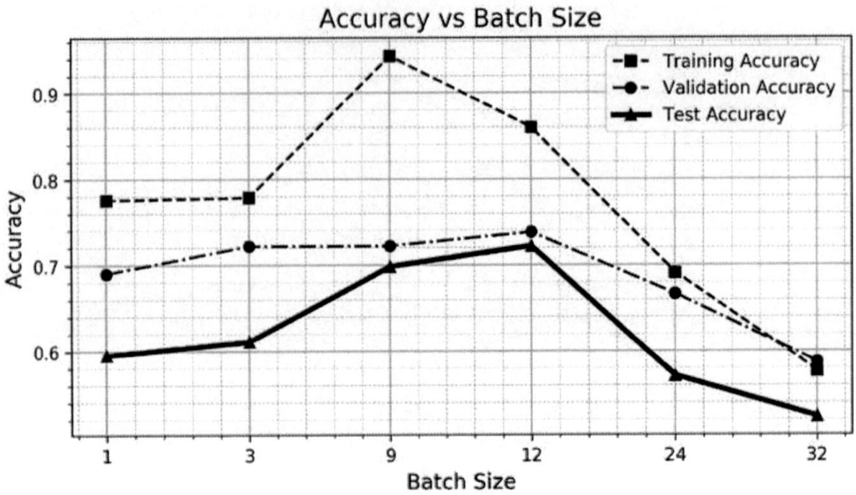

Fig. 5 Accuracy vs. batch size

Another hyperparameter studied was the *batch size* of the network. We chose to examine batch steps in multiples of three, given that we have three classes. A graph of accuracy over this search can be seen in Fig. 5. This graph shows that for this network, batch sizes smaller than the number of classes adversely affected accuracy. An increasing batch size improved accuracy up until a batch size of twelve at which point the accuracy started to decrease again. Therefore we used a batch size of 12 for the rest of the training runs.

The final hyperparameter studied for the Feedforward network was the learning rate. We started with a low learning rate to ensure the network did not make substantial weight changes and miss the global loss minima. Once a good test accuracy had been achieved, we investigated the possibility of shortening training time by increasing the learning rate while maintaining accuracy. We swept over the range from 0.001 to 0.1. The accuracy graph of this search is available in Fig. 6. There was an inverse relationship between learning rate and accuracy, the higher the learning rate, the lower the accuracy. Therefore we chose to continue with a learning rate of **0.001**.

K-Fold Cross-Validation and Confusion Matrix Analysis

Once a search over network design and hyperparameter choices had been performed, we moved onto k-fold cross-validation and confusion matrix analysis of the best performing feedforward network design. The goal was to evaluate how useful this type of network was at the given task of lymphoma biopsy classification.

Tenfold cross-validation was performed on feedforward model 2C; this was the 128-64-3 neuron network that had resulted in the best test accuracy of 73.02%. We

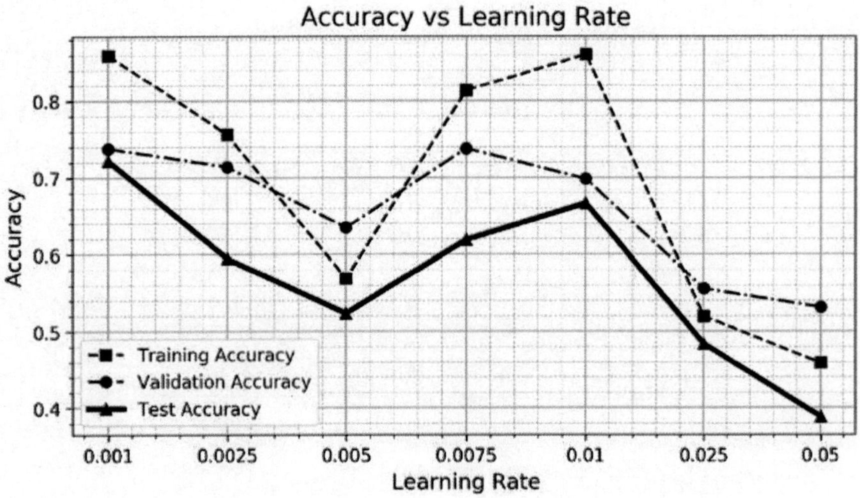

Fig. 6 Accuracy vs. learning rate

CLL (True)	259	51	110
FL (True)	64	318	38
MCL (True)	31	82	307
	CLL (Pred)	FL (Pred)	MCL (Pred))

Fig. 7 Tenfold cross-validation confusion matrix

created ten separate datasets, each consisting of training and test data. Each dataset had a separate 1/10th of the images to be used as test data, and ten separate networks were trained and evaluated. To avoid introducing bias to the results by averaging, we summed the confusion matrices and performed the analysis of the resulting data. That matrix is available below in Fig. 7. There were 42 members of each class in the test datasets. Given that there were ten separate folds, 420 members of each class were classified.

From this confusion matrix, we calculated several values that allowed us to evaluate how effective this classifier was at the task. The key metrics that we examined are *Sensitivity*; this represents the proportion of each class that was correctly identified by the network. Another is *Specificity* that measures the proportion of true-negatives that are correctly identified. Along with the *false-negative* and *false-positive rate*, these are critical metrics for medical diagnosis, particularly in this biopsy classification task when the cost of misdiagnosis is so high. The calculated values for this network are available in Fig. 8.

From this table we can see that the test accuracy for this network using Tenfold cross-validation was **70.16%**. A more revealing metric is the calculated Kappa value, which compares the classifier with random chance and the correct classifications. The Kappa metric ranges in value from −1 to 1. A kappa value below

Network Metric	Value		
Accuracy	70.16%		
Error	29.84%		
Kappa	0.5524		
Class Metrics	**CLL**	**FL**	**MCL**
Accuracy	79.68%	81.34%	79.23%
Area under ROC Curve	75.18%	79.94%	77.74%
Sensitivity	61.67%	75.71%	73.09%
Specificity	88.69%	84.17%	82.38%
False-Positive Rate	11.31%	15.83%	17.62%
False-Negative Rate	38.33%	24.28%	26.91%

Fig. 8 Confusion matrix metrics

zero would indicate the classifier was performing worse than random chance, and 1 indicates it is in complete agreement with the correct data labels [12]. Therefore the kappa value of 0.5524 for this network indicates it is performing around 55% better than if the network was randomly assigning the values; however, in the medical community a diagnostic test is only considered valuable if it has a Kappa value above 0.8 and ideally above 0.9 [13].

Another critical metric is the ROC Curve values, which calculate the area under the curve of values generated by plotting the true-positive rate against the false-positive rate. This is a plot of Sensitivity, vs (1-specificity) so it takes into account several metrics. Again for a diagnostic test to be considered of good quality, it would need to be above 0.9 [14], and this network ranges from 0.75 to 0.77, placing it in the "fair" range, but not suitable for reliable diagnostic tests. The ROC curves for this feedforward network are available in the appendix.

Evaluating the Sensitivity of the classifier, it performs best on Mantle Cell lymphoma correctly identifying it 73.09% of the time. It performs worst on Chronic Lymphocytic Leukaemia, only correctly classifying it 61.67% of the time. Evaluating the Specificity of the classifier shows that it performs best on CLL, correctly identifying when a sample is not CLL 88.69% of the time and worst on MCL at only 82.38%. These specificity values are much closer to the medical standards for Sensitivity and Specificity of greater than 0.9 [15].

Analysing the false-positive and negative rate of this classifier reveals that it incorrectly classifies a sample as MLC in 17.62% of cases, the highest false-positive rate, and identifies it as not MCL in only 26.91% of cases the lowest false-negative rate. This shows that the classifier is biased towards predicting MCL and biased against CLL, which has the lowest false-positive rate at 11.31% and the highest false-negative rate of 38.33%.

5.2 Convolutional Network

For the CNN, normalisation was investigated by the creation of two datasets for comparison. We used our base 8-layer network for this test. The un-normalised data resulted in a maximum test accuracy of **33.33%**, which is equivalent to random chance on a three-class dataset. The normalised dataset produced an accuracy of **89.68%**. Therefore we chose to normalise the dataset for the rest of the training sessions.

Kernel Size was investigated by sweeping over a range of values. We started with 1×1 kernels, and we initially wanted to sweep up to 24×24; however, we again ran into graphics memory limitations at 4×4 filters. A graph of training, validation and test accuracy over this search can be seen in Fig. 9.

The accuracy steadily increased with a larger filter size; we attribute this to the way convolutional networks recognise features. They do this through the filters recognising small image features in upper layers and building more abstract concepts as information is passed down through the layers. Given the relatively large dimensions of these images, this process worked better over a larger number of pixels. This improvement happens as while the biopsy features are small, the high pixel density of these images means the pertinent features range over many pixels. Therefore larger kernel sizes can more effectively learn features within the image. The best test accuracy of **93.65%** resulted from a **4x4** kernel; therefore, this was the kernel size we used in the rest of our network designs.

For the CNN, the batch size was examined in multiples of three, ranging from 1 to 33. A graph of accuracy over batch size is available in Fig. 10. An increased accuracy up to a batch size of 6 was observed, then decreasing after

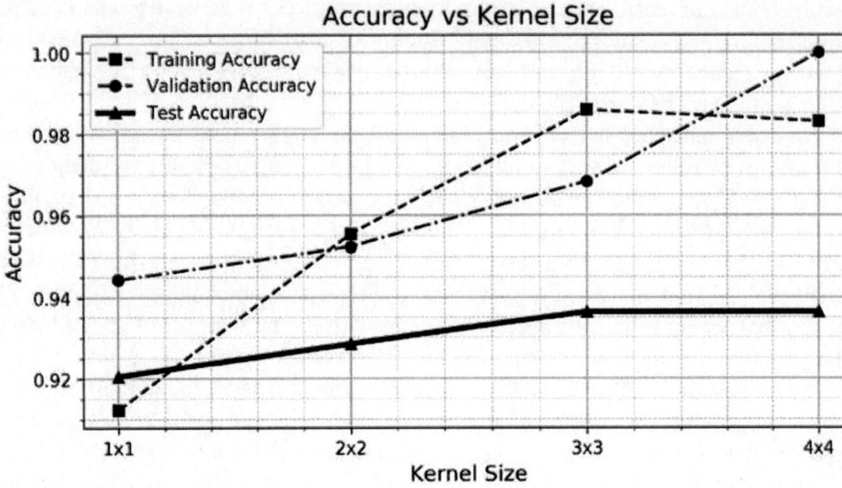

Fig. 9 Accuracy vs. Kernel size

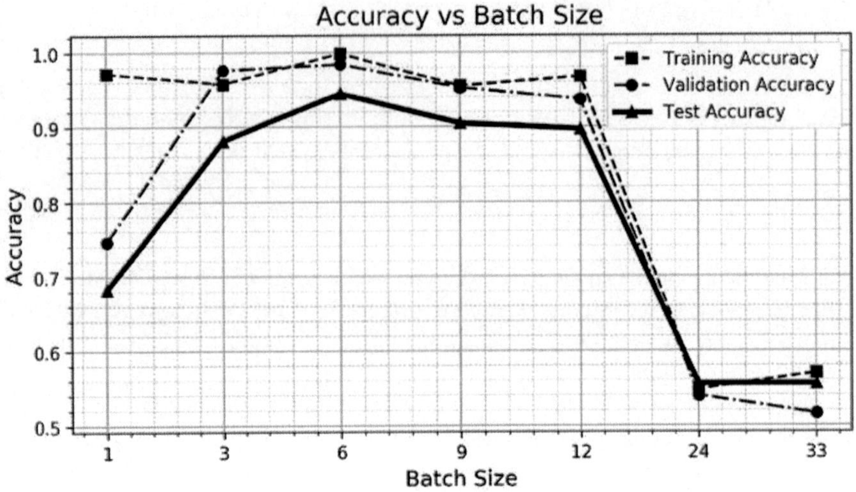

Fig. 10 Accuracy vs. batch size

that. Interestingly this is half the batch size of a Feedforward network; this suggests that smaller steps during backpropagation are crucial for the Convolutional Neural Network to learn effectively. Therefore we used a batch size of **6** for the rest of our training runs.

Sampling type was investigated by creating two datasets, a stratified *oversampled* and stratified *undersampled* one. The undersampled dataset reached a test accuracy of **94.44%** and the oversampled dataset reached **96.83%**. As with the feedforward network, we attribute this improvement to the larger number of training samples available within each epoch. The networks seemed to generalise better with oversampling, indicating that a small amount of it to balance class sample sizes does not induce overfitting and can improve results. Therefore, we implemented oversampling in the rest of the datasets.

Convolutional Neural Networks train most effectively with many layers, with the number of filters increasing in subsequent layers [16]. Therefore we decided to investigate how the number of filters per layer affects accuracy by using one filter in the first layer and doubling the number of filters every two layers. We created six models in total with 1 through 32 filters in the first layer and 8 to 128 in the final layer. A graph of accuracy over these models is available in Fig. 11. This graph shows that accuracy steadily increased along with the number of filters, including the largest model that our graphics card could successfully train. This network had 32-32-64-64-96-96-128-128 filters. It produced the best test accuracy of the CNN alone at **96.03%**. This result suggests that a larger number of filters and a deeper network are more effective up until overfitting occurs. In this case, we ran into graphics memory limitations before the filters became numerous enough to induce overfitting.

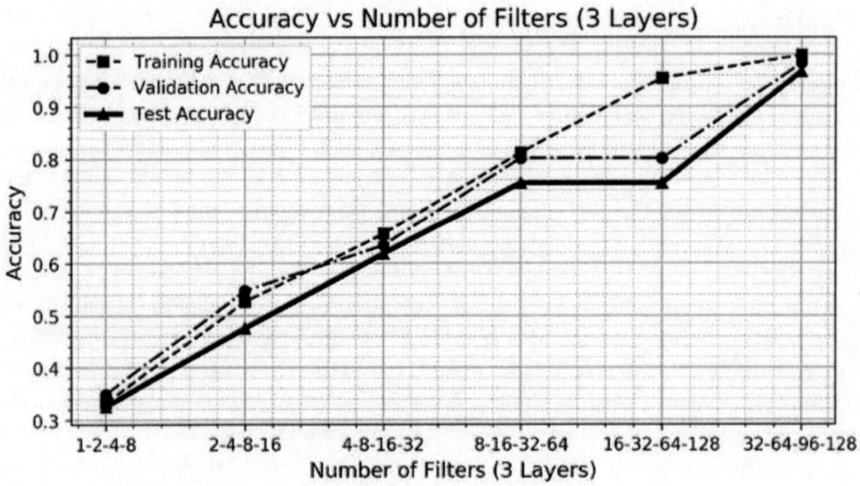

Fig. 11 Accuracy vs. number of filters

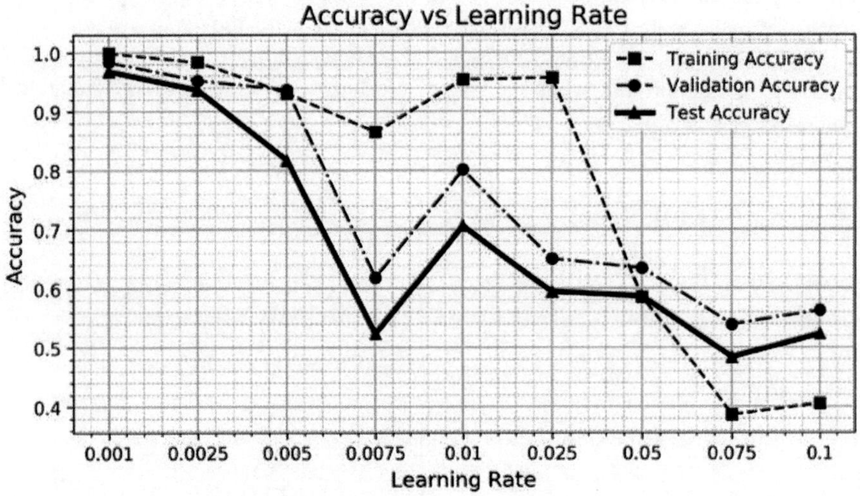

Fig. 12 Accuracy vs. learning rate

For the CNN, a low learning rate was used to ensure the network was not making too significant a change to its weights and missing a global loss minima. Now that a good test accuracy had been established, we wanted to investigate the possibility of reducing training time by increasing the learning rate while maintaining accuracy. We swept over the range from 0.001 to 0.1. The accuracy graph of this search is available in Fig. 12. There was an inverse relationship between learning rate and accuracy, the higher the learning rate, the lower the accuracy. Therefore we chose to continue with a learning rate of **0.001**.

K-Fold Cross-Validation and Confusion Matrix Analysis

Once an optimised network design had been created, we carried out k-fold cross-validation and confusion matrix analysis. The aim of this was to evaluate how useful this network would be at the given task of lymphoma biopsy classification.

Tenfold cross-validation was performed on convolutional model 2E; this was the 32-32-64-64-96-96-128-128 filter network that had resulted in the best test accuracy of 96.03%. We created ten separate datasets, each consisting of training and test data. Each dataset had a separate 1/10th of the images to be used as test data, and ten separate networks were trained and evaluated. To avoid introducing bias to the results by averaging, we summed the confusion matrices and performed the analysis of the resulting data. That confusion matrix is available below in Fig. 13. There were 42 members of each class in the test datasets. Given that there were ten separate folds, 420 members of each class were classified for this evaluation.

From this confusion matrix, we calculated several values that allowed us to evaluate the effectiveness of this classifier. The key metrics that we examined were *Sensitivity*; this represents the proportion of each class that was correctly identified by the network. Another is *Specificity*; it measures the proportion of true-negatives that are correctly identified. These, along with the *False-Negative* and *False-Positive rate*, are critical metrics for medical diagnosis, particularly in this biopsy classification task when the cost of misdiagnosis is so high. The calculated values for this network are available in Fig. 14.

CLL (True)	373	7	40
FL (True)	0	405	15
MCL (True)	26	9	385
	CLL (Pred)	FL (Pred)	MCL (Pred)

Fig. 13 Tenfold cross-validation confusion matrix

Network Metric	Value
Accuracy	92.30%
Error	7.69%
Kappa	0.8845

Class Metrics	CLL	FL	MCL
Accuracy	91.21%	97.54%	92.86%
Area under ROC Curve	92.85%	97.26%	92.56%
Sensitivity	88.81%	96.43%	91.67%
Specificity	96.91%	98.10%	93.45%
False Positive Rate	3.10%	1.91%	6.54%
False Negative Rate	11.19%	3.57%	8.33%

Fig. 14 Confusion matrix metrics

The test accuracy for this network calculated from tenfold cross-validation was **92.30%**. A Kappa value below zero would indicate the classifier was performing worse than random chance, and 1 indicates it is in perfect agreement with the correct data labels [12]. Therefore the kappa value of 0.8845 for this network indicates it is performing around 88% better than if the network was randomly assigning the class values. In the medical community, a diagnostic test is considered valuable if it has a Kappa value above 0.8 and ideally above 0.9 [13].

Another key metric is the area under the ROC Curve. Again for a medical diagnostic test to be considered of good quality, it should have an area under the curve above 0.9 [14] or 90%. This networks ROC curve areas range from 92.56 to 97.26%, placing it in the "Excellent" range, suitable for reliable diagnostic tests.

When evaluating Sensitivity, the classifier performed best on Follicular Lymphoma (FL), correctly identifying it 98.10% of the time. It performed worst on Chronic Lymphocytic Leukaemia (CLL), only correctly classifying it 88.81% of the time. Evaluating the Specificity of the classifier shows that it performs best on FL, correctly identifying when a sample is not FL 98.10% of the time and worst on Mantle Cell Lymphoma (MCL) at only 93.45%. The medical standards for Sensitivity and Specificity are that a test is reliable when it has values for each, higher than 0.9 or 90% [15]. Therefore all but one value meets this threshold. Only the CLL Sensitivity value is below 90%. It is interesting to note that this is the class with the least amount of original examples in the dataset.

Analysing the false-positive and -negative rate of this classifier reveals that it incorrectly classifies a sample as CLL in 6.54% of cases, the highest false-positive rate. It identifies a sample as not CLL in 11.19% of cases the highest false-negative rate. This outcome shows that the classifier is biased in predicting MCL, and biased against CLL. It is worth noting that this is the same result as was discovered in the Feedforward network.

5.3 Evolutionary Algorithm: Genetic Algorithm

The following describes the work we carried out for the optimisation of the genetic algorithm. To ensure consistency, we used the same set of starting weights and the same dataset for all parameter investigations. We also always evolved convolutional model 2E with a kernel size of 4.

A range of mutation rates were investigated, and each network was repeatedly evolved using each rate and the results averaged. A graph of percentage increase in test accuracy after evolution is available in Fig. 15. The accuracy increase improved with lower mutation rates down to 0.005, then at 0.00025, it worsened. The 0.001 and 0.0005 mutation rates resulted in the best increase in accuracy at a 4.87% improvement. We attribute the improved accuracy with a lower mutation rate to the fact that the network was pre-trained. Therefore only slight variations in the weights

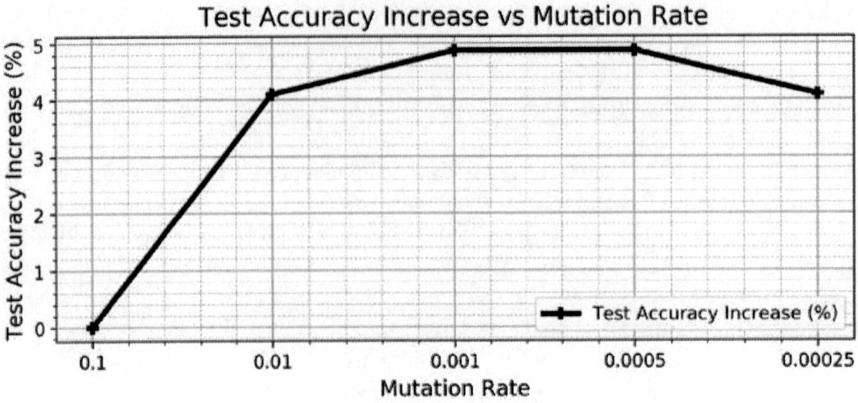

Fig. 15 Test accuracy increase vs. mutation rate

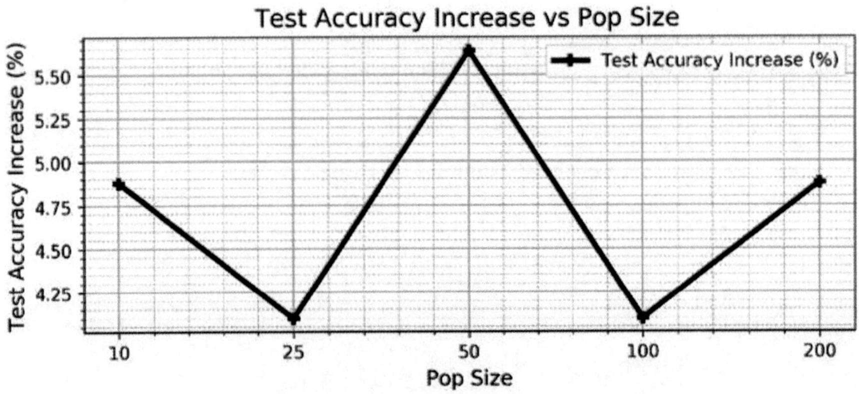

Fig. 16 Test accuracy increase vs. population size

were necessary to improve accuracy; significant changes would adversely affect it. The decrease in accuracy with a mutation rate smaller than 0.00025 is presumably because the lower rate was not altering the weights by a sufficient amount within the allotted number of generations. Given the length of time demanded by the evolutionary process, we settled on the highest mutation rate with the best accuracy at 0.001.

The effect of population size was studied by iterating over a range of population sizes and repeatedly evolving the network over each size and averaging the results. A graph of percentage increase in test accuracy after each evolution is shown in Fig. 16. There was not a correlation between population size and accuracy. Accuracy fluctuated over the range; therefore, we used the best performing population size of 50 for the rest of the evolutions.

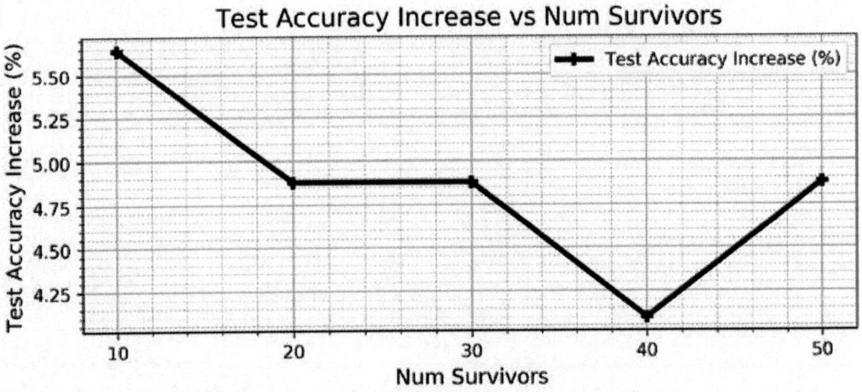

Fig. 17 Test accuracy increase vs. number of survivors per generation

A range of survivors per generation were investigated, and each network was repeatedly evolved using varying numbers, and the results averaged. A graph of accuracy increase vs the number of survivors is shown in Fig. 17.

In this instance, there was a correlation. The improvement in accuracy decreased with an increased number of survivors per generation. We attribute this result to increased survivor numbers reducing the number of new "paths" a solution could take by increasing the number of individuals that have already reduced their loss by changing their weights in a certain way. An increased number of individuals surviving into the next generation reduces the number of children and therein that generations ability to mutate in a desirable direction on the cost curve. Therefore we used the best performing value and only allowed 10% of survivors into the next generation.

It should also be noted that we attempted to evolve the convolutional network weights from entirely random weight values to see if evolutionary algorithms could train the network without gradient descent. However, the test accuracy of these networks never reached far above 50%. We only left each test running for less than 24 h, so it is possible that given time they would have reached a higher accuracy. However, we found that the most efficient approach was to train first with gradient descent then optimise with the genetic algorithm.

K-Fold Cross-Validation and Confusion Matrix Analysis

With the optimised genetic algorithm, we evolved the ten sets of weights from the tenfold cross-validation on the CNN and performed confusion matrix analysis. The aim of this was to evaluate if evolutionary algorithms were a viable optimisation method for an Artificial Neural Network constructed for lymphoma biopsy classification.

CLL (True)	402	2	16
FL (True)	0	409	11
MCL (True)	20	6	394
	CLL (Pred)	FL (Pred)	MCL (Pred)

Fig. 18 Tenfold cross-validation confusion matrix

Fig. 19 Confusion matrix metrics

Network Metric	Value		
Accuracy	95.64%		
Error	4.36%		
Kappa	0.9345		
Class Metrics	**CLL**	**FL**	**MCL**
Accuracy	96.98%	98.49%	95.79%
Area under ROC Curve	96.67%	98.21%	95.29%
Sensitivity	95.71%	97.38%	93.81%
Specificity	97.61%	99.04%	96.78%
False Positive Rate	2.38%	0.95%	3.21%
False Negative Rate	4.28%	2.62%	6.19%

We evaluated the test accuracy using only the original datasets corresponding to each set of weights. By partnering the weights with their original datasets, we ensured that no evolved weights had their test accuracy evaluated on any data to which they had already been exposed. To avoid introducing bias to any of the results by averaging, we summed the confusion matrices for all of the evolutionary runs. The analysis was performed on the resulting matrix. That confusion matrix is available below in Fig. 18. There were 42 members of each class in the test datasets. Given that there were ten separate folds, 420 members of each class were classified for this evaluation.

From this confusion matrix, we calculated several values that allowed us to evaluate the effectiveness of this classifier. The key metrics that we examined were *Sensitivity*; this represents the proportion of each class that was correctly identified by the network. Another is *Specificity*; it measures the percentage of true-negatives that are correctly identified. These, along with the *False-Negative* and *False-Positive rate*, are critical metrics for medical diagnosis, particularly in this biopsy classification task when the cost of misdiagnosis is so high. The calculated values for this network are available in Fig. 19.

The test accuracy after evolution was **95.64%**. The Kappa value calculated was 0.9345. This value compares how the classifier performed compared with random chance and the correct classifications. Therefore this value means it is performing around 93.45% better than if the evolved network was randomly assigning the class values. In the medical community, a diagnostic test is considered valuable if it has a Kappa value above 0.8 and excellent if the value is above 0.9 [13].

Another critical metric is the area under the ROC Curve, a graph generated by plotting the true-positive rate against the false-positive rate. This is a plot of Sensitivity, vs (1-specificity) so it takes into account several metrics. Again for a medical diagnostic test to be considered of good quality, it should have an area under the curve above 0.9 [14] or 90%. This evolved networks had ROC curve areas ranging from 92.29 to 98.21%, placing it in the "Excellent" range, and therefore deemed suitable for reliable diagnostic tests. The ROC curves for this evolved network are available in the appendix.

When evaluating Sensitivity; the classifier performed best on Follicular Lymphoma (FL), correctly identifying it 97.38% of the time, this is slightly lower than the purely convolutional network, so it seems some individual class accuracy has been sacrificed for overall accuracy here. It performed worst on Mantle Cell Lymphoma (MCL), only correctly classifying it 93.81% of the time. Evaluating the Specificity of the classifier shows that it performs best on FL, correctly identifying when a sample is not FL 99.04% of the time and worst on Mantle Cell Lymphoma (MCL) at only 96.78%. The medical standards for Sensitivity and Specificity are that a test is reliable when it has values for each that are greater than 0.9 or 90% [15]. Therefore all values for this evolved network are well above that threshold.

Analysing the false-positive and negative rate of this classifier reveals that it incorrectly classifies a sample as MCL 3.21% of the time, the highest false-positive rate. It identifies a sample as not MCL in 6.19% of cases the highest false-negative rate. This outcome shows that evolving the network weights has reduced the bias towards predicting MCL and also reduced the bias against CLL.

5.4 Statistical Significance Testing

Applying the *Wilcoxon Signed-Rank test* to the test accuracy before evolution vs after, results in a W+ of 55 and a W− of 0. The critical value of W is 5, at $N = 10$ with $\alpha = 0.05$. Therefore the smallest W is less than the critical value. The *p*-value is 0.00512, indicating that the result is statistically significant. We can reject our $H2_0$ null hypothesis for this network and accept the $H2_1$ alternative. In this case, the Evolved Classifier is significantly *better* than the original Convolutional Network alone. It resulted in an average improvement of 3.65%.

The *Wilcoxon Signed-Rank test* applied to the CNN test accuracy after evolution vs the mean human accuracy results in a W+ of 51 and a W− of 4. The critical value of W is 5, at $N = 10$ with $\alpha = 0.05$. Therefore the smallest W is less than the critical value. The *p*-value is 0.0164, indicating that the result is statistically significant. We can reject our $H1_0$ null hypothesis for this network and accept the $H1_1$ alternative. In this case, the Evolved CNN Classifier is significantly *better* than the mean human average.

6 Discussion

The goal of this work was to determine if it is possible to classify lymphoma biopsies at a similar accuracy to human pathologists, between 92 and 95%. The Feedforward class of ANN could not meet this standard. It was significantly worse than the average human accuracy. However, it did demonstrate that ANNs are capable of learning features of these biopsies, performing better than random chance. This outcome suggested the use of an ANN with the ability to learn image features without being fully connected, reinforcing our choice to use a Convolutional Neural Network in the second stage of this work which has a similar Feedforward architecture but with locally connected filters rather than fully connected neurons.

The best Convolutional Network architecture reached a test accuracy just above the lower end of the human range at 92.30% when evaluated with tenfold cross-validation. The best single run exceeded the upper range at 96.03%. The network Kappa, ROC curve, sensitivity and specificity values were all above or very close to medical standards. However, the results were not significantly better or worse than the mean human accuracy. We sought to determine if an increase was possible with some refinement of the network. This result led to the use of evolutionary algorithms to evolve pre-trained network weights in an attempt to increase test accuracy.

The lowest single run of the evolved Convolutional Network was 91.26%, just below the human range. The highest was 98.41%, well above human accuracy. When evaluated with tenfold cross-validation, the CNN reached a test accuracy of 95.64%, just above our human benchmark. The Kappa, ROC curve, sensitivity and specificity values were all well above the minimum for medical standards. Statistical analysis of the results showed it to be significantly better than average human accuracy, therein allowing rejection of our $H1_0$ null hypothesis and to accept the $H1_1$ alternative: that ANNs can classify the subtype of a non-Hodgkin's Lymphoma biopsy at a validation accuracy greater than experienced human pathologists.

The average increase in test accuracy after weight evolution was 3.65%. All other network metrics also improved from the previous stage. Statistical analysis showed it to be a significant improvement and this validated our $H2_1$ alternative hypothesis that Evolutionary Algorithms can improve the network metrics of ANNs designed to classify non-Hodgkin's lymphoma, and allowed the rejection of the $H2_0$ null hypothesis.

7 Conclusion

Lymphoma is a common disease that does not easily fit into the standards developed for diagnosing solid cancer biopsies [2]. The goal of this work was to answer the question: "Can Artificial Neural Networks classify lymphoma biopsies at a similar accuracy to humans?". We sought to provide a proof of concept for a future system that could ease the burden on healthcare systems through automation. The dataset of three Lymphoma subtypes published by the National Institute on Aging was used to evaluate the performance of two ANNs at this task. Evolutionary algorithms were then applied to the weights of the best performing network. The results gathered in this work suggest that Convolutional Neural Networks can classify a Lymphoma subtype at an accuracy similar to experienced human pathologists. Further to this, the Evolutionary Algorithm consistently improved test accuracy, increasing the CNN's test accuracy above the human range. This suggests that they are a strong optimisation technique on pre-trained convolutional network weights. Potential future work includes evaluating our method on larger datasets and applying it to the diagnosis of a more diverse range of Lymphoma subtypes.

References

1. D.S. Dojcinov, D.B. Wilkins, D.M. Calaminici, Standards for specialist laboratory integration for the histopathological reporting of lymphomas. The Royal College of Pathologists, Technical Report (2015)
2. S.H. Swerdlow, E. Campo, S.A. Pileri, N.L. Harris, H. Stein, R. Siebert, R. Advani, M. Ghielmini, G.A. Salles, A.D. Zelenetz, E.S. Jaffe, The 2016 revision of the world health organization classification of lymphoid neoplasms. Blood **127**(20), 2375–2390 *2016*. http://www.bloodjournal.org/content/127/20/2375
3. L. Nanni, S. Brahnam, S. Ghidoni, A. Lumini, Bioimage classification with handcrafted and learned features. IEEE/ACM Trans. Computat. Biol. Bioinf. **16**, 874–885 (2018). https://ieeexplore.ieee.org/document/8328839/
4. G. Liang, H. Hong, W. Xie, L. Zheng, Combining convolutional neural network with recursive neural network for blood cell image classification. IEEE Access **6**, 36188–36197 (2018). https://ieeexplore.ieee.org/document/8402091/
5. V. Lessa, M. Marengoni, Applying artificial neural network for the classification of breast cancer using infrared thermographic images, in *International Conference on Computer Vision and Graphics* (2016), pp. 429–438. http://link.springer.com/10.1007/978-3-319-46418-3_38
6. E.S. Jaffe (National Cancer Institute), N. Orlov (National Institute on Aging). Malignant lymphoma classification. https://ome.grc.nia.nih.gov/iicbu2008/lymphoma/index.html
7. M. Agrawal, U. Shah, S. Mahajan, B. Garware, R. Tambe, Towards designing an automated classification of lymphoma subtypes using deep neural networks, in *CoDS-COMAD '19: Proceedings of the ACM India Joint International Conference on Data Science and Management of Data* (2019), pp. 143–149
8. L. Lu, Y. Zheng, G. Carneiro, L. Yang (Eds.) *Deep Learning and Convolutional Neural Networks for Medical Image Computing*, ser. Advances in Computer Vision and Pattern Recognition (Springer International Publishing, Cham, 2017). http://link.springer.com/10.1007/978-3-319-42999-1
9. Y. Zhou, S. Cahya, S.A. Combs, C.A. Nicolaou, J. Wang, P.V. Desai, J. Shen, Exploring tunable hyperparameters for deep neural networks with industrial ADME data sets. J. Chem. Inf. Model. **59**, 1005–1016 (2019)
10. A. Krizhevsky, I. Sutskever, G.E. Hinton, ImageNet classification with deep convolutional neural networks, in *Advances In Neural Information Processing Systems* (2012), pp. 1–9
11. S. Luke, *Essentials of Metaheuristics*, 2nd edn. (Lulu, 2013). http://cs.gmu.edu/~sean/book/metaheuristics/
12. R. Landis, G.G. Koch, The Measurement of Observer Agreement for Categorical Data.Biometrics **33**(1), 159–174 (2016). http://www.jstor.org/stable/2529310. Accessed 31 Marach 2016

13. T. McGinn, P.C. Wyer, T.B. Newman, S. Keitz, R. Leipzig, G. Guyatt, Tips for teachers of evidence-based medicine: 3. Understanding and calculating kappa (Canadian Medical Association Journal (2004) 171, 11). Cmaj **173**(1), 18 (2005)
14. L. Yin, J. Tian, Joint confidence region estimation for area under ROC curve and Youden index. Stat. Med. **33**(6), 985–1000 (2014)
15. D.M.W. Powers, Evaluation: From precision, recall and f-factor to ROC, informedness, markedness & correlation. Technical Report (2007)
16. K. O'Shea, R. Nash, An introduction to convolutional neural networks. CoRR **abs/1511.08458** (2015). http://arxiv.org/abs/1511.08458

Deep Convolutional Likelihood Particle Filter for Visual Tracking

Reza Jalil Mozhdehi and Henry Medeiros

1 Introduction

Particle filters are widely applied in visual tracking problems due to their ability to find targets in challenging scenarios such as those involving occlusions or fast motion. Recently, particle filters have been used in conjunction with deep convolutional neural networks (CNN) [6, 12] and correlation filters [2, 7, 11, 15]. The Hierarchical Convolutional Feature Tracker (HCFT) proposed by Ma et al. in [7] showed significant performance improvements over previous works, demonstrating the effectiveness of using convolutional features along with correlation filters. Correlation filters provide a map showing similarities between convolutional features corresponding to an image patch and the target [2, 3, 15]. Adding a particle filter to convolutional-correlation visual trackers can significantly improve their results as shown in [8–10, 14, 16]. In these methods, particle filters sample several image patches and calculate the weight of each sample by applying a correlation filter to the convolutional response maps.

In this work, we propose a novel convolutional-correlation particle filter for visual tracking which estimates likelihood distributions from correlation response maps. Sampling particles from likelihood distributions improve the accuracy of patch candidates because correlation response maps have an initial evaluation of the target location. Thus, they are more reliable proposal densities than transition distributions, commonly used in particle-correlation trackers such as [8, 10, 14, 16]. Additionally, these trackers calculate the posterior distribution based on the peaks of correlation maps without considering them in the computation of particle weights. Our particle filter solves this problem using a multi-modal likelihood distribution

R. J. Mozhdehi (✉) · H. Medeiros
Marquette University, Milwaukee, WI, USA
e-mail: reza.jalilmozhdehi@marquette.edu; henry.medeiros@marquette.edu

H. R. Arabnia et al. (eds.), *Advances in Computer Vision and Computational Biology*, Transactions on Computational Science and Computational Intelligence,
https://doi.org/10.1007/978-3-030-71051-4_2

to address challenging tracking scenarios. Our proposed algorithm also calculates a likelihood distribution with larger variances, which is useful in other challenging scenarios involving fast motion or background clutter because it expands the target search area. Additionally, this method decreases the number of required particles. Experimental results on the Visual Tracker Benchmark v1.1 (OTB100) [13] show that our proposed framework outperforms the state-of-the-art methods.

2 The Change of Support Problem in Convolution-Correlation Particle Filters

The particle weights in a particle filter are calculated by [1]

$$\omega_{x_t}^{(i)} \propto \omega_{x_{t-1}}^{(i)} \frac{p(y_t|x_t^{(i)})p(x_t^{(i)}|x_{t-1})}{q(x_t^{(i)}|x_{t-1}, y_t)}, \tag{1}$$

where $p(x_t^{(i)}|x_{t-1})$ and $p(y_t|x_t^{(i)})$ are the transition and likelihood distributions, and $q(x_t^{(i)}|x_{t-1}, y_t)$ is the proposal distribution used to sample the particles. The posterior distribution is then approximated by

$$\hat{Pr}(x_t|y_t) \approx \sum_{i=1}^{N} \varpi_{x_t}^{(i)} \delta(x_t - x_t^{(i)}), \tag{2}$$

where $\varpi_t^{(i)}$ are the normalized weights. However, particle filters used in correlation trackers generally sample particles from the transition distribution, i.e., $q(x_t^{(i)}|x_{t-1}, y_t) = p(x_t^{(i)}|x_{t-1})$. These methods also re-sample particles at every frame, which removes the term corresponding to previous weights $\omega_{x_{t-1}}^{(i)}$ from Eq. (1). Finally, the weight of each particle in these trackers is given by [16]

$$\omega_{x_t}^{(i)} \propto p(y_t|x_t^{(i)}), \tag{3}$$

where $p(y_t|x_t^{(i)})$ is a function of $R_{x_t^{(i)}}^{y_t} \in \mathbb{R}^{M \times Q}$, the correlation response map centered at $x_t^{(i)}$. In these trackers, particles are shifted to the peaks of correlation maps and the posterior distribution is then approximated by the particles' weights at the shifted locations, i.e.,

$$\hat{Pr}(x_t|y_t) \approx \sum_{i=1}^{N} \varpi_{x_t}^{(i)} \delta(x_t - \tilde{x}_t^{(i)}), \tag{4}$$

where $\tilde{x}_t^{(i)}$ is the peak of the correlation response map corresponding to the i-th particle. However, the posterior distribution using the shifted locations must consider the weights corresponding to the new support points, not the original locations of the particles. That is, the original locations are used in weight computation, but the shifted support is used to approximate the posterior distribution. To solve this, we sample particles from the likelihood distribution instead. Particle filters that sample from likelihood distributions generate more accurate particles, but sampling from the likelihood distribution is not always possible. Fortunately, convolutional-correlation trackers generate correlation maps that can be used in the construction of likelihood distributions.

3 Likelihood Particle Filter

Our algorithm generates an initial correlation response map for the current frame based on the previously estimated target state to calculate an initial likelihood distribution. That is, we generate a patch from the current frame based on the previous target state and use a CNN [12] to extract the convolutional features from this patch. We then compare these features with the target model to calculate the final correlation response map [7]. As seen in Fig. 1, in most scenarios (which we call "simple frames") the correlation response map corresponds to a sharp Gaussian

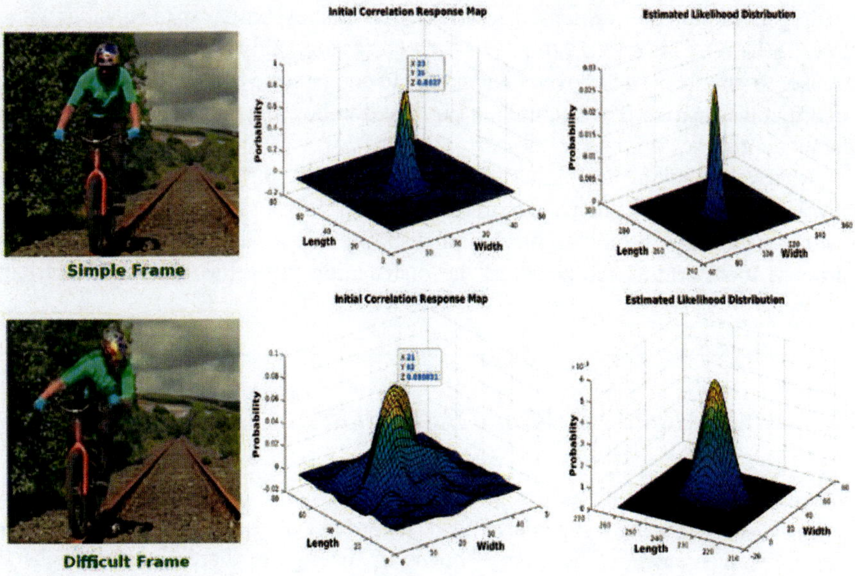

Fig. 1 Estimated likelihood distributions for common scenarios (simple frame) and a challenging scenario involving fast motion (difficult frame)

distribution with a prominent peak. In challenging scenarios ("difficult frames"), correlation maps are wider with less pronounced peaks. We need to estimate likelihood distributions consistently in both scenarios. To address this issue, we fit a Gaussian distribution to the correlation response maps while disregarding elements with probability lower than a threshold τ. By disregarding low probability elements, we mitigate the impact of the background on the computation of the model. We compute the mean of the correlation response map using

$$\mu \approx \frac{\sum_{i=1}^{u} q_i s_i}{\sum_{i=1}^{u} q_i}, \tag{5}$$

where s_i and q_i represent the elements of the correlation response map and their respective probabilities, and u is the number of elements with probability higher than τ. The variance of the response map is then given by

$$\sigma^2 \approx \frac{\sum_{i=1}^{u} q_i (s_i - \mu)^2}{\sum_{i=1}^{u} qi}. \tag{6}$$

Thus, our model assigns low probabilities to pixels that are likely to belong to the background while assigning relatively high probabilities to all the regions that might correspond to the target. As a result, our samples concentrate in regions where the target is more likely to be present.

Figure 1 shows our estimated likelihood distributions for two different frames of the *Biker* data sequence of the OTB100 benchmark. In the difficult frame, the target undergoes motion blur, which causes the correlation response map to be wider with a lower peak. Our estimated variance is then correspondingly higher, which helps our tracker to sample particles over a wider area to compensate for tracking uncertainties in difficult scenarios. The example in Fig. 2 shows how the variance increases as the target approaches difficult frames.

Although allowing for higher variances in challenging scenarios such as those involving fast motion helps our tracker address such issues, this strategy alone cannot handle multi-modal correlation response maps. To resolve this issue, we propose to determine the peaks of the distribution using the approach described below.

3.1 Multi-Modal Likelihood Estimation

The existence of multiple peaks in a correlation response map usually indicates the presence of confusing elements in the background of the frame, as the example in Fig. 3 illustrates. In the frame shown in the figure, there are two peaks in the correlation response map when partial target occlusion occurs. The peaks correspond to the woman on the left side of the image (the target) and the pole

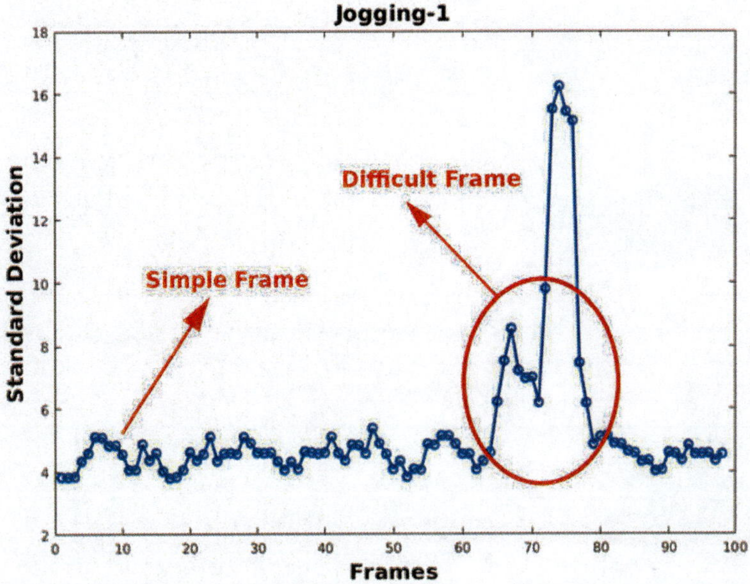

Fig. 2 Standard deviations of the estimated likelihood distributions in data sequence *Jogging-1* of the OTB-100 dataset

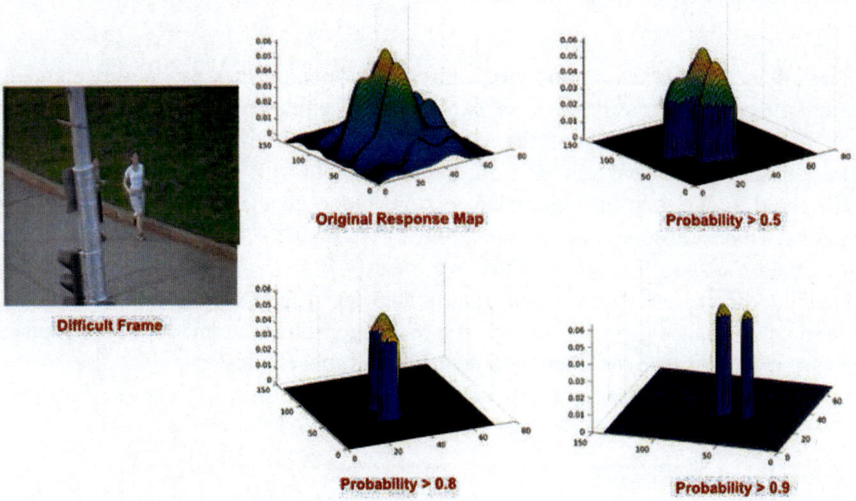

Fig. 3 A difficult frame including target occlusion. Its correlation response map has two peaks. By increasing the threshold to remove low probability elements, two clusters corresponding to the target and the pole are seen

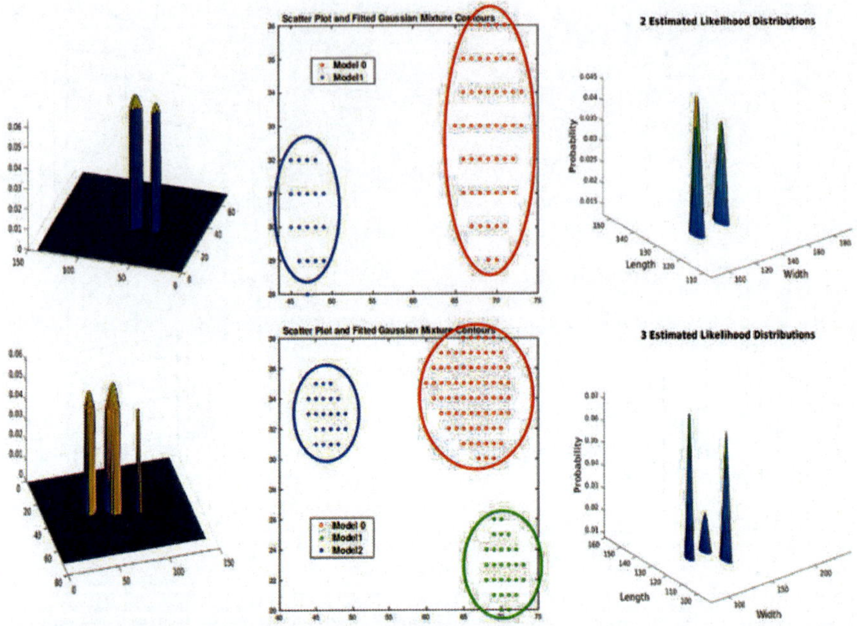

Fig. 4 Finding clusters; left: correlation response maps with two and three clusters, middle: clusters of the correlation response maps obtained by fitting a Gaussian mixture model, right: estimated likelihood distributions for each cluster

partially occluding her. By applying a threshold to remove low probability elements from the correlation response map, two clusters become apparent.

To identify the peaks of the correlation map while disregarding additional background clutter, we remove from the map points with probability lower than a threshold τ. We then fit a Gaussian mixture model to the remaining feature map points which clusters them into k groups [5]. Figure 4 shows two instances of correlation response maps in which we identify $k = 2$ and $k = 3$ clusters. The likelihood corresponding to each peak is then given by a normal distribution with mean and variance given by Eqs. (5) and (6). Algorithm 1 summarizes our proposed approach to estimate the likelihood distribution for each cluster.

3.2 *Particle Sampling*

We sample particles from the Gaussian likelihood distributions obtained from the correlation response maps in the current frame. The probability that a particle is sampled from the likelihood distribution is given by

Algorithm 1 Multi-modal likelihood estimation

Input: Current frame y_t and previous target state x_{t-1}
Output: One likelihood distribution for each correlation map cluster
1: Extract a patch from the current frame based on the previous target state
2: Extract the CNN features of the patch and calculate its correlation response map
3: Remove points with probability lower than τ
4: Fit a Gaussian mixture model to the map and find the clusters
5: Estimate the likelihood distribution of each cluster based on the mean and variance of its elements in the map according to Eqs. (5) and (6)

$$p(x_t^{(i)}|y_t) \propto \sum_{j=1}^{k} \mathcal{N}\left(x_t^{(i)}; \mu_j, \sigma_j\right), \tag{7}$$

where μ_j and σ_j are the mean and variance of the j-th mode of the likelihood. We generate a patch for each particle and extract its features using a CNN. After calculating the correlation response map for each particle, we shift the particles to the peaks of their respective correlation response maps. The peak of each correlation response map is the estimated target position based on the patch centered at the corresponding particle. Because each particle is shifted to the peak of the correlation response map, we consider $p(\tilde{x}_t^{(i)}|x_t^{(i)}) = 1$, where $\tilde{x}_t^{(i)}$ is the peak of the corresponding correlation response map. As a result, $p(x_t^{(i)}|y_t) = p(\tilde{x}_t^{(i)}|y_t)$.

3.3 Calculating the Weights and Posterior Distribution

By computing the weight of each shifted particle $\tilde{x}_t^{(i)}$, we can accurately estimate the posterior based on the shifted particles and their correct weights, which addresses the problem of incorrect support points observed in previous works. As discussed earlier, Eq. (1) corresponds to the weight of each particle before shifting. The weight of the shifted particles is then given by

$$\omega_{\tilde{x}_t}^{(i)} \propto \omega_{x_{t-1}}^{(i)} \frac{p(y_t|\tilde{x}_t^{(i)})p(\tilde{x}_t^{(i)}|x_{t-1})}{q(\tilde{x}_t^{(i)}|x_{t-1}, y_t)}, \tag{8}$$

where the term corresponding to the previous weight is removed because we perform resampling at every frame. Additionally, [1]

$$q(\tilde{x}_t^{(i)}|x_{t-1}, y_t) = p(\tilde{x}_t^{(i)}|y_t). \tag{9}$$

Thus, the weight of each shifted particle is

$$\omega_{\tilde{x}_t}^{(i)} \propto \frac{p(y_t|\tilde{x}_t^{(i)})p(\tilde{x}_t^{(i)}|x_{t-1})}{p(\tilde{x}_t^{(i)}|y_t)}. \tag{10}$$

Let the target state be defined as

$$z_{t-1} = \left[x_{t-1}, \dot{x}_{t-1}\right]^T, \tag{11}$$

where $\dot{x}_{t-1}$ is the velocity of x_{t-1}. We apply a first-order motion model to z_{t-1} according to

$$\bar{z}_{t-1} = Az_{t-1}, \tag{12}$$

where $\bar{z}_{t-1}$ represents the predicted target state and A is the process matrix defined by

$$A = \left[\begin{array}{c|c} I_4 & I_4 \\ \hline 0_{(4,4)} & I_4 \end{array}\right], \tag{13}$$

where I_4 is a 4×4 identity matrix and $0_{(4,4)}$ is a 4×4 zero matrix. We use a Gaussian distribution $\mathcal{N}(\bar{x}_{t-1}, \sigma^2)$ to find the probability of each estimated particle in the current frame $p(\tilde{x}_t^{(i)}|x_{t-1})$.

Additionally, $p(y_t|\tilde{x}_t^{(i)})$ is the likelihood of each shifted particle. Let $f_{x_t^{(i)}}(l, o)$ be the convolutional features of each particle $x_t^{(i)}$ where l and o represent the layers and channels of the network, respectively. The correlation response map is then calculated by [7]

$$R_{x_t^{(i)}}^{y_t}(x) = \sum_{l=1}^{L} \Upsilon_l \left(\mathfrak{F}^{-1}\left(\sum_{o=1}^{O} C_{t-1}(l, o) \odot \bar{F}_{x_t^{(i)}}(l, o)\right)\right), \tag{14}$$

where $\bar{F}_{x_t^{(i)}}(l, o)$ is the complex conjugate Fourier transform of $f_{x_t^{(i)}}(l, o)$, C_{t-1} is the model generated in the previous frame, $\odot$ represents the Hadamard product, $\mathfrak{F}^{-}1$ is the inverse Fourier transform operator, and Υ_l is a regularization term [7]. The peak of $R_{x_t^{(i)}}^{y_t}$ is then calculated by

$$\tilde{x}_t^{(i)} = \arg\max_{m,q} R_{x_t^{(i)}}^{y_t}(m, q), \tag{15}$$

where $m = 1, \ldots, M$ and $q = 1, \ldots, Q$. The likelihood of $\tilde{x}_t^{(i)}$ is calculated by [10]

$$p(y_t|\tilde{x}_t^{(i)}) = \frac{1}{M \times Q} \sum_{m,q} R_{\tilde{x}_t^{(i)}}^{y_t}(m, q). \tag{16}$$

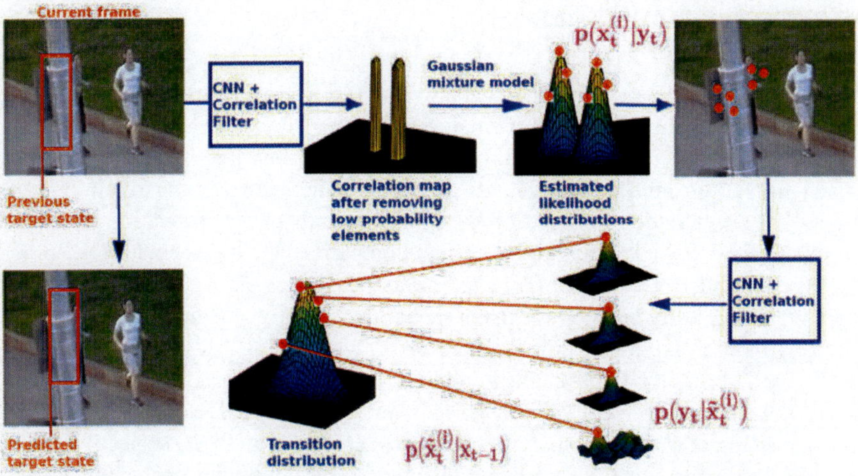

Fig. 5 Overview of the steps comprising the proposed DCPF-Likelihood visual tracker

---

Algorithm 2 DCPF-Likelihood visual tracker

Input: Current frame y_t and previous target state x_{t-1}
Output: Current target state x_t
1: Estimate a likelihood distribution for each cluster using Algorithm 1
2: Sample particles from the likelihood distributions $p(x_t^{(i)}|y_t)$
3: Extract the CNN features of the patches corresponding to each particle and calculate its correlation response map according to Eq. (14)
4: Shift the particles to the peaks of their correlation response maps based on Eq. (15)
5: Calculate the likelihood $p(y_t|\tilde{x}_t^{(i)})$ based on Eq. (16)
6: Calculate the transition probability $p(\tilde{x}_t^{(i)}|x_{t-1})$ according to Eqs. (11)–(13)
7: Compute the weight of each shifted particle $\omega_{\tilde{x}_t}^{(i)}$ according to Eqs. (8)–(10)
8: Calculate the posterior distribution according to Eq. (17)

The posterior distribution based on the shifted particles and their respective weights is then

$$\hat{Pr}(x_t|y_t) \approx \sum_{i=1}^{N} \varpi_{\tilde{x}_t}^{(i)} \delta(x_t - \tilde{x}_t^{(i)}), \tag{17}$$

where $\varpi_{\tilde{x}_t}^{(i)}$ is the normalized version of $\omega_{\tilde{x}_t}^{(i)}$. Figure 5 summarizes the steps of our method, and Algorithm 2 describes the details of our approach.

4 Experimental Results

We use the Visual Tracker Benchmark v1.1 (OTB100) to assess the performance of our tracker. This benchmark contains 100 video sequences, which include 11 challenging scenarios. Our results are based on the one-pass evaluation (OPE), which uses the ground truth target size and position in the first frame to initialize the tracker. Our evaluation is based on the precision and success measures, described in [13]. Figure 6 shows qualitative results comparing our tracker with DCPF [8], HCFT [7], and CNN-SVM [4]. In both data sequences shown in the figure, our method successfully handles occlusion scenarios. These results highlight the impact of using more reliable sampling distributions.

Figure 7 shows the OPE results for our tracker in comparison with DCPF, HCFT, and CNN-SVM. Our overall performance improvements over DCPF, the second best tracker, in terms of precision and success rates are 2.5% and 2%, respectively. Our method outperforms DCPF particularly in scenarios involving occlusions (+3%) and background clutter (+4.5%). DCPF uses the transition distribution as the proposal density, a common approach in particle-correlation trackers. Our results show that the likelihood is a more effective proposal distribution. In scenarios involving motion blur and fast motion, our performance improvements over DCPF are around 4.5% and 2%, respectively, because our tracker increases the variance of the likelihood distribution to spread out particles across a wider area. Our method also outperforms DCPF in scenarios involving illumination variation (+3%), out-of-plane rotation (+3.5%), and deformation (+3%). Our method also decreases the computational cost of the algorithm. Our tracker uses 100 particles, which is significantly less than the 300 particles used in DCPF.

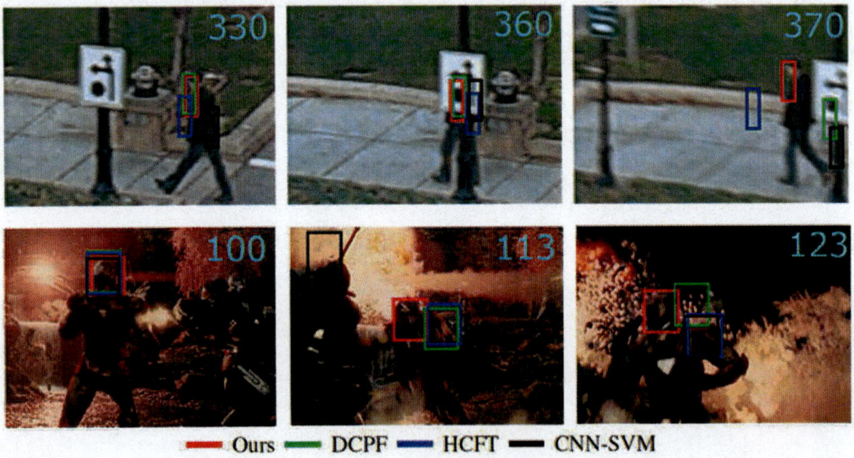

Fig. 6 Qualitative evaluation of our tracker against *DCPF*, *HCFT*, and *CNN-SVM* on two challenging sequences: *Human6* (top) and *Ironman* (bottom)

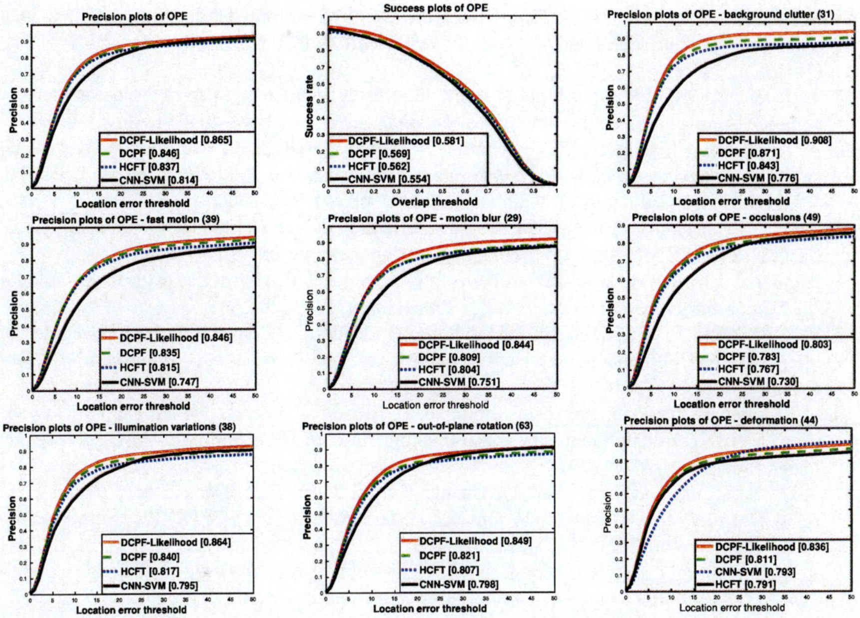

Fig. 7 One-pass evaluation of our tracker in comparison with three state-of-the-art approaches

5 Conclusion

In this work, we propose the DCPF-Likelihood visual tracker. Our method estimates a likelihood distribution as the proposal density for a particle filter based on correlation response maps. Correlation response maps provide an initial estimate of the target location, which results in more accurate particles. Furthermore, the resulting likelihood distribution has a wider variance in challenging scenarios such as fast motion and motion blur. Our particle filter also generates a likelihood distribution for each correlation map cluster in difficult scenarios such as target occlusions. Our results on the OTB100 dataset show that our proposed visual tracker outperforms the state-of-the-art methods.

References

1. M.S. Arulampalam, S. Maskell, N. Gordon, T. Clapp, A tutorial on particle filters for online nonlinear/non-gaussian Bayesian tracking. IEEE Trans. Signal Process. **50**(2), 174–188 (2002)
2. K. Dai, D. Wang, H. Lu, C. Sun, J. Li, Visual tracking via adaptive spatially-regularized correlation filters, in *Proceedings of the IEEE Conference on Computer Vision and Pattern Recognition* (2019), pp. 4670–4679
3. J.F. Henriques, R. Caseiro, P. Martins, J. Batista, High-speed tracking with kernelized correlation filters. IEEE Trans. Pattern Anal. Mach. Intell. **37**(3), 583–596 (2015)

4. S. Hong, T. You, S. Kwak, B. Han, Online tracking by learning discriminative saliency map with convolutional neural network, in *32nd International Conference on Machine Learning* (2015)
5. T. Kawabata, Multiple subunit fitting into a low-resolution density map of a macromolecular complex using a gaussian mixture model. Biophys. J. **95**(10), 4643–4658 (2008)
6. A. Krizhevsky, I. Sutskever, G.E. Hinton, Imagenet classification with deep convolutional neural networks, in *Advances in Neural Information Processing Systems 25*, ed. by F. Pereira, C.J.C. Burges, L. Bottou, K.Q. Weinberger (2012), pp. 1097–1105
7. C. Ma, J.B. Huang, X. Yang, M.H. Yang, Hierarchical convolutional features for visual tracking, in *IEEE International Conference on Computer Vision (ICCV)* (2015)
8. R.J. Mozhdehi, H. Medeiros, Deep convolutional particle filter for visual tracking, in *24th IEEE International Conference on Image Processing (ICIP)* (2017)
9. R.J. Mozhdehi, Y. Reznichenko, A. Siddique, H. Medeiros, Convolutional adaptive particle filter with multiple models for visual tracking, in *13th International Symposium on Visual Computing (ISVC)* (2018)
10. R.J. Mozhdehi, Y. Reznichenko, A. Siddique, H. Medeiros, Deep convolutional particle filter with adaptive correlation maps for visual tracking, in *25th IEEE International Conference on Image Processing (ICIP)* (2018)
11. Y. Qi, S. Zhang, L. Qin, H. Yao, Q. Huang, J. Lim, M.H. Yang, Hedged deep tracking, in *IEEE Conference on Computer Vision and Pattern Recognition (CVPR)* (2016), pp. 4303–4311. https://doi.org/10.1109/CVPR.2016.466
12. K. Simonyan, A. Zisserman, Very deep convolutional networks for large-scale image recognition, in *International Conference on Learning Representations (ICLR)* (2015)
13. Y. Wu, J. Lim, M.H. Yang, Online object tracking: a benchmark, in *IEEE Conference on Computer Vision and Pattern Recognition (CVPR)* (2013)
14. D. Yuan, X. Lu, Y. Liang, X. Zhang, Particle filter re-detection for visual tracking via correlation filters. Multimed. Tools Appl. **78**(11), 14277–14301 (2019)
15. M. Zhang, Q. Wang, J. Xing, J. Gao, P. Peng, W. Hu, S. Maybank, Visual tracking via spatially aligned correlation filters network, in *Proceedings of the European Conference on Computer Vision (ECCV)* (2018), pp. 469–485
16. T. Zhang, S. Liu, C. Xu, Correlation particle filter for visual tracking. IEEE Trans. Image Process. **27**(6), 2676–2687 (2018)

DeepMSRF: A Novel Deep Multimodal Speaker Recognition Framework with Feature Selection

Ehsan Asali, Farzan Shenavarmasouleh, Farid Ghareh Mohammadi, Prasanth Sengadu Suresh, and Hamid R. Arabnia

1 Introduction

Artificial Intelligence (AI) has impacted almost all research fields in the last decades. There exist countless number of applications of AI algorithms in various areas such as medicine [1, 2], robotics [3–5], multi-agent systems [6–8], and security and privacy [9]. Deep learning is, with no doubt, the leading AI methodology that revolutionized almost all computer science sub-categories such as IoT [10], Computer Vision, Robotics, and Data Science [11]. The field of Computer Vision has been looking to identify human beings, animals, and other objects in single photo or video streams for at least two decades. Computer vision provides variety of techniques such as image/video recognition [12, 13], image/video analysis, image/video segmentation [14], image/video captioning, expert's state or action recognition [15], and object detection within image/video [16, 17]. Object detection plays a pivotal role to help researchers find the most matching object with respect to the ground truth. The greatest challenge of object recognition task is the effective usage of noisy and imperfect datasets, especially video streams. In this paper, we aim to address this issue and propose a new framework to detect speakers.

E. Asali (✉) · F. Shenavarmasouleh · F. G. Mohammadi · P. S. Suresh · H. R. Arabnia
Department of Computer Science, University of Georgia, Athens, GA, USA
e-mail: ehsanasali@uga.edu; farzan.shenavarmasouleh@uga.edu; farid.ghm@uga.edu; ps32611@uga.edu; hra@uga.edu

H. R. Arabnia et al. (eds.), *Advances in Computer Vision and Computational Biology*, Transactions on Computational Science and Computational Intelligence,
https://doi.org/10.1007/978-3-030-71051-4_3

1.1 Problem Statement

Copious amount of research has been done to leverage single modality which is either using audio or image frames. However, very little attention has been given to multimodality based frameworks. The main problem is speaker recognition where the number of speakers is around 40. In fact, when the number of classes (speakers) proliferate to a big number and the dimension of extracted features becomes too high, traditional machine learning approaches may not be able to yield high performance due to the problem of curse of dimensionality [18, 19]. To explore the possibility of using multimodality, we feed the video streams to the proposed network and extract two modalities including audio and image frames. We aim to use feature selection techniques in two different phases in the proposed method.

Now this approach may prompt some questions: Why do we need multimodality if just single modality would give us a high enough accuracy? Is it always better to add more modalities or would an additional modality actually bring down the performance? If so, by how much? Bolstered by our experimental results, these are some questions we are going to delve into and answer in this paper. Let us start by looking at the potential impediments we could run into while using a single modality. Let us say, for instance, we just use audio-based recognition systems; in this case, we often face a bottleneck called SNR (Signal-to-Noise-Ratio) degradation, as mentioned in [20]. In short, when SNR is low in the input dataset, we observe our model efficiency plummets. On the other hand, image-based data is not unfettered by such predicaments as well. Images face problems like pose and illumination variation, occlusion, and poor image quality [21–24]. Thus, we hypothesize that combining the two modalities and assigning appropriate weights to each of the input streams would bring down the error rate.

1.2 Feature Selection

Feature selection is arguably one of the important steps in pre-processing before applying any machine learning algorithms. Feature selection or dimension reduction works based on two categories, including (1) filter-based and (2) wrapper-based feature selection. Filter-based feature selection algorithms evaluate each feature independent of other features and only rely on the relation of that feature with target value or class label. This type of feature selection is cheap, as it does not apply any machine learning algorithms to examine the features. On the contrary, wrapper-based feature selection algorithms choose subsets of features and evaluate them using machine learning algorithms. That is the main reason why wrapper-based feature selection algorithms are more expensive. Mohammadi and Abadeh [25, 26] applied wrapper-based algorithms for binary feature selections using artificial bee colony. In this study, we apply wrapper-based feature selection, as it yields a high performance on supervised datasets.

1.3 Contribution

Most of the speaker recognition systems currently deployed are based on modelling a speaker, based on single modality information, i.e., either audio or visual features. The main contributions of this paper are as following:

- Integration of audio and image input streams extracted from a video stream, forming a multimodality deep architecture to perform speaker recognition.
- Effectively identifying the key features and the extent of contribution of each input stream.
- Creating a unique architecture that allows segregation and seamless end-to-end processing by overcoming dimensionality bottlenecks.

The rest of the paper is arranged as follows: First, we touch base with the related work that has been done in this field, then we explain the overview working methodology of CNNs, followed by how we handle the data effectively. We also compare and contrast other classifiers that could be used instead of the built-in neural network of VGGNET. Then, we explain the experiments performed, compare the results with some baseline performance, and conclude with discussion, future work, and varied applications of the model developed in this paper.

2 Related Work

As explained before, most of the work done so far on speaker recognition is based on unimodal strategies. However, with the advancement of machine learning and deep learning in the past few years, it has been proven that multimodal architectures can easily surpass unimodal designs. Chetty and Wagner [20], Koda et al. [27], and Chibelushi et al. [28] were some of the very first attempts to tackle the task of person identity verification or speaker recognition while leveraging multiple streams to combine data collected from different sources such as clips recorded via regular or thermal cameras, and the varieties of corresponding features extracted from them via different external speech recognition systems, optical flow modules, and much more. After the features were extracted and fused, some basic machine learning models such as Hidden Markov Model (HMM), Latent Dirichlet Allocation (LDA), and Principal Component Analysis (PCA) were trained over them to act as the final classifier.

As impressive as these look, they can never beat the accuracy that one can achieve with deep learning models. Almost all of the architectures that are at the cutting edge in the modern tasks make use of two or more streams. Video action recognition is one example. Feichtenhofer et al. [29] and Rezazadegan et al. [30] both employ two parallel streams, one for capturing spatial data and the other for extracting temporal information from videos to classify the actions. Similarly, [31] uses two separate streams for RGB frame and sequence of different flows, whereas

[32] brings four modalities into play and makes use of 2D and 3D CNNs and their flows simultaneously. Another excellent work [15] that deals with multimodal inputs suggests a unique framework for recognizing robots' state-action pairs which uses two streams of RGB and Depth data in parallel. More creatively, [33] utilizes one slow and one fast stream, proving that the former is good to understand spatial semantics, and the latter, which is a lighter pathway, can be beneficial in finding out the temporal motion features. Also, [34] builds on top of this and adds one more stream to engage audios as well.

Tracking objects in videos, finding tampered images, and testing audio-visual correspondence (AVC) are some other tasks that parallel streams have been used for them to achieve the state-of-the-art performance. Feichtenhofer et al. [35] leverages two streams to jointly learn how to detect and track objects in the videos at the same time. He et al. [36] uses two parallel Siamese networks to do real-time object tracking and [37] employs face classification and patch triplet streams to investigate the possible alterations to the face images. Also, [38] and [39] both use parallel streams to enable their models to identify whether the input audio corresponds to a given video or not.

It can be perceived that an extensive amount of research has been done in the field of multimodal deep architectures. Nevertheless, to the best of our knowledge, [40] is the most related work that has been done for the task of speaker recognition and it only uses multimodality in the process of feature extraction. Additionally, it only uses audio data and tests on two datasets with 22 and 26 speakers, respectively. On the contrary, in this paper, we design our architecture to make use of video frames along with the audios in separate streams. On top of that, we create our custom dataset with 40 unique speakers and extend the scale of previous works.

3 Proposed Method

In this section, we propose a late-fusion framework using a dual-modality speaker recognition architecture using audios and frames extracted from videos. Firstly, we discuss challenges in speaker classification and recognition, then we talk about the bottlenecks of the architecture, and finally we present our model's architectural details.

3.1 Challenges

As the number of images and videos proliferate, the process of image/video classification becomes more challenging; so the task of real world computer vision and data analysis becomes crucial when the number of classes exceeds 10. The more the classes, the more time and computational power is required to do the task of classification. To learn a model to classify the speakers, we are required to have a proper dataset and a structured framework to do that. In this paper, the greatest challenge was to recognize 40 unique speakers. More so than that, since no standard dataset is available for our hypothesis, we had to create ours by subsampling from a combination of two other datasets. During the last 10 years, researchers have proposed different frameworks for deep learning using complex combination of neural networks such as ResNet [41] and GoogleNet [42] for image classification. These only focus on singular modality, either image or voice of the video, to do speaker recognition. In this paper, we address this problem and propose a new architecture leveraging VGGNET (VGG-16) [43] for speaker recognition task using multimodality to overcome all these limitations. The simple VGGNET, like other frameworks, suffers from having insufficient performance on speaker recognition. We provide three main steps consisting of combining two networks of VGGNET followed by feature selection and performing late-fusion on top of them.

Another common conundrum is on how to interpret the audio signals into a format which is suitable for VGGNET to work with. In general, in order to deal with audio streams, we have three options to choose from. One is to map the input audios to waveform images and feed the resultant diagrams to VGGNET as input. Another choice is to apply feature extraction to obtain a meaningful representation of the audio streams which is now a feature vector. The last but not the least, we can perform one more step on top of feature extraction by visualizing them as a two-dimensional image. Later in this paper we will see that the third choice has the best performance and is utilized in our final model.

3.2 Video Speaker Recognition

We present a base speaker recognition architecture that leverages two VGG16 networks in parallel; one for speakers' images and another for speakers' audio frames. We discuss generating speaker audio frames in the next subsection. Figure 1 illustrates the base speaker recognition architecture. VGGNET produces a 1-D vector of 4096 features for each input frame that could be used as an input to all common classification methodologies. Fusing these feature vectors yields to high dimensionality problem called curse of dimensionality (COD) [18, 19]. To reduce the problem's complexity, we apply feature selection as discussed earlier in Sect. 1.2.

Data Preparation We prepare a standard dataset of speaker images, along with speaker audios trimmed to 4 s, about which we discuss further in the dataset subsection under the experiment section. The dataset of the speakers' face images can be created quite easily; nevertheless, as previously mentioned, we should convert speaker voices into proper formats as well. To tackle this issue, we have tried various available methods to generate meaningful features out of input audio signals. There are a couple of choices which we have briefly mentioned previously and will investigate more in this section.

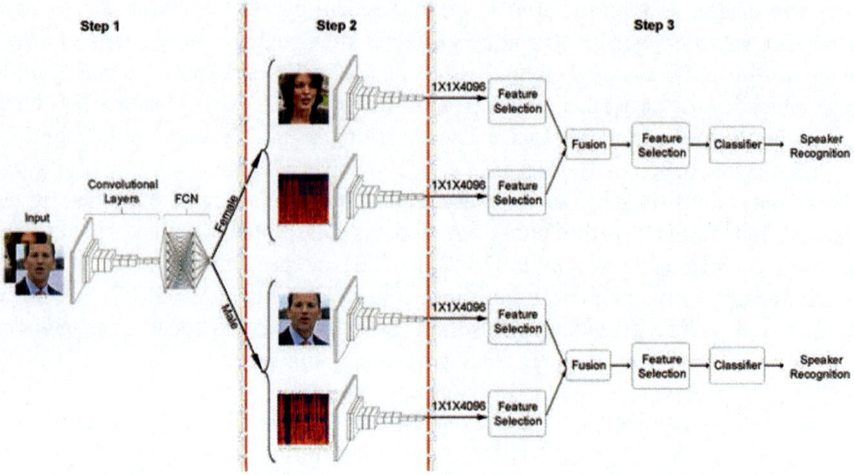

Fig. 1 DeepMSRF architecture. Step 1: A unimodal VGGNET takes the speaker's image as an input and detects the speaker's gender. Step 2: Based on the gender, the image and voice of the speaker is passed to the corresponding parallel multimodal VGGNETs to extract each modality's dense features. Step 3: Feature selection on each modality will be applied first; then, the resultant feature vectors are concatenated, and feature selection is performed again after concatenation. Eventually, a classifier is trained to recognize the speaker's identity

The first approach is to directly convert the audio files into wave form diagrams. To create such images, the main hurdle that we face is the frequency variation of the speakers' voices. To solve this issue, we plot them with the same y-axis range to have an identical axis for all the plots. Obviously, the y-axis length must be such that all wave form charts fall within its range. The generated images can directly be fed into VGGNET; nonetheless, later we will see that this approach is not really useful because of lacking sufficiently descriptive features.

Another approach is to extract meaningful and descriptive features of the audio streams instead of just drawing their waveform diagrams. Here, we have multiple options to examine; Mel-frequency cepstral coefficients (MFCCs), Differential Mel-frequency cepstral coefficients DMFCCs, and Filter Banks (F-Banks) are the algorithms reported to be effective for audio streams. MFCCs and DMFCCs can each extract a vector of 5200 features from the input audio file, while F-Banks can extract 10,400 features. Now we have the option of either using these feature vectors directly and concatenating them with the extracted feature vectors of the face images coming from VGGNET Fully Connected Layer 7 (so-called FC7 layer) or mapping them first to images and then, feeding them into the VGGNET. In the latter, we first need to fetch the flattened FC7 layer feature vector; afterwards, we have to perform the concatenation of the resultant vector with the previously learned face features. Spectrograms are another meaningful set of features we use in this paper. A spectrogram is a visual representation of the spectrum of frequencies of a signal (audio signal here) as it varies with time. We feed such images into VGGNET directly and extract the features from the FC7 layer. Later, we will see how beneficial each of the aforementioned approaches is to predict the speakers' identity.

Feature Selection The more features we have, the higher is the probability of occurring overfitting problems which is also known as Curse of Dimensionality. This can be resolved to some extent by making use of feature selection (FS) algorithms. Feature selection approaches carefully select the most relevant and important subset of features with respect to the classes (speakers' identities). We choose a wrapper-based feature selection by exploiting lib-SVM kernel to evaluate the subsets of features. After applying feature selection, the dimensionality of the dataset decreases significantly. In our work, we apply FS two times in the model; once for each of the models separately, and once again after concatenating them together (before feeding the resultant integrated feature vector to the SVM classifier.

3.3 Extended Video Speaker Recognition

To do the task of video speaker recognition we have divided our architecture into three main steps as presented in Fig. 1. The following sections explain each step in a closer scrutiny.

Step One Inevitably, learning to differentiate between genders is notably more straightforward for the network compared to distinguishing between the identities. The former is a binary classification problem while the latter is a multi-label classification problem with 40 labels (in our dataset). On the other hand, facial expressions and audio frequencies of the two genders differ remarkably in some aspects. For instance, a woman usually has longer haircuts, a smaller skull, jewelries, and makeup. Men, on the contrary, occasionally have a mustache and/or beard, colored ties, and tattoos. Other than facial characteristics, males mostly have deep, low pitched voices while females have high, flute-like vocals. Such differences triggered the notion of designing the first step of our framework to distinguish the speakers' genders.

Basically, the objective of this step is to classify the input into Male and Female labels. This will greatly assist in training specialized and accurate models for each class. Since the gender classification is an easy task for the VGGNET, we just use the facial features in this step. In fact, we pass the speakers' images to the VGGNET and based on the resultant identified gender class extracted from the model, we decide whether to use the network for Male speakers or Female ones. In our dataset, such a binary classification yields 100% accuracy on the test set. Later we will see the effect of this filtering step on our results.

Step Two In this step, we take the separated datasets of men and women as inputs to the networks. For each category, we apply two VGGNETs, one for speaker images and another for their voices. Thus, in total, we have five VGGNETs in the first and second steps. Indeed, we had one singular modality VGGNET for filtering out the speakers' genders in the first step, and we have two VGGNETs for each gender (four VGGNETs in total) in the second step. Note that the pipeline always uses the VGGNET specified for the gender recognition in the first step; afterwards, based on the output gender, it chooses whether to use the parallel VGGNET model for women or men, but not both simultaneously.

In the given dataset, we have 20 unique females and 20 unique males. Following this, we train the images and audios of males and females separately on two parallel VGGNETs and extract the result of each network's FC7 layer. Each extracted feature vector consists of 4096 features which is passed to the next step.

The second step may change a little if we use the non-visualized vocal features of either MFCCs, DMFCCs, or F-Bank approach. In this case, we only need VGGNET for the speakers' face images to extract the dense features; following this, we concatenate the resultant feature vector with the one we already have from vocal feature extractors to generate the final unified dataset for each gender.

Step Three After receiving the feature vectors for each modality of each gender, we apply a classifier to recognize the speaker. Since the built-in neural network of VGGNET is not powerful enough for identity detection, we try a couple of classifiers on the resultant feature vector of the previous step to find the best classifier for our architecture. Nonetheless, before we feed the data into the classifiers, we need to ensure the amount of contribution each modality makes to the final result. As the contribution of each modality on the final result can vary according to the density and descriptivity of its features, we need to filter out the unnecessary features from each modality. To do so, we apply feature selection on each modality separately to allocate appropriate number of features for each of them. Afterwards, we concatenate them together as a unified 1-D vector. We apply feature selection again on the unified vector and use the final selected features as input to the classifiers. The specific number of data samples, the number of epochs for each stage, and the results at each checkpoint are discussed in the Experiments section (Sect. 4).

4 Experiments

4.1 Dataset

We have used VoxCeleb2 dataset proposed in [44] which originally has more than 7000 speakers, 2000 h of videos, and more than one million utterances. We use an unbiased sub-sample [45] of that with 20,000 video samples in total, with almost 10,000 sample speakers per gender. The metadata of VoxCeleb2 dataset has gender and id labels; the id label is connected to the VGGFace2 dataset. The first step we have to go through is to bind the two metadata sets together and segregate the labels correctly. The way their dataset is arranged is that a celeb id is assigned to multiple video clips extracted from several YouTube videos which is almost unusable. Hence, we unfolded this design and assigned a unique id to each video to make them meet our needs.

As mentioned earlier, we selected 40 random speakers from the dataset which included 20 male and 20 female speakers. Thereupon, one frame per video was extracted where the speaker's face was clearly noticeable. The voice was also extracted from a 4-second clip of the video. Finally, the image-voice pairs shuffled to create training, validation, and test sets of 14,000, 3000, and 3000 samples, respectively, for the whole dataset, i.e., both genders together.

4.2 Classifiers

Random Forests Random forests [46] or random decision forests are an ensemble learning method for classification, regression, and other tasks that operates by constructing a multitude of decision trees at training time and outputting the class that is the mode of the classes (classification) or mean prediction (regression) of the individual trees. Random decision forests prevent the overfitting which is common in regular decision tree models.

Gaussian Naive Bayes Naïve Bayes [47] was first introduced in 1960s (though not under that name) and it is still a popular (baseline) method for classification problems. With appropriate pre-processing, it is competitive in the domain of text categorization with more advanced methods including support vector machines. It could also be used in automatic medical diagnosis and many other applications.

Logistic Regression Logistic regression is a powerful statistical model that basically utilizes a logistic function to model a binary dependent variable, while much more complicated versions exist. In regression analysis, logistic regression [48] (or logit regression) is estimating the parameters of a logistic model. Mathematically, a binary logistic model has a dependent variable with two possible values, such as pass/fail which is represented by an indicator variable, where the two values are labeled "0" and "1." In the logistic model, the log-odds (the logarithm of the odds) for the value labeled "1" is a linear combination of one or more independent variables ("predictors"); the independent variables can each be a binary variable (two classes, coded by an indicator variable) or a continuous variable (any real value). The corresponding probability of the value labeled "1" can vary between 0 (certainly the value "0") and 1 (certainly the value "1"), hence the labeling; the function that converts log-odds to probability is the logistic function, hence the name. The unit of measurement for the log-odds scale is called a logit, from logistic unit, hence the alternative names. Some applications of logits are presented in [49–51].

Support Vector Machine A Support Vector Machine [52] is an efficient tool that helps to create a clear boundary among data clusters in order to aid with the classification. The way this is done is by adding an additional dimension in cases of overlapping data points to obtain a clear distinction and then projecting them back to the original dimensions to break them into clusters. These transformations are called kernels. SVMs have a wide range of applications from finance and business to medicine[53] and robotics [54]. An example of its applications can be found in [55–57] where they detect the opponent team's formation in a Soccer 2D Simulation environment using various approaches including SVM. We use linear kernel in our experiments and we have Linear-SVM as a part of our proposed pipeline.

4.3 VGGNET Architecture

This section briefly explains the layers of our VGGNET architecture. Among the available VGGNET architectures, we have chosen the one containing the total of 13 convolutional and 3 Dense layers, framed as VGG-16 [58]. The architecture includes an input layer of size $224 \times 224 \times 3$ equal to a 2-D image with 224 pixels width and the same height including RGB channels. The input layer is followed by two convolutional layers with 64 filters each and a max pooling layer with a window of size 2×2 and the stride of 2. Then another pair of convolutional layers of size 112×112 with 128 filters each and a max pooling layer are implemented. Afterwards, in the next three stages, the architecture uses three convolutional layers and one pooling layer at the end of each stage. The dimension of the convolutional layers for these steps are $56 \times 56 \times 256$, $28 \times 28 \times 512$, and $14 \times 14 \times 512$, respectively. Finally, it has three dense layers of size $1 \times 1 \times 4096$ followed by a softmax layer. Since the output of the softmax layer specifies the output label (e.g., the speaker's name), its size must be equal to the number of classes. Also, notice that all convolutional and dense layers are followed by a ReLU function to protect the network from having negative values. Moreover, the first Dense layer is usually referred as FC7 layer (Fully Connected layer 7) that contains an extracted flattened feature vector of the input.

4.4 Implementation

In Sect. 4.1, we explained how we create the dataset and now we elucidate the steps taken to produce the results. In order to train the parallel VGGNET for each gender, we divide the dataset into two parts; the samples of the 20 Male speakers and the samples of the 20 Female speakers. Thereafter, each of the two partitions is fed into a dual-channel VGGNET consisting the image and audio streams. When the training process finishes, the architecture learns to extract meaningful features from the input data. Now, we can generate a new dataset for each gender by passing the face and Spectrogram's train, validation, and test images through their corresponding VGGNETs and fetch their FC7 layers' feature vectors.

Afterwards, using the linear-SVM feature extractor library in Scikit learn—Python, we are able to extract almost 1053 number of features for Male images, 798 features for Male voices, 1165 features for Female images, and 792 features for Female voices. Then, we concatenate the resultant feature vectors for each gender and feed it again to the same feature extractor to summarize it once more. The final size of the merged feature vectors for the Males is 1262 and for Females is 1383. Note that the reported number of voice features are related to the Spectrogram feature extractor which is the one we elected among the available options that were discussed earlier in Sect. 3.3. The last step is to train the Linear-SVM classifier and to get its result.

The very first baseline architecture that we are going to compare our results with, does not segregate genders, uses only one modality (i.e., either the face or the voice data), uses the plotted wave form of the voice data, and does not use any feature selection approach. To compare the effect of any changes to the baseline, we have accomplished an extremely dense ablation study process. The ablation study results are discussed in the next section.

4.5 Ablation Study

To check the effect of each contribution, we perform ablation study by training and testing the dataset in various conditions. The following sections briefly discuss the impact of each contribution on the final result.

Feature Extraction and Selection Feature Extraction (FE) is highly crucial in the learning process. The main contribution of deep learning pipelines over the classical machine learning algorithms is their ability to extract rich meaningful features out of a high dimensional input. Here, VGGNET plays this role for the face images of the speakers and also for the visualized vocal features. On the other hand, Feature Selection (FS) can prevent the model to be misled by irrelevant features. As previously mentioned, we have used linear-SVM feature selection in this work.

To evaluate the advantage of using FE and FS when dealing with audial data and also to compare the performance of diverse FE algorithms, we apply each algorithm on Male, Female, and the whole dataset. Then, we apply FS on top of it; then, we examine each algorithm with four different classification methods, including Random Forests, Naive Bayes, Logistic Regression, and Support Vector Machines. Finally, we compare the results for both cases of either using or not using FS. Table 1 shows the result for all the situations. As the results represent, the best test accuracy is achieved when we utilize Spectrogram feature extractor combined with linear-SVM feature selection approach.

To analyze the efficacy of FS on the face frames, we train VGGNET and extract the FC7 layer feature vector. We then apply FS and eventually, train on four different classifiers. Table 2 represents the test accuracy for each classifier with and without

Table 1 The accuracy for single/multimodality with/without feature selection

FE algorithm	Classifier RF	NB	LR	SVM
Spectogram(M) (%)	45.4	19.06	54.33	50.53
Spectogram(M) + FS (%)	45.93	25.93	52.86	**56.26**
Spectogram(F)(%)	44.26	21.53	52.26	48.46
Spectogram(F) + FS (%)	42.66	29.4	51.2	**53.3**
Spectogram(all)(%)	37.16	14.96	48.4	43.6
Spectogram(all) + FS (%)	38.03	21.6	46.5	**49.3**
Waveform(M)(%)	30.53	16.6	32.26	29.26
Waveform(M)(%) +FS	30.46	17.2	29.93	32.13
Waveform(F)(%)	22.06	14.08	27.73	21.4
Waveform(F)(%) +FS	22	13.93	23.26	23.6
MFCC(M)(%)	11.93	25.33	5.46	9.46
MFCC(M)(%) +FS	11.46	24.2	5.33	9.2
MFCC(F)(%)	10.8	21.86	5.93	9.46
MFCC(F)(%) +FS	10.8	21.53	5.93	9.73
Filter bank(M)(%)	32.33	19.13	42.06	36.6
Filter bank(M)(%) +FS	33	24	42.26	40.46
Filter bank(F)(%)	33.66	18.06	43.2	38.06
Filter bank(F)(%) +FS	33	25.46	41.93	41.06

Table 2 The accuracy of the speakers' face images for four different classifiers associated with different feature extractors with/without Feature Selection (FS)

FE	Classifiers RF	NB	LR	SVM
VGG(M) (%)	91	49.66	93.6	91.66
VGG(M) + FS (%)	91.26	66.73	92.53	**94.2**
VGG(F)(%)	86.26	55.33	90.93	87.33
VGG(F) + FS (%)	85.66	62.2	88.13	**91.26**
VGG(total) (%)	88.03	50.1	91.53	88.7
VGG(total) + FS (%)	88.06	58.43	90.4	**91.9**

FS. As the results demonstrate, the highest accuracy for each dataset is achieved for the case in which we have used FS on top of VGGNET and for the SVM classifier.

Gender Detection As discussed in Sect. 3.3 in details, the first step of our pipeline is to segregate speakers by their gender. Instead, we could train a model with 40 classes consisting of all men and women speakers. To see how the first step improves the overall performance of the model, we examined both cases and compared their results. The test accuracy of Male speakers, Female speakers, the average test accuracy of Male and Female speakers, and the test accuracy of the whole dataset (containing both genders) are reported in Table 3. The results show that the average accuracy increases when we perform gender segregation regardless of whether we use feature selection before and/or after concatenating the face and audio modalities or not. Also, notice that according to Table 3, we can achieve

Table 3 The accuracy of the whole dataset for SVM classifier associated with Spectrogram feature extractor combined with feature selection

	Samples			
Approach	Male	Female	Avg.	Total (genderless)
Simple concatenation	91.2	87.87	89.54	89.27
FS + concatenation	**95.13**	91.87	93.5	92.97
concatenation + FS	94.67	91.87	93.27	92.53
FS + concatenation + FS	95.07	**91.93**	**93.5**	**93.03**

Table 4 The accuracy for single/multimodality with/out feature selection

	Modality		
Result	Face frames	Audio (spectrogram)	Multimodality
Total (%)	88.7	43.6	89
Total + FS (%)	91.9	49.3	93.03

the highest accuracy when we perform feature selection, specifically before the concatenation step. According to the table, the average accuracy has been improved by almost 4% using our proposed method (the last row) compared to the baseline approach (the first row).

Single Modality Vs. Multimodality One of the greatest contributions of DeepMSRF is taking advantage of more than one modality to recognize the speaker efficiently. Each modality comprises of unique features that lead the model to distinguish different individuals. To show how multimodality can overcome the limitations of single modality, we carry out a comparison between the two, reported in Table 4. According to the results, using both visual and auditory inputs together can improve the accuracy of the task of speaker recognition.

4.6 Time Complexity

In Sect. 4.5, we saw the benefit of utilizing feature selection on the model's accuracy. Additionally, there exists one more criterion to consider which is the training time. Although the training process is being performed offline and in the worst case, training the SVM classifier over our dataset finishes in almost 20 min (for the whole dataset), it is noteworthy to see how feature selection can influence the training time. Figure 2 depicts the training time required for the SVM in the last step (step3) of our pipeline for the experiments shown in Table 3. According to Fig. 2, the required training time for each gender is approximately one third of the corresponding time required to train the whole dataset.

Nextly, the time required to accomplish the step 3 of DeepMSRF, including the time needed for feature selection and the training time, is reported in Table 5. The results can be discussed from two different points of view: (1) Among the examined

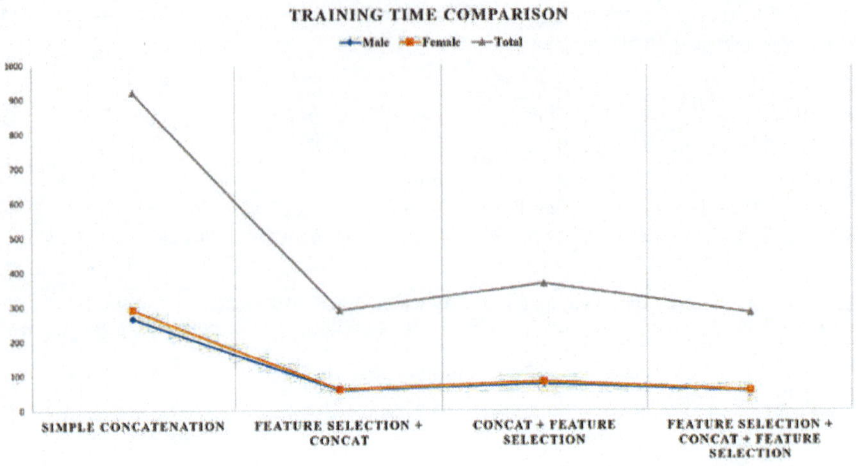

Fig. 2 Training time comparison (Male Vs. Female) for DeepMSRF with SVM classifier

Table 5 The accuracy of the whole dataset for SVM classifier associated with Spectrogram feature extractor combined with feature selection

	Samples		
Approach	Male	Female	Total (Genderless)
Simple concatenation	265.37	290.94	919.46
FS + concatenation	209.91	195.49	883.23
concatenation + FS	179.61	197.27	729.6
FS + concatenation + FS	296.93	291.56	1,208.52

methodologies, the least training duration is for the case in which we apply Feature Selection (FS) after the concatenation of the two modalities' feature vectors. On the contrary, the worst time performance is for the situation of applying FS before and after concatenation. (2) The time is significantly shorter when we segregate the genders. Each gender's dataset needs less than one third of the required time for the whole dataset. In fact, training two separate models (one per gender), together, requires lesser time than training a general model which contains both genders.

5 Future Work

The future work entails using multiple datasets to test the robustness of the system and adding more functionalities to the model such as recognizing the facial features of each individual person and predicting the extent of overlap between different people. Moreover, some aspects of the model can be investigated more. For instance, here we have used VGGNET; there remains a myriad of object detection pipelines to be tested. Another example of possible future probes is to try disparate approaches of feature selection. Altogether, this architecture has numerous applications beyond speaker recognition and are to be explored in the upcoming works.

6 Conclusion

This paper takes a trip down the novelty lane by adding multimodality to improve robustness of the recognition and overcomes the limitations of single modality performance. From the results of the experiments above, we can infer that the hypothesis made about the multimodality improving over the single modality results for person recognition using deep neural networks was nearly conclusive. Among other challenges, this paper also solves the dimensionality challenge arising from using multimodality input streams. Exploiting feature extraction has provided a deep insight into how significant features to train the network are to be extracted to obtain a well-trained model. We can see that although the images provide a high accuracy over speaker recognition, audio stream input reinforces the performance and provides an additional layer of robustness to the model. In conclusion, we state that the unique framework used in this paper, DeepMSRF, provides an efficient solution to the problem of speaker recognition from video streams. At last, DeepMSRF is a highly recommended framework for those researchers who deal with video analysis.

References

1. A. Afshar, I. Perros, H. Park, C. deFilippi, X. Yan, W. Stewart, J. Ho, J. Sun, Taste: temporal and static tensor factorization for phenotyping electronic health records, in *Proceedings of the ACM Conference on Health, Inference, and Learning* (2020), pp. 193–203
2. M. Sotoodeh, J.C. Ho, Improving length of stay prediction using a hidden Markov model. AMIA Summits Transl. Sci. Proc. **2019**, 425 (2019)
3. K.W. Buffinton, B.B. Wheatley, S. Habibian, J. Shin, B.H. Cenci, A.E. Christy, Investigating the mechanics of human-centered soft robotic actuators with finite element analysis, in *2020 3rd IEEE International Conference on Soft Robotics (RoboSoft)* (IEEE, Piscataway, 2020), pp. 489–496
4. H. Haeri, K. Jerath, J. Leachman, Thermodynamics-inspired modeling of macroscopic swarm states, in *Dynamic Systems and Control Conference*, vol. 59155 (American Society of Mechanical Engineers, New York, 2019), p. V002T15A001
5. E. Seraj, M. Gombolay, Coordinated control of UAVs for human-centered active sensing of wildfires (2020). Preprint, arXiv:2006.07969
6. M. Dadvar, S. Moazami, H.R. Myler, H. Zargarzadeh, Multiagent task allocation in complementary teams: a hunter-and-gatherer approach. Complexity **2020**, Article ID 1752571 (2020)
7. M. Etemad, N. Zare, M. Sarvmaili, A. Soares, B.B. Machado, S. Matwin, Using deep reinforcement learning methods for autonomous vessels in 2D environments, in *Canadian Conference on Artificial Intelligence* (Springer, Berlin, 2020), pp. 220–231

8. M. Karimi, M. Ahmazadeh, Mining robocup log files to predict own and opponent action. Int. J. Adv. Res. Comput. Sci. **5**(6), 1–6 (2014)
9. F. Tahmasebian, L. Xiong, M. Sotoodeh, V. Sunderam, Crowdsourcing under data poisoning attacks: a comparative study, in *IFIP Annual Conference on Data and Applications Security and Privacy* (Springer, Berlin, 2020), pp. 310–332
10. S. Voghoei, N.H. Tonekaboni, J. Wallace, H.R. Arabnia, Deep learning at the edge, in *Proceedings of International Conference on Computational Science and Computational Intelligence CSCI, Internet of Things" Research Track* (2018), pp. 895–901
11. F.G. Mohammadi, M.H. Amini, H.R. Arabnia, An introduction to advanced machine learning: meta-learning algorithms, applications, and promises, in *Optimization, Learning, and Control for Interdependent Complex Networks* (Springer, Berlin, 2020), pp. 129–144
12. S. Amirian, Z. Wang, T.R. Taha, H.R. Arabnia, Dissection of deep learning with applications in image recognition, in *Proceedings of International Conference on Computational Science and Computational Intelligence (CSCI 2018: December 2018, USA); "Artificial Intelligence" Research Track (CSCI-ISAI)* (2018), pp. 1132–1138
13. F.G. Mohammadi, H.R. Arabnia, M.H. Amini, On parameter tuning in meta-learning for computer vision, in *2019 International Conference on Computational Science and Computational Intelligence (CSCI)* (IEEE, Piscataway, 2019), pp. 300–305
14. Z. Wang, F. Li, T. Taha, H. Arabnia, 2d multi-spectral convolutional encoder-decoder model for geobody segmentation, in *2018 International Conference on Computational Science and Computational Intelligence (CSCI)* (IEEE, Piscataway, 2018), pp. 1193–1198
15. N. Soans, E. Asali, Y. Hong, P. Doshi, Sa-net: Robust state-action recognition for learning from observations, in *IEEE International Conference on Robotics and Automation (ICRA)* (2020), pp. 2153–2159
16. S. Ren, K. He, R. Girshick, J. Sun, Faster R-CNN: towards real-time object detection with region proposal networks, in *Advances in Neural Information Processing Systems* (2015), pp. 91–99
17. F. Shenavarmasouleh, H.R. Arabnia, DRDR: automatic masking of exudates and microaneurysms caused by diabetic retinopathy using mask R-CNN and transfer learning (2020). Preprint, arXiv:2007.02026
18. F.G. Mohammadi, M.H. Amini, Evolutionary computation, optimization and learning algorithms for data science, in *Optimization, Learning and Control for Interdependent Complex Networks* (Springer, Berlin, 2019)
19. F.G. Mohammadi, M.H. Amini, Applications of nature-inspired algorithms for dimension reduction: enabling efficient data analytics, in *Optimization, Learning and Control for Interdependent Complex Networks* (Springer, Berlin, 2019)
20. G. Chetty, M. Wagner, Robust face-voice based speaker identity verification using multilevel fusion. Image Vis. Comput. **26**(9), 1249–1260 (2008)
21. S.P. Mudunuri, S. Biswas, Low resolution face recognition across variations in pose and illumination. IEEE Trans. Pattern Anal. Mach. Intell. **38**(5), 1034–1040 (2015)
22. J.H. Shah, M. Sharif, M. Raza, M. Murtaza, S. Ur-Rehman, Robust face recognition technique under varying illumination. J. Appl. Res. Technol. **13**(1), 97–105 (2015)
23. H. Sellahewa, S.A. Jassim, Image-quality-based adaptive face recognition. IEEE Trans. Instrum. Meas. **59**(4), 805–813 (2010)
24. P. Li, L. Prieto, D. Mery, P. Flynn, Face recognition in low quality images: a survey (2018) . Preprint, arXiv:1805.11519
25. F.G. Mohammadi, M.S. Abadeh, Image steganalysis using a bee colony based feature selection algorithm. Eng. Appl. Artif. Intell. **31**, 35–43 (2014)
26. F.G. Mohammadi, M.S. Abadeh, A new metaheuristic feature subset selection approach for image steganalysis. J. Intell. Fuzzy Syst. **27**(3), 1445–1455 (2014)
27. Y. Koda, Y. Yoshitomi, M. Nakano, M. Tabuse, A facial expression recognition for a speaker of a phoneme of vowel using thermal image processing and a speech recognition system, in *RO-MAN 2009-The 18th IEEE International Symposium on Robot and Human Interactive Communication* (IEEE, Piscataway, 2009), pp. 955–960

28. C.C. Chibelushi, F. Deravi, J.S. Mason, Voice and facial image integration for person recognition (1994)
29. C. Feichtenhofer, A. Pinz, A. Zisserman, Convolutional two-stream network fusion for video action recognition, in *Proceedings of the IEEE Conference on Computer Vision and Pattern Recognition* (2016), pp. 1933–1941
30. D. Rezazadegan, S. Shirazi, B. Upcroft, M. Milford, Action recognition: from static datasets to moving robots, Jan 2017
31. X. Peng, C. Schmid, Multi-region two-stream R-CNN for action detection, in *European Conference on Computer Vision* (Springer, Berlin, 2016), pp. 744–759
32. X. Yang, P. Molchanov, J. Kautz, Multilayer and multimodal fusion of deep neural networks for video classification, in *Proceedings of the 24th ACM international conference on Multimedia* (2016), pp. 978–987
33. C. Feichtenhofer, H. Fan, J. Malik, K. He, Slowfast networks for video recognition, in *Proceedings of the IEEE International Conference on Computer Vision* (2019), pp. 6202–6211
34. F. Xiao, Y.J. Lee, K. Grauman, J. Malik, C. Feichtenhofer, Audiovisual slowfast networks for video recognition (2020). Preprint, arXiv:2001.08740
35. C. Feichtenhofer, A. Pinz, A. Zisserman, Detect to track and track to detect, in *Proceedings of the IEEE International Conference on Computer Vision* (2017), pp. 3038–3046
36. A. He, C. Luo, X. Tian, W. Zeng, A twofold Siamese network for real-time object tracking, in *Proceedings of the IEEE Conference on Computer Vision and Pattern Recognition* (2018), pp. 4834–4843
37. P. Zhou, X. Han, V.I. Morariu, L.S. Davis, Two-stream neural networks for tampered face detection, in *2017 IEEE Conference on Computer Vision and Pattern Recognition Workshops (CVPRW)* (IEEE, Piscataway, 2017), pp. 1831–1839
38. R. Arandjelovic, A. Zisserman, Look, listen and learn, in *Proceedings of the IEEE International Conference on Computer Vision* (2017), pp. 609–617
39. J. Cramer, H.-H. Wu, J. Salamon, J.P. Bello, Look, listen, and learn more: design choices for deep audio embeddings, in *ICASSP 2019-2019 IEEE International Conference on Acoustics, Speech and Signal Processing (ICASSP)* (IEEE, Piscataway, 2019), pp. 3852–3856
40. P. Dhakal, P. Damacharla, A.Y. Javaid, V. Devabhaktuni, A near real-time automatic speaker recognition architecture for voice-based user interface. Mach. Learn. Knowl. Extr. **1**(1), 504–520 (2019)
41. K. He, X. Zhang, S. Ren, J. Sun, Deep residual learning for image recognition, in *Proceedings of the IEEE Conference on Computer Vision and Pattern Recognition* (2016), pp. 770–778
42. C. Szegedy, W. Liu, Y. Jia, P. Sermanet, S. Reed, D. Anguelov, D. Erhan, V. Vanhoucke, A. Rabinovich, Going deeper with convolutions, in *Proceedings of the IEEE Conference on Computer Vision and Pattern Recognition* (2015), pp. 1–9
43. X. Zhang, J. Zou, K. He, J. Sun, Accelerating very deep convolutional networks for classification and detection. IEEE Trans. Pattern Anal. Mach. Intell. **38**(10), 1943–1955 (2015)
44. J.S. Chung, A. Nagrani, A. Zisserman, Voxceleb2: deep speaker recognition (2018). Preprint, arXiv:1806.05622
45. F. Shenavarmasouleh, H.R. Arabnia, Causes of misleading statistics and research results irreproducibility: a concise review, in *2019 International Conference on Computational Science and Computational Intelligence (CSCI)* (IEEE, Piscataway, 2019), pp. 465–470
46. T.K. Ho, Random decision forests, in *Proceedings of 3rd International Conference on Document Analysis and Recognition*, vol. 1 (IEEE, Piscataway, 1995), pp. 278–282
47. G.H. John, P. Langley, Estimating continuous distributions in Bayesian classifiers, in *Proceedings of the Eleventh conference on Uncertainty in Artificial Intelligence* (Morgan Kaufmann Publishers Inc., Burlington, 1995), pp. 338–345
48. D.G. Kleinbaum, K. Dietz, M. Gail, M. Klein, M. Klein, *Logistic Regression* (Springer, Berlin, 2002)
49. P.V. Amini, A.R. Shahabinia, H.R. Jafari, O. Karami, A. Azizi, Estimating conservation value of lighvan chay river using contingent valuation method (2016)

50. O. Karami, S. Yazdani, I. Saleh, H. Rafiee, A. Riahi, A comparison of Zayandehrood river water values for agriculture and the environment. River Res. Appl. **36**(7), 1279–1285 (2020)
51. A.R. Shahabinia, V.A. Parsa, H. Jafari, S. Karimi, O. Karami, Estimating the recreational value of Lighvan Chay River uses contingent valuation method. J. Environ. Friendly Process. **4**(3), 69 (2016)
52. M.A. Hearst, S.T. Dumais, E. Osuna, J. Platt, B. Scholkopf, Support vector machines. IEEE Intell. Syst. Appl. **13**(4), 18–28 (1998)
53. E. Maddah, B. Beigzadeh, Use of a smartphone thermometer to monitor thermal conductivity changes in diabetic foot ulcers: a pilot study. J. Wound Care **29**(1), 61–66 (2020)
54. R. Khayami, N. Zare, M. Karimi, P. Mahor, A. Afshar, M.S. Najafi, M. Asadi, F. Tekrar, E. Asali, A. Keshavarzi, Cyrus 2d simulation team description paper 2014, in *RoboCup 2014 Symposium and Competitions: Team Description Papers* (2014)
55. E. Asali, F. Negahbani, S. Tafazzol, M.S. Maghareh, S. Bahmeie, S. Barazandeh, S. Mirian, M. Moshkelgosha, Namira soccer 2d simulation team description paper 2018, in *RoboCup 2018* (2018)
56. E. Asali, M. Valipour, A. Afshar, O. Asali, M. Katebzadeh, S. Tafazol, A. Moravej, S. Salehi, H. Karami, M. Mohammadi, Shiraz soccer 2d simulation team description paper 2016, in *RoboCup 2016 Symposium and Competitions: Team Description Papers, Leipzig, Germany* (2016)
57. E. Asali, M. Valipour, N. Zare, A. Afshar, M. Katebzadeh, G.H. Dastghaibyfard, Using machine learning approaches to detect opponent formation, in *2016 Artificial Intelligence and Robotics (IRANOPEN)* (IEEE, Piscataway, 2016), pp. 140–144
58. K. Simonyan, A. Zisserman, Very deep convolutional networks for large-scale image recognition (2014). Preprint, arXiv:1409.1556

Deep Image Watermarking with Recover Module

Naixi Liu, Jingcai Liu, Xingxing Jia, and Daoshun Wang

1 Introduction

Images have been a main medium of information in the era of Internet. The popularity of smartphones has made it easier to create images and other digital work. Hundreds of millions of images are spreading on the net every day, which increases the difficulty of copyright management. Traditionally, visible watermark is added to digital content to declare its copyright. It is easy to be identified and removed and thus not so suitable for current complex Internet environment.

Digital watermarking is an effective strategy for digital copyright management. It declares copyright by adding related invisible watermark information, which is difficult to perceive but can be extracted by specific methods, to digital works, and is thus more safe and reliable. Meanwhile, digital watermarking requires resistance to certain attacks, such as cropping, noise addition, compression, etc. Most of the watermark information will be preserved in the covers after being attacked to a certain extent, so the robustness is also ensured. In this way, we create unique digital fingerprint similar to ID number as watermark information for each author. Application of digital watermarking will help establish and improve an open copyright management system. In this paper, we mainly aim at image watermarking.

This paper is submitted as: Regular Research Paper.

N. Liu · J. Liu · D. Wang (✉)
Department of Computer Science and Technology, Tsinghua University, Beijing, China

X. Jia
Department of Computer Science and Technology, Tsinghua University, Beijing, China

School of Mathematics and Statistics, Lanzhou University, Lanzhou, China
e-mail: jiaxx@lzu.edu.cn

H. R. Arabnia et al. (eds.), *Advances in Computer Vision and Computational Biology*, Transactions on Computational Science and Computational Intelligence,
https://doi.org/10.1007/978-3-030-71051-4_4

The LSB algorithm [1] is a classic spatial algorithm for image blind watermarking. The watermark information is embedded in the least significant bits of cover image, which will not significantly damage the image quality but is weak in resisting certain attacks. There are some other works based on statistical properties or image features, like color histogram [2, 3] and SVD [4]. Another type of methods embeds watermark information in the frequency domain, like DCT [5] and DWT [6]. These methods have shown great improvements in robustness toward attacks over those based on spatial domain. They all require handcraft features.

In recent years, the rapid development of deep learning in computer vision has also brought innovations in digital image watermarking. Actually, there have been some image steganography models based on deep learning. Though they do not show robustness against certain attacks [7–10], some ideas are adopted by image watermarking models. For image watermarking, Kandi et al. [11] proposed a learning-based auto-encoder convolutional network which outperforms previous work based on frequency domain in imperceptibility and robustness but is non-blind. Mun et al. [12] proposed a novel CNN-based framework for blind watermarking which consists of watermark embedding, attack simulation, and weight update. This scheme was declared to resist geometric and signal processing attacks. Zhu et al. [13] proposed HiDDeN, an end-to-end watermarking scheme, which contains an encoder for watermark embedding, a decoder for watermark extracting, and an attack layer for attack simulation. This work also adopts adversarial training to improve the visual quality of stego images. Ahmadi et al. [14] proposed ReDMark, which is also an end-to-end watermarking scheme but in DCT domain. Since JPEG compression is not differential, which will break the back propagation while training, both HiDDeN and ReDMark use approximate calculations. Liu et al. [15] proposed a two-stage separable blind watermarking model. On the first stage, the model is trained without noise attacks. On the second stage, weights for encoder are fixed, and the decoder is trained with attacks, in which the pure JPEG compression can be used without approximation. Wen et al. [16] proposed ROMark, which adopts the same architecture as HiDDeN but computes the attacked image in the worst case. Robustness to watermark attacks shows improvements over HiDDeN after training the framework.

In this work, we propose a novel architecture for image watermarking. Our main contributions are as follows:

1. We introduce recovery module, a novel component, to the framework. Since most of watermark information may be damaged during attack process, we try to recover the lost information and thus improve the accuracy of extracting.
2. Based on the existing methods, we proposed a new one, applying different JPEG compression approximation to different DCT frequency components. The combined approach can better approximate the real JPEG compression, thereby obtaining better robustness.
3. We use dilated convolution and other designs to increase the receptive field and utilization of feature maps so as to better resist cropping and attacks of other types.

The rest of this paper is organized as follows. Section 2 introduces some related work. Section 3 will give our proposed model in details. The experimental results will be illustrated in Section 4. We finally conclude this paper in Section 5.

2 Related Work

JPEG compression is a common type of attack in digital image watermarking. It mainly consists of forward DCT, quantization, and encoding. Among them, the quantization process introduces non-differentiable operations, which will break the back propagation during training. HiDDeN [13] and ReDMark [14] use different differentiable approximations to JPEG compression.

HiDDeN uses JPEG-Mask or JPEG-Drop. In JPEG-Mask, only the low-frequency DCT coefficients are kept, and the others are set to zero. In JPEG-Drop, random coefficients are set to zero, with higher probability in coarser quantization. The reason for this kind of approximation is that coefficients in higher frequency and coarser quantization are more likely to be set to zero during JPEG compression. However, other coefficients remain the same in JPEG-Mask and JPEG-Drop, which is far from the situation in real compression. In RedMark, the quantization is simulated by a uniform noise and related to the quantization matrix, which is thus a larger family of distortions than real JPEG. This approximation is more applicable to low-frequency coefficients, where elements of the quantization matrix is smaller. For high-frequency coefficients, the larger elements and thus the higher distortion will lead to more uncertainty to some extent, resulting in a gap between the approximating value and the real quantization value. In our opinion, a better approximation of JPEG compression is a flexible combination of these two kinds. More details will be illustrated in Section 3.

In previous works, digital watermarking frameworks based on deep learning have achieved quite good results but can be improved in some aspects. HiDDeN [13] is weak in resisting real JPEG compression attacks, while ReDMark [14] has poor performance against Gaussian filters. By the way, DCT-based methods always require image blocking. It is difficult to align the cropped watermarked image with the cover, which may easily lead to inconsistent blocking and thus inaccurate extraction. Zero error of extraction for ReDMark against cropping attacks may be under the assumption that cropped image and watermarked image have the same blocking. In our work, the cropped image is not required to be aligned with the watermarked image. The two-stage separable model [15] has shown improvement to former works. In this model, the watermark attacks are unseen to the encoder, so robustness against different attacks rely dependently on the decoder. We claim that the encoder can also play a role in the robustness to achieve better performance.

We propose a novel framework for digital image watermarking based on convolutional neural network. Experimental results show significant improvements against attacks of different type and different strengths. More details will be given in the rest of this paper.

3 The Proposed Method

In this section, we give our approximation of JPEG compression first and then the architecture and details of our proposed model. We introduce the loss function at the end.

3.1 Approximation of JPEG Compression

According to ReDMark [14], the quantization can be simulated as followed:

$$I_{\mathrm{DCT}*} = \left(\frac{I_{\mathrm{DCT}}}{Q} + \sigma\right) \times Q = I_{\mathrm{DCT}} + \sigma Q$$

where I_{DCT} and $I_{\mathrm{DCT}*}$ are the watermarked image and its approximated quantization, respectively, Q is quantization matrix, and σ is the uniform noise in the range of $[-0.5, 0.5]$. This approximation fit JPEG compression in a larger set of distortions, especially for low-frequency coefficients, where the corresponding values of quantization matrix are smaller. For high-frequency coefficients, the values are higher, and this approximation will introduce higher distortion, not always closed to zero. However, quantization results for real JPEG compression are always zero in higher-frequency DCT coefficients. On the other hand, quantization matrix is different in Y channel and U and V channel. JPEG compression keeps more information in Y channel and thus less zeros in quantization results.

Therefore, we used different approximation methods for different coefficients. We first set most of the coefficients with coarser quantization in higher frequency to be zeros, with different proportions in Y channel and U and V channels. Zeros in Y channel will be less than the other two channels. For the rest nonzero coefficients, we add a uniform noise related to the quantization matrix as mentioned above. In this way, we get a closer approximation to real JPEG compression and successfully train the proposed model to be more robust to JPEG compression than previous works.

3.2 Details of the Network

Our proposed model consists of five modules, namely, watermark embedding module, watermark attack module, watermark recover module, watermark extracting module, and watermark adversarial module. The whole model architecture is illustrated in Fig. 1.

Watermark Embedding Module This module embeds a bit string of certain length to a cover image with RGB channels. As is shown in Fig. 2, each bit of

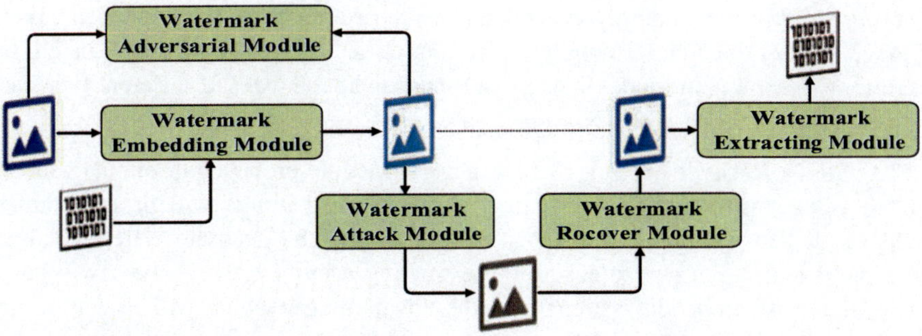

Fig. 1 Basic unit of the proposed model

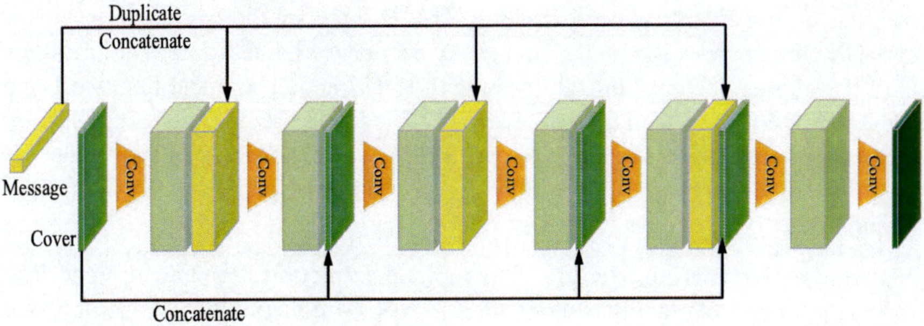

Fig. 2 Architecture of watermark embedding module

the watermark message is first duplicated in spatial to create a feature map with the same height and width as the cover image and then concatenated together. So number of the channels is equal to the length of the message. We apply a series of convolution operations with $3 \times 3 \times 64$ filters to the cover image. The duplicated message and the original cover are concatenated to the generated feature maps in turn. In this way, as much information is preserved in the watermarked or stego image as possible. For the last two layers, the feature maps concatenated with the duplicated message and the pure cover image are applied $3 \times 3 \times 64$ convolution and $1 \times 1 \times 3$ convolution, respectively. ReLU is used as the activation function in this model. We also adopt batch normalization [17].

For feature maps concatenated with pure cover image, we apply dilated convolutions [18] to increase the receptive fields. This method is supposed to strengthen robustness against watermark attacks like cropping, in which only a small proportion of the watermarked image is obtained while extracting.

Watermark Attack Module This module simulates possible attacks to the watermarked images. It takes the stego image as input and outputs the attacked noise image. Specially, we take "Identity" as one type of attack which do nothing to the stego image to increase the robustness while no attacks are applied. For each batch during training, we randomly select one attack type and apply it to the watermarked image. We set the attack strength in a certain range and vary in different batch. In this way, we train our model to be more robust against attacks of different type and different strength.

Watermark Recover Module This is a novel module proposed. From our aspect, some of the watermark message in the watermarked image will be lost during attacks, which will increase difficulty of extracting the accurate watermark bits for the decoder. Further, to ensure the extracting accuracy, the encoder will have to increase its embedding strength to the cover image, which will lead to more distortion to image quality. The recover module does not mean to restore the attacked image to the watermarked image, which would be a hard task for attacks unknown. The aim of this module, however, is to restore some lost watermark message during attacks as compensation. This will reduce the burden of decoder to extract accurate message and the strength of encoder to embed watermark message.

We use three deconvolutional layers with ReLU activation. The first two layers use $3 \times 3 \times 64$ filters, and the last layer uses $3 \times 3 \times 3$ filters. Batch normalization is also applied. For attacks like cropping which will change the size of image, we do not align the attacked image with watermarked image but continue with the pure outputs.

Watermark Extracting Module This module extracts watermark message from recovered image. We apply a series of $3 \times 3 \times 64$ convolutions (seven layers in experiment) to the recovered image with ReLU activation. Then, we use 3×3 convolution to change number of channels to the original message length and global adaptive average pooling to change the size of feature maps to 1×1. Finally, a linear transformation is applied. For bit string output in testing phase, the values are clipped to 0 or 1. We thus obtain the extracted binary bit string with the same length.

Watermark Adversarial Module This module is used in the training process to guide the embedding module to create more natural watermarked images compared to cover images. The idea is from GAN [19], a popular framework of generative adversarial network applying in many computer vision tasks. It is essentially a binary classifier to discriminate watermarked images from cover images. The network is similar to extracting module, but the linear transform generates values of one channel followed by Sigmoid activation to present the predicting probability. By adversarial training, the embedding module tends to generate a watermarked image visually and statically similar to the cover images.

3.3 Loss Function

For training the embedding module, the goal is to minimize the distance between cover image I_c and watermarked image I_w. For extracting module, it is to minimize the distance between the embedded watermark message M and extracted message

$\overline{M}$. For the recover module, it is to minimize the distance between the watermarked image I_w and the recovered image I_r. We all use mean squared error as the distance metric:

$$\begin{aligned} L_E &= \text{MSE}(I_C, I_W) &&= \|I_C - I_W\| \quad /N \\ L_D &= \text{MSE}\left(M, \overline{M}\right) &&= \left\|M - \overline{M}\right\| /L \\ L_R &= \text{MSE}(I_W, I_r) &&= \|I_W - I_r\| \quad /N \end{aligned}$$

Specially, noise image after cropping attacks without alignment will not be equal in size to the watermarked image, and the metric is not applicable. In this case, we set the distance to zeros since the cropped area never change during attack, and an Identity transformation mode will be learned in the special "Identity" attack. During training, we use a combined loss function:

$$L_W = \lambda_E L_E + L_D + \lambda_R L_R + \lambda_A L_A$$

where λ_E, λ_R, λ_A are weights for each component. And L_A is the adversarial loss for generator to decrease the visual distortion of generated watermarked image:

$$L_A = -\log(A(I_W))$$

where $A(_*)$ is the predicted probability. So for adversarial module, which aims to increase its capability to identify watermarked image from covers, the loss function would be:

$$L_{adv} = -\log(A(I_C)) - \log(1 - A(I_W))$$

In this way, we make the generator, mainly the embedding module, and discriminator, mainly the adversarial module, to compete against each other. The ultimate goal is to improve the naturalness of the generated watermarked image while the discriminator will be abandoned after training.

4 Experiment Result

We train our model on COCO 2014 datasets [20]. We use a subset of 10000 images in RGB format for the training set. For evaluation, we use 1000 images unseen during training. All the images are randomly cropped to $128 \times 128 \times 3$. A length of 30-bit string is embedded to the cover images. For a fair comparison, we use Cropout, Dropout, Gaussian, JPEG, and Crop as attack types as HiDDeN does. Cropout and Dropout attacks generate the noise image by taking a percentage p of pixels from watermarked image and the rest from cover image, while the former chooses each pixels independently and the latter takes a random square crop from

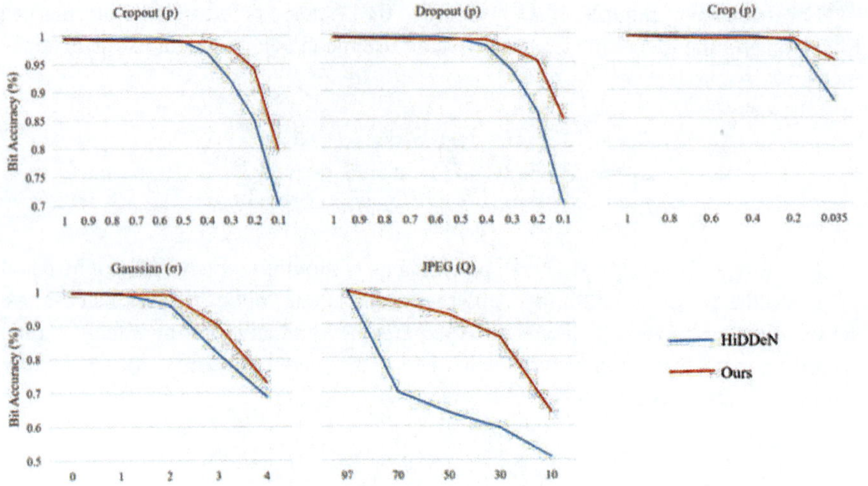

Fig. 3 Bit accuracy under attacks of different type and different strengths for HiDDeN and our proposed model. Data for HiDDeN are directly from the paper

watermarked image. Gaussian attack blurs the watermarked image with a Gaussian kernel with width σ, and JPEG attack applies JPEG compression with quality factor of Q. Crop attack take a percentage p of random square crop from watermarked image. By modifying the parameter p, σ, and Q, we apply attacks of different strength. For loss function, we set λ_E, λ_R, λ_A to be 0.7, 0.1, and 0.001.

For evaluating metrics, we use bit accuracy to test the performance of extracting watermark message. As is shown in Fig. 3, HiDDeN and our proposed model show similar performance and reach very high bit accuracy under low embedding strength. As embedding strength improves, the accuracy slides down. However, our model keeps relatively high accuracy in very high embedding strength and better than HiDDeN. This result shows that our model has stronger robustness against different types of attacks with different strength.

Among all the attacks tested, robustness against JPEG compression performs the worst. This is one of the hardest attacks to resist, for its complex computation and non-differentiable property, which needs approximation during training. For HiDDeN, bit accuracy drops to 50% with quality factor of 10. Our proposed model demonstrates a significant improvement in this case, which shows the effectiveness of our proposed approximation approach to JPEG compression to some extent.

Table 1 shows the bit accuracy of the proposed model and other previous work. For attack type of Cropout ($p = 0.3$), Dropout ($p = 0.3$), and Gaussian ($\sigma = 2$), our model has slight or no improvement since previous work has done quite well in these types. For JPEG ($Q = 50$), our model shows a significant improvement compared with the state of the art. For Crop ($p = 0.035$), our model performs the best except ReDMark. However, as previously analyzed, ReDMark has to align the cropped image with the watermarked image before extracting to reach this accuracy. The

Table 1 Bit accuracy of our proposed model compared with the state of the art. Red and blue color represent the highest accuracy and the second, respectively

Noise Type	HiDDeN	ReDMarK	Liu's	Ours
Cropout (p=0.3)	94%	92.5%	**97.3%**	**97.8%**
Dropout (p=0.3)	93%	92%	**97.4%**	**97.4%**
Gaussian (σ=2)	96%	50%	**98.6%**	**98.8%**
JPEG (Q=50)	63%	74.6%	**76.2%**	**92.6%**
Crop (p=0.035)	88%	**100%**	89%	**95.2%**

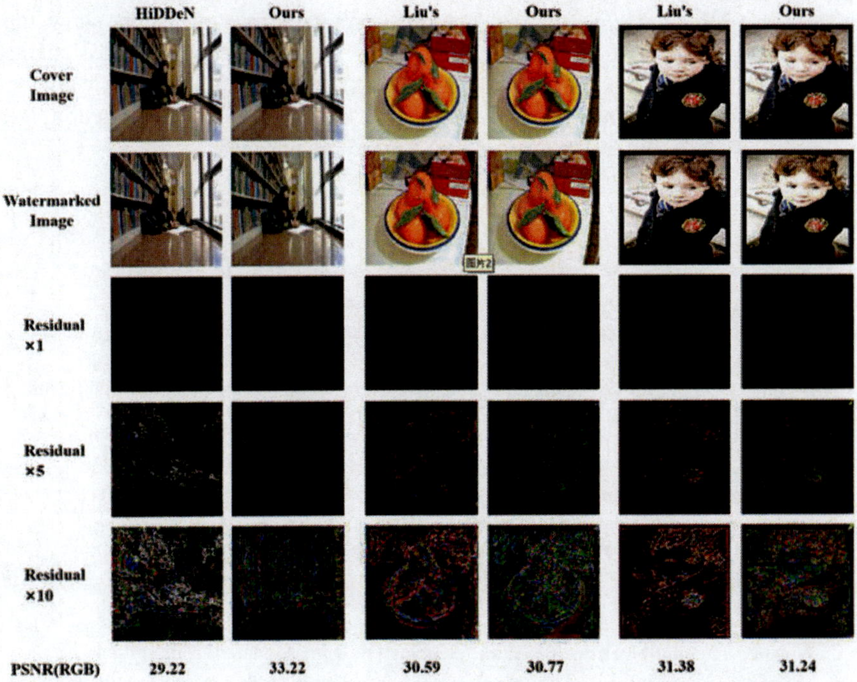

Fig. 4 Some sample cover and watermarked images for our model compared with HiDDeN and Liu's model

proposed model can directly extract watermark message from the cropped image, which will have wider applications in real use.

For watermarked image quality, we use PSNR and residual to evaluate the distance between cover image and watermarked image. As is shown in Fig. 4, image distortion for our model is no more severe than previous work. This indicates that our model can reach higher robustness against attacks of different types and different strength under the premise that image quality does not deteriorate and even improve in some case.

5 Conclusion

In this paper, we propose an image watermarking framework that embeds a watermark message of a fixed length into an RGB color image. We introduce the recover module into the network to compensate the damaged watermark information during attacks, which helps to improve the bit accuracy of extracting while not increasing the strength of watermark embedding. For JPEG compression which is non-differentiable during back propagation in training, we proposed a new approximation approach based on previous methods used in HiDDeN and ReDMark to get a result more close to real compression. Experimental results show that compared with the state of the art, our proposed method is more robust against attacks of different type and strength, especially significant in some case while not posing more distortion to watermarked image. The quality of our generated images is in a relatively high level compared with some previous work.

References

1. R.G. Van Schyndel, A.Z. Tirkel, C.F. Osborne, A digital watermark [C], image processing, 1994. Proceedings. ICIP-94., IEEE international conference. IEEE **2**, 86–90 (1994)
2. T. Zong, Y. Xiang, I. Natgunanathan, et al., Robust histogram shape-based method for image watermarking [J]. IEEE Transactions on Circuits and Systems for Video Technology **25**(5), 717–729 (2015)
3. W. Zheng, S.D. Li, X.H. Zhao, et al., Histogram based watermarking algorithm resist to geometric attacks [C], in *Advanced Information Management, Communicates, Electronic and Automation Control Conference (IMCEC)*, (2016), pp. 1438–1441
4. T.L. Kuang, W.D. Shun, S. Li, et al., Analysis and improvement of singular value decomposition-based watermarking algorithm [C], in *International Conference on Electric Information and Control Engineering (ICEICE)*, (2011), pp. 3976–3979
5. S.A. Parah, J.A. Sheikh, N.A. Loan, et al., Robust and blind watermarking technique in DCT domain using inter-block coefficient differencing [J]. Digit. Signal Proc. **53**, 11–24 (2016)
6. J.M. Guo, Y.F. Liu, J.D. Lee, et al., Blind prediction-based wavelet watermarking [J]. Multimed. Tools Appl. **76**(7), 9803–9828 (2017)
7. D. Volkhonskiy, B. Borisenko, E. Burnaev, Generative adversarial networks for image steganography [J]. 2016
8. J. Hayes, G. Danezis, Generating steganographic images via adversarial training [C]. Adv. Neural Inf. Proces. Syst., 1954–1963 (2017)
9. S. Baluja, Hiding images in plain sight: Deep steganography [C]. Adv. Neural Inf. Proces. Syst., 2069–2079 (2017)
10. A.u. Rehman et al., End-to-end trained CNN encoder-decoder networks for image steganography [C], in *Proceedings of the European Conference on Computer Vision (ECCV)*, (2018), pp. 723–729
11. H. Kandi, D. Mishra, S.R.K.S. Gorthi, Exploring the learning capabilities of convolutional neural networks for robust image watermarking [J]. Comput. Secur. **65**, 247–268 (2017)
12. S.M. Mun, S.H. Nam, H.U. Jang, et al., A robust blind watermarking using convolutional neural network [J]. arXiv preprint arXiv:1704.03248, 2017
13. J. Zhu, R. Kaplan, J. Johnson, F.-F. Li, HiDDeN: Hiding Data with Deep Networks [C], in *Proceedings of the European Conference on Computer Vision (ECCV), 2018*, (2018), pp. 657–672

14. M. Ahmadi, A. Norouzi, S.M. Soroushmehr, et al., ReDMark: framework for residual diffusion watermarking on deep networks [J]. arXiv **preprint arXiv**, 1810.07248 (2018)
15. Y. Liu, M. Guo, J. Zhang, et al., A novel two-stage separable deep learning framework for practical blind watermarking [C], in *Proceedings of the 27th ACM International Conference on Multimedia*, (2019), pp. 1509–1517
16. B. Wen, S. Aydöre, ROMark: A robust watermarking system using adversarial training. ArXiv **Preprint ArXiv**, 1910.01221 (2019)
17. S. Ioffe, C. Szegedy, Batch normalization: Accelerating deep network training by reducing internal covariate shift [C], in *Proceedings of The 32nd International Conference on Machine Learning*, (2015), pp. 448–456
18. F. Yu, V. Koltun, Multi-scale context aggregation by dilated convolutions [C], in *International Conference on Learning Representations (ICLR)*, (2016)
19. I. Goodfellow et al., Generative adversarial nets. Adv. Neural Inf. Proces. Syst. **3**, 2672–2680 (2014)
20. T.Y. Lin, M. Maire, S. Belongie, et al., *Microsoft COCO: Common Objects in Context. European Conference on Computer Vision* (2014), pp. 740–755

Deep Learning for Plant Disease Detection

Matisse Ghesquiere and Mkhuseli Ngxande

1 Introduction

Plant diseases can significantly decrease production of agriculture crops, where 20–30% of crop production per year is still lost [19]. These cause a major deficit in food supply where at least 800 million people are underfed [9]. In order to combat this problem, the plant disease has to be detected so remedies can be applied. Typical examples of destructive plant diseases include early blight and late blight [22]. Early detection is vital in order to prevent a disease from spreading throughout the rest of the crops [3]. Continuous monitoring by experts of all the different leaves is not a feasible approach, so different automated techniques need to be researched and tested. Several studies have been carried out with promising results and they all relied on machine learning and image processing techniques [5, 16, 18]. While these research papers offer excellent results, there is a trade-off between accuracy and computation time. In this project we try to minimize this gap by experimenting with different training approaches by systematic freezing of neural network layers at a predefined step (Fig. 1).

Computer vision has made a lot of progression in recent years, especially due to the ImageNet Large Scale Visual Recognition Challenge (ILSVRC) [20]. ImageNet is a large publicly available dataset containing approximately 14 million images and around 21,000 object classes [7]. This annual challenge is based on image classification performed on a subset of the data. In 2012, a convolutional neural network (CNN) named AlexNet achieved a top-5 error of 15.3% on the ImageNet Challenge, compared to the second place top-5 error rate of 26.2% [15]. This is seen as a major milestone in the deep learning community, because this model proved

M. Ghesquiere (✉) · M. Ngxande
Stellenbosch University, Western Cape, Stellenbosch, South Africa
e-mail: ngxandem@sun.ac.za

H. R. Arabnia et al. (eds.), *Advances in Computer Vision and Computational Biology*, Transactions on Computational Science and Computational Intelligence,
https://doi.org/10.1007/978-3-030-71051-4_5

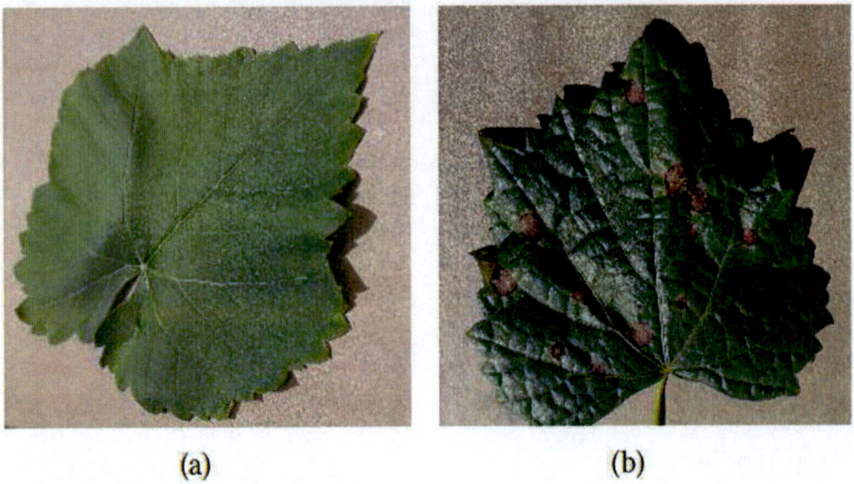

Fig. 1 Side by side comparison of a healthy grape leaf with a black rot grape leaf [12]. (**a**) Healthy grape leaf. (**b**) Grape with black rot

that CNN's actually work and often outperform more conventional techniques. Since then, other models have outperformed AlexNet on the ILSVRC by taking a different architectural approach [23, 25]. InceptionV3 [24], ResNet50V2 [10], and DenseNet201 [11]have been studied in this paper, these were chosen based on their high top-5 accuracy and their limited amount of parameters.

Machine learning is a hot topic and rightfully so. It has a wide range of applications, there is continuous improvement and no need for human intervention. Data is the fuel of every machine learning technique. So the main disadvantage of machine learning is the need of a sufficiently large dataset to prevent overfitting. This happens when the models fail to generalize from training data to testing data. Before the PlantVillage dataset [12], identifying plant diseases through machine learning was difficult, because data collection needs to be done manually. There was not enough data to accurately predict a disease. The PlantVillage dataset consists of 54,306 images, so it became possible to create a deep learning classifier.

Because of the complexity of deep learning models, they are often depicted as black boxes. Even if the results are accurate, the features on which the classifier predicts its decision are not known most of the time. If we want to evaluate our outcome and gather information for future predictions, it is important to visually see which features are a decisive factor. This is where saliency maps enter the picture [21]. A visualization is generated based on the output layer of the CNN. This is not only important for training purposes but also for real time evaluations by farmers. If they recognize a certain feature on a leaf that has a high chance of becoming a disease, they can act quickly and try to stop the spreading through the rest of their crops.

2 PlantVillage Dataset

Before 2015, there was no publicly available dataset of plant diseases large enough to be used for deep learning purposes. But then the PlantVillage project emerged, creating a dataset of 54,304 images classifying 26 diseases and 14 crop species [12]. This gives a total of 38 plant disease combinations. All these images have the correct disease and crop label and are resized to 256×256 pixels. This standardized format is necessary for equal input in our first neural network layers. We used the colored images for this project, because this has proven to perform well in a deep learning model [18]. This is also closest to real life images by farmers, taken with their smartphone, for example. 54,304 images are a lot, but a dataset this size is still prone to overfitting. We programmatically created data augmentation like rotation, zoom, rescaling..., so more features can be extracted from the same photos. Otherwise there is some inherent bias to the original images (Table 1).

3 Deep Learning Approach

3.1 Convolutional Neural Network

A convolutional neural network is a type of deep neural networks most commonly used for image classification. Traditional fully connected networks have a hard time extracting the right features to classify an image on and they are more computationally expensive. CNNs have some extra layers specifically made for these tasks. The first layer after the input layer is a convolution layer. This layer applies different kind of filters over the original image, so features like edges or curves are detected. Then we have the pooling layer. This layer reduces the dimensions of the data by extracting only the dominant features, so less computations are needed. Finally we feed the data into the fully connected layers, who try to combine the obtained features and a classification is made with the output layer. The main advantage with a deep learning approach is that it is fully automated. Feed in an image through the network and a classification is made without human intervention. Several studies have been conducted to detect plant diseases using traditional machine learning techniques [1, 2, 6]. This relies on manual feature engineering so there is less automation. Deep learning often outperforms conventional techniques so that is why we opted for this approach.

3.2 Transfer Learning

Image recognition with deep learning neural networks was improved a lot due to classification challenges. The most influential one was the ImageNet Large Scale

Table 1 The PlantVillage dataset

Plant	Disease	Nr. of images
Apple	Apple scab	630
	Black rot	621
	Cedar apple rust	275
	Healthy	1645
Blueberry	Healthy	1502
Cherry	Healthy	854
	Powdery mildew	1052
Corn	Cercospora/gray leaf spot	513
	Common rust	1192
	Healthy	1162
	Northern leaf blight	985
Grape	Black rot	1180
	Esca (black measles)	1383
	Healthy	423
	Leaf blight	1076
Orange	Haunglongbing (citrus greening)	5507
Peach	Bacterial spot	2297
	Healthy	360
Bell pepper	Bacterial spot	997
	Healthy	1478
Potato	Early blight	1000
	Healthy	152
	Late blight	1000
Raspberry	Healthy	371
Soybean	Healthy	5090
Squash	Powdery mildew	1835
Strawberry	Healthy	456
	Leaf scorch	1109
Tomato	Bacterial spot	2127
	Early blight	1000
	Healthy	1591
	Late blight	1909
	Leaf mold	952
	Septoria leaf spot	1771
	Spider/two-spotted spider mite	1676
	Target spot	1404
	Tomato mosaic virus	373
	Tomato yellow leaf curl virus	5357

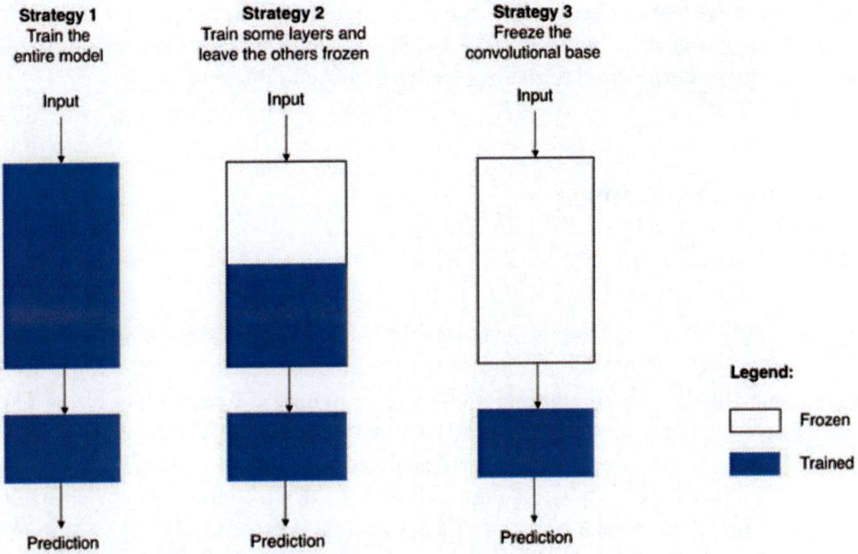

Fig. 2 Types of transfer learning [17]

Visual Recognition Challenge, or ILSVRC. Industry leaders and academics tried developing neural network architectures to classify 1000 different image classes based on the ImageNet dataset. In this project we used the best performing models and try to classify our PlantVillage dataset through transfer learning.

Transfer learning is the re-use of a model trained on another similar task [13]. For our purpose the models are trained on the ImageNet dataset, so they already recognize certain features, like edges, shapes... If we replace the output layer with a custom layer based on the different plant diseases, we can re-train this network on our new data. There are three main strategies as seen in Fig. 2. In the first strategy you're training the entire model, so the whole architecture will be trained. This requires longer training times and more resources. This is a type of transfer learning if the weights from pre-trained models are used, for example, the ImageNet weights. In the second strategy you can choose to freeze some layers. The first layers are mostly extracting general features, while subsequent layers are being more and more specific. The third strategy freezes the base model and only trains the fully connected layers. So you are dependent on the base model for feature extraction, but because there is fewer layers to train, it will speed up computations.

4 Keras

For this project we made use of Keras, a high-level deep learning library [4]. Keras is beginner friendly and easy to use for prototypes. Because of the tensorflow backend support, GPU training is possible, which is very useful for heavy image processing like in the PlantVillage dataset. There is also support for models pre-trained on the ImageNet dataset, data augmentation, regularization techniques like dropout... All of these features are very intuitive and become of use in this project.

5 Image Processing

5.1 *Preprocessing*

Because a neural network relies on numbers as input, we need to transform an image into something readable for our deep learning models. All images are 256×256 pixels, but different deep learning architectures require different input sizes. The InceptionV3 model, for example, has an input size of 299×299 pixels, while DenseNet has an input size of 224×224 pixels [11, 24]. So the first step when importing images is changing the dimensions to the desired input. An image can be seen as a two-dimensional array, with each value representing a number between 0 and 255 (for the intensity of our channel). Because we used colored images, we obtain a three-dimensional array. So our array is of the shape (width, height, channel). Data needs to be loaded in batches, so we added an additional dimension for the number of samples. The shape becomes (samples, width, height, channel). The intensity values for our images are still a number between 0 and 255. Each model re-scales these numbers, this is necessary so each image contributes evenly to the total loss. Rescaling values are different for each model, some are between 0 and 1, others between -1 and $+1$. Luckily Keras provides these functions for each supported model [4]. Now we have the desired input shape.

5.2 *Augmentation*

54,304 images taken from the PlantVillage dataset may seem like a lot, but this is still prone to overfitting. With more data, our model will be able to generalize more, so new unseen images will be correctly classified as well. With data augmentation techniques we can artificially expand our dataset by transforming our current images. This way, it will be better at picking up the right traits of a disease, instead of relying on features which are irrelevant. A leaf image from the testing dataset can have a different rotation, zoom or light intensity than the images the model has been trained on. If we want our model to handle these cases correctly, we need to provide training data that takes these conditions into account. Some of the operations used in this project are depicted in Fig. 3 and they are:

- Rotating
- Vertical and horizontal flipping
- Brightness intensity

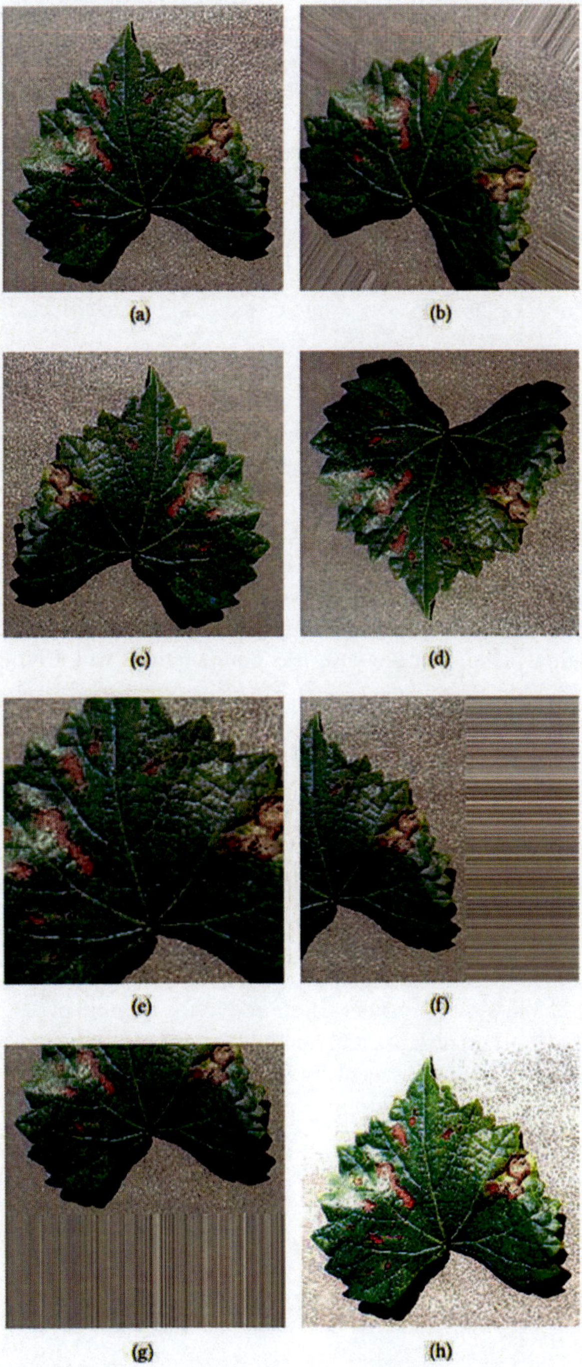

Fig. 3 Image data augmentation performed on the PlantVillage dataset [12]. (**a**) Original grape black measles. (**b**) Rotation. (**c**) Horizontal flip. (**d**) Vertical flip. (**e**) Zoom adjustment. (**f**) Width shift. (**g**) Height shift. (**h**) Brightness adjustment

- Width and height shift
- Zoom intensity

6 Implementation

6.1 Architectures

Three well known CNN architectures are tested on the PlantVillage dataset:

- InceptionV3 [24]
- ResNet50V2 [10]
- DenseNet201 [11]

These were chosen based on their excellent results on the ILSVRC and are supported by the Keras framework.

InceptionV3 is 48 layers deep with less than 25 million parameters and makes use of inception modules. An inception module combines sets of convolution and pooling layers which are then concatenated, so features are captured in parallel. This allows convolutions to perform on the same level, the network gets wider, not deeper. Inception modules make sure less computations and a limited amount of parameters are used.

ResNet50V2, on the other hand, has 50 layers and around 23 million parameters and makes use of residual components, containing a skip connection. This connection does not have any parameters and is used for bypassing layers. While InceptionV3 avoids a deeper network by making it wider, ResNet does this by skipping layers.

DenseNet201 is an extension of ResNet with 201 layers and approximately 20 million parameters. In contrast to ResNet, it connects every layer to every forward layer with skip connections, so each layer has a collective knowledge of the previous ones. This reduces the computations and parameters needed. For more information on the used architectures, the reader is referred to the original papers [10, 11, 24].

We removed the output layer and applied another max-pooling layer. Then we added a 1024 node fully connected layer, with a 0.5 dropout regularization. The output layer is now a softmax output layer, classifying our 38 crop-disease pairs.

6.2 Training Types

There are four different types of training types used in this project:

1. Scratch
2. Deep

3. Shallow
4. Hybrid

Training from scratch means that we used the previously discussed architectures with a random weight initialization. This way, our neural network will not have learned anything, so everything will depend on the dataset.

In the deep training approach, we used the architectures trained on the ImageNet dataset, while still training the whole network. This means that it already has learned some image specific features, like edge detection, for example, which means the network learns faster. These first two methods do need the most computation time, because it trains the full network.

In the shallow approach we froze the convolutional base initialized with the ImageNet weights. This is an example of fixed feature extraction. The purpose of this training method is to combine the extracted features with our custom layer. This requires the least computation, but is more prone to overfitting. That is why we also used a hybrid approach.

The hybrid training method trained the whole network like the deep approach for a few epochs, then we froze the convolutional base and continued shallow training. This way, we made the network recognize dataset-specific features so the fully connected layers could combine these. This is a trade-off between computation time and performance.

6.3 Parameters

All the models were trained with the same parameters for comparing purposes. These are:

- Optimizer: Stochastic Gradient Descent
  - Initial Learning rate: 0.001
  - Momentum: 0.9
  - Weight decay: 0.0001
- Batch Size: 32
- Epochs: 30
- Epochs Hybrid Pre-training: 2

These were chosen based on short test runs while experimenting with the parameters. The final parameters used have the best average performance over the different models and training types.

7 Results

We evaluate the performance based on the mean F1-score. This is a better metric for this project than the overall accuracy, because it takes the false negatives and false positives into account. The results are seen in Table 2.

When we trained the models from scratch, it is clear that each model is able to correctly classify the data in almost all cases, with a minimum F1-score of 95.60%. The deep approach is performing slightly better and ResNet50V2 is able to catch up compared to training from scratch. When using transfer learning, the general goal is to have a higher start, slope, and asymptote on the training/performance curve. When plotting our accuracy for each type, we notice that the training accuracy after one epoch reaches between 20 and 30% when training from scratch, while the deep approach reaches a minimum of 75% after one only epoch, due to the ImageNet weight initialization. It has more time to fine-tune, which explains the improved results in the deep training type method.

The shallow approach suffers from overfitting, because it was not able to extract the necessary dataset-specific disease features, due to the fixed feature extraction approach. Combining the recognized ImageNet features was not enough to gain a high enough F1-score. ResNet50V2 performs almost 15% better than the other models here. The DenseNet architecture is an extension of ResNet, but there is a big difference. The ResNet architecture receives output from the previous layer, while DenseNet receives output from every previous layer, mimicking a global feature learning memory. This does seem to perform worse when using fixed feature extraction. After tinkering with the parameters, such as changing the batch size, the learning rate, and the amount of fully connected layers, there was not much improvement. One solution could be to only freeze parts of the convolutional base, so dataset-specific features could be recognized. In this project, we opted for a hybrid training approach.

Table 2 The mean F1-score by training type and model

Training type	Model	F1-score (%)
Scratch	InceptionV3	98.40
	ResNet50V2	95.60
	DenseNet201	98.11
Deep	InceptionV3	99.70
	ResNet50V2	99.40
	DenseNet201	99.50
Shallow	InceptionV3	51.60
	ResNet50V2	64.00
	DenseNet201	51.20
Hybrid	InceptionV3	98.70
	ResNet50V2	88.60
	DenseNet201	96.50

The hybrid approach seems to be a good trade-off between computation time and performance. The results are getting near the deep-trained models, but not elevating them, as expected. ResNet is again getting different results, but this time performing worse than the other architectures. DenseNet and Inception are able to extract the right features faster than ResNet, while ResNet is better at combining these, as seen in the shallow approach. For Resnet to perform the same as the others in the hybrid training type, the amount of epochs in the deep pre-training phase needs to be increased.

In Fig. 4 we can very clearly see the effect of transfer learning applied on the InceptionV3 architecture. Training from scratch starts off with a low accuracy and gradually increases, whereas the deep training type reaches a very high accuracy after just one epoch. There is also no need to increase the amount of epochs while using transfer learning. For all accuracy plots, we refer to the GitLab repository [8].

8 Visualization

In order to evaluate the results and see if the neural networks are picking up the right disease features, a visualization is made of the neural network. Suppose we try to predict a new type of leaf having a certain disease with our models. When using training data it performs very well, but after showing a new leaf type, it makes poor predictions. This could be due to our model picking up the wrong features. It could make its judgment solely based on the leaf shape, instead of also taking the disease spots into account, for example. Luckily there is a way to visualize our trained neural network by using saliency maps [21].This is done by computing the gradient of the output category after feeding in our input image. These gradients are used to highlight pixel regions that cause the most change in the output. This can be done with the Keras Visualization toolkit [14]. The output layer's activation is set to linear and we supply the output category and the input image. We only back-propagate the positive gradients through our network, so only positive activations are highlighted. The results are plotted in Fig. 5.

The healthy raspberry leaf seen in Fig. 5a triggers a global activation across the whole leaf. There are no disease bounded spots, but rather an overall recognition of the leaf type. The peach leaf diagnosed with the bacterial spot disease, seen in Fig. 5b, triggers the gradients more locally. On top of the leaf there is a colored spot, for which we can clearly see the activation that picks up on this disease trait. This means our model is picking up the correct features and correctly classifying the disease.

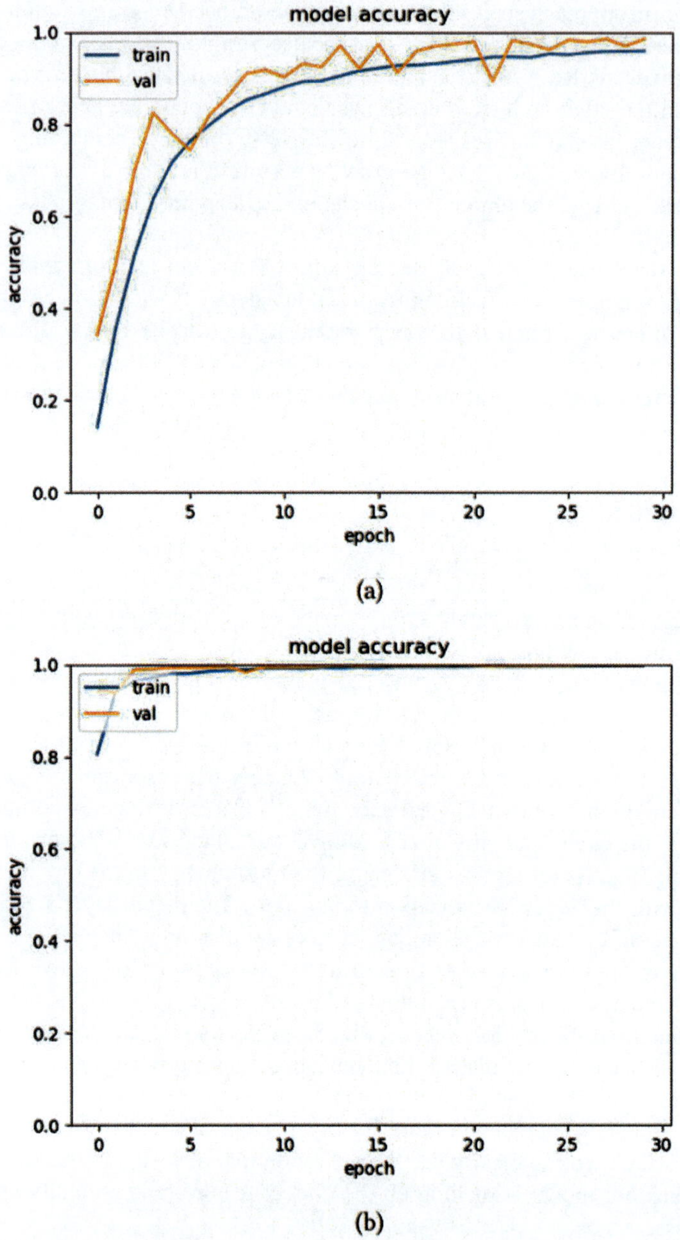

Fig. 4 InceptionV3 accuracy plot. (**a**) Scratch training type. (**b**) Deep training type

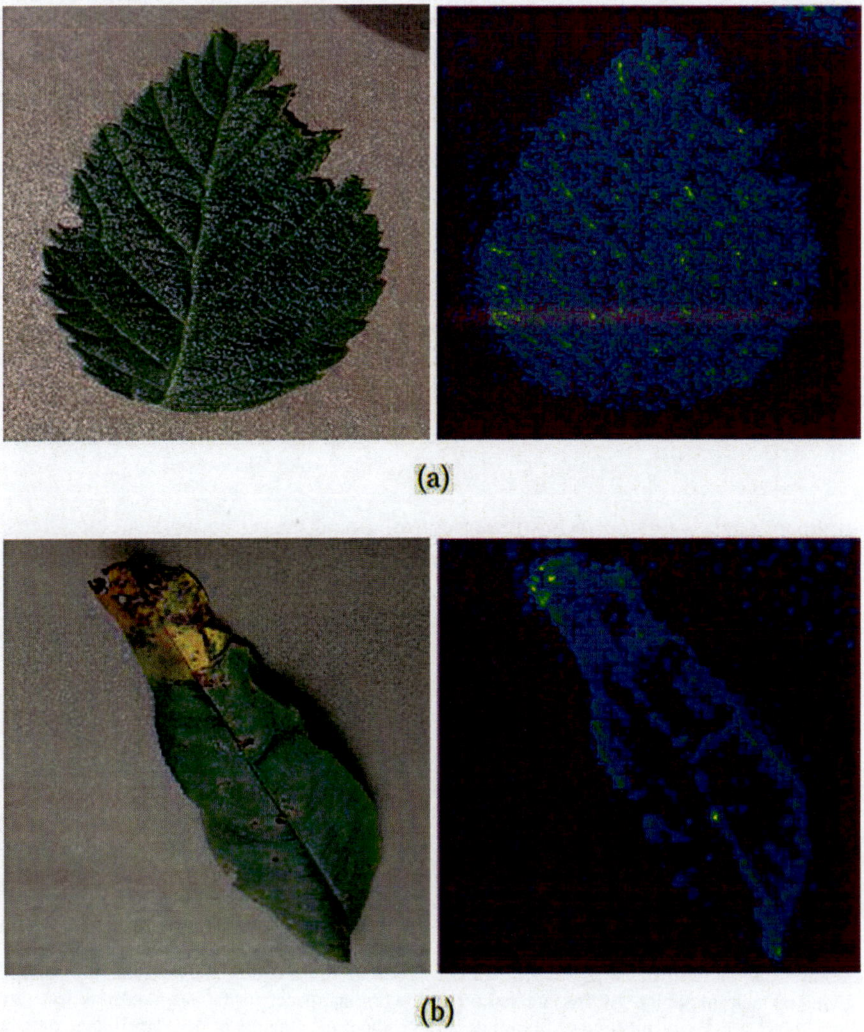

Fig. 5 Visualization of the output layer of a ResNet50V2 deep-trained model from plants taken from the PlantVillage dataset [12]. (**a**) Healthy Raspberry leaf. (**b**) Peach leaf with bacterial spot

9 Future Work

9.1 Leafroll Disease

The Stellenbosch Agriculture Department is preparing a dataset to predict leafroll disease in vineyards. Because of the similarities with using the PlantVillage dataset, we can perform transfer learning again, but this time with the leafroll disease data.

The models would already have learned the PlantVillage data specific features, so in theory the detection of leafroll should be straightforward.

9.2 Smartphone Application

The PlantVillage data contains images taken in optimal conditions. If farmers would like to classify diseases for their crop types, we would need a lot more data taken in suboptimal conditions. But this project proves that there is definitely an opportunity for smartphone-assisted detection on a global scale.

10 Conclusion

In this project, we evaluated different convolutional neural network architectures, designed for the ILSVRC, on how they performed in classifying different plant diseases based on the PlantVillage dataset. Our experimental results indicate that the architectures perform very well, especially when the convolutional base can be re-trained on the new dataset. When not using transfer learning, the models need more training time in order to reach its highest accuracy. If the convolutional base is used as a fixed feature extractor, the models would need more data in order to avoid overfitting. The hybrid training approach reduces the gap between computation time and performance, so it is the preferred approach. A saliency map was used to evaluate our models by visualizing the output layer. These indicate that the network was picking up the right disease traits. The trained models can be used as a base for detecting other plant disease types, if data can be provided. In the future, a smartphone-based application is also in our interests.

Acknowledgments I thank my supervisor Mr. Ngxande for assisting me with this project and giving me helpful advice. I thank the authors of the original paper for the inspiration to base my project on [18]. This project was also not possible without the creators of the PlantVillage dataset [12].

References

1. A. Akhtar, A. Khanum, S.A. Khan, A. Shaukat, Automated Plant Disease Analysis (APDA): performance comparison of machine learning techniques, in *2013 11th International Conference on Frontiers of Information Technology*, pp. 60–65 (2013)
2. H. Al-Hiary, S. Bani-Ahmad, M. Ryalat, M. Braik, Z. Alrahamneh, Fast and accurate detection and classification of plant diseases. Int. J. Comput. Appl. **17**(03) (2011). https://doi.org/10.5120/2183-2754

3. W.C. Chew, M. Hashim, A.M.S. Lau, A.E. Battay, C.S. Kang, Early detection of plant disease using close range sensing system for input into digital earth environment, in *IOP Conference Series: Earth and Environmental Science*, vol. 18 (2014), p. 012143. https://doi.org/10.1088/1755-1315/18/1/012143
4. F. Chollet et al., Keras (2015). https://keras.io
5. A. Cruz, Y. Ampatzidis, R. Pierro, A. Materazzi, A. Panattoni, L. De Bellis, A. Luvisi, Detection of grapevine yellows symptoms in Vitis vinifera L. with artificial intelligence. Comput. Electron. Agric. **157**, 63–76 (2019)
6. Y. Dandawate, R. Kokare, An automated approach for classification of plant diseases towards development of futuristic Decision Support System in Indian perspective, in *2015 International Conference on Advances in Computing, Communications and Informatics (ICACCI)* (2015), pp. 794–799
7. J. Deng, W. Dong, R. Socher, L.-J. Li, K. Li, F.-F. Li, ImageNet: a large-scale hierarchical image database, in *2009 IEEE Conference on Computer Vision and Pattern Recognition*, pp. 248–255 (2009)
8. N. Ghesquiere, Deep Learning for Plant Disease Detection (2020). https://git.cs.sun.ac.za/24541702/deep-learning-for-leafroll-disease-detection
9. C.A. Harvey, Z.L. Rakotobe, N.S. Rao, R. Dave, H. Razafimahatratra, R.H. Rabarijohn, H. Rajaofara, J.L. MacKinnon, Extreme vulnerability of smallholder farmers to agricultural risks and climate change in Madagascar. Philos. Trans. R. Soc. B Biol. Sci. **369**(1639), 20130089 (2014). https://doi.org/10.1098/rstb.2013.0089
10. K. He, X. Zhang, S. Ren, J. Sun, Identity mappings in deep residual networks, in *CoRR*, abs/1603.05027 (2016). arXiv:1603.05027. http://arxiv.org/abs/1603.05027
11. G. Huang, Z. Liu, K.Q. Weinberger, Densely connected convolutional networks, in *CoRR*, abs/1608.06993 (2016). arXiv:1608.06993. http://arxiv.org/abs/1608.06993
12. D.P. Hughes, M. Salathé, An open access repository of images on plant health to enable the development of mobile disease diagnostics through machine learning and crowdsourcing, in *CoRR*, abs/1511.08060 (2015). arXiv:1511.08060. http://arxiv.org/abs/1511.08060
13. M. Hussain, J. Bird, D. Faria, A study on CNN transfer learning for image classification, in *UK Workshop on computational Intelligence* (Springer, Cham, 2018), pp. 191–202
14. R. Kotikalapudi et al., Keras-vis (2017). https://github.com/raghakot/keras-vis
15. A. Krizhevsky, I. Sutskever, G.E. Hinton ImageNet classification with deep convolutional neural networks, in *Advances in Neural Information Processing Systems 25*, ed. by F. Pereira, C.J.C. Burges, L. Bottou, K.Q. Weinberger (Curran Associates, Red Hook, 2012), pp. 1097–1105. http://papers.nips.cc/paper/4824-imagenet-classification-with-deep-convolutional-neural-networks.pdf
16. B. Kusumo, A. Heryana, O. Mahendra, H. Pardede, Machine learning-based for automatic detection of corn-plant diseases using image processing (2018), pp. 93–97. https://doi.org/10.1109/IC3INA.2018.8629507
17. P. Marcelino, Transfer learning from pre-trained models (2018). https://miro.medium.com/max/1400/1*9t7Po_ZFsT5_lZj445c-Lw.png [Online; Accessed 07 May 2020]
18. S.P. Mohanty, D.P. Hughes, M. Salathé, Using deep learning for image-based plant disease detection, in *CoRR*, abs/1604.03169 (2016). arXiv:1604.03169. http://arxiv.org/abs/1604.03169
19. E.-C. Oerke, H.-W. Dehne, Safeguarding production—losses in major crops and the role of crop protection. Crop Prot. **23**(04), 275–285 (2004). https://doi.org/10.1016/j.cropro.2003.10.001
20. O. Russakovsky, J. Deng, H. Su, J. Krause, S. Satheesh, S. Ma, Z. Huang, A. Karpathy, A. Khosla, M. Bernstein, A.C. Berg, L. Fei-Fei, ImageNet large scale visual recognition challenge. Int. J. Comput. Vis. **115**(3), 211–252 (2015). https://doi.org/10.1007/s11263-015-0816-y
21. K. Simonyan, A. Vedaldi, A. Zisserman, Deep inside convolutional networks: visualising image classification models and saliency maps, in *CoRR*, abs/1312.6034 (2014)

22. W. Stevenson, W. Kirk, Z. Atallah, Management of foliar disease, early blight, late blight and white mold, in *Potato Health Management* (APS Press, St. Paul, 2007), pp. 209–222
23. C. Szegedy, W. Liu, Y. Jia, P. Sermanet, S.E. Reed, D. Anguelov, D. Erhan, V. Vanhoucke, A. Rabinovich, Going deeper with convolutions, in *CoRR*, abs/1409.4842 (2014). arXiv:1409.4842. http://arxiv.org/abs/1409.4842
24. C. Szegedy, V. Vanhoucke, S. Ioffe, J. Shlens, Z. Wojna, Rethinking the inception architecture for computer vision, in *CoRR*, abs/1512.00567 (2015). arXiv:1512.00567. http://arxiv.org/abs/1512.00567
25. M.D. Zeiler, R. Fergus, Visualizing and understanding convolutional networks, in *CoRR*, abs/1311.2901 (2013). arXiv:1311.2901. http://arxiv.org/abs/1311.2901

A Deep Learning Framework for Blended Distortion Segmentation in Stitched Images

Hayat Ullah, Muhammad Irfan, Kyungjin Han, and Jong Weon Lee

1 Introduction

In recent years, the rising popularity of immersive media technology such as Virtual Reality (VR), Augmented Reality (AR), and Mixed Reality (MR) has attracted plentiful attention of the computer vision research community. These immersive technologies provide the user with realistic experience via wide field of view images known as panoramic images. Panoramic images are typically obtained by stitching multiple images captured from different view angles with sufficient overlapping region. To obtain high-quality panoramic image, various image stitching algorithms have been proposed [1, 2]. However, each stitching algorithm causes different types of stitching distortions while creating panoramas (i.e., geometric distortion and photometric distortion) that significantly affect the visual quality of resultant panorama.

Different from classical 2D image distortion, these stitching relevant distortions cannot be captured with traditional image quality assessment metrics. Numerous SIQA methods have been proposed for measuring the quality of stitched images. These SIQA method areas are mainly categorized into two parts: Full-Reference SIQA (FR-SIQA) and No-Reference SIQA (NR SIQA) algorithms.

In FR-SIQA algorithms, the quality of stitched image is objectively evaluated by comparing the SIQA score of stitched images and unstitched images using quality assessment metrics including Structure Similarity Index (SSIM) and Peak Signal-to-Noise Ratio (PSNR). For instance, Jia et al. [3] proposed SIQA algorithm which evaluates the stitched regions of omnidirectional images. They used three different region quality assessment metrics (histogram features, perceptual hash,

H. Ullah · M. Irfan · K. Han · J. W. Lee (✉)
Department of Software Convergence, Sejong University, Seoul, Korea
e-mail: jwlee@sejong.ac.kr

H. R. Arabnia et al. (eds.), *Advances in Computer Vision and Computational Biology*, Transactions on Computational Science and Computational Intelligence,
https://doi.org/10.1007/978-3-030-71051-4_6

and sparse reconstruction) for measuring the local relation of stitched images with its corresponding cross-reference images. In other work, Yang et al. [4] proposed content-aware SIQA method for capturing the geometric and structure inconsistency error in stitched images by computing optical flow field and chrominance of stitched and reference images.

On the other hand, NR-SIQA methods evaluate the quality of panoramic images without any reference image by analyzing the actual content of distorted images. For example, Ling et al. [5] suggested an NR-SIQA algorithm based on Convolutional Sparse Coding (CSC). Their proposed approach used convolutional filters and trained kernels to locate the distorted region and measure the effect of specific distortion. Similarly, Sun et al. [6] proposed a CNN-assisted quality assessment framework for 360° images. Their proposed method first extracts features from intermediate layers which are then regressed by regression layer at the tail of MC-CNN network.

This paper proposed a novel blended distorted region segmentation approach, which segments the blended distortion in stitched images and generates the binary mask for segmented region. The following are the key contributions of our work:

- To the best of our knowledge, there is no learning-based approach for segmenting the stitching relevant distorted region, i.e., blended distortion. We present first deep learning-based method that segments blended distortion in panoramic image.
- The proposed method precisely extracts the distorted specific region using end-to-end learnable network.
- The proposed system can significantly improve the performance of stitching methods by segmenting the blended distortion and eliminating the distortion using segmented region.

The remainder of this paper is arranged as follows. The proposed methodology is described in Section II, where experimental results are discussed in Section III. Finally, we conclude this paper with possible future directions in Section IV.

2 Method

In this section, we discuss the proposed method and its main components in detail. Our proposed method is based on Mask R-CNN architecture [7] originally proposed for object instance segmentation, which can efficiently detect objects and generate high-quality binary mask for the segmented objects. For better understanding, we divide the proposed methodology into six sections including (a) backbone architecture, (b) region proposal, (c) ROI pooling and alignment, (d) box prediction and classification, and (e) mask generation. Fig. 1 illustrates the outline of the overall proposed system.

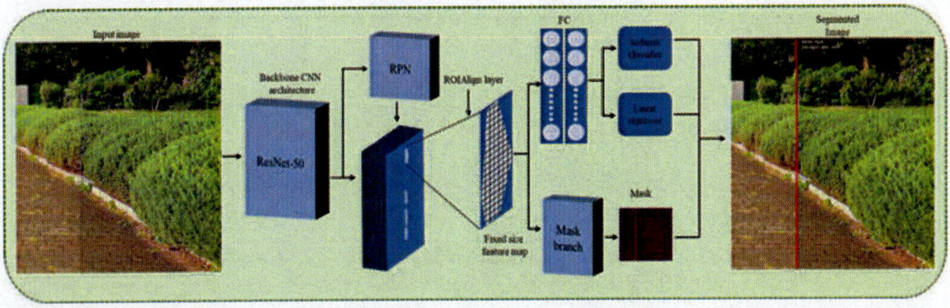

Fig. 1 Framework of our proposed method for blended distortion segmentation

2.1 *Backbone Architecture*

Originally, Mask R-CNN is used with different CNN architectures for semantic segmentation task. In this paper, we select ResNet50 [8] architecture as a backbone network of the proposed method, which extracts deep features from the input distorted image using last convolution layer. After feature extraction process, the extracted feature maps are then forwarded to the next module that randomly generates bounding boxes using the salient regions of the feature maps.

2.2 *Region Proposal*

The region proposal process involves a fully CNN network called Region Proposal Network (RPN) that takes an image as input and produce multiple boxes/anchors by examining the salient regions in the feature maps. The RPN network first extracts features from each region proposal and then forward the extracted features to the two distinct layers called rpn_cls_score and rpn_bbox_pred layer. The first layer classifies the anchor either foreground or background, while the second layer predicts the coordinates of the anchors.

2.3 *ROI Pooling and Alignment*

The region proposals generated by the RPN network have nonuniform dimensionality, whereas the fully connected layer only accepts the data with fixed dimensionality. This nonuniformity is removed by the ROIPool layer, which quantizes the input region proposal to fixed size by doing max pooling. However, the quantization process introduces misalignment between the feature maps and region proposals that have negative impacts on binary mask prediction. This problem is solved using ROIAlign layer that removes the severe quantization produced by the ROIPool layer.

The use of ROIAlign layer significantly improves the mask generation (pixel-to-pixel binary classification) performance. After pooling and alignment process, the refine ROIs are then forwarded to two distinct modules including box prediction and classification module and segmentation mask generation module.

2.4 *Box Prediction and Classification*

The outputs of the ROIPool and ROIAlign are then interpreted by a fully connected layers which are then forwarded to two distinct output heads, i.e., classification head and regression head. The classification head classifies the class of the object inside the region proposal, whereas the regression head predicts the coordinates for each region proposal.

2.5 *Mask Generation*

The last step of the proposed system is to predict the binary masks for all ROIs. The mask branch network processes the fixed size refine ROIs feature maps and generates high-quality binary masks. The final segmented image is obtained by applying the estimated binary masks on its corresponding regions. The obtained binary masks can be further used to retrieve the specific object in the image.

3 Experimental Results

This section presents the detail about the implementation of experimental evaluation of our proposed framework. The proposed framework is implemented in python language version 3 using deep learning library TensorFlow on a machine equipped with NVIDIA GTX 1060 6GB GPU and Intel Core i7 processor of 3.60 GHz. For training the proposed blended distortion segmentation framework, we adopt two main changes in the original implementation of Mask R-CNN. First, we squeezed all the network layers and train only the network head on our blended distortion dataset using pretrained COCO weights for 20 epochs. Second, we replace the classification layer of original Mask R-CNN layer with new classification layer having classes $N + 1$. Where N represents the number of classes, in our case, we have only one class "blended distortion," and 1 is added for the background class. Furthermore, we initialized the training of Mask R-CNN with the following hyper-parameters: batch size $= 32$, learning rate $= 0.0001$, images per GPU $= 1$, and iterations per epochs $= 100$.

The quantitative results are generated using well-known segmentation performance evaluation metrics including Mean Average Precision (mAP), Mean

Table 1 The obtained quantitative results on our blended distortion dataset

Evaluation stage	mAP	mAE	MIoU
Validation	0.84	0.17	0.81
Test	0.82	0.18	0.79

Absolute Error (mAE), and Mean Intersection Over Union (MIoU). Mathematically, these metrics can be expressed as

$$\text{mAP} = \frac{1}{n}\sum_{i=1}^{n}\text{AP}_i \tag{1}$$

where n is the total number of test images, and AP_i is the ith average precision.

$$\text{mAE} = \frac{\sum_{i=1}^{n}|y_i - x_i|}{n} \tag{2}$$

where y_i is the predicted pixel class, i.e., foreground/background, and x_i is the ground truth that represents the actual class of ith pixel.

$$\text{MIoU} = \frac{1}{k+1}\sum_{i=0}^{k}\frac{P_{ii}}{\sum_{j=0}^{k}P_{ij} + \sum_{j=0}^{k}\left(P_{ji} - P_{ii}\right)} \tag{3}$$

where k is the total number of classes, P_{ij} is the number of pixels that are from class i but misclassified as class j, while P_{ii} is the number of pixels that are correctly classified. The obtained segmentation results of 170 test images are given in Table I, where the proposed framework achieved reasonable results that satisfy the reliability of blended distortion segmentation.

Besides quantitative evaluation, we also validate the effectiveness of our proposed framework through qualitative evaluation. Fig. 2 illustrates the obtained segmentation results, where it can observe that the proposed framework generates three different output for the input stitch image that includes mask map, distortion-specific image, and final segmented image. The obtained visual results confirm that the proposed framework can be used to capture, extract, and segment the blended distortion in stitched images.

4 Conclusion

The quality assessment of stitched image is an ill-posed problem that is actively studied by the research community. Numerous SIQA methods are presented by different studies till date, most of them estimate the quality of stitched image using 2D image quality assessment metrics or using deep learning networks. These methods adopted computationally expensive strategies for estimating the quality of

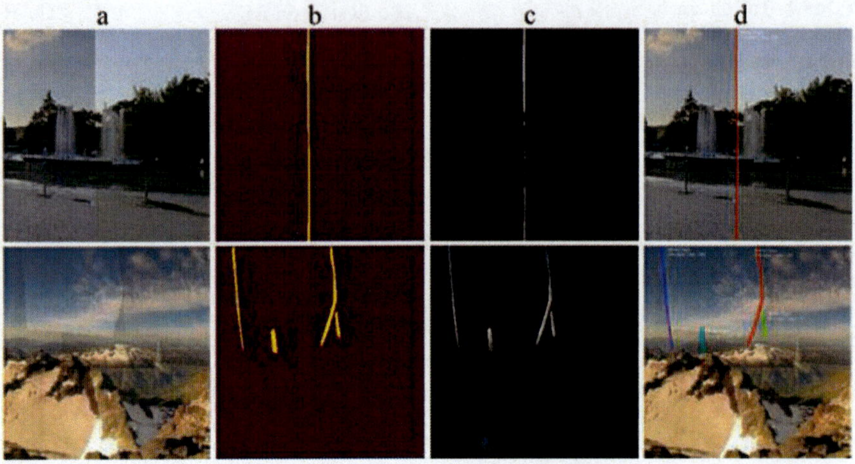

Fig. 2 The obtained visual results: (**a**) input blended distorted image, (**b**) generated segmentation mask, (**c**) distortion-specific image, and (**d**) final segmented image

stitched images. Further, these approaches are limited to quality estimation only without knowing the actual location and magnitude of stitching distortion. With these motivations, a segmentation-based approach for quality assessment of stitched image is proposed in this paper. Our proposed method first captures the blended distortion and then segments the distorted region using binary mask. The segmented regions are then used to compute the quality of panoramic image by counting the number of distorted pixels.

Acknowledgment This research was supported by the MSIT (Ministry of Science and ICT), Korea, under the ITRC (Information Technology Research Center) support program (IITP-2020-2016-0-00312) supervised by the IITP (Institute for Information and communications Technology Planning and Evaluation).

References

1. Y. Li, M. Tofighi, V. Monga, Robust alignment for panoramic stitching via an exact rank constraint. IEEE Transact Image Proc **28**, 4730–4745 (2019)
2. J. Zheng, Y. Wang, H. Wang, B. Li, H.-M. Hu, A novel projective-consistent plane based image stitching method. IEEE Transact. Multimedia **21**, 2561–2575 (2019)
3. J. Li, K. Yu, Y. Zhao, Y. Zhang, and L. Xu, "Cross-Reference Stitching Quality Assessment for 360° Omnidirectional Images," in Proceedings of the 27th ACM International Conference on Multimedia, 2019, pp. 2360–2368
4. L. Yang, Z. Tan, Z. Huang, G. Cheung, A content-aware metric for stitched panoramic image quality assessment, in *Proceedings of the IEEE International Conference on Computer Vision Workshops*, (2017), pp. 2487–2494

5. S. Ling, G. Cheung, P. Le Callet, No-reference quality assessment for stitched panoramic images using convolutional sparse coding and compound feature selection, in *2018 IEEE International Conference on Multimedia and Expo (ICME)*, (2018), pp. 1–6
6. W. Sun, X. Min, G. Zhai, K. Gu, H. Duan, S. Ma, MC360IQA: A multi-channel CNN for blind 360-degree image quality assessment. IEEE J. Selected Topics Signal Proc (2019)
7. K. He, G. Gkioxari, P. Dollár, R. Girshick, Mask r-cnn, in *Proceedings of the IEEE International Conference on Computer Vision*, (2017), pp. 2961–2969
8. K. He, X. Zhang, S. Ren, J. Sun, Deep residual learning for image recognition, in *Proceedings of the IEEE Conference on Computer Vision and Pattern Recognition*, (2016), pp. 770–778

Intraocular Pressure Detection Using CNN from Frontal Eye Images

Afrooz Rahmati, Mohammad Aloudat, Abdelshakour Abuzneid, and Miad Faezipour

1 Introduction

1.1 Background and Motivation

Glaucoma is an international disease causing vision loss for many patients around the world. A gradual increase of intraocular pressure (IOP) and missing early diagnoses might cause blindness forever. However, preventative measures and actions can be taken if high IOP is detected at the very early stages of glaucoma.

Observing IOP generally requires the patient's presence at a healthcare facility where ophthalmologists or nurses evaluate the eye pressure through different medical tests. In some cases, the healthcare professional anesthetizes the eye by dropping a numb liquid which would take at least 6 hours to totally wear off from the eyes and irritate the patient.

Anatomically, one of the main causes of glaucoma is due to the expansion of pressure inside the eye (IOP). The eye fluid called aqueous humor builds up in the front layer of the eye. This extra fluid develops eye pressure and progresses into the anterior chamber between the iris and cornea [1]. At the same time, the frontal view

A. Rahmati · A. Abuzneid
Department of Computer Science & Engineering, University of Bridgeport, Bridgeport, CT, USA

M. Aloudat
Applied Science University, Amman, Jordan
e-mail: m.aloudat@asu.edu.jo

M. Faezipour (✉)
Department of Computer Science & Engineering, University of Bridgeport, Bridgeport, CT, USA

Department of Biomedical Engineering, University of Bridgeport, Bridgeport, CT, USA
e-mail: mfaezipo@bridgeport.edu

H. R. Arabnia et al. (eds.), *Advances in Computer Vision and Computational Biology*, Transactions on Computational Science and Computational Intelligence,
https://doi.org/10.1007/978-3-030-71051-4_7

of the eye may appear altered by a dilated, droopy shaped pupil and/or red areas in the sclera. The excess pressure inside the eye could damage the entire optic nerve. This damage might cause eventual blindness.

Accessing regular eye checkup services would decrease the risk of developing glaucoma. IOP is generally measured by a healthcare professional at health facilities through different examinations such as the tonometry test and gonioscopy test [2]. All these tests require the patient's presence. Sometimes, ophthalmologists anesthetize the eyes by numb drops to gently touch the iris surface and measure IOP. This action irritates the patients' eye. On the other hand, highly accurate, noninvasive, and noncontact methods are more convenient. To this end, computer vision-based techniques that rely on eye images have grabbed much attention in healthcare facilities.

1.2 Related Work

Many computer vision-based studies have been conducted on detecting glaucoma and measuring IOP at an early stage. However, most of these studies analyze the fundus eye images that reflect the optic nerves [3, 4]. We have identified only one research group whose work is based upon evaluating frontal eye images [5–7]. In a recent work, Aloudat et al. [5] proposed a novel risk assessment framework of IOP on frontal eye images and applied a fully conventional network (FCN) to separate the iris and sclera area. Six different features were then extracted, and a decision tree classifier was designed to distinguish eye images with high IOP and glaucoma from the normal eye pressure cases.

2 Proposed Methodology

We build upon our prior work [5] and propose a computer vision and deep learning-based approach toward distinguishing normal (healthy) IOP cases from high IOP cases using frontal eye images to automate the feature selection process.

2.1 CNN

We are proposing a solution to utilize convolutional neural network (CNN) for the process of extracting eye features and determining high IOP.

The proposed CNN system receives frontal eye images as input, assigns weights and biases to differentiate eye segments, uses ConvNet to filter images, pools layers to extract dominant features, and finally classifies the output with a regular neural network [8]. The structure or the proposed CNN is depicted in Fig. 1.

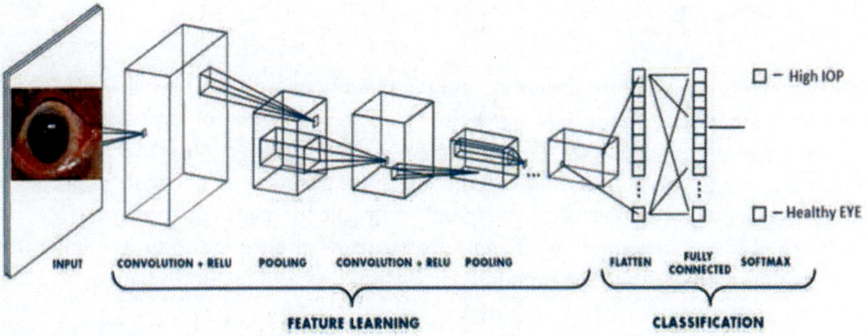

Fig. 1 Structure of proposed CNN

2.2 *Dataset*

Image data for this work was gathered from a hospital in Jordan with 473 patients. Two hundred frontal eye images were collected from high-eye pressure patients, and the rest 273 images were taken from healthy patients with normal IOP. Both male and females participated in the frontal eye image database. The IOP value for each patient's eye was recorded by ophthalmologists. The range of IOP measures of the normal (healthy) eye pressure cases were 11–21 mmHg, while the high IOP measured cases were in the range of 22–30 mmHg [9, 10]. The images were all taken in a range of 20 cm distance between the camera and the participant's face. The model of the camera used for data collection was Canon model T6 K1 with a resolution of 3241 × 2545, and the lighting condition for all the images in the dataset was consistent.

IRB approval was obtained at Princess Basma Hospital for the human subject samples. Authors formally requested access to the dataset.

2.3 *Training and Test Data*

In the ongoing research work presented here, our preliminary training dataset contains 100 images from high IOP and 100 normal eye pressure cases. The remaining 273 images are considered for testing purposes.

For the purpose of training deep learning models that require large number of instances and to improve the accuracy of the high IOP detection system, we are working closely with few hospitals in the Middle East to increase the number of images in the dataset.

3 Expected Outcome

This research is a work in progress, and the outcomes are yet to be observed. The weights and biases of the CNN structure will be adjusted for best performance results in terms of accuracy. We anticipate that with the proposed deep learning method using CNN, high IOP cases can be distinguished from normal eye pressure ones with accuracies above 90% using only frontal eye images as the input.

The proposed ideas are significant efforts made in an attempt to automate the determination of the onset of high IOP and vision loss as a result of glaucoma, at an early stage from only frontal eye images.

Nowadays, smartphones offer convenient platforms for a variety of smart healthcare monitoring systems, given their user-friendly interfaces, connectivity, and processing capabilities [11–13]. The ideas proposed in this paper can be further personalized for patients by embedding the techniques into smartphone devices. Frontal eye images captured from the smartphone camera can be used as the input image to the proposed CNN-based high-IOP detection system.

References

1. A.A. Salam, M.U. Akram, K. Wazir, S.M. Anwar, M. Majid, Autonomous Glaucoma detection from fundus image using cup to disc ratio and hybrid features, in *Proc. IEEE Int. Symp. Signal Process. Inf. Technol. (ISSPIT)*, (Abu Dhabi, 2015), pp. 370–374
2. R. Sorkhabi, M.B. Rahbani, M.H. Ahoor, V. Manoochehri, Retinal nerve fiber layer and central corneal thickness in patients with exfoliation syndrome. Iranian J. Ophthalmol. **24**(2), 40–46 (2012)
3. K.R. Martin, K. Mansouri, R.N. Weinreb, R. Wasilewicz, C. Gisler, J. Hennebert, D. Genoud, T. Shaarawy, C. Erb, N. Pfeiffer, G.E. Trope, Use of machine learning on contact lens sensor–derived parameters for the diagnosis of primary open-angle glaucoma. Am. J. Ophthalmol. **194**, 46–53 (2018)
4. S. Maetschke, B. Antony, H. Ishikawa, G. Wollstein, J. Schuman, R. Garnavi, A feature agnostic approach for glaucoma detection in OCT volumes. PLoS One **14**(7), e0219126 (2019)
5. M. Aloudat, M. Faezipour, A. El-Sayed, Automated vision-based high intraocular pressure detection using frontal eye images. IEEE J. Transl. Eng. Health Med. (IEEE J-TEHM) **7**(1) Article No. 3800113, 1–13 (2019)
6. M. Aloudat, M. Faezipour, A. El-Sayed, High intraocular pressure detection from frontal eye images: a machine learning based approach, in *Proceedings of the IEEE International Engineering in Medicine and Biology Society Conference, (IEEE EMBC'18)*, (Jul. 2018), pp. 5406–5409
7. M. Al-Oudat, M. Faezipour, A. El-Sayed, A smart intraocular pressure risk assessment framework using frontal eye image analysis. EURASIP J. Image Video Proc. **90**, 1–15, Springer (2018)
8. S. Saha, (2018). A comprehensive guide to convolutional neural networks — the ELI5 way. Retrieved from towards Data Science: Accessed 24 Mar 2020. [Online]. https://towardsdatascience.com/a-comprehensive-guide-to-convolutional-neural-networks-the-eli5-way-3bd2b1164a53
9. M.C. Leske, The epidemiology of open-angle glaucoma: A review. Amer. J. Epidemiol. **118**(2), 166–191 (1983)

10. C. Tsai, High eye pressure and glaucoma. Glaucoma Research Foundation. Accessed 24 Mar 2020. [Online]. Available: https://www.glaucoma.org/gleams/high-eye-pressure-and-glaucoma.php
11. M. Faezipour, A. Abuzneid, Smartphone-based self-testing of COVID-19 using breathing sounds. Telemed. e-Health (2020). https://doi.org/10.1089/tmj.2020.0114
12. A. Abushakra, M. Faezipour, Augmenting breath regulation using a mobile driven virtual reality therapy framework. IEEE J Biomed. Health Inform. **18**(3), 746–752 (2014)
13. O. Abuzaghleh, B.D. Barkana, M. Faezipour, Noninvasive real-time automated skin lesion analysis system for melanoma early detection and prevention. IEEE J. Transl.. Eng. Health Med. **3**, Article No. 4300212, 1–12 (2015)

Apple Leaf Disease Classification Using Superpixel and CNN

Manbae Kim

1 Introduction

Plants in the farms serve as a backbone to sustain the environment. Plants suffer from diseases, which affects the normal growth. Detection of such plant diseases is an important task to perform. Currently, the identification and classification of diseases are carried out by humans. Plant experts observe the plant diseases by monitoring over a period of time, which is time-consuming. Therefore, to monitor the plant disease at an early stage, an automatic detection method can be beneficial. Apple leaf disease recognition is an essential research topic in the field of plant agriculture, where the key task is to find an effective way to classify the diseased leaf images.

The apple leaf diseases are generally classified into three categories: (1) *apple scab*, (2) *black rot*, and (3) *cedar apple rust*, which are shown in Fig. 1. In addition, healthy leaves are included for classification purpose.

In general, the classification methods are categorized into two areas. One method is to use the segmentation of the infected regions of a leaf [1, 2]. Then, statistical features are derived and analyzed by diverse machine learning methods for recognizing disease types. The other approach is directly to use a neural network in the form of end-to-end learning [3]. For an image, CNN (convolutional neural network) is usually adopted for their superior representation performance.

The demerit of end-to-end learning can be observed in Fig. 2. The leaf image in Fig. 2a feeds into a neural network; however, as shown in Fig. 2b, in practice, a camera might capture a large region including the leaf of interest. In this situation,

M. Kim (✉)
Department of Computer and Communications Engineering, Kangwon National University, Chunchon, Republic of Korea
e-mail: manbae@kangwon.ac.kr

H. R. Arabnia et al. (eds.), *Advances in Computer Vision and Computational Biology*, Transactions on Computational Science and Computational Intelligence,
https://doi.org/10.1007/978-3-030-71051-4_8

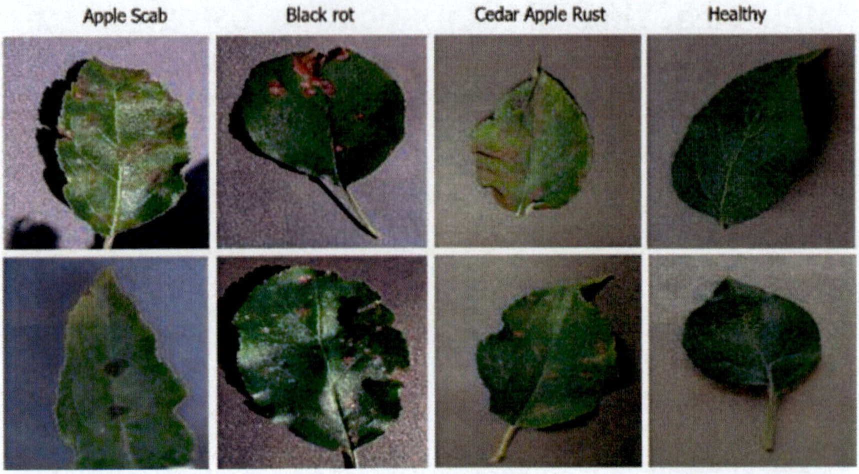

Fig. 1 Leaves with three kinds of diseases and healthy leaves

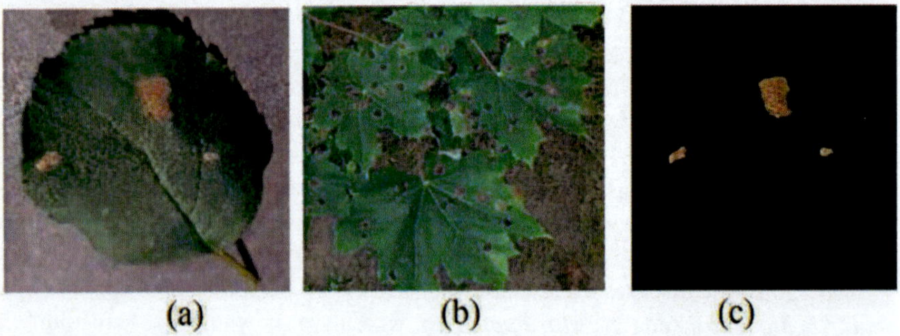

Fig. 2 Shows the demerits of end-to-end learning as well as segmentation in practice. (**a**) Input leaf, (**b**) an image acquired by a camera, and (**c**) segmentation of diseased region

the training images and test images could be different, resulting in the incorrect classification by CNN inference. As well, the segmentation is difficult to achieve satisfactory performance as shown in Fig. 2c. Further, in the farm, a dense growth of trees contains many leaves, preventing the accurate image acquisition of a single leaf. To solve the aforementioned problems, we propose a superpixel-based CNN method that focuses on apple disease classification.

2 Proposed Method

Figure 3 shows an overall flow of the proposed method. Firstly, a leaf image is decomposed by superpixel segmentation. Then we build a bounding box enclosing

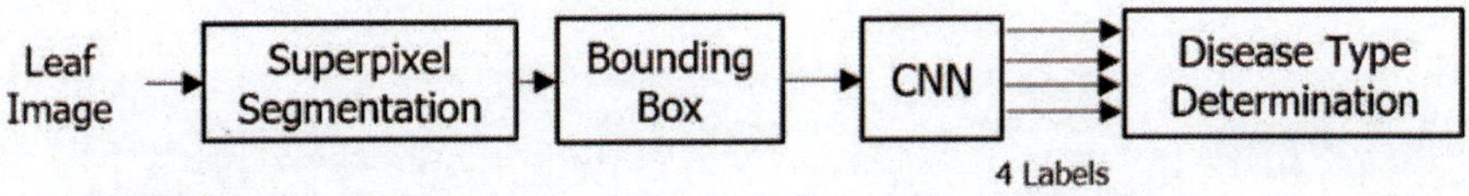

Fig. 3 Overall block diagram of the proposed method

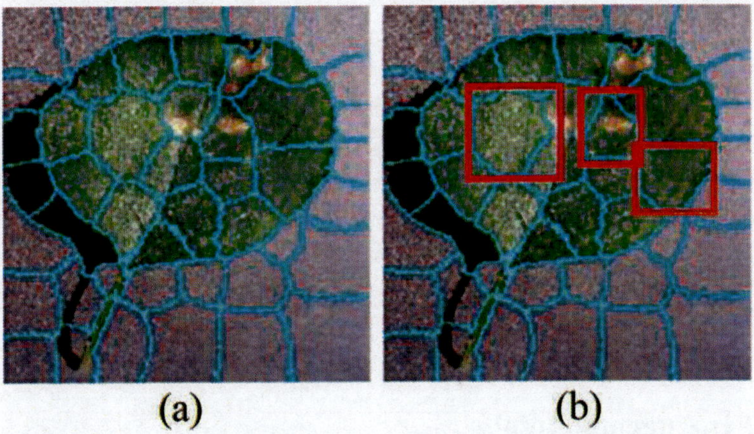

Fig. 4 Superpixel segmentation and bounding box. (**a**) Superpixel segmentation and (**b**) bounding box marked in red

a superpixel. Train data are composed of the bounding boxes with their associated labels.

Our methodology consists of building a data set containing labeled images of four types of diseases. For each leaf image, SLIC [4] is carried out for image segmentation. Figure 4a shows the result of superpixel segmentation. Then since only a rectangular image feeds into the input of CNN, we transform an arbitrary-sized superpixel into a bounding-box image (red boxes in Fig. 4b).

3 CNN Architecture

Since the main objective of this work is to investigate the feasibility of superpixel-based learning ability compared with full image, we adopt a shallow network, which can meet the purpose of this work.

The network in Fig. 5 consists of only few convolutional layers with few filters per layer, followed by two fully connected layers, and ends with a softmax normalization. We train the shallow network of three convolutional layers. Each convolutional layer has 16 filters of size 5×5 and a Rectified Linear Unit (ReLU) activation. All layers are followed by a 2×2 max-pooling layer, except for the last convolutional layer. The first fully connected layer has 64 nodes with a ReLU

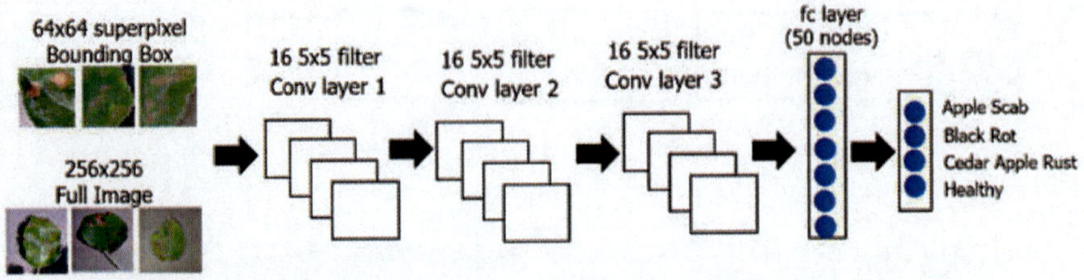

Fig. 5 CNN model. Superpixel bounding boxes feed into the network. For performance comparison, original full images are also examined by the identical network

activation and is followed by a dropout layer with a dropout ratio of 50%. The last fully connected layer has four outputs associated with the four classes. The softmax layer calculates the probability output and decides a predicted class.

For full image and superpixels, an identical CNN model is used for a fair comparison.

4 Experimental Results

The proposed work was implemented on MATLAB 2018b. Images used in the experiment are available in the public PlantVillage data set [5]. The PlantVillage is an open-access database of healthy and diseased crops. We selected the color images of apple leaf with *scab*, *black rot*, *cedar apple rust,* and *healthy*. Image resolution is 256 × 256 pixels. All pixel values are divided by 255 to be compatible with the CNN network's initial values.

The performance evaluation of the proposed work is evaluated using *F1 score* that is based on a *confusion table*. The number of leaf images for *apple scab*, *black rot*, *cedar apple rust*, and *heathy* is 630, 621, 275, and 1,645, respectively. For each leaf image, a bounding-box image is made from superpixel segmentation. In the experiment, the number of subpixels that we want to create was set to 20. Since bounding boxes contain disease and healthy parts, we manually separated them into their associated classes. The number of bounding-box images is 693, 1000, 985, and 522 for the four classes, respectively. Since the resolution of bounding-box images is different, we scaled them into 64x64 resolution. The examples of bounding-box images are shown in Fig. 6.

The data set was randomly partitioned into training and test subsets. The training subset was used to train and optimize a CNN model and fully connected layers. The test set was then used to assess the performance of the classifier.

The classification accuracy of CNN train and test is shown in Table 1. Train and test accuracy of full image are 99.38 and 98.29, respectively, and train and test accuracy of superpixel are 97.76 and 92.43, respectively.

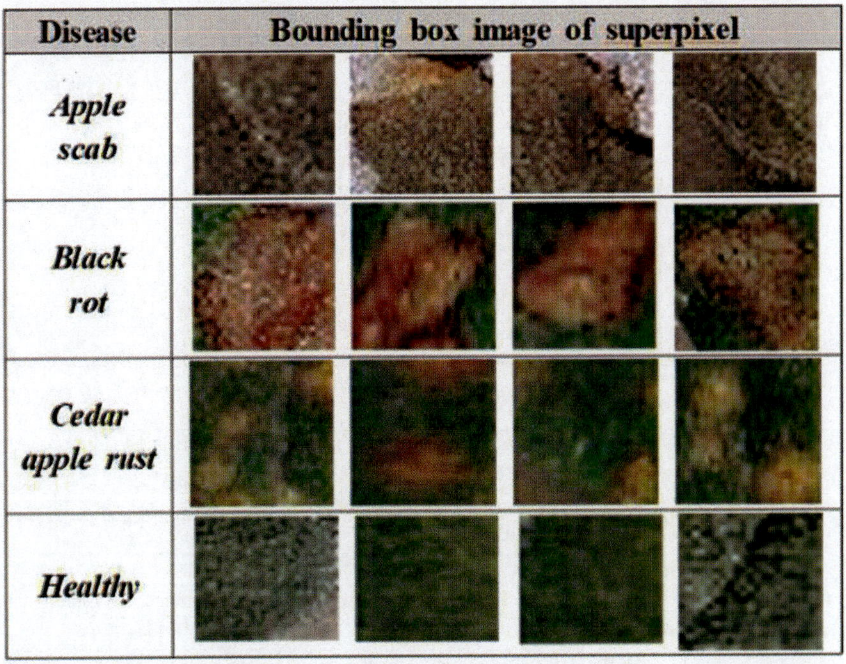

Fig. 6 Superpixel mages used in the experiment

Table 1 Classification accuracy of full image and superpixel from CNN inference

	Classification accuracy	
Image type	Train	Test
Full image	99.38%	98.29%
Superpixel	97.76%	92.43%

Table 2 Confusion matrix

		Ground truth	
		Pos	Neg
Prediction result	Pos	TP	FP
	Neg	FN	TN

To compute F1 score of the classifier, a confusion table in Table 2 is used, where four components of TP (true positive), TN (true negative), FP (false positive), and FN (false negative) are computed. In the multi-class classifier, the four components are derived in the separate manner. Then precision (PRE) and recall (REC) are computed by

$$\mathrm{PRE} = \frac{\sum_{k=1}^{K} \mathrm{TP}_k}{\sum_{k=1}^{K} \mathrm{TP}_k + \sum_{k=1}^{K} \mathrm{FP}_k} \tag{1}$$

Table 3 Confusion matrix of *train* superpixel image

		Ground truth			
		Scab	Black rot	Cedar rust	Healthy
Classification result	Scab	567	1	15	0
	Black rot	20	771	15	2
	Cedar rust	3	0	753	0
	Healthy	1	0	0	353

Table 4 Confusion matrix of *test* superpixel image

		Ground truth			
		Scab	Black rot	Cedar rust	Healthy
Classification result	Scab	96	1	12	1
	Black rot	9	171	10	2
	Cedar rust	3	7	219	1
	Healthy	4	2	1	161

Table 5 Confusion matrix of *train* full image

		Ground truth			
		Scab	Black rot	Cedar rust	Healthy
Classification result	Scab	509	7	0	3
	Black rot	0	496	0	0
	Cedar rust	0	0	226	0
	Healthy	4	0	0	1154

$$\text{REC} = \frac{\sum_{k=1}^{K} \text{TP}_k}{\sum_{k=1}^{K} \text{FN}_k + \sum_{k=1}^{K} \text{TP}_k} \tag{2}$$

where K is the number of classes. Subsequently, F1 score is computed by

$$\text{F1} = 2 \times \frac{\text{PRE} \times \text{REC}}{\text{PRE} + \text{REC}} \tag{3}$$

Tables 3, 4, 5, and 6 show the confusion tables generated by the CNN model. Tables 3 and 4 show the confusion table of train and test of superpixel image. F1 scores of the four classes are 0.87, 0.92, 0.93, and 0.97. F1 score of four classes derived by Eq. (3) is 0.93. For the full image, the confusion tables of train and test are shown in Tables 5 and 6. F1 score of each class is 0.95, 0.98, 0.97, and 0.98 producing F1 score of 0.98 in four classes. The F1-score of the full image outperforms that of the superpixel only by 0.05, indicating that the performance of superpixel is comparable to that of full image.

Experimental results show that the performance of superpixels is slightly lower than that of full images. The reasons are twofold: (1) The difference between train and test accuracy indicates the problem of data shortage. Thus, we need

Table 6 Confusion matrix of *test* full image

		Ground truth			
		Scab	Black rot	Cedar rust	Healthy
Classification result	Scab	111	2	0	3
	Black rot	2	116	0	0
	Cedar rust	0	0	45	1
	Healthy	4	0	0	412

more superpixel data. (2) The selection process of diseases and healthy superpixels requires more precise work. Some superpixels may contain regions of partial disease or full infection, resulting in lower accuracy and F1 score.

5 Conclusion

The plant diseases are harmful to plant and can affect the growth of the plant. To solve two problems such as unreliable segmentation and the impractical adaptation of full images to real applications, we have proposed superpixel-based CNN for classification of apple leaf diseases. The results, when compared with full image, show that the proposed method achieves satisfactory performance in terms of classification accuracy and F1 score. In future, this work can be extended to work on different diseases with dissimilar characteristics.

Acknowledgment This research was supported by the MSIT (Ministry of Science and ICT), Korea, under the ITRC (Information Technology Research Center) support program **(IITP-2020-2018-0-01433)** supervised by the IITP (Institute for Information and communications Technology Promotion).

References

1. S. Chouhan, A. Kaul, U. Singh, S. Jaini, Bacterial foraging optimization based Radial Basis Function Neural Network (BRBFNN) for identification and classification of plant leaf diseases: an automatic approach towards plant pathology. IEEE Access (2018). https://doi.org/10.1109/ACCESS.2018.2800685
2. M. Khan, I. Lali, M. Sharif, K. Javed, K. Aurangzeb, S. Haider, A. Altmarah, T. Akram, An optimized method for segmentation and classification of apple diseases based on strong correlation and genetic algorithm based feature selection. IEEE Access (2019). https://doi.org/10.1109/ACCESS.2019.2908040
3. G. Wang, Y. Sun, J. Wang, Automatic image-based plant disease severity estimation using deep learning. Hindawi Comput. Intell. Neurosci., 2917536, 8 pages (2017, 2017). https://doi.org/10.1155/2017/2917536

4. R. Achanta, A. Shaji, K. Smith, A. Lucchi, P. Fua, S. Susstrunk, SLIC superpixels compared to state-of-the-art superpixel methods. IEEE Trans. Pattern Anal. Mach. Intell. **34**(11), 2274–2281 (2012)
5. D. Hughes, M. Salathe, An open access repository of images on plant health to enable the development of mobile disease diagnostics through machine learning and crowdsourcing. CoRR **abs/1511.08060** (2015). [Online]. Available: http://arxiv.org/abs/1511.08060

Part II
Imaging Science – Detection, Recognition, and Tracking Methods

Similar Multi-Modal Image Detection in Multi-Source Dermatoscopic Images of Cancerous Pigmented Skin Lesions

Sarah Hadipour, Siamak Aram, and Roozbeh Sadeghian

1 Introduction

About 4% of all skin cancers are malignant melanoma which is a serious type of skin cancer. About 75% of skin cancer patients die from malignant melanoma worldwide. Risk factors for developing melanomas are both genetic and environmental. They range from being sensitive to sun or having light colored skin to excessive exposure to sun [1]. Family history of melanoma as well as patient's history of skin cancer are also important factors. Just like any other disease, treating this disease and reducing mortality rate starts with early detection. First step towards detection is to take medical images, which conventionally used to be with digital cameras, from the affected area in order to distinguish between benign and malignant types of pigmented skin lesions. However, often times these pictures are taken multiple times and stored in the image base with different modalities. This duplication causes issues in detecting cancerous images that is discussed in detail in Sect. 2. This will bring us to the subject of finding similar or near duplicate images in the image set of the pigmented skin lesions. To get an idea of how these images look, Fig. 1 shows four different examples of skin lesions taken from ISIC 2018 [2] and [3] image set.

S. Hadipour
Northeastern University, Boston, MA, USA
https://ece.northeastern.edu/
e-mail: hadipour.s@northeastern.edu

S. Aram (✉) · R. Sadeghian
Harrisburg University of Science and Technology, Harrisburg, PA, USA
https://harrisburgu.edu/profile/siamak-aram/
https://harrisburgu.edu/profile/roozbeh-sadeghian/
e-mail: SAram@harrisburgu.edu; RSadeghian@harrisburgu.edu

H. R. Arabnia et al. (eds.), *Advances in Computer Vision and Computational Biology*, Transactions on Computational Science and Computational Intelligence,
https://doi.org/10.1007/978-3-030-71051-4_9

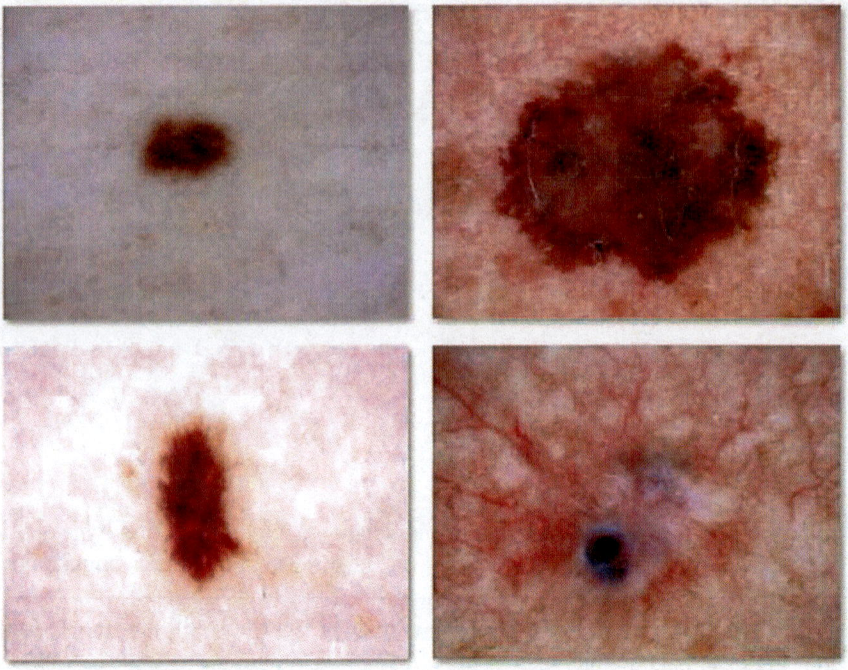

Fig. 1 Example images of four skin lesions

Historically speaking, image similarity detection has been the most sought after subject in analyzing images [4]. To accomplish the similarity detection between two images we need to first define the feature space which in our case is the histogram domain. This similarity manifests itself in the image histogram. The histograms as image feature are discussed in Sect. 4 in detail. The main role of histogram features in computer vision is to transform visual information into the vector space. This gives us opportunity to perform our similar image test on them, for example finding the minimum difference in their features which leads us to finding similar image in our medical image base [5].

2 Similar Image Detection

While we often assume that images in an image set are independent and identically distributed, that is rarely the case when dealing with medical scans. In our case of pigmented skin lesion image set, the ultimate goal is to detect the malignant cases which is initiated by designing and training a Convolutional Neural Network (CNN) model. That is where it would be possible to remove those duplicate images before training our CNN model. But trying to manually detect duplicate images

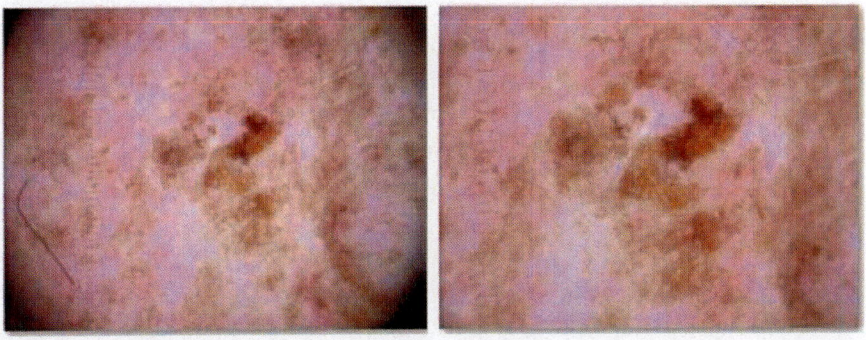

Fig. 2 Example images of similar skin lesions with different modality

in an image set is extremely time-consuming and error-prone and it also does not scale easily. Therefore a method is needed to automatically detect and remove duplicate images from our Deep Learning image set. Another key point to keep in mind is that our model has to be able to generalize to any unseen skin lesion that might show up in future image sets. By including multiple identical or near identical images in our training image set, our neural network is allowed to see and learn patterns from that image multiple times per epoch. Our network could become biased toward patterns in those duplicate images, giving our Deep Neural Network (DNN) additional opportunities to learn patterns specific to the duplicates and making it less likely to generalize to new images. This impacts the ability of our model to generalize to new images outside of what it was trained on. Bias and ability to generalize are a big deal in Machine Learning and can be hard to combat specially when working with skin lesion image set. The duplication issue can clearly be seen in Fig. 2 that shows images of a pigmented skin lesion in the same spot with two different modalities.

3 Literature Review

Similarity is basically measured by the means of distance in particular distance between the histogram derived from a grey-scale image. The use of histograms as main features is discussed in prior works such as [6]. Image distances have been applied to image histograms in so many ways. Six of these distances that are commonly used and defined in the literature are fully described in Sect. 3.1 through Sect. 3.6. Their inadequacy when they are used to calculate the distance between image histograms such as histograms of pigmented skin lesion is considered.

The histogram distance is defined as the element-wise distance between two images that come directly from the skin lesion image set. Given two images we are looking for the least amount of distance between two images. In the following sections, six common methods of calculating the histogram distances are discussed. Other methods such as Hellinger distance, Tsallis divergence, Euclidean distance, or Mahalanobis distance have been considered but for the purpose of this paper we keep it to the six methods discussed below. Then the results and introduction to the best method for our application are discussed in Sect. 3.7.

3.1 Intersection Distance

Histogram intersection calculates the similarity of two discretized probability distributions (histograms). Histogram intersection works equally well on categorical data, for instance the different categories of skin cancer. The histogram intersection algorithm was proposed by Swain and Ballard [7]. They have introduced the intersection distance as the following:

$$\text{Distance}\,(H_1, H_2) = \sum_I \min\,(H_1(I), H_2(I)) \tag{1}$$

where $H(I)$ represents the histogram of input image I.

The result of the intersection is the number of pixels from the model image that has corresponding pixels of the same colors in the reference image. However, one issue with the intersection method is that the intersection depends on how the bins have been selected.

3.2 Bhattacharyya Distance

One of the ways to find the similarity of two discrete probability distributions or two images is the Bhattacharyya distance [8]. The Bhattacharyya distance formula is shown in equation below :

$$\text{Distance}\,(H_1, H_2) = 1 - \frac{1}{\sqrt{\sum H_1 \sum H_2}} \sum_I \sqrt{H_1(I) \cdot H_2(I)} \tag{2}$$

Since the Bhattacharyya distance is normalized it provides a similarity detection method that is easier to use. It also offers other useful features [9].

3.3 Chi-Square Distance

The chi-square of two images is once again based on their histograms. The number of bins in two image histograms should be equal. The definition of the chi-square of two images is that the number of occurrences reported in each bin should be close in two similar images. The formula for the chi-square distance is defined as below:

$$\text{Distance}\,(H_1, H_2) = \sum_I \frac{(H_1(I) - H_2(I))^2}{H_1(I) + H_2(I))} \tag{3}$$

In our experiment we chose a 256 bin histogram which is appropriate for our image sets [10].

3.4 Pearson Correlation Distance

Pearson correlation distance is a statistic that measures linear correlation between two image histograms H_1 and H_2. The correlation distance formula is shown here [ref here]:

$$\text{Distance}\,(H_1, H_2) = \frac{\sum_I \left(H_1(I) - \overline{H}_1\right)\left(H_2(I) - \overline{H}_2\right)}{\sqrt{\sum_I \left(H_1(I) - \overline{H}_1\right)^2 \sum_I \left(H_2(I) - \overline{H}_2\right)^2}} \tag{4}$$

where

$$\overline{H}_k = \frac{1}{N} \sum_J H_k(J) \tag{5}$$

One important point is that, under heavy noise conditions, extracting the correlation distance between two image histograms is nontrivial. Later, we will see how this method compares to others.

3.5 Kullback–Leibler (K–L) Distance

The K–L in literature is also called KL divergence [11, 12], relative entropy information gain, or information divergence and is a way to compare differences between two image histograms $H_1(I)$ and $H_2(I)$. Equation below shows how this divergence is calculated:

$$\text{Distance}\,(H_1, H_2) = \sum_I H_2(I) \log \frac{H_2(I)}{H_1(I)} \tag{6}$$

3.6 Earth Mover's Distance (EMD)

The Earth Mover's Distance (EMD) was introduced by Rubner and Guibas [13]. They came up with a method to fix the issue with the image histograms that do not overlap completely. This gap is called an earth mover's distance. It basically describes the amount of work that needs to be done in order to turn one histogram into another by moving the mass of the distribution by solving a linear optimization problem.

The Earth mover's distance is a type of distance where the position and weight of the points in the image histogram are very critical. The formula on how to calculate the EMD is described briefly below:

$$\begin{gathered}\text{Distance}(H_1, H_2) = \min_{F=\{F_{ij}\}} \frac{\sum_{i,j} F_{ij} D_{ij}}{\sum_i F_{ij}} \\ \text{s.t: } \sum_j F_{ij} \leq H_1 \\ \sum_i F_{ij} \leq H_2 \\ \sum_{i,j} F_{ij} = \min\left(\sum H_1, \sum H_2\right) \\ F_{ij} \geq 0\end{gathered} \tag{7}$$

3.7 Methodology Comparison

Six methods of image similarity detection were discussed in Sect. 3.1 through Sect. 3.6. These methods have also been found useful in other applications involving histograms [14]. We put all these six methods to test to find out which one is suitable for our task and works well with our skin lesion image set. Since we know the ground truth, we can now design a test to accomplish two goals. First, to find out which one of these tests correctly identifies the near duplicate image(s) and second, which one would provide the best margin and also is easier to implement. In order to do that, we randomly picked ten images and used image 4 as our reference image. As mentioned, we know the ground truth, therefore, we know that image 3 is a scaled version of image 4 with some changes in the pigmented lesion. Image 3 also has a black frame which is a prominent feature of the image. Figure 3 shows the comparison of various distance methods.

Inspecting each of the six methods, we come to the conclusion that all six methods to some degree are performing as they should and all are pointing to the fact that image 3 is the near duplicate found in this set. However, the other factors such as a good margin and implementation simplicity lead us to choose Chi-square method as our guide going forward. In Sect. 4, the experimental results and the final pair-wise comparison of every single image in the image set are discussed. Also, in future we will look into a hybrid method of combining the above distance methods.

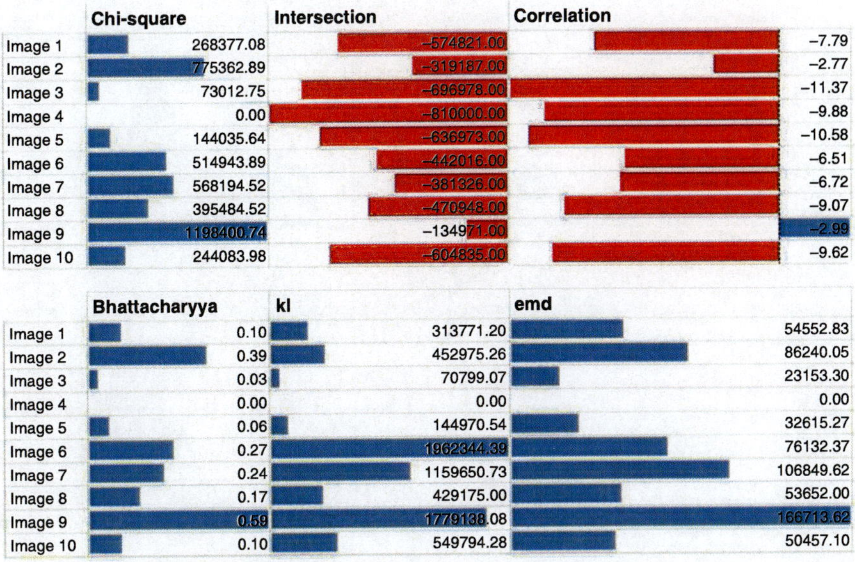

Fig. 3 Comparison of various distance methods

4 Experimental Results

As it has already been mentioned above, the most meaningful feature of the image for the application of image similarity detection is a histogram. What makes histograms an ideal candidate for feature extraction is the fact that they are invariant to translation and change slowly under different view angles, scales, and in presence of occlusions. Now that we have chosen the similarity method, it is time for implementation. In this section we will first create the histogram plots of the two cases: First the four distinct images (Fig. 4) and then the two semi-identical images (Fig. 5). As it can be seen below, the four distinct images shown in Fig. 1 have very different distribution. Keep in mind that the peaks are referring to concentration of a specific color range in the image. This kind of distribution is expected in the pigmented skin lesion images. Figure 4 shows the image histogram of four different examples of skin lesions shown in Fig. 1.

Figure 5 shows the image histogram of similar skin lesions with different modality that are shown in Fig. 2. In this case that the two histograms come from similar images, we see some similarities in the distributions. The rough distribution mass centered around bin 200 and similar amount of energy are two examples of their similarities.

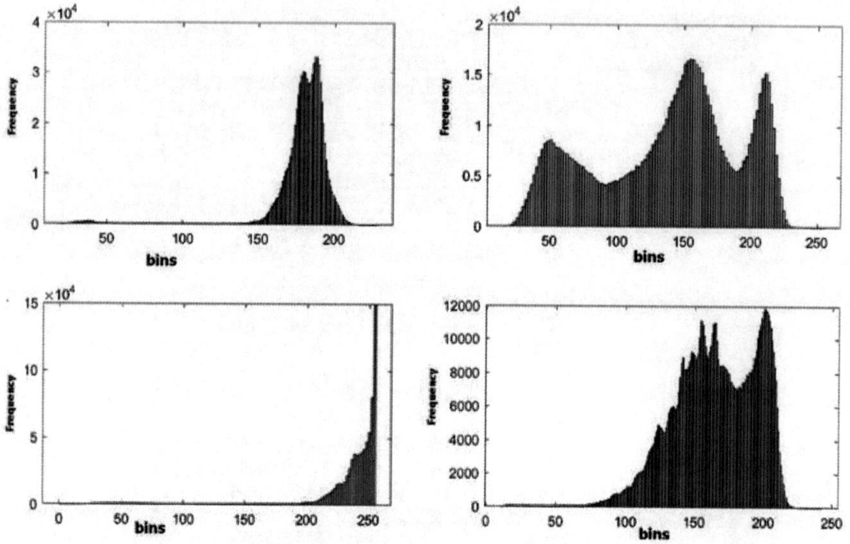

Fig. 4 Image histogram of four different examples of skin lesions

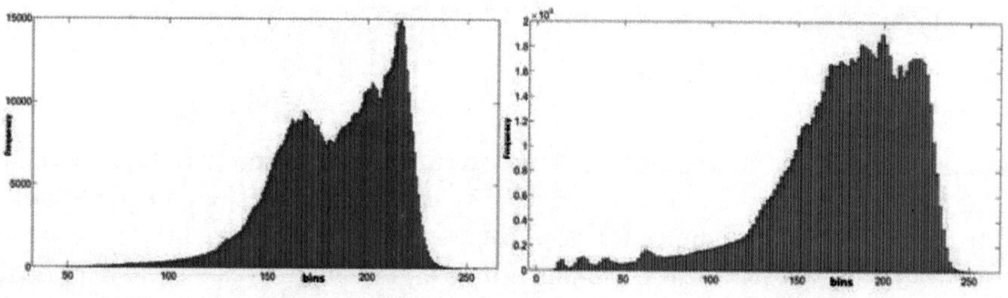

Fig. 5 Example image histograms of similar skin lesions with different modality

4.1 Setting the Threshold and Numerical Results

We performed a chi-square two-sample test and now in order to identify the closest match(es) we have to set a threshold. Having tested the Chi-square method on multiple two-combination of images we have come to conclusion that a threshold, specific to our application, somewhere between 75,000 and 100,000 should enable our algorithm to find as many semi-identical images as possible. Figure 6 shows the Chi-Square distance of ten images in comparison with image 4 and threshold line. Anything left of the threshold line will be called a close enough image to be considered a copy.

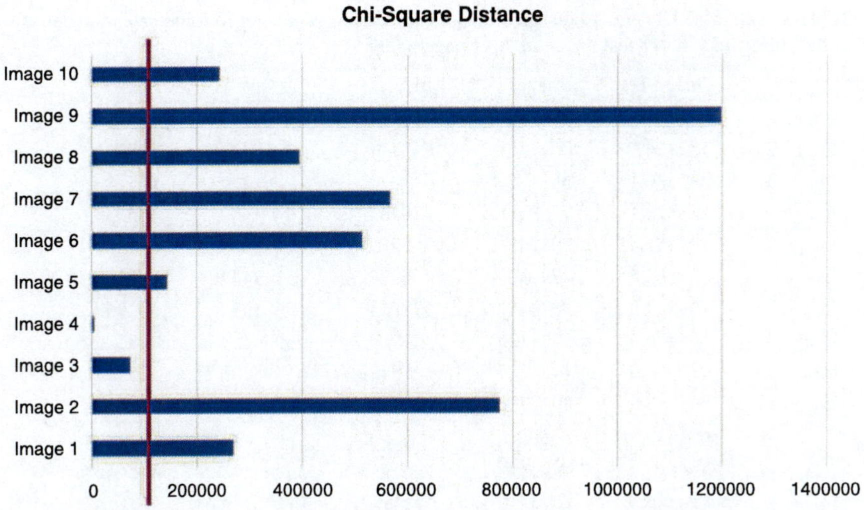

Fig. 6 Chi-Square distance of ten images in comparison with image 4. Also depicted: *the similarity line*

As it can be seen the bars for image 4 and image 3 fall to the left of the line which matches our ground truth. Now that we have developed our testing algorithm and have set a reasonable threshold, we can now expand our search window and look for any two combinatorial sets of images. All the numerical results are shown in Table 1. The values in the table are the pair-wise chi-square distances between every possible two combination of the two images in this sample image set.

Again, any numeric value that falls below our 75,000 threshold would be declaring a match for resemblance. This matrix is obviously symmetrical as expected as the distance between two images does not change based on which one is selected as the reference image.

5 Conclusion and Future Work

The Chi-square method is shown to be an effective and efficient method to do similar image detection. In this image set of pigmented skin lesion the threshold of 75,000 has shown to work well in identifying the closest match to an identical or near identical image. This method could be used as a pre-processing method in detection of various cancerous cases in our image set. Developing a Neural Network for diagnostic purposes of pigmented skin lesions was negatively influenced by the similar images with different modalities in the image pool. Deployment of our distance-

Table 1 Pair-wise Chi-square distance image comparison. The bold font indicates the detection of the closest match to a test image in this image pool

	Image 1	Image 2	Image 3	Image 4	Image 5
Image 1	0	1221246.7	237329.1	268377.1	197350.4
Image 2	1221247.7	0	653171.1	775362.9	908241.1
Image 3	237330.1	653172.1	0	**73012.8**	96527.9
Image 4	268378.1	775363.9	**73013.8**	0	144035.6
Image 5	197351.4	908242.1	96528.9	144036.6	0
Image 6	946583.4	479440.4	466628.3	514944.9	542512.5
Image 7	768959.9	1074653.7	538815	568195.5	502967
Image 8	709786.6	322112.9	303969.2	395485.5	448226.3
Image 9	970033.9	1430227.9	1078120.2	1198401.7	1062351.4
Image 10	635369.8	394777.7	221435.4	244085	423810.3

	Image 6	Image 7	Image 8	Image 9	Image 10
Image 1	946582.4	768958.9	709785.6	970032.9	635368.8
Image 2	479439.4	1074652.7	322111.9	1430226.9	394776.7
Image 3	466627.3	538814	303968.2	1078119.2	221434.4
Image 4	514943.9	568194.5	395484.5	1198400.7	244084
Image 5	542511.5	502966	448225.3	1062350.4	423809.3
Image 6	0	490656.7	548978.3	1427105.6	353270.5
Image 7	490657.7	0	882481.4	1425996	574760
Image 8	548979.3	882482.4	0	1227724.1	290028.8
Image 9	1427106.6	1425997	1227725.1	0	1370853.1
Image 10	353271.5	574761	290029.8	1370854.1	0

based tool could increase the diagnosis rate significantly in dermatoscopic images collected from skin cancer patients. A Deep Learning algorithm in conjunction with our similar image detection tool would be able to categorize and diagnose cancerous pigmented lesions [15].

Acknowledgments The data used in this study is from a Kaggle competition ISIC 2018: Skin Lesion Analysis Towards Melanoma Detection [2] and [3].

References

1. Z. Apalla, A. Lallas, E. Sotiriou, E. Lazaridou, D. Ioannides, Epidemiological trends in skin cancer. Dermatol. Pract. Concept. **7**(2), 1 (2017)
2. N.C. Codella, D. Gutman, M.E. Celebi, B. Helba, M.A. Marchetti, S.W. Dusza, A. Kalloo, K. Liopyris, N. Mishra, H. Kittler, A. Halpern, Skin lesion analysis toward melanoma detection: a challenge at the 2017 International symposium on biomedical imaging (ISBI), hosted by the international skin imaging collaboration (ISIC), in *Proceedings - International Symposium on Biomedical Imaging* (2018)

3. P. Tschandl, C. Rosendahl, H. Kittler, Data descriptor: the HAM10000 dataset, a large collection of multi-source dermatoscopic images of common pigmented skin lesions. Sci. Data **5**(1), 1–9 (2018)
4. Z. Zhou, Q.J. Wu, F. Huang, X. Sun, Fast and accurate near-duplicate image elimination for visual sensor networks. Int. J. Distrib. Sens. Netw. **13**(2), 1550147717694172 (2017)
5. G. Pass, R. Zabih, Comparing images using joint histograms. Multimed. Syst. **7**(3), 234–240 (1999)
6. O. Chum, J. Philbin, M. Isard, A. Zisserman, Scalable near identical image and shot detection, in *Proceedings of the 6th ACM International Conference on Image and Video Retrieval, CIVR 2007* (2007), pp. 549–556
7. M.J. Swain, D.H. Ballard, Color indexing. Int. J. Comput. Vis. **7**(1), 11–32 (1991)
8. T. Kailath, The divergence and Bhattacharyya distance measures in signal selection. IEEE Trans. Commun. Technol. **15**(1), 52–60 (1967)
9. O. Michailovich, Y. Rathi, A. Tannenbaum, Image segmentation using active contours driven by the Bhattacharyya gradient flow. IEEE Trans. Image Process. **16**(11), 2787–2801 (2007)
10. V. Asha, V. Asha, N.U. Bhajantri, P. Nagabhushan, GLCM-based chi-square histogram distance for automatic detection of defects on patterned textures. Int. J. Comput. Vis. Robot. **2**(4), 302–313 (2011)
11. S. Kullback, R.A. Leibler, On information and sufficiency. Ann. Math. Stat. **22**(1), 79–86 (1951)
12. A. Renyi, On measures of entropy and information, in *Fourth Berkeley Symposium on Mathematical Statistics and Probability* (1961)
13. Y. Rubner, C. Tomasi, L.J. Guibas, Metric for distributions with applications to image databases, in *Proceedings of the IEEE International Conference on Computer Vision* (1998)
14. P.A. Marín-Reyes, J. Lorenzo-Navarro, M. Castrillón-Santana, Comparative study of histogram distance measures for re-identification (2016), pp. 3–8. Preprint, arXiv:1611.08134
15. R. Srivasta, M. Rahmathullah, S. Aram, R. Sadeghian, A deep learning approach to diagnose skin cancer using image processing, in *Conference of CSCE* (2020)

Object Detection and Pose Estimation from RGB and Depth Data for Real-Time, Adaptive Robotic Grasping

Shuvo Kumar Paul, Muhammed Tawfiq Chowdhury, Mircea Nicolescu, Monica Nicolescu, and David Feil-Seifer

1 Introduction

Current advances in robotics and autonomous systems have expanded the use of robots in a wide range of robotic tasks including assembly, advanced manufacturing, human-robot or robot-robot collaboration. In order for robots to efficiently perform these tasks, they need to have the ability to adapt to the changing environment while interacting with their surroundings, and a key component of this interaction is the reliable grasping of arbitrary objects. Consequently, a recent trend in robotics research has focused on object detection and pose estimation for the purpose of dynamic robotic grasping.

However, identifying objects and recovering their poses are particularly challenging tasks as objects in the real world are extremely varied in shape and appearance. Moreover, cluttered scenes, occlusion between objects, and variance in lighting conditions make it even more difficult. Additionally, the system needs to be sufficiently fast to facilitate real-time robotic tasks. As a result, a generic solution that can address all these problems remains an open challenge.

While classification [1–6], detection [7–12], and segmentation [13–15] of objects from images have taken a significant step forward—thanks to deep learning, the same has not yet happened to 3D localization and pose estimation. One primary reason was the lack of labeled data in the past as it is not practical to manually infer, thus as a result, the recent research trend in the deep learning community for such applications has shifted towards synthetic datasets [16–20]. Several pose estimation

S. K. Paul (✉) · M. T. Chowdhury · M. Nicolescu · M. Nicolescu · D. Feil-Seifer
Department of Computer Science and Engineering, University of Nevada, Reno, NV, USA
e-mail: shuvo.k.paul@nevada.unr.edu; mtawfiqc@nevada.unr.edu; mircea@cse.unr.edu; monica@cse.unr.edu; dave@cse.unr.edu

H. R. Arabnia et al. (eds.), *Advances in Computer Vision and Computational Biology*, Transactions on Computational Science and Computational Intelligence,
https://doi.org/10.1007/978-3-030-71051-4_10

methods leveraging deep learning techniques [21–25] use these synthetic datasets for training and have shown satisfactory accuracy.

Although synthetic data is a promising alternative, capable of generating large amounts of labeled data, it requires photorealistic 3D models of the objects to mirror the real-world scenario. Hence, generating synthetic data for each newly introduced object needs photorealistic 3D models and thus significant effort from skilled 3D artists. Furthermore, training and running deep learning models are not feasible without high computing resources as well. As a result, object detection and pose estimation in real-time with computationally moderate machines remain a challenging problem. To address these issues, we have devised a simpler pipeline that does not rely on high computing resources and focuses on planar objects, requiring only an RGB image and the depth information in order to infer real-time object detection and pose estimation.

In this work, we present a feature-detector-descriptor based method for detection and a homography based pose estimation technique where, by utilizing the depth information, we estimate the pose of an object in terms of a 2D planar representation in 3D space. The robot is pre-trained to perform a set of canonical grasps; a canonical grasp describes how a robotic end-effector should be placed relative to an object in a fixed pose so that it can securely grasp it. Afterward, the robot is able to detect objects and estimates their pose in real-time, and then adapt the pre-trained canonical grasp to the new pose of the object of interest. We demonstrate that the proposed method can detect a well-textured planar object and estimate its accurate pose within a tolerable amount of out-of-plane rotation. We also conducted experiments with the humanoid PR2 robot to show the applicability of the framework where the robot grasped objects by adapting to a range of different poses.

2 Related Work

Our work constitutes of three modules: object detection, planar pose estimation, and adaptive grasping. In the following sub-sections, several fields of research that are closely related to our work are reviewed.

2.1 *Object Detection*

Object detection has been one of the fundamental challenges in the field of computer vision and in that aspect, the introduction of feature detectors and descriptors represents a great achievement. Over the past decades, many detectors, descriptors, and their numerous variants have been presented in the literature. The applications of these methods have widely extended to numerous other vision applications such as panorama stitching, tracking, visual navigation, etc.

One of the first feature detectors was proposed by Harris et al. [26] (widely known as the Harris corner detector). Later Tomasi et al. [27] developed the KLT (Kanade-Lucas-Tomasi) tracker based on the Harris corner detector. Shi and Tomasi introduced a new detection metric GFTT [28] (Good Features To Track) and argued that it offered superior performance. Hall et al. introduced the concept of saliency [29] in terms of the change in scale and evaluated the Harris method proposed in [30] and the Harris Laplacian corner detector [31] where a Harris detector and a Laplacian function are combined.

Motivated by the need for a scale-invariant feature detector, in 2004 Lowe [32] published one of the most influential papers in computer vision, SIFT (Scale-Invariant Feature Transform). SIFT is both a feature point detector and descriptor. H. Bay et al. [33] proposed SURF (Speeded Up Robust Features) in 2008. But both of these methods are computationally expensive as SIFT detector leverages the difference of Gaussians (DoG) in different scales while SURF detector uses a Haar wavelet approximation of the determinant of the Hessian matrix to speed up the detection process. Many variants of SIFT [34–37] and SURF [38–40] were proposed, either targeting a different problem or reporting improvements in matching, however, the execution time remained a persisting problem for several vision applications.

To improve execution time, several other detectors such as FAST [41] and AGAST [42] have been introduced. Calonder et al. developed the BRIEF [43] (Binary Robust Independent Elementary Features) descriptor of binary strings that has a fast execution time and is very useful for matching images. E. Rublee et al. presented ORB [44] (Oriented FAST and Rotated Brief) which is a combination of modified FAST (Features from Accelerated Segment Test) for feature detection and BRIEF for description. S. Leutnegger et al. designed BRISK [45] (Binary Robust Invariant Scale Keypoint) that detects corners using AGAST and filters them using FAST. On the other hand, FREAK (Fast Retina Keypoint), introduced by Alahi et al. [46], generates retinal sampling patterns using a circular sampling grid and uses a binary descriptor, formed by a one bit difference of Gaussians (DoG). Alcantarilla et al. introduced KAZE [47] features that exploit non-linear scale-space using non-linear diffusion filtering and later extended it to AKAZE [48] where they replaced it with a more computationally efficient method called FED (Fast Explicit Diffusion) [49, 50].

In our work, we have selected four methods to investigate: SIFT, SURF, FAST+BRISK, AKAZE.

2.2 *Planar Pose Estimation*

Among the many techniques in literature on pose estimation, we focus our review on those related to planar pose estimation. In recent years, planar pose estimation has been increasingly becoming popular in many fields, such as robotics and augmented reality.

Simon et al. [51] proposed a pose estimation technique for planar structures using homography projection and by computing camera pose from consecutive images. Changhai et al. [52] presented a method to robustly estimate 3D poses of planes by applying a weighted incremental normal estimation method that uses Bayesian inference. Donoser et al. [53] utilized the properties of Maximally Stable Extremal Regions (MSERs [54]) to construct a perspectively invariant frame on the closed contour to estimate the planar pose. In our approach, we applied perspective transformation to approximate a set of corresponding points on the test image for estimating the basis vectors of the object surface and used the depth information to estimate the 3D pose by computing the normal to the planar object.

2.3 *Adaptive Grasping*

Designing an adaptive grasping system is challenging due to the complex nature of the shapes of objects. In early times, analytical methods were used where the system would analyze the geometric structure of the object and would try to predict suitable grasping points. Sahbani et al. [55] did an in-depth review on the existing analytical approaches for 3D object grasping. However, with the analytical approach it is difficult to compute force and not suitable for autonomous manipulation. Later, as the number of 3D models increased, numerous data driven methods were introduced that would analyze grasps in the 3D model database and then transfer to the target object. Bohg et al. [56] reviewed data driven grasping method methods where they divided the approach into three groups based on the familiarity of the object.

Kehoe et al. [57] used a candidate grasp from the candidate grasp set based on the feasibility score determined by the grasp planner. The grasps were not very accurate in situations where the objects had stable horizontal poses and were close to the width of the robot's gripper. Huebner et al. [58] also take a similar approach as they perform grasp candidate simulation. They created a sequence of grasps by approximating the shape of the objects and then computed a random grasp evaluation for each model of objects. In both works, a grasp has been chosen from a list of candidate grasps (Fig. 1).

The recent advances in deep learning also made it possible to regress grasp configuration through deep convolutional networks. A number of deep learning-based methods were reviewed in [59] where the authors also discussed how each element in deep learning-based methods enhances the robotic grasping detection. [60] presented a system where deep neural networks were used to learn hierarchical features to detect and estimate the pose of an object, and then use the centers of the defined pose classes to grasps the objects. Kroemer et al. [61] introduced an active learning approach where the robot observes a few good grasps by demonstration and learns a value function for these grasps using Gaussian process regression. Aleotti et al. [62] proposed a grasping model that is capable of grasping objects by their parts which learns new tasks from human demonstration with automatic 3D shape segmentation for object recognition and semantic modeling. Saxena et al. [63]

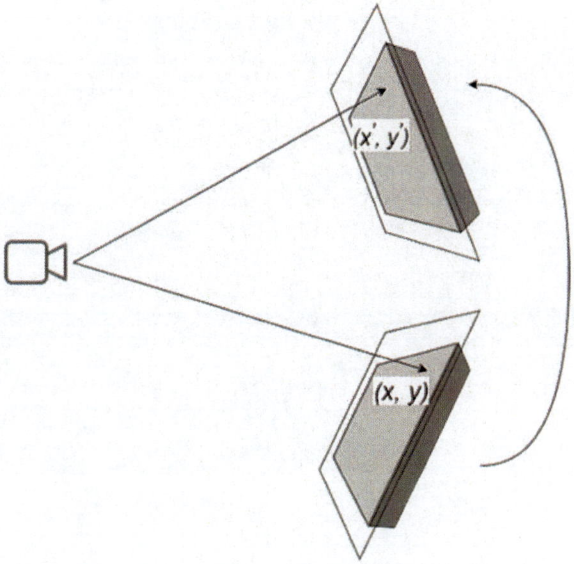

Fig. 1 Object in different orientation from the camera

and Montesano and Lopes [64] used supervised learning to predict grasp locations from RGB images. In [65], as an alternative to a trial-and-error exploration strategy, the authors proposed a Bayesian optimization technique to address the robot grasp optimization problem of unknown objects. These methods emphasized developing and using learning models for obtaining accurate grasps.

In our work, we focus on pre-defining a suitable grasp relative to an object that can adapt to a new grasp based on the change of position and orientation of the object.

3 Method

The proposed method is divided into two parts. The first part outlines the process of simultaneous object detection and pose estimation of multiple objects and the second part describes the process of generating an adaptive grasp using the pre-trained canonical grasp and the object pose. The following sections describe the architecture of the proposed framework (Fig. 2) in detail.

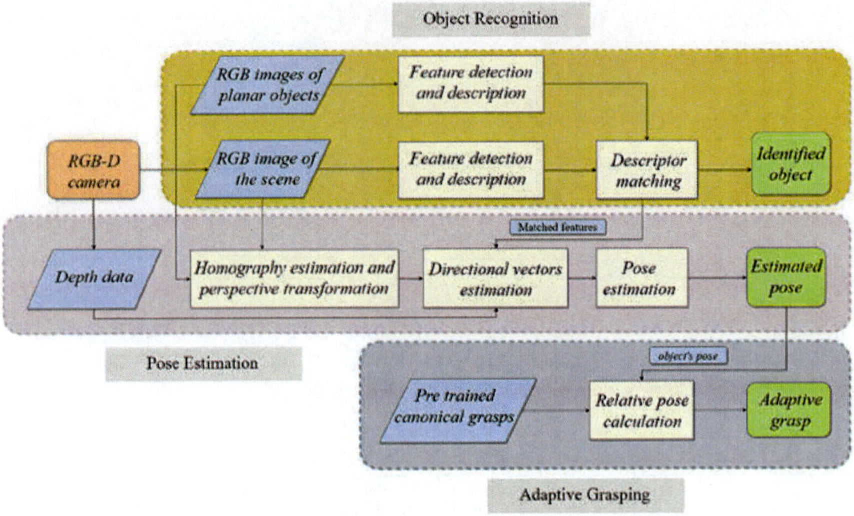

Fig. 2 System architecture

3.1 Object Detection and Pose Estimation

We present a planar pose estimation algorithm (Algorithm 1) for adaptive grasping that consists of four phases: (1) feature extraction and matching, (2) homography estimation and perspective transformation, (3) directional vectors estimation on the object surface, (4) planar pose estimation using the depth data. In the following sections, we will focus on the detailed description of the aforementioned steps.

Feature Extraction and Matching

Our object detection starts with extracting features from the images of the planar objects and then matching them with the features found in the images acquired from the camera. Image features are patterns in images based on which we can describe the image. A feature detecting algorithm takes an image and returns the locations of these patterns—they can be edges, corners or interest points, blobs or regions of interest points, ridges, etc. This feature information then needs to be transformed into a vector space using a feature descriptor, so that it gives us the possibility to execute numerical operations on them. A feature descriptor encodes these patterns into a series of numerical values that can be used to match, compare, and differentiate one feature to another; for example, we can use these feature vectors to find the similarities in different images which can lead us to detect objects in the image. In theory, this information would be invariant to image transformations. In our work, we have investigated SIFT [32], SURF [33], AKAZE [48], and

Algorithm 1: Planar pose estimation

```
Input: Training images of planar objects, I
Detector ← Define feature detector
Descriptor ← Define feature descriptor
/* retrieve feature descriptor                                          */
/* for each image in I                                                  */
for i in I do
    /* K is set of detected keypoints for image i                       */
    K ← DetectKeypoints(i, Detector)
    /* D[i] is the corresponding descriptor set for image i             */
    D[i] ← GetDescriptors( K, Descriptor)
end for
while camera is on do
    f ← RGB image frame
    PC ← Point cloud data
    /* K_F is set of detected keypoints for image frame f               */
    K_F ← DetectKeypoints(f, Detector)
    /* D_F is the corresponding descriptor set for rgb image f          */
    D_F ← GetDescriptors( K_F, Descriptor)
    for i in I do
        matches ← FindMatches( D[i], D_F)
        /* If there is at least 10 matches then we have the object
           (described in image i) in the scene                          */
        if Total number of matches ≥ 10 then
            /* extract matched keypoints pair (kp_i, kp_f) from the
               corresponding descriptors matches.                       */
            kp_i, kp_f ← ExtractKeypoints(matches)
            H ← EstimateHomography(kp_i, kp_f)
            p_c, p_x, p_y ← points on the planar object
            obtained using Eq. (3)
            p_c', p_x', p_y' ← corresponding projected points
            of p_c, p_x, p_y on image frame f
            estimated using equations
                    (1) and (2)
            /* c⃗ denotes the origin of the object frame with respect to the
               base/world frame                                         */
            c, x, y ← corresponding 3d locations
            of p_c', p_x', p_y' from point cloud PC
            /* shift x, y to the origin of the base or the world frame  */
            x ← x − c
            y ← y − c
            /* estimate the object frame in terms of three orthonormal
               vectors î, ĵ, and k̂.                                    */
            î, ĵ, k̂ ← from Eq. (4)
            /* compute the rotation φ_i, θ_i, ψ_i of the object frame î, ĵ, k̂ with
               respect to the base or the world frame X, Y, Z.          */
            φ_i, θ_i, ψ_i ← from Eq. (8)
            /* finally, publish the position and orientation of the object.
               */
            publish(c, φ_i, θ_i, ψ_i)

    end for
end while
```

BRISK [45] descriptors. SIFT, SURF, AKAZE are both feature detectors and descriptors, but BRISK uses FAST [41] algorithm for feature detection. These descriptors were selected after carefully reviewing the comparisons done in the recent literature [66, 67].

Once the features are extracted and transformed into vectors, we compare the features to determine the presence of an object in the scene. For non-binary feature descriptors (SIFT, SURF) we find matches using the Nearest Neighbor algorithm. However, finding the nearest neighbor matches within high dimensional data is computationally expensive, and with more objects introduced it can affect the process of updating the pose in real-time. To counter this issue to some extent, we used the FLANN [68] implementation of K-d Nearest Neighbor Search, which is an approximation of the K-Nearest Neighbor algorithm that is optimized for high dimensional features. For binary features (AKAZE, BRISK), we used the Hamming distance ratio method to find the matches. Finally, if we have more than ten matches, we presume the object is present in the scene.

Homography Estimation and Perspective Transformation

A homography is an invertible mapping of points and lines on the projective plane that describes a 2D planar projective transformation (Fig. 1) that can be estimated from a given pair of images. In simple terms, a homography is a matrix that maps a set of points in one image to the corresponding set of points in another image. We can use a homography matrix **H** to find the corresponding points using Eqs. (1) and (2), which defines the relation of projected point (x', y') (Fig. 1) on the rotated plane to the reference point (x, y).

A 2D point (x, y) in an image can be represented as a 3D vector $(x, y, 1)$ which is called the homogeneous representation of a point that lies on the reference plane or image of the planar object. In Eq. (1), **H** represents the homography matrix and $[x\ y\ 1]^T$ is the homogeneous representation of the reference point (x, y) and we can use the values of a, b, c to estimate the projected point (x', y') in Eq. (2).

$$\begin{bmatrix} a \\ b \\ c \end{bmatrix} = \mathbf{H} \begin{bmatrix} x \\ y \\ 1 \end{bmatrix} = \begin{bmatrix} h_{11} & h_{12} & h_{13} \\ h_{21} & h_{22} & h_{23} \\ h_{31} & h_{32} & h_{33} \end{bmatrix} \begin{bmatrix} x \\ y \\ 1 \end{bmatrix} \tag{1}$$

$$\begin{cases} x' = \dfrac{a}{c} \\ y' = \dfrac{b}{c} \end{cases} \tag{2}$$

We estimate the homography using the matches found from the nearest neighbor search as input; often these matches can have completely false correspondences, meaning they do not correspond to the same real-world feature at all which can be a problem in estimating the homography. So, we chose RANSAC [69] to robustly estimate the homography by considering only inlier matches as it tries to estimate the underlying model parameters and detect outliers by generating candidate solutions through random sampling using a minimum number of observations.

While the other techniques use as much data as possible to find the model parameters and then pruning the outliers, RANSAC uses the smallest set of data point possible to estimate the model, thus making it faster and more efficient than the conventional solutions.

Finding Directional Vectors on the Object

In order to find the pose of a planar object, we need to find the three orthonormal vectors on the planar object that describe the object coordinate frame and consequently, the orientation of the object relative to the world coordinate system. We start by estimating the vectors on the planar object that form the basis of the plane, illustrated in Fig. 3. Then, we take the cross product of these two vectors to find the third directional vector which is the normal to the object surface. Let us denote the world coordinate system as XYZ, and the object coordinate system as xyz. We define the axes of the orientation in relation to a body as:

$$\begin{aligned} x &\rightarrow \text{right} \\ y &\rightarrow \text{up} \\ z &\rightarrow \text{towards the camera} \end{aligned}$$

First, we retrieve the locations of the three points p_c, p_x, p_y on the planar object from the reference image using Eq. (3) and then locate the corresponding points $p_c^{'}, p_x^{'}, p_y^{'}$ on the image acquired from the Microsoft Kinect sensor. We estimate the locations of these points using the homography matrix $\mathbf{H}$ as shown in Eqs. (1) and (2). Then we find the corresponding 3D locations of $p_c^{'}, p_x^{'}, p_y^{'}$ from the point cloud data also obtained from the Microsoft Kinect sensor. We denote them as vectors **c**,**x**, and **y**. Here, **c** represents the translation vector from the object frame to the world frame and also the position of the object in the world frame. Next, we subtract **c** from **x**, **y** which essentially gives us two vectors **x** and **y** centered at the origin of the world frame. We take the cross product of these two vectors **x**, **y** to find the third axis **z**. But, depending on the homography matrix the estimated axes **x** and **y** might not be exactly orthogonal, so we take the cross product of **y** and **z** to recalculate the vector **x**. Now that we have three orthogonal vectors, we compute the three unit vectors $\hat{i}$, $\hat{j}$, and $\hat{k}$ along the **x**, **y**, and **z** vectors, respectively, using Eq. (4). These three orthonormal vectors describe the object frame. These vectors were projected onto the image plane to give a visual confirmation of the methods applied; Fig. 4 shows the orthogonal axes projected onto the object plane.

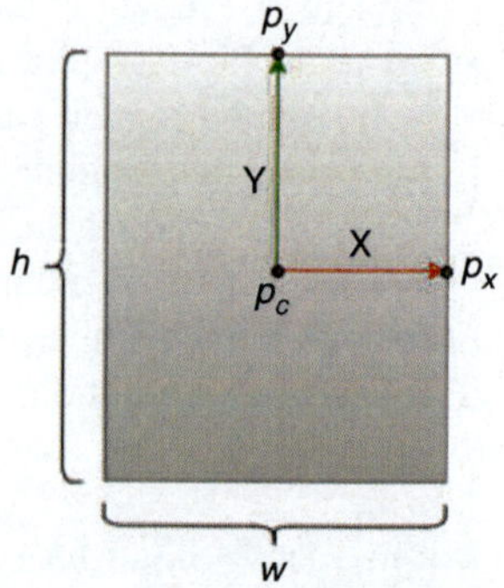

Fig. 3 Axis on the reference plane

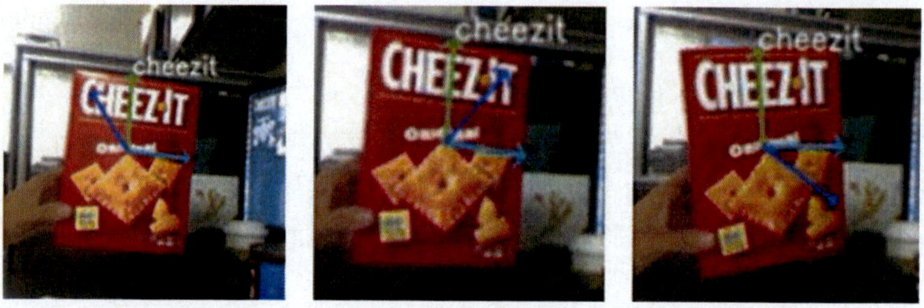

Fig. 4 Computed third directional axis projected onto image plane

$$\begin{cases} p_c = (w/2, h/2) \\ p_x = (w, h/2) \\ p_y = (w/2, 0) \end{cases} \tag{3}$$

$$\begin{aligned} \hat{j} &= \frac{\mathbf{y}}{|\mathbf{y}|} = [j_X \;\; j_Y \;\; j_Z] \\ \hat{k} &= \frac{\mathbf{x} \times \mathbf{y}}{|\mathbf{x} \times \mathbf{y}|} = [k_X \;\; k_Y \;\; k_Z] \\ \hat{i} &= \frac{\mathbf{y} \times \mathbf{z}}{|\mathbf{y} \times \mathbf{z}|} = [i_X \;\; i_Y \;\; i_Z] \end{aligned} \tag{4}$$

Planar Pose Computation

We compute the pose of the object in terms of the Euler angles. Euler angles are three angles that describe the orientation of a rigid body with respect to a fixed coordinate system. The rotation matrix **R** in Eq. (5) rotates X axis to $\hat{i}$, Y axis to $\hat{j}$, and Z axis to $\hat{k}$.

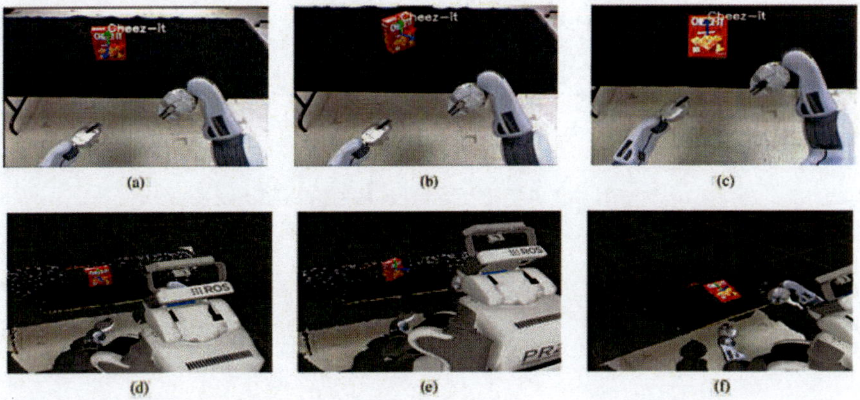

Fig. 5 (**a**), (**b**), (**c**) are recovered poses from robot's camera and (**d**), (**e**), (**f**) are corresponding poses visualized in RViz

$$\mathbf{R} = \begin{bmatrix} i_X & j_X & k_X \\ i_Y & j_Y & k_Y \\ i_Z & j_Z & k_Z \end{bmatrix} \tag{5}$$

Euler angles are combinations of the three axis rotations (Eq. (6)), where ϕ, θ, and ψ specify the intrinsic rotations around the X, Y, and Z axis, respectively. The combined rotation matrix is a product of three matrices: $\mathbf{R} = \mathbf{R}_z\ \mathbf{R}_y\ \mathbf{R}_x$ (Eq. (7)); the first intrinsic rotation rightmost, last leftmost (Fig. 5).

$$\begin{cases} \mathbf{R}_x = \begin{bmatrix} 1 & 0 & 0 \\ 0 & \cos\phi & -\sin\phi \\ 0 & \sin\phi & \cos\phi \end{bmatrix} \\ \mathbf{R}_y = \begin{bmatrix} \cos\theta & 0 & \sin\theta \\ 0 & 1 & 0 \\ -\sin\theta & 0 & \cos\theta \end{bmatrix} \\ \mathbf{R}_z = \begin{bmatrix} \cos\psi & -\sin\psi & 0 \\ \sin\psi & \cos\psi & 0 \\ 0 & 0 & 1 \end{bmatrix} \end{cases} \tag{6}$$

$$\mathbf{R} = \begin{bmatrix} c\theta c\psi & s\phi s\theta c\psi - c\phi s\psi & c\phi s\theta c\psi + s\phi s\psi \\ c\theta s\psi & s\phi s\theta s\psi + c\phi c\psi & c\phi s\theta s\psi - s\phi c\psi \\ -s\theta & s\phi c\theta & c\phi c\theta \end{bmatrix} \tag{7}$$

In Eq. (7), c and s represents cos and sin, respectively.

Solving for ϕ, θ, and ψ from (5) and (7), we get,

$$\begin{cases} \phi = \tan^{-1}\left(\frac{j_Z}{k_Z}\right) \\ \theta = \tan^{-1}\left(\frac{-i_Z}{\sqrt{1-i_Z^2}}\right) = \sin^{-1}(-i_Z) \\ \psi = \tan^{-1}\left(\frac{i_Y}{i_X}\right) \end{cases} \tag{8}$$

3.2 *Training Grasps for Humanoid Robots*

To ensure that the robot can grasp objects in an adaptive manner, we pre-train the robot to perform a set of canonical grasps. We place the object and the robot's gripper close to each other and record the relative pose. This essentially gives us the pose of the gripper with respect to the object. Figure 6 illustrates the training process in which the robot's gripper and a cracker box have been placed in close proximity and the relative poses have been recorded for grasping the objects from the side.

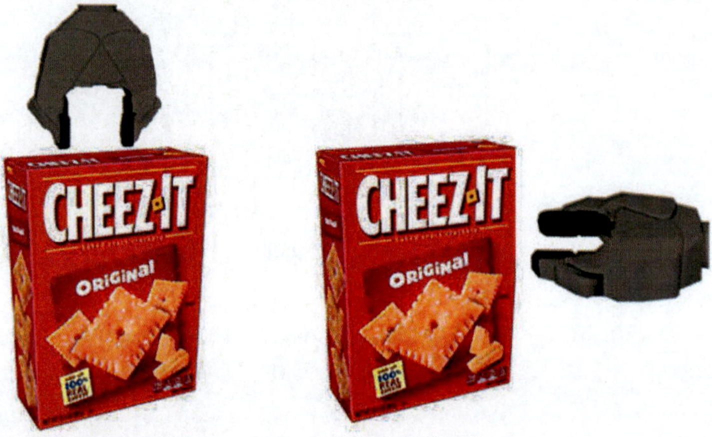

Fig. 6 Pre-training canonical grasp

$$\mathbf{T}_s^d = \begin{bmatrix} \mathbf{R}_s^d & P_s^d \\ 0 & 1 \end{bmatrix} = \begin{bmatrix} r_{11} & r_{12} & r_{13} & X_t \\ r_{21} & r_{22} & r_{23} & Y_t \\ r_{31} & r_{32} & r_{33} & Z_t \\ 0 & 0 & 0 & 1 \end{bmatrix} \tag{9}$$

Equation (9) outlines the structure of a transformation matrix $\mathbf{T}_s^d$ that describes the rotation and translation of frame d with respect to frame s; $\mathbf{R}_s^d$ represents the rotation matrix similar to Eq. (7) and $P_s^d = [X_t, Y_t, Z_t]^T$ is the translation matrix which is the 3D location of the origin of frame d in frame s.

During the training phase, we first formulate the transformation matrix $\mathbf{T}_b^o$ using the rotation matrix and the object location. We take the inverse of $\mathbf{T}_b^o$ which gives us the transformation matrix $\mathbf{T}_o^b$. We then use the Eq. (10) to record the transformation $\mathbf{T}_o^g$ of the robot's wrist relative to the object.

$$T_o^g = T_o^b \times T_b^g \text{ where } T_o^b = (T_b^o)^{-1} \tag{10}$$

In the Eq. (10), b refers to the robot's base, o refers to the object, and g refers to the wrist of the robot to which the gripper is attached. Once we record the matrix, we get a new pose of the object from the vision in the testing phase and generate the final matrix using the Eq. (11) that has the new position and orientation of the robot's wrist in matrix form .

$$T_b^g = T_b^o \times T_o^g \tag{11}$$

We then extract the rotational angles γ, β, α (roll, pitch, yaw) of the grasp pose from matrix $\mathbf{T}_b^g$ using Eq. (12)

$$\begin{cases} \gamma = tan^{-1}(r_{32}/r_{33}) \\ \beta = tan^{-1}\dfrac{-r_{31}}{\sqrt{r_{32}^2 + r_{33}^2}} \\ \alpha = tan^{-1}(r_{21}/r_{11}) \end{cases} \tag{12}$$

4 Evaluation

The proposed object recognition and pose estimation algorithm was implemented on an Ubuntu 14.04 platform equipped with 3.0 GHz Intel R Core(TM) i5-7400 CPU and 8GB system memory. The RGB-D camera used in the experiments was a Microsoft Kinect sensor v1. We evaluated the proposed algorithm by comparing the accuracy of object recognition, pose estimation, and execution time of four different feature descriptors. We also validated the effectiveness of our approach for adaptive grasping by conducting experiments with the PR2 robot.

4.1 Object Detection and Pose Estimation

Without enough observable features, the system would fail to find good matches that are required for accurate homography estimation. Consequently, our object detection and pose estimation approach has a constraint on the out-of-plane rotation θ, illustrated in Fig. 7. In other words, if the out-of-plane rotation of the object is more than θ, the system would not be able to recognize the object. Fast execution is also a crucial aspect to facilitate multiple object detection and pose estimation for real-time applications. We experimented with four different descriptors on several planar objects and the comparative result is shown in Table 1. The execution time was measured for the object detection and pose estimation step. AKAZE and BRISK had much lower processing time for detection and pose estimation, thus would have a better frame rate, but SIFT and SURF had larger out-of-plane rotational freedom.

We also compared the *RMS* difference ϵ (Eq. (13)) of re-calculated $\mathbf{x}$ to original $\mathbf{x}$ ($\mathbf{x}'$ in the equation) for increasing out-of-plane rotation of the planar objects to assess the homography estimation. Ideally, the two estimated vectors $\mathbf{x}$ and $\mathbf{y}$, which

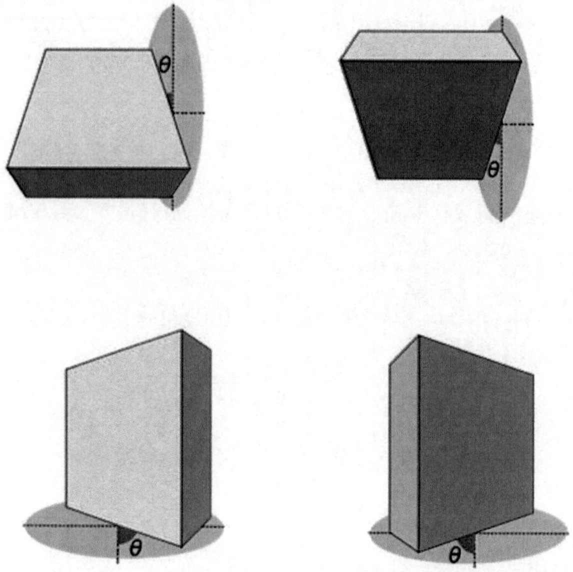

Fig. 7 Out-of-plane rotation

Table 1 Comparison of feature descriptors

Descriptor	Maximum out-of-plane rotation (degree)	Execution time (second)
SIFT	$48 \pm 2°$	0.21 s
SURF	$37 \pm 2°$	0.27 s
AKAZE	$18 \pm 1°$	0.05 s
BRISK	$22 \pm 2°$	0.06 s

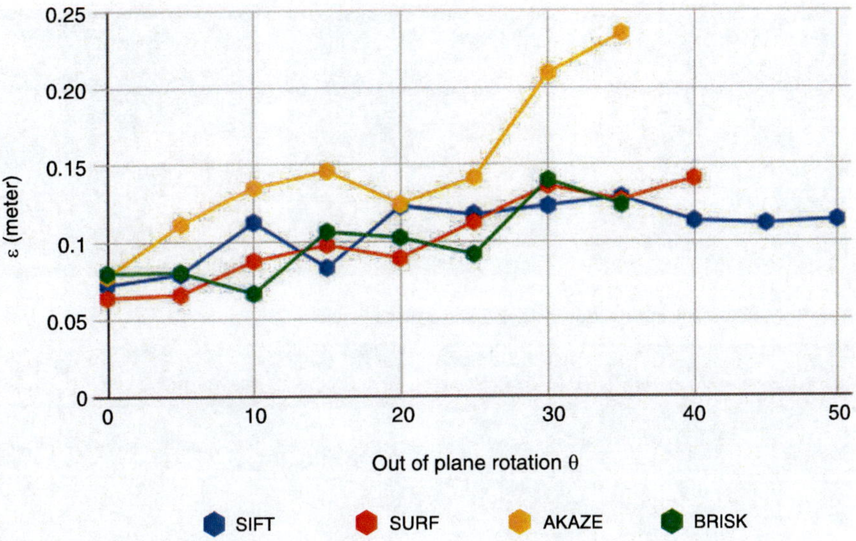

Fig. 8 Out-of-plane rotation vs ϵ

Table 2 Execution time of SIFT and SURF for multiple object detection

Number of Objects	Detection time (second)	
	SIFT	SURF
1	0.06 s	0.09 s
2	0.11 s	0.17 s
3	0.17 s	0.26 s
4	0.22 s	0.35 s
5	0.28 s	0.45 s
6	0.34 s	0.54 s

describe the basis of the plane of the planar object, should be orthogonal to each other, but often they are not. So, the values of ϵ in Fig. 8 give us an indication of the average error in homography estimation for different out-of-plane rotations. In Fig. 8, we can see AKAZE has much higher ϵ values while the rest remained within a close range. This tells us AKAZE results in a much larger error in estimating the homography than the other methods.

We chose SIFT and SURF to evaluate how the execution time for detection scales up while increasing the number of objects. From Table 2, which shows the mean processing time for object detection, we can see that SURF had a detection time around 50% more than SIFT in all the cases. This outcome coupled with the previous results prompted us to select SIFT for the subsequent experiments.

The system was capable of detecting multiple objects in real-time and at the same time could estimate their corresponding poses. Figure 9 shows detected objects with estimated directional planar vectors. We can also observe that the system was robust to in-plane rotation and partial occlusion.

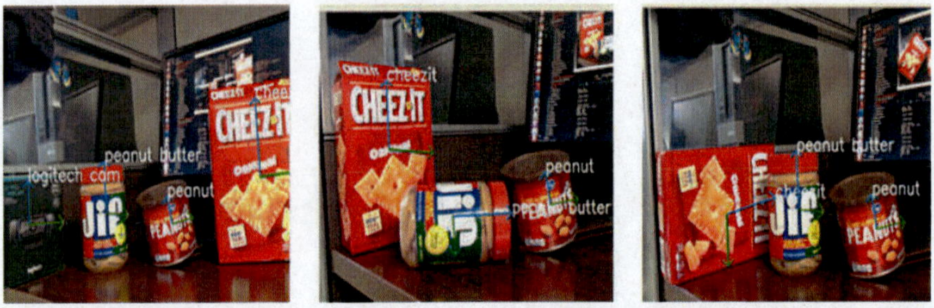

Fig. 9 Multiple object detection with estimated planar vectors

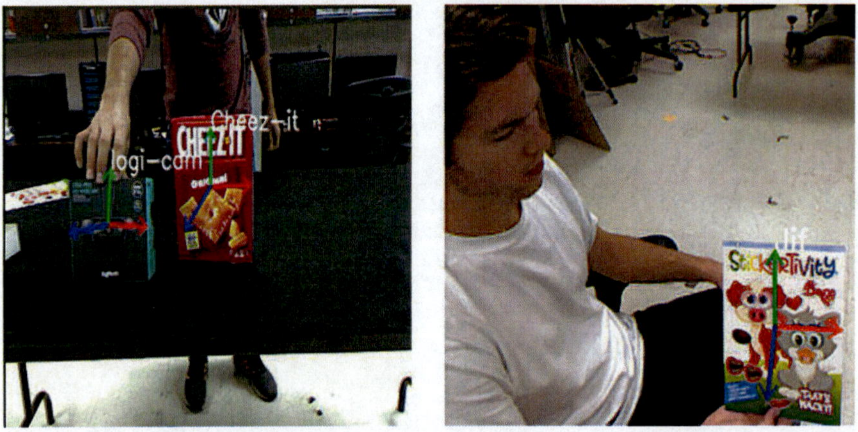

Fig. 10 (**a**) Pose estimation of multiple objects (**b**) Estimated pose of an object held by a human

We used RViz, a 3D visualizer for the Robot Operating System (ROS), to validate the pose estimation. The calculated directional axes were projected onto the image and the estimated poses were visualized in RViz. As shown in Fig. 5, we qualitatively verified the accuracy of the detection and the estimated pose by comparing the two outputs. We can see that both the outputs render similar results. We conducted experiments with multiple objects and human held objects as well. Figure 10 illustrates the simultaneous detection and pose estimation of two different boxes and an object held by a human, respectively.

$$\epsilon = \frac{1}{N}\sum_{i=1}^{N} ||\mathbf{x_i'} - \mathbf{x_i}||, \text{ where N is the number of frames} \tag{13}$$

4.2 Adaptive Grasping

We assessed our approach for adaptive grasping keeping two different aspects of the robotic application in mind; robotic tasks that require (1) interacting with a static environment, and (2) interacting with humans.

We first tested our system for static objects where the object was attached to a tripod. Next, we set up experiments where the object was held by a human. We used a sticker book and a cartoon book and evaluated our system on a comprehensive set of poses. In almost all the experiments, the robot successfully grasped the object in a manner consistent with its training. There were some poses that were not reachable by the robot—for instance, when the object was pointing inward along the X axis in the robot reference frame, it was not possible for the end-effector to make a top grasp. Figures 11 and 12 show the successful grasping of the robot for both types of experiments.

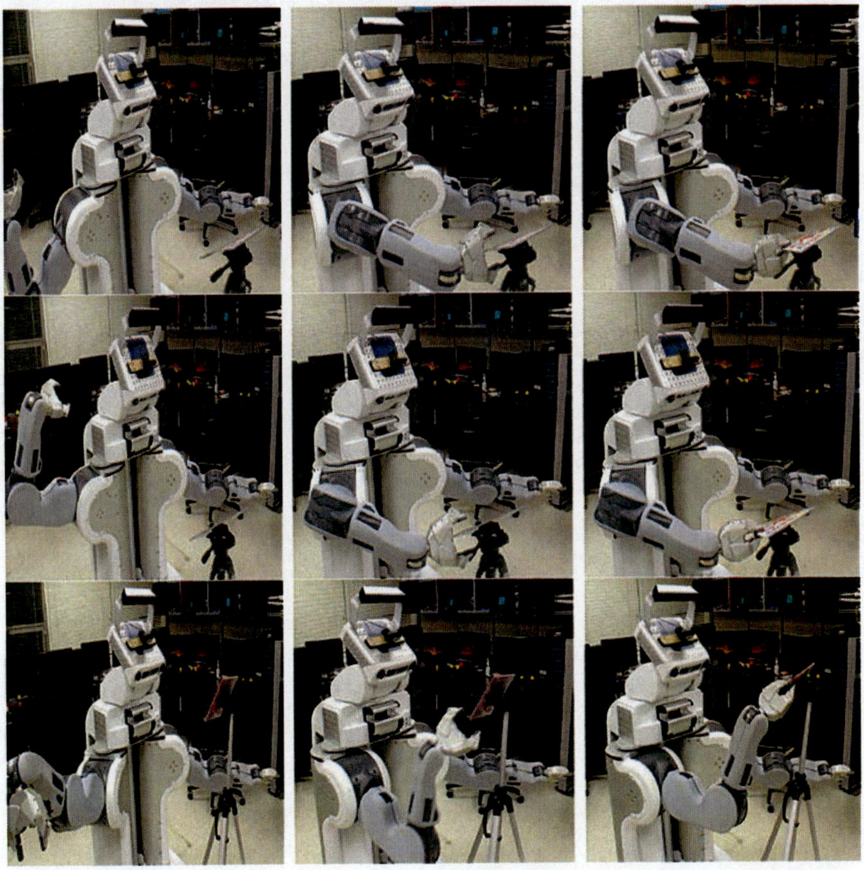

Fig. 11 Robot grasping an object from a tripod. Left: initial position of the robot's gripper, middle: gripper adapting to the object's pose, right: grasping of the object

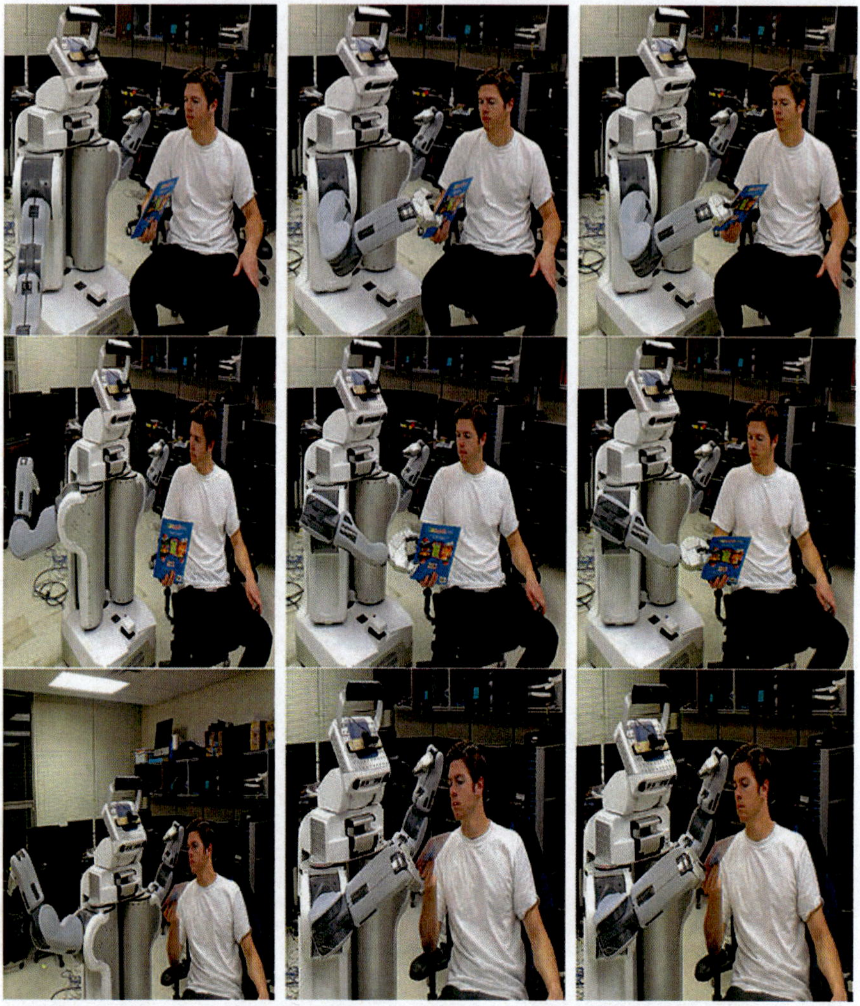

Fig. 12 Robot grasping an object held by a human. Left: initial position of the robot's gripper, middle: gripper adapting to the object's pose, right: grasping of the object

5 Conclusion and Future Work

This work presents an approach that enables humanoid robots to grasp objects using planar pose estimation based on RGB image and depth data. We examined the performance of four feature-detector-descriptors for object recognition and found SIFT to be the best solution. We used FLANN's K-d Tree Nearest Neighbor implementation, and Bruteforce Hamming to find the keypoint matches and employed RANSAC to estimate the homography. The homography matrix was used to approximate the three orthonormal directional vectors on the planar object using perspective transformation. The pose of the planar object was estimated from the three directional vectors. The system was able to detect multiple objects and estimate the pose of the objects in real-time. We also conducted experiments with the humanoid PR2 robot to show the practical applicability of the framework where the robot grasped objects by adapting to a range of different poses.

In the future, we plan to add GPU acceleration for the proposed algorithm that would further improve the overall computational efficiency of the system. We would like to extend the algorithm to automatically prioritize certain objects and limit the number of objects needed for detection based on different scheduled tasks. Finally, we would like to incorporate transferring grasp configuration for familiar objects and explore other feature matching technique, e.g., multi probe LSH, hierarchical k-means tree, etc.

Acknowledgments This work has been supported in part by the Office of Naval Research award N00014-16-1-2312 and US Army Research Laboratory (ARO) award W911NF-20-2-0084.

References

1. K. He, et al., Deep residual learning for image recognition, in *Proceedings of the IEEE Conference on Computer Vision and Pattern Recognition* (2016), pp. 770–778
2. S. Liu, W. Deng, Very deep convolutional neural network based image classification using small training sample size, in *2015 3rd IAPR Asian Conference on Pattern Recognition (ACPR)* (2015), pp. 730–734
3. C. Szegedy, et al., Going deeper with convolutions, in *Proceedings of the IEEE Conference on Computer Vision and Pattern Recognition* (2015), pp. 1–9
4. D.C. Ciresan, et al., Flexible, high performance convolutional neural networks for image classification, in *Twenty-Second International Joint Conference on Artificial Intelligence* (2011)
5. P. Sermanet, et al., Overfeat: integrated recognition, localization and detection using convolutional networks, in *2nd International Conference on Learning Representations (ICLR 2014), Conference Date: 14-04-2014 Through 16-04-2014* (2014)
6. K. He, et al., Spatial pyramid pooling in deep convolutional networks for visual recognition. IEEE Trans. Pattern Anal. Mach. Intell. **37**(9), 1904–1916 (2015)
7. R. Girshick, Fast R-CNN, in *Proceedings of the IEEE International Conference on Computer Vision* (2015), pp. 1440–1448
8. S. Ren, et al., Faster R-CNN: towards real-time object detection with region proposal networks, in *Advances in Neural Information Processing Systems* (2015), pp. 91–99
9. W. Liu, et al., SSD: single shot multibox detector, in *European Conference on Computer Vision* (Springer, Berlin, 2016), pp. 21–37
10. J. Redmon, et al., You only look once: unified, real-time object detection, in *Proceedings of the IEEE Conference on Computer Vision and Pattern Recognition* (2016), pp. 779–788
11. J. Redmon, A. Farhadi, Yolo9000: better, faster, stronger, in *Proceedings of the IEEE Conference on Computer Vision and Pattern Recognition* (2017), pp. 7263–7271
12. T.-Y. Lin, et al., Focal loss for dense object detection, in *Proceedings of the IEEE International Conference on Computer Vision* (2017), pp. 2980–2988
13. V. Badrinarayanan, et al., Segnet: a deep convolutional encoder-decoder architecture for image segmentation, IEEE Trans. Pattern Anal. Mach. Intell. **39**(12), 2481–2495 (2017)

14. K. He, et al., Mask R-CNN, in *Proceedings of the IEEE International Conference on Computer Vision* (2017), pp. 2961–2969
15. O. Ronneberger, et al., U-net: convolutional networks for biomedical image segmentation, in *International Conference on Medical Image Computing and Computer-Assisted Intervention* (Springer, Berlin, 2015), pp. 234–241
16. D.J. Butler, et al., A naturalistic open source movie for optical flow evaluation, in *Computer Vision – ECCV 2012*, ed. by A. Fitzgibbon et al. (Springer, Berlin, 2012), pp. 611–625
17. N. Mayer, et al., A large dataset to train convolutional networks for disparity, optical flow, and scene flow estimation, in *Proceedings of the IEEE Conference on Computer Vision and Pattern Recognition* (2016), pp. 4040–4048
18. W. Qiu, A. Yuille, Unrealcv: connecting computer vision to unreal engine, in *European Conference on Computer Vision* (Springer, Berlin, 2016), pp. 909–916
19. Y. Zhang, et al., Unrealstereo: a synthetic dataset for analyzing stereo vision (2016, preprint). arXiv:1612.04647
20. J. McCormac, et al., Scenenet RGB-D: can 5m synthetic images beat generic imagenet pre-training on indoor segmentation? in *The IEEE International Conference on Computer Vision (ICCV)* (2017)
21. Y. Xiang, et al., Posecnn: a convolutional neural network for 6d object pose estimation in cluttered scenes, in *Robotics: Science and Systems (RSS)* (2018)
22. J. Tremblay, et al., Deep object pose estimation for semantic robotic grasping of household objects, in *Conference on Robot Learning (CoRL)* (2018)
23. E. Brachmann, et al., Learning 6d object pose estimation using 3d object coordinates, in *European Conference on Computer Vision* (Springer, Berlin, 2014), pp. 536–551
24. C. Wang, et al., Densefusion: 6d object pose estimation by iterative dense fusion, in *Proceedings of the IEEE Conference on Computer Vision and Pattern Recognition* (2019), pp. 3343–3352
25. Y. Hu, et al., Segmentation-driven 6d object pose estimation, in *Proceedings of the IEEE Conference on Computer Vision and Pattern Recognition* (2019), pp. 3385–3394
26. C.G. Harris, et al., A combined corner and edge detector, in *Alvey Vision Conference*, vol. 15 (Citeseer, 1988), pp. 10–5244
27. C. Tomasi, T. Kanade, Detection and tracking of point features. School of Computer Science, Carnegie Mellon University, Pittsburgh (1991)
28. J. Shi, et al., Good features to track, in *1994 Proceedings of IEEE Conference on Computer Vision and Pattern Recognition* (IEEE, Piscataway, 1994), pp. 593–600
29. D. Hall, et al., Saliency of interest points under scale changes, in *British Machine Vision Conference (BMVC)* (2002), pp. 1–10
30. T. Lindeberg, Feature detection with automatic scale selection. Int. J. Comput. Vis. **30**(2), 79–116 (1998)
31. K. Mikolajczyk, C. Schmid, Indexing based on scale invariant interest points, in *Proceedings Eighth IEEE International Conference on Computer Vision (ICCV 2001)*, vol. 1 (IEEE, Piscataway, 2001), pp. 525–531
32. D.G. Lowe, Distinctive image features from scale-invariant keypoints. Int. J. Comput. Vis. **60**, 91–110 (2004)
33. H. Bay, et al., SURF: speeded up robust features, in *Computer Vision – ECCV 2006*, ed. by A. Leonardis, et al. (Springer Berlin, 2006), pp. 404–417
34. Y. Ke, R. Sukthankar, PCA-sift: a more distinctive representation for local image descriptors, in *Proceedings of the 2004 IEEE Computer Society Conference on Computer Vision and Pattern Recognition, (CVPR 2004)*, vol. 2 (IEEE, Piscataway, 2004), p. II
35. S.K. Lodha, Y. Xiao, GSIFT: geometric scale invariant feature transform for terrain data, in *Vision Geometry XIV*, vol. 6066 (International Society for Optics and Photonics, Bellingham, 2006), p. 60660L
36. A.E. Abdel-Hakim, A.A. Farag, CSIFT: a sift descriptor with color invariant characteristics, in *2006 IEEE Computer Society Conference on Computer Vision and Pattern Recognition (CVPR'06)*, vol. 2 (IEEE, Piscataway, 2006), pp. 1978–1983

37. J.-M. Morel, G. Yu, ASIFT: a new framework for fully affine invariant image comparison. SIAM J. Imag. Sci. **2**(2), 438–469 (2009)
38. P.F. Alcantarilla, et al., Gauge-surf descriptors. Image Vis. Comput. **31**(1), 103–116 (2013)
39. T.-K. Kang, et al., MDGHM-surf: a robust local image descriptor based on modified discrete Gaussian–Hermite moment. Pattern Recognit. **48**(3), 670–684 (2015)
40. J. Fu, et al., C-surf: colored speeded up robust features, in *International Conference on Trustworthy Computing and Services* (Springer, Berlin, 2012), pp. 203–210
41. E. Rosten, T. Drummond, Machine learning for high-speed corner detection, in *European Conference on Computer Vision* (Springer, Berlin, 2006), pp. 430–443
42. E. Mair, et al., Adaptive and generic corner detection based on the accelerated segment test, in *European Conference on Computer Vision* (Springer, Berlin, 2010), pp. 183–196
43. M. Calonder, et al., Brief: computing a local binary descriptor very fast. IEEE Trans. Pattern Anal. Mach. Intell. **34**(7), 1281–1298 (2011)
44. E. Rublee, et al., ORB: an efficient alternative to sift or surf, in *2011 International Conference on Computer Vision* (2011), pp. 2564–2571
45. S. Leutenegger, et al., Brisk: binary robust invariant scalable keypoints, in *2011 International Conference on Computer Vision* (IEEE, Piscataway, 2011), pp. 2548–2555
46. R. Ortiz, Freak: fast retina keypoint, in *Proceedings of the 2012 IEEE Conference on Computer Vision and Pattern Recognition (CVPR), CVPR'12, Washington* (IEEE Computer Society, Washington, 2012), pp. 510–517
47. P.F. Alcantarilla, et al., Kaze features, in *Computer Vision – ECCV 2012*, ed. by A. Fitzgibbon, et al. (Springer, Berlin, 2012), pp. 214–227
48. P.F. Alcantarilla, et al., Fast explicit diffusion for accelerated features in nonlinear scale spaces, in *British Machine Vision Conference (BMVC)* (2013)
49. J. Weickert, et al., Cyclic schemes for PDE-based image analysis. Int. J. Comput. Vis. **118**(3), 275–299 (2016)
50. S. Grewenig, et al., From box filtering to fast explicit diffusion, in *Joint Pattern Recognition Symposium* (Springer, Berlin, 2010), pp. 533–542
51. G. Simon, M. Berger, Pose estimation for planar structures. IEEE Comput. Graph. Appl. **22**(6), 46–53 (2002)
52. C. Xu, et al., 3D pose estimation for planes, in *2009 IEEE 12th International Conference on Computer Vision Workshops, ICCV Workshops* (2009), pp. 673–680
53. M. Donoser, et al., Robust planar target tracking and pose estimation from a single concavity, in *2011 10th IEEE International Symposium on Mixed and Augmented Reality* (2011), pp. 9–15
54. D. Nistér, H. Stewénius, Linear time maximally stable extremal regions, in *Computer Vision – ECCV 2008*, ed. by D. Forsyth et al. (Springer, Berlin, 2008), pp. 183–196
55. A. Sahbani, et al., An overview of 3d object grasp synthesis algorithms. Robot. Auton. Syst. **60**(3), 326–336 (2012)
56. J. Bohg, et al., Data-driven grasp synthesis–a survey. IEEE Trans. Robot. **30**(2), 289–309 (2013)
57. B. Kehoe, et al., Cloud-based robot grasping with the google object recognition engine, in *2013 IEEE International Conference on Robotics and Automation* (IEEE, Piscataway, 2013)
58. K. Huebner, et al., Minimum volume bounding box decomposition for shape approximation in robot grasping, in *2008 IEEE International Conference on Robotics and Automation* (IEEE, Piscataway, 2008)
59. S. Caldera, et al., Review of deep learning methods in robotic grasp detection. Multimodal Technol. Interact. **2**(3), 57 (2018)
60. J. Yu, et al., A vision-based robotic grasping system using deep learning for 3d object recognition and pose estimation, in *2013 IEEE International Conference on Robotics and Biomimetics (ROBIO)* (IEEE, Piscataway, 2013)
61. O. Kroemer, et al., Active learning using mean shift optimization for robot grasping, in *2009 IEEE/RSJ International Conference on Intelligent Robots and Systems* (IEEE, Piscataway, 2009)

62. J. Aleotti, S. Caselli, Part-based robot grasp planning from human demonstration, in *2011 IEEE International Conference on Robotics and Automation* (IEEE, Piscataway, 2011)
63. A. Saxena, et al., Robotic grasping of novel objects using vision. Int. J. Robot. Res. **27**(2), 157–173 (2008)
64. L. Montesano, M. Lopes, Active learning of visual descriptors for grasping using non-parametric smoothed beta distributions. Robot. Auton. Syst. **60**(3), 452–462 (2012)
65. J. Nogueira, et al., Unscented Bayesian optimization for safe robot grasping, in *2016 IEEE/RSJ International Conference on Intelligent Robots and Systems (IROS)* (IEEE, Piscataway, 2016)
66. E. Karami, et al., Image matching using sift, surf, brief and orb: performance comparison for distorted images, in *The 24th Annual Newfoundland Electrical and Computer Engineering Conference, NECEC* (2015)
67. S.A.K. Tareen, Z. Saleem, A comparative analysis of sift, surf, kaze, akaze, orb, and brisk, in *2018 International Conference on Computing, Mathematics and Engineering Technologies (iCoMET)* (IEEE, Piscataway, 2018), pp. 1–10
68. M. Muja, D.G. Lowe, Fast approximate nearest neighbors with automatic algorithm configuration, in *International Conference on Computer Vision Theory and Application VISSAPP'09)* (INSTICC Press, Lisboa, 2009), pp. 331–340
69. M.A. Fischler, R.C. Bolles, Random sample consensus: a paradigm for model fitting with applications to image analysis and automated cartography, Commun. ACM **24**(6), 381–395 (1981)

Axial Symmetry Detection Using AF8 Code

César Omar Jiménez-Ibarra, Hermilo Sánchez-Cruz, and Miguel Vázquez-Martin del Campo

1 Introduction

In both the arts and sciences, as well as in everyday life, symmetry is a characteristic that plays an important role in the recognition of objects. At the same time, a computational treatment of symmetry has the potential to play an important role in computer science [1]. Symmetry is a geometric characteristic very common in natural objects, particularly in living beings and, highly marked, in artificial objects; in particular, mirror symmetry is a relevant topic in fields such as computer vision and pattern recognition.

Lockwood and Macmillan [2] informally define that a geometric object is symmetric if there is a group of transformations under which the object does not change its general shape. Weyl [3] says that symmetric means something that is well proportioned and well balanced, and the symmetry denotes that type of agreement of several parts by which they are integrated in a whole. Karush [4] defines a symmetric relationship as "a relationship with the following properties: if one thing is in the given relationship to another, then the second is necessarily in the relationship given with the first."

Since symmetries are outstanding features to distinguish geometric structures from messy backgrounds, symmetry detection is a field of study for detection and recognition of objects. There have been several efforts to detect and represent symmetry, Li and Li [5] presented a method to detect reflection symmetry for shape analysis and object recognition; to solve this problem, the authors defined and solved a trigonometric system derived from directional and invariant moments of reflection.

C. O. Jiménez-Ibarra (✉) · H. Sánchez-Cruz · M. V.-M. del Campo
Universidad Autónoma de Aguascalientes, Aguascalientes, México
e-mail: omar.jimenez@edu.uaa.mx; hsanchez@correo.uaa.mx; al266176@edu.uaa.mx

H. R. Arabnia et al. (eds.), *Advances in Computer Vision and Computational Biology*, Transactions on Computational Science and Computational Intelligence,
https://doi.org/10.1007/978-3-030-71051-4_11

Bitsakos et al. [6] presented an algorithm to calculate bilateral symmetry of object silhouettes under perspective distortion exploiting the invariance of projective transformations.

Cornelius and Loy [7] introduced a method to detect local bilateral symmetries or global on flat surfaces under perspective projection on complex backgrounds; this method is based on feature descriptors, robust to related local distortion, and on quadruples of entities formed from pairs of symmetric entities. Michaelsen et al. [8] developed a mirror symmetry detection algorithm in 2D images based on the transformation algorithm of invariant characteristics of scale that detects a symmetric combinatorial set of higher order. Wang et al. [9] proposed a unified detection of rotation, reflection, and translation symmetries using related invariant contour features. Elawady et al. [10] proposed a global reflective symmetry detection scheme based on a feature based on edges extracted using Log-Gabor filters and a parameterized voting scheme by the textural neighborhood and corresponding color information of the image.

Although chain codes are a suitable technique to represent curves, a few works use them to detect symmetry in 2D images, for example, the ones proposed in [11–13]. In [12], the authors use the Freeman chain code of eight directions [14] to find local symmetries in the contours of isolated objects, and in [13], the authors use Slope Chain Code (SCC) [15] to detect local and global mirror symmetries, as well as multiple axes of symmetry.

Computational symmetry in real-world data turns out to be a challenge. A fully automated symmetry system remains an open field for real-world applications. In many practical cases through human vision, it can be clear to us where the axes of symmetry are; however, when the information is taken and stored as an image, an algorithm is required to recognize these symmetries even though the image contour has noise or simply malformations that human vision does not detect by the naked eye.

For the representation of shape contours, as well as the detection of axes and level of mirror symmetry, in this work, we use AF8 chain code [16].

This paper is organized as follows. In Sect. 2, the proposed method is described, whereas in Sect. 3 application of our method is shown. In Sect. 4, a comparison with other methods and objects, and then in Sect. 5, an analysis of our work is carried out. Finally, in Sect. 6, some conclusions are given.

2 Method

This section presents the preprocessing to which the objects are subjected, to later extract their contour, and finally to determine the equations that give us the axes and levels of symmetry.

2.1 Images Processing

From the database of MPEG7, http://www.dabi.temple.edu/ shape/MPEG7/dataset .html, we choose some objects to firstly preprocess with mathematical morphology, then to find axes of symmetry, and finally to propose a level of symmetry.

Once the objects were chosen, morphological operators are applied. The close operator is used on the object to eliminate noise, smooth contour, and fill gaps, which hinder or distort the contour. After removing the noise and smoothing, the erosion followed by a subtraction is used to extract the contour of the objects to obtain its AF8 chain code.

2.2 Contour Coding

AF8 is a code based on two vectors: one of reference and one of change, whose changes of direction are labeled by the symbols of the alphabet $\Sigma_{\mathrm{AF8}}= \{a, b, c, d, e, f, g, h\}$. See Fig. 2.

With all the contours, we proceed to use the AF8 chain code to represent them. For example, the AF8 chain code of Fig. 3 is S = *gcgcbbgbbchahcbbgbbc*.

Although there are different chain codes, the AF8 code was chosen because it is simple to encode, it correctly describes the contour, and it is invariant under translation and rotation; although the Slope Chain Code can be better adjusted to the curves, the AF8 code is chosen since we can visit all the pixels, and we prove to obtain more accurate results of the symmetries.

2.3 Proposed Energy Function to Obtain the Symmetry Level

The chain code obtained from the contour is formed by a number n of characters : $|AF8| = n$.

In this work, we define two kinds of symmetry functions: S_1 that depends on the symmetry of the chain code and S_2 that changes according to the frequency of appearance of chain code characters. In this way, we propose that the level of symmetry of the object is given by a linear combination S of these two energy functions.

For the first symmetry function, we start by comparing the first character with the $(n-1)$-th character of the chain code, then we compare the second character with the $(n-2)$-th character, and so on until we cover the entire chain, finally, if n is even, the n-th is compared to the $(n/2)$-th character. Then distance error, $error_p$, increases by 1 for each compared character that is different. This is repeated for the

Table 1 Results of the first energy functions for Fig. 4

Starting point	Chain code	error_p	E_p	S_1
1	gcgcbbgbbchahcbbgbbc	7	0.7	0.3
2	cgcbbgbbchahcbbgbbcg	7	0.7	0.3
3	gcbbgbbchahcbbgbbcgc	8	0.8	0.2
4	cbbgbbchahcbbgbbcgcg	1	0.1	0.9
5	bbgbbchahcbbgbbcgcgc	8	0.8	0.2
6	bgbbchahcbbgbbcgcgcb	7	0.7	0.3
7	gbbchahcbbgbbcgcgcbb	7	0.7	0.3
8	bbchahcbbgbbcgcgcbbg	8	0.8	0.2
9	bchahcbbgbbcgcgcbbgb	3	0.3	0.7
10	chahcbbgbbcgcgcbbgbb	8	0.8	0.2

following (*n*/2) − 1 chains that can be formed from the object (see Table 1). So, error_p is

$$\text{error}_p = \begin{cases} \text{error}_p + 1, & \text{if } AF8_{(i+1)} \neq AF8_{(n-i-1)} \\ \text{error}_p, & \text{if } AF8_{(i+1)} = AF8_{(n-i-1)} \end{cases}, \tag{1}$$

for *i* from 0 to (*n*/2) − 1 rounding down.

And also, if *n* is even,

$$\text{error}_p = \begin{cases} \text{error}_p + 1 & \text{if } AF8_{(n/2)} \neq AF8_{(n)} \\ \text{error}_p, & \text{if } AF8_{(n/2)} = AF8_{(n)} \end{cases} \tag{2}$$

We define that the energy required for the chain to be fully palindromic is proportional to the ratio between the error and the number of characters compared or

$$E_p = \begin{cases} \frac{2\text{error}_p}{n}, & if\ n \text{ even} \\ \frac{2\text{error}_p}{n-1}, & if\ n \text{ odd} \end{cases} \tag{3}$$

In [13], it is proposed that the degree of symmetry is the difference between the unit and the energy used. Something similar is proposed for this work using our energy function; therefore, our first symmetry level function is

$$S_1 = 1 - E_p \tag{4}$$

As an example, we apply (1) to (4) to Fig. 4, and the results shown in Table 1 are obtained.

As this error differs from the human eye, one more function is determined that helps to give us a more precise value of the level of symmetry of an object.

So for the second symmetry, we halve our AF8 chain code into two subchains, to the left, $L(C_{AF8})$, and to the right, $R(C_{AF8})$, of the midpoint and subtract the

Table 2 Results of the second energy function for Fig. 4

Starting point	Chain code	error_f	E_f	S_2
1	gcgcbbgbbchahcbbgbbc	2	0.4	0.6
2	cgcbbgbbchahcbbgbbcg	0	0	1
3	gcbbgbbchahcbbgbbcgc	0	0	1
4	cbbgbbchahcbbgbbcgcg	2	0.4	0.6
5	bbgbbchahcbbgbbcgcgc	2	0.4	0.6
6	bgbbchahcbbgbbcgcgcb	2	0.4	0.6
7	gbbchahcbbgbbcgcgcbb	2	0.4	0.6
8	bbchahcbbgbbcgcgcbbg	2	0.4	0.6
9	bchahcbbgbbcgcgcbbgb	2	0.4	0.6
10	chahcbbgbbcgcgcbbgbb	2	0.4	0.6

frequency of appearance of the characters of the subchains from each other. We have the frequency difference as following:

$$f\left(C_{\mathrm{AF8}}(x)\right) = \left|f\left(L\left(C_{\mathrm{AF8}}(x)\right)\right) - f\left(R\left(C_{\mathrm{AF8}}(x)\right)\right)\right| \tag{5}$$

where x is an AF8 chain code character.

Then we add a unit to the error_f if the frequency difference is greater than or equal to 10 % of n, i.e.,

$$\text{error}_f = \begin{cases} \text{error}_f + 1, & \text{if } f\left(C_{\mathrm{AF8}}(x)\right) \geq 0.1n \\ \text{error}_f, & \text{if } f\left(C_{\mathrm{AF8}}(x)\right) < 0.1n \end{cases} \tag{6}$$

We consider that the energy of frequency E_f is proportional to the ratio between the error error_f and the number m of different characters in the chain, or

$$E_f = \frac{\text{error}_f}{m} \tag{7}$$

Analogously to (4), we propose a second symmetry function as

$$S_2 = 1 - E_f \tag{8}$$

This symmetry is calculated for each point on the contour, as was also done in the first symmetry function.

Applying this second method, in Fig. 4, we obtain the results shown in Table 2.

Finally, we propose to make a linear combination with (4) and (8). For this, we use the parameters α and β, with $\alpha + \beta = 1$, and the proposed symmetry is given by (9).

$$S = \alpha S_2 + \beta S_1 \tag{9}$$

Table 3 Level of symmetry of Fig. 4

Starting point	S
1	0.48
2	0.68
3	0.96
4	0.44
5	0.48
6	0.48
7	0.44
8	0.64
9	0.44
10	0.48

So the object is totally symmetric in a point if $S = 1$ and totally asymmetric if $S = 0$, and the intermediate values give us its level of symmetry.

Finally, we compute the level of symmetry of Fig. 4, and Table 3 shows our result. Since the second symmetry function gives us a more accurate value of the level of symmetry, we use the values of $\alpha = 0.6$ and $\beta = 0.4$ to obtain this result.

As we can see from Table 3, the axis of symmetry starts in the third pixel and ends at the pixel it was compared to, in this case the 13th pixel of the object.

3 Results of the Method

Figure 5 shows the results of the method for the chosen objects (Fig. 1), marking with a red line the axes of symmetry and below each object its level of symmetry.

4 Comparison

This section is dedicated to comparing our method and results with other methods, other objects, and what people see.

4.1 Ground Truth

To analyze how our method worked by assigning a level of symmetry and finding an axis of symmetry, we compared it with the ground truth, and Table 4 shows the results.

To define the ground truth, we asked 50 subjects to assign a value of symmetry to the contours generated in the method; in addition, we ask the subjects to write down the global axis of symmetry in those contours.

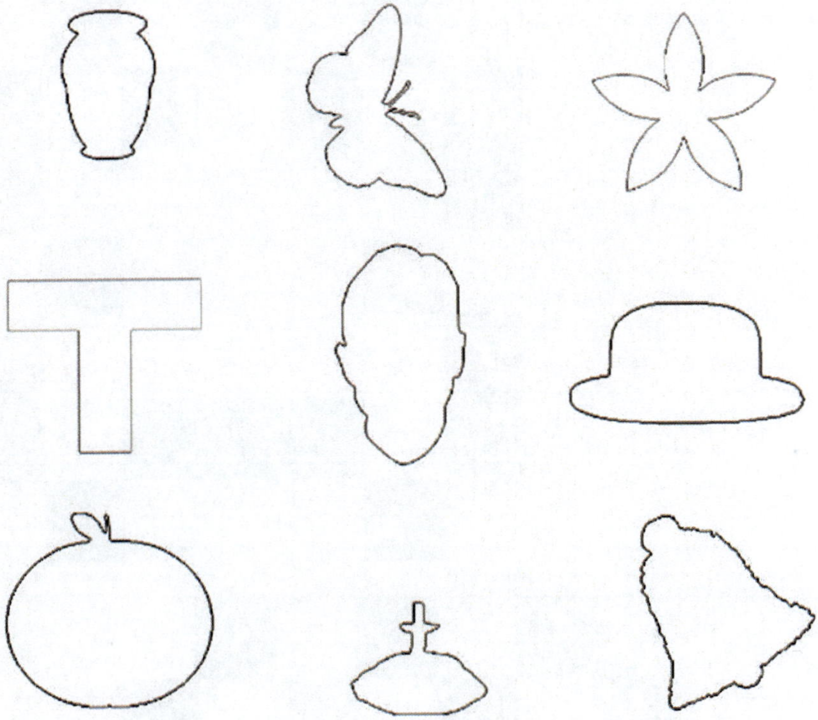

Fig. 1 Contours of the objects

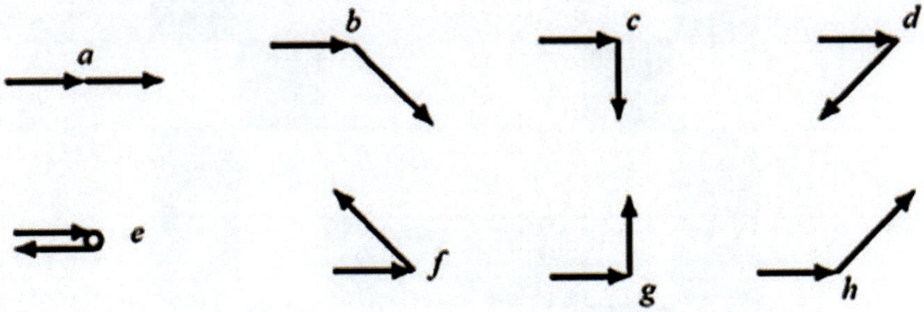

Fig. 2 AF8 symbols

Table 4 Results of the comparison with ground truth

Experiment	Level of agreement
Find axes of symmetry	1.00
Assign a level of symmetry	1.00

Under these considerations, our method performed with a precision equal to 1.00 and an accuracy equal to 1.00 (Table 4). This means that our method does coincide totally compared to human vision.

Fig. 3 In yellow, the AF8 vectors to coding the object

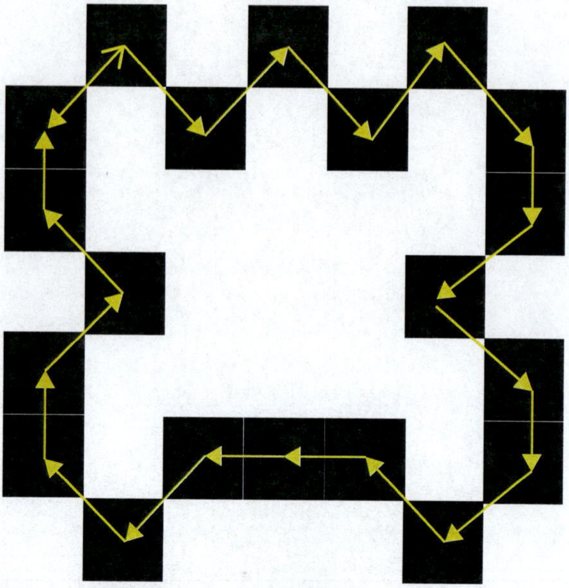

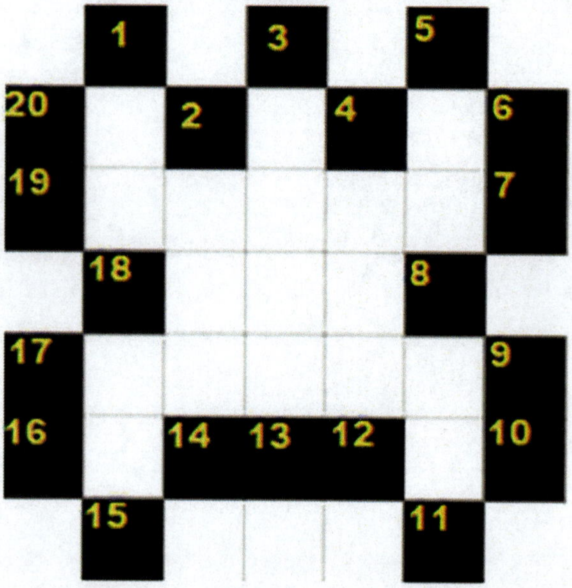

Fig. 4 Object with clockwise numbered pixels

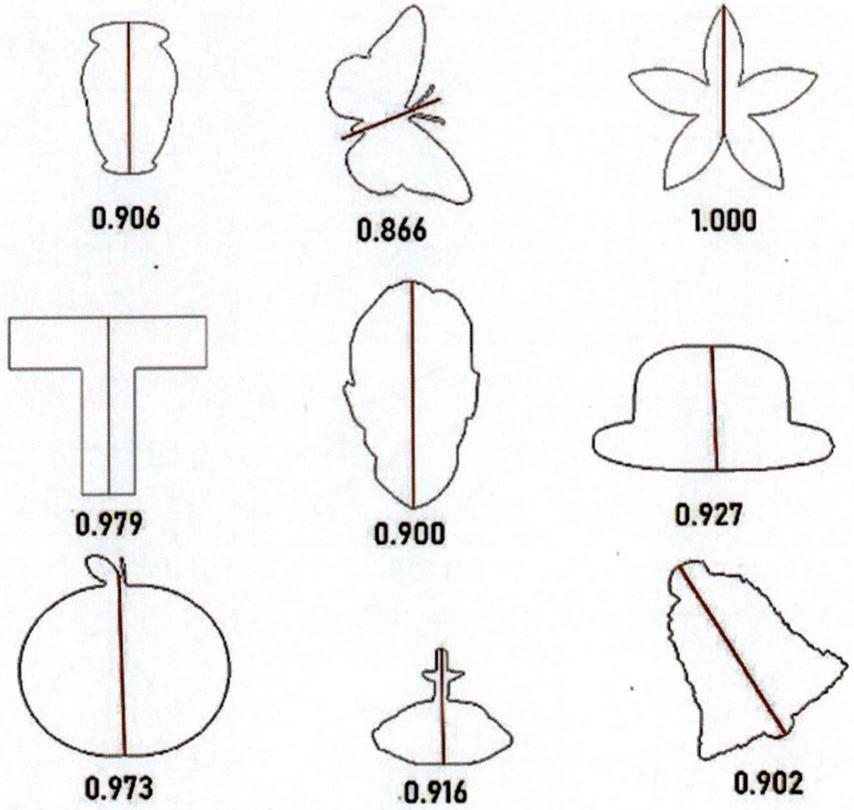

Fig. 5 Symmetry levels of an object. In red, its axes of symmetry

4.2 *Rotated Objects*

Now, a question arises: Are these methods invariant under intermediate rotations? These observations have not been reported by the recent works in literature. We make the experiment to rotate the objects to see if our method is invariant under intermediate rotations for seeing whether the level of symmetry of objects in Fig. 5 changes, and if it changes, why it does. If the symmetry level does not change for any rotation, we say that our method is isotropic; otherwise, we do an analysis why this happen and if only the level of symmetry changes or also the axes.

We then begin by rotating each object in Fig. 5 to different angles. Afterward, we apply our method to obtain the levels and axes of symmetry and be able to compare them with those obtained previously. All rotations were made counterclockwise, with angles of $\frac{\pi}{2}, \pi, \frac{3\pi}{2}, \frac{3\pi}{2}, \frac{\pi}{4}, \frac{3\pi}{2}, \frac{5\pi}{4}, \frac{3\pi}{2}$, and $-\frac{\pi}{6}$ rad for objects from 1 to 9, respectively. The results are shown in Fig. 6.

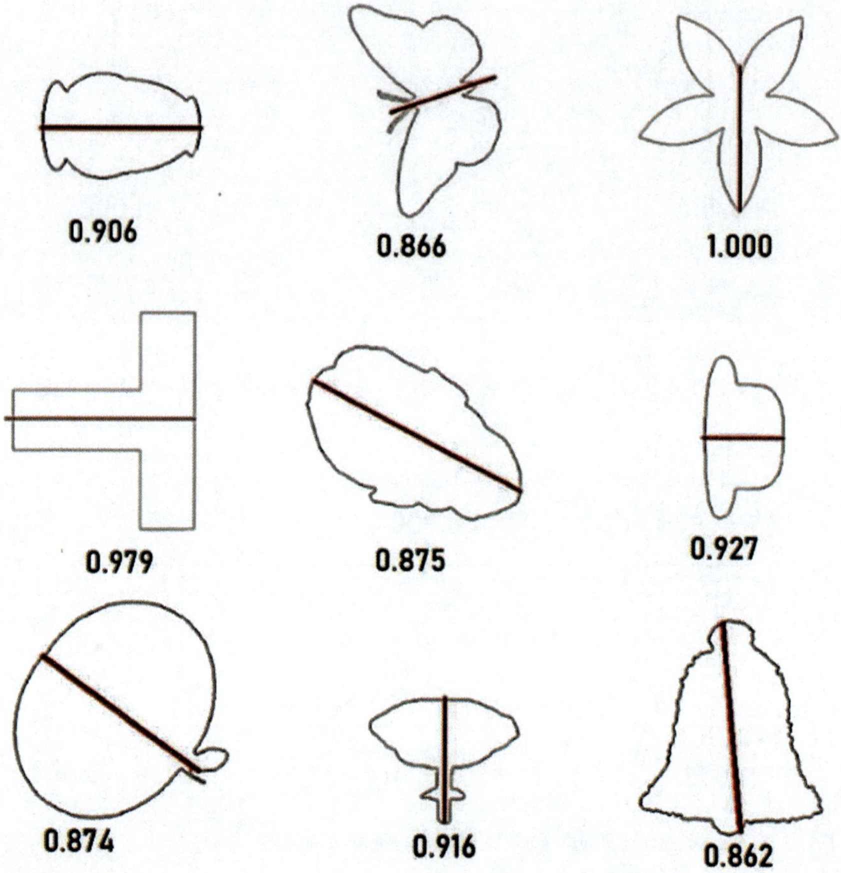

Fig. 6 Symmetry levels of rotated objects. In red, its axes of symmetry

If we look closely, we can see that the apple, the bell, and the face underwent slight changes since they widened a little. This deformation can be caused by the fact that the rotation angles of these objects are not multiples of $\frac{\pi}{2}$ and cause, in the discrete domain, the length of the lines that make up the objects to vary for the mentioned angles.

We can notice that the axes of symmetry do not change for the most part, except for the bell that moved a little. However, the symmetry levels in the face, the apple, and the bell do change more, and in all other objects, it remained the same.

These changes in symmetry levels can be attributed to the fact that the images vary according to their rotation. For objects that were rotated with multiples of $\frac{\pi}{2}$ angles, their symmetry did not change since the images does not change.

On the other hand, if the object is rotated with some other angle, the image undergoes some changes in the number of pixels and/or the way they are distributed

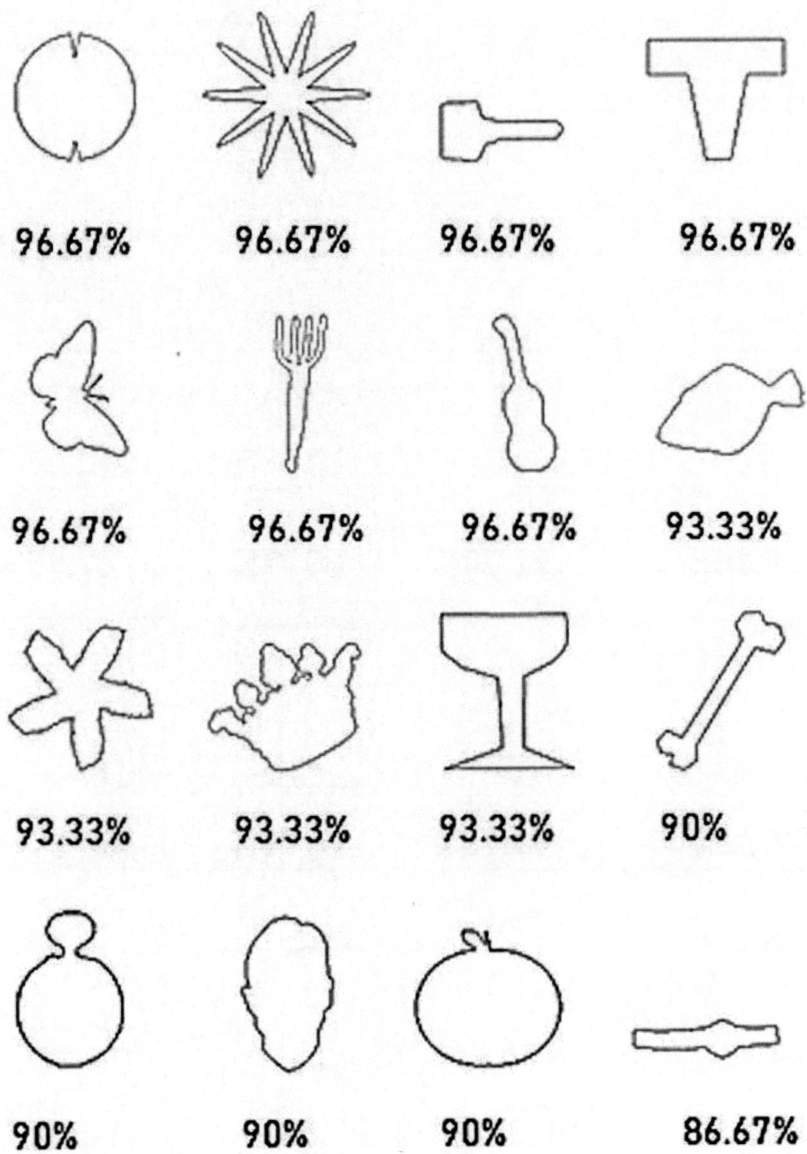

Fig. 7 Results of symmetry levels by Alvarado et al.

as mentioned above. These changes cause the level of symmetry to vary from the first; however, this can agree with human perception.

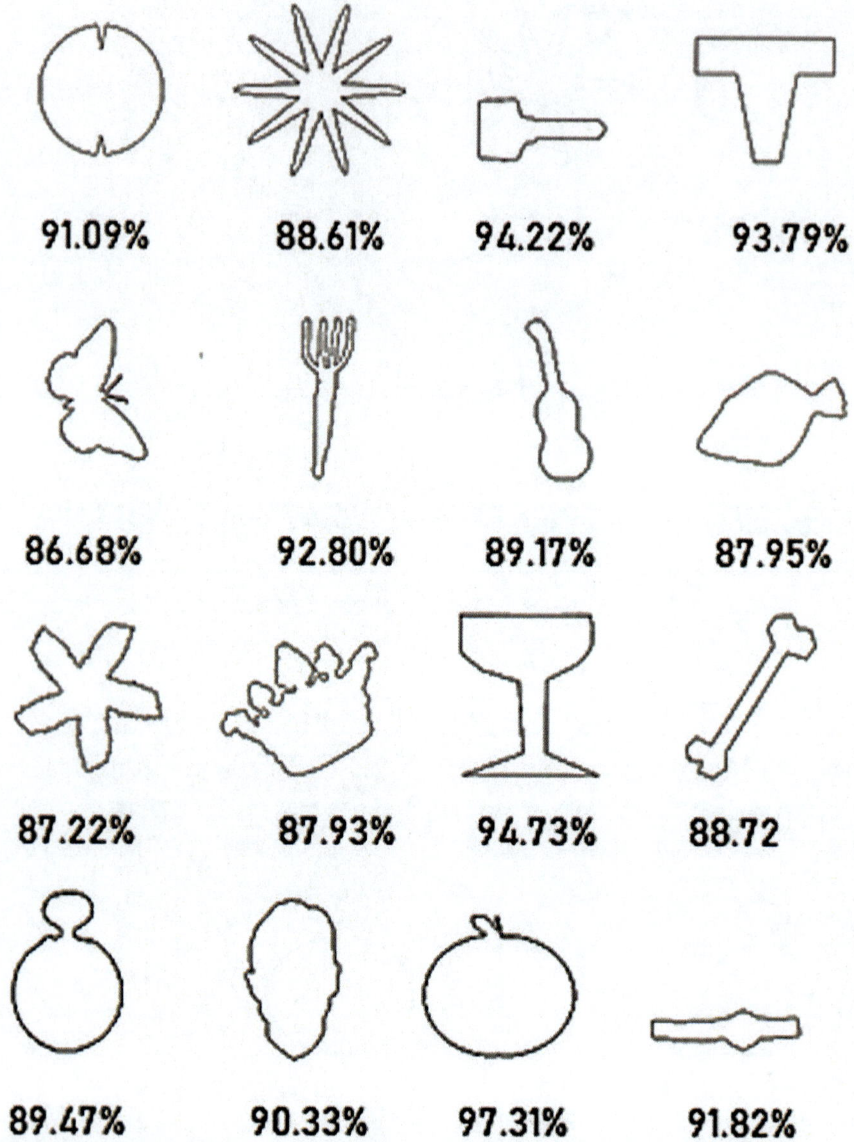

Fig. 8 Results of symmetry levels with our method in the objects used by Alvarado et al.

4.3 Slope Chain Code

This section is dedicated to the comparison of our method with that made by Alvarado et al. [13], where they used a chain code called a Slope Chain Code (SCC)

[15]. The purpose of this comparison is to see how much our results differ from theirs and to understand what this difference indicates and why it occurs.

Thus, Alvarado et al. make use of this chain code for the description of 2D objects, and they use approximately 200 line segments for the description of these. With this information, they proceeded to determine axes of symmetry and assigned a percentage of symmetry to the objects (Fig. 7).

On the other hand, we tested our method on the same objects (Fig. 8) to carry out the comparison.

The results are quite similar, and both methods detect a similar level of symmetry. Even so, there are notable differences in the results of some objects, and this could be due to the fact that, as previously mentioned, Alvarado's method is made with only 200 line segments for each figure. This means that the information of theirs images is different from ours. That is why there may be variations in the results.

In addition, it is difficult to determine an exact level of symmetry for each figure because it depends on the perception of each person although the results can be limited and thus establish a range of possible levels of symmetry.

5 Advantages

The main advantage is the simplicity of our algorithm since we only need the image to be encoded to carry out the entire procedure to give us the levels of symmetry. On the contrary, the method of Alvarado et al. requires, in addition to the image to be processed, that they need to analyze the number of straight-line segments to find the SCC and then proceed to recognize it to finally obtain axes and levels of symmetry.

We can also denote the fact that with the information of the whole pixels of the contour, we have accurate results and similar to those of Alvarado et al. who used less information of contour pixels due to the constant number of segments established initially by them.

The variation of our results is something to highlight because in general terms of what people see, it is very difficult for two different objects to have the same symmetry value. If we look at the first seven objects (considering the first two rows from Fig. 7), we can see that its symmetry level totally coincides, and the same happens with the following two groups of four objects. This does not happen in our method (Fig. 8). Then our method is more versatile in the results, which gives a more concrete idea of what is the perception of the levels of symmetry.

Then we have the independence of the starting point, which means that regardless of the first pixel that we read to encode the figure, the results in levels and axes of symmetry do not change. This is because our algorithm goes through all the pixels to assign them a level of symmetry. So even if it starts at a specific pixel, in the end, all the pixels are traversed.

Detecting multiple axes of symmetry is another advantage that our method gives us since there are objects like stars that have several axes of symmetry and must be marked as such. Just as there are objects with multiple axes of symmetry, there are others that do not since they are asymmetric objects. Our method gives the facility to recognize these objects, starting from a level that can be specified by the user to decide when an object is or is not symmetric.

As shown in Sect. 4.2, our method is invariant to rotations if the characteristics of the objects do not change, and if they change, this method identifies the changes and corrects the levels of symmetry.

We can see there are several advantages in the proposed method that helps to detect, classify, and measure symmetry of objects regardless of their shape, orientation, or direction.

As previously mentioned, the issue of symmetry detection is quite broad, and different authors have approached to it; however, few did it using chain codes. This work demonstrates that the AF8 chain code works correctly for symmetry detection.

To achieve this, we must propose several equations to properly define those of energy and symmetry and to improve the results. So we chose to have an equation that takes into account the shape of the contour (4), but also the characteristics of the chain code obtained (8), thus being able to combine both characteristics and units in an Eq. (9) that can also be manipulated by the user to obtain more real results.

The use of more than one symmetry equation, which in the end are combined, contributed to the results since each one analyzes different characteristics of the chain code. All this is observed in Sect. 4.1, where the results agree satisfactorily with the ground truth proposed.

Finally, the proposal can be applied to both robotics and artificial intelligence, for example, in the reconstruction, detection, separation or recognition of images, etc.

6 Conclusion

The proposed method achieves the objective of measuring the level of symmetry of an object, comparable to the human perspective, in addition to optimally detecting axes of symmetry.

Additionally, doing several experiments, we were able to realize that the method of detecting symmetries through palindromes (4) is not as efficient as it is through frequency appearance of characters (8). Thus, for future works, it is planned to give weight to this characteristic in the detection of symmetries and see how this affects the results.

References

1. W. Aguilar, E. Bribiesca, Symmetry detection in 3D chain coded discrete curves and trees. Pattern Recognit **48**(4), 1420–1439 (2015). https://doi.org/10.1016/j.patcog.2014.09.024

2. E.H. Lockwood, R.H. Macmillan, *Geometric symmetry* (Cambridge University Press, London, 1978)
3. Libro: Hermann Weyl. Symmetry. Princeton. University Press. 1952. 168 p'aginas
4. W. Karush, *Webster's New World Dictionary of Mathematics* (Simon Schuster, Inc., New York, 1989), p. 10023
5. E. Li, H. Li, Reflection invariant and symmetry detection. ArXiv e-prints (2017)
6. K. Bitsakos, H. Yi, L. Yi, C. Fermuller, Bilateral symmetry of object silhouettes under perspective projection, in *19th International Conference on Pattern Recognition*, (2008), pp. 1–4
7. H. Cornelius, G. Loy, Detecting bilateral symmetry in perspective, in *Conference on Computer Vision and Pattern Recognition Workshop (CVPRW'06), IEEE Computer Society, New York City, New York, USA*, (2006), p. 191
8. E. Michaelsen, D. Muench, M. Arens, Recognition of symmetry structure by use of Gestalt algebra, in *IEEE Conference on Computer Vision and Pattern Recognition Workshops*, (2013), pp. 206–210
9. Z. Wang, L. Fu, Y. Li, Unified detection of skewed rotation, reflection and translation symmetries from affine invariant contour features. Pattern Recognit **47**(4), 1764–1776 (2014)
10. M. Elawady, C. Ducottet, O. Alata, C. Barat, P. Colantoni, Wavelet-based reflection symmetry detection via textural and color histograms. ArXiv e-prints (2017)
11. S. Parui, D.D. Majumder, Symmetry analysis by computer. Pattern Recognit **16**(1), 63–67 (1983)
12. J. Inesta, M. Buend'ıa, M.A. Sarti, Local symmetries of digital contours from their chain codes. Pattern Recognit **29**(10), 1737–1749 (1996)
13. M. Alvarado-Gonzalez, W. Aguilar, E. Garduño, C. Velarde, E. Bribiesca, V. Medina-Bañuelos, Mirror symmetry detection in curves represented by means of the Slope Chain Code. Pattern Recognit **87**, 67–79., ISSN 0031-3203 (2019). https://doi.org/10.1016/j.patcog.2018.10.002
14. H. Freeman, Techniques for the digital computer analysis of chain-Encoded arbitrary plane curves. Proc. Natl. Electronics. Conf. **17**, 421–432 (1961)
15. E. Bribiesca, A measure of tortuosity based on chain coding. Pattern Recognit **46**(3), 716–724 (2013)
16. Y.K. Lui, B. Zalik, An efficient chain code with Huffman coding, Pattern Recognit. **38**, 553–557 (2005).

Superpixel-Based Stereoscopic Video Saliency Detection Using Support Vector Regression Learning

Ting-Yu Chou and Jin-Jang Leou

1 Introduction

Visual attention, an important characteristic of the human visual system (HVS), can rapidly detect and focus on salient regions in natural scenes. A number of saliency detection approaches are proposed for image, video, stereoscopic image, and stereoscopic video applications.

For image salient detection, Cheng et al. [1] proposed a global contrast-based image saliency detection approach using histogram-based and region-based contrast computations. Chen et al. [2] proposed an image saliency detection approach using Gabor texture cues. For video saliency detection, Li et al. [3] proposed a video saliency detection approach based on superpixel-level trajectories. Wang et al. [4] proposed a video saliency detection approach based on geodesic distance. Liu et al. [5] proposed a superpixel-based spatiotemporal saliency detection approach. For stereoscopic image saliency detection, Fang et al. [6] proposed a stereoscopic image saliency detection approach, in which the color contrast, luminance, texture, and depth features are extracted from discrete cosine transform (DCT) domain. Wang et al. [7] proposed a stereoscopic image saliency detection approach using spatial edges and disparity boundaries. Ju et al. [8] proposed a stereoscopic image saliency detection approach based on anisotropic center-surround difference. Liang et al. [9] proposed a stereoscopic salient object detection approach using RGB-D deep fusion. For stereoscopic video saliency detection, spatial, temporal, depth, and spatiotemporal features are extracted from different domains, which are integrated to generate the final saliency map using different fusion strategies.

T.-Y. Chou · J.-J. Leou (✉)
Department of Computer Science and Information Engineering, National Chung Cheng University, Chiayi, Taiwan
e-mail: ctyu105m@cs.ccu.edu.tw; jjleou@cs.ccu.edu.tw

H. R. Arabnia et al. (eds.), *Advances in Computer Vision and Computational Biology*, Transactions on Computational Science and Computational Intelligence,
https://doi.org/10.1007/978-3-030-71051-4_12

Banitalebi-Dehkordi, Pourazad, and Nasiopoulos [10] proposed a learning-based visual saliency prediction model for stereoscopic 3D video. Fang, Wang, and Lin [11] proposed a video saliency detection approach incorporating spatiotemporal cues and uncertainty weighting. Zhang et al. [12] proposed a stereoscopic video saliency detection approach based on spatiotemporal correlation and depth confidence optimization. Fang et al. [13, 14] proposed two stereoscopic video saliency detection approaches using two types of deep convolutional networks. In this study, a superpixel-based stereoscopic video saliency detection approach is proposed.

This paper is organized as follows. The proposed superpixel-based stereoscopic video saliency approach is addressed in Section 2. Experimental results are described in Section 3, followed by concluding remarks.

2 Proposed Approach

2.1 System Architecture

In this study, as shown in Fig. 1, a superpixel-based stereoscopic video saliency detection approach is proposed. Based on the input stereoscopic video sequences containing left-view and right-view video sequences, a sequence of right-to-left disparity maps are obtained. First, the simple linear iterative clustering (SLIC) algorithm [15] is used to perform superpixel segmentation on all video frames. Second, the spatial, temporal, depth, object, and spatiotemporal features are extracted from video frames to generate the corresponding feature maps. Third, all feature maps are concatenated and support vector regression (SVR) learning using LIBLINEAR tools is employed to generate the initial saliency maps of video frames. Finally, the initial saliency maps are refined by using the center bias map, the significant increased map, visual sensitivity, and Gaussian filtering.

2.2 SLIC Superpixel Segmentation

Let $L_n^r(x, y)$, $L_n^g(x, y)$, and $L_n^b(x, y)$, $n = 1, 2, \ldots, N$, $1 \leq x \leq W$, $1 \leq y \leq H$ be the R, G, and B components of the n-th left-view color video frame, where N is the number of left-view color video frames, and W and H are the width and height of video frames, respectively. Additionally, let $\mathrm{DM}_n(x, y)$, $n = 1, 2, \ldots, N$, be the corresponding n-th right-to-left disparity map.

The SLIC algorithm [15] is employed to perform superpixel segmentation on each video frame in CIELab color space. Let $\mathrm{sp}_{n,k}$, $n = 1, 2, \cdots, N$, $k = 1, 2, \cdots, K$ be the k-th superpixel of frame n, where K denotes the number of superpixels in the n-th left-view video frame.

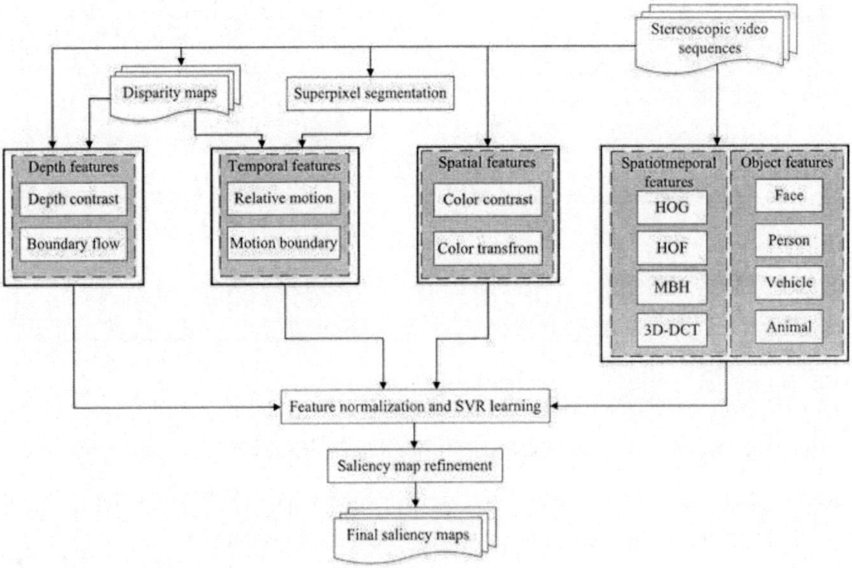

Fig. 1 Framework of the proposed approach

2.3 *Feature Extraction*

Spatial Features

In this study, each video frame is transformed from RGB color space into YCbCr color space. $L_n^{\mathrm{y}}(x, y)$, $L_n^{\mathrm{cb}}(x, y)$, and $L_n^{\mathrm{cr}}(x, y)$ denoting the corresponding Y, Cb, and Cr color components are divided into patches (8×8 pixels), and 64 discrete cosine transform (DCT) coefficients are extracted for each patch. For patch h_n^i of frame *n*, the three DC coefficients of Y, Cb, and Cr components and sum of all AC coefficients of *Y* component are extracted and denoted as $\mathrm{DC}_n^{\mathrm{y}}(h_n^i)$, $\mathrm{DC}_n^{\mathrm{cb}}(h_n^i)$, $\mathrm{DC}_n^{\mathrm{cr}}(h_n^i)$, and $A\mathrm{C}_{\mathrm{n}}^{\mathrm{y}}(h_n^i)$, respectively. For patch h_n^i of frame *n*, the color contrast feature is calculated as

$$\mathrm{FCC}_n\left(h_n^i\right) = \frac{1}{4}\left(\mathrm{CC}_n^{\mathrm{y}}\left(h_n^i\right) + \mathrm{CC}_n^{\mathrm{cb}}\left(h_n^i\right) + \mathrm{CC}_n^{\mathrm{cr}}\left(h_n^i\right) + \mathrm{AY}_n^{\mathrm{y}}\left(h_n^i\right)\right), \quad (1)$$

$$\mathrm{CC}_n^{\mathrm{y}}\left(h_n^i\right) = \sum\nolimits_{j\neq i} \exp\left(-d_s\left(h_n^i, h_n^j\right)/\sigma^2\right) \times T_{\mathrm{DC}}\left(\mathrm{DC}_n^{\mathrm{y}}\left(h_n^i\right), \mathrm{DC}_n^{\mathrm{y}}\left(h_n^j\right)\right), \quad (2)$$

$$\mathrm{CC}_n^{\mathrm{cb}}\left(h_n^i\right)=\sum\nolimits_{j\neq i}\exp\left(-d_s\left(h_n^i,h_n^j\right)/\sigma^2\right)\times T_{\mathrm{DC}}\left(\mathrm{DC}_n^{\mathrm{cb}}\left(h_n^i\right),\mathrm{DC}_n^{cb}\left(h_n^j\right)\right),\tag{3}$$

$$\mathrm{CC}_n^{\mathrm{cr}}\left(h_n^i\right)=\sum\nolimits_{j\neq i}\exp\left(-d_s\left(h_n^i,h_n^j\right)/\sigma^2\right)\times T_{\mathrm{DC}}\left(\mathrm{DC}_n^{\mathrm{cr}}\left(h_n^i\right),\mathrm{DC}_n^{\mathrm{cr}}\left(h_n^j\right)\right),\tag{4}$$

$$\mathrm{AY}_n^{y}\left(h_n^i\right)=\sum\nolimits_{j\neq i}\exp\left(-d_s\left(h_n^i,h_n^j\right)/\sigma^2\right)\times T_{\mathrm{AC}}\left(\mathrm{AC}_n^{y}\left(h_n^i\right),\mathrm{AC}_n^{y}\left(h_n^j\right)\right),\tag{5}$$

where $d_s\left(h_n^i,h_n^j\right)$ is the spatial (Euclidean) distance between patches h_n^i and h_n^j, σ is a parameter (set as 5), and $T_{\mathrm{DC}}\left(\mathrm{DC}_n^{y}\left(h_n^i\right),\mathrm{DC}_n^{y}\left(h_n^j\right)\right)$, $T_{\mathrm{DC}}\left(\mathrm{DC}_n^{\mathrm{cb}}\left(h_n^i\right),\ \mathrm{DC}_n^{\mathrm{cb}}\left(h_n^j\right)\right)$, $T_{\mathrm{DC}}\left(\mathrm{DC}_n^{\mathrm{cr}}\left(h_n^i\right),\mathrm{DC}_n^{\mathrm{cr}}\left(h_n^j\right)\right)$, and $T_{\mathrm{AC}}\left(\mathrm{AC}_n^{y}\left(h_n^i\right),\ \mathrm{AC}_n^{y}\left(h_n^j\right)\right)$ represent color differences between patches h_n^i and h_n^j of the DC coefficients of Y, Cb, and Cr components and sum of all AC coefficients of Y component, respectively [16]. Then the pixel-based color contrast feature map for frame n, $\mathrm{CCMap}_n(x, y)$, $1 \leq x \leq W$, $1 \leq y \leq H$, is defined as the color contrast feature value of the corresponding patch. The superpixel-level characteristic feature $\mathrm{CF}_n\left(\mathrm{sp}_n^i\right)$ is determined by the average normalized x and y coordinates; the average RGB, CIELab, and HSV color values; the RGB, CIELab, hue, saturation, and gradient histograms; the global and local contrasts; and the element compactness, area of superpixel, and superpixel singular value [17]. The initial classification feature $\mathrm{IC}_n\left(\mathrm{sp}_n^i\right)$ is computed by the characteristic feature by Otsu's thresholding, i.e.,

$$\mathrm{IC}_n\left(\mathrm{sp}_n^i\right)=\begin{cases}1, & \text{if } \mathrm{CF}_n\left(\mathrm{sp}_n^i\right)\geq \mathrm{th}_n,\\ 0, & \text{otherwise,}\end{cases}\tag{6}$$

where th_n is the 25-th superpixel of frame n sorted by initial classification feature values of superpixels of frame n. $\mathrm{IC}_n\left(\mathrm{sp}_n^i\right)=0, 1$ if superpixel sp_n^i is classified into background and foreground regions, respectively. In this study, 11 color features extracted from R, G, B, L^*, a^*, b^*, hue, and saturation components as well as color gradients of R, G, and B components (with gamma correction) are denoted as $\mathbf{CG}_n$, $\mathbf{CB}_n$, $\mathbf{CL}_n$, $\mathbf{Ca}_n$, $\mathbf{Cb}_n$, $\mathbf{CH}_n$, $\mathbf{CS}_n$, $\mathbf{CgR}_n$, $\mathbf{CgG}_n$, and $\mathbf{CgB}_n$. The color feature $\mathbf{CV}_n$ of frame n is a $K\times 44$ matrix defined as

$$\mathbf{CV}_n=\left[\mathbf{CR}_n\ \mathbf{CG}_n\ \mathbf{CL}_n\ \mathbf{Ca}_n\ \mathbf{Cb}_n\ \mathbf{CH}_n\ \mathbf{CS}_n\ \mathbf{CgR}_n\ \mathbf{CgG}_n\ \mathbf{CgB}_n\right].\tag{7}$$

For frame n, the color transform feature $\mathbf{fct}_n$, a $K\times 1$ vector, is computed as

$$\mathbf{fct}_n = \mathbf{CV}_n \cdot \boldsymbol{\alpha}_n, \tag{8}$$

$$\boldsymbol{\alpha}_n = \left(\mathbf{CVfg}_n{}^T \mathbf{CVfg}_n + \lambda \cdot \mathbf{I}\right)^{-1} \mathbf{CVfg}_n{}^T \cdot \mathbf{s}_n, \tag{9}$$

where $\boldsymbol{\alpha}_n$ is a 44×1 vector; $\mathbf{CVfg}_n$ is a $K \times 44$ matrix, in which each row vector is the initial classification feature vector (background or foreground) for $\mathbf{CV}_n$; λ is a parameter (set as 0.05); I is a 44×44 identity matrix; and $\mathbf{s}_n$ is a $K\times 1$ vector, in which each element is 1 (foreground region) and 0 (background region). The pixel-based color transform feature map for frame n, $\boldsymbol{CTMap}_n(x, y)$, $1 \le x \le W$, $1 \le y \le H$ is defined as the color transform feature value of the corresponding superpixel.

Temporal Features

In this study, $M_n^x(x, y)$, $M_n^y(x, y)$, and $M_n^z(x, y)$ denoting motions in x, y, and z directions for pixel (x, y) in frame n, respectively, are computed. $M_n^x(x, y)$ and $M_n^y(x, y)$ are computed by the fast correlation flow algorithm [18], and based on the N disparity maps, $\mathrm{DM}_n(x, y)$, $n = 1, 2, \cdots, N$, $M_n^z(x, y)$ is calculated as [10]

$$M_n^z(x, y) = \mathrm{DM}_{n+1}\left(x + M_x^t(x, y), y + M_y^t(x, y)\right) - \mathrm{DM}_n(x, y). \tag{10}$$

By averaging motion values over all pixels in superpixel sp_n^i of frame n, superpixel-level motions in x, y, and z directions are computed as $M_n^x\left(\mathrm{sp}_n^i\right)$, $M_n^y\left(\mathrm{sp}_n^i\right)$, and $M_n^z\left(\mathrm{sp}_n^i\right)$, respectively.

For superpixel sp_n^i of frame n, the relative planer and depth motion feature maps are calculated as [11]

$$\mathrm{RM}_n^{xy}\left(\mathrm{sp}_n^i\right) = \sum\nolimits_{j\neq i} \exp\left(-d_s\left(\mathrm{sp}_n^i, \mathrm{sp}_n^j\right)/\sigma^2\right) \times T_{x,y}\left(\mathrm{sp}_n^i, \mathrm{sp}_n^j\right), \tag{11}$$

$$\mathrm{RM}_n^z\left(\mathrm{sp}_n^i\right) = \sum\nolimits_{j\neq i} \exp\left(-d_S\left(\mathrm{sp}_n^i, \mathrm{sp}_n^j\right)/\sigma^2\right) \times T_z\left(\mathrm{sp}_n^i, \mathrm{sp}_n^j\right), \tag{12}$$

$$T_{x,y}\left(\mathrm{sp}_n^i, \mathrm{sp}_n^j\right) = \left[\left|M_n^{x,y}\left(\mathrm{sp}_n^i\right) - M_n^{x,y}\left(\mathrm{sp}_n^j\right)\right| / \left(\left|M_n^{x,y}\left(\mathrm{sp}_n^i\right)\right| + \left|M_n^{x,y}\left(\mathrm{sp}_n^j\right)\right|\right)\right] \times C, \tag{13}$$

$$M_n^{x,y}\left(\mathrm{sp}_n^i\right) = \sqrt{\left(M_n^x\left(\mathrm{sp}_n^i\right) + M_n^y\left(\mathrm{sp}_n^i\right)\right)^2}, \tag{14}$$

$$T_z\left(\mathrm{sp}_n^i, \mathrm{sp}_n^j\right) = \left[\left|M_n^z\left(\mathrm{sp}_n^i\right) - M_n^z\left(\mathrm{sp}_n^j\right)\right| / \left(\left|M_n^z\left(\mathrm{sp}_n^i\right)\right| + \left|M_n^z\left(\mathrm{sp}_n^j\right)\right|\right)\right] \times C, \tag{15}$$

respectively, where $d_s\left(\mathrm{sp}_n^i, \mathrm{sp}_n^j\right)$ is the spatial (Euclidean) distance between superpixels sp_n^i and sp_n^j, σ is a parameter (set as 5), and C is a small constant. The relative planer motion map and the relative depth motion feature map of frame n, denoted as $\mathrm{RMMap}_n^{x,y}(x, y)$ and $\mathrm{RMMap}_n^z(x, y)$, $1 \leq x \leq W$, $1 \leq y \leq H$, are defined as the relative planer and depth motion feature values of the corresponding superpixel, respectively.

The spatial edge map $E_n(x, y)$ can be obtained by the boundary detection algorithm [19], and the motion edge map $B_n(x, y)$ can be obtained by the fast correlation flow algorithm [18]. Then the spatial edge probability feature $\hat{E}_n\left(\mathrm{sp}_n^i\right)$ and motion edge probability feature $\hat{B}_n\left(\mathrm{sp}_n^i\right)$ for superpixel sp_n^i of frame n are computed as averaging over the pixels with the ten largest edge probabilities in sp_n^i from $E_n(x, y)$ and $B_n(x, y)$, respectively. For superpixel sp_n^i of frame n, the spatiotemporal edge feature is calculated as

$$\mathrm{STE}_n\left(\mathrm{sp}_n^i\right) = \hat{E}_n\left(\mathrm{sp}_n^i\right) \times \hat{B}_n\left(\mathrm{sp}_n^i\right). \tag{16}$$

For superpixel sp_n^i of frame n, the shortest geodesic distance [4] can be used to estimate the salient object probability from spatiotemporal edge feature of frame n as the intra-frame motion boundary feature, which is computed as

$$\mathrm{FMB}_n^{\mathrm{intra}}\left(\mathrm{sp}_n^i\right) = \min_{\mathrm{spe} \in \mathrm{spe}_n} d_g\left(\mathrm{sp}_n^i, \mathrm{spe}\right), \tag{17}$$

where spe_n denotes the superpixels of frame n connected to the edge of frame n; $d_g\left(\mathrm{sp}_n^i, \mathrm{spe}\right)$, the geodesic distance between superpixels sp_n^i and spe, is defined as

$$d_g\left(\mathrm{sp}_n^i, \mathrm{spe}\right) = \min_{d_p\left(\mathrm{sp}_n^i, \mathrm{spe}\right)} \sum\nolimits_{d_p\left(\mathrm{sp}_n^i, \mathrm{spe}\right) = 0,1} \left|Q_n\left(\mathrm{sp}_n^i, \mathrm{spe}\right) \times d_p\left(\mathrm{sp}_n^i, \mathrm{spe}\right)\right|, \tag{18}$$

$$Q_n\left(\mathrm{sp}_n^i, \mathrm{spe}\right) = \left\|\mathrm{STE}_n\left(\mathrm{sp}_n^i\right) - \mathrm{STE}_n(\mathrm{spe})\right\| \tag{19}$$

and $d_p\left(\mathrm{sp}_n^i, \mathrm{spe}\right)$ is the shortest distance between superpixels sp_n^i and spe by using Dijkstra's algorithm. The inter-frame motion boundary feature for superpixel sp_n^i of frame n is defined as

$$\mathrm{FMB}_n^{\mathrm{inter}}\left(\mathrm{sp}_n^i\right) = \min_{\mathrm{br} \in \mathrm{br}_n \cup \mathrm{br}_{n+1}} d_g\left(\mathrm{sp}_n^i, \mathrm{br}\right), \tag{20}$$

where br_n and br_{n+1} are the background regions of the intra-frame motion boundary features of frames n and $n + 1$, respectively, and br_n is the superpixels less than the mean value of all superpixels in the intra-frame feature of frame n and temporally connected to the background region of frame $n - 1$, i.e.,

$$d_g\left(\mathrm{sp}_n^i, \mathrm{br}\right) = \min_{d_p\left(\mathrm{sp}_n^i, \mathrm{br}\right)} \sum\nolimits_{d_p\left(\mathrm{sp}_n^i, \mathrm{br}\right)=0,1} \left| Q_n\left(\mathrm{sp}_n^i, \mathrm{br}\right) \times d_p\left(\mathrm{sp}_n^i, \mathrm{br}\right)\right|, \tag{21}$$

$$Q_n\left(\mathrm{sp}_n^i, \mathrm{br}\right) = \left\| \mathrm{STE}_n\left(\mathrm{sp}_n^i\right) - \mathrm{STE}_n\left(\mathrm{br}\right)\right\|. \tag{22}$$

The intra-frame and inter-frame motion boundary feature maps for frame n, $\boldsymbol{MBMap_n^{intra}(x, y)}$ and $\boldsymbol{MBMap_n^{inter}(x, y)}$, $\boldsymbol{1 \le x \le W, 1 \le y \le H}$, are defined as the intra-frame and inter-frame motion boundary feature values of the corresponding superpixel.

Depth Features

The DCT coefficients of patch h_n^i (8×8 in size) of disparity maps are computed, and then the DC coefficient $\mathrm{DC}_n^{\mathrm{dm}}\left(h_n^i\right)$ is extracted. The depth contrast feature for patch h_n^i of the n-th disparity map is computed as

$$\mathrm{DC}_n\left(h_n^i\right) = \sum\nolimits_{j \neq i} \exp\left(-d_s\left(h_n^i, h_n^j\right)/\sigma^2\right) \times T_{DC}\left(\mathrm{DC}_n^{\mathrm{dm}}\left(h_n^i\right), \mathrm{DC}_n^{\mathrm{dm}}\left(h_n^j\right)\right), \tag{23}$$

$$\begin{aligned} &T_{\mathrm{DC}}\left(\mathrm{DC}_n^{\mathrm{dm}}\left(h_n^i\right), \mathrm{DC}_n^{\mathrm{dm}}\left(h_n^j\right)\right) \\ &= \left[\left|\mathrm{DC}_n^{\mathrm{dm}}\left(h_n^i\right) - \mathrm{DC}_n^{\mathrm{dm}}\left(h_n^j\right)\right| / \left(\left|\mathrm{DC}_n^{\mathrm{dm}}\left(h_n^i\right)\right| + \left|\mathrm{DC}_n^{\mathrm{dm}}\left(h_n^j\right)\right|\right)\right] \times C, \end{aligned} \tag{24}$$

where σ is a parameter (set as 5), and C is a small constant. The depth contrast feature map for the n-th disparity map, $\mathrm{DCMap}_n(x, y)$, $1 \le x \le W$, $1 \le y \le H$, is defined as the depth contrast feature value of the corresponding patch.

Based on spatial edges and disparity boundaries [7], the edge-boundary map $\mathrm{EB}_n(x, y)$ for the n-th disparity map $\mathrm{DM}_n(x, y)$ is computed as

$$\mathrm{EB}_n\,(x, y) = \Theta\Big(E_n\,(x, y) \times (\beta + \Theta\,(\nabla \mathrm{DM}_n\,(x, y))\Big), \tag{25}$$

where $\Theta(\cdot)$ represents the dilation operation with radius =5 pixels, $E_n(x, y)$ is the spatial edge map of $\mathrm{DM}_n(x, y)$, β is a parameter (set as 0.2), and $\nabla\mathrm{DM}_n(x, y)$ is the gradient magnitude of $\mathrm{DM}_n(x, y)$. Based on $\mathrm{EB}_n(x, y)$, the boundary flow feature map $\mathrm{BFMap}_n(x, y)$, $1 \leq x \leq W$, $1 \leq y \leq H$, is calculated by the gradient flow method [20].

Object Features

In this study, the face detector [21] is used to generate human faces by generating the face bounding boxes, and the object detector [22] is used to generate person, vehicle, and animal bounding boxes. Based on these bounding boxes, the probability distribution of face, person, vehicle, and animal object regions are used to generate face, person, vehicle, and animal feature maps.

Spatiotemporal Features

In this study, based on the dense trajectories, spatiotemporal features containing HOG, HOF, and MBH features are extracted [23].

Before applying 3D-DCT transform, each video frame is transformed from RGB color space into YCbCr color space. 3D-DCT is applied on 3D sliding cubes (16×16×16 in size) with sliding steps being 8, 8, and 16 in x, y, and t directions, respectively. For the l-th 3D sliding cube CU_l, the three DC coefficients of Y, Cb, and Cr components, and sum of all AC coefficients of Y component denoted as $\mathrm{DC}^y(\mathrm{cu}_l)$, $\mathrm{DC}^{cb}(\mathrm{cu}_l)$, $\mathrm{DC}^{cr}(\mathrm{cu}_l)$, and $\mathrm{AC}^y(\mathrm{cu}_l)$, respectively, are extracted. The 3D-DCT feature for cu_l is calculated as [24]

$$\mathrm{FTDD}\,(\mathrm{cu}_l) = \frac{1}{4}\Big(\mathrm{CC}^y\,(\mathrm{cu}_l) + \mathrm{CC}^{\mathrm{cb}}\,(\mathrm{cu}_l) + \mathrm{CC}^{\mathrm{cr}}\,(\mathrm{cu}_l) + \mathrm{AY}\,(\mathrm{cu}_l)\Big), \tag{26}$$

$$\mathrm{CC}^y\,(\mathrm{cu}_l) = \sum\nolimits_{j \neq i} \exp\left(-d_{\mathrm{S}}\,(\mathrm{cu}_l, \mathrm{cu}_j)\,/\sigma^2\right) \times T_{\mathrm{DC}}\left(\mathrm{DC}^y\,(\mathrm{cu}_l), \mathrm{DC}^y\,(\mathrm{cu}_j)\right), \tag{27}$$

$$\mathrm{CC}^{\mathrm{cb}}\,(\mathrm{cu}_l) = \sum\nolimits_{j \neq i} \exp\left(-d_s\,(\mathrm{cu}_l, \mathrm{cu}_j)\,/\sigma^2\right) \times T_{\mathrm{DC}}\left(\mathrm{DC}^{\mathrm{cb}}\,(\mathrm{cu}_l), \mathrm{DC}^{\mathrm{cb}}\,(\mathrm{cu}_j)\right), \tag{28}$$

$$\mathrm{CC}^{\mathrm{cr}}\left(\mathrm{cu}_l\right) = \sum\nolimits_{j \neq i} \exp\left(-\mathrm{d}_s\left(\mathrm{cu}_l, \mathrm{cu}_j\right)/\sigma^2\right) \times T_{\mathrm{DC}}\left(\mathrm{DC}^{\mathrm{cr}}\left(\mathrm{cu}_l\right), \mathrm{DC}^{\mathrm{cr}}\left(\mathrm{cu}_j\right)\right), \tag{29}$$

$$\mathrm{AY}\left(\mathrm{cu}_l\right) = \sum\nolimits_{j \neq i} \exp\left(-d_s\left(\mathrm{cu}_l, \mathrm{cu}_j\right)/\sigma^2\right) \times T_{\mathrm{AC}}\left(\mathrm{AC}^{y}\left(\mathrm{cu}_l\right), \mathrm{AC}^{y}\left(\mathrm{cu}_j\right)\right), \tag{30}$$

where σ is a parameter (set as 5). The 3D-DCT feature map for the l-th cube cu_l denotes as $\mathrm{TDMap}_l(x, y, t)$, $1 \leq x \leq W$, $1 \leq y \leq H$, $1 \leq t \leq N$, and is defined as the 3D-DCT feature value of the corresponding cube.

2.4 *Feature Normalization and SVR Learning*

In this study, each feature map of frame n is scaled to [0,1], and a convex function is employed, which is defined as

$$\Phi\left(M_n\left(x, y\right)\right) = \exp\left(M_n\left(x, y\right)\right) - \mu_{M_n}, \tag{31}$$

where $\hat{M}_n\left(x, y\right)$ is the feature map of frame n, and μ_{M_n} is the mean value of $M_n(x, y)$. Then, each normalized feature map $\hat{M}_n\left(x, y\right)$ is computed as

$$\hat{M}_n\left(x, y\right) = \left(\Phi\left(M_n\left(x, y\right)\right) - \Phi_n^{\min}\right) / \left(\Phi_n^{\max} - \Phi_n^{\min}\right), \tag{32}$$

where $\Phi_n^{\min}$ and $\Phi_n^{\max}$ denoted the maximum and minimum values of $\Phi(M_n(x, y))$, respectively.

In this study, all extracted feature values of each pixel are concerned to a feature vector. Support vector regression (SVR) learning using LIBLINEAR tools [25] is used to train extracted feature vectors of stereoscopic video sequences.

2.5 *Saliency Map Refinement*

Based on the fact that the center regions of scenes are more salient than the surrounding regions, both the center bias map and the significant increased map [6] are used to refine the initial saliency maps. The refined saliency map of frame n is computed as

$$S_n^r\left(x, y\right) = \omega_1 \times S_n^t\left(x, y\right) + \omega_2 \times S_n^c\left(x, y\right) + \omega_3 \times S_n^m\left(x, y\right), \tag{33}$$

(a)

(b)

(c)

(d)

(e)

(f)

(g)

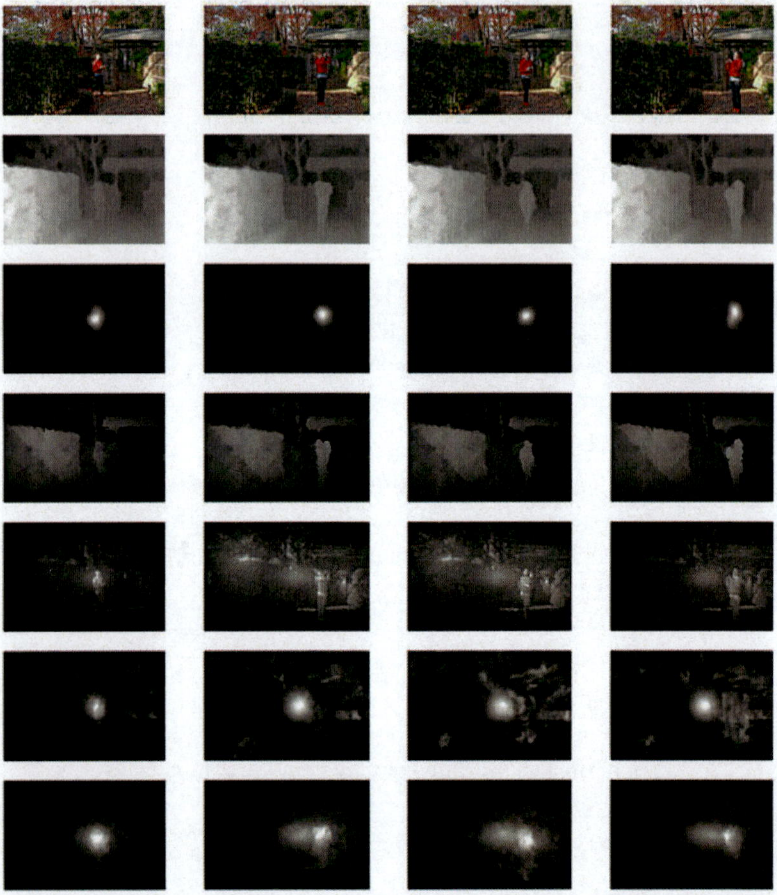

Fig. 2 Experimental results of frames 90, 180, 270, 360 of stereoscopic video "Okugai park falling leaves": (**a**) the original left view frames; (**b**) the corresponding disparity maps; (**c**) the ground truth; (**d–g**) the saliency maps by Ju et al.'s approach [8], Fang et al.'s approach [6], Banitalebi-Dehkordi et al.'s approach [10], and the proposed approach

where $S_n^t(x, y)$, $S_n^c(x, y)$, and $S_n^m(x, y)$ denote the initial saliency map, the center bias map, and the significant increased map of frame n, and ω_1, ω_2, and ω_3 are weight parameters (empirically set as 0.6, 0.3, and 0.1, respectively). Then the obtained saliency map is further enhanced by visual sensitivity with thresholding and Gaussian filtering.

Table 1 In terms of five average metrics, AUC, NSS, PLCC, SIM, and EMD, performance comparisons of the three comparison approaches and the proposed approach

Types	Approaches	AUC	NSS	PLCC	SIM	EMD
3D image	Ju et al. [8]	0.499	1.205	0.260	0.325	0.771
3D image	Fang et al. [6]	0.639	1.868	0.347	0.383	0.486
3D video	Banitalebi-Dehkordiet al. [10]	0.574	1.759	0.343	0.368	0.482
3D video	Proposed	**0.713**	**2.683**	**0.464**	**0.441**	**0.405**

3 Experimental Results

The proposed approach is implemented on Intel Core i7-7700K CPU 4.20 GHz for 64-bit Microsoft Windows 10 platform with 32 GB main memory by using MATLAB 9.0.0 (R2016a). IRCCyN eye-tracking database [26] is employed, which contains 47 stereoscopic videos with spatial resolution 1080 × 1920, the right-to-left disparity map, and the corresponding ground truth. In this study, 80 percent stereoscopic video sequences are used for training, while the remaining 20 percent stereoscopic video sequences are used for testing.

To evaluate the effectiveness of the proposed approach, three comparison approaches including Ju et al.'s approach [8], Fang et al.'s approach [6], and Banitalebi-Dehkordi et al.'s approach [10] are employed. To evaluate the final saliency maps, five performance measures, namely, area under the receiver operating characteristics curve (AUC) [26], normalized scanpath saliency (NSS) [27], Pearson linear correlation coefficient (PLCC) [27], similarity (SIM) [25], and earth mover's distance (EMD) [25], are employed.

Experimental results of frames 90, 180, 270, 360 of stereoscopic video sequence "Okugai park falling leaves" by the three comparison approaches and the proposed approach are shown in Fig. 2. In terms of five average metrics, AUC, NSS, PLCC, SIM, and EMD, performance comparisons of the three comparison approaches and the proposed approach are listed in Table 1. Based on the experimental results obtained in this study, the performance of the proposed approach is better than those of three comparison approaches.

4 Concluding Remarks

In this study, a superpixel-based stereoscopic video saliency detection approach using SVR learning is proposed. Based on the experimental results obtained in this study, the performance of the proposed approach is better than those of three comparison approaches.

Acknowledgment This work was supported in part by Ministry of Science and Technology, Taiwan, ROC under Grants MOST 108-2221-E-194-049 and MOST 109-2221-E-194-042.

References

1. M.M. Cheng et al., Global contrast based salient region detection. IEEE Trans. Pattern Anal. Mach. Intell. **37**(3), 569–582 (2015)
2. Z.H. Chen et al., Image saliency detection using Gabor texture cues. Multimed. Tools Appl. **75**(24), 16943–16958 (2016)
3. J. Li et al., Spatiotemporal saliency detection based on superpixel-level trajectory. Signal Process. Image Commun. **38**(1), 100–114 (2015)
4. W. Wang, J. Shen, F. Porikli, Saliency-aware geodesic video object segmentation, in *Proceedings of 2015 IEEE Conference on Computer Vision and Pattern Recognition*, (2015), pp. 3395–3402
5. Z. Liu et al., Superpixel-based spatiotemporal saliency detection. IEEE Trans. Circuits Syst. Video Technol. **24**(9), 1522–1540 (2014)
6. Y. Fang et al., Saliency detection for stereoscopic images. IEEE Trans. Image Process. **23**(6), 2625–2636 (2014)
7. W. Wang et al., Stereoscopic thumbnail creation via efficient stereo saliency detection. IEEE Trans. Vis. Comp. Graph. **23**(8), 2014–2027 (2016)
8. R. Ju et al., Depth saliency based on anisotropic center-surround difference, in *Proceedings of 2014 IEEE International Conference on Image Processing (ICIP)*, (2014), pp. 1115–1119
9. F. Liang et al., CoCNN: RGB-D deep fusion for stereoscopic salient object dectectin. Pattern Recogn. **104**, 1–14 (2020)
10. A. Banitalebi-Dehkordi, M.T. Pourazad, P. Nasiopoulos, A learning-based visual saliency prediction model for stereoscopic 3D video (LBVS-3D). Multimed. Tools Appl. **1**(1), 1–32 (2016)
11. Y. Fang, Z. Wang, W. Lin, Video saliency incorporating spatiotemporal cues and uncertainty weighting. IEEE Trans. Image Process. **23**(9), 3910–3921 (2014)
12. P. Zhang et al., Stereoscopic video saliency detection based on spatiotemporal correlation and depth confidence optimization. Neurocompting **377**, 256–268 (2020)
13. Y. Fang et al., Deep3DSaliency: Deep stereoscopic video saliency detection model by 3D convolutional networks. IEEE Trans. Image Process. **28**(5), 2305–2318 (2019)
14. Y. Fang et al., Visual attention prediction for stereoscopic video by muti-module fully convolutional network. IEEE Trans. Image Process. **28**(11), 5253–5265 (2019)
15. R. Achanta et al., SLIC superpixels compared to state-of-the-art superpixel methods. IEEE Trans. Pattern Anal. Mach. Intell. **34**(11), 2274–2282 (2012)
16. Y. Fang et al., Saliency detection in the compressed domain for adaptive image retargeting. IEEE Trans. Image Process. **21**(9), 3888–3901 (2012)
17. L. Breiman, Random forests. Mach. Learn. **45**(1), 5–32 (2001)
18. M. Drulea, S. Nedevschi, Motion estimation using the correlation transform. IEEE Trans. Image Process. **22**(8), 3260–3270 (2013)
19. M. Leordeanu, R. Sukthankar, C. Sminchisescu, Efficient closed-form solution to generalized boundary detection, in *Proceedings of 12th European Conference on Computer Vision*, (2012), pp. 516–529
20. W. Wang, J. Shen, L. Shao, Consistent video saliency using local gradient flow optimization and global refinement. IEEE Trans. Image Process. **24**(11), 4185–4196 (2015)
21. P. Viola, M. Jones, Rapid object detection using a boosted cascade of simple features, in *Proceedings of 2001 IEEE Conference on Computer Vision and Pattern Recognition*, (2001), pp. 511–518
22. P.F. Felzenszwalb et al., Object detection with discriminatively trained part-based models. IEEE Trans. Pattern Anal. Mach. Intell. **32**(9), 1627–1645 (2010)
23. H. Wang, L. Schmid, Actopn recognition with improved trajectories, in *Proceedings of 2013 IEEE International Conference on Computer Vision (ICCV)*, (2013), pp. 3551–3558
24. X. Li, Q. Guo, X. Lu, Spatiotemporal statistics for video quality assessment. IEEE Trans. Image Process. **25**(7), 3329–3342 (2016)

25. R.E. Fan et al., LIBLINEAR: A library for large linear classification. J. Mach. Learn. Res. **9**, 1871–1874 (2008)
26. Y. Fang et al., An eye tracking database for stereoscopic video, in *Proceedings of 2014 the Sixth International Workshop on Quality of Multimedia Experience (QoMEX)*, (2014), pp. 51–52
27. A. Borji, D.N. Sihite, L. Itti, Quantitative analysis of human-model agreement in visual saliency modeling: A comparative study. IEEE Trans. Image Process. **22**(1), 55–69 (2013)

Application of Image Processing Tools for Scene-Based Marine Debris Detection and Characterization

Mehrube Mehrubeoglu, Farha Pulukool, DeKwaan Wynn, Lifford McLauchlan, and Hua Zhang

1 Introduction

Floating debris of varying sizes can have major impacts on the marine environments and can adversely affect marine animals. Examples of debris include plastic bags, fishing lines, shopping bags, plastic bottles, microplastics, and straws [1, 2]. Microplastics and other marine debris pose a threat for the marine environment as well as many types of marine wildlife including mammals, fish, and turtles that may encounter marine debris [3–9]. Seals can become entangled in discarded fishing lines or nets [3]. Turtles, for example, have been found with straws caught in their nose [4]. Other animals have been found with plastic soda can holders around their necks [5]. It is, therefore, important to develop methods to detect and remove floating debris from bodies of water.

Plastic pollution is one of today's main environmental problems, threatening marine species, posing potential human health risks, and reducing the capacity of urban drainage networks [10–12]. Without improvements in waste management infrastructure or strategies, the cumulative quantity of environmental plastic waste is predicted to increase by an order of magnitude by 2025 [13]. Global estimates of plastic waste mass to enter oceans annually are several orders of magnitude greater than the estimated mass of floating plastic debris in high-concentration ocean

M. Mehrubeoglu (✉) · H. Zhang
Texas A&M University-Corpus Christi, Department of Engineering, Corpus Christi, TX, USA
e-mail: ruby.mehrubeoglu@tamucc.edu

F. Pulukool · D. Wynn
Texas A&M University-Corpus Christi, Department of Computing Sciences, Kingsville, TX, USA

L. McLauchlan
Texas A&M University-Kingsville, Department of Electrical Engineering and Computer Science, Kingsville, TX, USA

H. R. Arabnia et al. (eds.), *Advances in Computer Vision and Computational Biology*, Transactions on Computational Science and Computational Intelligence,
https://doi.org/10.1007/978-3-030-71051-4_13

gyres, resulting in the so-called missing plastics [14, 15], indicating a fundamental knowledge gap in the transport of marine debris from land.

There is an urgent need for improved, quantitative understanding of river plastic load from coastal urban regions. This is particularly needed for macroplastics (>5 cm) as they account for the majority of debris mass and are the current and predicted future major source of microplastics [16]. Quantification of floating macroplastics has relied on visual inspection, which could yield large uncertainties due to difference in survey protocols between different groups or the difficulty in estimating the debris size [17, 18]. This may lead to significant bias in estimating the total quantity and mass of floating debris. Methods for detection and quantification of floating macroplastics will enhance the assessment of land-based plastic sources and offer critical evidence to identify neglected sinks and controls of the plastic life cycle for finally resolving the mystery of global plastic discrepancy.

The focus of this paper is the detection of man-made water pollutants that are at macroscale. In particular, detection methods for three kinds of floating water debris have been investigated, including plastic bags, bottles, and a cup. Detection of debris is important to facilitate debris removal. Research into unmanned aerial systems and autonomous underwater vehicles to perform automated debris detection has been conducted by multiple groups [19–24]. Valdenegro-Toro describes the use of three labels to classify detected objects in images as plastic, man-made, or biological [20]. Bao et al. utilize thresholding in the green and blue bands to segment beach images [24]. Other research groups have used image processing techniques to segment debris in images: Li et al. describe the use of mathematical morphology applied to space images for debris detection [25]. Harjoko et al. apply edge detection and thresholding to video frames to estimate debris flow rate [26]. Mahankali et al. also use morphological operations to segment debris images in video frames [27]. In this paper, we combine a multitude of low- and high-level image processing tools in a flexible image processing chain to detect man-made marine debris in different scenarios.

This paper discusses debris detection for different cases of floating debris in freely accessible images. The Methods section covers image samples and the detailed description of the applied image processing tools and techniques. Debris detection and characterization results are presented in the so-named section that follows Methods. A brief discussion of results is introduced under Discussion section. Conclusions are presented in Sect. 5.

2 Methods

In this section, selected images with man-made debris and image processing operations are described. All image processing operations and algorithms are implemented using MATLAB 2019b (The MathWorks, Inc.) software tool.

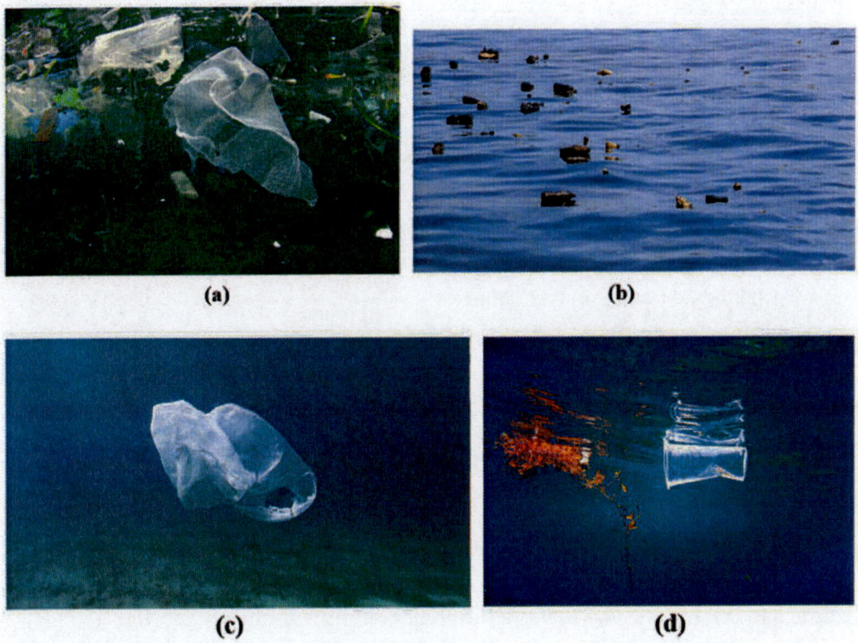

Fig. 1 (**a**) Case I: Multiple submerged floating debris [28]. (**b**) Case II: Multiple floating surface debris [29]. (**c**) Case III: Single submerged floating debris [30]. (**d**) Case IV: Single near-surface floating debris [31]

2.1 Images of Floating Man-Made Debris

Several image scenes have been considered demonstrating man-made debris in water. Images were selected from free online resources to reflect a variety of cases with floating debris including those with underwater view, semi-submerged view, and surface view (Fig. 1a–d).

2.2 Image Processing

Debris detection is achieved through the image processing chain shown in Fig. 2, which includes image preprocessing.

HSV Color Model

Each input color image is first converted from red, green, and blue (RGB) color space to hue, saturation, and value (HSV) color space, also known as hue, saturation,

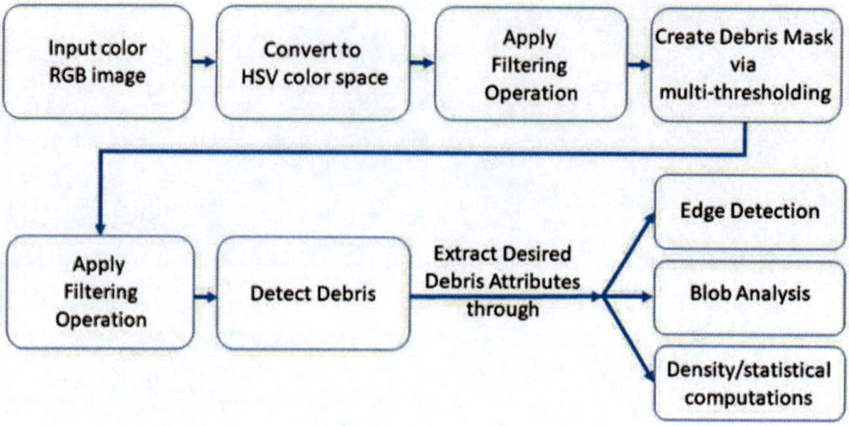

Fig. 2 Image processing chain for debris detection and characterization

and intensity (HSI) [23]. HSV color space offers an alternative way to represent colors in an image with its three components that describe the colors in terms of shade and brightness, and offers a different contrast for object detection.

The HSV color wheel can be depicted as a cone or cylinder. Six colors, or hue representations, exist as red, yellow, green, cyan, blue, and magenta [32]. Each color falls into a given range in the HSV cylinder. The formulas used to transform the RGB color model to HSV color model can be found in [32].

Debris Mask

Debris mask is created by applying multilevel thresholding separately in H, S, and V frames to separate man-made debris from its background and other objects in the scene. Threshold sandwich is applied to select the optimal range of pixel values that represent the man-made debris in each image. To bring the debris objects to the forefront, selection of one of the channels (e.g., hue, saturation, or value) may be sufficient, depending on the scene. For complex scenes with a variety of man-made objects and materials, the following threshold selection scheme is applied:

HSV pixel, $I(x,y)$, located at 2D Cartesian coordinates, (x,y), belongs to debris if the following conditions are satisfied for all color frames:

$$I(x, y) \in \mathbf{D}, \text{if} \begin{cases} t_{H1} < I(x, y, H) \leq t_{H2} \\ t_{S1} < I(x, y, S) \leq t_{S2} \\ t_{V1} < I(x, y, V) \leq t_{V2} \end{cases}, \tag{1}$$

where **D** is a set of pixels that belongs to man-made debris, and t_{X1} and t_{X2} are the lower and upper threshold limits representing the range of debris values for $X \in \{H, S, V\}$. If $I(x,y) \in \mathbf{D}$, then $I(x,y) = 1$; otherwise, $I(x,y) = 0$.

Once appropriately filtered, the mask is used to extract debris regions from the original image by masking the background as well as unwanted regions. In addition, the mask is used in blob analysis and debris characterization.

Filtering Operations

To remove noise as well as unwanted details, a 3x3 median filter was applied to digital images before processing. Median filtering was accomplished prior to converting the HSV image into binary image.

Additional filtering operations were implemented as needed after thresholding to the resultant binary images as morphological opening (erosion followed by dilation) and closing (dilation followed by erosion) operations. Three different structuring elements, se_x, where $x \in \{1, 2, 3\}$, were used depending on the size of debris and details in the image as follows:

$$se_1 = \begin{bmatrix} 0\,1\,0 \\ 1\,1\,1 \\ 0\,1\,0 \end{bmatrix}, se_2 = \begin{bmatrix} 0\,0 & 1\,0 & 0 \\ 0\,1 & 1\,1 & 0 \\ 1\,1 & 1\,1 & 1 \\ 0\,1 & 1\,1 & 0 \\ 0\,0 & 1\,0 & 0 \end{bmatrix}, se_3 = \begin{bmatrix} 0\,0\,0\,1\,1\,1\,0\,0\,0 \\ 0\,0\,1\,1\,1\,1\,1\,0\,0 \\ 0\,1\,1\,1\,1\,1\,1\,1\,0 \\ 1\,1\,1\,1\,1\,1\,1\,1\,1 \\ 1\,1\,1\,1\,1\,1\,1\,1\,1 \\ 1\,1\,1\,1\,1\,1\,1\,1\,1 \\ 0\,1\,1\,1\,1\,1\,1\,1\,0 \\ 0\,0\,1\,1\,1\,1\,1\,0\,0 \\ 0\,0\,0\,1\,1\,1\,0\,0\,0 \end{bmatrix}.$$

Edge Detection

Edge detection is a powerful tool for characterizing the shape, size, as well as contour of objects of interest. Edge detection provides both qualitative and quantitative analysis of objects. Canny edge detector was applied to images for qualitative analysis in this work.

Blob Analysis

Blob analysis involves identifying the connected regions within the binary image that is not part of the background, followed by investigating each blob's attributes as desired. In the cases presented in this paper, after thresholding and filtering, blob analysis is performed to detect the pieces of man-made debris, count the number of debris pieces, identify their location within the scene, and find the largest piece of debris.

Statistical Computations

The statistical computations applied in the presented debris scenes include percent area of debris cover of the scene and the size distribution of the detected debris in the case of multiple debris objects. Equation (2) is used to determine the total number of pixels belonging to the debris identified using the appropriate debris mask for the given scene:

$$c = \sum_{m=0}^{M-1} \sum_{n=0}^{N-1} I_b\,(m, n)\,, \tag{2}$$

where I_b represents the binary mask, *(m,n)* represents the mth row and n^{th} column in the binary mask, and $I_b(m,n)$ is the mask's pixel value (1 or 0) located at *(m,n)*. *M* and *N* are the number of rows and columns in the image, respectively, and *c* represents the total number of pixels that belong to debris.

Percent debris in the scene, *d*, is computed using Eq. (3):

$$d = \frac{100c}{(MN)}. \tag{3}$$

Size distribution of debris pieces is determined by first counting the total number of pieces detected as debris and then sorting these pieces into bins based on their area represented by the total number of pixels in each piece. This is accomplished through a histogram plot. The histogram plot can be converted into a probability density function by dividing the number of objects in the corresponding size bin by the total number of objects identified in the scene, as in Eq. (4).

$$p(s) = \frac{f}{T}, \tag{4}$$

where *p(s)* is the probability of debris pieces in the scene being in the predetermined size range, *s*; *f* is the frequency of occurrence (number) of pieces whose size falls in the range represented by *s* (e.g., 1–200 pixels for bin 1); and T is the total number of pieces detected as debris.

3 Debris Detection and Characterization Results

Four different cases are presented here, each following the general processing chain represented in Fig. 2, with minor adaptations to achieve the optimum results in man-made debris detection. As mentioned before, the four cases investigated include multiple floating submerged debris (Case I, Fig. 1a), multiple floating surface debris

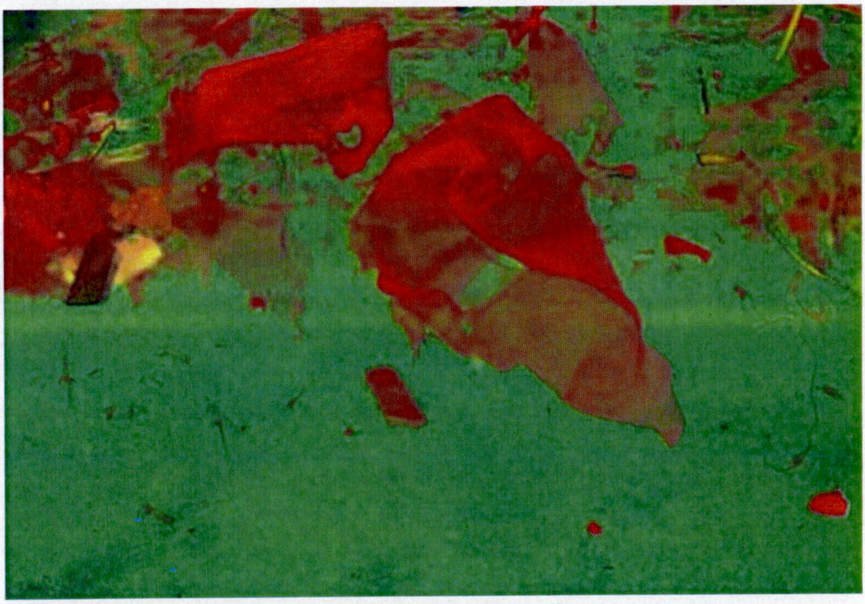

Fig. 3 Multiple floating debris image represented in HSV color space

(Case II, Fig. 1b), single submerged floating debris (Case III, Fig. 1c), and single near-surface floating debris (Case IV, Fig.1d).

3.1 Case I: Multiple Submerged Floating Debris

The original RGB image is first transformed to HSV color space (Fig. 3).

The HSV color space offers good contrast between the marine environment and the man-made plastic debris shown. To distinguish the debris from its marine environment, hue, saturation, and values are investigated. As can be seen in the HSV image, water is selectively represented in green and debris in red. Applying a set of binary thresholds as described in Eq. 1 to separate these two HSV color model representations, the binary mask in Fig. 4 (left) is created. In this case, only V frame is used for the segmentation of the foreground and background. Pixels with a value of 1 (white pixels) represent the areas of debris. Pixels with a value of 0 (black pixels) show the water and other unwanted objects such as seagrass blades.

Once the mask is created, further analysis can be performed on abundance, size distribution, shape, as well as other attributes related to the debris as required. To visually validate the detection of the debris, the mask in Fig. 4 (left) is multiplied pixel by pixel by the original image in Fig. 1a to obtain the debris image in Fig. 4 (right). No additional filtering was performed on the mask in Case I.

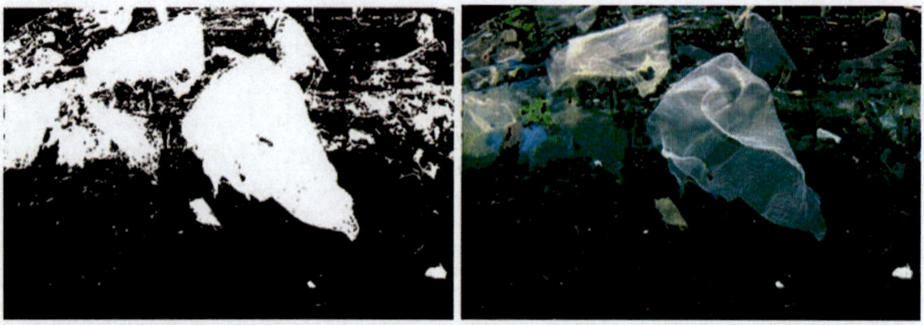

Fig. 4 (Left) Debris mask from HSV image. (Right) Extracted debris from the original image (Fig. 1a) using the debris mask

A simple edge detector (Canny) is applied to the mask to qualitatively represent the shape and size distribution of pieces of debris in the scene. Size distribution could be a valuable indicator of deterioration of petroleum-based pollutants in the water and could potentially be used to estimate how long the debris has been in the water.

This debris scene represents objects with no particular or standard shape. Beyond being man-made petroleum product-based debris, other physical attributes of interest include density or percent volume of debris within the scene. Since the digital image is a 2D representation of a 3D scene, one meaningful way to quantify debris is to compute its percentage in the image. Using Equations (2) and (3), the percent debris cover in the scene is computed as 35%.

3.2 Case II: Multiple Floating Surface Debris

To analyze floating debris imaged over the surface of the water, the same image processing chain as described in Fig. 2 is followed. First, the original color image is converted to HSV color space, demonstrated in false colors in Fig. 5.

As can be seen in Fig. 5, overlap exists in HSV color model for debris and water surface. To minimize misclassification of pixels representing debris, thresholding was achieved using Eq. 1 (t_{h2}<139, t_{v2}<160), followed by morphological opening and closing as previously described in Methods section. Resulting debris mask is shown in Fig. 6 (left). The debris mask is applied on the original image to obtain a visualization of the detected debris. In this case, because the debris in the original scene represents dark objects, the background is set to white to increase contrast (Fig. 6 (right)).

Canny edge detector algorithm applied on the masked debris produces the edge image. This information can be used to assess debris contours.

It is noted that the surface reflection of debris appears as joint pieces with the actual debris, affecting the size and distribution thereof. However, since each piece is

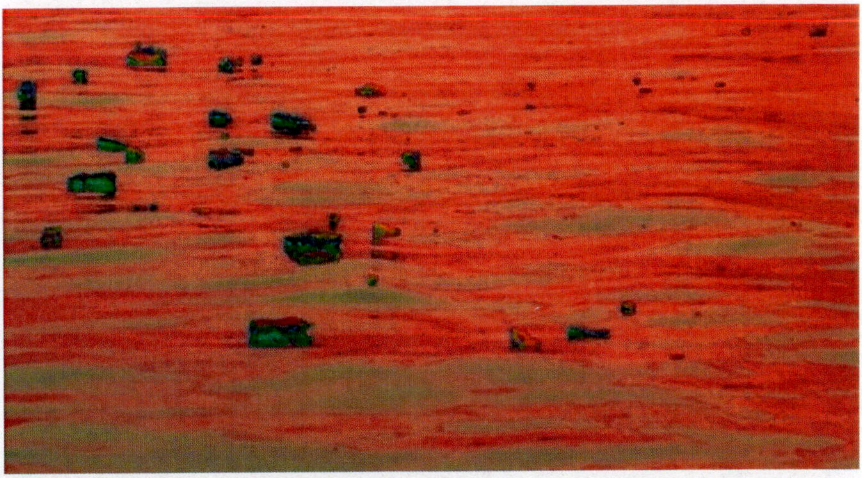

Fig. 5 HSV color transform of original image in Fig. 1b

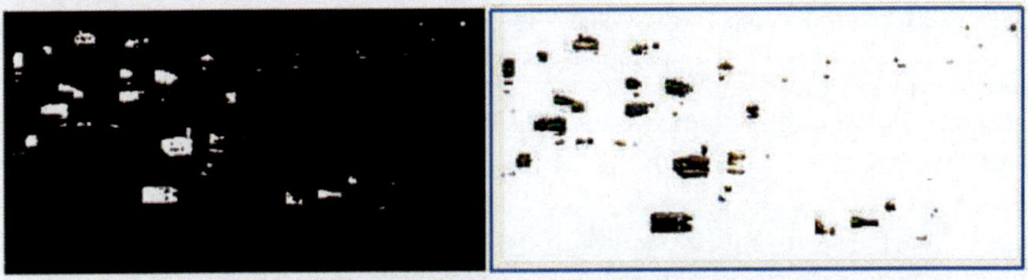

Fig. 6 (Left) Mask for the floating surface debris of Fig. 1b. (Right) Extracted debris from the original image (Fig. 1b) using the debris mask with white background for enhanced contrast

expected to be affected similarly, probability density function for debris size should keep the same model and shape.

In this scene, 51 pieces of surface debris are detected. Size distribution in pixels is shown in Fig. 7 with its probability density function. Over 75% (first three bins) of the debris pieces have an area of 300 pixels or less.

3.3 *Case III: Single Submerged Floating Debris*

This case shows a plastic bag that is captured underwater as single submerged floating debris. Light reflection and noise are apparent in the original image (Fig 1c). After applying HSV conversion as before, Fig. 8 is obtained. The overlap of color between the plastic debris and water, as well as between the bag and the bottom surface, can easily be seen.

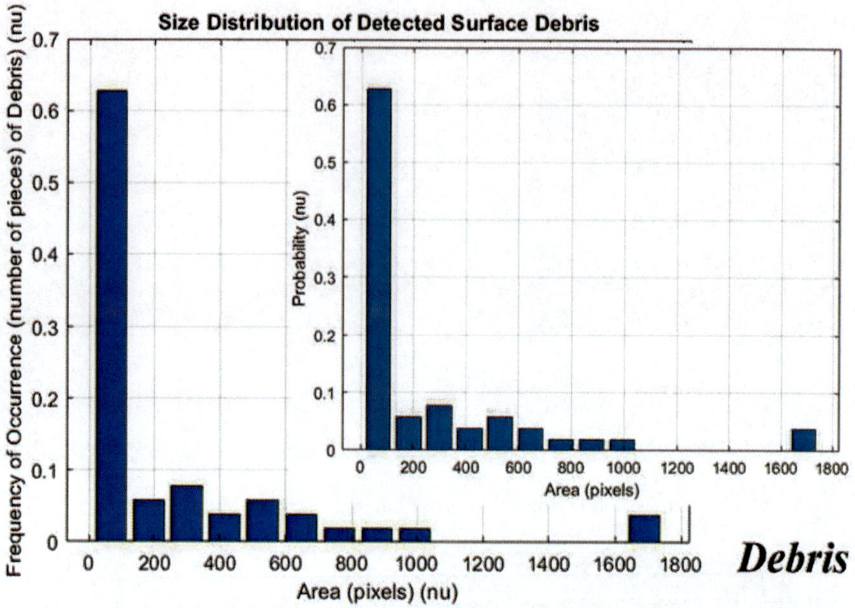

Fig. 7 Size distribution of surface debris in pixels (not corrected for perspective effects on size) (nu: no units)

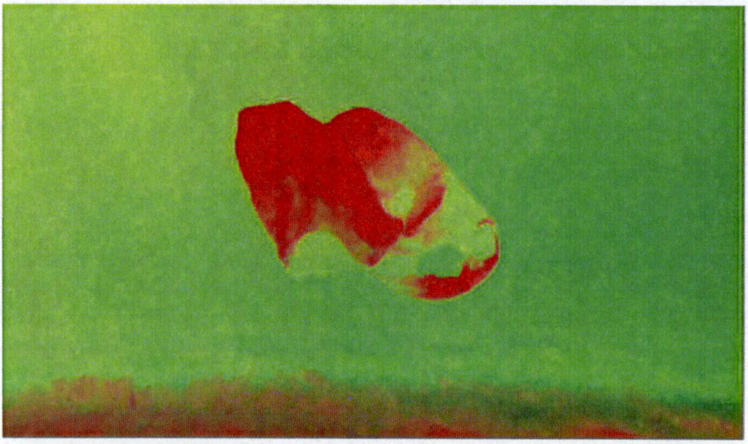

Fig. 8 Original image of Fig. 1c in HSV color space

Morphological operations (opening and closing) are applied to the debris mask to remove the noise in the image and close some of the holes on the debris mask, resulting in the improved debris mask shown in Fig. 9 (left). When the mask is overlaid with the original image via pixel-by-pixel multiplication, Fig. 9 (right) is obtained, highlighting the debris and residual reflections from the seabed.

Fig. 9 (Left) Improved debris mask after morphological operations. (Right) Identifying single large piece of debris object using the binary mask

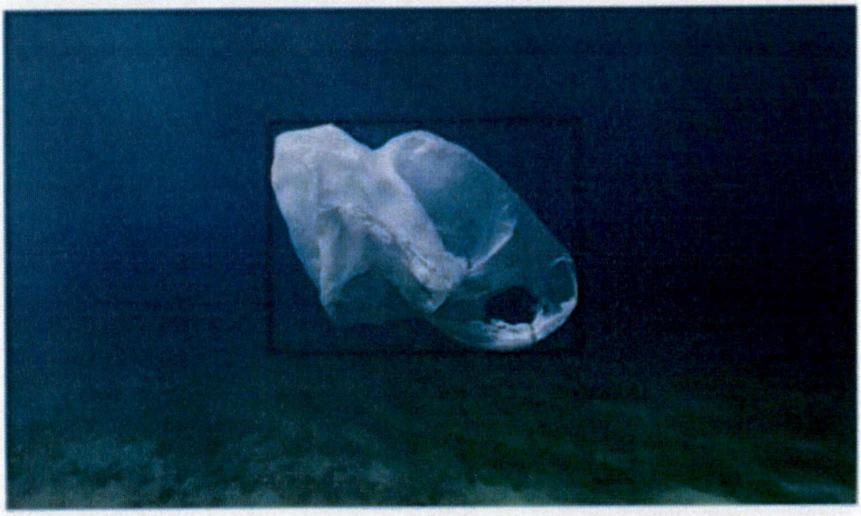

Fig. 10 Identifying single debris object using maximum-sized bounding box in binary mask

Although some parts of the plastic bag are missing, the bigger challenge in the debris mask is the unwanted illumination effects captured in the lower part of the scene that belong to the seabed and not debris.

In this case, with single debris in the scene, the unwanted effects due to lighting, scattering, and reflection can be further minimized by finding the bounding box on the largest connected object in the masked image and ignoring all other mask pixels. The result is shown in Fig. 10.

3.4 Case IV: Single Near-Surface Submerged Floating Debris

Another challenging case was presented in Fig. 1d for a single near-surface submerged floating debris. In this case, the image suffers from effects of surface

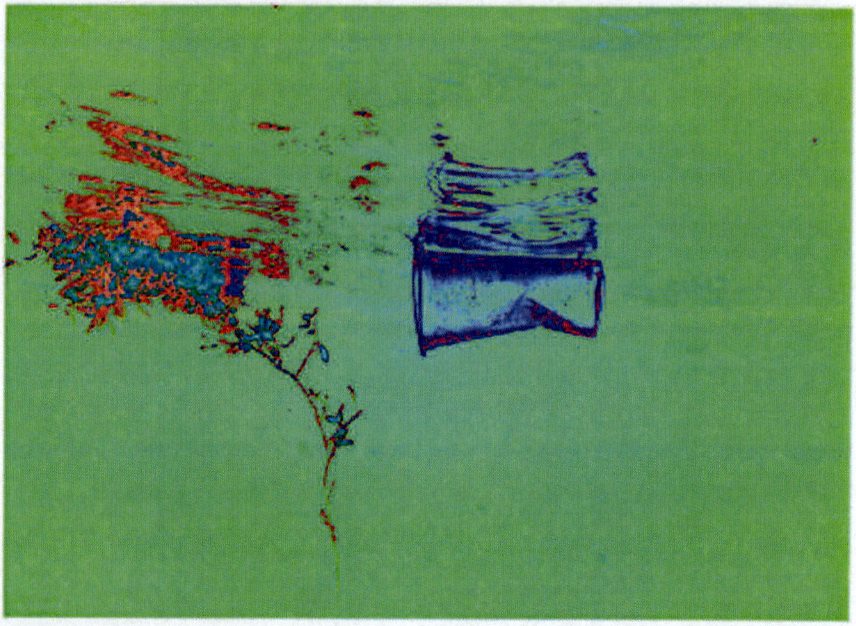

Fig. 11 HSV color space representation of plastic cup, its reflection at the water surface, as well as natural debris and its reflection.

reflection, which renders the debris piece larger than it really is. Similarly, glint in the form of image noise is visible in the natural debris (Fig. 1d).

HSV color model represents the image such that contrast between object of interest and background water is improved (Fig. 11). However, glint causes algorithmic problems in differentiating debris from its underwater surface reflection.

Multilevel thresholding is applied to the HSV image to obtain the binary mask, followed by morphological opening and closing to turn the objects into connected regions or blobs (Fig. 12 (left)). Man-made debris is detected as the blob with the largest area (see bounding box, Fig. 12 (left), (right)).

4 Discussion

It is shown that different scenes require similar but slightly adapted image processing chain to identify and characterize man-made marine debris. Contributing factors to chosen image processing tools include whether the images are captured above or under water, weather conditions during image capture, contrast between

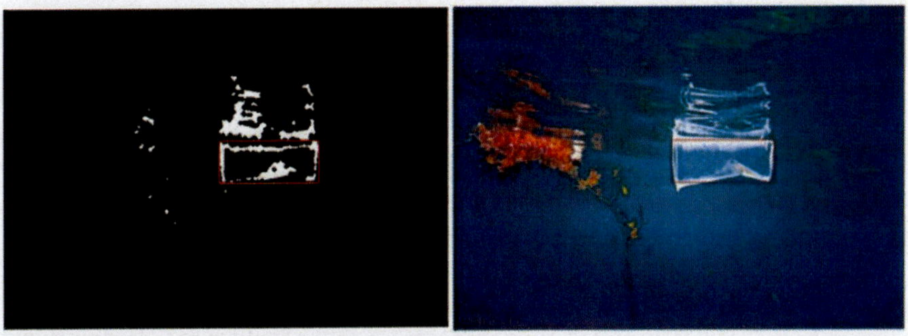

Fig. 12 (Left) Thresholding and morphological image processing to reduce the area of interest with man-made debris. (Right) Detection of plastic cup as the largest blob, with a bounding box

the debris and its environment as well as other objects in the scene, the number and size of objects in the scene, occlusions and overlaps within the scene, as well as illumination, reflection, scattering, and other effects, to list a few.

In the first case that was presented, debris consisted mainly of parts of plastic bags that have deteriorated and included a variety of dimensions with high overlap. In this scene, it is not practical to separately identify the pieces of debris. We chose to represent the amount of debris based on the percentage of the scene it occupied compared to its background and other objects not considered as debris.

In the second case, the debris on water surface was countable and easily separable. In such a scene, the number of pieces of debris can be counted, and size distribution determined. It is noted that perspective vision due to camera lens, viewing angle, and associated geometric distortion were not corrected when computing debris size distribution. A more realistic approach would account for perspective vision and geometric distortion, which can be achieved by estimating the size of standard objects, such as plastic bottles, at different distances.

In the third case, a single submerged plastic bag was detected. This object had relatively low contrast with respect to its environment partly due to its translucent nature. The debris was detected by using blob analysis and identifying the largest bounding box representing this single debris piece.

In the fourth case, additional challenges introduced by glint had to be addressed. Glint removal and reduction has been a topic of previous work, particularly in remote sensing and multispectral imagery [33, 34]. In this case, the effects of glint were avoided by similar techniques introduced in Case III, by multi-thresholding and morphological image processing tools such as opening and closing to reduce the area of interest that included the plastic cup. The plastic cup was detected as being the largest connected object after morphological operations.

5 Conclusion

Four different scenarios of floating debris, both on the surface and under the surface of water, have been presented. Different debris scenes allow different debris attributes to be extracted for qualitative as well as quantitative analysis.

In the first scenario, the underwater debris is quantified as the percent cover of the scene. In the second scenario, debris on the water surface is individually detected and counted and size distribution determined. In the third scenario, a single large piece of debris is detected and localized using the largest bounding box among what was detected. The fourth scenario represented another challenging case with both man-made and natural debris. The man-made debris was isolated based on its size but suffered the effects of glint from the surface of the water.

Beyond detection, identification (labeling) of debris can be achieved by shape and size determination of standardized man-made objects, such as bottles and plastic cups, or even plastic bags. Other more complex sensors, such as hyperspectral imagers, may be necessary to differentiate different materials of which the debris is made. This is particularly the case when debris pieces exhibit similar visual properties to the naked eye and do not represent visually recognizable shapes when they are deformed, damaged, or otherwise deteriorated.

Classical image processing tools and techniques described for marine debris detection and characterization are valuable, as these tools are able to extract meaningful features and attributes that may be lost in deep learning solutions. Debris detection and characterization could not only help researchers in identifying different kinds of debris in bodies of water and how they deteriorate and spread but also assist in removal technologies as vision solutions. More recent techniques in detection and classification of debris are underway. These techniques use artificial intelligence and machine learning methods to process thousands of images.

Acknowledgment This project has been supported in part by a grant from Texas A&M University-Corpus Christi: TCRF 2016-2017 *Integrated Characterization and Simulation System for Microplastics in Coastal Watersheds.*

References

1. United States Environmental Protection Agency, Sources of aquatic trash., https://www.epa.gov/trash-free-waters/sources-aquatic-trash
2. National Oceanic and Atmospheric Administration, What is marine debris?., https://oceanservice.noaa.gov/facts/marinedebris.html
3. E. Jepsen, P. de Bruyn, Pinniped entanglement in oceanic plastic pollution: Global review. Mar. Pollut. Bull. **145**, 295–305 (2019)
4. J. Lee, How did sea turtle get a straw up its nose? Natl. Geogr. (2018) https://www.nationalgeographic.com.au/animals/how-did-sea-turtle-get-a-straw-up-its-nose.aspx
5. University of Exeter, Marine turtles dying after becoming entangled in plastic rubbish. ScienceDaily (2017) http://www.sciencedaily.com/releases/2017/12/171218154235.htm

6. F. Yaghmour, M. Bousi, B. Whittington-Jones, J. Pereira, S. García-Nuñez, J. Budd, Marine debris ingestion of green sea turtles, *Chelonia mydas*, (Linnaeus, 1758) from the eastern coast of the United Arab Emirates. Mar. Pollut. Bull. **135**, 55–61 (2018)
7. C. Evans-Pughe, All at sea cleaning up the Pacific garbage. Eng. Technol. **12**(1) (2017)
8. N.J. Beaumont, M. Aanesen, M.C. Austen, T. Börger, et al., Global ecological, social and economic impacts of marine plastic. Mar. Pollut. Bull. **142**, 189–195 (2019)
9. E. Duncan, J. Arrowsmith, C. Bain, A. Broderick, J. Lee, et al., The true depth of the Mediterranean plastic problem: Extreme microplastic pollution on marine turtle nesting beaches in Cyprus. Mar. Pollut. Bull. **136**, 334–340 (2018)
10. M.Z. Alam, A.H.F. Anwar, D.C. Sarker, A. Heitz, C. Rothleitner, Characterising stormwater gross pollutants captured in catch basin inserts. Sci. Total Environ. **586**, 76–86 (2017)
11. M. Cole, P. Lindeque, C. Halsband, T. Galloway, Microplastics as contaminants in the marine environment: A review. Mar. Pollut. Bull. **62**(12), 2588–2597 (2011). https://doi.org/10.1016/j.marpolbul.2011.09.025
12. P. Dauvergne, Why is the global governance of plastic failing the oceans? Glob. Environ. Chang. **51**, 22–31 (2018). https://doi.org/10.1016/j.gloenvcha.2018.05.002
13. J. Jambeck et al., Plastic waste inputs from land into the ocean. Science **347**(6223), 768–771 (2015). https://doi.org/10.1126/science.1260352
14. C. Schmidt, T. Krauth, S. Wagner, Export of plastic debris by rivers into the sea. Environ. Sci. Technol. **51**(21), 12246–12253 (2017). https://doi.org/10.1021/acs.est.7b02368
15. R. Thompson et al., Lost at sea: Where is all the plastic? Science **304**(5672), 838 (2004). https://doi.org/10.1126/science.1094559
16. L. Goddijn-Murphy, S. Peters, E. van Sebille, N. James, S. Gibb, Concept for a hyperspectral remote sensing algorithm for floating marine macro plastics. Mar. Pollut. Bull. **126**, 255–262 (2017). https://doi.org/10.1016/j.marpolbul.2017.11.011
17. C. Lebreton et al., Evidence that the Great Pacific Garbage Patch is rapidly accumulating plastic. Sci. Rep. **8**(1), 4666 (2018). https://doi.org/10.1038/s41598-018-22939-w
18. P. Ryan, C. Moore, J. van Franeker, C. Moloney, Monitoring the abundance of plastic debris in the marine environment. Philos. Trans. R. Soc. Lond. Ser. B Biol. Sci. **364**, 1999–2012 (2009). https://doi.org/10.1098/rstb.2008.0207
19. M. Fulton, J. Hong, M. Islam, J. Sattar, Robotic detection of marine litter using deep visual detection models. Int. Conf. Robot. Automation (ICRA), 5752–5758 (2019)
20. M. Valdenegro-Toro, Submerged marine debris detection with autonomous underwater vehicles. Int. Conf. Robot. Automation Humanitarian Apps. (RAHA) (2016)
21. G. Gonçalvesa, U. Andriolob, L. Pintoc, D. Duarteb, Mapping marine litter with Unmanned Aerial Systems: A showcase comparison among manual image screening and machine learning techniques. Mar. Pollut. Bull. **155** (2020)
22. G. Gonçalves, U. Andriolo, L. Pinto, F. Bessa, Mapping marine litter using UAS on a beach-dune system: a multidisciplinary approach. Sci. Total Environ. **706** (2020)
23. K. Topouzelis, A. Papakonstantinou, S. Garaba, Detection of floating plastics from satellite and unmanned aerial systems (Plastic Litter Project 2018). Int. J. Appl. Earth Obs. Geoinf. **79**, 175–183 (2019)
24. Z. Bao, J. Sha, X. Li, T. Hanchiso, E. Shifaw, Monitoring of beach litter by automatic interpretation of unmanned aerial vehicle images using the segmentation threshold method. Mar. Pollut. Bull. **137**, 388–398 (2018)
25. K. Li, Q. Zhang, Z. Guo, J. Yuan, C. Zhao, K. Xu, Space debris detection algorithm based on mathematical morphology. Int. Conf. AI Comput. Intell., 178–180 (2009)
26. A. Harjoko, L. Awaludin, R.M. Hujja, The flow rate of debris estimation on the Sabo Dam area with video processing. Int. Conf. Signals Syst., 57–61 (2017)
27. S. Mahankali, S.V. Kabbin, S. Nidagundi, R. Srinath, Identification of illegal garbage dumping with video analytics. Int. Conf. Adv. Comp. Commun. Inform., 2403–2407 (2018)
28. R. McLendon, What is the Great Pacific ocean garbage patch?, (2019). https://www.mnn.com/earth-matters/translating-uncle-sam/stories/what-is-the-great-pacific-ocean-garbage-patch. Photo: Rich Carey, Shutterstock

29. A.P. Stevens, Environment: Plastic trash rides ocean currents to the Arctic, in *Science News for Students*, (2017). Photo: Chepe Nicoli. https://www.sciencenewsforstudents.org/article/plastic-trash-rides-ocean-currents-arctic
30. Australia's Plastic Bag Ban; A cause for cheer, 2018. https://www.perthbinhire.com.au/australias-plastic-bag-ban-a-cause-for-cheer/
31. Why do sea turtles eat ocean plastics? New research points to smell. in UNC University Communications, 2020
32. R.C. Gonzalez, R.E. Woods, *Digital Image Processing*, 4th edn. (Pearson, New York, 2018), pp. 541–545
33. J.D. Hedley, A.R. Harborne, P.J. Mumby, Technical note: Simple and robust removal of sun glint for mapping shallow-water benthos. Int. J. Remote Sens. **26**(10), 2107–2112 (2005)
34. C.J. Legleiter, Removing sun glint from optical remote sensing images of shallow rivers. Earth Surf. Proc. Landforms **42**(2), 318–333 (2016)

Polyhedral Approximation for 3D Objects by Dominant Point Detection

Miguel Vázquez-Martin del Campo, Hermilo Sánchez-Cruz, César Omar Jiménez-Ibarra, and Mario Alberto Rodríguez-Díaz

1 Introduction

The demand in applications that use the treatment of objects in the domain of two and three dimensions is a challenge for artificial intelligence, especially for computer vision, to simplify the information the descriptors of the images are used since they represent the entire object with the least possible redundant information.

The descriptors of the images may vary. They may come from inside of the figures, for example, the skeleton [1, 2], or from the surface or contour [3, 4]. In both cases, the original object can be partially or totally recovered. One of the contour representations is based on the chain codes [5–8]. They describe an object by a symbol sequence that means a segment of straight line of unit size with an orientation. There are several chain codes for objects in two and three dimensions. They can be relative, such as 3OT and AF8, or absolute, such as F4 and F8. It means the chain code may vary or not if the object is rotated [9].

The polygonal approximation is another representation of *two-dimensional* (2D) objects [10–13]. In the case of *three-dimensional* (3D) objects, the approximation is polyhedral, in which, from a set of contour points called dominant points, selected strategically, they are joined by straight lines, thus forming a polyhedron, which visually represents the original object. Since the contour is approximated by straight segments, even where the contour has more details, this method is tolerable to a

M. V.-M. del Campo (✉) · H. Sánchez-Cruz · C. O. Jiménez-Ibarra
Universidad Autónoma de Aguascalientes, Aguascalientes, México
e-mail: al266176@edu.uaa.mx; hsanchez@correo.uaa.mx; omar.jimenez@edu.uaa.mx

M. A. Rodríguez-Díaz
Instituto Tecnológico de Aguascalientes, Aguascalientes, México
e-mail: mario.rd@aguascalientes.tecnm.mx

H. R. Arabnia et al. (eds.), *Advances in Computer Vision and Computational Biology*, Transactions on Computational Science and Computational Intelligence,
https://doi.org/10.1007/978-3-030-71051-4_14

certain error because although the approximated polyhedron and the original object are visually similar, they are not strictly identical.

Along the contour, we can see corners, lines, and inflection points, but it is in the inflection points and corners where there is more information about the original shape. Hence, the dominant points are located in these regions. The development of a method that allows to find the set of dominant points is not an easy task; however, several works have previously been presented about it. Attneave did one of the first proposal [14] in 1954, which was based on the assumption that any corner should be a dominant point. The algorithms to find the dominant points can be classified by their approach, which have three large groups: sequential, split and merge, and heuristic [15].

In the sequential approach, Masood [15] proposed a set of initial breakpoints, in which there is a change of direction in the contour, to later eliminate, in each iteration, a point and evaluate the error until the tolerable error is reached. Ray and Ray [16] determine the longest possible line segments with the minimum possible error. Kurozumi and Davis [17] proposed a method that derives the approximated segments by minimizing the maximum distance between a given set of points and the corresponding segment. Teh and Chin [18] determined the region of support for each point, based on their local properties and calculation of their relative importance (curvature), to finally detect dominant points through a non-maximum suppression process.

In the approach of split and merge, Ramer [19] presented an iterative method to produce polygons that begins with a segmentation of initial limits, and in each iteration, the segment is divided in the point that has the furthest distance from the corresponding segment until the approximation error exceeds the tolerable error. Held et al. [20] proposed a method where the segments are split using the difference of slope and merged on the criteria of perceptual significance.

For the heuristic search approach, dynamic algorithms [21, 22], genetic algorithms [23, 24], Tabu search [25], and ant colony [24] have been used, and in one of the most recent researches, Fernández García [26] proposes an automatic and nonparametric method for polygonal approaches. Based on a new symmetrical version of the known Ramer's method, he develops a method with an adaptive threshold to obtain the dominant points.

As far as we know, although there are methods of polyhedron representation for 3D objects [27], there are not methods that generate the polyhedron from a cloud of dominant points.

Processing of 3D objects is much more difficult than the 2D case; however, taking advantage of the fact that a 3D object can be represented by slices, we propose to use the context-free grammar method [28] to obtain a point cloud, which are joined to form the polyhedron.

This paper is organized as follows. In Section 2, the proposed method is described, whereas in Section 3 experimental results are shown. Finally, in Section 4, some conclusions are given.

2 Proposed Method

The proposed method consists of several steps, starting with the slice selection of a voxelized object, continuing processing each slice to find its set of dominant points in order to obtain a point cloud of the entire object. Finally, we join the points to create the polyhedron and calculate the error committed.

2.1 Slice Selection and Connected Components

The proposed method starts with a voxelized 3D object. In Fig. 1, a voxelized brain can be observed.

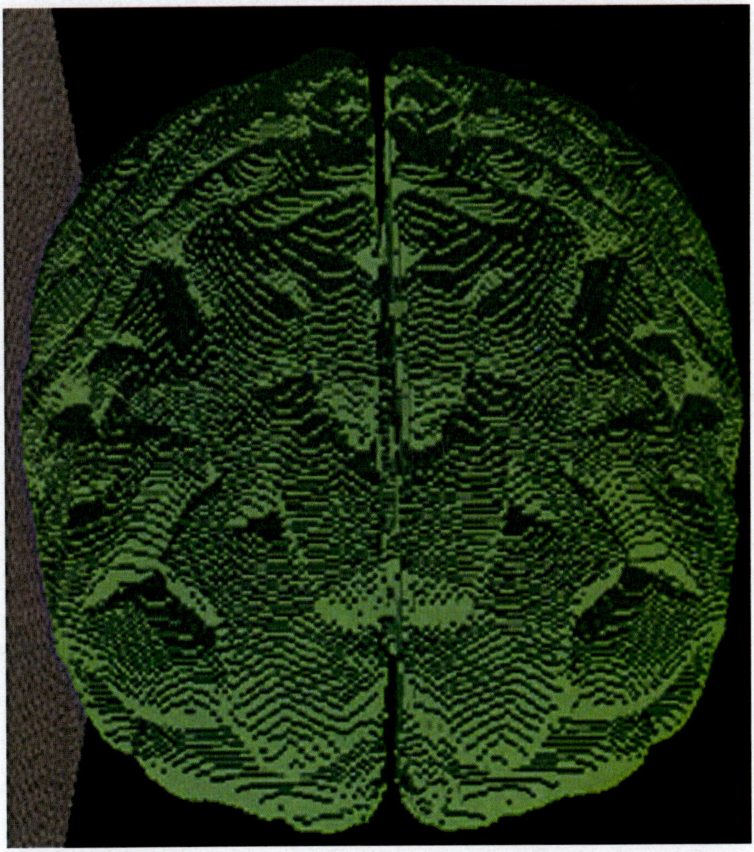

Fig. 1 Voxelized brain

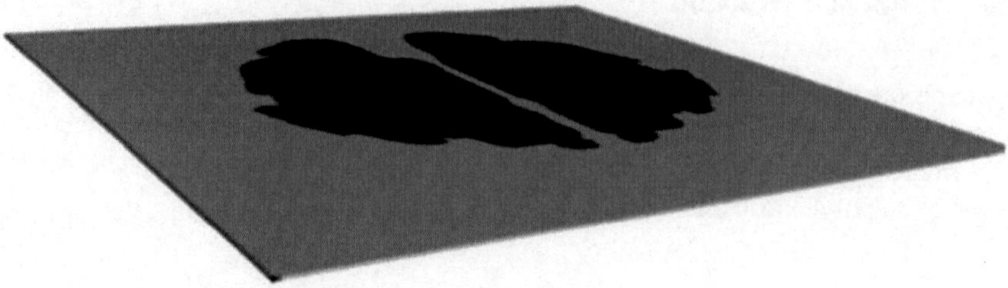

Fig. 2 The third slice of the voxelized brain

A voxelized object is treated like a closed box containing 1-voxels (part of the object) and 0-voxels (background), organized by slices on the Z axis, so the object is traversed from the bottom looking for the first 1-voxel. All voxels in this level are part of the first slice. The following slices are chosen by traveling upward in intervals of N slices, getting one slice every N slices traveled, which is calculated with the closest integer number to the value of $\sqrt{(\text{number of voxels per side})}$, and the remainder of (1) has to be zero.

$$\frac{(\text{Number of voxels per side})}{N} \tag{1}$$

In our case, the number of voxels is 128, so $\sqrt{128} = 11.31$, the closest integer numbers upward are 12, 13, 14, 15, and 16, and downward are 11, 10, 9, and 8. These possible values of N are evaluated, but the only values that the remainder of (1) is zero are 8 and 16, so N could be 8 or 16. For this work, we used $N = 8$. In Fig. 2, the third slice of the brain can be observed.

Once the object is represented by slices, each slice is treated such an object in 2D grid composed of r rows and c columns, where each cell, called pixel, can take two values in its intensity, 0 and 1. It is 1 if it is part of the figure and 0 if it is part of the background.

The slice requires a processing to identify the connected components in the image. For this, the flood fill algorithm was used to identify them. In Fig. 3, we can see the two connected components, and each component is processed separately.

2.2 *Selection of the Set of Dominant Points*

In our proposal, to make the selection of the dominant points, it is necessary to obtain the AF8 chain code of the contour of each component. AF8 is an invariant chain code under transformations of rotation and translation based on two vectors:

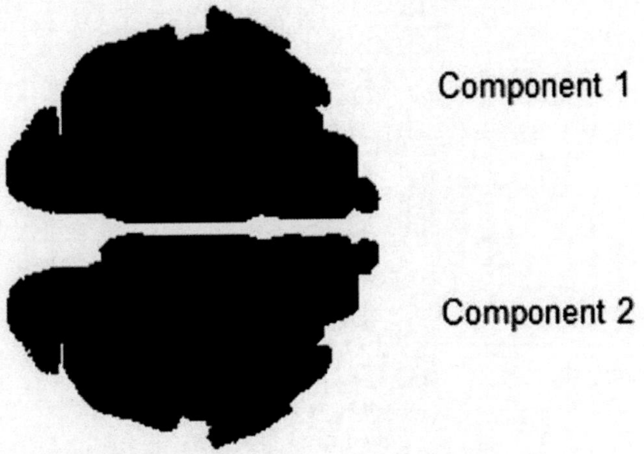

Fig. 3 Two connected components in the third slice of the brain

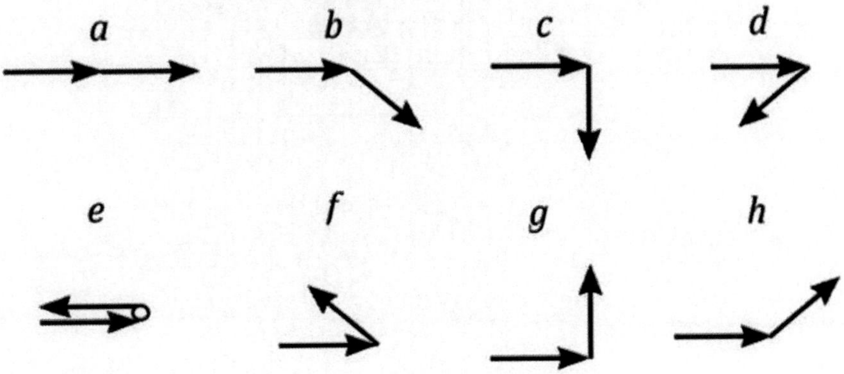

Fig. 4 AF8 symbols

a reference vector and a change vector. It has eight directions of change (see Fig. 4) labeled by a symbol of the alphabet $\sum_{AF8} = \{a, b, c, d, e, f, g, h\}$.

For the explanation of this part of the method, we used Fig. 5.

Using the code of Fig. 4 in the contour of Fig. 5, we obtain the following AF8 chain code:

$$C_{AF8} = aaaabbhbahbacabhhgabhabbhaabcaahabbahbaaabhhbaabab.$$

In Table 1 is shown the frequency of each symbol of the abovementioned chain code. As can be observed, the most common symbols are a, b, and h.

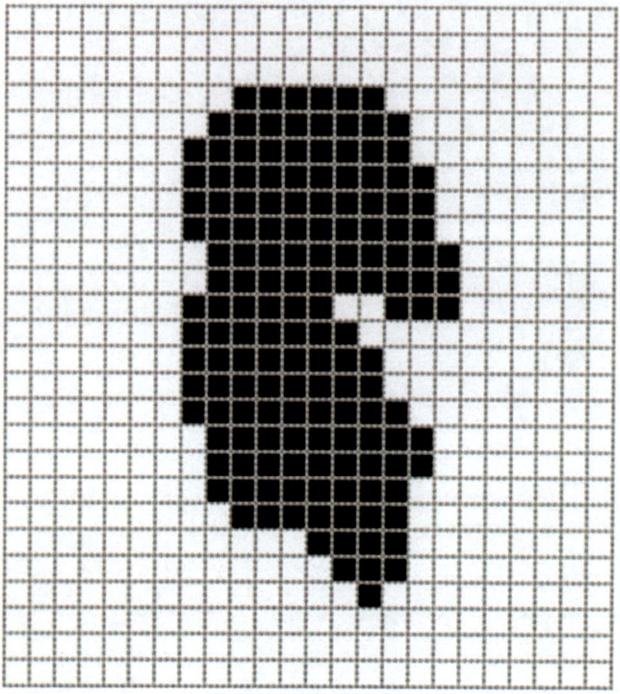

Fig. 5 Simple image in 2D grid

Table 1 Frequency of AF8 chain code symbols

Symbol	Frequency
a	21
b	16
c	2
d	0
e	0
f	0
g	1
h	10
Total:	50

The symbol a by itself represents a straight line, but a combination with the other two, b and h, can create what visually speaking is a line. It is the target of the method to find what appears to be a digital straight segment (DSS) [28].

In order to find the DSS from the contour, it is necessary to know the point where it begins and ends. It means dominant points. For that, the chain code C of each figure is evaluated for the language L of (2).

$$L = \left\{xa^{p}\left(bha^{q}\right)^{r}, xa^{p}\left(hba^{q}\right)^{r} | x \in \{a, b, c, d, e, f, g, h\}\right\}, \qquad (2)$$

Table 2 DSSs and their values of *p*, *q*, and *r*

DSS	Equivalence	*p*	*q*	*r*
xaaa	xa^3	3	0	0
xbh	$xa^0(bha^0)^1$	0	0	1
xahba	$xa^1(hba^1)^1$	1	1	1
xabh	$xa^1(bha^0)^1$	1	0	1
x	xa^0	0	0	0
xabha	$xa^1(bha^1)^1$	1	1	1
xbhaa	$xa^0(bha^2)^1$	0	2	1
x	xa^0	0	0	0
xaa	xa^2	2	0	0
xa	xa^1	1	0	0
x	xa^0	0	0	0
xahbaaa	$xa^1(hba^3)^1$	1	3	1
x	xa^0	0	0	0
xhbaa	$xa^0(hba^2)^1$	0	2	1
xa	xa^1	1	0	0
x	xa^0	0	0	0
	Maximum:	3	3	1

where x represents the beginning of one DSS. It means a dominant point. p, q, r represent the maximum values of times. The symbol or symbols set in parentheses are presented in the whole chain code, and a, b, $\ldots$, h are symbols of the AF8 alphabet [28].

L is a subset of a language generated by the context – free grammar G, giving for the 4 – tuple $G = (V, \Sigma_{\mathrm{AF8}}, S, P)$, where V and Σ_{AF8} are disjoint sets, $S \in P$, and P is a set of production rules given by

$$S \rightarrow xAB \mid xAC$$

$$B \rightarrow bhAB \mid \epsilon$$

$$C \rightarrow hbAC \mid \epsilon$$

$$A \rightarrow aA \mid \epsilon.$$

After the chain code C_{AF8} was evaluated in (2), it can be written in this way:

$$C_{\mathrm{AF8}} = xaaaxbhxahbaxabhxxabhaxbhaaxxaaxaxxahbaaaxxhbaaxax,$$

where each DSS has different values of p, q, and r. In Table 2, we can see the value of each of them.

The dominant points for this slice are shown in Fig. 6. The red points indicate where they are located.

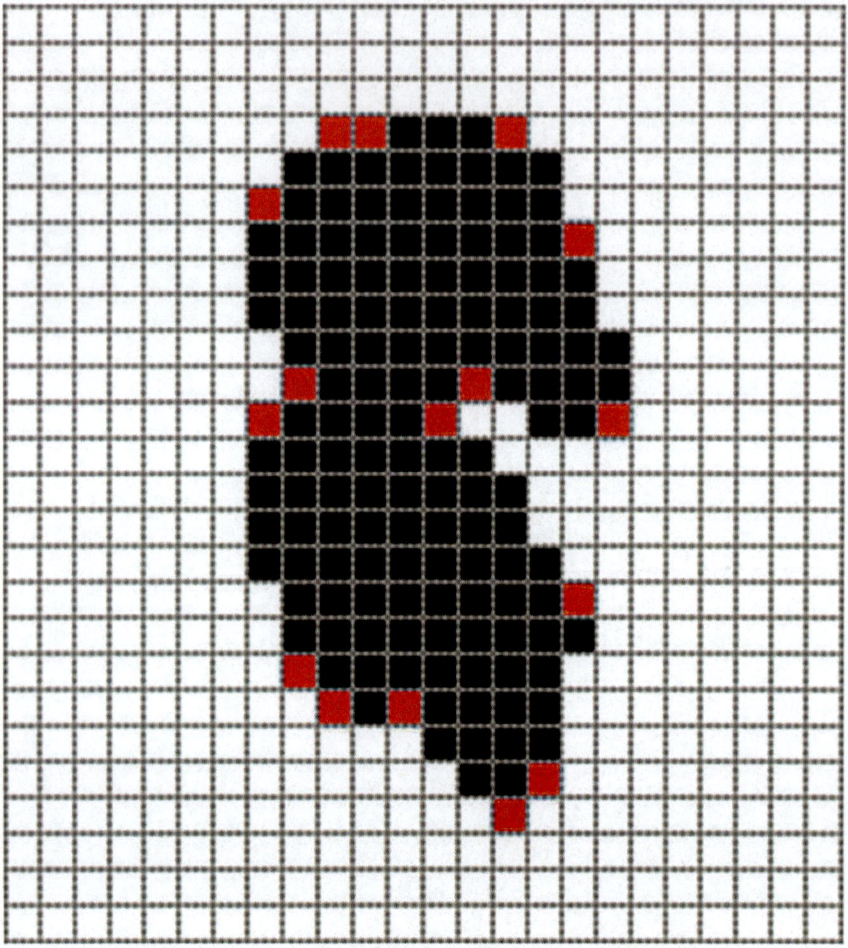

Fig. 6 Dominant points

Now, see a real case of the brain. The AF8 chain code of the component 2 of Fig. 3 is

$C_{AF8} =$ *aaaaabhaaaaaaaaaaaaaaaaaaaaaaaaaaaaaaaaaaaaaaaabhabh*
aaaahbaaahbaaaaabhaaaaaaaahbaaaabhabbhhahababhabbaaaaaabaah
caaahhaaaaaaaaaaaababhbhbahbahbhhaaabaaghaaabbaaaabhbhbabha
aabhbhaaaahhbbbhbhabhabhbhbhbaahbahacgbahbhbbbhachabghchhaaa
aabhbgahbhchbaaabhabhabhbhabhaaabhabhaabhbhbaaaaabhbhaabhbhb
aaaaaaaahghaaaaaabhaacabgchbabhbhbahgdhbhhbbhabahbaaaaaaaabh
aabaaacghcahbaahbahbaaaaaaaaaaaahbhbahhaahcaaabahbaah.

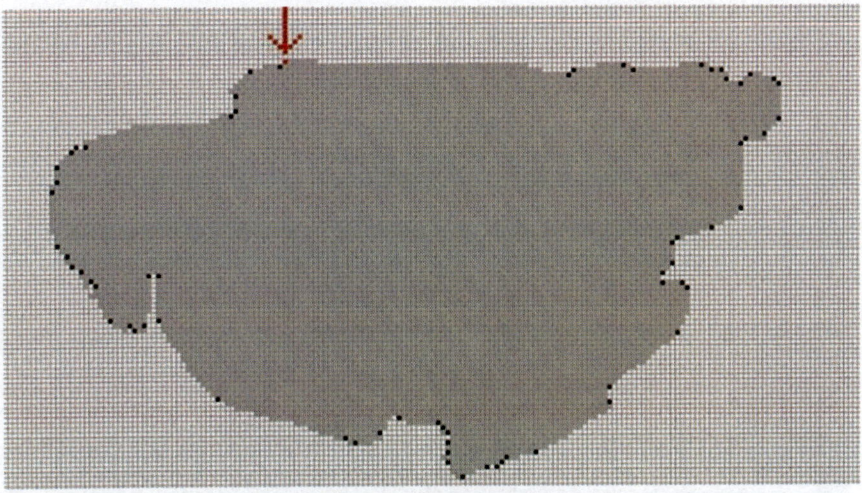

Fig. 7 Dominant points of the component 2 of the third slice

In Fig. 7, the dominant points of the component 2 of Fig. 3 can be observed, and the red arrow indicates the beginning of the figure. We do the same for each component of each slice of the object.

2.3 Creation of the Polyhedron

When we have the cloud of dominant points, the next step is to create the polyhedron. We join the dominant points in two different ways. The first one is in the same slice, joining all the dominant points of each component in order to create its polygon. In consequence, if there are two components in the same slice, then there are two polygons in this level. In Fig. 8, the polygon of the component 2 of the third slice is observed.

The second way of joining dominant points is between slices, where all the points are traversed for each polygon of each slice, taking two contiguous dominant points i and j, and the closest dominant point k is searched in both the upper and lower slice, thus forming a triangular plane. In Fig. 9, it can be seen how the slice z joins the slice $z + 1$ from the points i, j, and k. An example of joining dominant points between slices in the object of the brain is seen in Fig. 10.

When all the dominant points are joined, the result is the final polyhedron. In Fig. 11a, the obtained polyhedron of the brain is observed, and in Fig. 11b, it can be seen from another viewpoint.

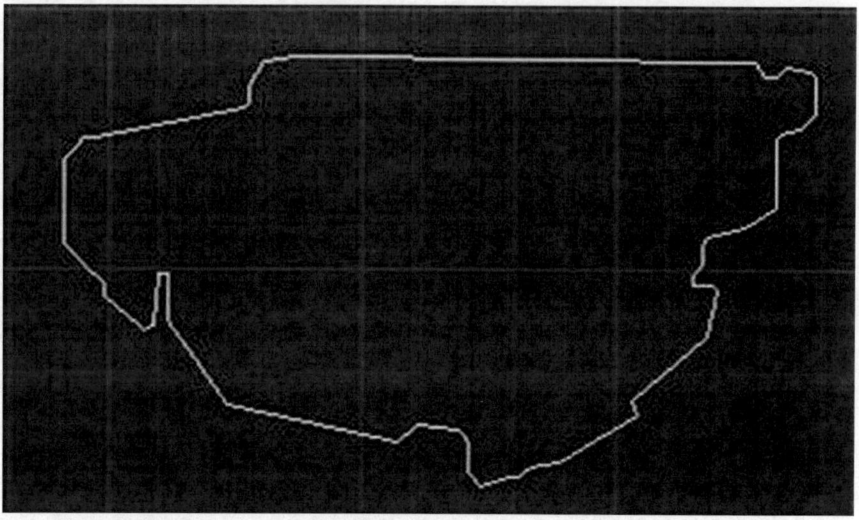

Fig. 8 Polygon from the component 2 of the third slice

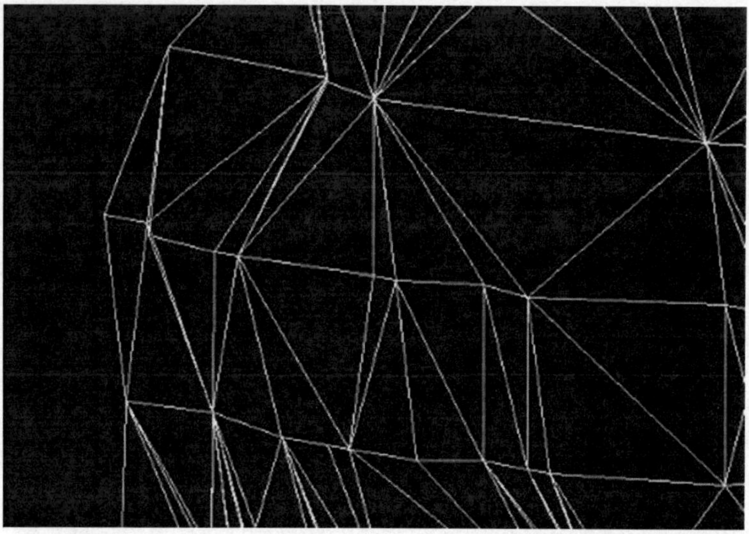

Fig. 9 Slices joining

2.4 Error Calculation

It is necessary to evaluate the polyhedron obtained to know how good the method is, that is, how different the polyhedron is from the original object and how much information was reduced. Typically, the Integral Square Error (ISE) is the sum of

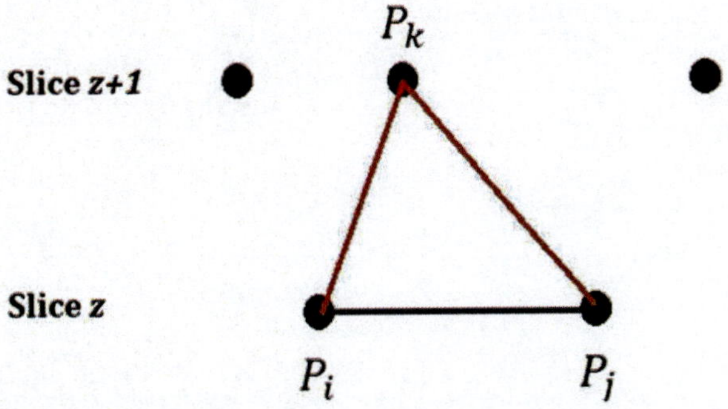

Fig. 10 Linking the dominant points (vertices) of different slices with edges

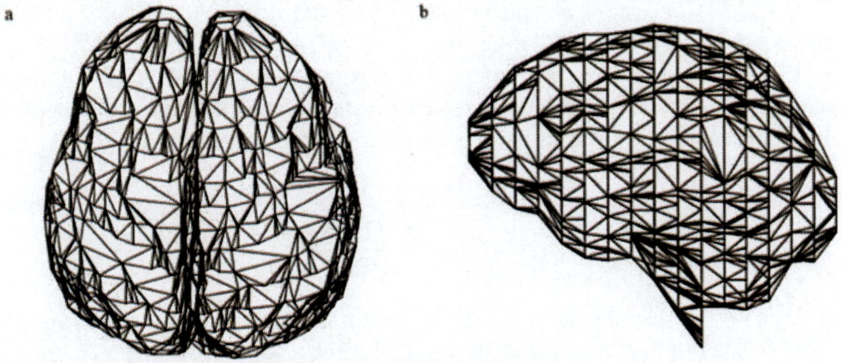

Fig. 11 Polyhedron of the brain from different viewpoints

all perpendicular distances of a contour to the approximate polygon. It gives the total distortion caused by the polygonal approximation; thus, it must be as small as a tolerable error for a good polygon. It is usually given by ISE $= \sum d_i$, where d_i is calculated by (3), but in this case, the distance is not from a point to the line of a polygon, but from a point X to a face of a polyhedron, that is, to a plane π with the three points P, Q, and R.

$$d_i\,(X, \pi) = \frac{|(Ax_x + By_x + Cz_x + D)|}{\sqrt{A^2 + B^2 + C^2}}, \tag{3}$$

where $X = (x_x, y_x, z_x)$, is a point from the original object surface. A, B, C, and D are components from general equation of the plane π and they are calculated by (4–7):

$$A = \begin{vmatrix} y_r - y_p & z_r - z_p \\ y_q - y_p & z_q - z_p \end{vmatrix}, \tag{4}$$

$$B = -\begin{vmatrix} x_r - x_p & z_r - z_p \\ x_q - x_p & z_q - z_p \end{vmatrix}, \tag{5}$$

$$C = \begin{vmatrix} x_r - x_p & y_r - y_p \\ x_q - x_p & y_q - y_p \end{vmatrix}, \tag{6}$$

$$D = -x_p \begin{vmatrix} y_r - y_p & z_r - z_p \\ y_q - y_p & z_q - z_p \end{vmatrix} - y_p \begin{vmatrix} x_r - x_p & z_r - z_p \\ x_q - x_p & z_q - z_p \end{vmatrix} - z_p \begin{vmatrix} x_r - x_p & y_r - y_p \\ x_q - x_p & y_q - y_p \end{vmatrix}, \tag{7}$$

where $P = (x_p, y_p, z_p)$, $Q = (x_q, y_q, z_q)$, and $R = (x_r, y_r, z_r)$ are points in the plane π. Equations (4)–(7) can be obtained by using the plane equations and looking for the distance from a given point X to the plane.

There is another error criterion called *compression ratio* (CR). This criterion shows how much information was reduced from the original object to the polyhedron. The value of CR means the smaller the nDP, the greater the CR. This criterion is given by the formula:

$$\text{CR} = \frac{n\text{VOX}}{n\text{DP}}, \tag{8}$$

where nVOX is the number of voxels on the surface of the original object, and nDP is the number of dominant points of the polyhedron.

Both ISE and CR constitute different error criteria, but if the method is evaluated, using only one of them is not enough since there is a trade-off between them, that is, a polyhedron with a high level of compression has a higher distortion, and a polyhedron with low distortion has a very low compression level. Sarkar, in 1993 [29], proposed another error criterion that relates the two previous ones called *figure of merit* (FOM) given by

$$\text{FOM} = \frac{\text{CR}}{\text{ISE}}. \tag{9}$$

These error criteria (ISE, CR, and FOM) have been widely used in the literature to make polygonal approximation; however, a work developed to polyhedron approximation obtaining the error criteria properly has not been published at the time of writing this work. As part of a new definition of error criteria, we consider for the 3D case, another characteristic provided by the number of faces of the polyhedron (nF), which, in our experiments, is approximately twice the nDP.

3 Experimental Results

The method was applied to several voxelized objects with size 128×128×128 voxels; thus, $N = 8$. In Fig. 12, the sample objects we used are shown.

Using our method, in Fig. 13, the obtained polyhedra from the set of objects of Fig. 12 are shown. The error criteria are shown in Table 3.

We changed the value of N to the other possible value, $N = 16$, and we did the same steps. The results for the same figures are shown in Table 4.

As we can see, nDP changes inversely proportional to N, and ISE, CR, and nF change directly proportional to N. FOM remains relatively the same because ISE doubled and nDP halved approximately.

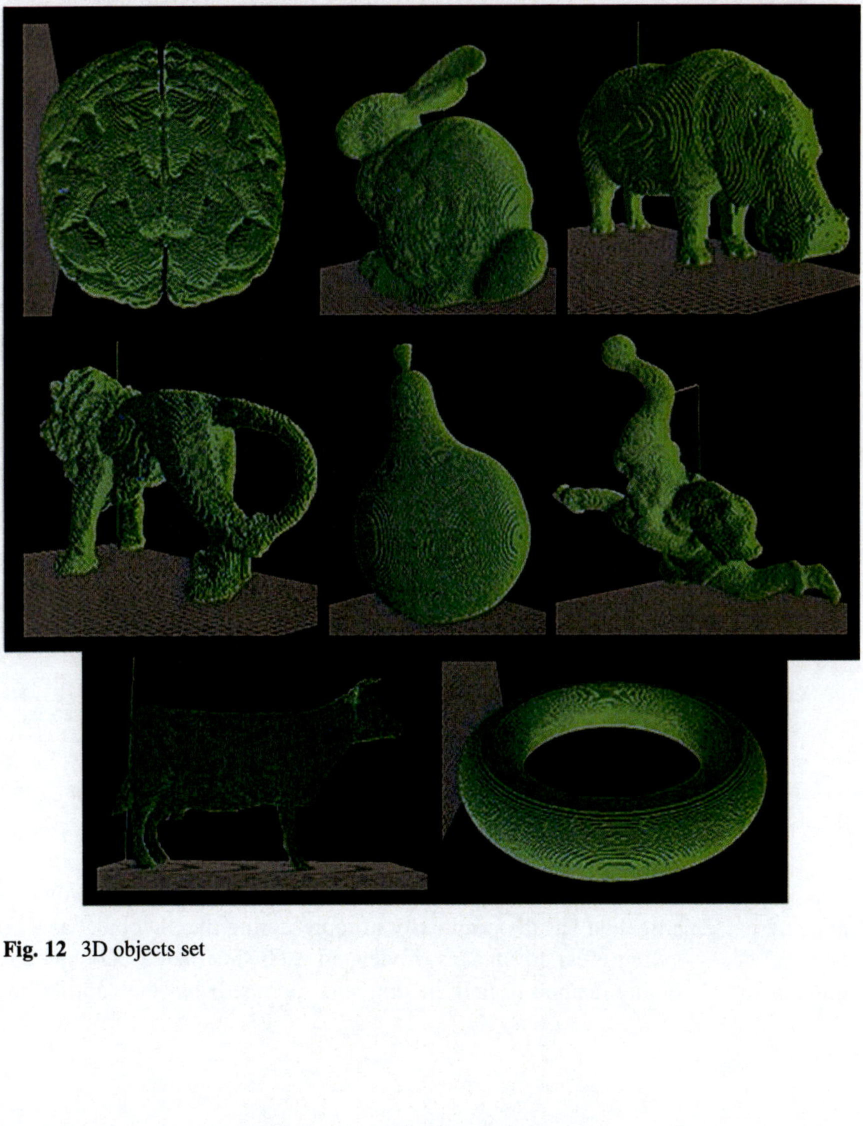

Fig. 12 3D objects set

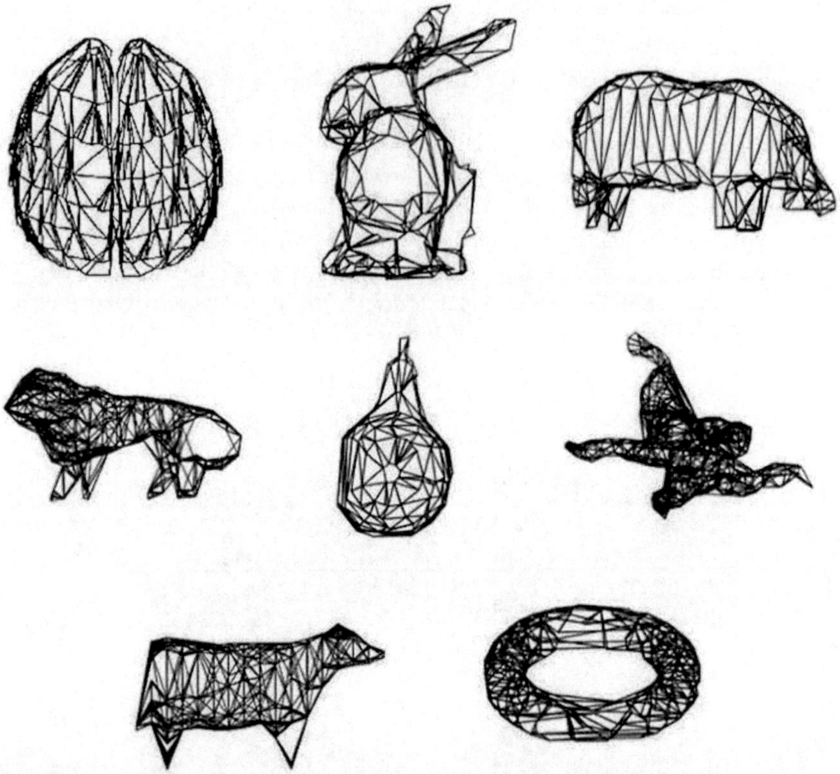

Fig. 13 Polyhedra set

Table 3 Results of the error criteria with $N = 8$

Object	ISE	nDP	CR	FOM	nF
Brain	35,919	1380	36.06	0.0010	2706
Bunny	31,839	536	61.77	0.0019	1045
Hippo	13,631	289	54.70	0.0040	563
Lion	10,632	350	35.40	0.0033	672
Pear	17,479	240	87.45	0.0050	461
Santa	12,307	384	41.67	0.0039	736
Cow	14,640	262	50.17	0.0034	512
Torus	23,936	328	65.71	0.0027	628

4 Conclusion

This paper presented a method for the representation of 3D objects through a polyhedron. This method has the peculiarity of representing the 3D object as a set of voxel slices, giving great advantages of viewing each slice like a 2D object, to implement an existing method to find the dominant points. It has the contribution

Table 4 Results of the error criteria with $N = 16$

Object	ISE	nDP	CR	FOM	nF
Brain	66,342	710	70.09	0.0010	1368
Bunny	65,883	274	120.83	0.0018	536
Hippo	20,771	146	108.29	0.0052	274
Lion	18,060	170	72.882	0.0040	330
Pear	27,209	125	167.92	0.0062	232
Santa	44,250	184	86.97	0.0020	356
Cow	28,044	117	112.36	0.0040	220
Torus	41,624	179	120.42	0.0029	330

of creating a polyhedron from a point cloud and the new adaptation of ISE and therefore the CR, FOM, and, furthermore, the definition of one more: nF.

For future work, although the fact we can see what object is, we can still adjust the method to reduce the ISE. An option would be to decrease the N. Another future work is to implement learning techniques to allow recognition.

References

1. H. Blum, A transformation for extracting new descriptors of the shape, in *Models of the Perception of Speech and Visual Forms*, ed. by W. Whaten-Dunn, (MIT Press, Cambridge, 1967), pp. 362–380
2. J.J. Koenderink, A.J. van Doorn, The internal representation of solid shape with respect to vision. Biol. Cybern. **32**, 211–216 (1979)
3. B. Kartikeyan, A. Sarkar, Shape description by time series. IEEE Trans. Pattern Anal. Mach. Intell. **11**, 977–984 (1989)
4. R. Kashyap, R. Dhellapa, Stochastic models for closed boundary analysis: Representation and reconstruction. IEEE Trans. Inf. Theory **27**, 627–637 (1981)
5. T. Kaneko, M. Okudaira, Encoding of arbitrary curves based on the chain code representation. IEEE Trans. Commun. **33**, 697–707 (1985)
6. J. Koplowitz, On the performance of chain codes for quantization of the line drawings. IEEE Trans. Pattern Anal. Mach. Intell. **3**, 180–185 (1981)
7. D. Neuhoff, K. Castor, A rate and distortion analysis of chain codes for line drawings. IEEE Trans. Inf. Theory **31**, 53–68 (1985)
8. J. Saghri, H. Freeman, Analysis of the precision of generalized chain codes for the representation of planar curves. IEEE Trans. Pattern Anal. Mach. Intell. **3**, 533–539 (1981)
9. H. Sanchez-Cruz, H.H. Lopez-Valdez, Equivalence of chain codes. J. Electron. Imag. **23**(1), 013031 (2014)
10. C.P. Chau, W.C. Siu, New nonparametric dominant point detection algorithm. Vision Image Signal Proc. **148**(5), 363–374 (2001)
11. T.M. Cronin, A boundary concavity code to support dominant points detection. Pattern Recogn. Lett. **20**, 617–634 (1999)
12. M. Marji, P. Siy, A new algorithm for dominant points detection and polygonization of digital curves. Pattern Recogn. **36**, 2239–2251 (2003)
13. H. Park, J.H. Lee, Error-bounded B-spline curve approximation based on dominant point selection. IEEE Int. Conf. Comp. Imag. Vision: New Trends, 437–446 (2005)
14. F. Attneave, Some informational aspects of visual perception. Psychol. Rev. **61**, 183–193 (1954)

15. Masood, S.A. Haq, A novel approach to polygonal approximation of digital curves. J. Vis. Commun. Image Represent. **18**(3), 264–274 (2007)
16. B.K. Ray, K.S. Ray, Determination of optimal polygon from digital curve using L1 norm. Pattern Recogn. **26**, 505–509 (1993)
17. Y. Kurozumi, W.A. Davis, Polygonal approximation by the minimax method. Comp. Grap. Image Proc. **19**, 248–264 (1982)
18. C. Teh, R. Chin, On the detection of dominant points on digital curves. IEEE Trans. Pattern Anal. Mach. Intell. **8**, 859–873 (1989)
19. U. Ramer, An iterative procedure for the polygonal approximation of plane curves. Comp. Graph. Image Proc. **1**, 244–256 (1972)
20. K. Held, C.A. Abe, Towards a hierarchical contour description via dominant point detection. IEEE Transact. Syst. Man Cybern. **24**(6), 942–949 (1994)
21. J.G. Dunham, Optimum uniform piecewise linear approximation of planar curves. IEEE Trans. Pattern Anal. Mach. Intell. **8**, 67–75 (1986)
22. Y. Sato, Piecewise linear approximation of plane curves by perimeter optimization. Pattern Recogn. **25**, 1535–1543 (1992)
23. E. Goldberg, *Genetic Algorithms in Search Optimization and Machine Learning* (Addison, Reading, 1989)
24. C. Huang, Y.N. Sun, Polygonal approximation using genetic algorithms. Pattern Recogn. **32**, 1409–1420 (1999)
25. P.Y. Yin, Genetic algorithms for polygonal approximation of digital curves. Int. J. Pattern Recognit. Artif. Intell. **13**, 1–22 (1999)
26. N.L. Fernández-García, L. Del-Moral Martínez, A. Carmona-Poyato, F.J. Madrid Cuevas, R. Medina-Carnicer, A new thresholding approach for automatic generation of polygonal approximations. J. Vis. Commun. Image Represent., 155–168 (2016)
27. T. Lafarge, B. Pateiro-López, A. Possolo, J.P. Dunkers, R implementation of a polyhedral approximation to a 3D set of points using the a-shape. J. Stat. Softw. **56**, 4 (2014)
28. H. Sánchez-Cruz, O.A. Tapia-Dueñas, F. Cuevas, Polygonal approximation using a multiresolution method and a context-free grammar, in *Pattern Recognition. MCPR 2019. Lecture Notes in Computer Science*, ed. by J. Carrasco-Ochoa, J. Martínez-Trinidad, J. Olvera-López, J. Salas, (Springer, Cham, 2019)
29. D. Sarkar, A simple algorithm for detection of significant vertices for polygonal approximation of chain-coded curves. Pattern Recognit. Lett. **14**, 959–964 (1993)

Multi-Sensor Fusion Based Action Recognition in Ego-Centric Videos with Large Camera Motion

Radhakrishna Dasari, Karthik Dantu, and Chang Wen Chen

1 Introduction

Over the past two decades, there has been a significant amount of research directed towards action recognition in videos. Current State-of-the-art approaches use convolutional networks trained on hundreds of thousands of videos. The videos of these datasets are predominantly sourced from video platforms like YouTube which host diverse video content captured mostly from a third-person perspective using a stable camera. The technological advancement in the area of wearable devices, which are capable of acquiring and processing video from a first-person perspective, have generated significant interest in ego-centric action recognition [1]. The focus of these large ego-centric video datasets is to recognize the actions of the first person wearing the camera. There are very few ego-centric video datasets that try to incorporate ego-motion into the framework of recognizing human actions from a first-person viewpoint [2]. To our knowledge, there are no video datasets that captured human actions, synchronized with other sensory information like audio, inertial measurements and GPS signals. We worked on bridging that gap. Our multi-sensory video dataset mimics KTH dataset [3], which pioneered research in human action recognition.

We collected a video dataset with over 25 subjects performing seven actions—*wave, walk, jog, sit, stand, box*, and *clap* (Fig. 1). We intentionally recorded the actions *sit* and *stand* in the same space with the same subject. Our understanding is that it would help test the temporal (not just spatial) perceptiveness of action recognition algorithms. To quantify the impact of camera translation and rotation on action recognition algorithms, we captured the same subject performing the same

R. Dasari (✉) · K. Dantu · C. W. Chen
Department of Computer Science and Engineering, University at Buffalo, Buffalo, NY, USA
e-mail: radhakri@buffalo.edu; kdantu@buffalo.edu; chencw@buffalo.edu

H. R. Arabnia et al. (eds.), *Advances in Computer Vision and Computational Biology*, Transactions on Computational Science and Computational Intelligence,
https://doi.org/10.1007/978-3-030-71051-4_15

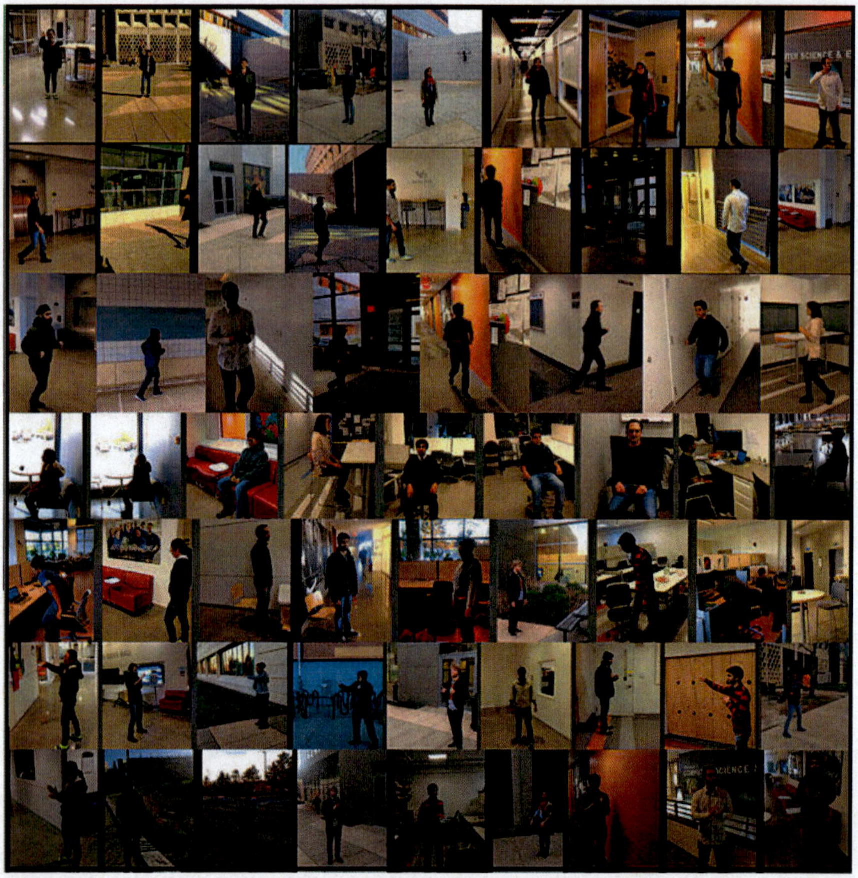

Fig. 1 Dataset snapshot with actions—wave, walk, jog, sit, stand, box, and clap

action in three different scenarios—normal camera motion, large camera rotation and a mix of both rotation and translation. In our study, we intend to evaluate the performance of visual, inertial, and multi-sensor fusion video stabilization techniques on action recognition performance.

Large camera motion incorporates great deal of motion information in the videos which is not related to the action being performed by another person. This results in feature representations which capture the essence of global motion rather than the representations of the actual human action. Stabilizing the videos before training and testing the action recognition classifier is known to improve the overall accuracy [4]. Our dataset presents an opportunity to study and evaluate the performance of visual, inertial, and visual-inertial stabilization in terms of accuracy and run time.

2 Preliminary Experiments and Results

We use dense trajectories [4] for evaluating action recognition performance on our dataset. Given the small size of the dataset, using convolutional neural networks is impractical. The videos are resized from 1920×1080 to 640×320 before extracting the dense trajectory features. A dictionary of dense trajectory features is built by randomly choosing features from normal camera motion, large camera motion and both rotation and translation, separately. This gives three dictionaries per visual stabilization technique. The videos are classified by building a histogram of the dense trajectory features obtained from the dictionary, using a Linear SVM with one-vs-all classification approach. The number of entries in the dictionary is set as 4000 as in [4].

The accuracy is reported in Table 1, comparing the performance with Inertial sensor stabilized video data [5] and visual stabilization using L1 camera paths [6]. Stabilizing the videos shows a clear trend of increase in recognition accuracy in both the scenarios with large camera motion. The next step is to run this pipeline on Videos stabilized using real-time SVO [7] and inertial sensor data based stabilization [8]. A joint visual-inertial technique for stabilization will be explored, which will be evaluated using motion capture system Fig. 2. Our intention is to broaden this action recognition framework to include other sensors—GPS for location context and ambient light sensor for indoor/outdoor context for smoothing the action predictions.

Table 1 Linear support vector machine based classification on dense trajectory features [4] (I-inertial sensor based stabilization, V-visual stabilization). The bold value signifies better performing technique (visual vs inertial stabilization) on that specific action

Action	Normal (I)	Normal (V)	Rotation (I)	Rotation (V)	Rot and trans (I)	Rot and trans (V)
Box	80%	**88%**	32%	**72%**	64%	**84%**
Jog	**64%**	60%	44%	**52%**	36%	36%
Wave	32%	**36%**	40%	**60%**	36%	**44%**
Walk	**72%**	64%	64%	**72%**	**60%**	52%
Clap	**40%**	36%	20%	**28%**	20%	**44%**
Sit	**80%**	60%	60%	**72%**	64%	**68%**
Stand	72%	72%	64%	**80%**	68%	**76%**
Total	**62.9%**	59.4%	46.3%	**62.3%**	49.7%	**57.7%**

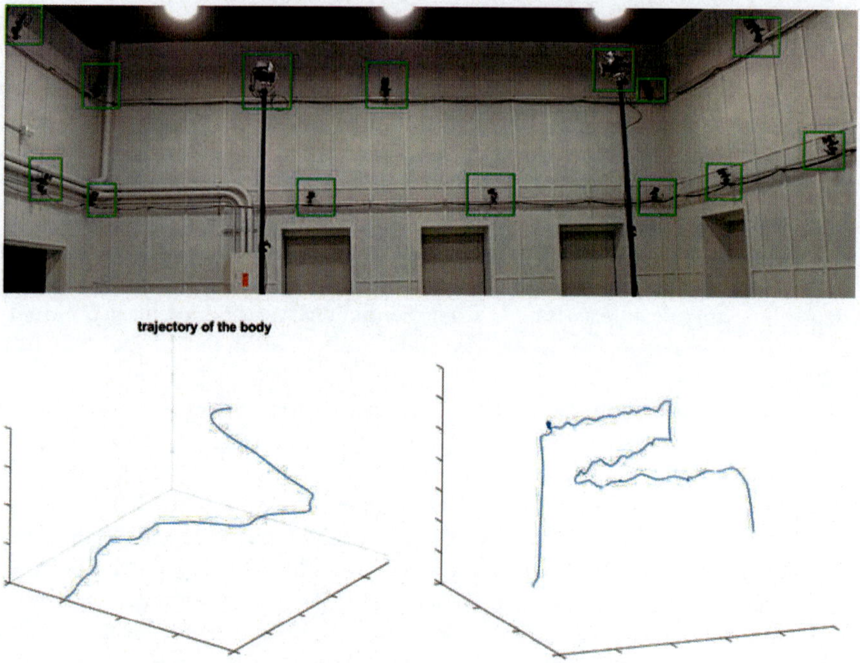

Fig. 2 Motion Capture System to validate performance of visual-inertial fusion

References

1. D. Damen, et al., Scaling egocentric vision: the epic-kitchens dataset, in *Proceedings of the European Conference on Computer Vision (ECCV)* (2018)
2. M.S. Ryoo, L. Matthies, First-person activity recognition: what are they doing to me? in *Proceedings of the IEEE Conference on Computer Vision and Pattern Recognition* (2013)
3. C. Schuldt, I. Laptev, B. Caputo, Recognizing human actions: a local SVM approach, in *Proceedings of the 17th International Conference on Pattern Recognition, ICPR 2004*, vol. 3 (IEEE, Piscataway, 2004)
4. H. Wang, et al., Action recognition by dense trajectories, in *IEEE Conference on Computer Vision & Pattern Recognition CVPR 2011* (IEEE, Piscataway, 2011)
5. R. Dasari, C.W. Chen, A joint visual-inertial image registration for mobile HDR imaging, in *2016 Visual Communications and Image Processing (VCIP)* (IEEE, Piscataway, 2016)
6. M. Grundmann, V. Kwatra, I. Essa, Auto-directed video stabilization with robust l1 optimal camera paths, in *IEEE Conference on Computer Vision & Pattern Recognition CVPR 2011* (IEEE, Piscataway, 2011)
7. C. Forster, M. Pizzoli, D. Scaramuzza, SVO: fast semi-direct monocular visual odometry, in *2014 IEEE International Conference on Robotics and Automation (ICRA)* (IEEE, Piscataway, 2014)
8. G. Hanning, et al., Stabilizing cell phone video using inertial measurement sensors, in *2011 IEEE International Conference on Computer Vision Workshops (ICCV Workshops)* (IEEE, Piscataway, 2011)

Part III
Image Processing and Computer Vision – Novel Algorithms and Applications

Sensor Scheduling for Airborne Multi-target Tracking with Limited Sensor Resources

Simon Koch and Peter Stütz

1 Overview

Situational awareness in the context of this work means knowledge about the presence, location, and other characteristics of certain moving objects of interest (referred to as the *target objects* or *targets* in short) in the mission area. We primarily consider visual (electro-optical and infrared) sensors although the proposed methods could be applied to other means of perceiving the environment as well. In the mentioned exemplary use cases, it is essential that multiple, spatially scattered targets can be tracked simultaneously. However, it is generally not always possible to observe all relevant targets at the same time. This leads to a challenging decision problem commonly referred to as the sensor scheduling or the view planning problem [1–3]. The sensor coverage provided by a single UAV is not large enough to accommodate all of the targets due to their many possible geometric constellations within the mission area. One possible solution would be to distribute the task to multiple UAVs, leading to a considerable coordination effort. Instead of increasing sensor coverage by the sheer number of sensors, we pursue a different idea and relax the requirement for truly concurrent observations to actively managed, quasi-simultaneous ones. An appropriately planned sequence of target observations, feedback control loops to reposition and reorient the sensor as needed, and sophisticated state estimation filters can be sufficient in many cases. To what degree this assumption is adequate and how individual aspects of computer vision, tracking, and scheduling algorithms contribute to the overall surveillance performance are central research objectives for a series of upcoming studies to which this one marks the starting point.

S. Koch (✉) · P. Stütz
University of the Bundeswehr Munich, Neubiberg, Germany
e-mail: simon.koch@unibw.de; peter.stuetz@unibw.de

H. R. Arabnia et al. (eds.), *Advances in Computer Vision and Computational Biology*, Transactions on Computational Science and Computational Intelligence,
https://doi.org/10.1007/978-3-030-71051-4_16

In previous research [4], we demonstrated that model-based adaptive algorithm selection can improve the surveillance performance of UAVs. Now, we aim to transfer the knowledge gained there and generalize the findings for every relevant aspect of the proposed architecture. Hence, we briefly present the overall structure of our concept in the following before we dedicate the remainder of this paper to the discussion of scheduling schemes for target observations and provide some preliminary simulation experiments.

2 Conceptual Design

Structurally, we conceive four distinct components of our system that form a functional decision cycle, depicted in Fig. 1.

The first module incorporates different object recognition computer vision algorithms. As mentioned in [4], we established that the object detection performance of an airborne surveillance system (using the same set of visual sensors) can be increased by using models to predict which, out of multiple available CV algorithms, yields the highest performance with regard to geometric and environmental characteristics of the scene. We revisit the same idea plan to extend it to the other system components as well.

The module outputs object detections to the second tracking stage. Although it is a very important part of our system, we will not discuss it in great detail because we want to emphasize the scheduling component. For these intents, it suffices to abstract away the details of filter design and assume that data association, track

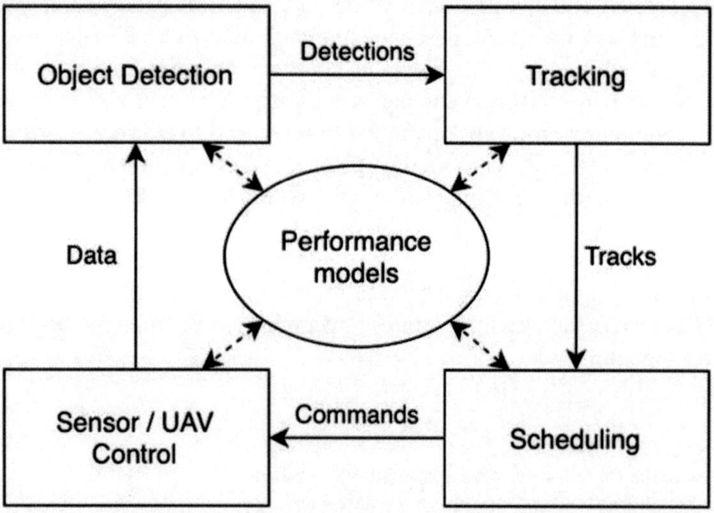

Fig. 1 Overview of the proposed functional design

maintenance, estimation filtering, and gating problems are handled here (i.e., by employing a multi-target capable form of unscented Kalman or particle filters). The expected outputs of tracking algorithms are the estimated target states along with correspondent uncertainties for all targets that have been observed so far (even those that are not located in the current sensor footprint).

In the general case, as discussed, there may be more targets than will fit into a single sensor footprint – implying that based on the state estimates, a schedule must be created which is expressed as a sequence of targets to be observed next. The schedule can be derived through various means, i.e., by applying a scheduling policy that maximizes a defined criterion. Other approaches that will be examined in future work include various techniques from the field of reinforcement learning, i.e., deep Q-learning. A learning agent could potentially be trained to infer suitable observation sequences from the own and the target states [5].

Finally, a set of control algorithms is required to execute the determined schedule, thus closing the feedback loop and providing image data to the detection algorithms. Control can potentially be exerted in every degree of freedom that the UAV and its sensor equipment offer. In other words, translational and rotational adjustments to the sensor pose (and the resulting modification of the sensor footprint) are carried out by various control algorithms that can take into account kinematic constraints of the flight hardware and mission-specific factors.

In any case, performance models present a promising approach to increase the respective performance of each individual component (apart from CV for which this property has already been demonstrated) with regard to mission requirements, as well as environmental circumstances (e.g., affecting visibility) and geometric relationships between the observing UAV and the targets. Consider the extremely large search space that covers all possible target state permutations. It is clear that in certain situations, there will be performance differences between different planning algorithms, and it is unlikely that the same algorithm will lead to the highest performance in all scenarios. Rather, it seems plausible that an adaptive system combining the advantages of a group of scheduling policies is a reasonable strategy to solve the scheduling problem. To explore this idea in more detail, we need to find appropriate means of planning target observations, analyze their properties, and identify situations in which they are particularly suitable. These characteristics can then be stored in performance models and exploited during the mission.

3 Sensor Scheduling

Given the established goal of tracking multiple targets with a single sensor, it is obvious that it is not always possible to observe all relevant targets simultaneously. This leads to a challenging decision problem commonly referred to as the sensor scheduling or the view planning problem.

Scheduling problems appear in many technical and nontechnical domains (i.e., Operations Research), with lots of recent research being done on them [6–8].

The family of periodic scheduling problems are proven to be NP-hard in [9]. Consequently, most research studies probabilistic or deterministic heuristics as a solution strategy. Yavuz and Jeffcoat [3] reduce a periodic scheduling problem to a problem similar to the one at hand: What is the optimal schedule for a sensor to follow if (1) only *one* target can be measured at a time, (2) each observation takes exactly one timestep, and (3) sensor movement happens instantaneously (in other words, a different object can be measured at each timestep). Costello et al. [10] provide insight into active vision systems, which they use to track people with Pan-Tilt-Zoom (PTZ) cameras. They evaluate the performance of their system against the number of people that are viewed only once and the number of people viewed multiple times in a given simulated scenario. Ward and Naish [11] compile and propose suitable scheduling policies they incorporate into a multi-target tracking system, albeit one that utilizes multiple cameras mounted together in an array. A comprehensive survey on active vision in the fields of surveillance, tracking, search, exploration, and more is given in [12].

For our purposes, the sensor scheduling problem translates into the task of deciding which target(s) should be observed when. To achieve that, a tuple of sensor-related settings (i.e., sensor position and orientation, zoom level, etc.) must be provided at a given time to the subsequent control loop, which in turn adjust the sensor settings. A visual example of the problem is shown in Fig. 2. Given the instantaneous sensor parameters, only two of the five target objects shown in the figure can be observed. Colored in blue is the target that will be observed next, according to the scheduling policy in place. The remaining two targets (illustrated in red) could, for instance, be prioritized lower because the control effort required to observe them is larger or their last measurement is more recent than that of the blue one. While a target is not being observed, its state can only be estimated. Intuitively, the uncertainties in these estimations grow larger with every timestep a target is not observed. However, the rate at which the estimation error grows is unique to each single target as their dynamic properties and levels of activity may all be different from one to another. Every time a target is observed, the estimation error is minimal with regard to the geometric constellation, the measurement properties, and the employed tracking algorithm.

3.1 Scheduling Policies

There is an abundance of research on scheduling policies for all kinds of applications in which sparse resources must be assigned a timeslot [13–15]. In this paper, we demonstrate our evaluation environment of four common, easy to implement schedule policies [10].

- Random

  This simplest of all policies randomly selects a target to be observed next, regardless of its last time of measurement.

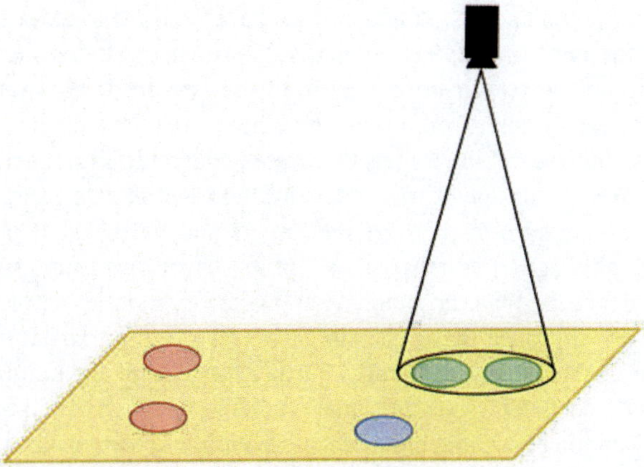

Fig. 2 Example of a situation with five targets: two of them are being observed (green), while three others are scheduled with different priorities (blue/red)

- Round-robin
  The sequence of target observations is determined by the order of which the targets first were detected.
- Earliest deadline first
  This policy considers the time since an object has been measured last. It selects the target which has the least recent last measurement.
- Least effort
  The least effort policy always selects the target next that requires the least amount of gimbal activity to achieve a target lock.

3.2 Quality Measures and Discussion of Challenges

To study the effects of different scheduling schemes in experiments, a measure to quantify the performance of the system is needed. A straightforward approach we use in our initial experiments is the mean elapsed time without observation, which makes it easy to get an intuition for the systems performance. It can be interpreted as the mean time between two observations of the same target.

However, there are many other options as well: Throughout the field of scheduling problems, performance is often expressed as raw throughput of the system or the utilization of available capacity. An equivalent to our problem would be the number targets that can be tracked quasi-simultaneously. While that is an important metric, for the use case of target tracking (which implies some form of reidentification), the residual deviation of the estimated target states must be eventually considered as well. For that purpose, criteria like the Mean Squared Error (MSE) or the Normalized Estimation Error Squared (NEES) [16] seem suitable. In any case, both metrics need to be balanced and adapted to the mission task before a quantitative evaluation of the performance can be made. Consider the following aspect (which was not mentioned so far) of initialization of the system: If the number of targets in the mission area is unknown, a portion of the available sensor observation time must be dedicated to searching targets that were not acquired yet, analogous to track-while-scan (TWS) radar operating modes. Matters complicate further when taking into account kinematic properties of the targets and the UAV. It is reasonable to expect that a highly agile UAV that can adapt its sensor pose very quickly would be able to execute a more dynamic schedule and possibly more effective schedule than a slower one. To approach these questions, we restrict the translational degrees of freedom of the UAV in this initial study. Further, we assume the number of targets to track as known and fixed. One additional challenge is that experiments to evaluate performance cannot be conducted with prerecorded sensor data. Therefore, they must be performed in simulations as it would be otherwise impossible to create repeatable scenarios for testing scheduling schemes. In other words, the system must be evaluated online since it reacts to the actions of the targets.

4 Evaluation Environment

For the development and evaluation of the concept, we introduce simplifications for the targets and components of the system other than the scheduling module. Their respective behaviors are modeled with probabilistic methods.

For the inertial frame, we assume a cartesian ECEF coordinate system. Further, our work is based on a constant timestep discretization. We aim to provide accurate tracking of targets located on the ground plane. More specifically, tracking formally means the measurement of the kinematic target state vector $\overrightarrow{x}$, which encodes the object's instantaneous location in x and y coordinates along with its orientation ψ and velocity v. At each timestep, the target velocity and yaw rate are updated, resulting in the trajectories that are displayed in Fig. 3. We provide the scheduler with approximate guesses of the initial target states (marked with "x").

The number of targets within the environment ultimately shall be variable, since target objects may enter or leave the mission area at any point in time. In this study though, we assume the number of targets n_t in the environment as known and constant throughout the simulation. Further, we restrict the UAV from translational movement, hence mimicking a loitering maneuver. In this case, only gimbal commands have to be scheduled. Additionally, we assume first-order gimbal movement behavior, meaning gimbal movements occur with a constant rotational velocity of ω_g. To compensate for CV challenges such as motion blur, we assume that the target detection algorithm only outputs valid data, when the sensor is locked onto a target, in other words not moving to acquire a target. We use ray tracing to determine whether an object is in view. Possible misclassifications are accounted for by dropping virtual frames with a probability of p_e. As stated before, tracking details are extremely simplified – every successfully detected object is considered

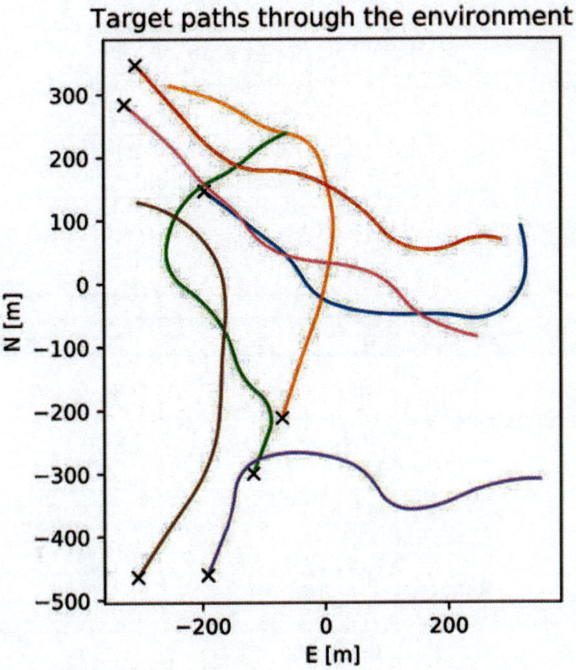

Fig. 3 Exemplary target paths through the environment. Notice the initial target locations marked with "x"

to be tracked when observable for at least $f_{\min}$ continuous frames. Estimated target states are simulated from the ground truth data and hence are subject to an additional random measurement error $\boldsymbol{R}$.

5 Experimental Demonstration

The preliminary experiments were conducted as a plausibility check and to illustrate performance differences that can possibly be exploited in the future development of a model-based, active scheduler. The only metric considered at present is therefore the mean elapsed time between measurements.

Table 1 summarizes important parameters in the simulation runs. In the simulation experiments, the UAV is placed centrally above the mission area, in which the targets are initialized at random starting positions. The targets are modeled as point masses. To prevent statistical artifacts, each policy is evaluated in a Monte-Carlo fashion over one thousand random scenarios.

Figure 4 displays the resulting mean values for the interval between measurements. No significant performance difference can be determined between random

Table 1 Simulation parameters

Number of scenarios per policy	1000
Duration of a scenario	60 s
Probability of misclassification p_e	10 %
Min. #frames to generate detections $f_{\min}$	30
Number of tracked targets n_t	7
Max. gimbal speed ω_g	180 °/s
Sensor FOV	45°
UAV altitude	50 m

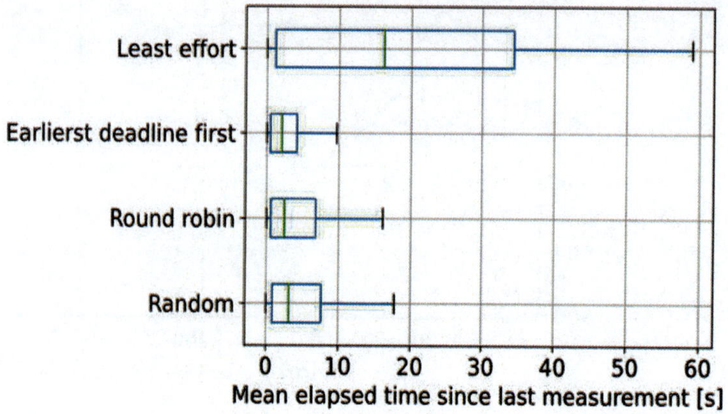

Fig. 4 Simulation results for different scheduling algorithms

and round-robin scheduling. Their mean intervals between measurements are 5.5 s and 5.7 s, with standard deviations of 6.8 s and 8.3 s, respectively. At times though, schedule policies that does not take into account the target states (as these two do) can be hard to follow by the control loop, which leads to long reacquiring phases and large outliers. The earliest deadline first policy performs the highest, with a mean interval of only 3.1 s of simulated time between measurements and a standard deviation of 3.6 s. This is expected as the whole purpose of this policy is to prioritize the oldest measurements, thus keeping the average low. A least effort approach, at least as implemented at this stage, often loses targets who are not in close proximity to the current one because it gets trapped on clusters of close-by targets. Unsurprisingly, its mean interval between observations of 19.8 s and 18.1 s standard deviation is both much larger than those of the other policies.

This does not generally rule out such a type of scheduling policy per se for the purpose of multi-target tracking with a single sensor since in some situations, this behavior may be beneficial under other mission restrictions (i.e., limited energy resources).

6 Conclusion and Future Work

A concept for a UAV-based, single-sensor, multi-target tracking system has been presented. After a short overview of the system components, especially the challenging aspect of sensor scheduling was elaborated in more detail. A simulation environment was developed that allows for easy testing of similar setups and following research.

Four different scheduling policies were subject to initial simulation experiments, in which quite a difference in scheduling performance, measured as the mean elapsed time since the last measurement was attested. These results may lead to similar performance models as have been presented for object detections algorithms in [4]. It seems plausible that different scheduling policies better suited for different situations than others – creating opportunities to successfully apply performance models.

While it performed well in these experiments, the earliest deadline first policy could deliver less admirable results in scenarios where targets interact with each other and purposefully try to evade tracking by moving strategically. These and many more details will have to be studied in future research so they can be stored and actively exploited using performance models.

Among other things, a complete implementation of the detection algorithms and tracking filters will reduce the influence of simplifications that were used here. A realistic initialization with an unknown and variable number of target objects will help to create a system that is applicable on real-world data as well. Restrictions that have been imposed here for simplicity will be loosened (and complicate matters even further, i.e., by opening up the whole field of path planning). Finally, alternative and more sophisticated means for the scheduling aspect should be examined, i.e., by utilizing deep reinforcement learning-based schedulers.

References

1. P. Wang, R. Krishnamurti, K. Gupta, View planning problem with combined view and traveling Cost, in *Proceedings 2007 IEEE International Conference on Robotics and Automation, Rome, Italy*, (2007), pp. 711–716. https://doi.org/10.1109/ROBOT.2007.363070
2. C. Rusu, J. Thompson, N.M. Robertson, Sensor scheduling with time, energy, and communication constraints. IEEE Trans. Signal Process. **66**(2), 528–539 (2018). https://doi.org/10.1109/TSP.2017.2773429
3. M. Yavuz, D. Jeffcoat, An analysis and solution of the sensor scheduling problem, in *Advances in cooperative control and optimization*, ed. by P. M. Pardalos, R. Murphey, D. Grundel, M. J. Hirsch, vol. 369, (Springer Berlin Heidelberg, Berlin, Heidelberg, 2007), pp. 167–177
4. C. Hellert, S. Koch, P. Stütz, Using algorithm selection for adaptive vehicle perception aboard UAV, in *16th IEEE International Conference on Advanced Video and Signal Based Surveillance (AVSS)*, (Taipei, 2019, 2019), pp. 1–8. https://doi.org/10.1109/AVSS.2019.8909862
5. J.Z. Stadlan, To follow the targets, follow the reward: A reinforcement learning approach to multi-target tracking with a multi-function radar, 4

6. H. Xu, S. Koenig, T.K.S. Kumar, Towards effective deep learning for constraint satisfaction problems, in *Principles and Practice of Constraint Programming*, ed. by J. Hooker, vol. 11008, (Springer International Publishing, Cham, 2018), pp. 588–597
7. S. Amizadeh, S. Matusevych, M. Weimer, PDP: A general neural framework for learning constraint satisfaction solvers. ArXiv190301969 Cs Stat (2019)., Accessed: 14 Apr 2020. [Online]. Available: http://arxiv.org/abs/1903.01969
8. Y. Xu, D. Stern, H. Samulowitz, Learning adaptation to solve constraint satisfaction problems, 5
9. A. Bar-Noy, R. Bhatia, J. (Seffi) Naor, B. Schieber, Minimizing service and operation costs of periodic scheduling. Math. Oper. Res. **27**(3), 518–544 (Aug. 2002). https://doi.org/10.1287/moor.27.3.518.314
10. C.J. Costello, C.P. Diehl, A. Banerjee, H. Fisher, Scheduling an active camera to observe people, in *Proceedings of the ACM 2nd international workshop on Video surveillance & sensor networks - VSSN '04*, (NY, USA, New York, 2004), p. 39. https://doi.org/10.1145/1026799.1026808
11. C.D.W. Ward, M.D. Naish, Scheduling active camera resources for multiple moving targets, in *2009 Canadian Conference on Electrical and Computer Engineering*, (St. John's, NL, Canada, 2009), pp. 528–532. https://doi.org/10.1109/CCECE.2009.5090187
12. S. Chen, Y. Li, N.M. Kwok, Active vision in robotic systems: A survey of recent developments. Int. J. Robot. Res. **30**(11), 1343–1377 (Sep. 2011). https://doi.org/10.1177/0278364911410755
13. M. Shahsavari, M.F. Nadeem, S.A. Ostadzadeh, Z. Al-Ars, K. Bertels, Task Scheduling Policies in General Distributed Systems: A Survey and Possibilities, 19
14. A. Gantman, P. Guo, J. Lewis, and F. Rashid, Scheduling real-time tasks in distributed systems: A survey
15. A. Banerjee, F. Esposito, A survey of scheduling policies in software defined networks, in *2017 IEEE International Conference on Advanced Networks and Telecommunications Systems (ANTS)*, (Bhubaneswar, 2017), pp. 1–6. https://doi.org/10.1109/ANTS.2017.8384177
16. Y. Bar-Shalom, X.-R. Li, *Estimation and Tracking: Principles, Techniques, and Software* (Artech House, Boston, 1993)

Superpixel-Based Multi-focus Image Fusion

Kuan-Ni Lai and Jin-Jang Leou

1 Introduction

Due to the finite depth of field of optical lenses, it is difficult to make all objects in an image sharp and clear. Only objects within the depth of field are in focus and sharp, while the others are defocus and blurred. The common solution, namely, multi-focus image fusion, is to extract the focus parts of two or more multi-focus source images in same scene and combine the focus parts into a single fused image.

Multi-focus image fusion approaches can be roughly divided into three categories, namely, transform domain based, spatial domain based, and learning based. For transform domain-based approaches, each multi-focus source image is transformed into some transform domain with transform coefficients. Some fusion rules are applied on the transform coefficients. The fused image is obtained by applying the inverse transform. The commonly used transforms include discrete wavelet transform (DWT) [1, 2], stationary wavelet transform (SWT) [3], complex wavelet transform (CWT) [4], dual-tree complex wavelet transform (DT-CWT) [5], dual-tree discrete wavelet transform (DT-DWT) [6], contourlet transform (CT) [7], non-subsampled contourlet transform (NSCT) [8, 9], etc.

For spatial domain-based approaches, focus regions from multi-focus source images are directly selected and fused. Spatial domain-based approaches can be roughly divided into three categories: pixel-based, block-based, and region-based. For pixel-based approaches, Aslantas and Toprak [10] proposed a pixel-based multi-focus image fusion approach using point spread function (PSF). Li et al. [11] proposed a multi-focus image fusion approach for dynamic scenes using image

K.-N. Lai · J.-J. Leou (✉)
Department of Computer Science and Information Engineering, National Chung Cheng University, Chiayi, Taiwan
e-mail: lkn104m@cs.ccu.edu.tw; jjleou@cs.ccu.edu.tw

H. R. Arabnia et al. (eds.), *Advances in Computer Vision and Computational Biology*, Transactions on Computational Science and Computational Intelligence,
https://doi.org/10.1007/978-3-030-71051-4_17

matting. Li, Kang, and Hu [12] proposed a multi-focus image fusion approach using guided filtering. Guo, Yan, and Qu [13] proposed a multi-focus image fusion approach using self-similarity and depth information. Liu, Liu, and Wang [14] proposed a multi-focus image fusion approach using dense SIFT.

For block-based approaches, De and Chanda [15] proposed a multi-focus image fusion approach using the morphology-based focus measure in a quad-tree structure. Rahman et al. [16] proposed a multi-focus image fusion approach using degree of focus and fuzzy logic. For region-based approaches, Yang and Guo [17] proposed a superpixel-based fusion and demosaicing approach for multi-focus Bayer images. Duan, Chen, and Chen [18] proposed a multi-focus image fusion approach using superpixel segmentation and mean filtering. Zhang, Bai, and Wang [19] proposed a boundary finding-based multi-focus image fusion approach using multi-scale morphological focus measure.

For learning-based approaches, Mustafa, Yang, and Zareapoor [20] proposed a multi-scale convolutional neural network for multi-focus image fusion, in which a Siamese multi-scale feature extraction module is employed. Yang et al. [21] proposed a multilevel features convolutional neural network architecture for image fusion. Zhao, Wang, and Lu [22] proposed an end-to-end deep convolutional neural network for multi-focus image fusion. In this study, a superpixel-based multi-focus image fusion approach is proposed.

The paper is organized as follows. The proposed multi-focus image fusion approach is described in Sect. 2. Experimental results are addressed in Sect. 3, followed by concluding remarks.

2 Proposed Approach

2.1 System Architecture

As shown in Fig. 1, the proposed approach contains three main stages. First, each multi-focus source image is performed superpixel segmentation, and the saliency, depth, and difference image information are computed. Second, each superpixel is classified into one of three (focus, defocus, and undefined) types, and each undefined superpixel is determined as focus or defocus by sum-modified-Laplacian (SML). The initial focus maps are estimated and then refined by matting Laplacian-based image interpolation. Third, the boundaries between focus and defocus regions are employed to generate the weighting maps, followed by fused image generation.

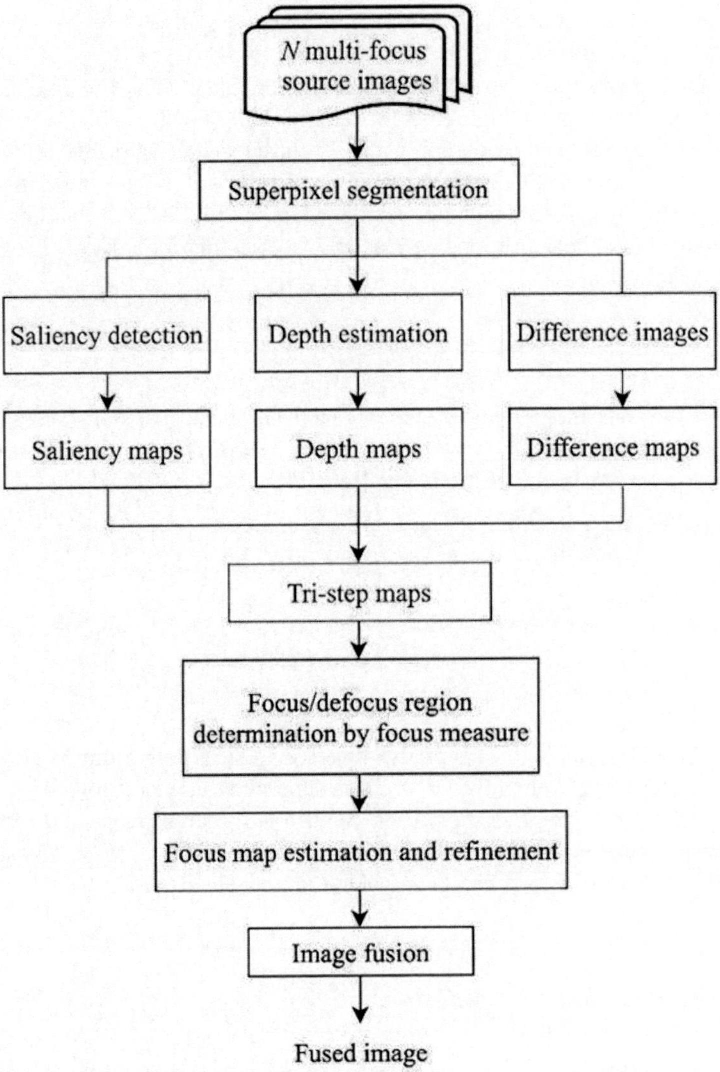

Fig. 1 Framework of the proposed approach

2.2 *Superpixel Segmentation*

Assume that there are N multi-focus source images of size $W \times H$ $L_n(x, y)$, $n = 1$, $2, \ldots, N$, $1 \leq x \leq W$, $1 \leq y \leq H$. In this study, each multi-focus source image is transformed from RGB color space to CIE-Lab color space. Here, pixel (x, y) in the n-th multi-focus source image can be represented as a five-dimensional (5D) vector:

$$C_n(x, y) = [l_n\ a_n\ b_n\ x\ y]^T, n = 1, 2, \ldots, N, 1 \leq x \leq W, 1 \leq y \leq H, \quad (1)$$

where l_n, a_n, and b_n denote the CIE-Lab color component values of pixel (x, y).

Because pixels having high-gradient values usually lie on the boundary between focus and defocus regions or noise, the K cluster centers are selected as pixels having small gradient values. Neighboring pixels with high similarities (short distances) to any cluster center are searched all pixels in a 2w × 2w sliding window and grouped into the corresponding cluster. Distance (dissimilarity) D between two pixels is defined as

$$D = \sqrt{d_c^2 + (d_s/w)^2 m^2}, \quad (2)$$

where m is a constant [23], and d_c and d_s denote color and spatial distances between pixels $C_n(x,y) = [l_n\ a_n\ b_n\ x\ y]^T$ and $C_n'(x', y') = [l_n'\ a_n'\ b_n'\ x'\ y']^T$ in the n-th multi-focus source image, respectively. Here, d_c and d_s are defined as

$$d_c = \sqrt{\left(l_n - l_n'\right)^2 + (a_n - a_n')^2 + \left(b_n - b_n'\right)^2}, \quad (3)$$

$$d_s = \sqrt{(x - x')^2 + (y - y')^2}. \quad (4)$$

In this study, simple linear iterative clustering (SLIC) algorithm [23] based on K-means clustering is employed to perform superpixel segmentation.

After all pixels are classified, each multi-focus source image will contain K superpixels, denoted as $Sp_{n,k}$, $k = 1, 2, \ldots, K, n = 1, 2, \ldots, N$. In this study, on the average, each superpixel will contain approximately 60 pixels.

2.3 *Information Computation*

In the study, the saliency, depth, and difference image information are computed and used to classify superpixels into three types (focus, defocus, and undefined). After performing Fourier transform on each multi-focus source image $L_n(x, y)$, the spectral residual $\text{Residual}_n(u, v)$ and phase spectrum $\text{Phase}_n(u, v)$ for frequency component (u, v) will be obtained [24]. The saliency value of pixel (x, y) is computed as

$$\text{Saliency}_n(x, y) = g * \mathfrak{F}^{-1}\left[\exp\left(\text{Residual}(u, v) + \text{Phase}(u, v)\right)\right]^2, \quad (5)$$

where $\mathfrak{F}^{-1}(\bullet)$ denotes the inverse Fourier transform, g denotes the Gaussian filter, and * denotes the convolution operation.

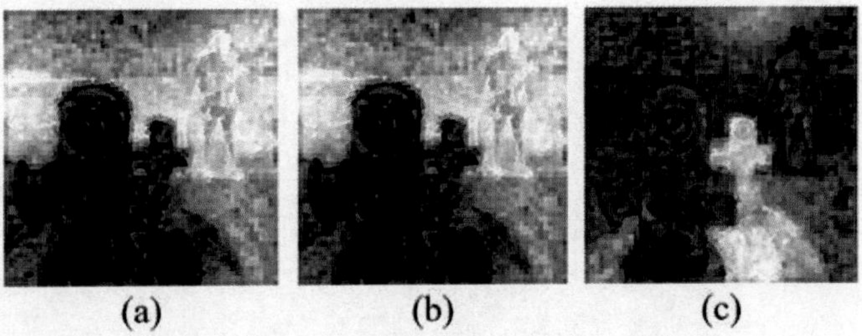

Fig. 2 (**a–c**) Superpixel-based saliency detection maps of three illustrated multi-focus source images

The average value of the saliency values of all pixels within a superpixel is used as the saliency value $\text{SpSaliency}_{n,k}$ of superpixel $\text{Sp}_{n,k}$, i.e.,

$$\text{SpSaliency}_{n,k} = \frac{1}{\left|\text{Sp}_{n,k}\right|} \sum_{(x,y)\epsilon \text{Sp}_{n,k}} \text{Saliency}_n\,(x, y)\,, \tag{6}$$

where $|\text{Sp}_{n,k}|$ denotes the number of pixels in superpixel $\text{Sp}_{n,k}$. The superpixel-based saliency maps of three illustrated multi-focus source images are shown in Fig. 2. In this study, the depth estimation method proposed in Zhuo and Sim [25] is employed. First, the sparse depth map $\hat{d}_n\,(x, y)$ of the n-th multi-focus source image is obtained by using Canny edge detector [26] and joint bilateral filtering (JBF) [27]. Then by using matting Laplacian-based image interpolation [28], the depth map $d_n(x, y)$ of the n-th multi-focus source image can be obtained by minimizing

$$\begin{aligned} E\,(d_n\,(x, y)) = {} & d_n(x, y)^T M_{L,n} d_n\,(x, y) \\ & + \lambda\Big(d_n\,(x, y) - \hat{d}_n\,(x, y)\Big)^T \text{Diag}\,\Big(d_n\,(x, y) - \hat{d}_n\,(x, y)\Big)\,, \end{aligned} \tag{7}$$

where $M_{L,n}$ denotes matting Laplacian matrix, λ denotes a smoothness parameter, and Diag denotes a diagonal matrix with each main diagonal element being set to 1 for edge position and 0 otherwise.

The average value of the depth values of all pixels within a superpixel is used as the depth value $\text{SpDepth}_{n,k}$ of superpixel $\text{Sp}_{n,k}$, i.e.,

$$\text{SpDepth}_{n,k} = \frac{1}{\left|\text{Sp}_{n,k}\right|} \sum_{(x,y)\in \text{Sp}_{n,k}} d_n\,(x, y)\,. \tag{8}$$

Superpixel-based depth maps of three illustrated multi-focus source images are shown in Fig. 3.

Inspired by the approaches in Aslantas and Toprak [10] and Yan et al. [29], difference image of two images with different blurring can be used to detect image texture. In this study, Gaussian filter is applied on the intensity image $I_n(x, y)$ of

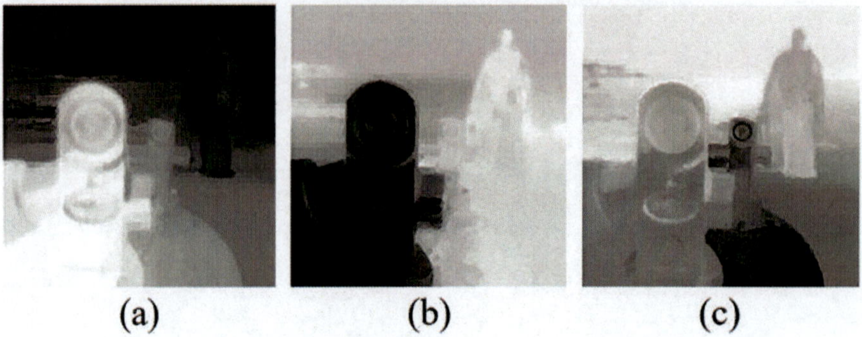

Fig. 3 (a–c) Superpixel-based depth maps of three illustrated multi-focus source images

each multi-focus source image $L_n(x, y)$ to obtain the corresponding blurred image $B_n(x, y)$. The difference image $\mathrm{dif}_n(x, y)$ of the n-th multi-focus image is defined as

$$\mathrm{dif}_n(x, y) = I_n(x, y) - B_n(x, y). \tag{9}$$

The intensity variance $\mathrm{IV}_n(x, y)$ [29] of the n-th difference image $\mathrm{dif}_n(x, y)$ is defined as

$$\mathrm{IV}_n(x, y) = \frac{1}{r \times r} \sum\nolimits_{i=-r}^{r} \sum\nolimits_{j=-r}^{r} \left(\mathrm{dif}_n(x+i, y+j) - \mu_n\right)^2, \tag{10}$$

where μ_n denotes the average pixel value of the n-th difference image $\mathrm{dif}_n(x, y)$. Similarly, the difference image variance value $\mathrm{SpIV}_{n,k}$ of superpixel $\mathrm{Sp}_{n,k}$ is defined as

$$\mathrm{SpIV}_{n,k} = \frac{1}{|\mathrm{Sp}_{n,k}|} \sum_{(x,y) \in \mathrm{Sp}_{n,k}} \mathrm{IV}_n(x, y). \tag{11}$$

Superpixel-based difference image maps of three illustrated multi-focus source images are shown in Fig. 4.

2.4 Foreground and Background Label Estimation

Based on $\mathrm{SpSaliency}_{n,k}$, the saliency map $\mathrm{SaliencyMap}_{n,k}$ for superpixel $\mathrm{Sp}_{n,k}$ is defined as

$$\mathrm{SaliencyMap}_{n,k} = \begin{cases} 1 \text{ (focus)}, \text{ if } \mathrm{SpSaliency}_{\mathrm{n,k}} > t^{l}_{n,k}, \\ 0 \text{ (defocus)}, \text{ otherwise}, \end{cases} \tag{12}$$

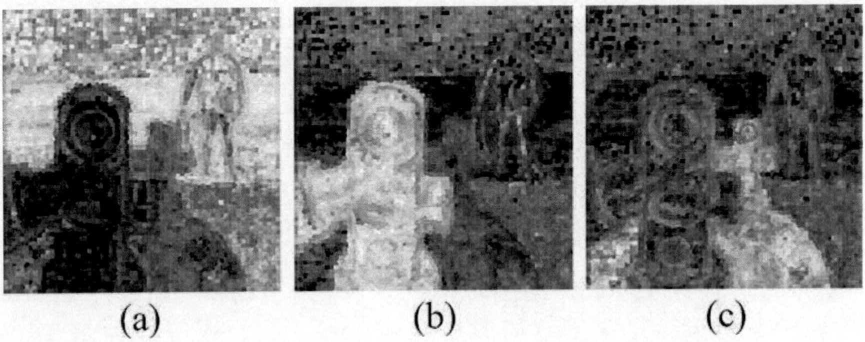

Fig. 4 (**a–c**) Superpixel-based difference image maps of three illustrated multi-focus source images

where threshold $t_{n,k}^{l}$ is computed by

$$t_{n,k}^{l} = \frac{1}{N \times \left|\mathrm{Sp}_{n,k}\right|} \sum_{n=1}^{N} \sum_{(x,y)\epsilon \mathrm{Sp}_{n,k}} \mathrm{Saliency}_n(x, y). \tag{13}$$

The depth map $\mathrm{DepthMap}_{n,k}$ for each superpixel $\mathrm{Sp}_{n,k}$ is defined as

$$\mathrm{DepthMap}_{n,k} = \begin{cases} 1 \text{ (focus) , if } \mathrm{SpDepth}_{n,k} < t_{n,k}^{2}, \\ 0 \text{ (defocus) , otherwise,} \end{cases} \tag{14}$$

where threshold $t_{n,k}^{2}$ is computed as

$$t_{n,k}^{2} = \frac{1}{N \times \left|\mathrm{Sp}_{n,k}\right|} \sum_{n=1}^{N} \sum_{(x,y)\epsilon \mathrm{Sp}_{n,k}} d_n(x, y). \tag{15}$$

The difference map $\mathrm{DiffMap}_{n,k}$ for superpixel $\mathrm{Sp}_{n,k}$ is defined as

$$\mathrm{DiffMap}_{n,k} = \begin{cases} 1 \text{ (focus) , if } \mathrm{SpIV}_{n,k} > t_{n,k}^{3}, \\ 0 \text{ (defocus) , otherwise,} \end{cases} \tag{16}$$

where threshold $t_{n,k}^{3}$ is computed as

$$t_{n,k}^{3} = \frac{1}{N \times \left|\mathrm{Sp}_{n,k}\right|} \sum_{n=1}^{N} \sum_{(x,y)\in \mathrm{Sp}_{n,k}} IV_n(x, y). \tag{17}$$

Based on $\text{SaliencyMap}_{n,k}$, $\text{DepthMap}_{n,k}$, and $\text{DiffMap}_{n,k}$, the tri-step map $\text{TriMap}_{n,k}$ for superpixel $\text{Sp}_{n,k}$ is defined as

$$\text{TriMap}_{n,k} = \begin{cases} 1\ (\text{focus}),\ \text{if SaliencyMap}_{n,k} \\ \qquad +\text{DepthMap}_{n,k} + \text{DiffMap}_{n,k} = 3, \\ 0.5\ (\text{undefined}),\ \text{if } 1 \le \text{SaliencyMap}_{n,k} \\ \qquad + \text{DepthMap}_{n,k} + \text{DiffMap}_{n,k} < 3, \\ 0\ (\text{defocus}),\ \text{otherwise}. \end{cases} \tag{18}$$

To deal with undefined superpixels, sum-modified-Laplacian (SML) [30] is employed. Here, modified Laplacian $\text{ML}_n(x, y)$ of pixel (x, y) can be defined as

$$\begin{aligned} \text{ML}_n(x, y) = &\left|2I_n(x, y) - I_n(x-1, y) - I_n(x+1, y)\right| \\ &+ \left|2I_n(x, y) - I_n\big(x, y-1\big) - I_n\big(x, y+1\big)\right|. \end{aligned} \tag{19}$$

Then sum-modified-Laplacian $\text{SML}_n(x, y)$ is defined as

$$\text{SML}_n(x, y) = \sum_{i=x-r}^{x+r} \sum_{j=y-r}^{y+r} \text{ML}_n(i, j), \tag{20}$$

where r is empirically set to 3. SML value of superpixel $\text{Sp}_{n,k}$ is defined as

$$\text{SML}_{n,k} = \frac{1}{\left|\text{Sp}_{n,k}\right|} \sum_{(x,y)\in \text{Sp}_{n,k}} \text{SML}_n(x, y). \tag{21}$$

The initial focus map is defined as

$$\text{IniFocusMap}_{n,k} = \begin{cases} 1\ (\text{focus}),\ \text{if TriMap}_{n,k} = 1 \text{ or } \text{SML}_{n,k} > t^4_{n,k}, \\ 0\ (\text{defocus}),\ \text{otherwise}, \end{cases} \tag{22}$$

where $t^4_{n,k}$ is defined as

$$t^4_{n,k} = \frac{1}{N \times \left|\text{Sp}_{n,k}\right|} \sum_{n=1}^{N} \sum_{(x,y)\in \text{Sp}_{n,k}} \text{SML}_n(x, y). \tag{23}$$

To refine initial focus maps, matting Laplacian-based image interpolation and Otsu's thresholding [31] are successively employed to obtain the focus map $\text{FocusMap}_{n,k}$. Additionally, for multi-focus images, boundaries between focus and defocus regions may be not clear, which should be refined. The weight $\text{WBoundary}_n(x, y)$ of boundary area $\text{Boundary}_n(x, y)$ in $\text{FocusMap}_{n,\,k}$ is defined as

$$\text{WBoundary}_n\,(x, y) = \text{Boundary}_n\,(x, y) \times \text{Dist}_n\,(x, y) \times \text{SML}_n\,(x, y)\,, \qquad (24)$$

where $\text{Dist}_n(x, y)$ denotes the distance between pixel (x, y) and the nearest neighbor focus pixel in $\text{FocusMap}_{n,\,k}$.

2.5 *Image Fusion*

The weighting maps of the fused image are computed as

$$\text{WeightMap}_n\,(x, y) = \left(\text{WBoundary}_n\,(x, y) + \text{FocusMap}_n\,\,(x, y)\right) / \text{SumMap}\,(x, y)\,, \qquad (25)$$

where

$$\text{SumMap}\,(x, y) = \sum_{n=1}^{N} \left(\text{WBoundary}_n\,(x, y) + \text{FocusMap}_n\,\,(x, y)\right). \qquad (26)$$

The fused image is generated as.

$$F\,(x, y) = \sum_{n=1}^{N} \text{WeightMap}_n\,(x, y)\, L_n\,(x, y)\,. \qquad (27)$$

3 Experimental Results

In this study, the proposed approach is implemented by Matlab 9.0 (R2016a) on Intel Core i7-6700 K CPU 4.0GHz-Microsoft Windows 7 platform with 32GB main memory. To evaluate the performance of the proposed approach, five comparison approaches based on image matting (IM) [11], guided filtering (GF) [12], shared self-similarity and depth information (SSSDI) [13], dense SIFT (DSIFT) [14], and boundary finding (BF) [19] are employed. Two multi-focus image databases are employed in this study. The first database consists of ten gray multi-focus image pairs and seven color multi-focus image pairs. The second (Lytro) database [32] consists of twenty color multi-focus image pairs and four color multi-focus image sequences (three source images).

In this study, both subjective evaluation and objective image quality metrics are employed. Two multi-focus source images of the first database and the fused images of the five comparison approaches and the proposed approach are shown in Fig. 5,

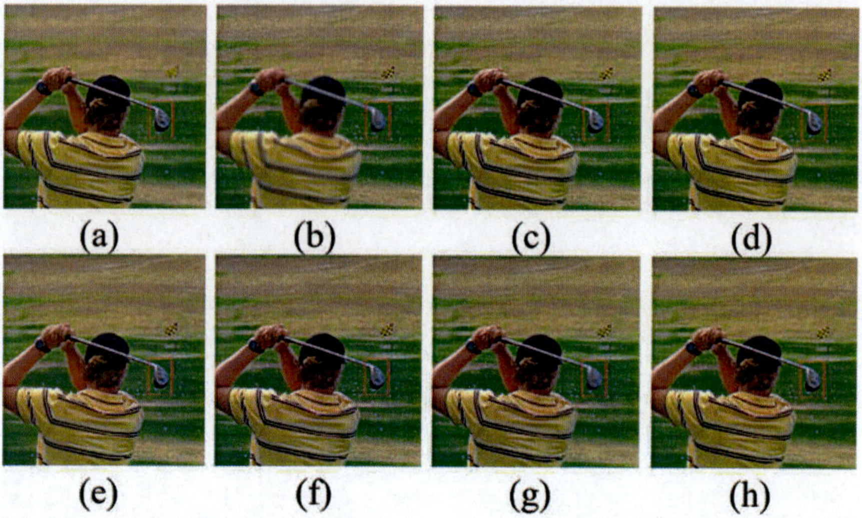

Fig. 5 Two multi-focus source images of the first database (**a**, **b**) and the fused images by (**c**) IM [11], (**d**) GF [12], (**e**) SSSDI [13], (**f**) DSIFT [14], (**g**) BF [19], and (**h**) proposed

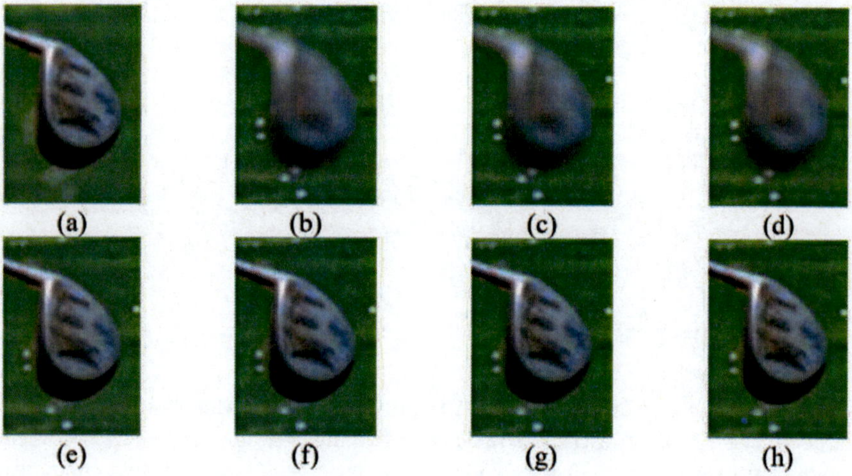

Fig. 6 Some detail parts of two multi-focus source images in Fig. 5 (**a**, **b**) and the fused images in Fig. 5 by (**c**) IM [11], (**d**) GF [12], (**e**) SSSDI [13], (**f**) DSIFT [14], (**g**) BF [19], and (**h**) proposed

while some detail parts of two multi-focus source images in Fig. 5 and the fused images in Fig. 5 are shown in Fig. 6. The image quality of the fused image by the proposed approach is better than those of the five comparison approaches.

In this study, four objective image quality metrics, namely, gradient-based fusion metric ($Q^{AB/F}$) [33], mutual information (MI) [34], nonlinear correlation information entropy (Q_{NCIE}) [35], and Yang's metric (Q_Y) [36], are employed.

Table 1 In terms of average $Q^{AB/F}$, MI, Q_{NICE}, and Q_Y, performance comparisons of the five comparison approaches and the proposed approach for the first database

Methods	Average $Q^{AB/F}$	Average MI	Average Q_{NICE}	Average Q_Y
IM [11]	0.736	8.199	0.840	0.970
GF [12]	0.735	7.630	0.835	0.956
SSSDI [13]	0.734	8.145	0.840	0.967
DSIFT [14]	0.744	8.367	0.841	0.971
BF [19]	0.743	8.358	0.841	0.987
Proposed	**0.747**	**8.484**	**0.843**	**0.990**

Table 2 In terms of average $Q^{AB/F}$, MI, Q_{NICE}, and Q_Y, performance comparisons of the five comparison approaches and the proposed approach for the second (Lytro) database

Methods	Average $Q^{AB/F}$	Average MI	Average Q_{NICE}	Average Q_Y
IM [11]	0.754	8.575	0.840	0.986
GF [12]	0.761	8.241	0.838	0.985
SSSDI [13]	0.759	8.535	0.841	0.988
DSIFT [14]	0.762	8.892	0.844	0.991
BF [19]	0.754	8.743	0.844	0.994
Proposed	**0.765**	**8.921**	**0.846**	**0.997**

Table 3 In terms of average $Q^{AB/F}$ and MI, performance comparisons of the five comparison approaches and the proposed approach for the second (Lytro) database

Methods	Average $Q^{AB/F}$	Average MI
IM [11]	0.632	10.407
GF [12]	0.642	10.223
SSSDI [13]	0.640	10.488
DSIFT [14]	0.642	10.838
BF [19]	0.645	10.760
Proposed	**0.648**	**10.915**

In terms of the four objective image quality metrics, the average performance comparisons between the five comparison approaches and the proposed approach for the two databases are listed in Tables 1, 2, and 3.

4 Concluding Remarks

In this study, a superpixel-based multi-focus image fusion approach is proposed. Based on the experimental results obtained in this study, in terms of both subjective evaluation and objective image quality metrics, the performance of the proposed approach is better than those of five comparison approaches.

Acknowledgments This work was supported in part by Ministry of Science and Technology, Taiwan, ROC under Grants MOST 108-2221-E-194-049 and MOST 109-2221-E-194-042.

References

1. M. Abdipour, M. Nooshyar, Multi-focus image fusion using sharpness criteria for visual sensor networks in wavelet domain. Comput. Electr. Eng. **51**, 74–88 (2016)
2. D. Xiao et al., Multi-focus image fusion and robust encryption algorithm based on compressive sensing. Opt. Laser Technol. **91**, 212–225 (2017)
3. Y. Liu, F. Yu, An automatic image fusion algorithm for unregistered multiply multi-focus images. Opt. Commun. **341**, 101–113 (2015)
4. J.J. Lewis et al., Pixel-and region-based image fusion with complex wavelets. Inform. Fusion **8**(2), 119–130 (2007)
5. S. Wei, W. Ke, A multi-focus image fusion algorithm with DT-CWT, in *Proceedings of 2007 International Conference on Computational Intelligence and Security*, (2007), pp. 147–151
6. J. Saeedi, K. Faez, A classification and fuzzy-based approach for digital multi-focus image fusion. Pattern. Anal. Applic. **16**(3), 365–379 (2013)
7. S. Yang et al., Image fusion based on a new contourlet packet. Inform. Fusion **11**(2), 78–84 (2010)
8. A.L. Da Cunha, J. Zhou, M.N. Do, The nonsubsampled contourlet transform: Theory, design, and applications. IEEE Trans. Image Process. **15**(10), 3089–3101 (2006)
9. J. Adu, S. Xie, J. Gan, Image fusion based on visual salient features and the cross-contrast. J. Vis. Commun. Image Represent. **40**, 218–224 (2016)
10. V. Aslantas, A.N. Toprak, A pixel based multi-focus image fusion method. Opt. Commun. **332**, 350–358 (2014)
11. S. Li et al., Image matting for fusion of multi-focus images in dynamic scenes. Inform. Fusion **14**(2), 147–162 (2013)
12. S. Li, X. Kang, J. Hu, Image fusion with guided filtering. IEEE Trans. Image Process. **22**(7), 2864–2875 (2013)
13. D. Guo, J. Yan, X. Qu, High quality multi-focus image fusion using self-similarity and depth information. Opt. Commun. **338**, 138–144 (2015)
14. Y. Liu, S. Liu, Z. Wang, Multi-focus image fusion with dense SIFT. Inform. Fusion **23**, 139–155 (2015)
15. I. De, B. Chanda, Multi-focus image fusion using a morphology-based focus measure in a quad-tree structure. Inform. Fusion **14**(2), 136–146 (2013)
16. M.A. Rahman et al., Multi-focal image fusion using degree of focus and fuzzy logic. Digital Signal Proc. **60**, 1–19 (2017)
17. B. Yang, L. Guo, Superpixel based fusion and demosaicing for multi-focus Bayer images. Optik-Int. J. Light Elect. Opt. **126**(23), 4460–4468 (2015)
18. J. Duan, L. Chen, C.P. Chen, Multifocus image fusion using superpixel segmentation and superpixel-based mean filtering. Appl. Opt. **55**(36), 10352–10362 (2016)
19. Y. Zhang, X. Bai, T. Wang, Boundary finding based multi-focus image fusion through multi-scale morphological focus measure. Inform. Fusion **35**, 81–101 (2017)
20. H.T. Mustafa, J. Yang, M. Zareapoor, A multi-scale convolutional neural network for multi-focus image fusion. Image Vis. Comput. **85**, 26–35 (2019)
21. Y. Yang et al., Multilevel features convolutional neural network for multifocus image fusion. IEEE Trans. Comput. Imag. **5**(2), 262–273 (2019)
22. W. Zhao, D. Wang, H. Lu, Multi-focus image fusion with a natural enhancement via a joint multi-level deeply supervised convolutional neural network. IEEE Trans. Circ. Syst. Video Technol. **29**(4), 1102–1115 (2019)
23. R. Achanta et al., SLIC superpixels compared to state-of-the-art superpixel methods. IEEE Trans. Pattern Anal. Mach. Intell. **34**(11), 2274–2282 (2012)
24. X. Hou, L. Zhang, Saliency detection: a spectral residual approach, in *Proceedings of 2007 IEEE Conference on Computer Vision and Pattern Recognition*, (2007), pp. 1–8
25. S. Zhuo, T. Sim, Defocus map estimation from a single image. Pattern Recogn. **44**(9), 1852–1858 (2011)

26. J. Canny, A computational approach to edge detection. IEEE Trans. Pattern Anal. Mach. Intell. **8**(6), 679–698 (1986)
27. G. Petschnigg et al., Digital photography with flash and no-flash image pairs. ACM Trans. Graph. **23**(3), 664–672 (2004)
28. A. Levin, D. Lischinski, Y. Weiss, A closed-form solution to natural image matting. IEEE Trans. Pattern Anal. Mach. Intell. **30**(2), 228–242 (2008)
29. X. Yan et al., Multi-focus image fusion using a guided-filter-based difference image. Appl. Opt. **55**(9), 2230–2239 (2016)
30. S.K. Nayar, Y. Nakagawa, Shape from focus. IEEE Trans. Pattern Anal. Mach. Intell. **16**(8), 824–831 (1994)
31. N. Otsu, A threshold selection method from gray-level histograms. IEEE Trans. Syst. Man Cybern. **9**(1), 62–66 (1979)
32. M. Nejati, S. Samavi, S. Shirani, Multi-focus image fusion using dictionary-based sparse representation. Inform. Fusion **25**, 72–84 (2015)
33. C. Xydeas, V. Petrovic, Objective image fusion performance measure. Electron. Lett. **36**(4), 308–309 (2000)
34. G. Qu, D. Zhang, P. Yan, Information measure for performance of image fusion. Electron. Lett. **38**(7), 313–315 (2002)
35. Q. Wang, Y. Shen, J.Q. Zhang, A nonlinear correlation measure for multivariable data set. Physica D: Nonlinear Phenomena **200**(3–4), 287–295 (2005)
36. C. Yang et al., A novel similarity based quality metric for image fusion. Inform. Fusion **9**(2), 156–160 (2008)

Theoretical Applications of Magnetic Fields at Tremendously Low Frequency in Remote Sensing and Electronic Activity Classification

Christopher Duncan, Olga Gkountouna, and Ron Mahabir

1 Introduction

While the utilization of the standard electrical spectrum for purposes of remote sensing has been common place for a long time, the magnetic spectrum has typically been relegated to measurements of polarization in the detection of surface condition and changes [3]. The fact remains, however, that where energy exists, so does a magnetic field and the magnetic field has a host of different properties and behaviors, and an entirely different propagation. It stands to reason that if the magnetic field behaves differently than the electrical field, then perhaps there is more information to be gained by analyzing the magnetic field, particularly that of the near-field at approximately 0.159 times the wavelength of the electrical field [5] and is reactive to the electrical field, while the far-field propagates indefinitely until attenuation.

In 1990, this general premise was validated by the detection of underground nuclear testing occurring on Novaya Zemlya Island, by the Russian satellite Intercosmos 24, which registered the magnetic variations a few minutes after the detonation, on the magnetic tape [2]. While it is possible that the recordings on the magnetic tape were anomalies or changes in pressure, the paper points to the possibility of renewed utility of the magnetic spectrum in the field of remote sensing. Further, satellites have also been used to detect variances in tidal flow by measuring variances in the secondary magnetic fields generated by the movement of the ocean tides from space [4].

The purpose of this research is to explore the possibility and feasibility of these potential applications of the magnetic spectrum, independently from the associated electrical fields. The testing attempts to validate that magnetic fields are

C. Duncan (✉) · O. Gkountouna · R. Mahabir
George Mason University, Computational and Data Sciences, Fairfax, VA, USA
e-mail: cduncan9@masonlive.gmu.edu

H. R. Arabnia et al. (eds.), *Advances in Computer Vision and Computational Biology*, Transactions on Computational Science and Computational Intelligence,
https://doi.org/10.1007/978-3-030-71051-4_18

collectable and distinguishable from the electrical fields altogether, particularly so in environments non-permissive to electrical field transmission in order to demonstrate the possibility of collection of the magnetic field at a distance from the electrical field of origin.

2 The Testing Environment

The methods used to conduct the collection of radio and magnetic signals, as well as the routines used for data analysis are discussed below.

2.1 The Setup

In order to test the hypothesis of whether or not magnetic fields could be collected and reasonably applied toward the advancement of remote sensing, an experiment was established in order to validate that magnetic signals could be remotely sensed in radio frequency prohibitive environments and potentially from inside of man-made structures. The two most obvious ways to conduct this research would be to conduct the study in an area with a high level of electromagnetic activity, or from within a structure designed to prohibit the transmission of signals. In order to create a realistic environment, a combination of the two options was employed.

The test was conduct by setting up a Faraday cage with a radio frequency transmitter inside. The Faraday cage was assembled in downtown Easton, Maryland, a city with a population of approximately 16,100 people on the eastern shore, and within five miles of the Easton Airport. Outside of the Faraday cage were two antennas. A six-axis magnetic loop antenna connected by fiber optic cable and staged inside an RF shield box approximately 50 feet from the Faraday cage and 100 feet from the digital signal processing computers. Approximately 15 feet from the magnetic loop antenna was a copper dipole antenna of approximately 100 feet in length, suspended twenty feet into the air.

Two battery powered Linux powered computers dedicated to digital signal processing were located, with one computer dedicated to collections in Radio Frequency and the other dedicated to the magnetic field. The decision to power the computers by battery was made in order to eliminate interference from AC electric power, and for the ability to seal the batteries inside RF shield boxes. Fiber optic cable was used to minimize signal interference from transmission from the antenna to the computers.

The research was conducted inside an engineering firm warehouse where aside from the on-going experiment, normal daily activity patterns occurred. The collection cycle would be established to collect the ambient noise in both the

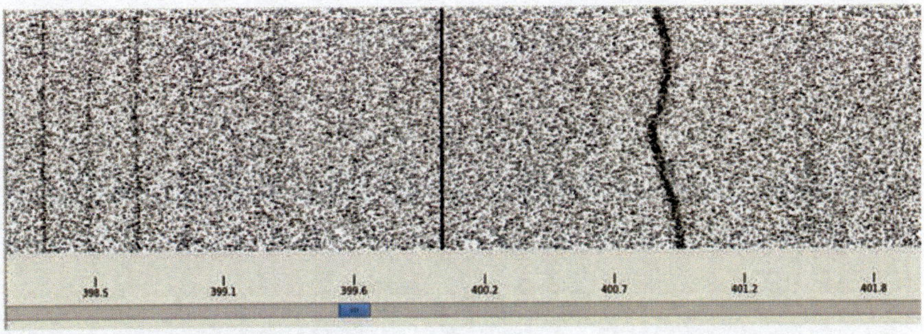

Fig. 1 The live signal waterfall collection screen view from the digital signal processing computers. The display shows a live feed from the antennas in the entire band, with darker colors indicating stronger signals. The x axis indicates frequency while the y axis is time, with the current time being at the top of the screen. The darker lines signify a strong signal detected in the frequency (*x* axis)

magnetic and RF spectrum, and then the transmitter would be placed inside the Faraday cage to broadcast signals. The door to the Faraday cage would be sealed and attempts to detect the signal would be made in both the RF spectrum and the magnetic spectrum. Although the primary focus for this research was in the Tremendously Low Frequency (TLF) designated portion of the electromagnetic spectrum, collection of broadcasts at that level of low frequency in the RF spectrum was not possible due to antenna size requirements [1]. The same antenna size requirements did not apply to the magnetic field. To compensate for the inability to compare spectrum collections, the research was expanded to include frequencies as high as 1 MHz (Fig. 1).

2.2 *Signal Broadcast*

To enable an RF broadcast from within the Faraday cage, an oscilloscope was connected to an RF antenna with a frequency broadcasting kit that enabled the operator to select frequencies to generate an artificial signal for broadcast. Varying frequencies were chosen for two basic reasons. First, larger wavelengths are more likely to pass through walls and physical barriers, which would possibly enable detection of the signal in the RF spectrum. Second, a varying frequency would create a visually distinguishable pattern on the digital signal processing waterfall display that would enable the operator to easily verify the collection of the desired transmission from the various other signals present in the ambient noise floor from regular activity. A test was conducted to ensure the desired effect was achieved, with the transmitter outside of the Faraday cage (Fig. 2).

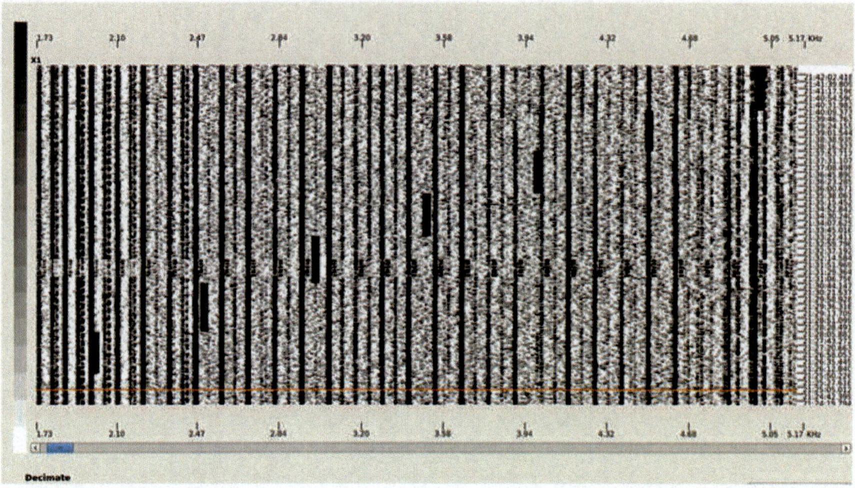

Fig. 2 The digital signal processing display waterfall clearly showing induced frequency change patterns in the magnetic field amongst ambient noise, broadcast from the RF transmitter outside of the Faraday cage. The transmitter patterns go from bottom left to upper right, in smaller high-density bars

2.3 Sensor Calibration

To ensure the proper calibration of the sensors and software in the magnetic field, a standard two coil Helmholtz coil was used, spaced apart approximately 3 feet. The coils were powered by uniform frequency electricity to create a uniform magnetic field between the two coils. The sensor was placed between the coils while inside the radio frequency shield box and calibration adjustments were made to ensure the frequency of the detected uniform magnetic field matched the frequency of electricity powering the coils. Sensors were calibrated each day before the tests were conducted.

2.4 Ambient Collections

So signal collection can be clearly identified, the first part of the test each day was a 30 min collection of the ambient noise in RF and the magnetic spectrum. Again, the RF spectrum collection was limited in the primary area of focus, but the magnetic spectrum ambient noise was available. The ambient collection, like the rest of the collection, was plotted in a power spectral density (PSD) plot to show the spectral power at each frequency across the band. The expected result was a varying PSD as the local daily activity varied during the work week. Ultimately, however, the ambient collections proved to be nearly identical every day (Fig. 3).

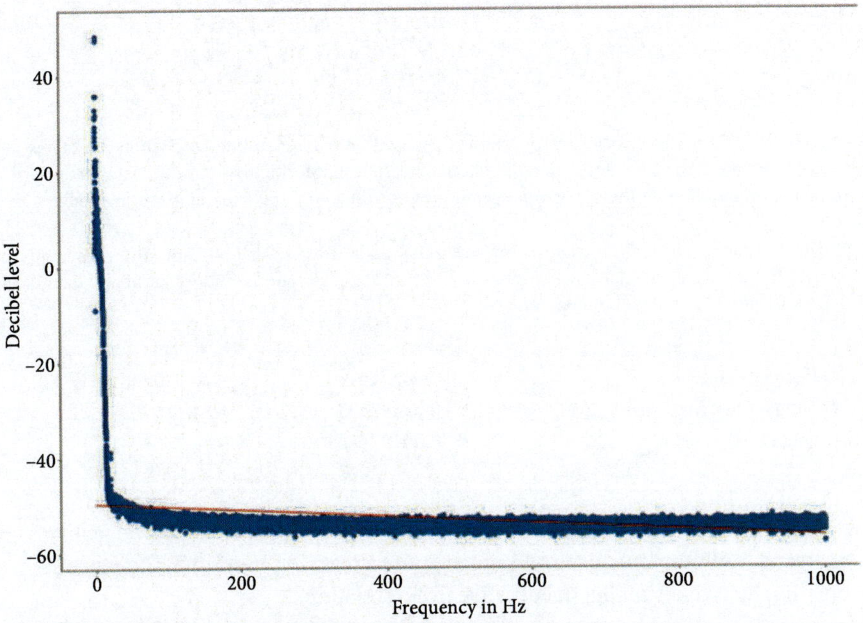

Fig. 3 The power spectral density plot of ambient noise in the TLF spectrum on a test day, including a linear regression line to baseline the standard trend. With the x axis being the frequency, from 0 to 1 Hz and the *Y* axis representing the decibel level of the given frequency ranging from −60 to 60 dB. The regression indicates a slope of −0.00697686 with an intercept of −49.7162045. Although unconventional, the linear regression proves useful to analyze the trend of PSD beyond visual assessment

2.5 *Data Collection and Handling*

The data collected from the sensors, both RF and magnetic, is stored in binary format, as raw data in MIDAS BLUE file formats. The MIDAS format essentially consists of a header with collection and sample rate, as well as other information, followed by the raw data in binary. The file sizes for these tests average approximately 5 gigabytes of raw binary data. In order to effectively render and process the data, a data handling script was written in Python 3.7 to read and unpack the data from binary into its true form, store the raw data in a PostgreSQL database, and then process the data through a Fast Fourier Transform and Welch's Method as shown in Fig. 4, to convert the signal data from the time domain to the signal domain and to estimate and generate the Power Spectral Density, storing it in a separate table as well as generating comparative plots using supervised and unsupervised algorithms. The database for collection of the data was created with the intent to limit the amount of times the files must be accessed, as the size of the data after decompressed and stored into a database went from approximately 5 gigabytes or more, to no more than 100 megabytes for all data stored in a single file.

$$\hat{S}_x^W(\omega_k) \triangleq \frac{1}{K} \sum_{m=0}^{K-1} P_{x_{m1}} M(\omega k)$$

Fig. 4 Welch's method for estimating power spectral density. Handled by Python packages, this converted data in the time domain to the frequency domain, producing plot-able data that was able to be manipulated, with the *x* axis representing frequency and the y axis representing decibel level

Table 1 Linear regression analysis of the PSD data revealed significant differences in the magnetic field transmission from within the Faraday cage, despite including anomalic data in the RF transmitter field, due to human error

	Slope	Intercept (dB)
Transmitter B field	−.00032167	−16.930933521
RF transmitter (incl. anomalies)	−0.02842537	−34.13376558
B field noise floor	0.00697686	−49.7162045

Finally, the script allowed the data, both raw and processed, to be statistically analyzed by both supervised and unsupervised learning algorithms to generate not only qualitative visual but quantitative differentiation.

3 Data Analysis and Evaluation of Classification Algorithms

In general, the data collected is presumed to be of *n* dimensionality in a PSD. Basic dimensions include, but are not limited to: frequency, time, decibel level, as well as audiometric dimensions and because of this, that data should be explored through as many algorithms as possible to identify those best fit for *n* dimensionality, for future research. Data including collection errors were included in the analysis, as the errors validated the methodology and will be explained in Sect. 4.

3.1 *Linear Regression Analysis*

Although unconventional, a linear regression analysis was run against the collections of the magnetic field ambient collection, the RF collection with transmitter on, and the magnetic field with transmitter on. The analysis displayed the differences in spectral density, in three states of the test process, and served to quantify those differences, showing differences in slope and intercept of the spectrum density over frequency (instead of time) (Table 1).

3.2 T-Distributed Stochastic Neighbor Embedding (tSNE)

The tSNE clustering method is primarily used as a qualitative method of visualizing data of low dimensional. Consequently, the algorithm produced mostly useless results, with the only exception being when data was reduced. The overall number of points per PSD was approximately 100,000. When randomly selecting 5000 points or less the algorithm typically identified 3 specific clusters. Beyond 5000 points, the algorithm progressively became less accurate.

3.3 Dendrogram

The dendrogram algorithm proved to be useful, although it also demonstrated it was resource intensive. After approximately 90 min of processing, the algorithm clearly produced two clusters, one with significantly more data than the other, which is likely the ambient magnetic and RF noise collection which were quite similar outside of error induced anomalies. The other was likely the transmitter collection in the magnetic field (Fig. 5).

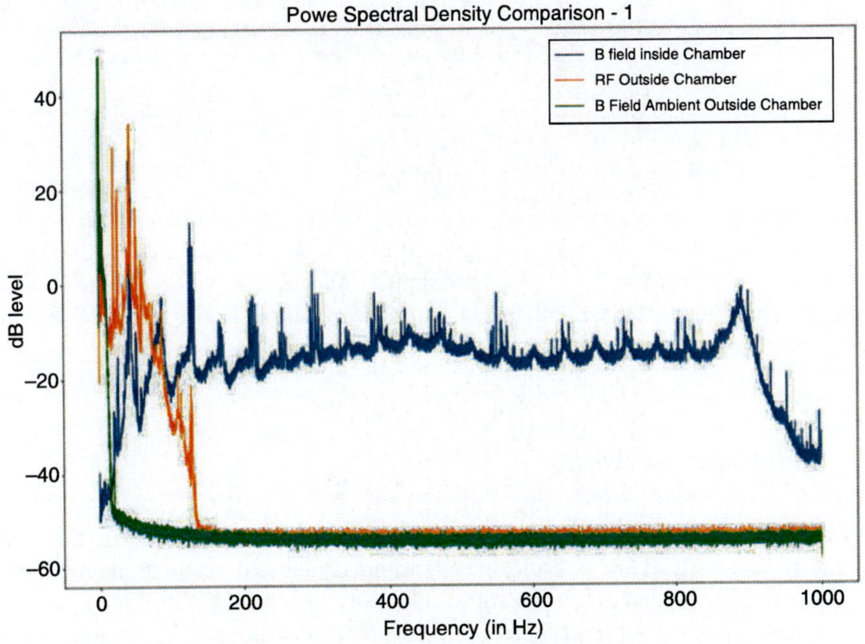

Fig. 5 The variances of spectral density displayed with green indicating the collection of ambient magnetic field, yellow indicating RF collection with transmitter on and inside the Faraday cage, and blue indicating magnetic field with transmitter on and inside the Faraday cage

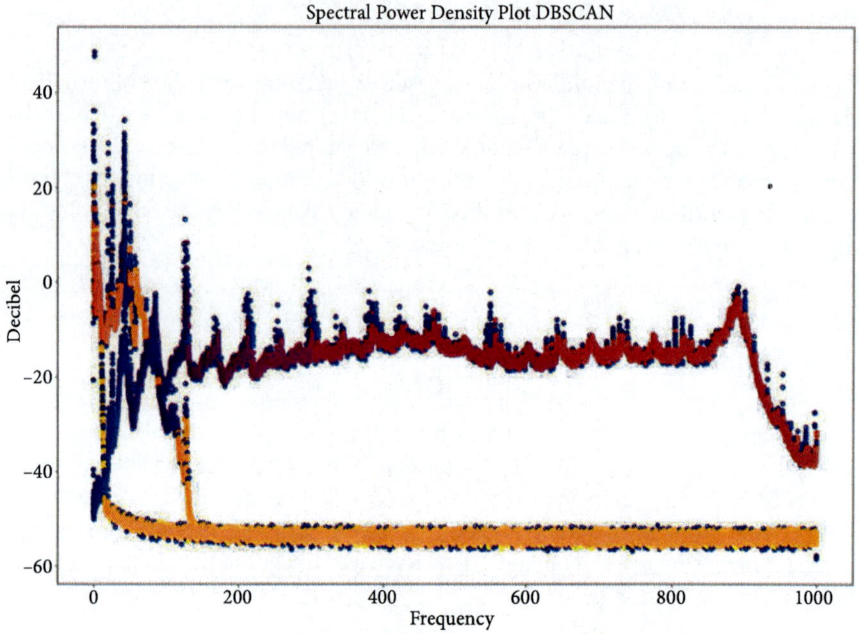

Fig. 6 The DBSCAN algorithm clearly demonstrated the variance in ambient and RF noise versus the magnetic field, as well as highlighting anomalies and border points. Overall, the results simplified and plotted at basic peaks in both the magnetic and RF spectrum appear in Fig. 7

3.4 DBSCAN

The DBSCAN algorithm proved unusually effective at clearly identifying the various data types. The DBSCAN appeared to identify both the ambient magnetic field, the RF field, the magnetic field transmitter collection, as well as anomalies and border points that could fall into several categories as shown in Fig. 6. The algorithm was also far less resource intensive.

4 Summary of Results

The results of both the plots of the post processing data, as well as the visualization of statistical analysis and classification algorithms, indicated a clear detection of the magnetic transmission even from within a Faraday cage at TLF and above.

Despite the clear visual distinction in Fig. 5, there were anomalous results the first day of testing. In Fig. 5 the anomalous results are overlaid in yellow to highlight the differences. The errors occurred when the Faraday cage was assembled but improperly sealed. The lack of proper sealing with copper tape caused hairline

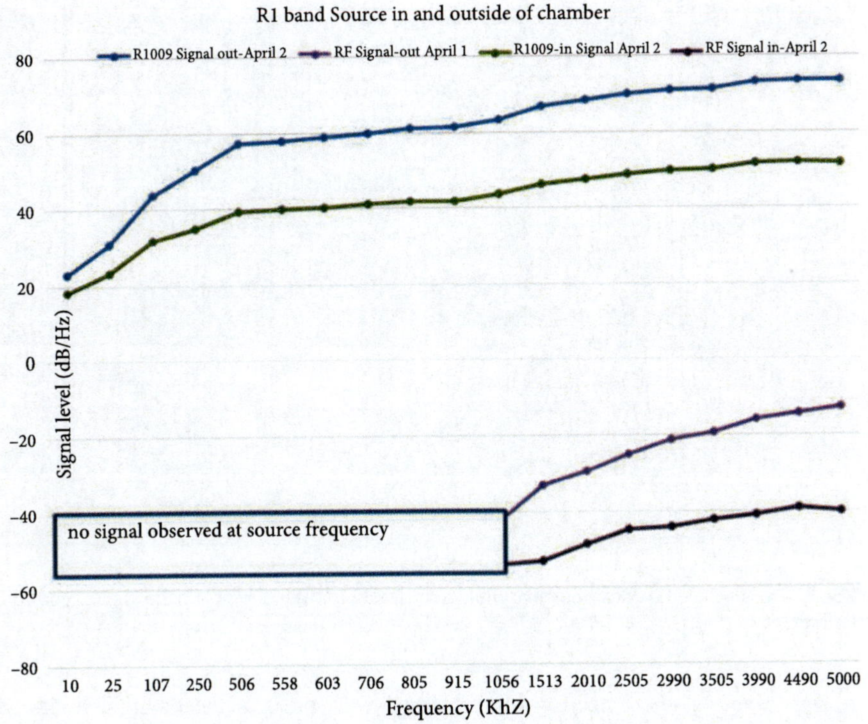

Fig. 7 The overall results indicate a significant shift in the RF versus magnetic field. The top two lines show an elevated magnetic field density with the transmitter inside and out of the Faraday cage, with the bottom lines showing the magnetic field density the RF spectrum. The magnetic field displays significant spectral density regardless of the placement of the transmitter, although there is a small shift when placed inside the Faraday cage, while the RF displays an increase in density only when the transmitter is outside the Faraday cage

cracks to allow signals to leak from the cage, producing anomalous readings and spikes in both the RF and magnetic spectrum, although the antenna height should have been prohibitive to collection of radio frequency at such low frequencies. Once the error was discovered and the cage was properly sealed, these anomalies ceased. This validated the functioning of the Faraday cage in both states; properly sealed and improperly sealed.

Further, throughout the collection, other anomalies were observed that were demonstrative of the ability to remotely sense via the magnetic field. While taking samples in other bands, visual displays appeared to display visualization of modulation of the magnetic field, indicating the collection was likely the near-field due to the near-field reactivity to the source electrical field [1]. Upon audiometric analysis, the signal was revealed to be a radio station located north of Baltimore. Although not entirely unheard of to detect a radio station from that distance in the AM band, it is primarily performed at night when distances are at their greatest.

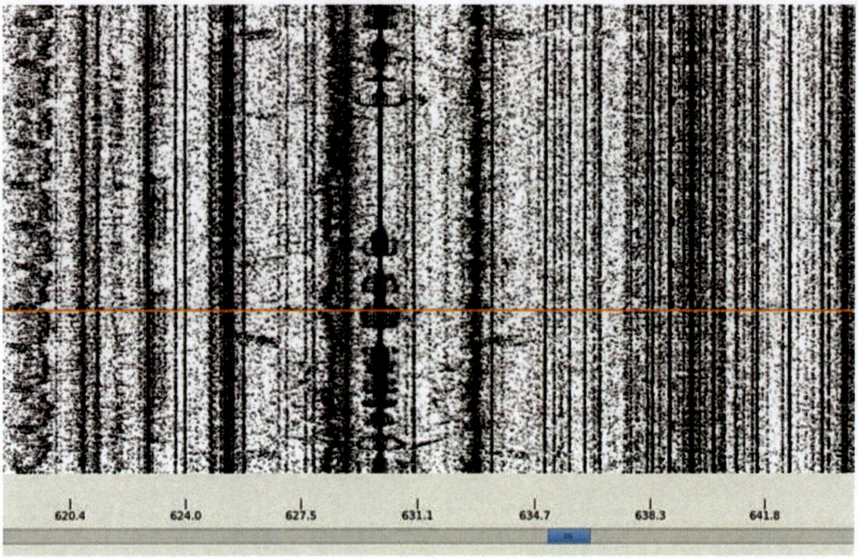

Fig. 8 The displayed modulations that ultimately were discovered to be a radio station north of Baltimore

In this example, the detection of the signal was made in the daylight hours at approximately 1430 eastern standard time (Fig. 8).

After analysis of the preliminary results, including error induced anomalies, comparison PSD plots were generated to further analyze and determine the effectiveness of the Faraday cage at attenuating the magnetic field, when the associated electrical field is attenuated to the point of no noticeable increase in local spectral density. The results of this analysis are in Figs. 9 and 10, but indicate virtually no attenuation in the magnetic field, suggesting that even in environments where the electrical field is undetectable it could be possible to make similar detections in the magnetic field, thus providing a signal for use in remote sensing and detection. This particular example demonstrates a potential for identification of electrical activity from within urban areas or abandoned buildings, such as identifying if power is running to a building, or in certain use cases, it may be possible to detect land and building use based on electromagnetic signature, if the ability to classify activities were well enough defined.

5 Conclusions and Further Research

The test results show a significant increase in spectral density in the magnetic field, while there is little to no density increase the electrical field spectrum, when the transmitter is located within a Faraday cage. These results provide preliminary

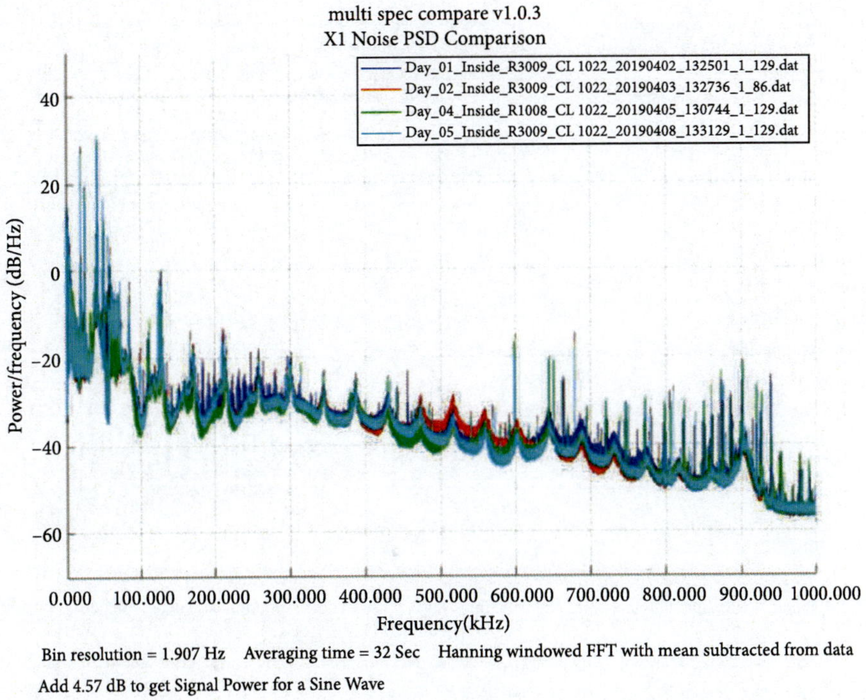

Fig. 9 Plot of the magnetic signature of the frequency transmitter located inside the Faraday cage as detected by the magnetic loop antenna located outside of the cage. Naming convention indicates the day, the location of the transmitter, the band (r3), and axis

validation of the hypothesis that there is a relevant utility in monitoring magnetic fields in remote sensing. This is especially true when the intention of the remote sensing application is hoping to identify electrical or magnetic activity, or any activities that may produce a magnetic field. Although it is not known whether the ability to detect increases in spectral density are frequency dependent, there have been similar incidental detections and results, such as that with Mikhailov [2].

The approach for further research into the utility of magnetic fields would be the application of band pass filter-like functions isolating individual frequencies for signal analysis in the time domain. Accompanied by machine learning algorithms a multi-dimensional analysis to catalog and classify devices and activity based upon emitted magnetic signature in a given frequency against a given set of targets to test the potential feasibility as well as achievable resolution of magnetic detections from the standard ambient noise floor would provide catalogs for future classification. Analysis of the spectral density proved valuable in gauging the overall increase in detected signals across the band spectrum, however, the ability to analyze single frequency signals in the time domain would provide a greater ability to potentially

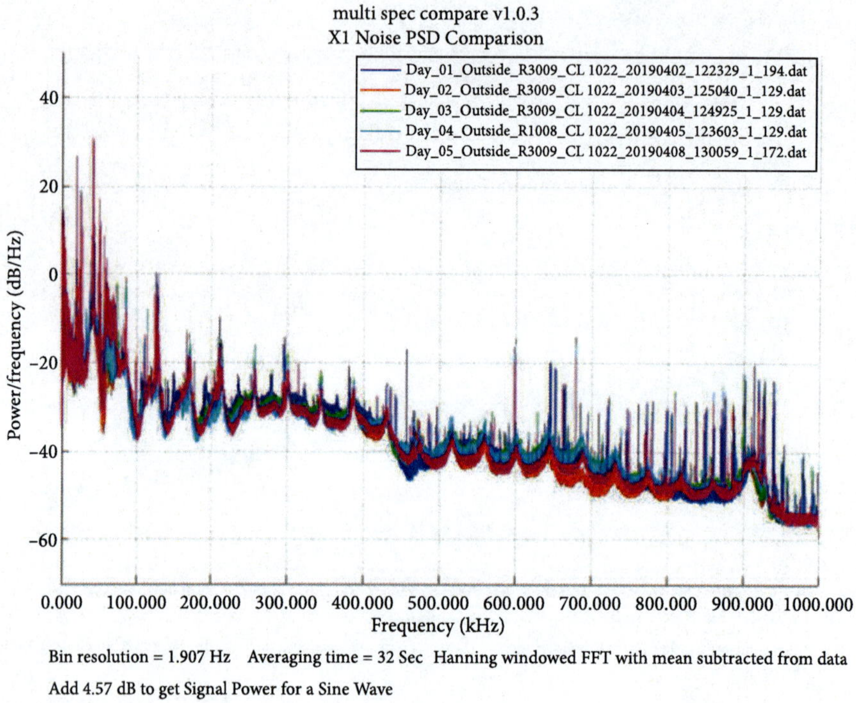

Fig. 10 Plot of the magnetic signature of the frequency transmitter located outside of the Faraday cage as detected by the magnetic loop antenna also located outside of the cage. Showing a near identical detection pattern to when the transmitter was located within a sealed Faraday cage. Naming convention indicates the day, the location of the transmitter, the band (r3), and axis

characterize signals to a point of being able to classify them based on signal dimensions. This ability, if confirmed by further research, expands the field of remote sensing by opening the doors to pattern detection and classification in the magnetic field that before was just considered to be noise.

References

1. R. Barr, D. Jones, C. Rodger, ELF and VLF radio waves. J. Atmos. Solar-Terrestrial Phys. **62**(17–18), 1689–1718 (2000)
2. Y. Mikhailov, G. Mikhailova, O. Kapustina, VLF effects in the outer ionosphere from the underground nuclear explosion on Novaya Zemlya Island on 24 October, 1990 (Intercosmos 24 satellite data). Phys. Chem. Earth C Solar Terrestrial Planet. Sci. **25**(1–2), 93–96 (2000)
3. G. Rondeaux, M. Herman, Polarization of light reflected by crop canopies. Remote Sens. Environ. **38**(1), 63–75 (1991)

4. R.H. Tyler, Satellite observations of magnetic fields due to ocean tidal flow. Science **299**(5604), 239–241 (2003)
5. United States Department of Labor, Occupational safety and health administration. https://www.osha.gov/SLTC/radiofrequencyradiation/electromagnetic_fieldmemo/electromagnetic.html.section_6. Accessed 11 May 2019

Clustering Method for Isolate Dynamic Points in Image Sequences

Paula Niels Spinoza, Andriamasinoro Rahajaniaina, and Jean-Pierre Jessel

1 Introduction

In the robotics field, the Simultaneous Localization and Mapping (SLAM) technique is used to know the position of the robot by exploiting the position of the static reference points in the environment where the robot evolves. In reality, there may be dynamics objects in this environment, and this could distort the estimate of the robot's pose. Therefore, to reduce these errors, it is essential to use a method of grouping the dynamics points in an image in order to isolate their later. This approach requires a technique capable of selecting and tracking objects in the real scene like [13] and then modified by Shi and Tomasi [16] who is called Kanade-Lucas-Tomasi (KLT). Once the points are extracted and tracked by this technique, it is important to distinguish among the tracking points those which correspond to 3D points carried by dynamics objects. To group these points, grouping or clustering techniques can be proposed, but most of them require a priori knowledge of the number of groups to find in the scene as in K-means [8] and mean shift [6]. The success of these methods strongly depends on these initialization parameters [1]. Encountered a problem for the analysis of short video sequences. In fact, the author presented a grouping algorithm based on an a-contrario method, which does not need any parameter or initial information on the scene to find in a sequence of images groups of points projections of 3D points carried by dynamics objects. To overcome these problems, in this chapter, we propose an improvement of the

P. N. Spinoza · A. Rahajaniaina (✉)
Department of Mathematics, Computer Science and Applications, University of Toamasina, Toamasina, Madagascar

J.-P. Jessel
IRIT, REVA, Paul Sabatier University, Toulouse, France
e-mail: jessel@irit.fr

H. R. Arabnia et al. (eds.), *Advances in Computer Vision and Computational Biology*, Transactions on Computational Science and Computational Intelligence,
https://doi.org/10.1007/978-3-030-71051-4_19

technique of grouping a-contrario by using the technique of probabilistic measure of quality [7].

The remainder of the chapter is organized as follows. Section 2 summarizes the various previous works. Section 3 discusses the contribution and Sect. 4 explains the experimental results. We end the chapter with a brief conclusion and perspective.

2 Previous Works

In this section, we will see the various works relating to the tracking and distinction of dynamic objects by knowing their speed, their position, and their orientation [3] studied computer vision techniques for autonomous cars. As for [4], the authors proposed a technique for real-time monitoring of vehicles and pedestrians. Then [18] adopted a technique of tracking human objects in real time for intelligent surveillance. These approaches are based on an off-line tracking technique. Once the scene is disturbed or the camera encounters a difficult situation such as lighting problem, partial or total occlusion, motion blur, etc., it is important to follow an object online [5, 12, 17]. There are also different techniques that focus on the use of visual data [4, 9, 15]. The performance of such systems depends on a reliable and efficient object tracking algorithm.

In general, visual tracking of objects is a major computer vision problem, above all, when the objects or events to be detected are multiple, of variable forms, and poorly understood. In this case, these approaches that we list above need other methods that allow them to efficiently group the pixels of the image according to their local texture [8]. Ref. [2] shows a correct alignment detection which depends on the amount of masking in the texture, the bilateral local density of the alignment, internal regularity and reduction of redundancy. Other author searches another method for establishing correspondences on deformable objects for single target object tracking [14]. These different approaches offer advantages such as a minimum amount of background pixels [11], tighter data sets, obtaining an orientation of the object in the image plane. Despite these positive points, there are still problems to be solved: calculation of rotation angle and scale estimation. Many researchers tried to give a solution to this problem, but there are still limits in terms of tracking speed or accuracy [10, 15].

3 Contribution

The presence of dynamic objects in an uncontrolled environment could distort the topological map of SLAM. It will be necessary to adopt a grouping technique capable of grouping these mobile objects and optimizing static objects. To solve this problem, we chose the "a-contrario" technique.

3.1 *Evaluation of the Background Model*

The objective of the a-contrario grouping method is to group points of interest having a coherent movement along a short sequence of images. Here, the consistency criterion refers to motion vectors (tracklets) which have roughly similar magnitudes and directions for all points in the group of a binary tree. The method receives a set V of input vectors $(x, y, v, \ominus \mid t)$, such that x and y represent the magnitude and v the orientation which is defined in R^4. The latter contains the scattered optical flow accumulated points of interest over time. In the vector V, the variable t is added just to indicate the moment when these points were selected (start of selection and tracking of interest points); this recalls the temporal nature of the data.

The first objective consists in evaluating, which elements of V have a particular distribution and contrary to that established by the background model. To avoid element-by-element evaluation, a binary tree is constructed with the elements of V, using the single-link method to have all the groups that can be formed from these elements.

In the root of the binary tree, we find the group which integrates all the elements of V; on the leaves of the tree, we find the elements individually where each group contains a single point. Each node in the tree represents a candidate group of points $G\ (x, y, v, \ominus \mid t) \subset V$ which will be compared with the background model using a set of regions preestablished in R^4. In the latter, these regions are hyper-rectangles whose size is a function of the values of the points on each dimension.

Then a set of test regions H is established in order to evaluate the distribution function of each group G of tracked points resulting from the accumulation of the optical flow, where $G \subset V$. The space of H regions is used to calculate the probability that the distribution of each group in the binary tree is similar to the distribution of a model for background objects.

In the background model, a random organization of the observations is distributed in an identical and independent manner and which follow a p distribution. This distribution is obtained by the product of four independent distributions, one for each component in the data.

Thus, for the dimensions corresponding to the positions of the points and the velocities orientations, their distribution is uniform because the position and direction of movement of the dynamic object are arbitrary. No information about the initial position or the orientation of dynamic object movement is known. The magnitude distribution of the velocity is obtained directly from the empirical histogram of the observed data. Then each time the region is centered on a different point $X \in G$, its distribution will change according to the dynamic points it contains. This search for the best region which will make it possible to identify the test group G as significant compared to the background model.

To detect and distinguish the mobile groups, all the nodes in the binary tree as well as the space of the H regions are analyzed in order to evaluate the following hypothesis:

Hypothesis 1: Any group of pixels which does not follow the random distribution of the background model is considered to be a group with independent movement. In order to obtain a quantitative value for the evaluation of this hypothesis, we use a measure called Number of False Alarms (NFA) as in [2] for each group in the binary tree. It is obtained by the following equation:

$$\mathrm{NFA}(G) = N^2 * |H| \min_{\substack{x \in G \\ h \in H \\ G \in H_x}} B\left(N-1, n-1, p\left(H_x\right)\right) \tag{1}$$

In this equation, N represents the number of elements of the initial vector of the data V, $| H |$ is the cardinality of the regions, and n is the number of elements in the test group G.

The term that appears in the minimum function is the accumulated binomial law, which represents the probability that at least n points including the point X (x, y, v_x, v_y) center of the region are inside the region h_X where $h \in H$. A group G is said to be significant (it can correspond to a dynamic object on the scene) if the quantity NFA (G) ≤ 1. Then a second evaluation taking into account only the groups significant will be made. After a validation of the first hypothesis, it is necessary to design a technique capable to distinguish the groups, which correspond to the static objects of the background model with the groups considered mobile by NFA. Hence, the intervention of the M_{GK} technique.

3.2 M_{GK} Concept

The intuitive meaning of an $X \rightarrow Y$ association rule is as follows: "Whenever the X pattern appears, the Y pattern also with a certain degree of confidence" or even "any object that has the X pattern has tendency to also have the Y pattern with an estimated degree of confidence." Consequently, to facilitate the interpretation of a rule (see Fig. 1), the normalization of the normalized measure associated with μ would consist in bringing its values back over the interval [−1, 1] so that:

- −1 value corresponds to the incompatibility.
- Values strictly between −1 and 0 correspond to repulsion or negative dependence.
- 0 value corresponds to independence.

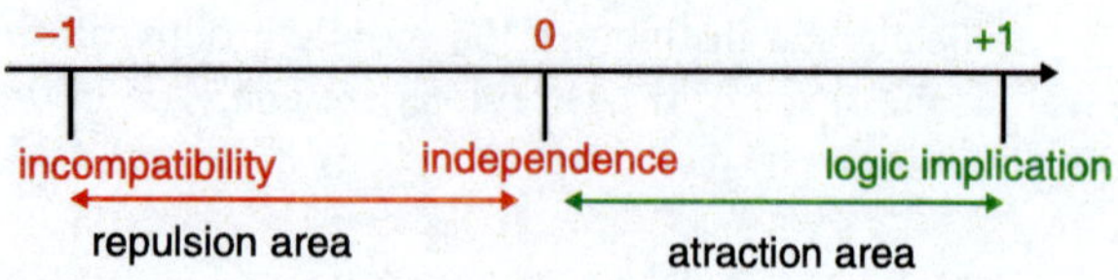

Fig. 1 Distribution of probabilistic quality measure normalization values

- Values strictly between 0 and 1 correspond to the attraction or oriented positive dependence.
- 1 value corresponds to the logical implication between the premise and the consequence of a rule $X \rightarrow Y$.

X and Y are two patterns for a data mining context. We define the measure M_{GK} by

$$M_{\mathrm{GK}}(X \rightarrow Y) = \begin{cases} \dfrac{P\left(Y' | X'\right) - P\left(Y'\right)}{1 - P\left(Y'\right)}, & \text{if } X \text{ favors } Y \\ \dfrac{P\left(Y' | X'\right) - P\left(Y'\right)}{P\left(Y'\right)}, & \text{if } X \text{ disfavors } Y \end{cases} \quad (2)$$

For two non-independent patterns X and Y, two cases can arise: (1) either there is mutual attraction; in this case, the dependence is positive. (2) Either there is repulsion; therefore, there is a positive dependence between X and $\overline{Y}$; hence, $X \rightarrow \overline{Y}$, on the one hand, then between X and Y. In this case, we have $X \rightarrow Y$, on the other hand. In both cases, we will always have to consider a positive dependence. Then decompose the measure M_{GK} as follows:

$$M_{\mathrm{GK}}(X \rightarrow Y) = \begin{cases} M^{f}_{\mathrm{GK}}, & \text{if } X \text{ favors } Y \\ M^{d}_{\mathrm{GK}}, & \text{if } X \text{ disfavors } Y \end{cases} \quad (3)$$

Thus, the favorable component will guide the semantics of M_{GK}. These properties allow the quality measure M_{GK} to select fewer rules if one confines oneself to positive rules. It also makes it possible to measure jointly the difference in independence and the degree of statistical implication between two reasons. Its coherence with the attraction and repulsion between two patterns makes it less ambiguous and more intelligible. In addition, the M_{GK} measure is favorably more discriminating.

3.3 M_{GK} and A-Contrario

Static objects and dynamic objects have different characteristics in a scene. If we consider that the group in the binary tree is static (distribution of static primitives in the scene), a new hypothesis must be verified.

Hypothesis 2: Any group which respects the NFA criterion and validates by measurement $\mathrm{M_{GK}}$ is considered as a group which represents a salient object in the scene.

To answer this hypothesis, we consider the two reasons for the following association rule: X, either the group in the binary tree is static; Y, i.e., the group is considered mobile by NFA, where $X, Y \in h_X$.

We calculate the distribution p composed of four independent distributions of each region h_X, which can contain a mobile or static group.

We determine $M^f_{\text{GK}}(X \rightarrow Y)$ and $M^f_{\text{GK}}(Y \rightarrow X)$, and then we compare the results obtained. Then we choose what is larger and closer to 1. To do this, we choose to use the formula of the favoring component of M^f_{GK} following:

$$M^f_{\text{GK}}(X \rightarrow Y) = \frac{p_X(Y) - p(Y)}{1 - p(Y)} \tag{4}$$

and

$$M^f_{\text{GK}}(Y \rightarrow X) = \frac{p_Y(X) - p(X)}{1 - p(X)} \tag{5}$$

Proposal: After the test, we take α as the final value of M^f_{GK}. Two cases are possible for validation:

- If α is between [0.95, 1], then we accept that groups that have a value NFA $(G) \leq \alpha$ are accepted as mobile.
- Otherwise, we accept the first evaluation NFA$(G) \leq 1$.

At this threshold, group G is considered mobile, and the information it contains represents the dynamic points on the stage. So we send it to the probability map which is used to track dynamic objects in the tracking process. All groups that do not meet this condition are considered static. In this case, it is considered as static points in the scene.

Indeed, these well-refined points could use as data, which feeds the location and mapping module in real time.

Figure 2 shows how to integrate our work with that carried out elsewhere on SLAM and Moving Objects Tracking (MOT). The functions that should be added to implement the SLAM-MOT are the numbers 4 and 5.

3.4 Klt Module

This module is dedicated to the analysis of images acquired by the camera of the smartphone (see Fig. 2). The result obtained from this module is a set of points of interest characterized in R^4 obtained from the partial results of the functions:

- Feature Selection: Give the position (x, y) of the N best points of interest in the image.

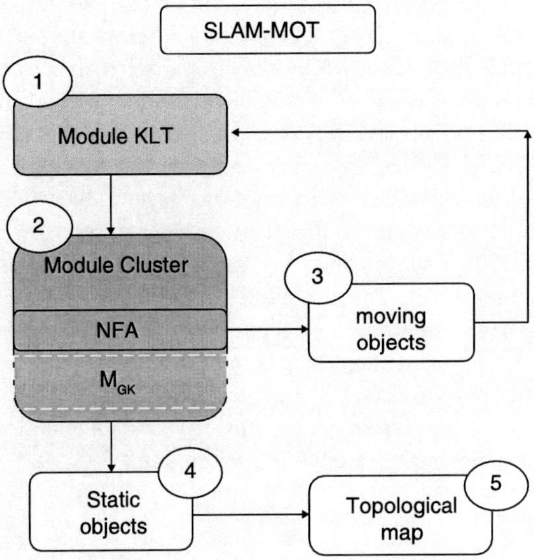

Fig. 2 Diagram of our approach combined with SLAM

- Tracking features: Find the position (x, y) of the points in the next image, and get their speed in the x and y directions (v_x, v_y).
- Probability map: Keep the cell position centered on each detected point of interest (x, y) in the image. A pixel value p_{ij} is assigned to each pixel in the cell according to a two-dimensional Gaussian distribution and its state over time. This map is reset every two tracking times.

These three functions are not performed for each image sequence. Feature Selection works only at the start of each tracking, while the other two functions are executed for each image (from the second image for the tracking features function).

Execution parameters: For each tracking, we use 150 points of interest to select in the image. The points found must be separated by at least ten pixels.

In order to select the points, which will be processed by the cluster module, these points must be tracking for at least four consecutive images and at the same time that the speeds v_x and v_y are greater than one pixel.

3.5 *Cluster Module*

This module analyzes the points of interest characterized as the quadruplets (x, y, v_x, v_y), which give their respective positions and velocities along the tracking time. It returns the same set but characterized as (x, y, v_x, v_y, C) where C represents the identifier of the group to which this point belongs. If $C = 0$, then the point is not part of an object, with a coherent or defined movement.

This module is executed at the end of each tracking module. This corresponds to the same frequency as the Feature Selection function. The computed time of this module depends on the number of points received at each execution. Using the ticker functions of the *C* identifier, the execution time is 1 ms to process 40 points, but this value increases to a few seconds from 300 points received as input.

Execution parameters: The a-contrario grouping method does not need parameters to settle; that is its big advantage. However, certain values must be defined before its execution, like the number and the sizes of the regions that we want to test. This involves selecting various sizes of regions to test all groups of points in the binary tree. The execution time depends directly on this parameter, but it should not be too small because the results are also dependent on this one.

So a good compromise is to set different sizes per dimension so that we go from a minimum size (we chose the smallest of ten pixels) to the size of the image. Thus, 20 sizes are chosen per dimension; the data being expressed in a four-dimensional space, this makes a total of 204 regions.

4 Experience and Results

After testing our grouping algorithm on a sequence of 35 images taken by a smartphone worn by a user, the results are as follows:

First, the points of interest accumulated in R^4 are represented in separate two-dimensional spaces. The x and y coordinates in the image are represented in pixels, the magnitude of the velocity in pixels/image and in degrees for the orientation of the velocity.

4.1 First Case: Environment with Rigid Mobile Object

This experiment is focused on the detection of rigid dynamics objects.

Figure 3 shows a scene where a car enters the field of view of the camera of our mobile user. Initially, 150 points of interest are detected (shown in yellow in Fig. 3). Then these points are followed along six consecutive images. Figure 4 shows in blue the position in the image of all the accumulated points and in green the only group of mobile points identified as a dynamic object.

The position of these points corresponds exactly to the position of the points on the car, which enters the field of view.

Figure 5 shows the magnitude and orientation of the velocity of the points. The green dots that correspond to the detected object all have the same orientation value since the orientation is around 0 and 360 degrees. Therefore, they correspond to the same direction.

The time required for the detection of a dynamic object in the image is a function of the number of images used for tracking points, six in the case presented. The

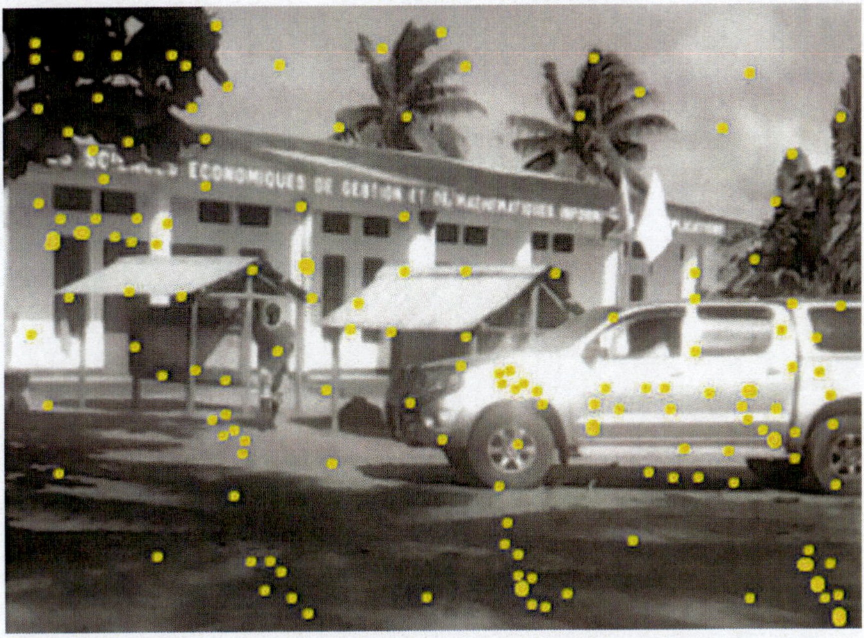

Fig. 3 Initial image

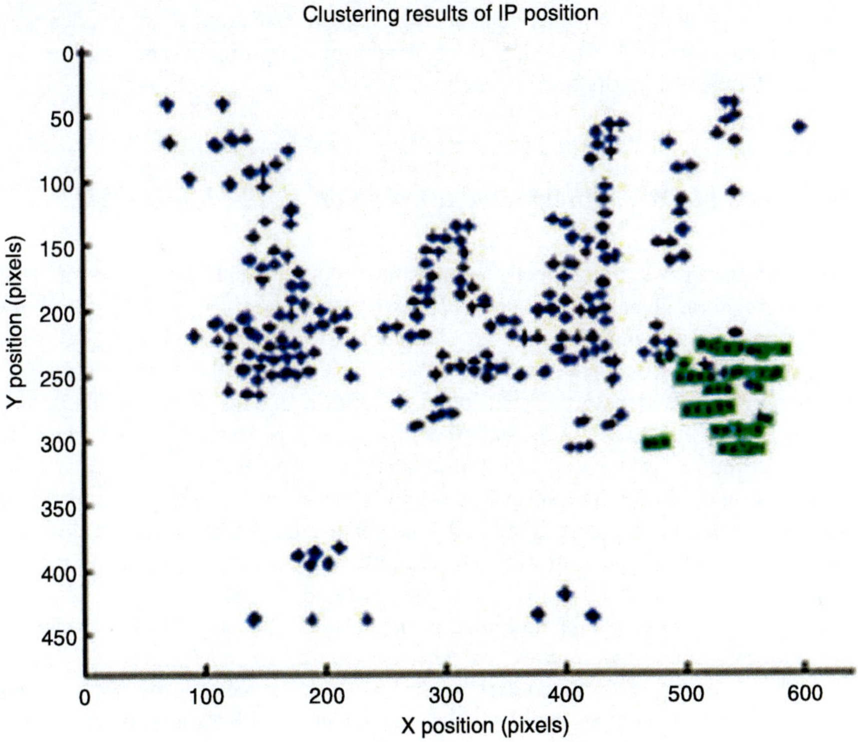

Fig. 4 Grouping positions

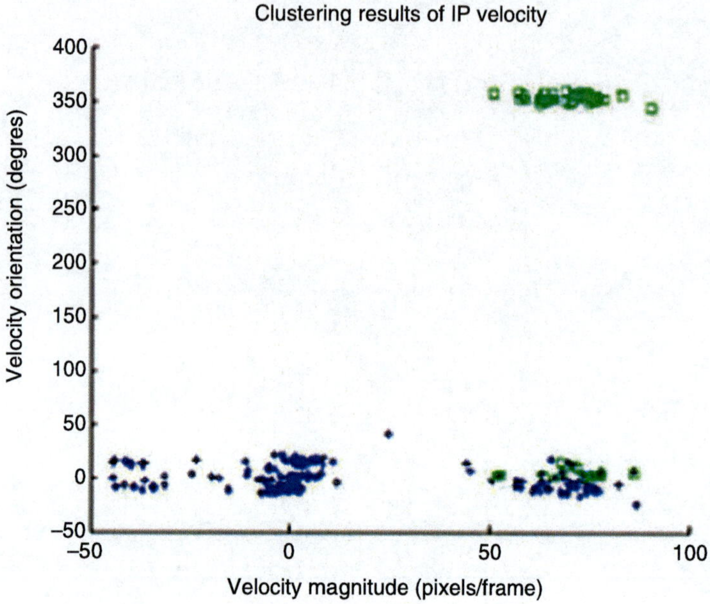

Fig. 5 Grouping velocities

detection went well even if there is a delay due to the detection of independent and coherent movements. Despite this, the detection of a rigid mobile object does not exceed 15 images after its first appearance.

4.2 *Second Case: Environment with Non-rigid Mobile Objects*

The detection of dynamic objects becomes more complicated with the presence of non-rigid mobile objects (for example, pedestrians) on the user's trajectory.

For this test, we initially selected 150 points of interest, which were followed for 20 consecutive images (See Fig. 6). The positions of the points as well as the two groups of dynamic points found are shown in Figs. 7 and 8. Thus, two groups are found despite the fact that there is only one pedestrian in the scene. The person's head and body are identified as a single object, shown in cyan, and the legs are detected as another object, which appears in green. By analyzing this result, we find that the points corresponding to the upper part of the body have different directions of movement from those corresponding to the lower part. The positions of the two groups in the image are not related due to the lack of points of interest on the person's trunk and the proximity of the person to the user's camera; this also prevents group merging.

It should be noted that to detect rigid objects, the processing of eight images is sufficient. On the other hand, in the case of non-rigid objects, more images

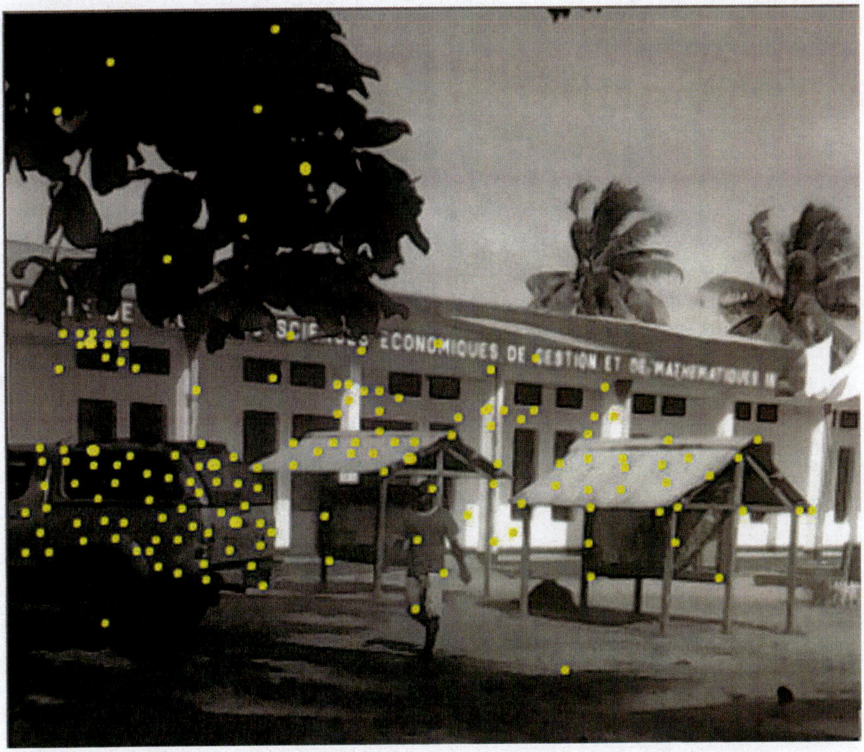

Fig. 6 Initial image

are necessary in order to properly represent the tracks. In particular, the case of pedestrians is more complicated because of the back-and-forth movement of the feet.

5 Conclusion and Future Work

The grouping technique presented in this chapter does not require any prior knowledge of the real scene or any prior information on the dynamic objects present in the scene. First, we used a scattered optical flow method by exploiting the KLT technique which allowed us to select and track the dynamics points in the scene in order to distinguish them from static objects using a probabilistic measurement technique M_{GK}. By comparing to previous work, we were able to take a small step to solve the problem of speed of tracking objects in an uncontrolled scene because the sequences presented in this chapter were acquired at 15 Hz, which is a 4 s as tracking time.

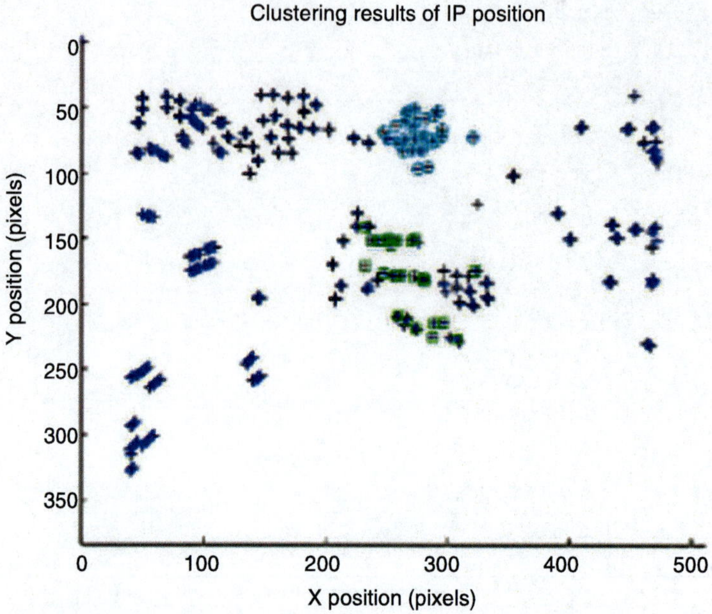

Fig. 7 Grouping positions

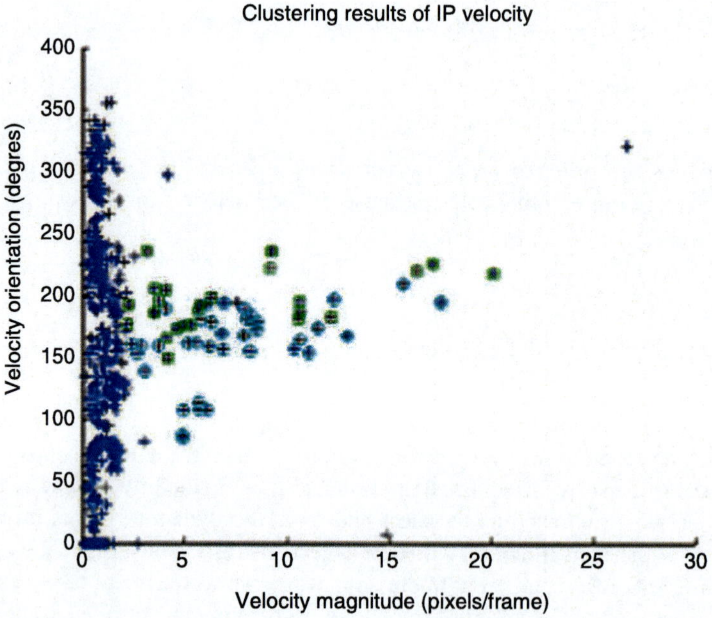

Fig. 8 Grouping velocities

In the future, we plan to improve our result, on the one hand, by incorporating a motion compensation technique to overcome the disturbance problems and, on the other hand, by using the method of measuring dissimilarity between correspondences to solve the problem of detection and tracking of deformable objects [14].

References

1. M. Ammar, S.L. Hégarat-Mascle, M. Vasiliu, R. Reunaud, An a-contrario approach for object detection in video sequence. Int. J. Pure Appl. Math **LXXXIX**(2), 173–201 (2013)
2. A. Gomez, G. Randall, R.G. Von Gioi, A contrario 3d point alignment detection algorithm. IPOL J. Image Proc. Line **VII**, 399–417 (2017)
3. N. Agarwal, C.-W. Chiang, A. Sharma, A study on computer vision techniques for self-driving cars, in *International Conference on Frontier Computing*, (Springer, 2018), pp. 629–634
4. A. Buyval, R. Gabdullin, I. Mustafin, I. Shimchik, Realtime vehicle and pedestrian tracking for didi udacity self-driving car challenge, in *2018 IEEE international conference on robotics and automation (ICRA)*, (2018), pp. 2064–2069
5. B.X. Chen, J.K. Tsotsos, Fast visual object tracking with rotated bounding boxes, in *2019 IEEE/cvf international conference on computer vision (ICCV) workshop*, (2019), pp. 629–634
6. D. Comaniciu, V. Ramesh, P. Meer, Real-time tracking of non-rigid objects using mean shift, in *Proc. IEEE conference on computer vision and pattern recognition (CVPR 2000)*, vol. II, pp. 142–149
7. D.R. Feno, J. Diatta, A. Totohasina, A basis for the association rules of a valid binary context within the meaning of the mgk quality measure, in *Proc. of the 13'eme rencontre de la société francophone de classification*, (2006), pp. 105–109
8. R. Giraud, Y. Berthoumieu, Texture Superpixel Clustering from patch-based nearest neighbor matching, in *27th european signal processing conference (EUSIPCO)*, (2019), pp. 1–5
9. Q. Guo, W. Feng, C. Zhou, C.-M. Pun, B. Wu, Structure-regularized compressive tracking with online data-driven sampling. IEEE Trans. Image Proc. **26**(12), 5692–5705 (2017)
10. Y. Hua, K. Alahari, C. Schmid, Online object tracking with proposal selection, in *proceedings of the IEEE international conference on computer vision*, (2015), pp. 3092–3100
11. M. Kristan, A. Leonardis, J. Matas, M. Felsberg, R. Pflugfelder, L. Čehovin Zajc, T. Vojir, G. Häger, A. Lukežič, A. Eldesokey, G. Fernandez, et al., The seventh visual object tracking vot2019 challenge results. Int. Conf. Comp. Vision (ICCV) Workshop, 639–654 (2019)
12. Y.-G. Lee, Z. Tang, J.-N. Hwang, Online-learning-based human tracking across nonoverlapping cameras. IEEE Trans. Circ. Syst. Video Technol **28**(10), 2870–2883 (2017)
13. B.D. Lucas, T. Kanade, An iterative image registration technique with an application to stereo vision, in *Proc. DARPA Image Understanding Workshop*, (1981), pp. 121–130
14. G. Nebehay, R. Pflugfelder, Clustering of static-adaptive correspondences for deformable object tracking, in *Proceedings of the IEEE Conference on Computer Vision and Pattern Recognition*, (2015), pp. 2784–2791
15. L. Rout, D. Mishra, R.K.S.S. Gorthi, et al., Rotation adaptive visual object tracking with motion consistency, in *2018 IEEE winter conference on applications of computer vision (WACV)*, (2018), pp. 1047–1055
16. J. Shi, C. Tomasi, Good features to track, in *Proc. IEEE international conference on computer vision and pattern recognition (CVPR 1994)*, (1994), pp. 593–600
17. Q. Wang, L. Zhang, L. Bertinetto, W. Hu, P.H. Torr, Fast online object tracking and segmentation: a unifying approach. 2019 IEEE Conf. Comp. Vision Pattern Recogn. (CVPR) (2019). https://doi.org/10.1109/CVPR.2019.00142
18. R. Xu, S.Y. Nikouei, Y. Chen, A. Polunchenko, S. Song, C. Deng, T.R. Faughnan, Realtime human objects tracking for smart surveillance at the edge, in *2018 IEEE international conference on communications (ICC)*, (2018), pp. 1–6

Computer-Aided Industrial Inspection of Vehicle Mirrors Using Computer Vision Technologies

Hong-Dar Lin and Hsu-Hung Cheng

1 Introduction

Vehicle mirrors allow light to be reflected so that the objects behind the car can be seen. Curved vehicle mirrors can make driver's rear view more widely. The side and rear vehicle mirrors are among the most important safety features on our vehicles. In manufacturing stages of vehicle mirrors, certain tasks, for example, baking, electroplating, and edging, operated unusually will cause producing scratches, chips, pinholes, bubbles, and damaged edges, the general surface and profile defects on vehicle mirrors. These appearance defects sometimes will severely have an impact on standard of the vehicle mirror reflection and grow the steering hazard. At traditional examination of vehicle mirrors in manufacturing process, almost all works are performed by human examiners. Manual examination is simple to be disturbed by foreign objects reflected on the mirror surfaces and arouse causing mistaken determinations of defect examination. Fig. 1 shows a side-view mirror and a rear-view mirror of vehicle.

General vehicle mirrors manufactured of transparent glass with aluminum- or chromium-coated materials have good ability of high reflectance, and they with curved and convex shapes have wider field of view. Regular appearance defects of vehicle mirrors comprise scratch, bubble, chip, and pinhole, belonging to the surface defect type, and broken edges and burrs, belonging to the profile defect type. The appearance defects influence not only the visual quality of mirror parts but also their performance, effectiveness, structural strength, etc. The defect sizes of usual vehicle mirrors should be detected and are leastwise 0.20 mm and 0.26 mm

H.-D. Lin (✉) · H.-H. Cheng
Department of Industrial Engineering and Management, Chaoyang University of Technology, Taichung, Taiwan
e-mail: hdlin@cyut.edu.tw

H. R. Arabnia et al. (eds.), *Advances in Computer Vision and Computational Biology*, Transactions on Computational Science and Computational Intelligence,
https://doi.org/10.1007/978-3-030-71051-4_20

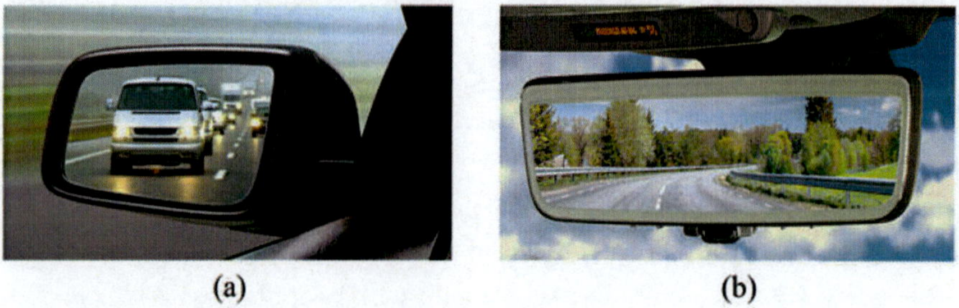

Fig. 1 (**a**) A side-view mirror. (**b**) A rear-view mirror

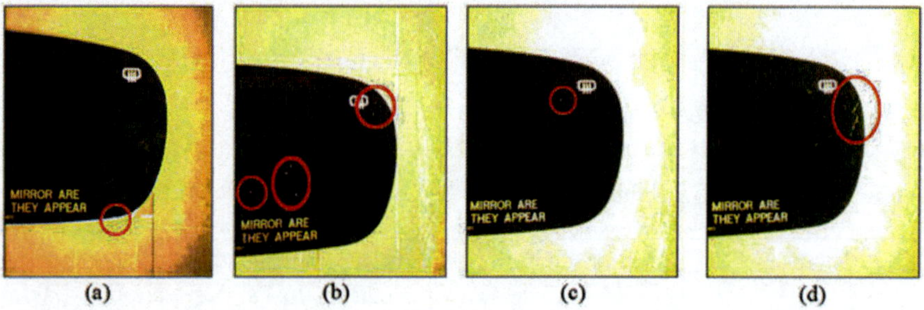

Fig. 2 Some general sorts of appearance defects on vehicle mirrors: (**a**) broken edge, (**b**) pinhole, (**c**) chip, and (**d**) scratch

for the surface defect type and the profile defect type, respectively. A workpiece of vehicle mirror has two equal size images captured from a testing sample. Two laser marks, including a sketch and some texts, are located on the mirror workpiece. The mirror workpiece having 18.1 cm in length, 10.71 cm in width, and 0.2 cm in thickness needs to be scanned into two images to obtain better image resolution for further process to reach the industry standard requirement in appearance inspection of vehicle mirrors. Appearance defects on curved surfaces are hard to be censored for practical examiners owing to not only defect attributes but also light reflection on mirror exteriors. Fig. 2 illustrates some general sorts of appearance defects on vehicle mirrors: broken edge, pinhole, chip, and scratch.

Visual examination by operators is boring, laborious, and highly dependent on the inspectors' expertise. Mistaken discernments are simply made owing to inspectors' eye exhaustion and subjectivity. Because vehicle mirrors have high reflective appearances, these reflected lightings cause the defect inspection work more difficult when appearance defects are embedded on the uneven exteriors of vehicle mirrors. Higher reflection on uneven exteriors grows the difficulty of differentiating the appearance defects on vehicle mirrors. The suitable lighting control technique of acquiring images provides the possibility to execute automatic defect inspection. Thence, this study conducts an automated appearance defect detection system of vehicle mirrors to substitute visual examination workers from inspection works of vehicle mirrors. This study recommends a defect enhancement technique based on Fourier high-pass filtering and the convex hull arithmetic to examine appearance defects on curved mirrors of vehicles.

Automated visual inspections of surface flaws have changed into pivotal tasks for manufacturers endeavoring to promote product quality and manufacturing efficiency [1, 2]. Lin, Chiu, and Lin [3] proposed using image reconstruction method based on cosine transform to inspect small appearance variations on capacitor chips of electronic elements. Park et al. [4] modelled lots of parameter combinations for deep learning networks with distinct depths and layer nodes to take proper configuration for automated inspection of exterior blemishes on textured and non-textured elements. Lin et al. [5] utilized some novel convolutional neural network models having deep learning skills to inspect flaws on light-emitting diode (LED) chips.

Several investigations report the automatic appearance flaw detection of glass-related products. Lin and Tsai [6] introduced a rebuilt scheme based on Fourier domain to detect linear flaws on capacitive touch panels. Li, Liang, and Zhang [7] used the principal components analysis theory to detect visual defects on the cover glass of mobile phones. Lin and Li [8] implemented a defect inspection system with wavelet domain-based filtering method to detect area flaws on touch panels. Chiu and Lin [9] integrated Hotelling's distance function and gray theory based on discrete cosine domain to detect surface defects on transparent lenses of LEDs. Lin and Chen [10] incorporated the partial least squares theory in the wavelet packet domain for surface flaw inspection on textured LED lenses.

Certain research even more concentrated on exploring the visual defect detection of mirror goods. Chiu, Lo, and Lin [11] developed an optical distortion detection skill based on Hough domain for automatic flaw detection on clear glass of vehicle mirrors. Lin and Hsieh [12] implemented a visual inspection system having small-shift detection schemes to find display deviations on convex vehicle mirrors. Chiu, Lin, and Lin [13] proposed the image models based on Fourier descriptors to detect profile flaws on vehicle mirrors. From the previous commentary of articles, most of the present studies concentrate on automatic flaw detections of transparent glass, optical lenses, and mirrors. Those optical inspection systems focus mostly on the distortion and profile blemish detections. Since appearance defects sometimes have an impact on not only the visual quality of industrial parts but also their functionality, efficiency, structural strength, etc. [14], the degree of harm even more than the distortion and profile defects. Less studies explore appearance inspections with attributes of little flaws on curved surfaces of vehicle mirrors. Consequently, we apply the Fourier high-pass filtering and convex hull arithmetic to inspect appearance defects on high reflective surfaces of vehicle mirrors.

Fourier transform is insensitive to noises and unvarying to translation, rotation, and scaling, which causes it be a perfect selection for automatic flaw inspection in the production process. Chan and Pang [15] defined two diagrams, the central spatial and frequency spectrums, based on the Fourier transform to analyze fabric defects. Da et al. [14] developed a quantitative inspection method in Fourier domain applying directed ultrasonic waves for efficiently detecting flaws in pipeline structures. He et al. [16] used an optical measurement method based on Fourier transform profilometry to recover the rail profile and flaws on the rail web. Tsai and Huang [17] introduced an image rebuilt method in Fourier domain to inspect and locate little flaws in homogeneous pattern images of electronic surfaces. The flaw inspection arithmetic used in the spatial images are normally reactive to noises, lighting changes, and geometric variations. The Fourier transform-based rebuilt method is a sturdy means for defect inspection in uniform mode, random texture, and periodical pattern surfaces covering most of workpieces in electronic industry. Consequently, this study presents an image rebuilt scheme using Fourier high-pass filtering with cross-shaped filter and convex hull arithmetic to inspect small appearance defects on vehicle mirror images.

2 Proposed Methods

This study proposes an image rebuilt technique based on Fourier high-pass filtering and convex hull arithmetic to inspect appearance defects for vehicle mirrors. Five steps are developed to accomplish the procedure of appearance defect inspection. Firstly, image preprocessing is executed to remove laser marks and background region and produce an ROI and a merged image to reduce the obstruction of non-mirror regions in further frequency analyses. Secondly, the merged image is transformed to Fourier domain, and the appearance message of the trial mirror is converted to frequency spectrum. Thirdly, by selecting a proper filtering width in frequency domain, the high-frequency parts outside the central cross-shaped region are retained, and the remainders are given to zero for reconstructing the object appearance. There is detailed message regarding defects and edges in the preserved high-frequency elements than those in the low-frequency elements. Fourthly, the filtered frequency image is executed by the inverse Fourier transform to make a reconstructed image. Thus, a defect-enhanced image could be reconstructed from the frequency domain for contrasting with the preprocessed image. Fifthly, the convex hull arithmetic is applied to remove noises for detecting appearance defects. Therefore, the appearance defects on the curved vehicle mirrors can be exactly identified and located by the proposed approach.

For acquiring finer image resolution and defect inspection manifestation, a testing trial is partitioned into two portions for image capture. Thus, the whole testing trial is evenly acquired into two testing images to obviously exhibit the contents of object surfaces and boundaries on both images. The two parts of laser marks at fixed locations are first removed from the testing image. In this study, we define an ROI (region of interest) in a square block including the objects will be explored. The adoption of ROI avoids unconcerned regions from obstructing neighborhood calculations or mathematical transformations. If an image having unconcerned districts is converted to a frequency domain, the unrelated regions can notably obstruct the frequency analysis of the interested objects. Therefore, after we capture the image of mirror and background, we produce a mask to depict the mirror area. Then, we acquire a merged image by integrating the mirror area with an operated background (average intensity of the mirror area) to decrease the obstruction of the initial background. This merged image could be applied as the source for Fourier transformation.

Fourier transform possesses the advantageous attributes of noise resistivity and increase of periodic properties [15, 18]. The Fourier domain portrays the textured image expressed as frequency parts. These entire textured patterns are simply discernible as gathering of low-frequency coefficients with large energy in the spectrum. Suppose $f(x, y)$ be an intensity located at coordinates (x, y). If an image with size of $M \times M$ pixels, the two-dimensional DFT (discrete Fourier transform) of $f(x, y)$ can be defined as [18]

$$F(u, v) = \frac{1}{M^2} \sum_{x=0}^{M-1} \sum_{y=0}^{M-1} f(x, y)\, e^{-j2\pi(ux+vy/M)} \tag{1}$$

where $j = \sqrt{-1}$, (u, v) are frequency variables and $u, v = 0, 1, 2, \ldots, M\text{-}1$. The DFT is a complex function, denoted as $F(u, v) = R(u, v) + jI(u, v)$, where $R(u, v)$ and $I(u, v)$ are the real and imaginary parts of $F(u, v)$, that is,

$$R(u, v) = \frac{1}{M^2} \sum_{x=0}^{M-1} \sum_{y=0}^{M-1} f(x, y) \cdot \cos[2\pi(ux + vy/M)] \tag{2}$$

$$I(u, v) = \frac{1}{M^2} \sum_{x=0}^{M-1} \sum_{y=0}^{M-1} f(x, y) \cdot \sin[2\pi(ux + vy/M)] \tag{3}$$

The size of the transformation is concentrated on the origin of the Fourier-frequency image. The directional attributes of an intensity image obviously correlate with low-frequency coefficients having high energy, which are dispersed on the unbent stripes in the Fourier-frequency image with orientations orthogonal to their equivalents in the spatial domain image. If a mirror image with the vertical and horizontal edges of mirror boundary is converted to Fourier domain, two major stripes with low-frequency coefficients having high energy cross at the middle of Fourier spectrum image.

Low-frequency coefficients having high energy are related with regular line patterns and may arise about the major stripes in the Fourier-frequency image. For entirely removing all homologous line modes in the spatial domain image, not merely the frequency coefficients placing on the major stripes but those frequency coefficients in the vicinity of the major stripes as well need to be eliminated from the Fourier-frequency image. These frequency coefficients dropping in the vicinity of the major stripes in the Fourier-frequency image are essentially filtrated through assigning these coefficients to zero. After filtering the specified stripe regions, we conduct inverse Fourier transform to obtain a filtrated reconstructed image in the spatial domain.

The filtered rebuilt image has consistent intensities for pixels pertaining to homologous regions of object and operated background, but it also produces notably distinct intensities for pixels pertaining to nonhomologous defect areas. The gray level changes in homologous districts could be very little, while the intensity changes in nonhomologous regions could be big contrast to the whole rebuilt image. Thence, this study can determine a threshold for distinguishing defects from mirror area in the rebuilt image. The rebuilt image will be approximately a consistent intensity image if a non-defect appearance image is tested. The upper limit T_U for intensity changes in the rebuilt image is expressed by $T_U = \mu + N\sigma$, where μ and σ are the mean and standard deviation of the intensities of the rebuilt image $f'(x, y)$, and N is a controlled parameter decided by experiments. The binary defect image $D(x, y)$ for defect separation is

$$D(x, y) = \begin{cases} 255, \text{ if } f'(x, y) \leq (\mu + N\sigma) \\ 0, \text{ otherwise.} \end{cases} \tag{4}$$

If a pixel with the intensity is less than the upper limit T_U, the pixel is categorized as a homologous element. On the contrary, it is categorized as a defect element. When the defect sizes to be detected are usually very little contrast to the whole appearance image, the μ and σ can be counted straight from the rebuilt image of an initial image to tolerate the illumination changes in the examination circumstance.

The binarized rebuilt image $D(x, y)$ may have many false alarm pixels due to the inaccurate estimates of parameters μ and σ. Since the testing mirrors have near-convex shapes, the convex hull arithmetic is utilized to produce a convex hull image of the rebuilt image for removing the pixels of detecting usual districts as defects. Convex hull of a shape is the smallest convex set containing it, and it has extensive implementations in image processing and object recognition [19]. The convex hull arithmetic [20] is applied in this research to the binary image to produce a convex hull image. Then an XOR image obtained from the differences of taking exclusive OR operations between the convex hull image and binarized rebuilt image will significantly reduce the false alarm pixels.

3 Experiments and Analyses

To mathematically confirm the representation of the recommended technique, we compare the results of our experiments against those provided by professional inspectors (ground truth). The expression guides, (1-α) and (1-β), are used to express proper inspection assessments; the larger the two guides, the more precise the inspection outcomes. False alarm mistake (α, regarding usual districts as defects) divides the regions of usual districts inspected as defects by the regions of actual

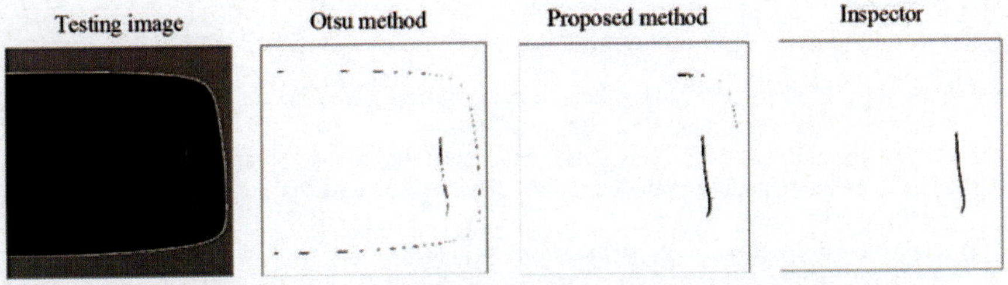

Fig. 3 Partial detection results of the Otsu method, proposed methods, and inspector

usual districts to gain the mistake. Missing alarm mistake (β, unsucceeding to alarm actual defects) divides the regions of uninspected actual defects by the regions of all actual defects to obtain the mistake. For the both mistakes, the lower the guide values, the better the detection outcomes.

One existing scheme usually applied to anomaly detection is contrast to the recommended approach to differentiate effects of appearance defect inspection. To indicate the defect inspection outcomes of a testing image, Fig. 3 demonstrates fractional outcomes of inspecting appearance defects by the Otsu method [21], the recommended method, and the ground truth provided by inspectors, separately. The Otsu method produces many erroneous judgments in missing alarms on appearance defect inspection. The suggested method inspects most of the appearance defects and produces less erroneous judgments. Therefore, the suggested technique surpasses the Otsu method in the appearance defect detection of vehicle mirrors with high reflective surfaces.

4 Conclusions

This research suggests a defect enhancement technique based on Fourier high-pass filtering and the convex hull arithmetic to the optical inspection of appearance defects on high reflective surfaces of vehicle mirrors. Through self-comparing the testing image with the corresponding convex hull image, the suggested method does not need any standard pattern for template matching, and there is no need the accurate positioning of mirror workpieces in jigs. Trial outcomes present that the proposed approach achieves a higher probability of correctly discriminating appearance defects from normal regions and a lower probability of erroneously detecting normal regions as defects on reflective exteriors of vehicle mirrors. This research contributes a solution to a common appearance defect detection problem of vehicle mirrors with high reflective surfaces.

Acknowledgments This work was partially supported by the Ministry of Science and Technology, Taiwan (R.O.C.), for the financial support through the Grant MOST 107-2221-E-324-016.

References

1. E.M. Taha, E. Emary, K. Moustafa, Automatic optical inspection for PCB manufacturing: A survey. Int. J. Sci. Eng. Res. **5**(7), 1095–1102 (2014)
2. C.F.J. Kuo, C.H. Lai, C.H. Kao, C.H. Chiu, Integrating image processing and classification technology into automated polarizing film defect inspection. Opt. Lasers Eng. **104**, 204–219 (2018)
3. H.D. Lin, Y.P. Chiu, W.T. Lin, An innovative approach for detection of slight surface variations on capacitor chips. Int. J. Innov. Comput. Inform. Contr. **9**(5), 1835–1850 (2013)
4. J.K. Park, B.K. Kwon, J.H. Park, D.J. Kang, Machine learning-based imaging system for surface defect inspection. Int. J. Precision Eng. Manufact.-Green Technol. **3**(3), 303–310 (2016)
5. H. Lin, B. Li, X.G. Wang, Y.F. Shu, S.L. Niu, Automated defect inspection of LED chip using deep convolutional neural network. J. Intell. Manuf. **30**(6), 2525–2534 (2019)
6. H.D. Lin, H.H. Tsai, Automated quality inspection of surface defects on touch panels. J. Chinese Inst. Indust. Eng. **29**(5), 291–302 (2012)
7. D. Li, L.Q. Liang, W.J. Zhang, Defect inspection and extraction of the mobile phone cover glass based on the principal components analysis. Int. J. Adv. Manuf. Technol. **73**, 1605–1614 (2014)
8. H.D. Lin, J.M. Li, An innovative quality system for surface blemish detection of touch panels. Int. J. Appl. Eng. Res. **12**(21), 11523–11531 (2017)
9. Y.P. Chiu, H.D. Lin, An innovative blemish detection system for curved LED lenses. Expert Syst. Appl. **40**(2), 471–479 (2013)
10. H.D. Lin, H.L. Chen, Detection of surface flaws on textured LED lenses using wavelet packet transform based partial least squares techniques. Int. J. Innov. Comput. Inform. Contr. **15**(3), 905–921 (2019)
11. Y.P. Chiu, Y.C. Lo, H.D. Lin, Hough transform based approach for surface distortion flaw detection on transparent glass. Int. J. Appl. Eng. Res. **12**(19), 8150–8159 (2017)
12. H.D. Lin, K.S. Hsieh, Detection of surface variations on curved mirrors of vehicles using slight deviation control techniques. Int. J. Innov. Comput. Inform. Contr. **14**(4), 1407–1421 (2018)
13. Y.P. Chiu, Y.K. Lin, H.D. Lin, Effective image models for inspecting profile flaws of car mirrors with applications. J. Appl. Eng. Sci. **18**(1), 81–91 (2020)
14. Y. Da, G. Dong, B. Wang, D. Liu, Z. Qian, A novel approach to surface defect detection. Int. J. Eng. Sci. **133**, 181–195 (2018)
15. C.H. Chan, G.K.H. Pang, Fabric defect detection by Fourier analysis. IEEE Trans. Ind. Appl. **36**, 1267–1276 (2000)
16. S. He, J. Li, X. Gao, L. Luo, Application of FTP in flaw detection of rail web. Optik **126**(2), 187–190 (2015)
17. D.M. Tsai, C.K. Huang, Defect detection in electronic surfaces using template-based Fourier image reconstruction. IEEE Trans. Compon. Packag. Manuf. Technol. **1**(9), 163–172 (2019)
18. R.C. Gonzalez, R.E. Woods, *Digital Image Processing*, 4th edn. (Pearson, New York, 2017)
19. M.A. Jayaram, H. Fleyeh, Convex hulls in image processing: A scoping review. Am. J. Intell. Syst. **6**(2), 48–58 (2016)
20. R.L. Graham, An efficient algorithm for determining the convex hull of a finite planar set. Inf. Process. Lett. **1**(4), 132–133 (1972)
21. N. Otsu, A threshold selection method from gray level histogram. IEEE Trans. Syst. Man Cybern. **9**, 62–66 (1979)

Utilizing Quality Measures in Evaluating Image Encryption Methods

Abdelfatah A. Tamimi, Ayman M. Abdalla, and Mohammad M. Abdallah

1 Introduction

Image quality measures are essential in evaluating the efficacy of algorithms used in image processing and computer vision. The quality assessment may be computed objectively and automatically or through subjective user evaluation. Although the users' viewpoint is important for many applications, it is not very useful for applications sensitive to the minor changes invisible to humans. Furthermore, it is infeasible to use a large group of users for testing many cases involving dozens of images. Therefore, most researchers focus on objective metrics rather than relying on subjective metrics obtained from human users. Nonetheless, many researchers, such as [1–5], only used some metrics and overlooked the others.

Image quality measurements are often made by comparing a modified image to the original image. Nonetheless, the goals of making such comparisons differ with different applications. Generally, the changes made onto an image can be categorized into two categories based on the purposes of these changes. One category aims at obtaining an image very similar to the original for applications such as denoising, restoration, steganography, and compression. The other category aims at distorting the image to make it unrecognizable, usually for cryptography applications. Previous work on quality measurement, such as [6–10], mostly focused on the first goal. Alternatively, this paper will focus on the latter, that is, using quality metrics for cryptography. Little previous work focused on image quality from that point of view. Recently, [11] proposed a new metric, called a Contrast Sensitivity Function, to measure the degradation of compressed and encrypted

A. A. Tamimi (✉) · A. M. Abdalla · M. M. Abdallah
Faculty of Science and Information Technology, Al-Zaytoonah University of Jordan, Amman, Jordan
e-mail: drtamimi@zuj.edu.jo

H. R. Arabnia et al. (eds.), *Advances in Computer Vision and Computational Biology*, Transactions on Computational Science and Computational Intelligence,
https://doi.org/10.1007/978-3-030-71051-4_21

image sequences. However, this new metric is more suited for image sequences than individual images. On the other hand, quality measures used for evaluating image encryption can also be used for evaluating audio encryption, as done by [12]. Furthermore, many image encryption algorithms apply to three-dimensional objects [13–15].

Additionally, since cryptography produces images unrecognizable by humans, and their visual analyses require experts to recognize possible patterns, this paper will not consider subjective quality metrics. Nonetheless, it is not practical to rely on a small set of metrics to evaluate any given method. A collection of different quality measurement techniques must be used to cover the encryption strength in resisting different types of attacks.

In lossless encryption methods, the decrypted image must be identical to the original. On the other hand, lossy encryption methods recover an imperfect decrypted image. The quality of this decrypted image can be evaluated with the same tools used for recovered and denoised images because it is desired to be very similar to the original. Therefore, decrypted image quality is not in the focus of this paper.

2 Statistical Analysis Measures

The use of statistical analysis measures for a cryptography technique can help in evaluating its resistance to various attacks, especially statistical attacks. This section will discuss common statistical measures employed in image cryptography.

2.1 Keyspace

The keyspace of an encryption algorithm is the set of all possible keys that can be used to encrypt the data. A sufficiently large keyspace prevents brute-force attacks and increases the difficulty for other attacks that try to guess the secret key used in encryption

2.2 Mean Absolute Error

When Mean Absolute Error (MAE) is used in comparing a plain image with its encrypted image, a high MAE value is desired to indicate more difference between the image and its encryption and thus better encryption. MAE is computed with (1).

$$\text{MAE} = \frac{1}{mn} \sum_{i=1}^{m} \sum_{j=1}^{n} \left| A\,[i,j] - B\left[i,j\right] \right| \tag{1}$$

2.3 MSE and PSNR

Similar to MAE, the mean squared error (MSE) indicates the difference between two given images. Therefore, large values are desired when MSE is computed for an image and its encryption. MSE for two images, stored in matrices A and B, is computed as in (2):

$$\text{MSE} = \frac{1}{mn} \sum_{i=1}^{m} \sum_{j=1}^{n} \left(A\,[i,j] - B\,[i,j]\right)^2 \tag{2}$$

For image quality measurement, Peak Signal to Noise Ratio (PSNR) is preferred more than MSE. It is computed based on MSE as in (3):

$$\text{PSNR} = 10 \log_{10} \left(\frac{\text{MAX}^2}{\text{MSE}} \right) \tag{3}$$

where MAX is the maximum pixel value in the image. PSNR, measured in decibels, is focused on the unchanged values in the image rather than on the noise. Therefore, a better encryption technique should produce lower PSNR values to indicate having less unaltered values and, consequently, more resistance to attacks.

2.4 Entropy

The randomness of the pixel values, indicated by entropy, should increase after encryption to increase the encrypted image resistance against different attacks. The increase in randomness can be measured by computing the entropy ratio, that is, the rate of increase in entropy. Entropy is given by (4):

$$H = -\sum_{i=1}^{\text{MAX}} \left(P(i) \log_2 \left(P(i)\right) \right) \tag{4}$$

where:

MAX is the maximum pixel value of the image, and
$P(i)$ is the probability of the occurrence of pixel value i.

2.5 Correlation and Neighbors Correlation

The resemblance of one image to another can be measured with correlation, as given by (5), where $\overline{A}$ and $\overline{B}$are mean values for matrices A and B, respectively:

$$r = \frac{\sum_{i=1}^{m}\sum_{j=1}^{n}\left(A[i,j]-\overline{A}\right)\left(B[i,j]-\overline{B}\right)}{\sqrt{\left(\sum_{i=1}^{m}\sum_{j=1}^{n}\left(A[i,j]-\overline{A}\right)^2\right)\left(\sum_{i=1}^{m}\sum_{j=1}^{n}\left(B[i,j]-\overline{B}\right)^2\right)}} \tag{5}$$

For encryption techniques, it is desirable to have very low correlation values to show stronger encryption.

In addition to the above correlation indicator, the correlation between the neighboring pixels in the encrypted image can be measured and compared with that of the original image. A good indicator of neighbors' correlation is the Value Difference Degree (VDD). To compute VDD, start with computing Value Difference (VD) of each pixel value $P(i, j)$ at position (i, j) as in (6):

$$\mathrm{VD}(i,j) = \frac{1}{4}\sum_{i',j'}\left[P(i,j)-P\left(i',j'\right)\right]^2 \tag{6}$$

where the neighborhood of the pixel at position (i, j) is $(i', j') = \{(i-1, j), (i+1, j), (i, j-1), (i, j+1)\}$. Then, compute the Average Value Difference (AVD) for the whole image. Finally, VDD can be obtained by computing the difference of AVD values for the original image and the encrypted image, divided by their sum, as in (7). The value of VDD should be a number between -1 and 1 where a value near 1 indicates strong encryption.

$$\mathrm{VDD} = \left(\mathrm{AVD}_{\mathrm{original}}-\mathrm{AVD}_{\mathrm{encrypted}}\right) / \left(\mathrm{AVD}_{\mathrm{original}}+\mathrm{AVD}_{\mathrm{encrypted}}\right) \tag{7}$$

2.6 SSIM and MSSIM

As the image is encrypted, structural information should become degraded and distorted. In other words, the structural information of the encrypted image should be sufficiently different from that of the original image. The structural similarity index (SSIM) of an image is given by (8):

$$\mathrm{SSIM} = \frac{\left(2\mu_x\mu_y + c_1\right)\left(2\sigma_{xy} + c_2\right)}{\left(\mu_x^2 + \mu_y^2 + c_1\right)\left(\sigma_x^2 + \sigma_y^2 + c_2\right)} \tag{8}$$

where:

μ_x is the average of x,
μ_y is the average of y,
σ_x^2 is the variance of x,
σ_y^2 is the variance of y,
σ_{xy} is the covariance of x and y,
$c_1 = (k_1\ L)^2$ and $c_2 = (k_2\ L)^2$ are two variables to stabilize the division with weak denominator,
L is the dynamic range of the pixel values (typically, this is $2^{\text{bpp}} - 1$, *bpp* is bits per pixel), and
$k_1 = 0.01$ and $k_2 = 0.03$ by default.

To compare the overall structural quality of an encrypted image Y to the original image X, the Mean SSIM (MSSIM) value is computed as in (9):

$$\text{MSSIM}\,(X, Y) = \frac{1}{M}\sum_{j=1}^{M}\text{SSIM}\left(x_j - y_j\right) \tag{9}$$

For encrypted images, a low value of MSSIM is desired since it indicates less structural similarity and better encryption.

2.7 Histogram Analysis

An effective image encryption method should perform sufficient confusion and diffusion of the pixels. The encryption method needs confusion to permute the pixels and diffusion to change their values. However, many metrics of encryption could indicate that an encryption method is effective when it has a strong confusion component even when its diffusion component is weak or nonexistent. For an example, see [14, 15]. This problem creates a serious weakness for statistical attacks. Therefore, it is better to use histogram analysis, which is often effective in detecting weaknesses in image diffusion.

A simple and common method of histogram analysis is histogram visualization where the histogram of the original image is compared to the histogram of the encrypted image. The two histograms should appear different to indicate that the distribution of pixel values has changed after encryption. To indicate further resistance against statistical attacks, the histogram of the encrypted image should appear uniform and contain no distinctive peaks that could provide a weakness for the attacks.

For quantitative histogram analysis, the variance of histogram can be computed where a smaller variance value indicates less variation in values and a uniform histogram. The variance Var(V) of the histogram V stored as a one-dimensional array is given by (10) where v_i is the ith element of V and represents the frequency of gray value i in the image.

$$\mathrm{Var}(V) = \frac{1}{2n^2}\sum_{i=1}^{n}\sum_{j=1}^{n}\left(v_i - v_j\right)^2 \tag{10}$$

2.8 Balancedness

In addition to the above measures, encryption systems that employ cellular automata must examine their balancedness. That is, each generation of cellular automata must have nearly an equal number of ones and zeros. Failure to maintain this balance could undermine the efficacy of the whole encryption system. For examples of how this metric is used, see [14, 15].

3 Sensitivity Analysis Measures

The sensitivity of an encryption method to minor changes in the key or the input image makes it more effective, especially against differential attacks. Furthermore, this sensitivity keeps the rest of the secret key or the image secure if part of that information was revealed. Note that the lack of key sensitivity will also undermine the keyspace since many keys would become equivalent and should be excluded.

This sensitivity can be observed visually by making very small changes to the secret key or the input image and observing the result. However, better evaluations could be achieved using UACI and NPCR.

The Unified Averaged Changed Intensity (UACI) and the Number of Pixel Change Rate (NPCR) measure the strength of encryption techniques, especially their resistance against differential attacks. NPCR concentrates on the absolute number of pixels that change their values in differential attacks, while UACI focuses on the averaged difference between two paired encrypted images.

The desired UACI and NPCR values vary with the type and size of the image. A set of benchmark images with tables of theoretically computed upper and lower bounds for UACI and NPCR values have been provided by [16]. They showed through theoretical analysis and practical experiments that their computed theoretical values provide better measures of encryption quality than simple comparisons to other encryption methods.

4 Distortion Robustness Measures

Part of the encrypted image could be lost or distorted with different types of noise during transmission or storage. Therefore, an effective encryption system should be able to recover a meaningful recognizable image after it suffered from added noise or when part of it was occluded. This can be tested with visual observations or with measures of image quality.

To test the robustness of an encryption system with noise, sample encrypted images can be modified by adding noise of different types and intensities. Occlusion can be tested by replacing portions of the image with a single color such as black or white. If the decryption method recovers meaningful images similar to the original, this indicates that the system robustness can tolerate the tested distortion levels. Some of these types of tests were utilized by [14, 15].

5 Complexity Analysis

Space and time efficiency of the encryption system are important factors in determining the suitability of the system implementation for integration into various applications and hardware systems. The time and space requirements of most encryption algorithms are linear functions of the input size. However, the actual running time of these algorithms can vary significantly. Therefore, time and memory space required by the encryption technique should be estimated theoretically and measured empirically. The theoretical analysis should indicate the best, worst, and average cases. The practical experiments should provide the details of the implementation environment, such as the hardware and software specifications, the types and sizes of test data, etc.

6 Conclusion

The goals of image quality measurement differ according to application. This paper focused on image cryptography applications where the quality measurement goal is to ensure having noisy encrypted images with very low visual quality. Different metrics should be used for the encryption technique to ensure its robustness against various types of attacks such as brute-force, statistical, and differential attacks and to demonstrate its suitability for practical applications. Furthermore, these metrics can be used for making comparisons among various encryption techniques.

References

1. A. Yahya, A. Abdalla, *An AES-Based Encryption Algorithm with Shuffling, 2009 International Conference on Security and Management (SAM '09), Las Vegas, NV, USA, in Security and Management* (Eds, CSREA Press, H.R. Arabnia and K. Daimi, 2009), pp. 113–116
2. A. Tamimi, A. Abdalla, A double-shuffle image-encryption algorithm, 2012 international conference on image Processing, computer vision, and pattern recognition (IPCV '12), Las Vegas, NV, USA, in *Image Processing, Computer Vision, and Pattern Recognition*, (CSREA Press, H.R. Arabnia and K. Daimi, 2012), pp. 496–499
3. A. Abdalla, A. Tamimi, Algorithm for image mixing and encryption. Int. J. Multimedia Appl. **5**(2), 15–21 (2013)
4. A. Tamimi, A. Abdalla, An image encryption algorithm with XOR and S-box, in *19th International Conference on Image Processing, Computer Vision, and Pattern Recognition (IPCV '15), Las Vegas, NV, USA*, (2015), pp. 166–169
5. A. Tamimi, A. Abdalla, A variable circular-shift image-encryption algorithm, in *Proceedings of the International Conference on Image Processing, Computer Vision, and Pattern Recognition (IPCV '17)*, (Las Vegas, 2017), pp. 33–37
6. Z. Wang, H.R. Sheikh, E.P. Simoncelli, Image quality assessment: From error visibility to structural similarity, IEEE trans. Image Proc. **13**(4), 1–14 (2004)
7. K.-H. Thung, P. Raveendran, *A survey of image quality measures. 2009 International Conference for Technical Postgraduates (TECHPOS), Kuala Lumpur, Malaysia* (2009). https://doi.org/10.1109/TECHPOS.2009.5412098
8. Z. Wang, A.C. Bovik, *Modern Image Quality Assessment* (Morgan & Claypool, 2006). https://doi.org/10.2200/S00010ED1V01Y2005081VM003
9. B.W. Keelan, *Handbook of Image Quality: Characterization and Prediction* (Marcel Dekker, 2002)
10. R.R. Choudhary, V. Goel, G. Meena, Survey paper: Image quality assessment, proceedings of international conference on sustainable computing in science, technology and management (SUSCOM), Jaipur, India, February 26-28. (2019, 2019). https://doi.org/10.2139/ssrn.3356307
11. N. Khlif, M. Ben Amor, F. Kammoun, N. Masmoudi, A new evaluation of video encryption security with a perceptual metric. J. Test. Eval. **48**. (in press) (2020). https://doi.org/10.1520/JTE20160456
12. A. Tamimi, A. Abdalla, An audio shuffle-encryption algorithm. International Conference on Internet and Multimedia Technologies (ICIMT '14), San Francisco, CA, USA, in *Proceedings of the World Congress on Engineering and Computer Science, vol. I, 2014*, (2014), pp. 409–412
13. M. Mizher, R. Sulaiman, *Robotic Movement Encryption Using Guaranteed Cellular Automata. 2018 Cyber Resilience Conference (CRC), Putrajaya, Malaysia* (2018). https://doi.org/10.1109/CR.2018.8626820
14. M.M. Mizher, R. Sulaiman, A. Abdalla, M.M. Mizher, A simple flexible cryptosystem for meshed 3D objects and images. J. King Saud Univ.-Comp. Inform. Sci.. (in press) (2019). https://doi.org/10.1016/j.jksuci.2019.03.008
15. M.M. Mizher, R. Sulaiman, A. Abdalla, M.M. Mizher, An improved simple flexible cryptosystem for 3D objects with texture maps and 2D images. J. Inform. Secur. Appli. **47C**, 390–409 (2019). https://doi.org/10.1016/j.jisa.2019.06.005
16. Y. Wu, J.P. Noonan, S. Agaian, NPCR and UACI randomness tests for image encryption. Cyber J.: Multidiscip. J. Sci. Technol., J. Select. Areas Telecommun. (JSAT) **1**(2), 31–38 (2011)

Part IV
Novel Medical Applications

Exergames for Systemic Sclerosis Rehabilitation: A Pilot Study

Federica Ferraro, Marco Trombini, Matteo Morando, Marica Doveri, Gerolamo Bianchi, and Silvana Dellepiane

1 Introduction

Systemic Sclerosis (SSc) is a rare autoimmune rheumatic disease characterized by vascular injury, immune dysfunction, and an excessive production and accumulation of collagen, called fibrosis, that can affect the skin and internal organs including lungs, gastrointestinal tract and cardiovascular system [1, 2]. One of the major impairments, caused by skin induration and joint and muscle involvement, is the gradual loss of mobility which substantially affects the quality of life [3]. In particular, hand disabilities in SSc are frequent and contribute to the manifestation of diseases such as inflammatory arthritis, tendon friction rubs, tendonitis/tendinosis, puffy hands, skin sclerosis, calcinosis, acro-osteolysis, Raynaud's phenomenon, and digital ulcers [4]. Furthermore, finger flexion and extension are the most impaired aspects of hand mobility in SSc patients [5]. Indeed, severe skin thickness in the hands can cause deformity in the flexion of the fingers, leading to the loss of flexion at the metacarpophalangeal (MCP) joints, the loss of extension of the proximal interphalangeal (PIP) joints, and the loss of thumb abduction. Moreover, the distal interphalangeal (DIP) joint may also become fixed in mid-range flexion. These impairments cause a claw-type deformity of MCP extension, PIP flexion, and thumb adduction.

F. Ferraro · M. Trombini (✉) · M. Morando · S. Dellepiane
Department of Electrical, Electronic, Telecommunications Engineering and Naval Architecture (DITEN), Università degli Studi di Genova, Genoa, Italy
e-mail: marco.trombini@edu.unige.it; silvana.dellepiane@unige.it

M. Doveri · G. Bianchi
Azienda Sanitaria Locale 3, Division of Rheumatology, Department of Locomotor System, Genoa, Italy
e-mail: marica.doveri@asl3.liguria.it; gerolamo.bianchi@asl3.liguria.it

H. R. Arabnia et al. (eds.), *Advances in Computer Vision and Computational Biology*, Transactions on Computational Science and Computational Intelligence, https://doi.org/10.1007/978-3-030-71051-4_22

As for skin ulcerations, they generally occur over joint contractures due to increased skin pressure in areas of bony prominences and reduced blood flow to the skin from scleroderma vasculopathy [4]. Focusing on the hands, small joint contractures yield dissatisfaction with appearance, social embarrassment, and difficulties in carrying out work activities, thus resulting in a significant drawback for SSc patients [4, 5].

These various manifestations of hand impairment can result in reduced mobility, dexterity, and grip strength, recognize them is essential, although there is no definitive medical treatment options yet [4]. In patients with SSc, hand rehabilitation aims at improving hand mobility, functionality and strength as well as increasing involvement in daily living activities [3]. The role of rehabilitation treatment is crucial and involves a multidisciplinary team consisting of physicians, physiotherapists, and occupational therapists. Even though most therapists recognize the importance of rehabilitation for SSc, there is currently minimal awareness and SSc rehabilitation therapy is not widespread [5].

In this work, a phase of an ongoing research project on SSc patients is described. Such a study is jointly being conducted by the Department of Electrical, Electronic, Telecommunications Engineering and Naval Architecture (DITEN) of Università degli Studi di Genova and the Department of Locomotor System, Division of Rheumatology of Azienda Sanitaria Locale 3, with the support of the ReMoVES[1] system [6, 7]. ReMoVES is a tele-rehabilitation platform that provides a set of services to support the motor and cognitive recovery through exergames [8].

The term *exergames* refers to a category of video games which combine virtual support with physical exercise. They are usually performed via sensors which also record actual movements. Exergames have recently gained large popularity and proved scientific reliability, thus overcoming their original purpose of entertainment. Indeed, they are frequently used in physiotherapy, occupational therapy, psychotherapy, and also in rehabilitation, since they provide engaging versions of standard activities, which entice patients in practicing, thus enabling the continuity of care. These types of video games are designed and developed under the supervision of medical staff, who certifies the correctness of movements that will be made during the games.

In the present work, patients interact with the game via the Leap Motion [9], thus without wearing sensors, markers, or controllers in hand. The data-acquisition capabilities of the ReMoVES platform are based on such a device which delivers an accurate informative content related to patients' movements. As a result, therapists are enabled to monitor the patient's activity and progress also without directly supervising them.

Movement analysis via ReMoVES system is personalized and makes it easy to explain some particular behavior related to the patient's impairment. Furthermore, patient's conditions can be automatically assessed by leveraging on machine learning algorithm. In particular, the sequential data collected by ReMoVES are

[1]numip.it/removes.

here studied by using a Long-Short Term Memory (LSTM) [10] Recurrent Neural Network (RNN) [11].

An informed consensus was obtained from participants prior to the beginning of the activity and the principles of the Declaration of Helsinki were followed.

2 Materials and Methods

2.1 *ReMoVES for Remote Monitoring and Rehabilitation*

The ReMoVES platform is a flexible tele-rehabilitation system developed at the Department of Electrical, Electronic, Telecommunications Engineering and Naval Architecture (DITEN) of Università degli Studi di Genova [7].

It is based on a multi-client/server architecture which allows for both the collection and access to information from different locations. As a result, ReMoVES is a support tool for the rehabilitation process both in clinical centers, with the assistance of therapists and doctors, and at patient's home, thus enabling the continuity of care also after de-hospitalization.

The medical team is provided with reliable data, including automated data processing methods [12].

ReMoVES is designed as support for both motor and cognitive recovery via exergames performed using Microsoft Kinect, Leap Motion and touchscreen.

Only the four exergames used in the patient's hand rehabilitation process are here presented, even though the ReMoVES platform includes other eleven activities. Patients interact with the system via the Leap Motion sensor, which is also the responsible for data acquisition. The position of hand joints in Fig. 1 is recorded at a frequency of 10 Hz, so that patients' movement can be accurately studied.

2.2 *Hand Exergames*

In this section, the used exergames are presented. All the activities are conceived as rehabilitation exercises which deliver task-oriented training by requiring patients to perform particular movements so that consecutive and repetitive tasks are fulfilled. The major benefit of this approach consists on the re-acquisition of skills to be involved in real life activities or, at least, on the maintenance of the current patient's condition.

As for the duration of the games, one of them (Finger Tap) lasts 60 s, while the others last 90 s. Features are extracted from game sessions, in order to analyze them and find patterns in patients' movements. In this way, each performance can be evaluated. To this purpose, at the end of each game session a log-file is created, which is populated with features values at a particular time.

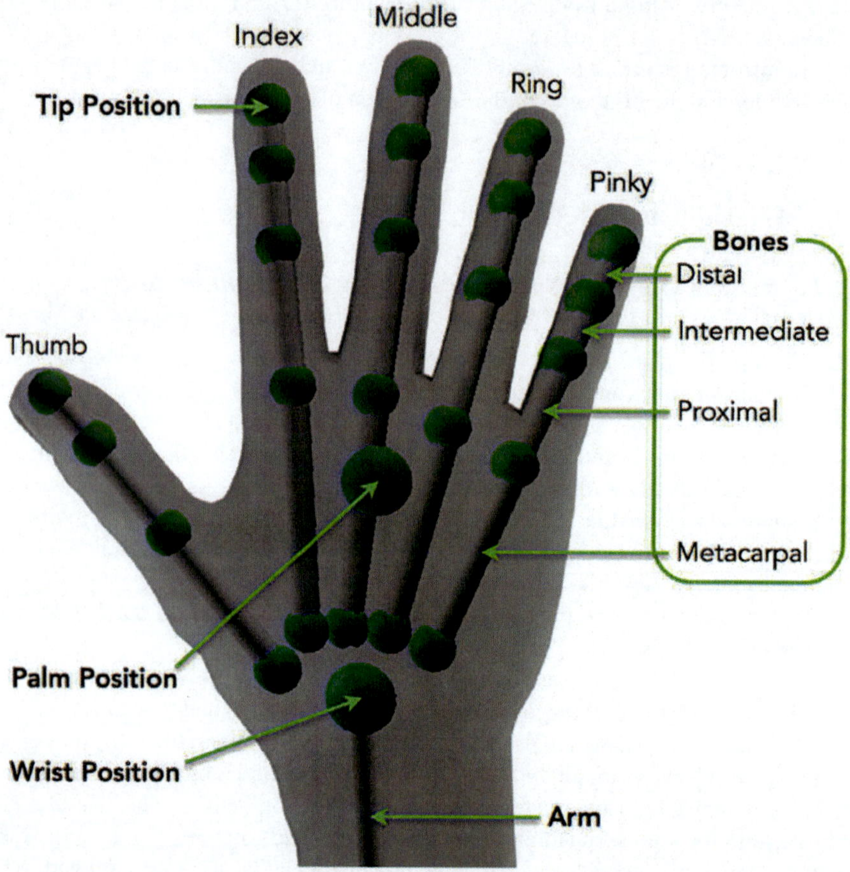

Fig. 1 Hand joint locations and names as captured by the Leap Motion sensor, on the coronal plane. The hand is composed of 3D coordinates for each of its 26 joints

The log-file is a JavaScript Object Notation (JSON) file consisting of an array that collects temporal events. There are keyvalue pairs in each element of the array that provide the data. Some keys are common to all exergames, i.e., *time* of recording in milliseconds (ms), *leap motion* joints position, and in-game *score*.

Further features describing the game session depend on the activity and are described in the following. Table 1 summarizes all the features for each exergame.

In addition to the aforementioned features, which are tracked by the ReMoVES system, others are later computed on the basis of the joint positions. They refer to three over the four exergames (Floating Trap, Endless Zig and City Car) and represent the range of motion (ROM) of the peculiar gesture. In particular, they are Opening ROM (Floating Trap), Yaw ROM (Endless Zig), and Pitch ROM (City Car), and will be discussed in the section referring to the corresponding exergames.

Table 1 Features for each exergame

	Finger tap	Floating trap	Endless zig	City car
Feature 1	Time	Time	Time	Time
Feature 2	Leap motion	Leap motion	Leap motion	Leap motion
Feature 3	Score	Score	Score	Score
Feature 4	Hand	Sphere	Speed	Speed
Feature 5	Wrong finger	Wrong target	Dead counter	Wrong path
Feature 6	Correct index	Correct target	Correct target	Forced restart
Feature 7	Correct middle	Bubble position	Block generated	
Feature 8	Correct ring			
Feature 9	Correct pinky			
Feature 10	Distance green			
Feature 11	Distance yellow			
Feature 12	Distance red			
Feature 13	Distance blue			
Feature 14	Miss green			
Feature 15	Miss yellow			
Feature 16	Miss red			
Feature 17	Miss blue			
Feature 18	Ball color			

Table 2 Opposition movements for each colored marble, for right and left hand

Marble color	Right hand	Left hand
Green	Thumb—Index	Thumb—Pinky
Yellow	Thumb—Middle	Thumb—Ring
Red	Thumb—Ring	Thumb—Middle
Blue	Thumb—Pinky	Thumb—Index

Finger Tap In Finger Tap exergame, the patients perform the finger opposition exercise, namely they are required to touch with the thumb other fingers, one finger at a time. The scene of the game represents a neck of a four-string guitar, where patients pretend to play the instrument. Some colored marbles sequentially fall off the strings. The color sequence is green, yellow, red, and blue, corresponding to fingers from left to right. The exergame self-adapts to both left and right hands, by defining the correct correspondence finger opposition—color, as specified in Table 2.

To stop the falling marbles, patients must pluck the right string, by opposing the right finger, at the correct timing. The goal of the game is to stop the marble when it is in the corresponding colored ring. The more precise is the stop, the more the score increases. If the patient misses some marbles or touches the wrong finger, the score decreases. In Fig. 2, the game set and the peculiar gesture are shown.

The specific features for this exergame are:

- Hand: either Left or Right;

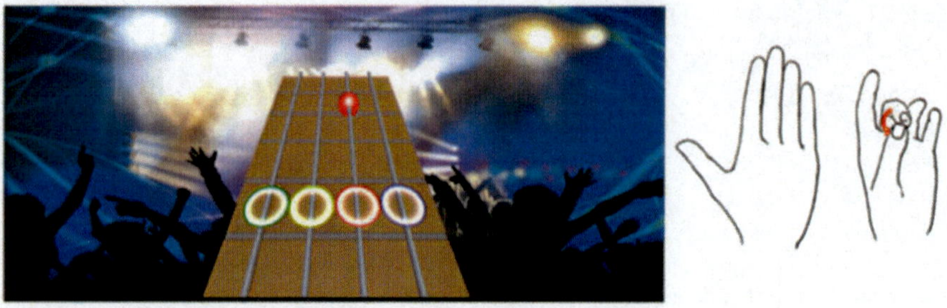

Fig. 2 Finger tap screenshot captured during activity and corresponding thumb opposition movement

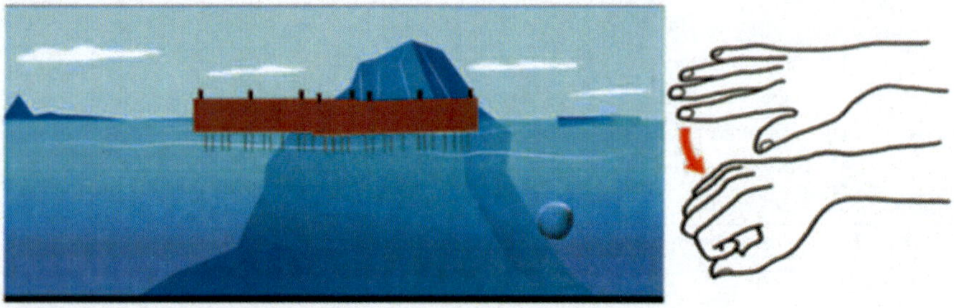

Fig. 3 Floating trap screenshot captured during activity and corresponding finger flexion-extension movement

- Wrong Finger: number of marbles stopped with the wrong finger;
- Correct+*finger*: number of correctly stopped marbles;
- Distance+*color*: distance between the stopped marble and the corresponding colored ring;
- Miss+*color*: number of missed marbles;
- Ball Color: color of the marble at the time instant considered.

Floating Trap The aim of the present activity is to stimulate the finger flexion-extension movement. The patient is led to open his hand and make a fist alternatively. Consequently, two floating rafts move accordingly to the flexion-extension of the fingers. In the meantime, a bubble of air rises towards the surface of the water. The bubbles must not hit the rafts, or they will explode, causing loss of in-game score. Figure 3 shows the game scenario and the specific movement to be performed.

This exergame has the following characteristic features:

- Sphere: length of the radius of a virtual sphere contained in the hand palm (it measures the finger extension);
- Wrong Target: number of exploded bubbles;
- Correct Target: number of emerged bubbles;

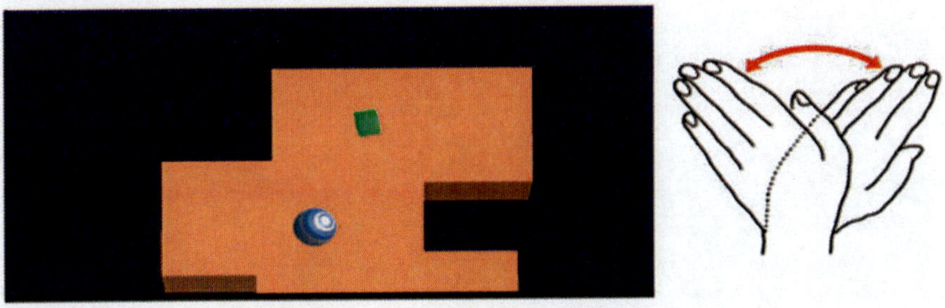

Fig. 4 Endless Zig screenshot captured during activity and corresponding radial-ulnar deviation movement

- Bubble Position: position where the bubbles appear, either left, right, or center;
- Opening ROM: difference between the maximum and minimum of Sphere field.

Endless Zig In this exergame, the patient moves a marble along a *zigzag* path that appears on the screen, hence practicing the radial-ulnar deviation movement. Going out of the boundaries causes score loss. In order to increase the score, the patient must take the bonus gems that appear along the path. The game set and the peculiar gesture are depicted in Fig. 4.

In this exergame, the peculiar features are:

- Speed: ball speed;
- Dead Counter: number of times the ball falls off the course;
- Correct Target: number of bonus gems correctly taken;
- Block Generated: number of blocks generated to build the path;
- Yaw ROM: difference between the maximum and the minimum angle of the line joining the Wrist and the Palm positions (Fig. 1) on the coronal plane. It measures the radial-ulnar deviation.

City Car Flexion-extension of the wrist is stimulated in City Car exergame. Consequently, patients drive a car along a randomly generated road. The speed of the car increases progressively and returns to the initial condition as soon as the player goes out of the carriageway, introducing a penalty in the score. Figure 5 depicts the game scenario and the characteristic movement of the present game.

This exergame presents the following peculiar features:

- Speed: car speed;
- Wrong Path: number of times the car has gone out of the carriage;
- Forced Restart: number of times the car has been replaced in the carriage;
- Pitch ROM: difference between the maximum and the minimum angle of the line joining the Wrist and the Palm positions (Fig. 1) on the sagittal plane. It measures the wrist flexion-extension.

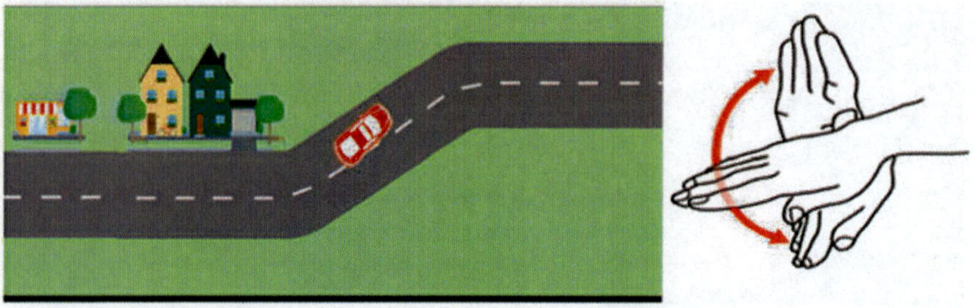

Fig. 5 City car screenshot captured during activity and corresponding wrist flexion-extension movement

Table 3 Number of sessions for each exergame

Exergame	Group
Finger tap	Patients: 19
	Control: 16
Floating trap	Patients: 19
	Control: 16
Endless zig	Patients: 18
	Control: 15
City car	Patients: 18
	Control: 14

2.3 Participants

The involved population consisted on nineteen SSc patients referring to La Colletta Hospital (Genoa) and sixteen other subjects, including medical staff and other hospitalized patients. A written informed consent was obtained from all the participants to the trial. Patients and subjects are uniquely marked by a numerical code to make the data collected on the ReMoVES database anonymous.

Under the supervision of medical staff, all SSc patients followed the traditional rehabilitative treatment for systemic sclerosis combined with the use of exergames for hand rehabilitation. Table 3 resumes the number of persons involved in this study, based on the exergames. All the patients and members from control group performed both Finger Tap and Floating Trap activities, while one patient and one subject and one patient and two subjects did not participate to Endless Zig and City Car activities, respectively.

The exergames performed with the ReMoVES platform should not be considered as a substitute for traditional rehabilitation but as an integration for entertainment and evaluation purposes.

2.4 Intervention

The schedule of use of the ReMoVES system followed a general procedure but was adapted to all patients, based on their conditions. Furthermore, data analyzed in the present work refers to the first time patients and subjects experienced ReMoVES activities, since this paper is focused on the assessment of SSc.

The admission of patients to each game session was determined by the judgment of the clinical staff, who evaluated the willingness to participate and the general conditions of the patient at that particular time.

The treatment plan was divided on the basis of finger and wrist movements, in particular it consisted on:

- one session for stimulating thumb opposition (Finger Tap);
- one session for stimulating finger flexion-extension (Floating Trap);
- one session for stimulating radial-ulnar deviation (Endless Zig);
- one session for stimulating wrist flexion-extension (City Car).

All the games were performed with the dominant hand.

Patients feedback related to ReMoVES was extremely positive and all of them were willing to repeat the activities.

3 Experimental Results

The work here presented aims at assessing patients' conditions on the basis of the activities delivered by ReMoVES. Since the present is the preliminary phase of the study, the number of subjects involved is limited. However, features extracted from games sessions prove to be significant to discriminate SSc patients and control group members.

Indeed, in order to compare the sessions performed by patients and control group, the Kruskal-Wallis test was used. Such a test focused only on one feature for each exergames. In particular, the number of correct targets was considered for Finger Tap, Opening ROM for Floating Trap, Yaw ROM for Endless Zig, and Pitch ROM for City Car. The resulting p-values prove that the considered features are significantly different in the two groups, with respect to all the activities (Table 4).

Table 4 p-values from the Kruskall-Wallis tests

Exergame	p-value
Finger tap	0.0001
Floating trap	0.0019
Endless zig	0.0028
City car	0.0001

In addition to the aforementioned analysis, an LSTM RNN was developed and tested, in order to provide an automatic evaluation of game sessions. Such an approach was applied only to Finger Tap, because of the nature of the movement involved. Indeed, thumb opposition is a small movement and hence, one can consider short sub-sessions which still depict appropriately the hand gesture. On the contrary, all finger flexion-extension, radial-ulnar deviation, and wrist flexion-extension are wide movements that can be accurately described only taking into consideration the whole game session.

To sum up, each Finger Tap session was divided into 5 segments. To avoid errors due to incorrect hand positioning either at the beginning or end, such starting and final frames were removed (1.5 s at the beginning and 1.5 s at the end). As a result, for each patient and subject, 5 segments collecting 114 extracted features each were fed in the network. Training, validation, and test sets were defined by splitting the data with percentage of 80, 10, and 10%, respectively, hence enabling tenfold cross-validation, in order to control for over-fitting. The network was trained from scratch. To account for randomness, cross-validation was performed on 15 permutations and the average overall accuracy was 86.31%.

4 Conclusion

Even though rehabilitation is of fundamental importance to improve the quality of life of SSc patients, it is often underappreciated in the management of SSc.

Indeed, also due to the small number of patients and members in the control group, the efficacy and safety of rehabilitation for SSc is currently poorly supported.

The need for evidence in favor of rehabilitation in SSc led to design the study here presented.

In this work the standard practice was supported by the ReMoVES platform, delivering activities in the form of exergames.

Movements that are typically impaired for SSc patients, such as thumb opposition, finger flexion-extension, radial-ulnar deviation, and wrist flexion-extension, are stimulated by ReMoVES exergames, which help to entice patients in practicing the rehabilitation activity.

The present paper refers to the first phase of the study, focused on the disease assessment. Patients and control group participated and significant differences are detected on the basis of ReMoVES feedback. Also the preliminary attempt for automatic staging of the disease, leveraging on deep learning techniques, yielded promising results.

ReMoVES exergames are currently involved for the rehabilitation treatment of SSc patient. In the near future, a feedback on its effectiveness and reliability will be provided.

References

1. L. Kwakkenbos, T.A. Sanchez, K.A. Turner, L. Mouthon, M.E. Carrier, M. Hudson, C.H.M. van den Ende, A.A. Schouffoer, J.J.K.C. Welling, M. Sauvé, B.D. Thombs; The SPIN Investigators. The association of sociodemographic and disease variables with hand function: a scleroderma patient-centered intervention network cohort study. Clin. Exp. Rheumatol. **36** Suppl 113(4), 88–94 (2018). Epub 2018 Sep 29. PMID: 30277865. https://pubmed.ncbi.nlm.nih.gov/30277865/
2. A. Del Rosso, S. Maddali Bongi, F. Sigismondi, I. Miniati, F. Bandinelli, M. Matucci-Cerinic, The Italian version of the hand mobility in scleroderma (hamis) test: evidence for its validity and reliability. Clin. Exp. Rheumatol. **28**(5), S42 (2010)
3. S. Parisi, C. Celletti, M. Scarati, M. Priora, A. Laganà, C. Peroni, F. Camerota, G. La Torre, D. Blow, E. Fusaro, Neuromuscular taping enhances hand function in patients with systemic sclerosis: a pilot study. La Clinica Terapeutica **168**(6), e371–e375 (2017)
4. A. Young, R. Namas, C. Dodge, D. Khanna, Hand impairment in systemic sclerosis: various manifestations and currently available treatment. Curr. Treat. Options Rheumatol. **2**(3), 252–269 (2016)
5. N. Mugii, Y. Hamaguchi, S. Maddali-Bongi, Clinical significance and usefulness of rehabilitation for systemic sclerosis. J. Scleroderma Rel. Disorders **3**(1), 71–80 (2018)
6. S. Ponte, S. Gabrielli, J. Jonsdottir, M. Morando, S. Dellepiane, Monitoring game-based motor rehabilitation of patients at home for better plans of care and quality of life, in *2015 37th Annual International Conference of the IEEE Engineering in Medicine and Biology Society (EMBC)* (IEEE, Piscataway, 2015), pp. 3941–3944
7. M. Morando, S. Ponte, E. Ferrara, S. Dellepiane, Definition of motion and biophysical indicators for home-based rehabilitation through serious games. Information **9**(5), 105 (2018)
8. Y. Oh, S. Yang, Defining exergames & exergaming, in *Proceedings of Meaningful Play* (2010), pp. 1–17
9. A. Colgan, How does the leap motion controller work? http://blog.leapmotion.com/hardware-to-software-how-does-the-leap-motion-controller-work/
10. S. Hochreiter, J. Schmidhuber, Long short-term memory. Neural Comput. **9**(8), 1735–1780 (1997)
11. I. Goodfellow, Y. Bengio, A. Courville, *Deep Learning* (MIT Press, Cambridge, 2016)
12. M. Morando, M. Trombini, S. Dellepiane, Application of SVM for evaluation of training performance in exergames for motion rehabilitation, in *Proceedings of the 2019 International Conference on Intelligent Medicine and Image Processing* (ACM, New York, 2019), pp. 1–5

Classification of Craniosynostosis Images by Vigilant Feature Extraction

Saloni Agarwal, Rami R. Hallac, Ovidiu Daescu, and Alex Kane

1 Introduction

Craniosynostosis is a congenital disability that affects about one in 3500 newborns. It stems from premature fusion of the skull sutures resulting in asymmetric and abnormal craniofacial shape [14]. We group subtypes of craniosynostosis that lack dysmorphisms and challenging to recognize as non-syndromic synostosis [10]. The most common forms of non-syndromic craniosynostosis are metopic, sagittal, and unicoronal [22], illustrated in Fig. 1. These subtypes are associated with several cranial features. The features are visually identifiable and often used to diagnose patients with craniosynostosis. Although currently CT scans are used to confirm premature fusion of the skull, they are expensive imaging technology. Moreover, early detection of disease is critical because progression could lead to blindness and impede the development of a child's brain. This study aims to develop accessible and affordable tools to detect craniosynostosis automatically and classify its manifestation into metopic, sagittal, or unicoronal based on multiview (front face view and top head view) 2D photographs [20].

In recent years, convolutional neural networks (CNNs) have made remarkable advances in the field of computer vision [12, 17]. However, despite their success, they usually require a large dataset for training [3]. In sub-specialized medicine, such as plastic surgery, data acquisition results in small-scale datasets. Hence, we have a small digital image dataset for craniosynostosis from various views. Overcoming small data size problem often relies on the popular technique of transfer

S. Agarwal (✉) · O. Daescu
University of Texas at Dallas, Richardson, TX, USA
e-mail: saloni.agarwal1@utdallas.edu

R. R. Hallac · A. Kane
UT Southwestern Medical Center, Dallas, TX, USA

H. R. Arabnia et al. (eds.), *Advances in Computer Vision and Computational Biology*, Transactions on Computational Science and Computational Intelligence,
https://doi.org/10.1007/978-3-030-71051-4_23

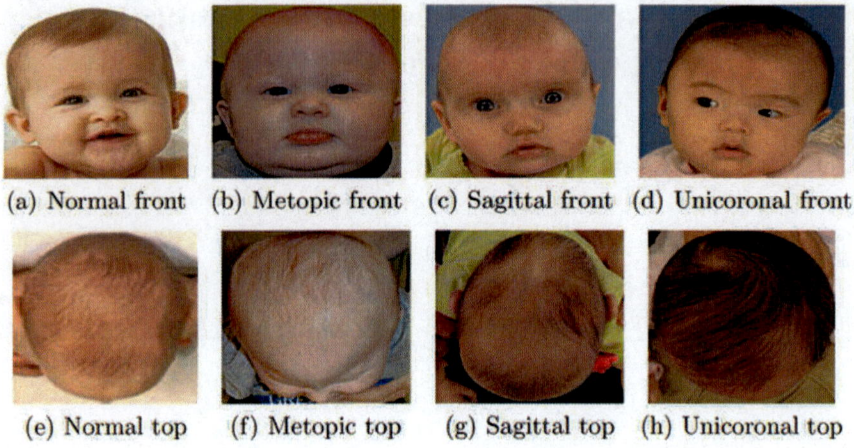

Fig. 1 Front and top view images of a healthy child (a), (e) and children with various types of craniosynostosis—metopic, (b), (f); sagittal (c), (g); and unicoronal (d), (h)

learning [18]. In this approach, a CNN model is pre-trained on a large dataset, and the model weights are then adapted for the given application. In our case, in the presence of a small dataset, we freeze the weights of initial layers and fine-tune later layers. The fact that earlier layers of a CNN learn generic features while later layers learn task-specific features is the motivation behind freezing initial and fine-tuning later layers. One of the most commonly used datasets for pre-training is ImageNet [8], which contains images from a thousand general categories. Due to its large diversity of classes, we can adapt a model pre-trained on ImageNet for various digital image-based general-purpose computer vision tasks. Similar to ImageNet, VGGFace2 [2] is a recent dataset containing 3.31 million facial images of 9,131 subjects. One can use VGGFace2 for pre-training models in facial applications, much like ImageNet is used in general-purpose tasks.

However, there are limitations to the method of transfer learning. First, it could be challenging to find a large dataset suitable for pre-training models for a given task. For example, a large dataset having the front face and top head images of each subject will be ideal for craniosynostosis classifier model pre-training. However, to our knowledge, there is no large dataset comprising both front and top view images of the human head, in general, and newborns in particular. Second, the application dataset might not be sufficiently large enough for fine-tuning later layers and learning class-specific details. For craniosynostosis, we have under a hundred images for fine-tuning final layers, which is a small dataset in comparison to the size of the dataset used in such studies [16].

In the absence of large-scale human head and face dataset for craniosynostosis model building, we handle the first challenge of transfer learning by using two different datasets for model pre-training. Specifically, we use a model pre-trained on the VGGFace2 dataset for front view classification and another model pre-trained on

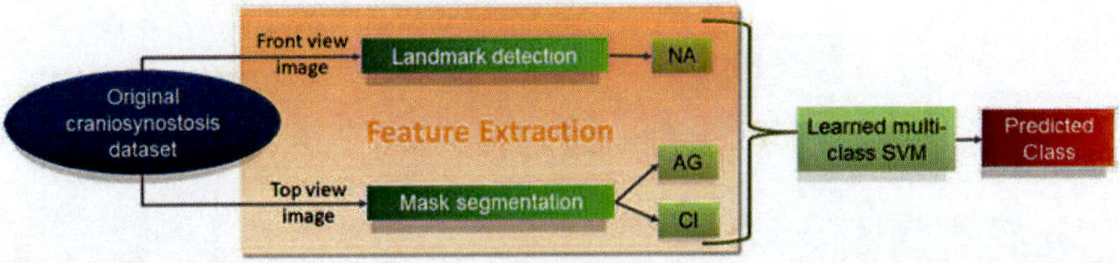

Fig. 2 The proposed ML model pipeline for craniosynostosis classification using original craniosynostosis dataset. We extract Nose Angle (NA) using landmark detection from the front view image. Next, we obtain the Average Gradient (AG), and Cranial Index (CI) features from a segmented mask of the top view image. Finally, we train a multiclass SVM model on these features that outputs the predicted class

the ImageNet dataset for top view classification. Front and top view craniosynostosis dataset for respective pre-trained model fine-tuning are small, and we overcome the second challenge by augmenting them with web scrapped images. Moreover, we further train the pre-trained models for a few epochs to avoid overfitting. In the presence of a small dataset, we build a traditional machine learning (ML) model based on cranial features. Further, we compare the results of the ML model with the results of the CNN model extensively.

The main contributions of this work are:

- We peruse the geometric characteristics of craniosynostosis subtypes [20] and propose the extraction of three robust features from the front and top view images. These are three class differentiating features that reflect the pediatrician's way of identifying craniosynostosis subtypes. Further, we build an ML model (see Fig. 2) by training multiclass SVM on the extracted features for craniosynostosis classification.
- Next, we build a multiview CNN model by extending the original dataset by adding web scrapped images [11]. We use transfer learning from two different datasets (VGGFace2 and ImageNet) for front and top view ResNet50 [13] models pre-training, respectively, as shown in Fig. 3. We fine-tune the final layers of the pre-trained networks for four-class classification—metopic(M), normal(N), sagittal(S), and unicoronal(U). We combine the results from the front and top view models for final predictions.

2 Related Work

In traditional machine learning approaches, feature extraction taking domain knowledge input from human experts takes a lot of effort. Due to difficulty in extracting features from images, researchers designed general handcrafted feature extraction techniques for building image-based machine learning models. Most widely used

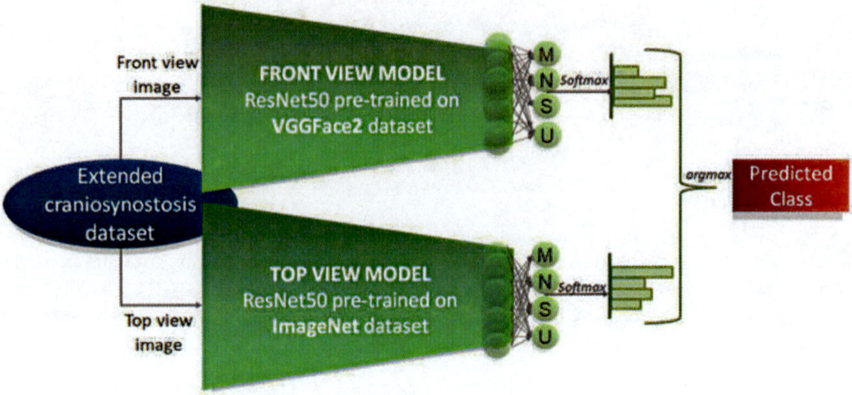

Fig. 3 Overview of our CNN model. The front view model and top view model are pre-trained on VGGFace2 and ImageNet, respectively, and the final layers are modified. While testing, the model outputs the class corresponding to the maximum of eight predicted probabilities (four from each view model)

handcrafted features are Histogram of Oriented Gradients [7], Scale-Invariant Feature Transform(SIFT) , Speeded Up Robust Feature(SURF), and Haar Cascades [23]. These general handcrafted feature extraction techniques reduce the feature space from input image size to the number of such features extracted. Due to the availability of limited images for craniosynostosis, the general handcrafted feature space is still large for significant training of a machine learning model. Hence, we carefully examine class properties and develop class-specific handcrafted feature extraction techniques for building an ML-based craniosynostosis classifier.

In 2014, the authors of [15] proposed an ensemble of gradient boosting regression trees model for face landmark estimation. We obtain the facial landmark points from front view images using this model. Further, we process these landmark points and head shapes for the ML model feature extraction. As shown in Fig. 1, the head shape for various classes of craniosynostosis differs. We capture the differences in head shape by fitting an ellipsoid using [9] on head contour points. We detail these class-specific handcrafted features for the classification of craniosynostosis further in the paper.

In the study [21], the authors demonstrate that multiple CNNs, one for each view with the same model architecture, can be combined at a middle layer to form a multiview CNN model. In this study, the authors fuse output from an intermediate layer of all the single-view models using a view pooling layer (performing the max-pooling operation). The rest of the layers in multiview CNN after view pooling layer are the same as those from a single-view model architecture. We design a two-view CNN classifier taking inspiration from this multiview model.

To the best of our knowledge, there is only one previous work [1] on the classification of craniosynostosis using 2D photographs. We update the base models from [1] and use deeper models in classifier construction—ResNet50 pre-trained on VGGFace2 for front face images, and ResNet50 pre-trained on ImageNet for top head images, opposed to AlexNet pre-trained on ImageNet for both views in [1]. We use two different datasets for pre-training because (a) VGGFace2 dataset is enormous containing human face images and appropriate for front view model pre-training. (b) The pre-trained facial features of a model trained on the VGGFace2 dataset do not help in the top view image classification of craniosynostosis. Therefore, we use a model pre-trained on ImageNet, having a variety of more general object classes, for top view classification. Further, we balance the craniosynostosis dataset, with around a hundred images per class, but the dataset used in [1] is highly imbalanced. The dataset used in [1] contains very few images for unicoronal subtype and top view of the normal category.

3 Our Approach

In this section, we describe the handcrafted class-specific features and models for craniosynostosis classification. These models take front and top view images of a subject as input and predict one of the categories (Normal, Metopic, Sagittal, or Unicoronal) as output class. We pre-process the images by roughly centering and cropping all the images. We align and rotate the top view images such that the head is not tilted and frontal head faces downwards.

3.1 Features for ML Model

The main challenge in designing an ML model for craniosynostosis classification is the extraction of features related to class-specific cranial properties from images. We received a detailed list of cranial properties associated with craniosynostosis's subtypes from the pediatrician in our team. For example, hypotelorism is one of the cranial properties of metopic craniosynostosis, where the distance between the eyes decreases. Nevertheless, it is difficult to extract this feature from an image due to the large variability in facial measurements. After rigorous analysis, we find three robust craniosynostosis subtype differentiating features, one for each class, and formulate their method of extraction from images. We describe these three features below.

Average Gradient (AG) Metopic craniosynostosis contains a rigid triangular structure at the center of the frontal head [4, 5], as shown in Fig. 4b. We design a feature called Average Gradient (AG) to capture this property. We extract this feature by segmenting the head from top view image and generating a head mask. Then, we outline the contour of the generated head mask using points and fit two equations on each side of head ($y_1 = a_1 e^{b_1 x} + c_1$ on the right and $y_2 = a_2 e^{b_2 x} + c_2$ on the left), taking the bottom-most contour point as the origin. Thereafter, we compute the gradients ($y_1'(x_1) = a_1 b_1 e^{b_1 x_1}$, $y_2'(x_2) = a_2 b_2 e^{b_2 x_2}$) in tandem, at each

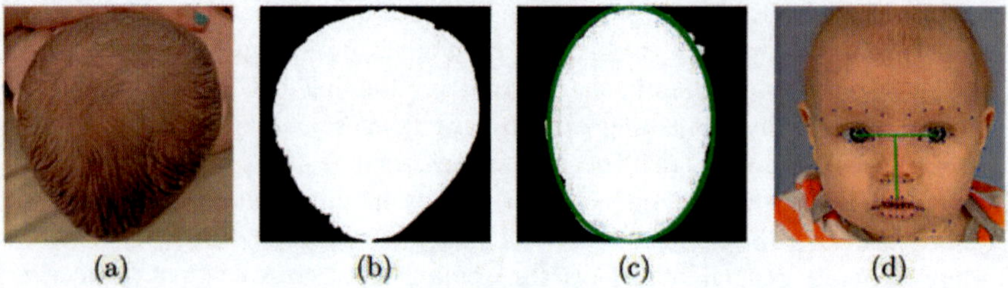

Fig. 4 Capturing craniosynostosis features from top and front view images. (**a**) Metopic top. (**b**) Metopic mask. (**c**) Sagittal ellipse. (**d**) Tilted nose

pixel on the x-axis, until the change in gradient is greater than 0.3 or 100th pixel is encountered. Let us say we compute gradients till m pixel points in each side, we can mathematically represent AG as follows:

$$AG = \frac{1}{2m}\left(\sum_{x_1=1}^{m} y_1'(x_1) + \sum_{x_2=1}^{m} y_2'(x_2)\right) \tag{1}$$

Cranial Index (CI) One of the defining properties of sagittal craniosynostosis is the elongation of the head, as observed in Fig. 4c. We can measure the extent of elongation using the percentage of the maximum width (side to side) to the maximum length (front to back) of the head, named Cranial Index (CI) [6]. We calculate CI from top view image by fitting an ellipse (E) on the segmented head mask using the ellipse fitting algorithm described in [9]. We calculate the maximum width and length of the head by computing the measurement of the minor axis ($\mathrm{mi}(E)$) and major axis ($\mathrm{MA}(E)$) of the fitted ellipse (E), respectively. Using these measurements, we define the Cranial Index (CI) as expressed in the Eq. (2). Since sagittal craniosynostosis has an elongated head, the width of the head is less as compared to the length. Hence, CI is lower for the sagittal class compared to the other classes.

$$\mathrm{CI} = 100 \times \frac{\mathrm{mi}(E)}{\mathrm{MA}(E)} \tag{2}$$

Nose Angle (NA) In the unicoronal craniosynostosis, the nose is deviated towards the affected side, as shown in Fig. 4d. Based on the nose's deviation, we design the third feature called Nose Angle (NA). We extract this feature using 68 facial landmark points, described in [15] and shown with blue dots in Fig. 4d. We process the landmark points on each eye's boundary to get an approximate point representing the center of the eyes. Then, we calculate the equation of the line passing through the centers (l_{eyes}). Subsequently, we determine the equation of the line joining the upper nose and center of the upper lip landmark points (l_{nose}). We define NA as the acute angle formed between the two lines (l_{eyes} and l_{nose}) and compute using the given formula:

$$NA = min\big(\angle(l_{eyes}, l_{nose}), 180 - (\angle(l_{eyes}, l_{nose}))\big) \quad (3)$$

3.2 Machine Learning Model

We extract the three features from the front and top view images of the original craniosynostosis dataset. After that, we normalize them by subtracting the mean and dividing by the standard deviation of the training dataset features. We use these normalized features for building three binary class classifiers, one feature per classifier. Each of these classifiers helps to analyze the differentiating capability of the respective feature. To categorize the individual class in the classifiers, we learn the threshold values of AG, CI, and NA from the training dataset. We test the subjects in the testing dataset and classifying them as sagittal if CI feature value is lower than the learned threshold value. In contrast, we classify the subjects as metopic and unicoronal, respectively, if AG and NA feature values are higher than the learned threshold values.

Additionally, we train an unsupervised k-means clustering algorithm on the normalized features. Since the original dataset contains only one data point for normal class, we remove it to avoid noise and cluster the rest around three centers. Each of these clusters in the feature space depicts a craniosynostosis subtype. Training this model gives insights into the compactness of intra-class data points and the looseness of inter-class data points in the feature space.

We build the proposed supervised multiclass Support Vector Machine (SVM) using all the three normalized features—AG, CI, and NA of the training dataset along with associated classes. We use one-vs-rest multiclass SVM because it scales well with the number of samples. While testing, we pass the normalized features corresponding to a subject as input, and the multiclass SVM predicts a class as the output.

3.3 CNN Based Model

Because the original dataset contains less than a hundred subjects' front and top view images, it is insufficient for training a CNN model. We extend the original craniosynostosis dataset using web-scrapping and use the extended dataset for building the CNN model. The CNN model comprises two sub-networks for front and top views, shown in Fig. 3. The sub-networks are trained separately for classifying the respective view images in the extended training set.

Cao et al. [2] proposed a new face dataset—VGGFace2 and trained a ResNet50 on it. We fine-tune this pre-trained ResNet50 on the front view craniosynostosis dataset, containing face images for craniosynostosis classification. We change the last layers of the pre-trained ResNet50 network for building a four-class craniosynostosis classifier. Further, we tune the model using fivefold cross-validation on the front extended craniosynostosis training dataset. We try different learning rates, optimization techniques, number of epochs, number of frozen initial layers, mini-batch sizes, and final layer learning rate for cross-validation. The best performing model has a $3e^{-4}$ learning rate optimized using stochastic gradient descent with momentum for six epochs. We freeze 100 initial layers of this model and train it with a mini-batch of size ten images and final layer learning rate of $30e^{-4}$. This ResNet50 pre-trained on **VGGFace2** is our **front** view classifier.

Similarly, we train and cross-validate various CNN models with different hyperparameters on top head images in the extended dataset. We change the final layer of the models for four-class classification. We obtain the best cross-validation accuracy by a ResNet50 model pre-trained on the ImageNet dataset with a learning rate of $3e^{-4}$ optimized using stochastic gradient descent for six epochs. This model contains 92 initial frozen layers and trained with a mini-batch of size ten images and the final layer learning rate of $30e^{-4}$. This ResNet50 pre-trained on **ImageNet** is our **top** view model.

We pass the front and top view images of a test subject as input to the respective sub-network and receive the output class. We combine the results of individual view by taking argmax of the probabilities from both the single-view CNN model's softmax layer, as in [1]. The class corresponding to the highest predicted probability in both the single-view models is our CNN classier output.

4 Experiments

4.1 Dataset

The original dataset consists of images collected over the years at the UT Southwestern Medical Center in Dallas. It contains images from 7 views for each subject (frontal, lateral, basal, top, and posterior views). By visually analyzing the images from all the views and comparing them with craniosynostosis class properties, we find that front and top view images hold maximum information. Hence, we use front and top view images for craniosynostosis analysis, and our dataset contains images from these two views. We randomly split the original dataset class-wise into 67% training and 33% testing subsets. We detail the distribution of the original dataset in Fig. 5a). Since there are only 72 subjects in the original dataset, we extend it by adding web scrapped images. We conduct a web search using keywords like craniosynostosis, metopic, sagittal, unicoronal, etc. to collect more images. The expert physicians in our team validate the correctness of class in the gathered images. Additionally, we append these verified images and their label in the original dataset to form an extended dataset.

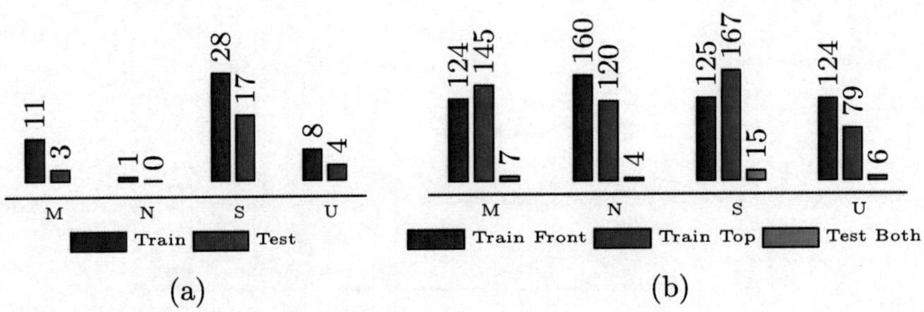

Fig. 5 Data distribution of original and extended datasets. (**a**) Original data distribution. (**b**) Extended data distribution

We divide the extended dataset into training and testing subsets. Moreover, the testing subset includes images from both (front and top) views for every subject. Due to the inclusion of web scrapped images in the training set, front and top view images are from different sets of subjects. The training set contains front and top view images as two separate subsets. Figure 5b shows the class-wise distribution of the front and top view images in the extended dataset. Due to our modeling technique, the multiclass SVM model requires both—front view and top view—images for every subject. While the CNN model simultaneously learns two separate sub-networks, one for each front and top view, and uses single-view images of a subject for training these sub-networks. Thus, we use two distinct datasets for training these models. We train and test the SVM and CNN models using the original and extended craniosynostosis datasets, respectively.

Pre-Processing We aligned all images such that the subjects were upright. During real-time utilization of the diagnostic tool, we will ensure that the images are correctly aligned using landmark points while acquiring photographs. We cropped the images in the original and extended dataset to 500×500 (arbitrarily chosen) and 224×224 (input layer size of pre-trained networks) pixels size, respectively. After initial processing, we segmented the top view images in the original dataset and generated head masks using Matlab's Image Segmenter GraphCut algorithm. The input to this algorithm consists of digital images of the head, with marking of foreground and background in them. This algorithm performs segmentation based on the provided marking on images and gives a segmented head as output, as shown in Fig. 4a, b. We extracted and normalized the features in the original dataset using front view images and top view segmented mask.

Further, we trained a multiclass SVM on the normalized features extracted from the original dataset's training set. We tested this multiclass SVM model on the testing split of the original image dataset. Similarly, we trained front and top view sub-networks on the extended dataset training subset. We measured multiview CNN model performance on the extended craniosynostosis testing subset by predicting class corresponding to the highest probability among eight output probabilities from both the single-view sub-networks.

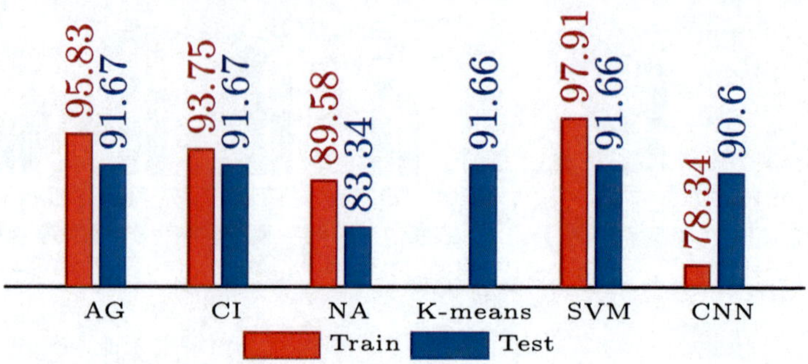

Fig. 6 Accuracy plot of various models in percentage

4.2 Results and Discussion

Figure 6 shows the results of classification using various classifiers. The training and testing accuracies for classification of the metopic and non-metopic classes using the learned threshold value of Average Gradient are 95.83 and 91.67%, respectively. Likewise, we classify sagittal versus non-sagittal at learned Cranial Index threshold value with a training accuracy of 93.75% and testing accuracy of 91.67%, and unicoronal and non-unicoronal images at learned Nose Angle threshold value with a training accuracy of 89.58% and testing accuracy of 83.34%. High classification accuracy using AG and CI suggests the superiority of these features for metopic and sagittal craniosynostosis classification, respectively. However, the lower value of accuracy for classification of unicoronal versus non-unicoronal samples is because we trained on only eight unicoronal samples versus 64 non-unicoronal samples.

The unsupervised k-means clustering forms three cluster centers—Cluster1: (1, 43, 1); Cluster2: (13, 1, 1); Cluster3: (0, 2, 10); with metopic, sagittal, and unicoronal images. Cluster1, Cluster2, and Cluster3 represent sagittal, metopic, and unicoronal classes, respectively. This unsupervised ML algorithm has a three-class classification accuracy of 91.66%. The data distribution in clusters indicates that Average Gradient, Cranial Index, and Nose Angle together have high inter-class separability and intra-class compactness.

Multiclass SVM trained on features extracted from 67% original dataset has 97.91% training accuracy and 91.67% test accuracy. We observe that both the training and testing accuracies of multiclass SVM are higher than single class classifiers. Thus, we infer that the classes are separated better in the feature space created by the three combined features instead of individual feature space. We plot the SVM receiver operating characteristic curves (ROCs) along with the associated area under the curve (AUC) values for each class, shown in Fig. 7a. From the single feature-based classification, we observed that the unicoronal class was not classified very well. However, the AUC value for unicoronal class in multiclass SVM is one, suggesting that the unicoronal class separates well in the combined feature space.

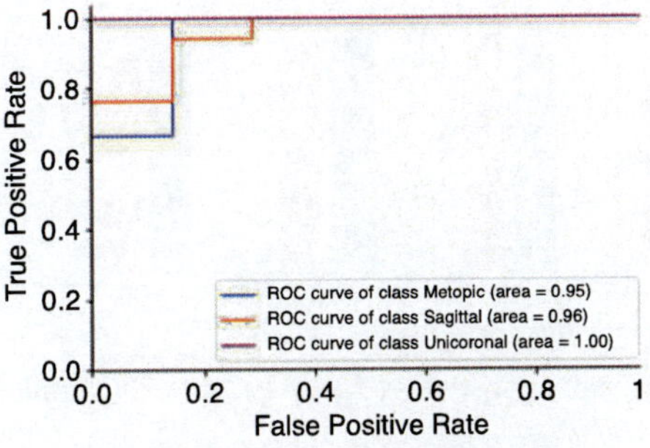

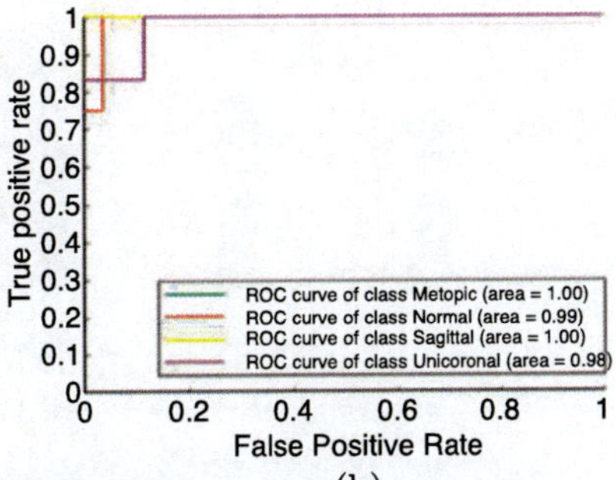

Fig. 7 Multiclass SVM and CNN classifier ROC curve and AUC values. (**a**) ROC curve for multiclass SVM. (**b**) ROC curve for CNN classifier

Given limitations in the size of the dataset, the accuracies and AUC values resulting from multiclass SVM are excellent.

The proposed CNN model has 90.6% test accuracy on the extended test dataset. The average training accuracy of each of the two views of the CNN model is 78.34%, lower than the multiview testing accuracy of 90.6%. Since we combine front and top models during testing this improves the prediction capability, compared to the performance of sub-networks on the single-view training dataset. Moreover, the test dataset contains higher quality images from the medical center compared to the image quality of web scrapped images in the training set. Further, we observe that the model could not predict older subjects correctly, and there is a medical reason for the miss-classification of older subjects. As an infant grows, the shape of the skull and face changes, which makes the identification of craniosynostosis features harder. We show the AUC values and ROC curve for four-class classification using the CNN model in Fig. 7b. The average AUC value for this model is 0.99, which is very high compared to the 0.84 results of the current state-of-the-art model mentioned in [1].

The CNN model's average training accuracy is 78.34–87.5% for the front view model and 68.8% for the top view model, and the normal class AUC is 0.99. The lower top view model training accuracy is because we obtain most of the normal class top view images from web-scrapping. These web scrapped top view images contain the infant's head held by someone. Possibly the hand in these images creates occlusion and decreases the top view model accuracy and normal class AUC value in the multiview CNN model performance. Moreover, the AUC value of unicoronal class is low in the given ROC curve because few unicoronal samples are present in the top dataset, as stated in Fig. 5b, and the top view sub-network is not trained sufficiently on unicoronal top view images.

We observe from the results of multiclass SVM and CNN models that feature extraction gives the ML model the upper hand. Although feature extraction is taxing compared to self-learned features in CNN, the ML features are explainable, which is very important in medical settings. The unicoronal type has AUC value 1 in the

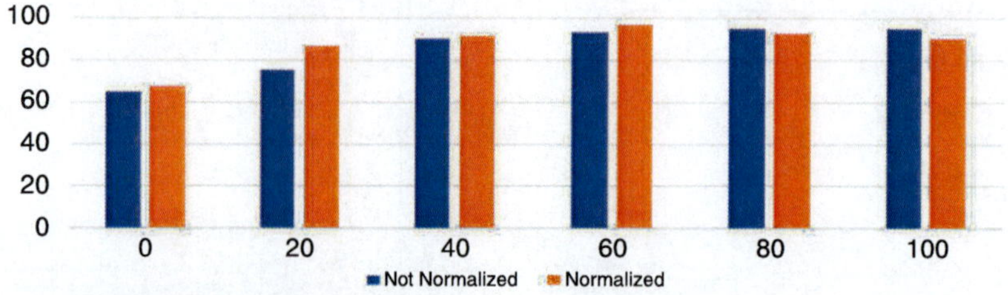

(a) Distribution of accuracy based on various percentage facial height additions.

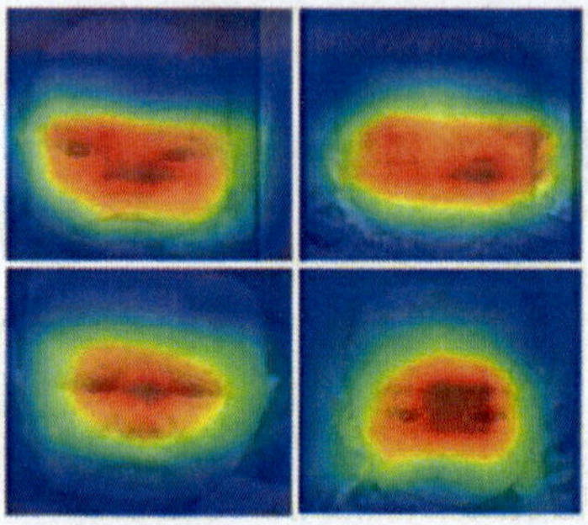

(b) Gradient weighted activation maps.

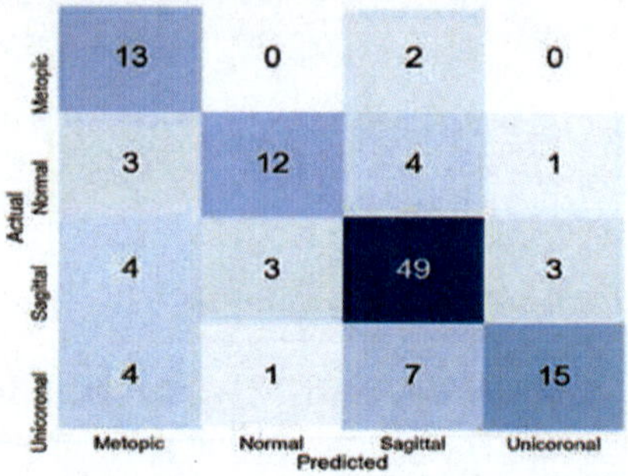

(c) CNN clinical data confusion matrix.

Fig. 8 Various facial height model accuracy plot (a); class activation maps for front view CNN model (b); front view CNN model performance on unseen clinical data (c)

SVM model, Metopic and Sagittal types have AUC value of 1 in the CNN model, and Normal class has near 1 AUC value in the CNN model. This high AUC values in one or the other models suggest that we might get a near-perfect classifier if we can combine both models' power.

We also analyze different face cropping for the CNN model building. We build models based on various facial heights. Suppose, h is the height of detected face, we add 0, 20, 40, 60, 80, and 100% of h region above the detected face. The different percentage of inclusion represents a varying amount of the forehead in the images. We use two types of ResNet50 pre-trained on the VGGFace2 dataset—normalized: with intensity values of the image normalized in the range between 0 to 1; and not normalized: without normalizing the intensity values of images, i.e., same as the pre-trained model. We can see from Fig. 8a that the accuracy of the model increases and eventually saturates at an additional 60% facial height. The saturation is because the image generated by the addition of 60% facial height above the detected face covers the entire forehead. The increase in accuracy suggests that the inclusion of the whole forehead in front view image is vital for craniosynostosis detection. Further, we also crop the forehead from front view images and train the model using just the forehead image. The performance of this model was inferior to the proposed CNN model. The lower performance of the model trained on forehead images suggests both face and forehead are essential for the classification of craniosynostosis, as suggested by the craniofacial specialists.

Further, we generate gradient weighted class activation maps [19] for front view images, as shown in Fig. 8b. We notice in these activation maps that the eyes and forehead regions of the face are highly activated. Hence, the CNN model makes predictions based on these regions. The importance of eyes and forehead in CNN prediction aligns with the practitioner's way of diagnosis as they use the distance of eyes and structure of the forehead for detecting craniosynostosis.

Trial on Unseen Clinical Data We tested the CNN model on completely unseen data at the UTSW medical center. The overall confusion matrix of the front view CNN model prediction is shown in Fig. 8c. We can see from the confusion matrix that the CNN model predicts 13 out of 15 metopic, 12 out of 20 normal, 49 out of 59 sagittal, and 15 out of 27 unicoronal cases correctly. It is interesting to note that the front view model can differentiate diseased craniosynostosis (metopic + sagittal + unicoronal) from normal cases with an accuracy of 90.08% (109 out of 121).

5 Conclusion

We extracted three powerful features—Average Gradient, Cranial Index, and Nose Angle, which separates the craniosynostosis subtypes decently in the feature space. These features have significance in the medical study; over ostensibly learned features of CNN models. The multiclass SVM build using these three extracted features has very high segregating power and performs better than the CNN model in a limited data setting. Both the multiclass SVM and CNN outperform the current state-of-the-art model for craniosynostosis classification.

Next, a smartphone application for craniosynostosis classification is in development and soon to be deployed at various clinical centers. In this application, we will send the front and top view images captured by a mobile camera to our server, and receive back the predicted class. Simultaneously, we are also improving the model by combining the extracted features with the CNN model for better performance. In the future, we will investigate the classification problem by keeping the few-shot learning paradigm in mind. Being aware that collecting more data will improve the prediction power of the CNN model, we are collecting more data. A larger dataset will open paths for incorporating more than two views, resulting in better prediction.

References

1. S. Agarwal, R.R. Hallac, R. Mishra, C. Li, O. Daescu, A. Kane, Image based detection of craniofacial abnormalities using feature extraction by classical convolutional neural network, in *2018 IEEE 8th International Conference on Computational Advances in Bio and Medical Sciences (ICCABS)* (IEEE, Piscataway, 2018)

2. Q. Cao, L. Shen, W. Xie, O.M. Parkhi, A. Zisserman, Vggface2: a dataset for recognising faces across pose and age, in *International Conference on Automatic Face and Gesture Recognition* (2018)
3. J. Cho, K. Lee, E. Shin, G. Choy, S. Do, How much data is needed to train a medical image deep learning system to achieve necessary high accuracy? (2015, preprint). arXiv:1511.06348
4. M. Cho, A. Kane, J. Seaward, R. Hallac, Metopic "ridge" vs. "craniosynostosis": quantifying severity with 3d curvature analysis. J. Cranio-Maxillo-Facial Surg. **44**(9), 1259–1265 (2016). https://doi.org/10.1016/j.jcms.2016.06.019
5. M.J. Cho, R.R. Hallac, M. Effendi, J.R. Seaward, A.A. Kane, Comparison of an unsupervised machine learning algorithm and surgeon diagnosis in the clinical differentiation of metopic craniosynostosis and benign metopic ridge. Sci. Rep. **8**(1), 6312 (2018)
6. S. Cronqvist, Roentgenologic evaluation of cranial size in children: a new index. Acta Radiologica. Diagnosis **7**(2), 97–111 (1968). https://doi.org/10.1177/028418516800700201
7. N. Dalal, B. Triggs, Histograms of oriented gradients for human detection, in *2005 IEEE Computer Society Conference on Computer Vision and Pattern Recognition (CVPR'05)*, vol. 1 (IEEE, Piscataway, 2005), pp. 886–893
8. J. Deng, W. Dong, R. Socher, L.J. Li, K. Li, L. Fei-Fei, ImageNet: a large-scale hierarchical image database, in *Conference on Computer Vision and Pattern Recognition CVPR09* (2009)
9. A. Fitzgibbon, M. Pilu, R.B. Fisher, Direct least square fitting of ellipses. IEEE Trans. Pattern Anal. Mach. Intell. **21**(5), 476–480 (1999)
10. R.M. Garza, R.K. Khosla, Nonsyndromic craniosynostosis, in *Seminars in Plastic Surgery*, vol. 26 (Thieme Medical Publishers, New York, 2012), pp. 053–063
11. R.R. Hallac, B.M. Dumas, J.R. Seaward, R. Herrera, C. Menzies, A.A. Kane, Digital images in academic plastic surgery: a novel and secure methodology for use in clinical practice and research. Cleft Palate-Craniofacial J. **56**(4), 552–555 (2019)
12. R.R. Hallac, J. Lee, M. Pressler, J.R. Seaward, A.A. Kane, Identifying ear abnormality from 2d photographs using convolutional neural networks. Sci. Rep. **9**(1), 1–6 (2019)
13. K. He, X. Zhang, S. Ren, J. Sun, Deep residual learning for image recognition, in *Proceedings of the IEEE Conference on Computer Vision and Pattern Recognition* (2016), pp. 770–778
14. D. Johnson, A.O. Wilkie, Craniosynostosis. Eur. J. Hum. Genet. **19**(4), 369–376 (2011)
15. V. Kazemi, J. Sullivan, One millisecond face alignment with an ensemble of regression trees, in *Proceedings of the IEEE Conference on Computer Vision and Pattern Recognition* (2014), pp. 1867–1874
16. S. Khan, N. Islam, Z. Jan, I.U. Din, J.J.C. Rodrigues, A novel deep learning based framework for the detection and classification of breast cancer using transfer learning. Pattern Recognit. Lett. **125**, 1–6 (2019)
17. W. Liu, Z. Wang, X. Liu, N. Zeng, Y. Liu, F.E. Alsaadi, A survey of deep neural network architectures and their applications. Neurocomputing **234**, 11–26 (2017)
18. S.J. Pan, Q. Yang, A survey on transfer learning. IEEE Trans. Knowl. Data Eng. **22**(10), 1345–1359 (2009)
19. R.R. Selvaraju, A. Das, R. Vedantam, M. Cogswell, D. Parikh, D. Batra, Grad-cam: why did you say that? Visual explanations from deep networks via gradient-based localization. CoRR **abs/1610.02391** (2016). http://arxiv.org/abs/1610.02391
20. J. Shillito, D.D. Matson, Craniosynostosis: a review of 519 surgical patients. Pediatrics **41**(4), 829–853 (1968)
21. H. Su, S. Maji, E. Kalogerakis, E. Learned-Miller, Multi-view convolutional neural networks for 3d shape recognition, in *Proceedings of the IEEE International Conference on Computer Vision* (2015), pp. 945–953
22. F. Ursitti, T. Fadda, L. Papetti, M. Pagnoni, F. Nicita, G. Iannetti, A. Spalice, Evaluation and management of nonsyndromic craniosynostosis. Acta Paediatr. **100**(9), 1185–1194 (2011)
23. P. Viola, M. Jones, Rapid object detection using a boosted cascade of simple features, in *Proceedings of the 2001 IEEE Computer Society Conference on Computer Vision and Pattern Recognition. CVPR2001*, vol. 1 (IEEE, Piscataway, 2001), p. I

DRDr: Automatic Masking of Exudates and Microaneurysms Caused by Diabetic Retinopathy Using Mask R-CNN and Transfer Learning

Farzan Shenavarmasouleh and Hamid R. Arabnia

1 Introduction

Diabetic retinopathy is a major cause of vision impairment, and eventually vision loss in the world; especially among working-aged individuals. Its diagnosis can be done by analyzing color fundus images by experienced clinicians to identify its presence and the significance of the damages that it has caused. Fundus images are the results of screenings. The procedure is easy and it can easily and safely be done via retinal photography in every clinic with the proper tools. If detected soon enough, diabetic retinopathy (DR) can be treated via laser surgeries. But, the demand is increasing much more rapidly than the supply. The annual number of patients is growing and each patient requires frequent screenings. Each of these images needs to be carefully analyzed by doctors. The task is innately time-consuming since the deficiencies are usually extremely small and require careful examination and the doctors need to find and weight countless features for each image. The thing is from all the patients being screened annually, only 25.2% have diabetic retinopathy and are referred to ophthalmologist [1] and it begs the question as to whether it is possible to use the time and resources more sufficiently?

Luckily, the answer to the above question is yes. During the past few years, Machine Learning and notably Deep Learning have shown high potential in helping health care and they can be used to aid doctors in detecting and predicting the development of various illnesses. In fact, machine learning and deep learning approaches have already helped numerous researchers to overcome some of the difficulties in the aforementioned task at hand. However, the majority of the previous work in this part lies in the machine learning section, and classification

F. Shenavarmasouleh (✉) · H. R. Arabnia
Department of Computer Science, University of Georgia, Athens, GA, USA
e-mail: fs04199@uga.edu; hra@uga.edu

H. R. Arabnia et al. (eds.), *Advances in Computer Vision and Computational Biology*, Transactions on Computational Science and Computational Intelligence,
https://doi.org/10.1007/978-3-030-71051-4_24

and especially binary classification was the primary subject of interest. In other words, previous work was mostly devoted to finding a way to automatically identify whether a patient has diabetic retinopathy or not.

Decencière et al. [2] leveraged a big dataset extracted from OPHDIAT [1], a teleophthalmology network, during 2008–2009 and the help of three experts to tackle this issue. They merged features extracted from images with the patients' contextual data such as age, weight, diabetic type, and the number of years of DR and altogether could predict whether the patient needs to be referred or not. Bhatia et al. [3] and Antal et al. [4] used ensembles of machine learning techniques, namely Decision Trees, Support Vector Machines (SVM), Adaboost, Naïve Bayes, and Random Forests, on Messidor dataset. Usher et al. [5] and Gardner et al. [6] employed Neural Networks to perform the task of classification for them. The former, utilized candidate lesions, their position, and their type as the inputs of the Neural Network and the latter used Neural Networks and pixel intensity values.

In Priya et al. [7], the authors explored Probabilistic Neural Networks (PNN) along with Naïve Bayes and SVM. They employed Adaptive Histogram Equalization, Discrete Wavelet Transform, Matched Filter Response, Fuzzy C-Means Segmentation, and Morphological Processing on top of the Green channel of the images for their preprocessing phase. The train/test split was questionable though, as out of 350 total images, the authors used 250 of them for test and only 100 for the training.

Sopharak et al. [8] made use of Naïve Bayes, SVM, and K Nearest Neighbors (KNN) classifiers to detect exudates in pixel level. This task was traditionally being dealt with by using region growing and thresholding [9–11]. They selected 15 handpicked features and operated on them. However, their dataset was extremely small with only 39 images.

Several attempts were made to extend the level of classification as well and drag the level of severity to this task too. Lachure et al. [12] utilized SVM and KNN to classify images of Messidor and DB-reet into 3 classes. Their model could tell whether a fundus image is normal or not; and if abnormal, whether it is grade 1 or 3. Roychowdhury et al. [13] used Gaussian Mixture Model (GMM), KNN, SVM, Adaboost along with feature selection to classify images of Messidor in 4 classes. Acharya et al. [14] and Adarsh et al. [15] also used SVM to deal with this problem and classified patients into 5 classes.

All of the forenamed approaches required an external feature extraction phase. Authors needed to manually perform multiple morphological operations, apply various filters to the images, and use techniques such as region growing and thresholding to extract features one by one and then fuse them with other contextual data, if any, and then use the resulting files as inputs for the different classifiers.

With the advancement of deep learning and specifically Convolutional Neural Networks (CNN), network architectures solely designed to enhance working with images, the task of feature extraction turned into an implicit phase instead. Gargeya et al. [16] made use of CNN to identify healthy and unhealthy patients using a huge dataset with 75 thousand images. Gulshan et al. [17] employed Inception V3, a more complex type of CNN, to classify images of EyePACS-1 and Messidor-2 into two categories. And finally, Pratt et al. [18] harnessed CNN and a huge publicly available Kaggle dataset to classify the fundus images into 5 classes.

In this paper, we approach the problem from another angle and address the problem of automatically identifying the deficiencies caused by diabetic retinopathy in fundus images together with their exact shape and location. We modify and leverage a CNN-based model that can identify and use the intricate features in the available images to detect, locate, and most importantly mask and label two important lesion types, namely microaneurysms and exudates. Due to the automatic behavior of our approach, it can easily fit into clinical systems and aid clinicians in the process of identifying unhealthy patients while saving them plenty of time. It has the potential to both be incorporated into retinal cameras and/or be used as a post-photography tool for optometrists and ophthalmologists.

The remainder of the paper is organized as follows: First, we touch base with the related works that are aligned with our interests. Then, we fully explain our methodology, including how we handle our limited available data effectively. Next, we show the experiments that we have performed and illustrate our results. Finally, we conclude with the discussion and future work.

2 Related Work

2.1 Convolutional Neural Networks

Computer Vision is the branch of computer science which its ultimate goal is to imitate the behavior and functionality of human eyes. It assists computers to analyze images and videos and ultimately understand objects that are present in them. Thanks to the advancement of Deep Learning in the past few years, we are now able to handle this task very well. Since AlexNet [19] won the ImageNet image classification competition in 2012, Convolutional Neural Networks (CNN) have become the go-to approach for any task that required dealing with images. In fact, nowadays, CNNs are so powerful that they even surpass humans' performance on the ImageNet challenge. Image captioning [20], Learning from Observation [21], and Embodied Question Answering [22], to name a few, are some of the very high-level tasks that implicitly use CNNs as one of their core components. Besides, researchers in the field of Meta-Learning and Neural Architecture Search (NAS) are constantly trying to find an innovative way to further improve the performance of these systems [23, 24].

Image classification, Object Localization, Object Detection, Semantic Segmentation, and Instance Segmentation are 5 main Computer Vision problems, sorted by their level of difficulty in ascending order. In Image Classification problem, usually exists an image with a single main object in it and the goal is to predict what category that image belongs to. A tad more challenging task is Object Localization. In object localization, the image usually contains one or more objects from the same category and the model's goal is to output the location of those objects as bounding boxes, a rectangular box around the object, besides predicting the category that they all are affiliated with.

As impressive as they look like, these tasks are not remotely as complex as what humans visual understanding and eyes are capable of doing.

Next is Object detection and recently a huge breakthrough has happened in it. CNNs work similarly to human eyes and they are able to detect edges and consequently define boundaries of the objects. Hence, they could be used to detect objects of different kinds in a given image. However, to do so, it is required to apply them to a massive number of locations with varieties of scales on each image, making it extremely time-consuming. As a result, an extensive amount of research has been done to tackle this issue.

R-CNN (Region-based CNN) [25] solves the aforementioned issue by making use of a region proposal module. This module proposes a collection of candidate bounding boxes, also known as Regions of Interests (ROIs), using the Selective Search technique. The pixels corresponding to each of these boxes are then fed into a pre-trained modified version of AlexNet to check if any object is present inside that box. On the very last layer of this CNN lies an SVM that judges whether the pixels represent an object or not and if yes, what is the category that goes with them. At last, if an object is found in the box, the box is tightened to best fit the object dimensions.

Training an R-CNN model is hard and time-consuming because approximately 2000 ROIs are proposed for every single image and all of them need to be fed to the CNN individually. Besides, three different networks are ought to be trained separately.

Fast R-CNN [26] solved both of these problems. Normally, many of the regions that are proposed for further examination overlap with each other and hence this causes the CNN phase to do so many redundant computations. Fast R-CNN overcomes this issue by using only one CNN per image to compute all the features at once. The result is then shared and used by all the 2000 proposals, reducing the computational time significantly. This technique is called Region of Interest Pooling (RoIPool) in the original paper.

To tackle the second issue, Fast R-CNN united all the three models into one single network to enable jointly training of all of them. The SVM classifier was exchanged with a Softmax layer to handle the task of classification and a regression layer was added in parallel to that to find and yield the best bounding box for each object.

However, Fast R-CNN still used the Region Proposal method using selective search to find the ROIs, which turned out to be the bottleneck of the overall process.

Faster R-CNN [27] was proposed to resolve this issue. The authors' main intention was to replace the selective search phase with something more efficient. They argued that the image feature maps that were already calculated with the forward pass of the CNN could be fed directly to a Fully Convolutional Network (FCN) on top of them to perform the task of region proposal instead of running a separate selective search algorithm. This newly added FCN was called Region

Proposal Network (RPN) in the paper and this way, ROIs could be proposed almost for free, fixing the last problem present in the system.

As wonderful as object detection is, it still could not understand and provide us the actual shape of the objects and stops at delivering the bounding box only. This task, however, is where Image Segmentation comes into play and tackles the issue by creating a pixel-wise mask for each object. The task of image segmentation itself can be done in two main ways. In Semantic Segmentation, every pixel in the image needs to be assigned to a predefined class. In addition, all the pixels corresponding to a class are treated the same and are given an identical color and thus the differences among different object instances that belong to one class are disregarded. By contrast, in Instance Segmentation, each instance of the same class is treated discretely and given a unique color and label.

Mask R-CNN [28] is a model developed for the task of image instance segmentation. It extends Faster R-CNN, goes one step further, and specializes in generating pixel-level masks for each object in excess of finding the bounding box and the class label. It, creatively, adds another FCN on top of RPN, altogether creating a new parallel branch to the Fast R-CNN model which outputs a binary mask for the object found in a given region. It is also worth noting that the authors needed to slightly modify the RoIPool to fix the problem of location misalignment caused by its quantization behavior. They called the modified technique RoIAlign.

2.2 Transfer Learning

Humans are really good at transferring their knowledge across tasks. We rarely learn a certain task from scratch and instead, we tend to leverage our previous knowledge that we have acquired in the past in some similar activity or topic. By doing so, we utilize and accelerate our new learning process. Traditional machine learning and deep learning algorithms are designed to work in insulation and learn to handle only a domain-specific task. To make a model work for another task or domain, the entire model has to be retrained from scratch, and thus not taking advantage of the previously learned task will result in consuming so much more time and resources than required, as plenty of redundant operations are needed to take place. Besides, often a huge amount of labeled data are required to learn a specific task in a supervised manner. Preparing such datasets is innately hard as it takes a long time to collect and then label them manually. And sometimes constructing them is nearly impossible for some domains.

Transfer learning is the proposed solution to overcome this issue and facilitate the knowledge sharing process among different tasks. It suggests reusing parts of the model which have been already trained on a similar task as the foundation for the new task at hand. This approach has proved to be extremely helpful in cases where no good or large enough dataset is available for the target domain, but a fairly good one exists for the source domain. In addition, it saves a lot of time and computational power as the pre-trained weights are employed and the model only needs to learn the last few layers and barely fine-tune the other ones if necessary.

3 Methodology

3.1 Dataset

Diabetic retinopathy causes different types of deficiencies in the patients' eyes such as exudates, hemorrhages, aneurysms, cotton wool spots, and abnormal growth of blood vessels to name a few. There are many publicly available datasets that could be found online, some small and some really huge. Often, big datasets are used for learning complex tasks to avoid overfitting and ensure the reproducibility of the research result [29]. However, we needed a dataset that could offer masks for the type of defect which it corresponds to. We came across the e-ophtha [2] which had two separate masked datasets: one for exudates and one for aneurysms; and both were manually annotated by ophthalmology experts. E-ophtha EX contains 47 images with exudates and 35 images with no lesion, while e-ophtha MA provides 148 images with microaneurysms or small hemorrhages and 233 images with no lesion.

We only made use of the images with lesions present in them, which altogether summed up to a total of 195 fundus pictures, all having another black and white image as their mask. We shuffled and splitted them into train, validation, and test sets with 155, 20, 20 images in each of them respectively.

3.2 Preprocessing

The images in the datasets were collected from different clinics with different fundus photography facilities and this had resulted in having varying lighting and pixel intensity values in them, collectively creating unimportant differences among pictures that would have been misleading for the CNN model if left unaltered. Hence, a preprocessing phase was required to counterbalance this issue.

First, we employed OpenCV [30] to crop the images and trim the extra blank space from them. Next, to make the dataset even more homogeneous, we morphed the eyes into perfect circles and removed the extra margins once more. The colors needed to be normalized and enhanced as well, so we performed a weighted sum, and for each image, we applied Gaussian blur (sigma $X = 20$) on it and added it to its original version. We assigned weights of 4 and -4 to the original and blurred images respectively. The gamma was also set to 128. Finally, the images were resized to 1024×1024 pixels (Figs. 1, 2 and 3).

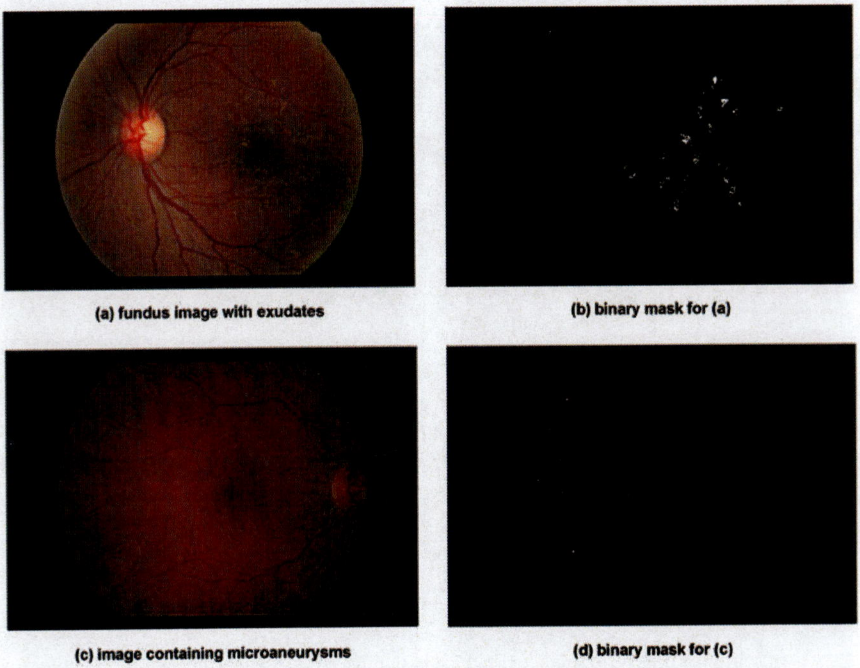

Fig. 1 (**a**) An image from e-ophtha EX containing exudates. (**b**) Binary mask showing the position of exudates in image (**a**). (**c**) An image from e-ophtha MA containing microaneurysms. (**d**) Binary mask showing the location of microaneurysms in picture (**c**)

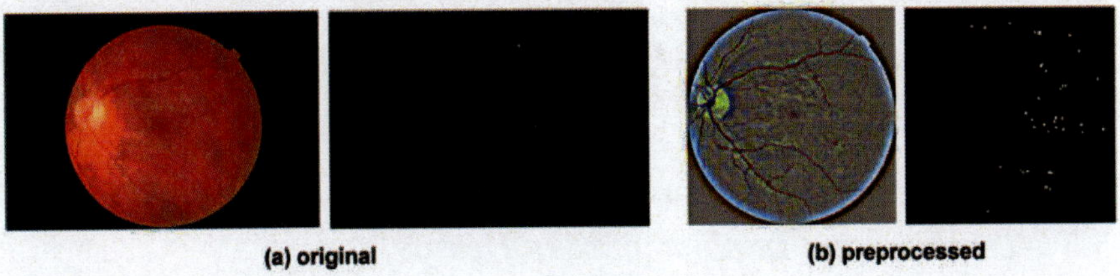

Fig. 2 (**a**) An example of the original image from e-ophtha MA and its mask. (**b**) Resulting image and its mask after the preprocessing phase

All of the above operations were concurrently applied to the masks as well, to preserve the exact scale and position that they signify in the image. But, the masks, especially the ones which corresponded to microaneurysms were extremely small and only consisted of a handful of pixels (between 1–5) as opposed to the total image dimension of 1024×1024. This would have been a tremendously hard task for the model to learn. To tackle this issue, the masks were dilated 2 times with a kernel size of 5×5 to make them big enough to be identifiable by the network.

Also, all the instances of a certain defect were shown in one single mask in the dataset. To make them usable, we needed to create a separate binary mask for each

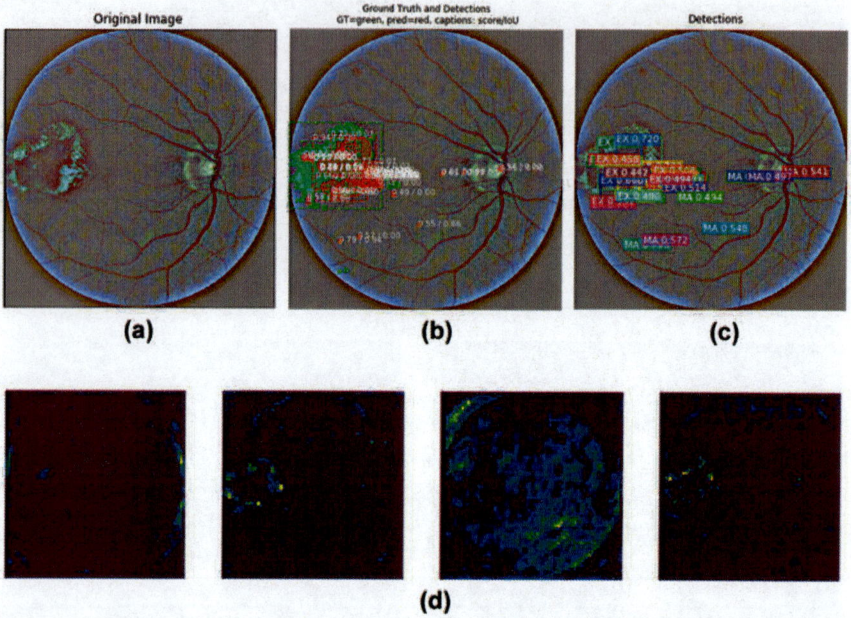

Fig. 3 (**a**) Original image (**b**) predicted masks, bounding boxes, their score, and IoU (**c**) types of the lesions detected and their scores. (**d**) Sample activations of a few layers of the model

instance present in the image. Thus, first, we found all the contours in a given mask. Then, we detached the instances and constructed an exclusive binary mask for each of them. Finally, class ids were assigned to the masks to indicate which defect each of them represents.

3.3 Training and Implementation Details

We started with the original implementation of Mask R-CNN for Keras which was made publicly available by its authors. By default, the model's hyperparameters were configured to find the medium to large objects in the image. However, as mentioned before, even after dilating the masks, they only consisted of a few pixels and were really small relative to the complete picture. Hence, we had to make alterations to the model to make it suitable for our task at hand. RPN anchor sizes had to be decreased to enable the model to find deficits as small as 8 pixels in size. Since lesions were small and could be found anywhere in the image, the number of anchors to be trained were increased from 256 to 512, the number of ROIs per image was raised to 512, and the maximum number of final detections was set to 256. Also, we needed to reduce the minimum confidence and threshold required for the model to accept a detection. We disabled the mini-mask feature to avoid any mask resize as we had enough memory and did not have to sacrifice accuracy for the memory load. Also, we defined the number of classes to be three; one for the background, and two more for exudates and microaneurysms. Adam optimizer was found to be more effective than the default stochastic gradient descent as well. So, it was employed instead to help the model converge to the optimal point faster.

We found out that Mask R-CNN can easily overfit the training set if used naively. As for our first way out, we made use of data augmentation. It comprised random vertical and horizontal flips, 90° clockwise and counterclockwise rotations, and translations and scalings along x and y axes; all of which been applied to the input training images on the fly with the help of the CPU, in parallel to the main training which was being done on our Nvidia 2080Ti GPU to accelerate the process even more.

Our dataset was small, and thus, because of the aforementioned reasons, the best way to counteract this was to employ transfer learning. We put the pre-trained weights of ResNet101 [31] which were originally been trained on Microsoft COCO dataset [32] into service. The model was then trained for 65 epochs with the learning rates of 0.0001, 0.00001, and 0.000001 for two 25, and one 15 epochs respectively to fine-tune all the initial weights and make them suitable for our new task. The process in total took about 15 h to finish.

4 Experiments and Results

It is conventional to evaluate and measure the performance of segmentation models with IoU and mAP. Intersection over Union (IoU) calculates the area of the overlap that happens between the predicted bounding box and the actual mask and then divides it to the area of the union of those two. A completely correct bounding box will result in IoU of 1. A threshold is also set to accept IoUs above it as correct predictions. The percentage of correct predictions out of all predicted bounding boxes is called precision. Recall, on the other hand, is the percentage of correct predictions out of all objects present in the image. As more and more predictions are made the precision will decrease due to false positives, but the recall will increase. These two are calculated for different thresholds and then averaged to find out the AP (average precision) for a given image. The mean of APs across all the images in the dataset is referred to as mAP (mean average precision).

To calculate the mAP for our model, we first needed to fix an issue. Our model was deliberately trained on both tasks simultaneously, giving it the ability to find both types of lesions in a given fundus image at the same time. However, the masks that we had from the datasets were only associated with one type of lesion and for the most part, there was no overlap between the two datasets. If used this way, it would have caused our model to get a lower mAP. The reason behind it was that in the test phase, given a fundus image, our model would have predicted and masked both types of lesions, but the mask that it was being compared to was only showing

Table 1 mAP for train, validation, and test sets created from e-ophtha EX and e-ophtha MA datasets

	mAP_{35}	mAP_{50}	m AP_{75}
Train	0.5408	0.5217	0.3032
Validation	0.5113	0.4780	0.2563
Test	0.4562	0.4370	0.2071

one type, altogether making the evaluation agent think that the lesions from the other type are all false positives and hence reduce the precision.

To fix this, when the predictions were made for a given image by our model, we passed them through a filter to only keep the ones that are associated with the type that is marked in the corresponding mask image. This enabled us to test our model in a fair way and see how accurate the exudates and microaneurysms are being predicted individually.

Due to the innate complexity of the task and the extremely small size of the lesions that had to be found, we had previously decreased our model's minimum prediction confidence hyperparameter to 35. Hence, we used it along with two more standard thresholds that are usually used in the task of instance segmentation. As a result, 35, 50, and 75 were chosen as our three thresholds to calculate the results with. Results of the evaluation can be found in Table 1.

To the best of our knowledge, our work is the first to employ instance segmentation models to identify and mask the lesions in the eye and help to diagnose the infamous diabetic retinopathy. Given the complexity of the task, our model performed extremely well and we call our result a success.

5 Conclusion and Future Work

We have presented a simple, yet efficient approach to detect, locate, and generate segmentation masks for exudates and microaneurysms which are two types of lesions that diabetic retinopathy causes in eyes. Unlike most of the previous work, our model is capable of automatically extracting useful features related to the scale of our work, and learn to perform the task in an end-to-end manner. Moreover, due to its fast predictions, it has the potential to be easily incorporated into health care facilities.

Future work should consider using our model to identify the severity of DR in patients' eyes, exploring other instance segmentation architectures and their ensembles, and creating a better and bigger dataset with more types of lesions.

6 Conflict of Interest

The authors declare that there is no conflict of interest regarding the publication of this article.

References

1. P. Massin, A. Chabouis, A. Erginay, C. Viens-Bitker, A. Lecleire-Collet, T. Meas, P.-J. Guillausseau, G. Choupot, B. André, P. Denormandie, Ophdiat©: a telemedical network screening system for diabetic retinopathy in the île-de-france. Diabetes Metab. **34**(3), 227–234 (2008)
2. E. Decencière, G. Cazuguel, X. Zhang, G. Thibault, J.-C. Klein, F. Meyer, B. Marcotegui, G. Quellec, M. Lamard, R. Danno, et al., Teleophta: Machine learning and image processing methods for teleophthalmology. Irbm **34**(2), 196–203 (2013)
3. K. Bhatia, S. Arora, R. Tomar, Diagnosis of diabetic retinopathy using machine learning classification algorithm, in *2016 2nd International Conference on Next Generation Computing Technologies (NGCT)* (IEEE, Piscataway, 2016), pp. 347–351
4. B. Antal, A. Hajdu, An ensemble-based system for automatic screening of diabetic retinopathy. Knowledge-Based Syst. **60**, 20–27 (2014)
5. D. Usher, M. Dumskyj, M. Himaga, T.H. Williamson, S. Nussey, J. Boyce, Automated detection of diabetic retinopathy in digital retinal images: a tool for diabetic retinopathy screening. Diabetic Med. **21**(1), 84–90 (2004)
6. G. Gardner, D. Keating, T.H. Williamson, A.T. Elliott, Automatic detection of diabetic retinopathy using an artificial neural network: a screening tool. British J. Ophthalmol. **80**(11), 940–944 (1996)
7. R. Priya, P. Aruna, Diagnosis of diabetic retinopathy using machine learning techniques. ICTACT J. Soft Comput. **3**(4), 563–575 (2013)
8. A. Sopharak, M.N. Dailey, B. Uyyanonvara, S. Barman, T. Williamson, K.T. Nwe, Y.A. Moe, Machine learning approach to automatic exudate detection in retinal images from diabetic patients. J. Modern Optics **57**(2), 124–135 (2010)
9. Z. Liu, C. Opas, S.M. Krishnan, Automatic image analysis of fundus photograph, in *Proceedings of the 19th Annual International Conference of the IEEE Engineering in Medicine and Biology Society.'Magnificent Milestones and Emerging Opportunities in Medical Engineering'(Cat. No. 97CH36136)*, vol. 2 (IEEE, Piscataway, 1997), pp. 524–525
10. B.M. Ege, O.K. Hejlesen, O.V. Larsen, K. Møller, B. Jennings, D. Kerr, D.A. Cavan, Screening for diabetic retinopathy using computer based image analysis and statistical classification. Comput. Methods Program Biomed. **62**(3), 165–175 (2000)
11. C. Sinthanayothin, J.F. Boyce, H.L. Cook, T.H. Williamson, Automated localisation of the optic disc, fovea, and retinal blood vessels from digital colour fundus images. British J. Ophthalmol. **83**(8), 902–910 (1999)
12. J. Lachure, A. Deorankar, S. Lachure, S. Gupta, R. Jadhav, Diabetic retinopathy using morphological operations and machine learning, in *2015 IEEE International Advance Computing Conference (IACC)* (IEEE, Piscataway, 2015), pp. 617–622
13. S. Roychowdhury, D.D. Koozekanani, K.K. Parhi, Dream: diabetic retinopathy analysis using machine learning. IEEE J. Biomed. Health Inf. **18**(5), 1717–1728 (2013)
14. R. Acharya, C.K. Chua, E. Ng, W. Yu, C. Chee, Application of higher order spectra for the identification of diabetes retinopathy stages. J. Med. Syst. **32**(6), 481–488 (2008)
15. P. Adarsh, D. Jeyakumari, Multiclass SVM-based automated diagnosis of diabetic retinopathy, in *2013 International Conference on Communication and Signal Processing* (IEEE, Piscataway, 2013), pp. 206–210
16. R. Gargeya, T. Leng, Automated identification of diabetic retinopathy using deep learning. Ophthalmology **124**(7), 962–969 (2017)
17. V. Gulshan, L. Peng, M. Coram, M.C. Stumpe, D. Wu, A. Narayanaswamy, S. Venugopalan, K. Widner, T. Madams, J. Cuadros, et al., Development and validation of a deep learning algorithm for detection of diabetic retinopathy in retinal fundus photographs. Jama **316**(22), 2402–2410 (2016)
18. H. Pratt, F. Coenen, D.M. Broadbent, S.P. Harding, Y. Zheng, Convolutional neural networks for diabetic retinopathy. Procedia Comput. Sci. **90**, 200–205 (2016)

19. A. Krizhevsky, I. Sutskever, G.E. Hinton, ImageNet classification with deep convolutional neural networks, in *Advances in Neural Information Processing Systems* (2012), pp. 1097–1105
20. S. Amirian, K. Rasheed, T.R. Taha, H.R. Arabnia, Image captioning with generative adversarial network, in *2019 International Conference on Computational Science and Computational Intelligence (CSCI)* (IEEE, Piscataway, 2019), pp. 272–275
21. N. Soans, E. Asali, Y. Hong, P. Doshi, SA-net: Robust state-action recognition for learning from observations, in *IEEE International Conference on Robotics and Automation (ICRA)* (2020), pp. 2153–2159
22. A. Das, S. Datta, G. Gkioxari, S. Lee, D. Parikh, D. Batra, Embodied question answering, in *Proceedings of the IEEE Conference on Computer Vision and Pattern Recognition Workshops* (2018), pp. 2054–2063
23. F.G. Mohammadi, H.R. Arabnia, M.H. Amini, On parameter tuning in meta-learning for computer vision, in *2019 International Conference on Computational Science and Computational Intelligence (CSCI)* (IEEE, Piscataway, 2019), pp. 300–305
24. S. Xie, A. Kirillov, R. Girshick, K. He, Exploring randomly wired neural networks for image recognition, in *Proceedings of the IEEE International Conference on Computer Vision* (2019), pp. 1284–1293
25. R. Girshick, J. Donahue, T. Darrell, J. Malik, Rich feature hierarchies for accurate object detection and semantic segmentation, in *Proceedings of the IEEE Conference on Computer Vision and Pattern Recognition* (2014), pp. 580–587
26. R. Girshick, Fast R-CNN, in *Proceedings of the IEEE International Conference on Computer Vision* (2015), pp. 1440–1448
27. S. Ren, K. He, R. Girshick, J. Sun, Faster R-CNN: Towards real-time object detection with region proposal networks," in *Advances in Neural Information Processing Systems* (2015), pp. 91–99
28. K. He, G. Gkioxari, P. Dollár, R. Girshick, Mask R-CNN, in *Proceedings of the IEEE International Conference on Computer Vision* (2017), pp. 2961–2969
29. F. Shenavarmasouleh, H. Arabnia, Causes of misleading statistics and research results irreproducibility: A concise review, in *2019 International Conference on Computational Science and Computational Intelligence (CSCI)* (2019), pp. 465–470
30. G. Bradski, The OpenCV Library, *Dr. Dobb's Journal of Software Tools* (2000)
31. K. He, X. Zhang, S. Ren, J. Sun, Deep residual learning for image recognition, in *Proceedings of the IEEE Conference on Computer Vision and Pattern Recognition* (2016), pp. 770–778
32. T.-Y. Lin, M. Maire, S. Belongie, J. Hays, P. Perona, D. Ramanan, P. Dollár, C.L. Zitnick, Microsoft coco: Common objects in context, in *European Conference on Computer Vision* (Springer, Berlin, 2014), pp. 740–755

Postoperative Hip Fracture Rehabilitation Model

Akash Gupta, Adnan Al-Anbuky, and Peter McNair

1 Introduction

Hip fracture is a global public health issue and a critical life-threatening injury. It has a serious long-term devastating impact on the physical functionality of the elderly people (aged 60 and above) and on their ability to remain independent [1]. As hip fracture is common among older population, it occurs mainly from a fall or due to medical conditions like osteoporosis and stress injuries [2]. When a hip fracture injury occurs, the injury is most likely in the neck of femur [3]. The fracture can be either in head and neck of the femur or between/below the greater and lesser trochanters. After the doctor's examination, patients undergo a surgical operation. Following that, patients are taken to a recovery unit where rehabilitation process begins within a day of the operation [4]. Evidence indicates that rehabilitation plays a guaranteeing role in recovery and boosting the quality of life [1]. Initially, the goal for the patient is to regain their functional mobility. Along with the improvement in the physical functionality, the event and related hospitalization period often result in muscle degradation. Therefore, improving and maintaining the muscle strength with the exercises involved during postoperative rehabilitation is essential.

Research shows that after hip fracture, around 5–6% of total lean body mass and 4–11% of gain in body fat mass are observed. Most of this occur especially during the first 2–4 months following the fracture [5]. According to a study by [5], it is reflected that loss of muscle strength leads to poorer mobility recovery a

A. Gupta (✉) · A. Al-Anbuky
School of Engineering, Computer and Mathematical Sciences, Auckland, New Zealand
e-mail: akash.gupta@aut.ac.nz; adnan.anbuky@aut.ac.nz

P. McNair
School of Clinical Sciences, Auckland University of Technology, Auckland, New Zealand
e-mail: peter.mcnair@aut.ac.nz

H. R. Arabnia et al. (eds.), *Advances in Computer Vision and Computational Biology*, Transactions on Computational Science and Computational Intelligence,
https://doi.org/10.1007/978-3-030-71051-4_25

Table 1 Exercise movements and muscle and related physical movement involvement

S.no	Movements	Muscles involved in each movement	Related physical movement
1	Hip flexion	Iliopsoas, rectus femoris, sartorius, pectineus	Lifting thigh upwards, lying on back, walking
2	Hip extension	Gluteus maximus, semimembranosus semitendinosus and bicep femoris (hamstring)	Leg movement (while sitting), lying on stomach, walking
3	Hip abduction	Gluteus medius and minimus, tensor fascia latae, and piriformis	Swinging leg to a side, walking
4	Hip adduction	Adductor longus, brevis and magnus, pectineus and gracilis	Mini squats, bridging, walking
5	Hip lateral rotation	Biceps femoris, gluteus maximus, piriformis assisted by obturators, gemilli, and quadratus femoris	Lying on stomach and lying on back, walking
6	Hip medial rotation	Anterior fibers of gluteus medius and minimus, tensor fascia latae	Lying on stomach and lying on back, walking

year following the fracture. As a result, understanding the interrelation between the muscles involved in each of the movement exercises while strengthening hip joint is significant for a more precise planning of the recovery process. Table 1 represents the particular muscles involved in each of these movements [6].

In summary, the movement activities of lifting thigh upward, lying on back, walking, leg movement (while sitting), lying on stomach, swinging leg to a side, mini squats, and bridging are considered the key activities for supporting these important muscles.

Another concern is increase in the mortality rate. This is 20–24% in the first year following the hip fracture despite continual patient follow-up. Contributing reasons are losing the ability to live independently, loss of physical function, 40% not able to walk independently, and 60% requiring assistance due to loss of confidence and motivation. As a result of these loses, 33% of them are completely dependent or reside in a nursing home a year following the hip fracture [7].

Findings reported a need for identification of the optimal strategies to improve the functional performance of the patients following the hip fracture surgery [1]. It has also indicated that patient should be provided with optimal, well-coordinated, and organized rehabilitation program following the surgery. This will support the needs for the well-coordinated and organized rehabilitation program [2]. Moreover, little is known about the effectiveness of the rehabilitation pathways in improving the patient outcomes. Considering all these circumstances in mind, it is evident for a requirement of a generic rehabilitation program that could be applicable to any person undergoing rehabilitation from such type of injuries.

This paper provides a preliminary framework by underlining and illustrating all the key parameters of interest required for the post hip fracture rehabilitation process to be followed in progressive stages. The paper is organized as follows: Next section discusses about the rehabilitation process structure. Section 3 represents the proposed rehabilitation program. Section 4 discusses the potential for the online implementation of the proposed rehabilitation program. Section 5 presents some conclusion remarks.

2 Rehabilitation Process Structure

Rehabilitation process starts by performing basic everyday functional tasks activities like sitting on a chair, standing on an uninjured leg with assistance, and bed mobility (turning or bridging, etc.). Following that, ambulatory- or gait-related exercises like walking (slow or fast) and stepping the stairs up and down are started after 4–8 days depending on the patient's ability to balance the body posture and bear full weight on the injured leg [8]. Apart from the everyday and ambulatory exercises, a tailored program that focuses on strengthening the fractured hip joint muscle is provided by a physiotherapist to the patient. In this program, the key involved exercises during lying are heel slide, hip abduction, bridging, and quadriceps strengthening. All these exercises focus on building and regaining range of motion and strengthening the hip joint, whereas the exercise involved while sitting are sit-to-stand and knee extension (leg movement while sitting). These exercises help patient to balance the posture and improve the range of motion. Importantly, exercises involved when patient is standing are hip extension, sideways stepping, hip flexion (lifting thigh upward), mini squats, and hip abduction (swinging leg to a side). These exercises mainly focus in strengthening the fractured hip joint muscle along with the mobility and posture balance to avoid further similar incidents.

The abovementioned exercises are supervised by a physiotherapist. Once patient performs all the exercises correctly, he or she can redo these exercises independently (living at home or in outside environment) and unsupervised. There is not much information available relevant to the process structure, stages involved, and related measurement used for indicating the progress in the process. Along with phases, how many repetitions, for how long, and how many times each of the exercises should be repeated by a patient for an effective recovery process are not defined clearly. Reference [3, 9] recommends that patient should aim to perform each of the exercises two to three times a day with 10–20 repetitions each, whereas reference [10] advises patient to exercise at least two times a day by repeating each exercise 5–10 times. As the injury improves, patients are then instructed to slowly increase and perform each exercise 4 times a day, repeating each exercise 30 times [10].

From the above discussion, it becomes clear that rehabilitation services are not well-defined resulting in supporting unsupervised implementation. The instructions toward implementation of exercises are either miscommunicated or wrongly implemented. This, in effect, results in prolonging the process and sometimes taking so long to be fatal. It is clear that when patient is at the hospital, the exercises are supervised and a have regular follow-up by the healthcare staff. However, the problem arises when patient is discharged and lives independently at home as exercises performed are unsupervised. Here, the transparency of what exercises the patient has performed is not precisely known to the healthcare personnel. As a result, there is a lack of transparency between the patient implementation of the rehabilitation process and the health caretaker. Hence, it is essential to lay out and understand the recovery progression stages involved during rehabilitation. Based on the information provided from the literature [3, 9, 10], with the help of physiotherapist and medical domain expert knowledge, this paper attempts to lay out the post hip fracture rehabilitation process patient has to undergo straight after the surgery. Three phases of rehabilitation are recognized from the existing practices:

1. Supervised rehab at hospital
2. Guided/unsupervised rehab at home
3. Unsupervised rehab at outdoor

Involvements of these three phases are discussed in the following section alongside the proposal for the overall rehabilitation process structure.

3 Propose Rehabilitation Program

Figure 1 represents the overall structural design of the postoperative hip fracture rehabilitation pathway in stages. It exhibits the number and name of stages involved; key involved activities type and name across each stage; how frequently the exercise should be practiced; which activity is supervised, unsupervised, or is a combination of both; time duration of a particular activity to be performed; and activity image illustrating the movement direction and pattern. The description of the involvement of three rehabilitation phases spread across four different stages is as follows:

3.1 Supervised Rehabilitation at Hospital

The objective of the rehab just after the operation at the hospital aim at improving patient's independence through attempting range of motion resulting with strengthening the muscle through bed mobility (turning or bridging), transfer (sit-to-stand), and ambulation (walking with a walking aid and climbing stairs). These movements are part of stages 1 and 2 of the rehabilitation processes as it helps in returning of their daily physical functionality allowing them to be safe ambulators within their home environment. Before discharging from hospital, a team of health professional consisting of nurses, social services, and therapy staff works closely with the patients to agree on the achievable goals for a safe discharge.

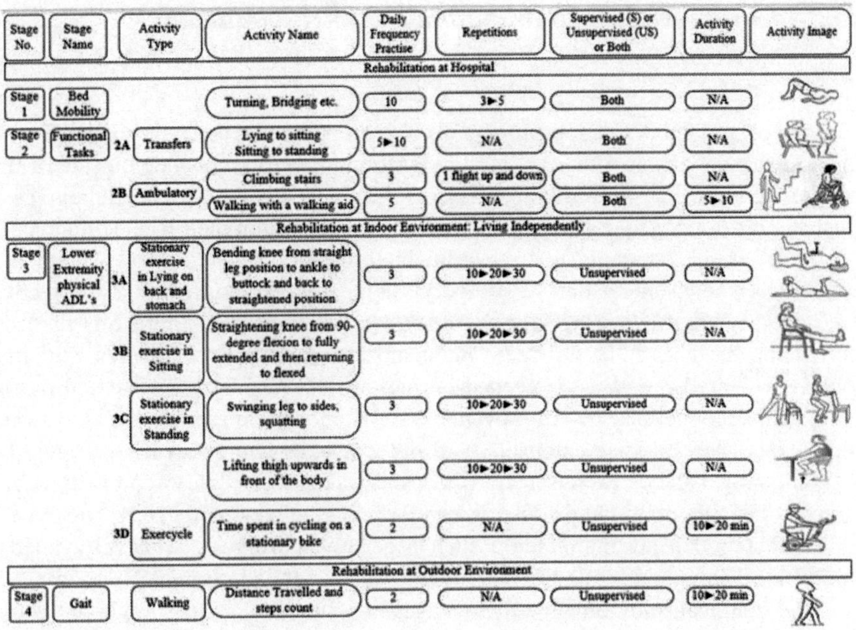

Fig. 1 Postoperative hip fracture rehabilitation pathway structural design in stages

3.2 Guided/Unsupervised Rehabilitation Exercise at Home: Living Independently

In stage 3 of the rehabilitation process, a hospital-based physiotherapist provides an exercise program for the patient to undertake at home. This is aimed at increasing joint range of motion, strength, and endurance with a view to improving lower extremity physical activities of daily living, particularly ambulation. It has been reported that home-based exercise programs with minimal supervision have a reasonable effect on improving physical functionality, mobility, and balance [11]. However, due to the lack of supervision, the patients' compliance to perform exercises and gait activities is not objectively quantified, and hence healthcare providers rely upon subjective commentary from the patient, its validity being questionable. The current implementation reflects random operation with significant uncertainty in expectation of outcome. The process if implemented correctly should help improve the mobility to the level of moving to the outdoor exercises. It could also help in identifying possibility to fine-tune the program to be more suitable to the particular person (i.e., personalization of the program).

3.3 Unsupervised Rehabilitation Exercise at Outdoor Environment

Stage 4 of the rehabilitation process aims to improve the patient's mental health along with the physical functionality by enabling them to ambulate outside of the home environment. In doing so, exercise programs can be advanced/progressed much more effectively, as is the ability to reintegrate within their local community.

Apart from the three key rehabilitation phases discussed above, there are situations where some patients get supervised rehabilitation once home irrespective of how they are progressing. The reason is exercise at home is limited by the lack of equipment that can be utilized. This is most relevant to strengthening exercises where increased resistance is needed in the form of weights or special equipment to obtain a more efficacious improvement. Resistance training exercises are needed for plantar flexors, knee extensors, and hip extensors and abductors particularly. Additionally, balance exercises are often undertaken in a supervised environment where the risk of a fall is less likely. Whether a patient receives supervised rehabilitation depends upon factors such as perceived progress, resources available in the local community, and provision within the patient's insurance program.

The significance of knowing these stages in systematic order is important while developing an automatic decision-making system model and fuzzy indicator based on the activity recognition. For instance, a system recognizes swinging leg to a side activity. Based on that recognition, system will automatically detect progression stage of the patient. This information will aid healthcare professionals in:

1. Actively monitoring the patient progression in a personalized manner
2. Accessing patient data remotely
3. Observing the vital changes taking place on a regular basis
4. Comprehending how slow or fast a patient is progressing and adjust the repetitions and exercise accordingly
5. Sending necessary feedback to the patients in case of emergency or for a follow-up.

Moreover, there are no evidences that discusses about the specific time frames of switching of the activity movements from one stage to another as the patients are generally elderly with a wide range of cognitive and physical ability. Prior to their fracture, some are very frail to start with while others exercise regularly. Similarly, their resilience, their confidence, and their anxiety levels vary, and this affects how they progress. Because it is so multifactorial, it is hard to discern exact milestones. However, the system in place and multiple patient data availability on these activity movements through the help of intelligent machine or artificial intelligence techniques could help researchers/clinicians in investigating the average amount of time required for a patient to switch from one activity to other.

4 Potential for Online Rehabilitation Program Implementation

The recent advancement in digital health could be leveraged upon in facilitating and remotely interacting with the above suggested rehabilitation program. Tracking, recording, and remotely monitoring can significantly help in following up the correct implementation of a predefined program. It can also merge the concurrent programs whether they are supervised or unsupervised, in effect helping people to be motivated for implementation wherever they are and correct any misperception toward the corrected ways of doing the exercises. The lockdown of COVID-19 offers a strong case for such a need and as it applies to elderlies.

The Internet of Things (IoT) is an important platform for such implementation. It is the technological revolution that allows subjects to be interconnected, related movement activities to be tracked, and online gathering of real-time and history data to be collected [12]. Furthermore, the ample resources at the remote service platform or the cloud allow for the integration of significant amount of intelligence that supports dynamic tracking, recognition, and alerting of important events. Figure 2 represents the IoT-based postoperative hip fracture rehabilitation care assistant system architecture. The architecture exhibits the significance and involvement of the three main layers, i.e., wireless sensing, gateway, and cloud layer in the overall movement monitoring process prescribed as part of the rehabilitation program.

In the architecture, human subject is the core part, and our earlier work [2] reported the use of system first layer, i.e., wireless wearable monitoring device in activity movement data collection, its placement at the ankle location, and its computational method for analysis and recognition of the activities involved during hip fracture rehabilitation. One approach for the activity recognition analysis is proposed by [2]. This is based on the frequency content within the integrated acceleration signals of the three axes using the Fast Fourier Transform (FFT) approach. This identifies the frequency content with maximum acceleration amplitude (f_{MA}) and the maximum acceleration amplitude (MA) parameters. Based on that approach, Fig. 3 portrays the sample activity detection of all the activities involved in the rehabilitation [2].

The raw activity movement data from monitoring device can be used for further analysis by sending its data to a nearby gateways (system second layer) that might be facilitated at hospitals, gym or exercise centers, rehabilitation homes, and residence place or could even be carried by patient as a mobile device when moving around. Therefore, after some level of processing at the gateway level, the data could be further subjected to the system third layer, i.e., cloud, where real-time, history, and knowledge data will be managed, visualized, modelled, and used for leveraging more advanced intelligent outcome. It will facilitate the key interaction with the healthcare service providers such as caretaker, physiotherapist, clinician, etc. An indicative example of visualizing the time domain of the subject activities from the data available within the cloud repository is shown by Fig. 4 [12]. This plot presents the overall summary of the different type of rehabilitation activity movements

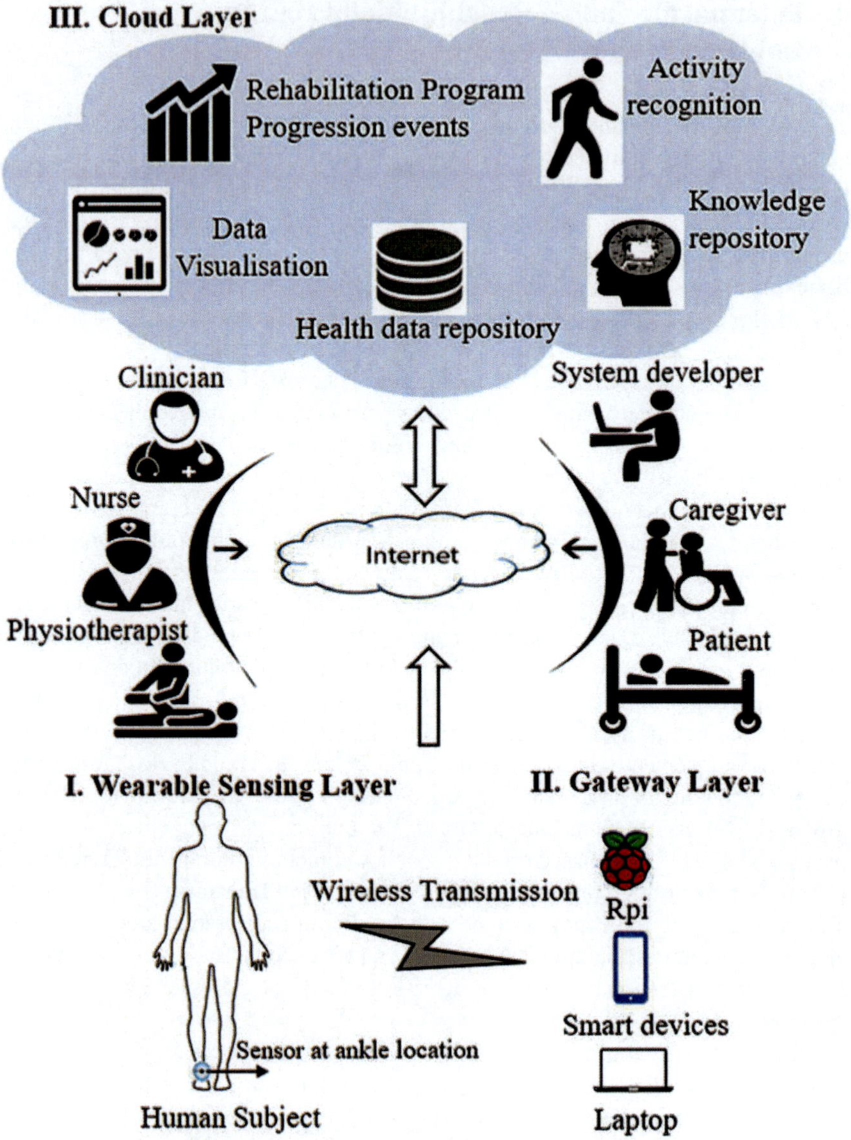

Fig. 2 Postoperative hip fracture rehabilitation care assistant system

performed by a subject over a specific time duration. Findings show that activities like lying on stomach, slow and fast walking, and lifting thigh upward have been performed by the patient where some of the activities were unrecognized. While this semi-raw data outcome may still need further processing to offer more precise and user-friendly information, this data presentation could help the multidisciplinary

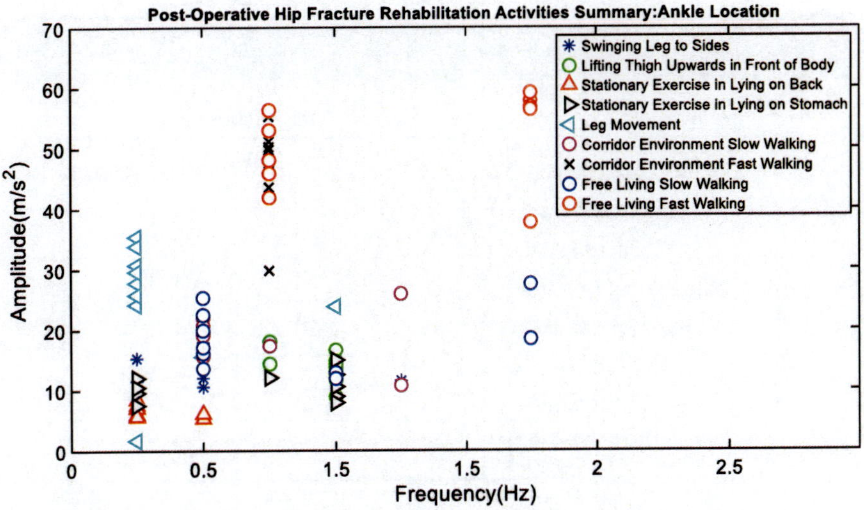

Fig. 3 Sample activity detection of the activities involved in hip fracture rehabilitation process

team. It may also be further specialized to target the purpose of each particular service whether of physiotherapist, social worker, occupational therapist, or nurse. It will be tailored according to their requirements in tracking and accomplishing patient goals of rehabilitation. It could also offer the flexibility of observing the overall day-to-day, week-to-week, and month-to-month performance of the patient's daily activities/exercises movements in real time from anywhere and at any time. This in effect can relate to the rehabilitation program progression stages stated by Fig. 1 and facilitate the necessary follow-up to the program implementation and any necessary dynamic maneuver for improving the effectiveness of the process.

Moreover, the stored data is available and managed at all the three levels, i.e., wearable monitoring device, gateway, and cloud level layer as a backup that could help researchers/clinicians for more intelligent computation and in making the system adaptable to a particular subject. Hence, this could further help in case of follow-up and in emergencies.

Another important aspect to reflect here is that of personalization based on activity recognition. Everyone has different physical fitness levels and may respond differently to the prescribed activities. In that case, a general-purpose solution that fits all users in recognizing activities may not offer precise solution. Herein, personalization can play a crucial role in reducing the degree of overlap among activities and allow for the recognition parameters to be trained for a particular subject. Moreover, it will also offer the flexibility in making the rehabilitation program adjustable based on the patient progression levels by healthcare staff.

An indicative example of such case is represented in Fig. 5. It shows the comparison between the general-purpose and the personalized subject range data

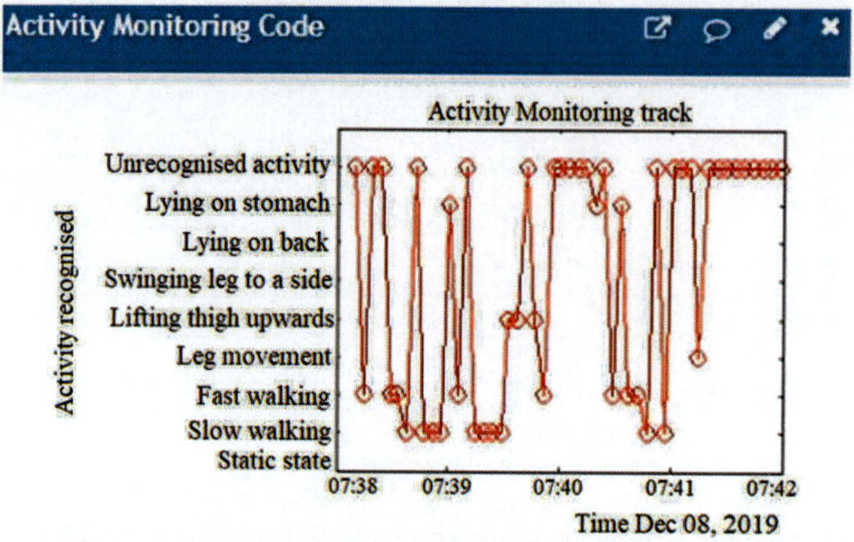

Fig. 4 Hip fracture rehabilitation activity movement monitoring track

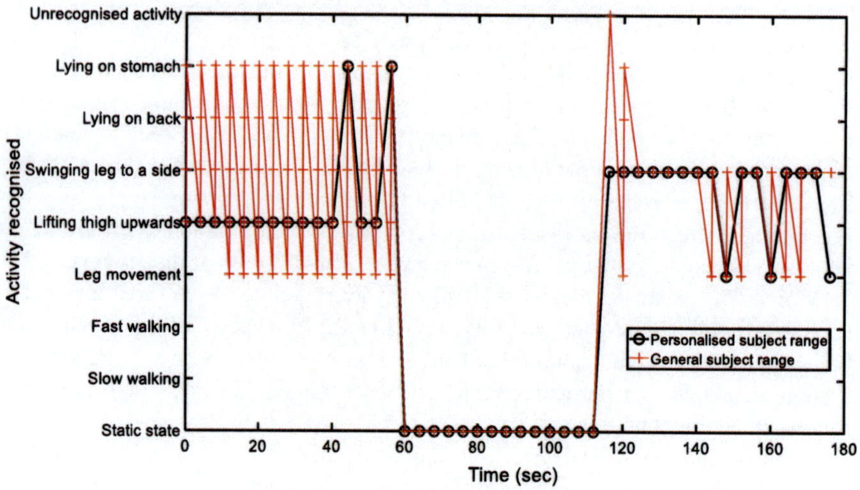

Fig. 5 Personalized vs. general subject activity recognition analysis comparison

analysis for three different activities, i.e., lifting thigh upwards, static state, and swinging leg to a side.

It clearly indicates that based on the general-purpose subject range, lifting thigh upward activity has high degree of overlap with the other four activities, i.e., swinging leg to a side, leg movement, and lying on back and stomach, whereas in case of personalized subject range, minimal overlap is observed and is only with lying on stomach. However, the static activity shows similar result as there is no movement from the subject. On the other hand, talking about swinging leg to a side activity, general-purpose approach again has high degree of overlap with leg movement activity and minimal overlap with lying on back and stomach activity, whereas with the personalized approach, swinging leg to a side activity is recognized with high precision, and there is a minimal overlap with leg movement activity. The minimal overlap could be avoided with the use of more intelligent computation and activity transition rules.

While the section reflects potential for the subject activity data to be collected online and processed remotely, further computational and interaction involvements will be needed for making full sense of the rehabilitation model stated in Sect. 3 above. Cloud-based environment like that of ThingSpeak [12] could offer the required resources for such solution.

5 Conclusion

This paper suggests a model for postoperative hip fracture rehabilitation process that facilitates stages for patients to undergo through straight after hospitalization. The model highlights the physiological interrelation between the rehabilitation process and affected muscles. It then relates the external physical or motor activities with the possible recovery of these affected muscles. While the program has emerged out analysis of existing recommendations within the science and practice of hip fracture rehabilitation process, it offers a ground for automating the process and allow for effective utilization of the modern digital environment. This in effect should help in evolving the solution with time and as further implementation data is made available. The ultimate target is the online rehabilitation program implementation that contains the key components to all detailed and abstracted data. These in effect should facilitate the environment for the various users for interaction with patient movement history and progress toward ultimate health.

References

1. J.-q. Wu, L.-b. Mao, J. Wu, Efficacy of balance training for hip fracture patients: A meta-analysis of randomized controlled trials. J. Orthop. Surg. Res. **14**(1), 83 (2019)
2. A. Gupta, A. Al-Anbuky, P. McNair, Activity classification feasibility using wearables: Considerations for hip fracture. J. Sens. Actuator Netw. **7**(4), 54 (2018)
3. P. H. N. F. Trust. Hip Fracture Information and exercises for patients. Available online: https://www.poole.nhs.uk/pdf/Hip%20fracture.pdf
4. MayoClinic. The Hip Fracture. Available online: https://www.mayoclinic.org/diseases-conditions/hip-fracture/diagnosis-treatment/drc-20373472
5. M. Visser et al., Change in muscle mass and muscle strength after a hip fracture: Relationship to mobility recovery. J. Gerontol. Ser. A Biol. Med. Sci. **55**(8), M434–M440 (2000)

6. T. Anatomy. The Hip Joint. Available online: https://teachmeanatomy.info/lower-limb/joints/hip-joint/
7. I. O. Foundation. Facts and Statistics. Available online: https://www.iofbonehealth.org/facts-statistics#category-16
8. P.A. Fenstemacher, P. Winn, *Long-Term Care Medicine: A Pocket Guide* (Springer Science & Business Media, 2010)
9. B. H. C. System. Hip Fracture Guide. Available online: https://www.baylorhealth.com/PhysiciansLocations/Dallas/SpecialtiesServices/Orthopaedics/Documents/Hip%20Fractures%20Guide_Web.pdf
10. A. Kania-Richmond, J. Werle, J. Robert, Bone and joint health strategic clinical network: Keeping Albertans moving. CMAJ **191**(Suppl), S10–S12 (2019)
11. N.K. Latham et al., Effect of a home-based exercise program on functional recovery following rehabilitation after hip fracture: A randomized clinical trial. JAMA **311**(7), 700–708 (2014)
12. A. Gupta, A. Al-Anbuky, K. Al-Naime, IoT based testbed for human movement activity monitoring and presentation, in *6th International Conference on Information and Communication Technologies for Ageing Well and e-health, 3-5 May*, (Prague, 2020), pp. 61–68. https://doi.org/10.5220/0009347800610068

ReSmart: Brain Training Games for Enhancing Cognitive Health

Raymond Jung, Bonggyn Son, Hyeseong Park, Sngon Kim, and Megawati Wijaya

1 Introduction

As human beings are getting older and living longer, the number of dementia patients is increasing. While dementia tends to degenerate cognitive abilities, recent evidence suggests that engaging in cognitively challenging activities can positively impact brain function, such that cognitive skills are improved following cognitive training. Recently, brain training activities are accessible through mobile platforms to keep elders' brains active and strengthen cognitive skills [2, 3].

However, training cognitive skills for special users require more attention in terms of two aspects: (1) a level of personalized brain training, (2) a lack of elders' self-motivation for technology use. First, since dementia patients experience different types of symptoms, brain training games require an understanding of individual responses in cognitive level. Also, senior citizens lack technology experiences, which reduces self-motivation to use technology. Although many researchers have introduced technologies aiming to improve cognitive health for elders [6, 7], enabling the use of technology without the support of dementia advisors or other staff can be impractical [1] (Fig. 1).

To enhance the cognitive abilities of elders, we propose a mobile platform called **ReSmart** which mainly depends on two features: *six distinct levels of the brain training task*, which covers five distributed cognitive areas (e.g., attention, coordination, memory, perception, and reasoning) to enable personalized brain training. Also, providing six brain training tasks are presented in a *game-like format*

R. Jung (✉) · B. Son · H. Park · S. Kim · M. Wijaya
AKA Cognitive Corp., Seoul, Republic of Korea
e-mail: rjung@akaintelligence.com; https://akaintelligence.com; daniel@akaintelligence.com; julie@akaintelligence.com; sgkim@akaintelligence.com; mega@akaintelligence.com

H. R. Arabnia et al. (eds.), *Advances in Computer Vision and Computational Biology*, Transactions on Computational Science and Computational Intelligence,
https://doi.org/10.1007/978-3-030-71051-4_26

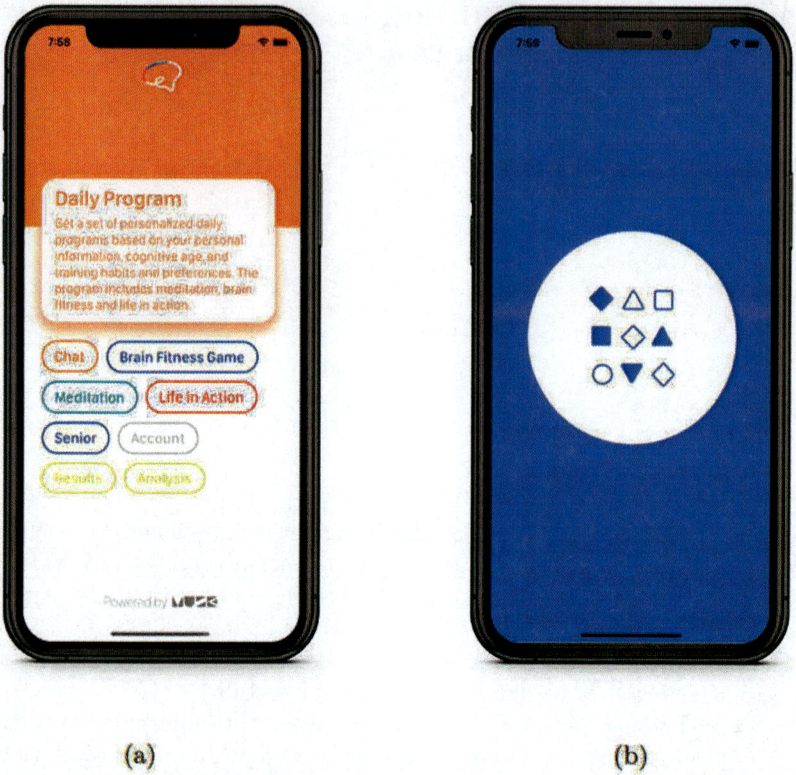

Fig. 1 ReSmart mobile application. (**a**) ReSmart landing page. (**b**) ReSmart brain fitness games

to not lose the elders' motivation for technology use and keeping interest. We address our research questions as below:

- RQ1: *To what extent, can our system improve the cognitive abilities of elders by providing personalized brain training games?*
- RQ2. *To what extent, can our system improve elders' motivation for technology use?*

We conducted our user study with elders, 79-91 years old, with their MMSE[1] score information.

[1]https://www.alzheimers.org.uk/about-dementia/symptoms-and-diagnosis/diagnosis/mmse-test.

2 Resmart

2.1 Implementation

ReSmart was built on the iOS framework, creating an application available on a mobile device or tablet, running the iOS operating systems. MySQL database stores user information along with an Amazon dynamoDB to store users' media.

2.2 Six Distinct Brain Training Games

Resmart is designed to enhance cognitive abilities based on two features: (1) personalized brain training games based on five diverse cognitive areas, (2) game-like format, inspired Lumosity [4] when game-playing can be an effective learning resource for elderly people [5]. We present six distinct brain training games along with five cognitive areas.

The five cognitive areas are explained by CogniFit[2] which designed cognitive assessment through monitoring the patient's cognitive rehabilitation process. **Memory** is the ability to retain new information and recover memories of the past. **Coordination** is the ability to efficiently perform precise and ordered movements. **Attention** is the ability to filter distractions and focus on relevant information. **Reasoning** is the ability to efficiently use (order, relate, etc.) the information acquired through the different senses, and **Perception** is the ability to interpret the stimuli of the environment.

- **Balloon Game:** Shown as Fig. 2a, when a ball and a button are given, a user can press as many buttons as possible, within the given time to make the ball bigger. The related cognitive areas are *Coordination, Reasoning, Attention.*
- **Letter Finding Game:** Shown as Fig. 2b, one consonant is given at the top while some multiple consonants at the bottom are shown on the same page. A user can tap all letters that are the same as the letter at the top. The related cognitive areas are *Perception.*
- **Shape Memory Game:** Shown as Fig. 2c, when the three different shapes are given, a user remembers the shape and order of each figure, then presses the button if it matches the pattern shown. The related cognitive areas are *Coordination, Reasoning, Perception.*
- **Ball tracking, and Color and Word Matching Game:** Shown as Fig. 2d, if the color and letters of the ball match, a user can press the button. If it does not match, the user is not allowed to press. The related cognitive areas are *Coordination, Reasoning, Attention, Perception.*

[2]https://www.cognifit.com/.

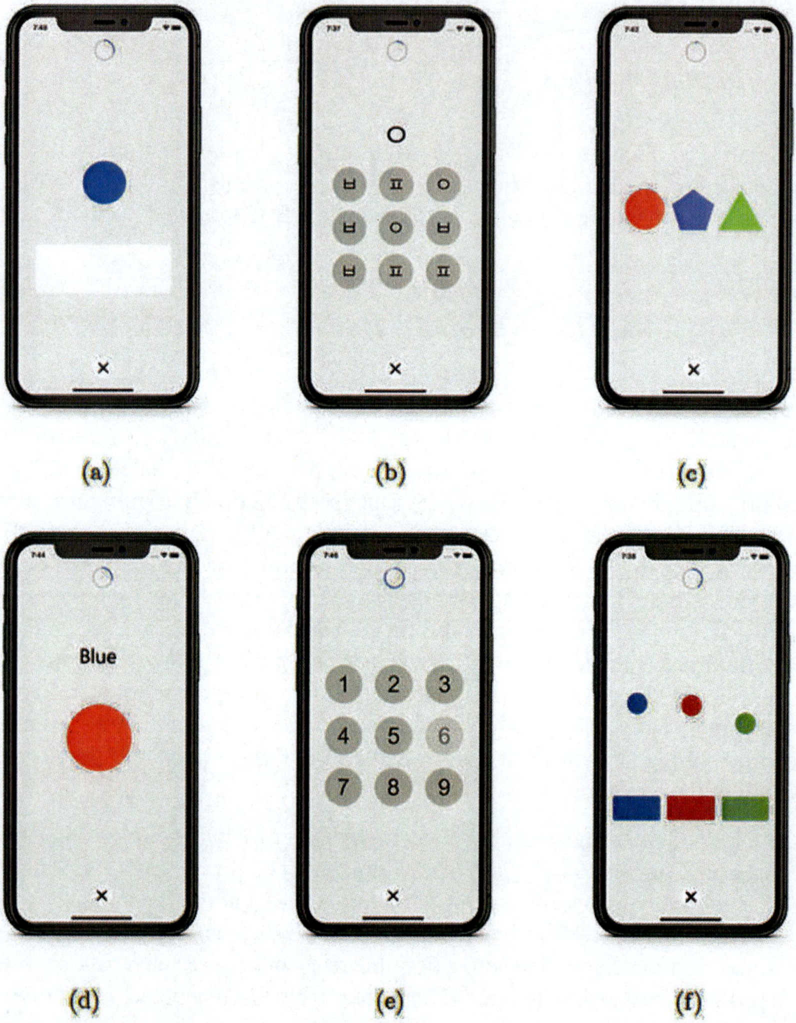

Fig. 2 Six brain training games. (**a**) Ballon. (**b**) Letter finding. (**c**) Shape memory. (**d**) Color/word matching. (**e**) Memorizing numbers. (**f**) Ball prediction

- **Memorizing Numbers:** Shown as Fig. 2e, when the several numbers are given in the sequence, a user remembers, and then presses the number button in the order in which they appear. The related cognitive areas are *Coordination, Reasoning, Memory*.
- **Ball Prediction Game:** Shown as Fig. 2f, when three balls with different colors are falling, a user can find the color of the ball that may reach to the square button. Then, he/she can press the square button. The relative cognitive areas are *perception, reasoning, coordination*.

3 User Study

3.1 Participants

There were 4 participating residents, all within the ages of 79–91, with moderate or severe dementia (MMSE score 17–27). Participants trained on up to six brain training games, that were presented in game-like formats. There were 3 volunteers (aged 25–30) with differing levels of experience of volunteering in care homes (from none to a regular visitor) and different levels of familiarity with the residents (from strangers to friends).

3.2 Apparatus

The experiment was conducted in the bed of the elderly where volunteers visited them. The volunteers installed ReSmart[3] to platforms (a version of iOS 11.0) where they can access the "Brain Games" section where listed up the games and explained task instruction until the senior citizens understand to play.

3.3 Procedure

Participants played the game in their room individually for 30-min. The tasks were followed with explanations from volunteers in the following order of brain game sessions. One volunteer explained how to play the game, while the other volunteer observed the behavior of elders and record it. We ran 30-min tasks for 3-days through ReSmart with participants to ensure the senior citizens understood the task instructions and how to use the mobile platform.

4 Discussion

We conducted the user study to observe the behavior of senior citizens in the usage of ReSmart. The findings from our studies are highlighted with two terms: (1) Personalization, (2) Motivation.

- **Personalized level of brain training games** We were able to monitor four participants in game play behaviors accurately by visiting their individual rooms through a 3-day period. Each participant showed a higher concentration in games

[3] https://appadvice.com/app/resmart/1463753511.

that a suitable match for them. For instance, One participant lacked memory ability had a feeling of uncomfortable to play games such as memorizing numbers. Another participant who weakened perception skills unable to understand in following games such as shape memory game and Ball tracking and color matching game. This suggests that the six distinct brain games can distinguish an individual's condition in their game play behaviors.

- **Motivation** Participants struggled to keep with using a mobile platform. They were unfamiliar with how to use the device. For example, each said *"I don't know where to press"*, *"The color is not clear because of the bright screen"*, *"It looks like a mobile phone, but it is too big to be uncomfortable"*. However, from using devices more and more, they enjoyed playing games, which result in the improvement of the playing. When the participants finished games, they experienced a sense of accomplishment that can positively impact on self-motivation.

5 Conclusion and Future Work

In this paper, we proposed a mobile platform called Resmart to enhance cognitive health, which embeds six distinct levels of the brain training in a game-like format. In the experiment, we observed positive effects of enhancing cognitive health by addressing two points of aspects such as personalized training, enhancing self-motivation. The six distinct brain training games found an individual's condition from different symptoms of dementia, which enables to cure the patients with personalized symptoms. Moreover, the game-like format enhanced self-motivation by enabling the enjoyment of cognitive training, avoiding the uncomfortable condition. In future work, we plan to deepen the study of measuring personalized cognitive health by improving the model with presenting personalized cognitive age analysis page, adjusting the difficulty level of games.

References

1. Alzheimer's society's view on assistive technology, https://www.alzheimers.org.uk/about-us/policy-and-influencing/what-we-think/assistive-technology. Accessed 2020 Jun 06
2. D. Coyle, H. van der Meulen, C. Tunney, P. Cooney, C. Jackman, Pesky gNATs: Using games to support mental health interventions for adolescents, in *The ACM SIGCHI Annual Symposium on Computer-Human Interaction in Play (CHI Play 2017)* (ACM, Amsterdam, 2017), pp. 15–18
3. M. Eisapour, S. Cao, J. Boger, Game design for users with constraint: Exergame for older adults with cognitive impairment, in *The 31st Annual ACM Symposium on User Interface Software and Technology Adjunct Proceedings* (2018), pp. 128–130
4. J.L. Hardy, R.A. Nelson, M.E. Thomason, D.A. Sternberg, K. Katovich, F. Farzin, M. Scanlon, Enhancing cognitive abilities with comprehensive training: a large, online, randomized, active-controlled trial. PloS One **10**(9), e0134467 (2015)
5. S. Oppl, C. Stary, Game-playing as an effective learning resource for elderly people: Encouraging experiential adoption of touchscreen technologies. Univ. Access Inf. Soc. **19**, 1–16 (2018)
6. L. Tabbaa, C.S. Ang, V. Rose, P. Siriaraya, I. Stewart, K.G. Jenkins, M. Matsangidou, Bring the outside in: Providing accessible experiences through VR for people with dementia in locked psychiatric hospitals, in *Proceedings of the 2019 CHI Conference on Human Factors in Computing Systems* (2019), pp. 1–15
7. D. Welsh, K. Morrissey, S. Foley, R. McNaney, C. Salis, J. McCarthy, J. Vines, Ticket to talk: Supporting conversation between young people and people with dementia through digital media, in *Proceedings of the 2018 CHI Conference on Human Factors in Computing Systems* (2018), pp. 1–14

ActiviX: Noninvasive Solution to Mental Health

Morgan Whittemore, Shawn Toubeau, Zach Griffin, and Leonidas Deligiannidis

1 Introduction

Millions of people are affected by mental health disorders each year. A study in 2018 found that 19.1% of adults and 16.5% of youth between the ages 6 and 17 in the United States suffered from mental health disorders [1]. The impact of an individual's poor mental health can be devastating and uproot their lives in an instant. Although treatments are available for mental health disorders, they are often expensive and have negative stigmas surrounding them [2, 3]. Because of this, only half of people afflicted seek treatment.

On the other hand, other studies show that only 30–50% of people who take antidepressants have an improvement in their mental health [4]. It is advised that people with depression [5] should seek more than pharmaceutical solutions which include having a good sleep schedule [6, 7] and practicing a healthy lifestyle. Self-care is especially important for people who are in the mild to moderate stages of depression because these non-pharmaceutical solutions can have drastic improvements [8].

2 Proposed Solution

ActiviX is a highly customizable solution that suggests positive lifestyle changes by monitoring user's completed tasks and mood self-evaluation. The user logs

M. Whittemore · S. Toubeau · Z. Griffin · L. Deligiannidis (✉)
Department of Computer Science and Networking, Wentworth Institute of Technology, Boston, MA, USA
e-mail: morganfwhittemore@gmail.com; griffinz@wit.edu; deligiannidisl@wit.edu

H. R. Arabnia et al. (eds.), *Advances in Computer Vision and Computational Biology*, Transactions on Computational Science and Computational Intelligence,
https://doi.org/10.1007/978-3-030-71051-4_27

completed tasks such as finishing homework or maintaining their hygiene, etc. This data is transmitted to a server that tracks the user's actions and encourages the user to complete them if they are not doing them. The user can use a mobile application where he/she/they can see their list of daily actions (shown in Fig. 1),

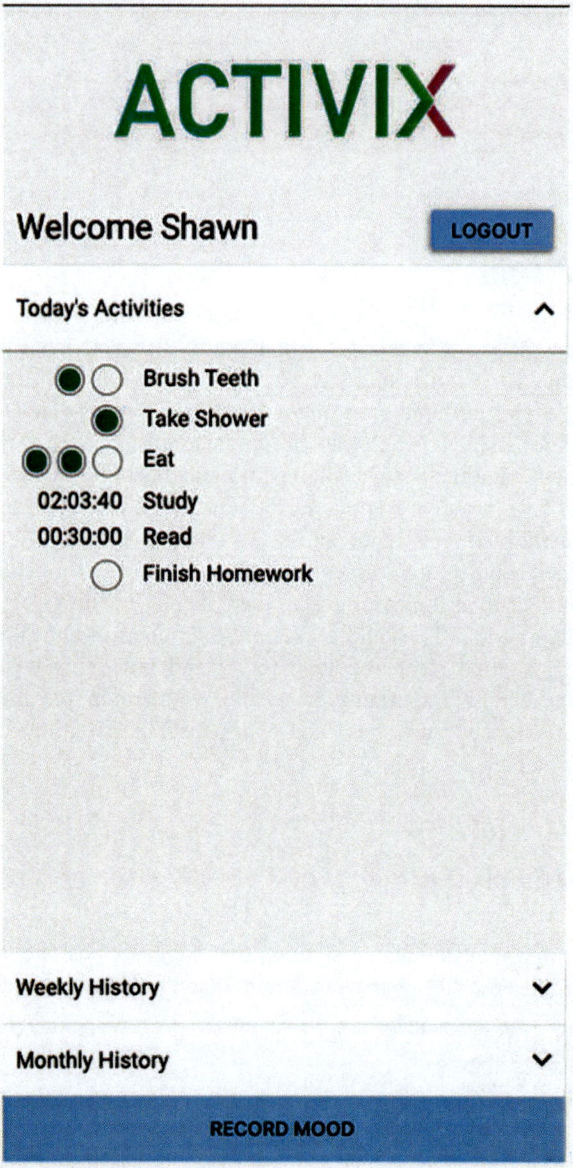

Fig. 1 Daily activities view and status for the user

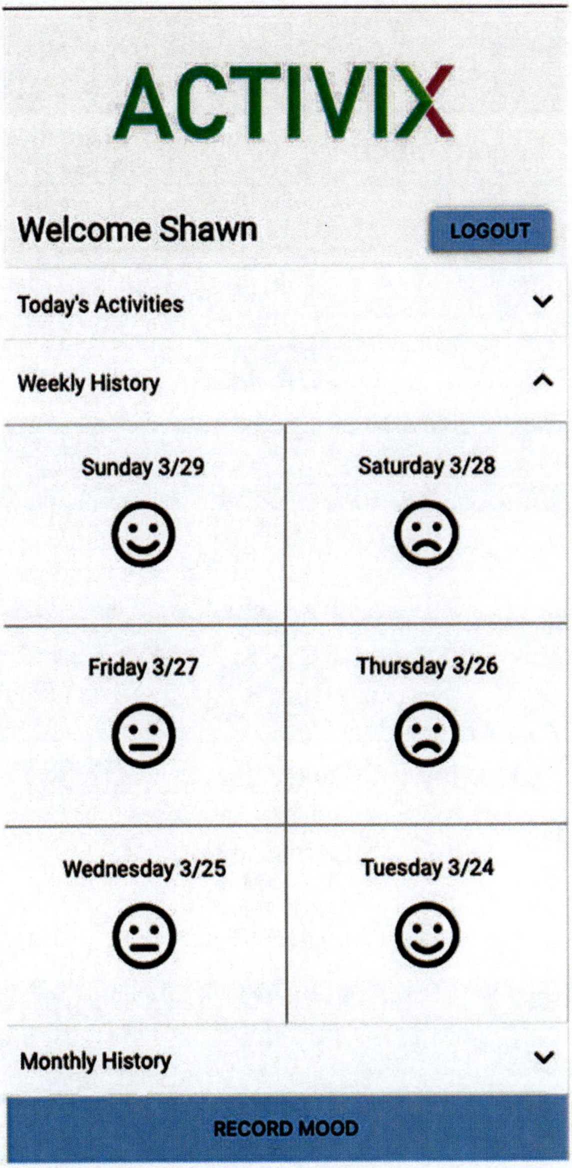

Fig. 2 Daily activities view and status for the user

their completion progress (shown in Fig. 2), and weekly and monthly history (shown in Fig. 3) and provide the ability to record their mood (shown in Fig. 4). By using both their action activity and mood scores, we can then use that information to

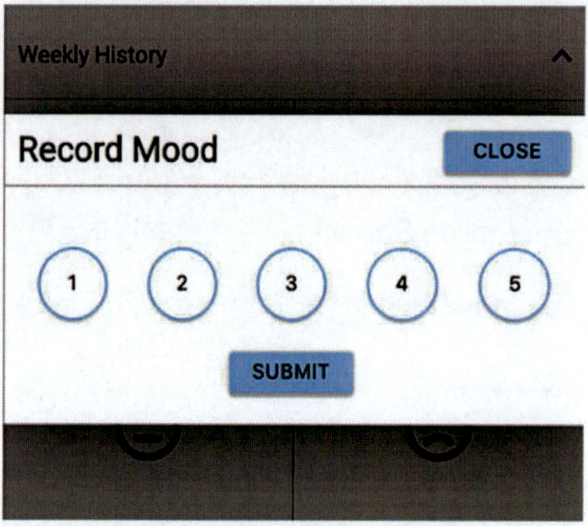

Fig. 3 Details of the user's mood history on a specific day

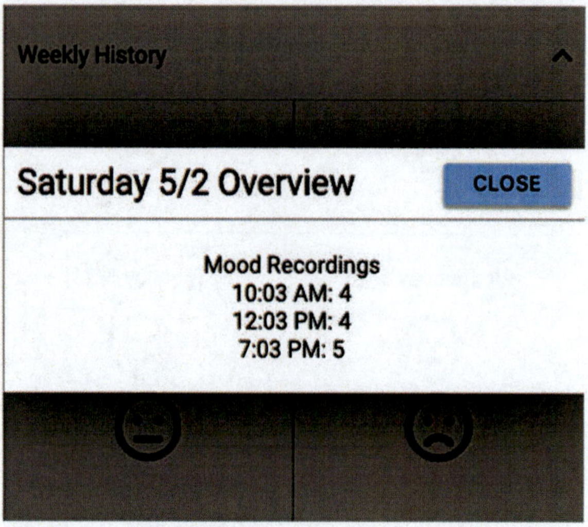

Fig. 4 Details of the user's mood history on a specific day

determine the well-being of the user and provide suggested actions, shown in Fig. 5, for them to complete in order to help them become happier and improve their life.

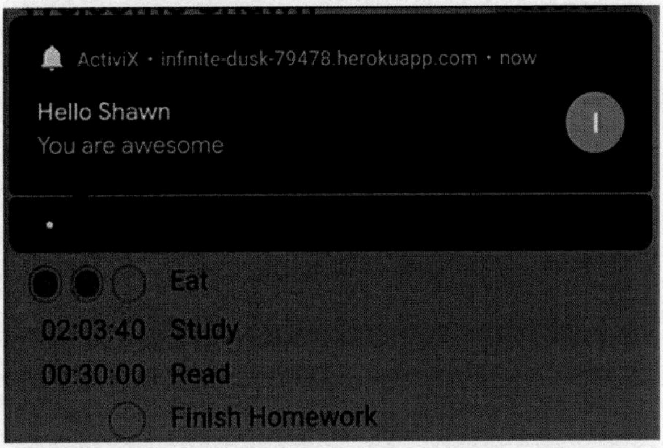

Fig. 5 Example notification on a mobile device

3 User Client

The client is a Progressive Web App (PWA) that is usable on both mobile and desktop devices through all major Internet browsers. The application showcases the user's mental health and productivity history, allows the user to input their mood, and sends reminders to complete missing activities if the user is forgetting to complete them. The benefit of making our client a PWA is that it provides the user a seamless experience regardless of Internet connection type and allows us to utilize push notifications to keep the user engaged.

In order to provide a simple and cohesive experience, we designed the client as one dashboard which houses all the information and functionality. By keeping our application as simple and intuitive as possible, we can offer a better user experience. Two components that helped make this possible were the modals and the accordion. The modals help highlight important details and actions to the user by emphasizing their importance and overshadowing everything else going on in the background. These are important because they add variation to the app but still make it feel as one fluent piece. The accordion allows us to quickly show and hide different sections that would normally be displayed as separate pages. Our mobile layout enables us to show a lot of different content but still be easy to navigate.

4 Application Back End

The back-end python application server includes services to calculate *productivity* and *mood* scores. The Django framework [9] is used for object-relational mapping, and the Django REST Framework is used for data retrieval and insertion. Django provides functionality to build out common features with minimum coding while

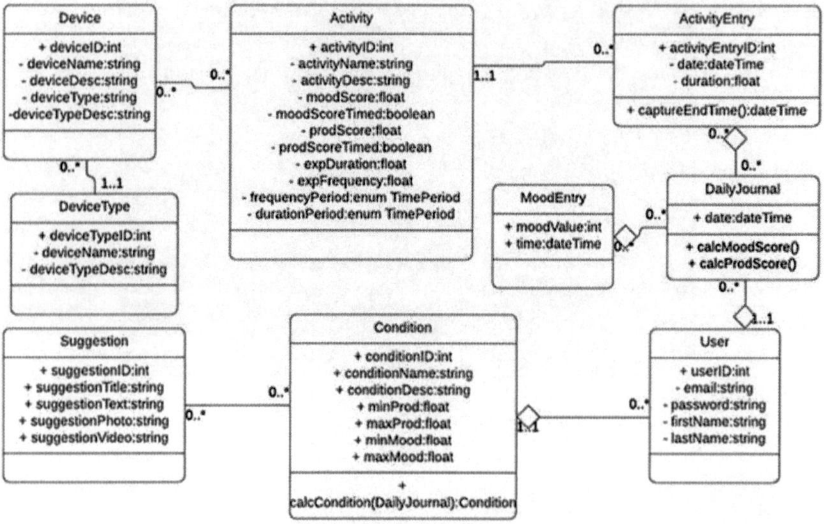

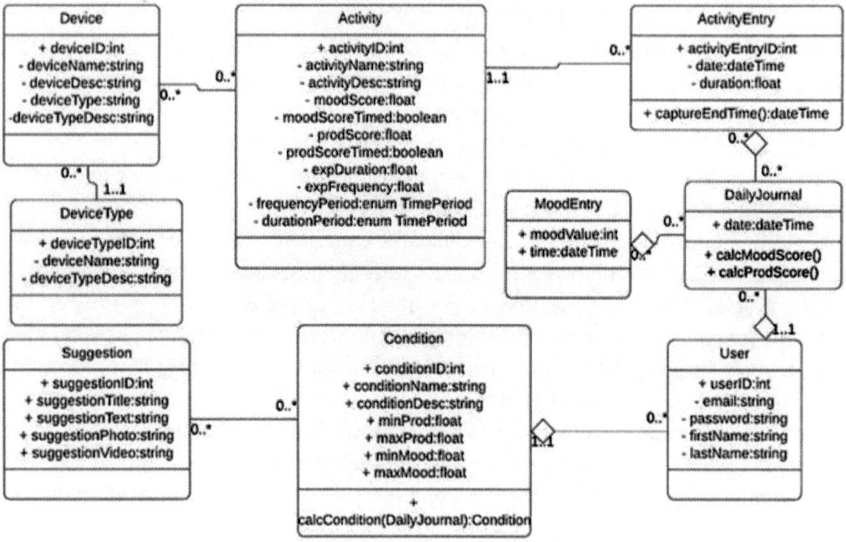

Fig. 6 UML diagram of the application server

allowing room for customization. The UML class diagram is shown in Fig. 6 to highlight the various elements used.

Device and *DeviceType* objects hold information about the hardware devices that are used to collect user data. An activity object represents an action a user can take, such as brushing their teeth, watching television, or going for a jog. *Conditions* describe stages of mental state such as mania or depression while incorporating both mood and productivity. *Suggestions* are the content of notifications which are delivered to the user, and *ConditionSuggestions* are the suggestions associated with the appropriate conditions.

The initial version of the ActiviX allows journals for a single day to be generated. However, all past activity entries are stored in the database, and thus journals or histories could be generated for any given period. *DailyJournal* is an aggregate of all activity entries for the current date. This is the point at which the mood score and productivity score are calculated, and this is the object from which they can be accessed.

5 Score Calculation

We use a couple of parameters from which inferences can be made. Every user has an ongoing mood and productivity score. These scores are generated based on a daily log. All entries of a user's activity from a date are gathered. The number of occurrences of a given activity, or the total duration of the activity, are then compounded to find a daily aggregate value.

Productivity and mood scores are calculated using the same formula (1). Either score can be dependent on duration or frequency of an activity. The resultant score is a positive number relative to the base score associated with each activity. We chose the base score values empirically, and they range from -1 to $+1$, though different ranges may yield better results.

$$s = b\frac{(x - E)}{E} \tag{1}$$

Deviation from an expected value, represented by $\boldsymbol{E}$ (i.e., expected duration of an activity throughout the day or expected frequency throughout a day), is found by dividing the difference between the actual duration or frequency value $\boldsymbol{x}$ and the expected value $\boldsymbol{E}$ by expected value $\boldsymbol{E}$. This value represents the magnitude to which the actual value deviates from the expected value and then reducing the value to be a fractional representation of the expected value. The base value $\boldsymbol{b}$ is the score if the actual value $\boldsymbol{x}$ equals the expected value $\boldsymbol{E}$. This is used as a multiplier in the formula to scale the score based on the deviation from the expected value. For nonzero actual values $\boldsymbol{x}$, the base value $\boldsymbol{b}$ must be added back to this value to correct for negative results when the desired value is a fraction of a positive base value. Otherwise, the preceding value is returned as the score.

The *Condition* score is based on the mood and productivity scores which are generated through the formula 7, as well as the manual mood entries given by the user. Various suggestions and encouragements are delivered to the user based on this calculated condition. These may include things like guided meditations, uplifting music, or gentle suggestions to perform activities that may improve the user's mental state and mood and encourage him/her, for example, to go for a walk. Ideally, these notifications, suggestions, and encouragements would be selected in concert with a mental health professional, as there are many considerations to how things may affect a user, and situations can vary greatly from person to person. This also allows for a possible future development of allowing a mental health professional to work directly with a client through the app to tailor their experience to a client's specific needs. For example, someone who is physically disabled may not have use for suggestions of physical activity and may even become upset at them. However, suggestions will be things which are scientifically proven to improve mood such as meditation [10], physical activity [11], and practicing gratitude [12, 13].

6 Communication Protocols

We utilized a Raspberry Pi [14] single-board computer running MQTT [15] to collect the data from the sensors and transmit the data to the back-end server. Physical interactions can be made with activity buttons placed throughout a space, and the action of pressing one can send information to the server including the action type and name and a timestamp. These buttons are placed where you want an activity to be tracked such as the bathroom sink for when you brush your teeth, etc. The Raspberry Pi acts as the main computer to handle sensor data input and Internet communication. The Pi will also be responsible in the future for directly connecting the service APIs such as existing smart lighting systems that are only accessible via a private (RFC1918-specified) address.

To handle growth, and manage costs, we also deployed our solution using cloud services. We decided to build two independent servers for two different purposes. The first is our application server where the user can access the front end and interact with the back end. The second machine is more of a marketing website. Our root DNS record (activixapp.com) points to this server and hosts information regarding the project. The DNS record of app.activixapp.com is pointed to the application server. Both machines are located behind an AWS Lightsail-managed firewall, restricting public access to ports 80 and 443. AWS S3 is used to store assets, data, and more information pertaining to the static usage of the site. Anything that does not need direct contact with the user data is stored here. The user data is stored with a managed RDS instance on AWS; during development, a MySQL server had been used.

7 Conclusion

We believe that ActiviX as a product could aid individuals who struggle with getting through their daily lives. Giving a user the ability to visualize and analyze their days could give them useful information that would otherwise be too cumbersome to gather themselves. With an informed approach to providing helpful suggestions and encouragement to a user, we could use that information to directly influence the user by providing them with options which could improve their mood and help with self-care.

References

1. National Alliance on Mental Illness, Mental health by the numbers (2019), https://www.nami.org/learn-more/mental-health-by-the-numbers. Accessed 19 Apr 2020
2. P.W. Corrigan, Mental health stigma as social attribution: Implications for research methods and attitude change. Clin. Psychol. Sci. Pract. **7**(1), 48–67 (2006). https://doi.org/10.1093/clipsy.7.1.48
3. P.W. Corrigan, D. Mittal, C.M. Reaves, et al., Mental health stigma and primary health care decisions. Psychiatry Res. **218**(1–2), 35–38 (2014). https://doi.org/10.1016/j.psychres.2014.04.028
4. G. Ell, Encouraging self-care and positive lifestyle changes in patients with depression. Pharm. J. (2020). https://doi.org/10.1211/PJ.2020.20207677
5. T. Vos, C. Allen, M. Arora, et al., Global, regional, and national incidence, prevalence, and years lived with disability for 310 diseases and injuries, 1990–2015: A systematic analysis for the Global Burden of Disease Study 2015. Lancet **388**(10053), 1545–1602 (2016). https://doi.org/10.1016/S0140-6736(16)31678-6
6. L.M. Paterson, D.J. Nutt, S.J. Wilson, NAPSAQ-1: National patient sleep assessment questionnaire in depression. Int. J. Psychiatry Clin. Pract. (2009). https://doi.org/10.1080/13651500802450498
7. Mental Health America, Get enough sleep (2020), https://www.mhanational.org/get-enough-sleep. Accessed 12 Apr 2020
8. S. McManus, P. Bebbington, R. Jenkins, et al., *Mental Health and Wellbeing in England: Adult Psychiatric Morbidity Survey 2014* (NHS Digital, Leeds, 2016)
9. Django Python Web Framework, Meet Django (2020), https://www.djangoproject.com/. Accessed 20 Apr 2020
10. M. Goyal, S. Singh, E.M.S. Sibinga, et al., Meditation programs for psychological stress and well-being: A systematic review and meta-analysis. JAMA Intern. Med. **174**(3), 357–368 (2014). https://doi.org/10.1001/jamainternmed.2013.13018
11. K.W. Choi, C.Y. Chen, M.B. Stein, et al., Assessment of bidirectional relationships between physical activity and depression among adults: A 2-sample Mendelian randomization study. JAMA Psychiat. **76**(4), 399–408 (2019). https://doi.org/10.1001/jamapsychiatry.2018.4175
12. A.M. Wood, J.J. Froh, A.W.A. Geraghty, Gratitude and well-being: A review and theoretical integration. Clin. Psychol. Rev. (2010). https://doi.org/10.1016/j.cpr.2010.03.005
13. W.L. Huberman, R.M. O'Brien, Improving therapist and patient performance in chronic psychiatric group homes through goal-setting, feedback, and positive reinforcement. J. Organ. Behav. Manag. **19**(1), 13–36 (1999). https://doi.org/10.1300/J075v19n01_04
14. Raspberry Pi. Raspberry Pi 4, https://www.raspberrypi.org/. Accessed 20 Apr 2020
15. MQ Telemetry Transport, MQTT (2019), http://mqtt.org/. Accessed 20 Apr 2020

Part V
Health Informatics and Medical Systems – Utilization of Machine Learning and Data Science

Visualizing and Analyzing Polynomial Curve Fitting and Forecasting of Covid Trends

Pedro Furtado

1 Introduction

Since a new coronavirus 2 (SARS-CoV-2) hit the world, first in Wuhan, China, and then spreading to the rest of the world, national governments have had to fight the outbreaks, and most of the world has had to come under movement and work restrictions to try to contain the virus spreading. The lack of prior immunity to the new virus and its high contagion rate (reproduction number r between 2 and 3 or even higher) were the two main drivers that caused such difficulties. Authorities in all the world were advised by epidemiologists, immunologists, virologists, and other medical experts to introduce emergency measures; physical distancing measures; closures of airports, businesses, and schools; and confinement of the population to slow the rate of spreading and that way relieve intensive care units from becoming overburdened with patients in serious condition.

The need for authorities to be alert, to keep track of the evolution of the outbreaks, and to manage restrictions resulted in daily reporting on the evolution of the crisis. Analysis of the evolution of the curves helps experts, authorities, and population in general understand that evolution and help contain the outbreaks as much as possible. Curve fitting can help draw a trend, forecast the short-term evolution, and understand if an outbreak is still in a dangerous exponential evolution or not. In this paper, we apply polynomial curve fitting to the problem, visualize the trends and short-term forecasts, and evaluate the quality of the results. In order to do so, we show how we transformed the data and applied curve fitting to help on this objective and how we discovered the most appropriate polynomial and the visualizations we got from all the alternatives.

P. Furtado (✉)
DEI/CISUC, University of Coimbra, Coimbra, Portugal
e-mail: pnf@dei.uc.pt

H. R. Arabnia et al. (eds.), *Advances in Computer Vision and Computational Biology*, Transactions on Computational Science and Computational Intelligence,
https://doi.org/10.1007/978-3-030-71051-4_28

2 Related Work

Polynomial regression of degree n is a fitting procedure that tries to approximate a given curve using a polynomial of degree n. Curve fitting in general is an important approach used to find a mathematical function that may describe some observed data. It is the process of curve construction based on a function, such that the curve may have a best fit to the data [1]. Reference [2] describes numerical methods for curve fitting. Curve fitting can be used to help data visualization or to infer values of a function where no data is available. Extrapolation or forecasting refers to using the discovered curve fitting function to extrapolate beyond the range of the observed data, subject to a degree of uncertainty. Regression analysis [3, 4] focuses especially in statistical inference related to curve fitting and associated uncertainty. These kinds of approaches can be helpful for abstracting trends and forecasting into the near future in the context of epidemiology as well.

In this work, we apply polynomial regression as an additional tool at the reach of anyone to visualize trends in the context of an epidemic, which is complementary to the main models used in epidemiology. Epidemiologists use well-known models to study the evolution of infections in a population [5–8] reviews the maths used to model infectious diseases. The famous SIR model models an epidemic using a set of differential equations [9], where S stands for Susceptible, I for Infectious, and R for Recovered, and the differential equations model the transition between those states. In that context, curve fitting is a possible aid and can be useful not only to fit those models to the actual curves but also to design the past and near future trends or to describe the curves using simpler functions. Simple polynomial or exponential functions can be fitted to the past observed data to visualize curve trends and possible near future evolution. References [10, 11] are examples of works on mathematical modeling of Covid-19.

Another important base concept in the context of epidemiology is population growth since it describes the spreading of an infection in general. In population growth theory, given a population of size N, the population growth is described as $dN/dt = r\,N$, r being the per capita rate of increase or rate of growth. The population growth is either exponential, if r is constant, or logistic (a.k.a. logarithmic), if r decreases as the population grows. Naturally, the main first objective of epidemic containment should be to turn the exponential growth into a sigmoid or logarithmic curve as soon as possible either through immunization, which is currently unavailable for the Covid-19 pandemic, or by social distancing. In that context, the transformation and analysis of evolution curves, and in particular the use of polynomial regression to fit and forecast short term, can help understand the current trend and whether the curves are turning from exponential into logarithmic or not.

3 Evolution

Figure 1 shows the evolution of Covid-19 up to the 27th of March in some of the worst hit countries. These are the initial input curves for transformation followed by polynomial regression analysis. Figures 2, 3, 4, and 5 illustrate the following steps in the transformation prior to curve fitting by polynomial regression. A prior step (not shown) aligns all curves on the first n (e.g., 50) cases. Figure 2 shows the first step which concerns smoothing the daily cases curves using moving averages (we applied two moving averages with 3- and 5-time units). Figure 3 differentiates the smoothed curve of Fig. 2 and computes the rate of change relative to the value, resulting in a chart of relative daily rates of change. Figure 4 cleans those rates of change to remove the initial peak from every curve (this is necessary because the first rates of change are huge because the daily number is still too small (e.g., the relative change from 0 to n is $n/0 = \text{inf}$). Figure 5 shows the last step which concerns further moving averages-based smoothing to remove peaks large than 100% of daily change. After these transformations, we were ready for applying polynomial regression. For comparison purposes, we applied polynomial regression to both the relative rates of change (outputs of Fig. 5) and to the smoothed daily cases (output of Fig. 2).

4 Polynomial Regression

Polynomial regression of degree n is a fitting procedure that tries to approximate a given curve using a polynomial of degree n. It searches for the best possible values of the polynomial coefficients that make the polynomial function as close as possible to the curve to be fitted. Eq. (1) shows the polynomial where some curve Y is to be approximated by the polynomial function Y_a with coefficients C_o to C_n,

$$Y_a = C_0 x^n + C_1 x^{n-1} + \cdots + C_{n-1} x + C_n \tag{1}$$

The fitting procedure itself is based on least squares method. The least squares method is an optimization method to minimize the sum of the squares of the residuals. Given each point Y_i in the curve and the corresponding estimation Y_{ai}, each residual is the error in the estimation $|Y_i - Y_{ai}|$. Given all points of the curve, the sum of squares of the residuals is to be optimized. In complex nonlinear problems, least squares optimization is obtained by gradient decent methods.

Polynomial regression is quite useful in many applications to fit curves and to estimate near future evolution. We applied it to the Covid-19 curves, with varying degrees.

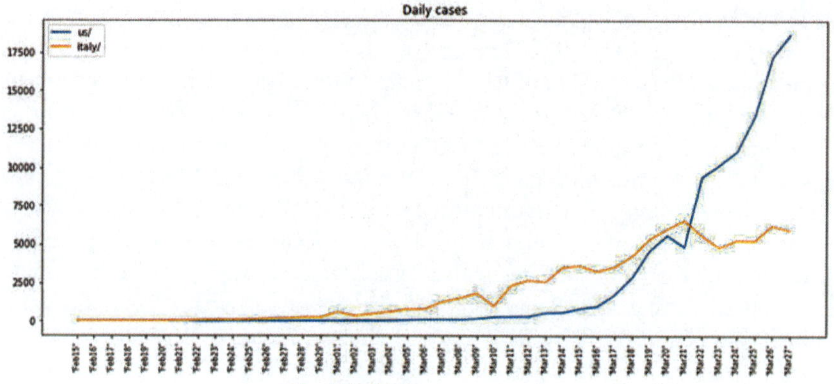

(a) US, Italy

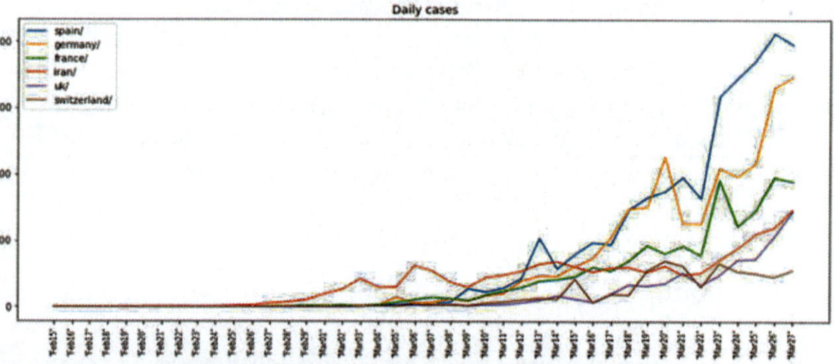

(b) Spain, Germany, France, Iran, UK, switzerland

Fig. 1 Evolution of Covid-19 daily curves in some of the most hit countries. (**a**) United States and Italy. (**b**) Spain, Germany, France, Iran, UK, and Switzerland

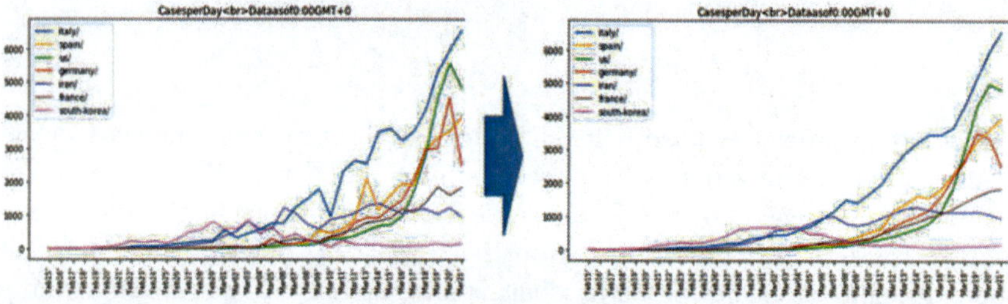

Fig. 2 Smoothing daily cases by moving averages

5 Visualizations of Regressions

Figures 6 and 7 show the visual results of polynomial regression on daily curves of United States, Italy, Spain, and Germany, including some possible continuation

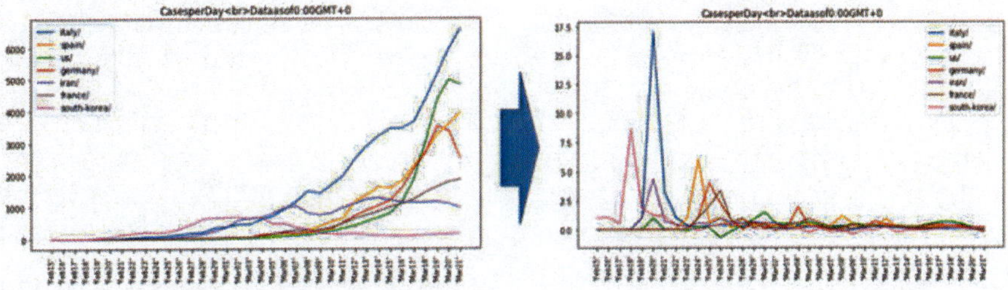

Fig. 3 Obtaining the daily rate of change

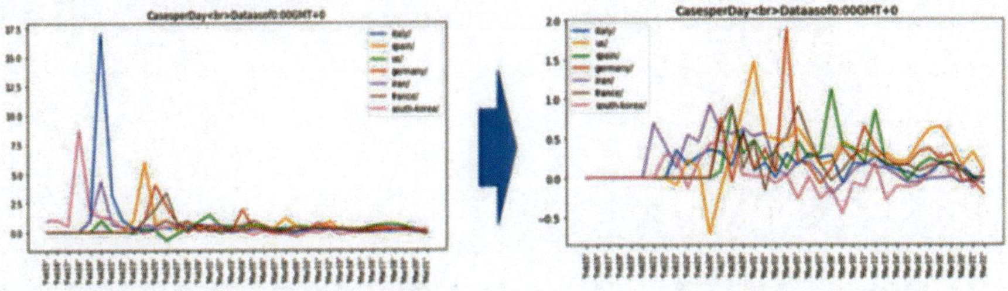

Fig. 4 Cleaning the daily rates of change

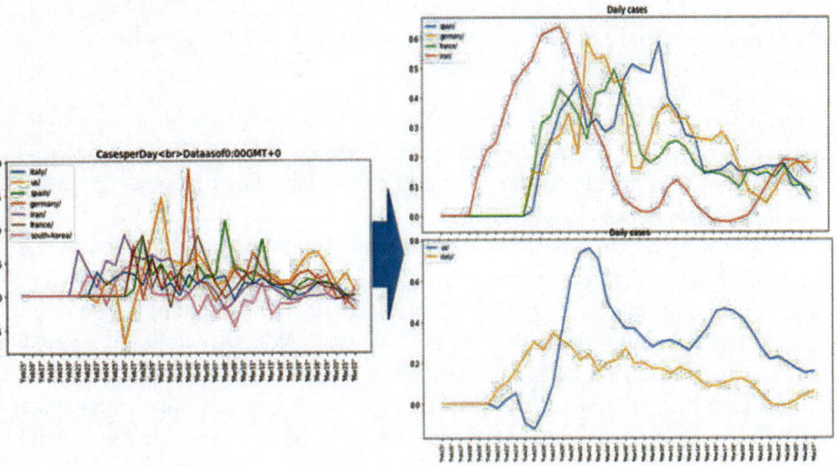

Fig. 5 Further smoothing the daily rate of change

of the curves. The results in Fig. 6 are for polynomial degree 6 and Fig. 7 is for polynomial degree 4. It is apparent that the polynomials fit the curves well in both cases. As an example of the differences, we can see that the polynomial of degree 4 forecasts a fast decay for Italy, which is not forecasted by the one with degree 6. This is as expected since the larger the degree of the polynomial, the more it fits details of the changes in the curves (note: we used a lower degree of smoothing in

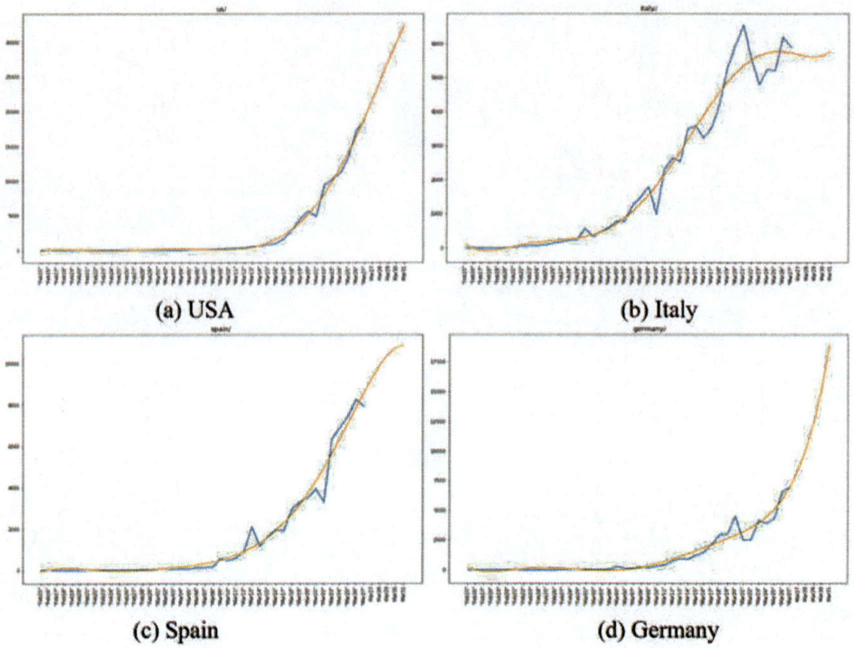

Fig. 6 Polynomial fitting of daily cases (degree $n = 6$). (**a**) United States, (**b**) Italy, (**c**) Spain, (**d**) Germany

the degree 6 curves). In our case in general, we do not want the approaches to fit all details of the curves because the daily curves vary due to Covid-19 testing and reporting issues by local authorities.

Figures 8, 9, and 10 show the results of applying polynomial regression to the rates of change. Figure 8 is an example of using a polynomial of degree 1 to approximate the China curve, while Figs. 9 and 10 show the fitting of United States (Fig. 9) and Italy (Fig. 10) with degrees 2, 3, and 4. Note that all polynomials fit the data adequately, and almost all polynomials indicate a decrease in the rate of change. This is very important since by then (27th of March), it was not clear whether the outbreaks would be controlled or not, and both these curves and the polynomial trends show that they were becoming under control.

6 Finding the Best Polynomials

In this section, we evaluate the quality of the approaches when forecasting. To find the best polynomials, we cut 15 days of the curves, fitted the polynomials, estimated the error for the next 15 days using those polynomials, and compared with the actual curve for those last 15 days.

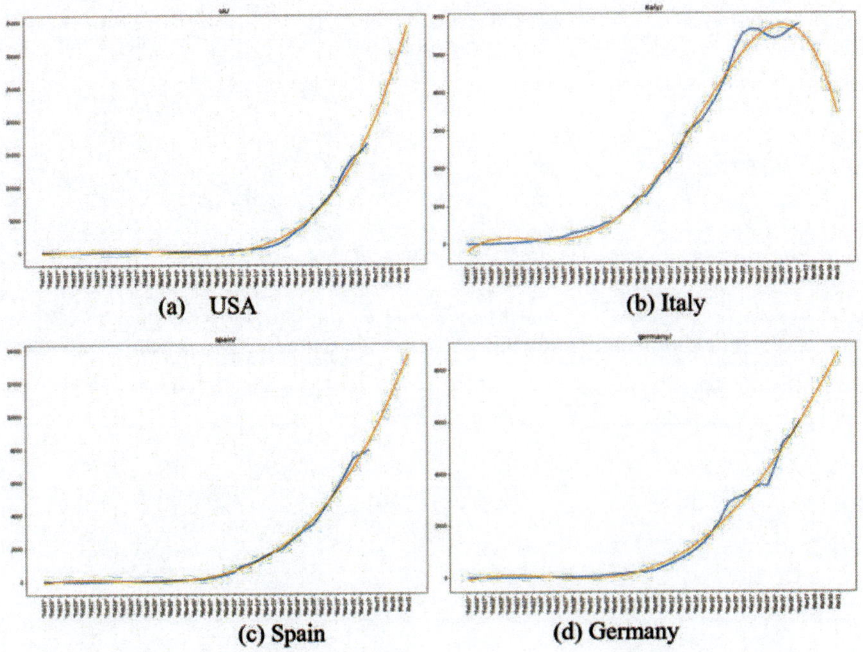

Fig. 7 Polynomial fitting of daily cases (degree $n = 4$). (**a**) United States, (**b**) Italy, (**c**) Spain, (**d**) Germany

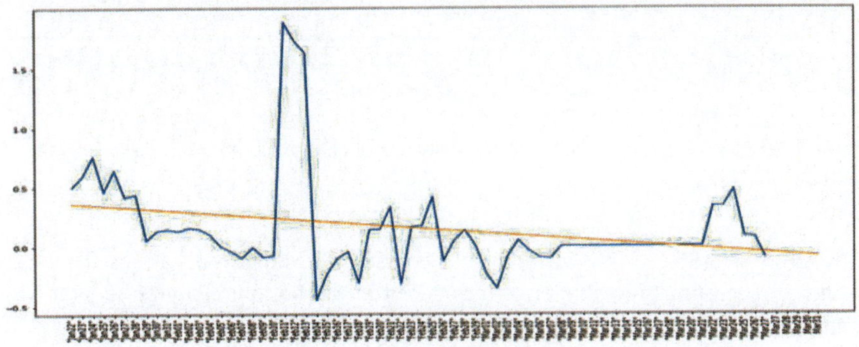

Fig. 8 Polynomial fitting of China: daily rate of change (degree 1)

For the daily rates of change (POL *d*), we created an algorithm for reconstruction and estimation of next few days based on the fitted rates of change. In Eq. (2), sz is the size of the known curve. The top equation produces the fit for the values before sz by as the sum of the actual value for the previous day (Y_{i-1}) and the amount of change estimated by the polynomial. The bottom equation for forecasting values beyond sz is similar, but instead of the actual value of the last day (Y_{i-1}), it uses the estimated value for the last day (Ye_{i-1}) because it is forecasting into the future;

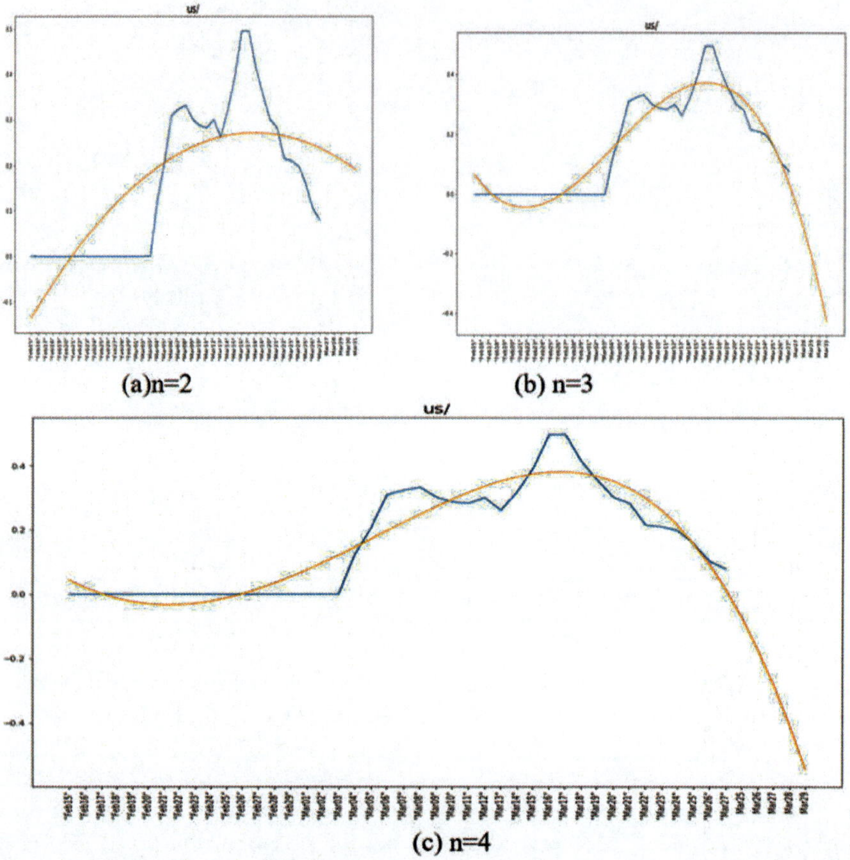

Fig. 9 Polynomial fitting of United States: daily rate of change (degree n). (**a**) $n = 2$, (**b**) $n = 3$, (**c**) $n = 4$

therefore, there is no known Y_{i-1}. Of course, this should only be used for near future forecasting since the error introduced in the bottom equation is larger and amplifies as we forecast further into the future.

$$\begin{cases} Y\mathrm{e}_i = Y_{i-1} \times \left[1 + \mathrm{POL}d(n)_i\right] \text{ iff } i <= \mathrm{sz} \\ Y\mathrm{e}_i = Y\mathrm{e}_{i-1} \times \left[1 + \mathrm{POL}d(n)_i\right] \text{ iff } i > \mathrm{sz} \end{cases} \tag{2}$$

The evaluation and comparison of the approaches were based on the average error using MAE relative to the values (MAEr) shown in Eq. (3).

$$\mathrm{MAEr} = \frac{\sum_{i=1}^{n} \left| \frac{Y_i - Y\mathrm{e}_i}{Y_i} \right|}{n} \tag{3}$$

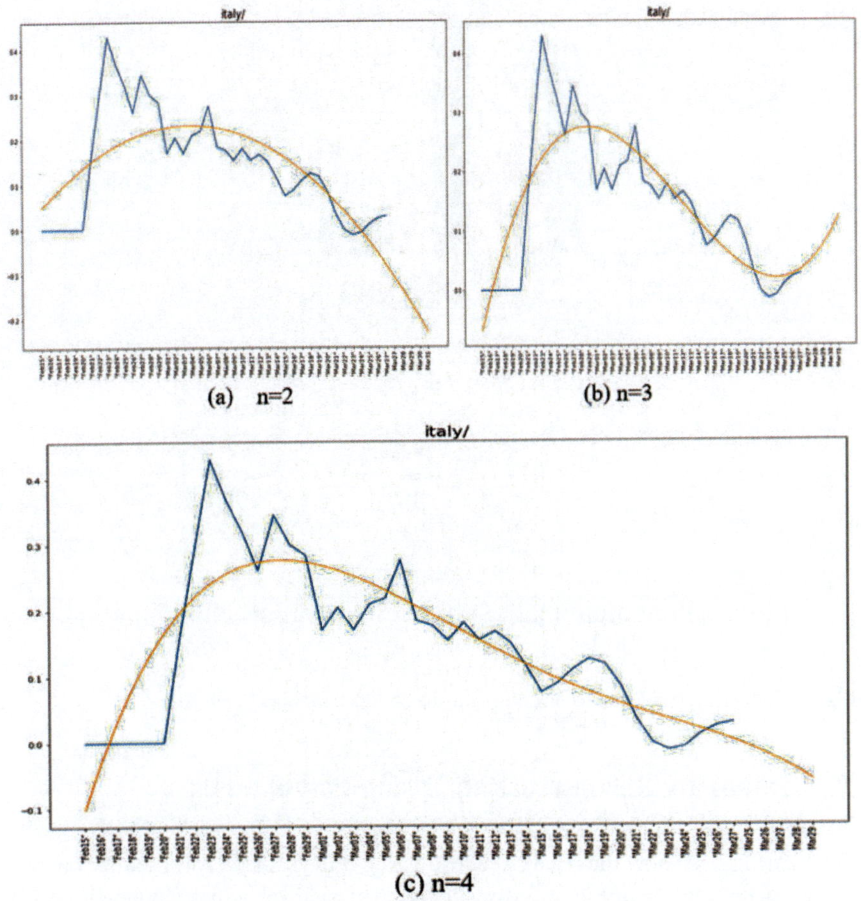

Fig. 10 Polynomial fitting of Italy: daily rate of change (degree n). (**a**) $n = 2$, (**b**) $n = 3$, (**c**) $n = 4$

Table 1 Average errors over the 20 top cases countries

POL(4)	POL(3)	POL(2)	POL(1)	POL d(4)	POL d(3)	POL d(2)
44%	28%	21%	49%	14%	11%	9%

Table 1 and Fig. 11 resume the results over the 20 countries with top number of Covid-19 cases on 27th of March. In that table, POL means polynomial over daily data, POL d means polynomial over daily rate of change (d = derivative), and the polynomial degree is shown inside the parenthesis.

The conclusions from this analysis are (1) polynomials of degree 2 or 3 on daily rates of change had the best results; (2) as the degree increased from 2 to 4, the error increased as well in both daily and daily rates of change; and (3) the polynomial of degree 1 was the worst of all.

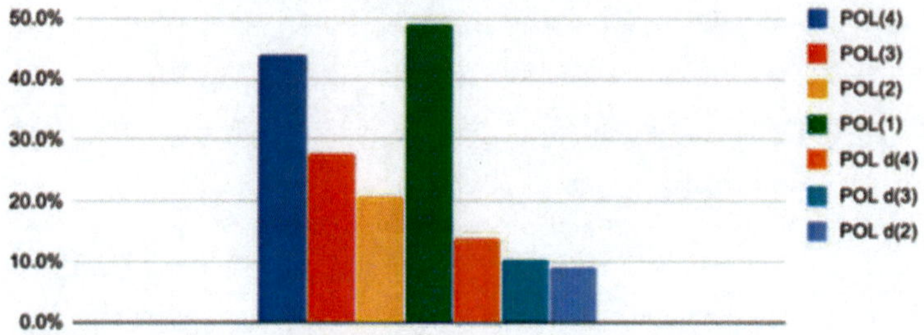

Fig. 11 Comparison of average error for different polynomials

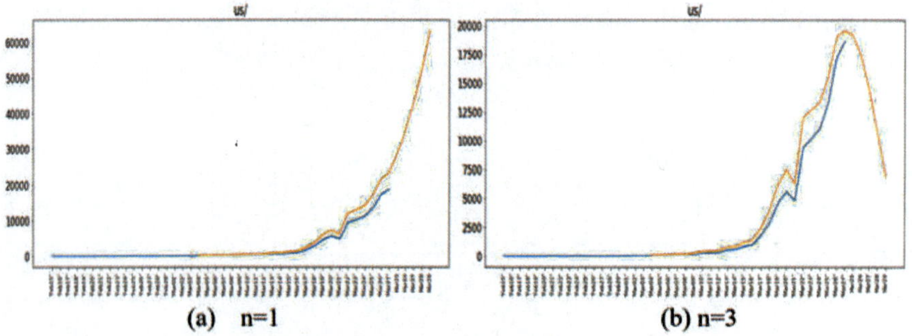

Fig. 12 United States: 5-day reconstruction using pol $d(n)$. (**a**) $n = 1$ and (**b**) $n = 3$

7 Visualizing Reconstructions Using Polynomials

The next figures show the results reconstructing 5 days ahead for a set of countries using polynomial degree 1 or 3 over the rates of change (which obtained the best results in Table 1). From the evaluation of the previous section, we already know the average errors incurred by each alternative (e.g., estimations using a polynomial of degree 3 have an average error of 11%, as seen in Table 1) (Figs. 12, 13, 14, and 15).

8 Conclusions

In this work, we studied and visualized the use of polynomial regression as a fitting mechanism for fitting, trend analysis, and short-term estimation on Covid-19 curves. We applied and tested the approaches over the 20 countries with most cases, obtained average error for each alternative, and visualized for some of the worst hit countries as of 27th of March. The conclusion is that polynomial regression can be useful indeed to estimate the short-term evolution of these curves. Our current and future work on this issue concerns applying curve fitting and forecasting to Covid-19

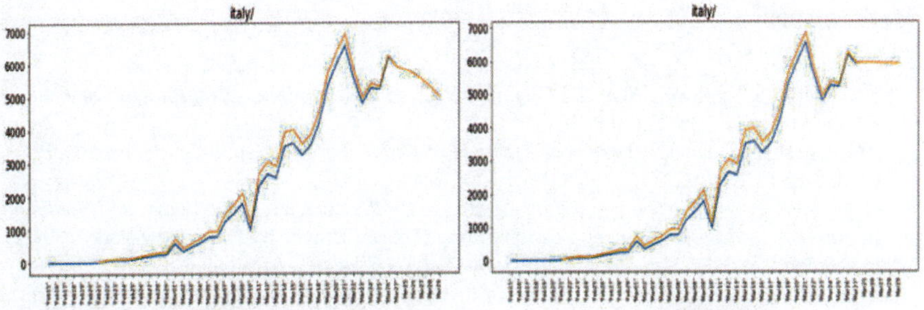

(a) n=1 (b) n=3

Fig. 13 Italy: 5-day reconstruction using pol $d(n)$. (**a**) $n = 1$ and (**b**) $n = 3$

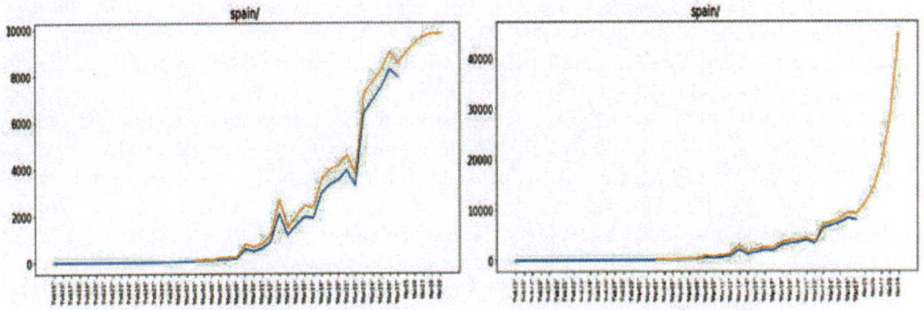

(a) n=1 (b) n=3

Fig. 14 Spain: 5-day reconstruction using pol $d(n)$. (**a**) $n = 1$ and (**b**) $n = 3$

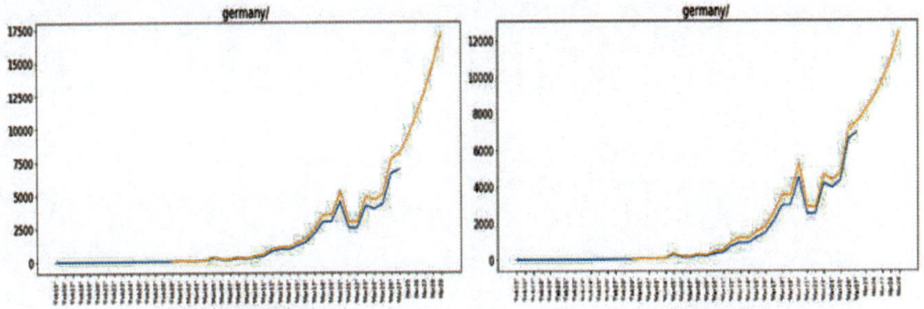

(a) n=1 (b) n=3

Fig. 15 Germany: 5-day reconstruction using pol $d(n)$. (**a**) $n = 1$ and (**b**) $n = 3$

using the SIR model, where we are noting that polynomial forecasting on the rates of change still achieves the best accuracies for short-term forecasting.

References

1. S.S. Halli, K.V. Rao, *Advanced Techniques of Population Analysis* (Springer Science & Business Media, New York, 2013)
2. P.G. Guest, P.G. Guest, *Numerical Methods of Curve Fitting* (Cambridge University Press, Cambridge, UK, 2012)
3. H. Motulsky, A. Christopoulos, *Fitting Models to Biological Data Using Linear and Nonlinear Regression: A Practical Guide to Curve Fitting* (Oxford University Press, New York, 2004)
4. R.J. Freund, W.J. Wilson, P. Sa, *Regression Analysis* (Elsevier, Amsterdam, 2006)
5. S. Altizer, C. Nunn, *Infectious Diseases in Primates: Behavior, Ecology and Evolution. Oxford Series in Ecology and Evolution* (Oxford University Press, Oxford/New York, 2006). ISBN 0-19-856585-2
6. R.M. Anderson, *Population Dynamics of Infectious Diseases: Theory and Applications* (Chapman and Hall, London/New York, 1982). ISBN 0-412-21610-8
7. N.T. Bailey, *The Mathematical Theory of Infectious Diseases and Its Applications*, 2nd edn. (Griffin, London, 1975). ISBN 0-85264-231-8
8. F. Brauer, C. Castillo-Chávez, *Mathematical Models in Population Biology and Epidemiology* (Springer, New York, 2001). ISBN 0-387-98902-1
9. W.O. Kermack, A.G. McKendrick, A contribution to the mathematical theory of epidemics. Proc. R. Soc. A **115**(772), 700–721 (1927). https://doi.org/10.1098/rspa.1927.0118
10. K. Prem, Y. Liu, T.W. Russell, A.J. Kucharski, R.M. Eggo, N. Davies, et al., The effect of control strategies to reduce social mixing on outcomes of the COVID-19 epidemic in Wuhan, China: A modelling study. Lancet Public Health **5**, e261–e270 (2020)
11. A.J. Kucharski, T.W. Russell, C. Diamond, Y. Liu, J. Edmunds, S. Funk, et al., Early dynamics of transmission and control of COVID-19: A mathematical modelling study. Lancet Infect. Dis. **20**, 553–558 (2020)

Persuasive AI Voice-Assisted Technologies to Motivate and Encourage Physical Activity

Benjamin Schooley, Dilek Akgun, Prashant Duhoon, and Neset Hikmet

1 Introduction

Chronic diseases – mainly cardiovascular diseases, cancers, chronic respiratory diseases, and diabetes – are the leading cause of death worldwide. More than 36 million people die annually from chronic diseases (63% of global deaths), including more than 14 million people who die too young between the ages of 30 and 70 [1]. Chronic diseases have become a focal point of public health worldwide with estimates of trillions of dollars in annual health-care cost. The Centers for Disease Control and Prevention (CDC) broadly define chronic diseases as conditions that last 1 year or more and require ongoing medical attention or limit activities of daily living or both [2]. More specifically, a chronic disease is slow in its progression and long in its continuance. Disease rates from these conditions are accelerating globally, advancing across every region, and pervading all socioeconomic classes [3]. Globally, chronic diseases have affected the health and quality of life of many citizens. As might be expected, the chronic diseases are among the most prevalent and costly health conditions in the United States. In fact, today, six in ten adults in the United States have a chronic disease like heart disease and stroke, cancer, or diabetes, and four in ten adults have two or more. They are the leading drivers of the United States' $3.5 trillion in annual health-care costs.

The prevalence of chronic diseases throughout the world has led scientists and health professionals to search various means of primary disease prevention and secondary disease treatment. As suggested by previous research studies, most

B. Schooley · P. Duhoon · N. Hikmet
University of South Carolina, Columbia, SC, USA

D. Akgun (✉)
University of South Carolina, Columbia, SC, USA
e-mail: Akgun@mailbox.sc.edu

H. R. Arabnia et al. (eds.), *Advances in Computer Vision and Computational Biology*, Transactions on Computational Science and Computational Intelligence,
https://doi.org/10.1007/978-3-030-71051-4_29

chronic diseases can be prevented by eating well, being physically active, avoiding tobacco and excessive drinking, and getting regular health screenings. Physical activity (PA) has long been associated with the chronic diseases. Indeed, according to the CDC, the rise of chronic diseases has been driven by primarily four major risk factors: one of which is the lack of physical activity [4]. The World Health Organization (WHO) defines physical activity as any bodily movement produced by skeletal muscles that require energy expenditure. Popular ways to be active are through walking, cycling, sports, and recreation and can be done at any level of skill and for enjoyment. As further research suggests, the incident rates of the chronic diseases continue to increase and this increase is heavily associated with an increase in physical inactivity. Insufficient physical activity can contribute to heart disease, type 2 diabetes, some kinds of cancer, and obesity [5].

PA has beneficial effects on an individual's health and well-being as a low-cost alternative to disease treatment and prevention and is also widely recognized as a means for the primary prevention of chronic diseases [6]. Despite this fact, the percentage of physically inactive adults in the United States and in the world continues to climb. In this context, making a change in behavior is needed in order to motivate and encourage people to be more physically active. However, persuading someone to change a behavior is not easy. When it comes to persuasion, there is no universally accepted definition even though philosophers and scholars have been examining it for at least 2000 years. Conventionally, persuasion means human communication designed to influence the autonomous judgments and actions of others [7]. The study of attitudes and persuasion remains a defining characteristic of contemporary social psychology [8]. When aiming at behavior change, it is important to fully understand which persuasion features lead to the success of an intervention. Human psychology poses significant challenges to understanding how to transform physical activity behavior changes into habits. Where technology interventions play a role, the process necessitates translation from behavioral science concepts into computer science and persuasive technologies and systems. These concepts, including user attitudes and behaviors, have been studied in the computer science field for many years [9].

In today's world, we are surrounded by technology tools and applications aiming to influence our short- and long-term behaviors. Persuasive technologies and systems have recently emerged as new research foci, with the potential to affect all aspects of the way in which people interact with computers. Persuasive technologies provide new capabilities for influencing a desired behavior, simulating compelling experiences to effectively persuade users, and creating relationships through a variety of cues to establish trust and support a desired change. Research in persuasive technologies and the associated usage of a computing system, device, or application intentionally designed to change a person's attitude or behavior in a predetermined way is showing the potential to assist in improving healthy living, reducing costs on the health-care system, and allowing elders to maintain a more independent life [10].

The health-care industry is one sector that is very likely to leverage persuasive technology. Persuasive technologies and systems can temper the burden on traditional health-care services when used to support healthy behaviors, for example, in the prevention and treatment of chronic diseases [11]. Today, a large number of interactive systems can be found that are designed to support health and promote healthier lifestyles. Indeed, there is a growing interest to design and/or use persuasive technologies in health care. In this study, we design one such system – an Artificial Intelligence Voice Assistant (AI VA) device (Echo Show/Alexa) – to incorporate behavioral change theory techniques to promote physical activity.

2 Motivation

Being physically active is one of the most important and beneficial actions for all people to improve their health no matter the age or risk level of developing chronic diseases. All bodily systems are functionally altered and improved by physical activity and exercise. Regular physical activity provides important health benefits for adults with chronic health conditions. Previous research has provided substantial evidence of the benefits for cancer survivors and people with osteoarthritis, hypertension, type 2 diabetes, dementia, multiple sclerosis, spinal cord injury, and other cognitive disorders. Among the many benefits of physical activity are (1) lower risk of early death, coronary heart disease, stroke, high blood pressure, high cholesterol or triglycerides, type 2 diabetes, metabolic syndrome, colon cancer, and breast cancer; (2) prevention of weight gain; (3) weight loss, particularly when combined with reduced calorie intake; (4) improved cardiorespiratory (aerobic) fitness and muscular strength; (5) prevention of falls; and (6) reduced depression [12–14]. Promoting and encouraging participation in PA is a global public health priority.

Previous studies have emphasized the health benefits of physical activity and exercise. PA is closely linked with health and well-being; however, only one in four US adults and one in five high school students meet the recommended physical activity guidelines, and about 31 million adults aged 50 or older are inactive, meaning that they get no physical activity beyond that of daily living according to factsheets published by the results from the CDC. According to the CDC's Behavioral Risk Factor Surveillance System (BRFSS) surveys for the years 2015–2018, all states and territories had more than 15 percent of adults who were physically inactive, and this estimate ranged from 17.3 to 47.7 percent [15]. In order to promote PA, a national CDC initiative called Active People, Healthy Nation^{SM} aims to help 27 million Americans become more physically active by 2027 [16]. The survey data shows that most US citizens still do not exercise the minimum recommended 150 minutes of moderate-intensity aerobic activity per week (Fig. 1). Furthermore, this lack of physical activity is linked to approximately $117 billion in annual health-care costs and about 10 percent of premature mortality in the United States. Previous research studies showed that physical inactivity is widespread and a major contributor to chronic disease, disability, and premature mortality in the United States [17].

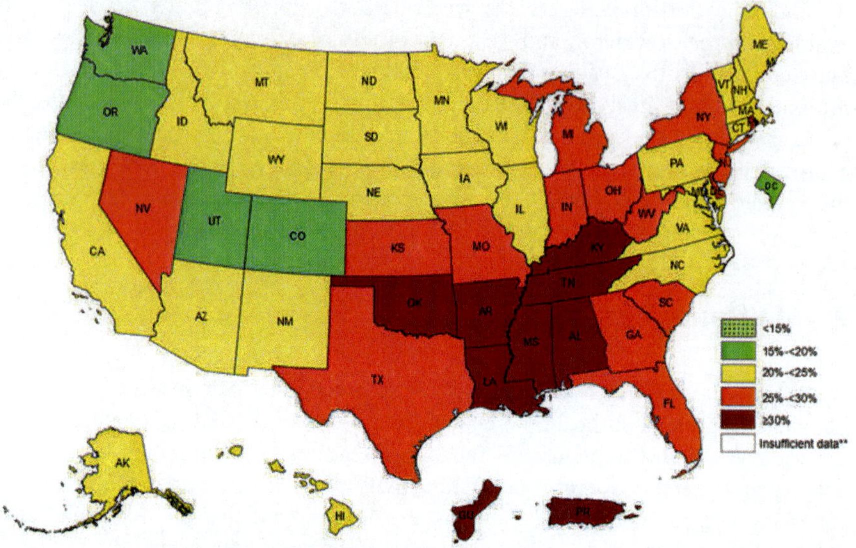

Fig. 1 Overall physical inactivity, prevalence of self-reported physical inactivity among US adults by state and territory, BRFSS, 2015–2018. (Source: Behavioral Risk Factor Surveillance System)

Despite the health benefits of regular physical activity which are well known and well publicized [18, 19], efforts to increase physical activity continue to fall short. Despite national and global efforts to promote physical activity, more is needed to motivate people to be more physically active and encourage the development of physical activity habits. The CDC recommends some strategies to overcome common barriers including lack of time, social support, lack of energy, lack of motivation, fear of injury, lack of skill, high costs and lack of facilities, and weather conditions [20]. The human psychology component of physical activity motivation is particularly important to understand for designing technologies that can act as support tools while motivating people to be physically active. Understanding these common barriers to physical activity and creating strategies to overcome them may promote physical activity to become an integral part of people's daily lives.

Previous research has emphasized the importance of using behavioral science theories to create exercise programs to aid in the transformation of short-term changes into long-term habits. Habitual behaviors, such as physical activity, are represented in associative memory and are experienced as low-effort, automatic actions independent of goals and intentions. People can easily build habits by repeating an action consistently in the same context [21, 22]. Several studies demonstrate the pervasive impact of habit and past behavior on physical activity adherence. In order to promote long-term and continuous participation in physical activity, interventions should seek to tap into processes linked to habit formation [23].

A wide range of stakeholders including health and wellness researchers and practitioners, technology designers, and public health and government agencies have increasing interest and investment in developing and using technology to promote health and wellness [24]. These technologies are often used to persuade users to maintain a healthy lifestyle, stop smoking, exercise more, be environmentally friendly, and increase physical activity participation aimed at chronic disease prevention. Indeed, a growing number of information technology systems, applications, and services are being developed with the purpose to change users' attitudes or behavior or both [25]. It is likewise important to communicate various approaches to how people may be, are being, and will be influenced through these information technology designs, including the pros and cons of technology-mediated behavior change. This is the motivation for the study described herein.

3 Theoretical Background

3.1 Physical Activity and Chronic Diseases

PA is a leading example of how lifestyle choices have a profound effect on health. The choices people make about other lifestyle factors, such as diet, smoking, and alcohol use, also have important and independent effects on their health. Research establishes that including PA and exercise into daily lifestyle activities provides multiple health benefits, promotes societal growth, and provides long-term chronic disease prevention and treatment while improving overall global health [26, 27]. The lack of physical activity is considered one of the most harmful risk factors for chronic medical conditions. Conditions such as cardiovascular disease, type 2 diabetes, obesity, and cancer are drastically improved when PA and exercise are part of a medical management plan [28]. Several studies suggest that PA and exercise are considered principal interventions for use in primary and secondary prevention of chronic diseases. Furthermore, regular PA is proven to help prevent and treat chronic diseases such as heart disease, stroke, diabetes, and breast and colon cancer. It also helps to prevent hypertension, overweight, and obesity and can improve mental health, quality of life, and well-being [29, 30].

PA clearly leads to increased physical fitness, exercise capacity, and risk reduction of a wide variety of pathological diseases and clinical disorders resulting in lower rates of morbidity, all-cause and cause-specific mortality, and increased life expectancy. Ample evidence clearly demonstrates that increased PA and exercise are associated with reduced chronic disease risk, and the lack of PA affects almost every cell, organ, and system in the body causing sedentary dysfunction and accelerated death. Comprehensive scientific evidence supports the importance of recommending that people should engage in regular PA to improve overall health and to reduce the risk of many health problems. Some research results show the incontrovertible evidence proving that regular physical activity contributes to the primary and secondary prevention of several chronic diseases and is associated with a reduced risk of premature death. These results present a gradual linear relation between the volume of physical activity and health status so that the most physically active people are at the lowest risk [31].

Lifestyle factors, such as physical inactivity, are heavily correlated with the development of many chronic diseases. A series of research studies has indicated that physical inactivity is a primary cause of most chronic diseases, major killers in the modern era [32]. There is growing evidence to suggest that there is a potential risk threshold for health related to the degree of activity or inactivity. Both physical inactivity and sedentary behavior contribute to the burden of chronic disease [33]. Physical inactivity (insufficient physical activity) is one of the leading risk factors for chronic diseases and death worldwide. To individuals, the failure to enjoy adequate levels of physical activity increases the risk of cancer, heart disease, stroke, and diabetes by 20–30% and shortens life span by 3–5 years. Moreover, physical inactivity burdens society through the hidden and growing cost of medical care and loss of productivity [34]. More specifically, physical inactivity increases the risk of coronary heart and cerebrovascular diseases, type 2 diabetes mellitus, hypertension, several cancers (e.g., lung, prostate, breast, colon, others), osteoporosis/fractures, and dementia, among others [35].

The realization of the importance of daily PA and regular exercise as a strategy in primary disease prevention has led many countries to develop national PA guidelines. Within this context, the Physical Activity Guidelines for Americans issued by the US Department of Health and Human Services (HHS) promotes daily PA and exercise as a part of everyday life. It focuses the importance of being physically active to promote good health and reduce the risk of chronic diseases [36]. In addition to the national PA guidelines, there is also the American College of Sports Medicine (ACSM) global initiative that is Exercise is Medicine™ focused on encouraging primary care physicians and other health-care providers to include exercise when designing treatment plans for patients [37]. Some authors have discussed that as more countries incorporate PA and exercise as part of primary and secondary prevention strategies, chronic diseases, such as CVD, type 2 diabetes, stroke, cancer, and many others, along with their health-care costs will be reduced while the quality of life is improved. However, prior research suggests that different types and doses of PA and exercise can be recommended depending on the type of chronic diseases while prescribing exercise as medicine in the treatment of chronic diseases [38].

As the authors note earlier, more work is necessary to better understand how different types of motivation contribute to exercise behavior and how to persuade and motivate people to exercise mainly with the use of technology. Future research needs a new approach to focus on the appropriate use of technology tools and methods to gain a better understanding of the impact of technology at the motivation for PA and exercise.

3.2 Physical Activity and Persuasive Technologies and Systems

Persuasive efforts become plentiful in a continuous attempt to shape, reinforce, or change attitudes, behaviors, feelings, or thoughts about an issue, object, or action. Changing behavior is difficult, but technology can assist through the application of several strategies, such as providing motivation to engage in healthier behaviors or creating awareness about a current behavior. In this context, technology becomes an especially powerful tool when it allows the persuasive techniques to be interactive rather than one way, that is, altering and adjusting the pattern of interaction based on the characteristics or actions of the persuaded party – the user's inputs, needs, and context [39]. The use of technologies to persuade and motivate behavior change has been an active domain for research. The use of technology tools and smart apps and devices shows a great deal of promise for measuring and promoting physical activity. These devices result in greater benefits when they are combined with behavioral strategies [40–42]. New behavioral models are also being designed having technology-based interventions in mind. One example is the Fogg Behavior Model which proposes that three elements must converge at the same moment for a behavior to occur: motivation, ability, and a prompt. The model asserts that at least one of those three elements is missing, in case a behavior does not occur [43, 44].

Humans are presumably the strongest persuaders. However, when it comes to persuasion, computers not only have an advantage over traditional media. The computers also have six distinct advantages over human persuaders: being more persistent than human beings; offering greater anonymity; storing, accessing, and managing huge volumes of data; using many modalities to influence; scaling easily; and being ubiquitous. Nowadays, computing technologies are designed not only to help human performing daily tasks, such as doing the administration work or teaching in the classroom, but also to take on a variety of roles as persuaders. These include the roles to persuade and motivate people to change an attitude or behavior toward issues or objects which were traditionally filled by teachers, coaches, clergy, therapists, doctors, salespeople, and so on. This advancement has led to the exploration of persuasive technology, defined as "an interactive product designed to change attitudes or behaviors or both by making a desired outcome easier to achieve through persuasion and social influence, but not through coercion nor deception" [45], and later of persuasive systems, defined as "computerized software or information systems designed to reinforce, change or shape attitudes or behaviors or both without using coercion or deception [46]."

In the 1970s and 1980s, some visionary people designed and developed a few computing systems to promote health and increase workplace productivity as spotting the earliest signs of persuasive technologies. A computer system named Body Awareness Resource Network, as one of the earliest examples, was developed in the late 1970s. This pioneering program aimed to teach adolescents about health issues such as smoking, drugs, exercise, and more, with an ultimate focus on enhancing teens' behaviors in these areas [47].

There is an abundance of applications that can be developed with the purpose of behavioral change. A behavior change support system was conceptualized evolving from and building upon the persuasive technologies. A behavior change support system is a sociotechnical information system with psychological and behavioral outcomes designed to form, alter, or reinforce attitudes, behaviors, or an act of complying without using coercion or deception [48]. Built by incorporating persuasive software features and expanding the research discipline of persuasive technologies, behavior change support systems are claimed as the primary focus of research in the area of persuasive technologies [49].

Apart from this, behavioral psychologist B.J. Fogg coined the term "captology" – an acronym based on the phrase "computers as persuasive technologies" which focuses on the design, research, and analysis of interactive computing products created for the purpose of changing people's attitudes or behaviors. With the functional triad framework conceptualized by Fogg, the field of persuasive technology emphasized the capacity of information systems and computing technologies as an instrument for persuasion where technology acts as a tool, as a medium, and as a social actor [45].

As suggested by the Fogg's study, interactivity gives computing technology a strong advantage over other persuasive media. When persuasion techniques are interactive, they are more effective. Persuasive technologies can adjust what they do based on user inputs, needs, and situations. They adjust their influence tactics as the situation evolves. The ability to use various modalities enables technology to match people's preferences for visual, audio, or textual experiences. Computing technologies can present data and graphics, rich audio and video, animation, simulation, or hyperlinked content to persuade [50]. By combining modes, such as audio, video, and data, during an interaction to produce the optimum persuasive impact, persuasive technologies also create a synergistic effect.

Several theories have been conceptualized and proposed for changing peoples' attitudes and behaviors. One is Social Influence Theory [51] which asserts that people can generally achieve a greater degree of attitude and behavior change working together than working alone. Another theory, one of the most popular and effective ways for changing attitudes and behaviors, is Social Learning Theory (relabeled social cognitive theory) [52] which provides a useful framework for changing behavior [53, 54], including exercise, and posits that learning occurs in a social context with a dynamic and reciprocal interaction of the person, environment, and behavior. Research on Social Learning Theory has shown that people learn new attitudes and behaviors by observing others' actions and then noting the consequences of those actions. People tend to observe and learn most when behavior is modeled by others who are similar to themselves but somewhat older or more experienced.

Persuasive technologies aim to influence user's behaviors. There is a useful framework as the Coventry, Aberdeen, and London–Refined (CALO-RE) taxonomy of behavior change techniques which builds on initial work on classifying psychological techniques used in intervention to change behavior [55]. The CALO-RE provides a common language and describes behavior change techniques which help people change particularly their physical activity and healthy eating behaviors [56]. However, it is important to identify what intervention components, known as behavior change techniques, to decide the combination of these components which work best for increasing physical activity, to incorporate them into the technology, and to associate with PA. Therefore, multiple behavior change strategies may be needed to have an impact with inactive individuals. As previous studies suggested, further research needs to be done to determine which motivational components and conditions using technology tools are most effective for facilitating long-term behavior change in the promotion of PA [57]. Behavior change techniques listed in this taxonomy such as goal setting, self-monitoring, feedback, rewards, social support, and coaching are included in physical activity interventions [40, 58]. These behavior change techniques seem to be especially helpful in increasing activity and healthy behaviors. Goal setting has been shown to be an effective strategy for changing behavior; therefore, applying goals in persuasive technologies may be an effective way to encourage behavior change [59]. And it is frequently included in physical activity interventions [60]. In fact, setting appropriate goals is a key determinant of the success of any persuasive technology. Several reviews have shown the importance of goal setting in technology-based behavior change interventions targeting the promotion of physical activity [61, 62]. Goal setting has been used as a strategy in healthy lifestyle interventions as well as in recent research on persuasive technologies to encourage physical activity.

A successful persuasive technology is able to persuade people to change from one state to a more well-known state. A persuasive technology should be designed in a way to elicit positive emotions in users by using different persuasion principles or strategies. The critical part is to make the users trust the technology which in turn will lead successfully persuasion of the users to the targeted attitude or behavior [63]. Furthermore, promoting and supporting confidence in users while using persuasive technologies give credence on the information presented or advices provided. These interactions consequently manifest themselves in the form of a change in attitude or behavior [64].

While persuasive technologies aim to modify user attitudes, intentions, or behavior through computer human dialogue and social influence, personalized technologies aim to enhance user experience by taking into account users' interests, preferences, and other relevant information. Some research studies suggest that if both persuasive and personalized systems are combined, the influence on user interaction and behavior could be significantly increased [65].

Psychologists have investigated the reasons and moderators that lead humans to break established patterns of action since long ago. Work from as far back as the beginning of the 1930s showed that within the sports of Northeastern University in the United States, improvement in physical fitness was more dependent on the instructor/coach than on the sport itself [66]. Previous research results point out that an external agent, in this case a human coach, can play a crucial role in the motivation of the individual to reach a desired behavior change. The use of embodied conversational agents in the support of Active and Healthy Ageing has been explored in diverse areas, one of which is coaching in real time to the performance of physical exercises [67].

There are many ways to influence and motivate people. Previous psychology research has shown that tailored information is more effective than generic information in changing attitudes and behaviors [68]. Tailoring is defined as "any of a number of methods for creating communications individualized for their receivers, with the expectation that this individualization will lead to larger intended effects of these communications [69]." Additionally, a tailoring technology is a computing product that provides information relevant to individuals to change their attitudes or behaviors or both. It is widely believed that tailoring, or personalization, helps increasing the adherence and effectiveness of technology promoting behavior change a lot since each individual has unique, different, and dynamic characters [70]. If information provided by computing technology is tailored to the individual's needs, interests, personality, usage context, or other factors relevant to the individual, it will be more persuasive. Persuasive technologies, like a tailor fitting a suit, can benefit from personalization or tailoring under the circumstances where each person receives an individually "tailored" plan for his or her need.

People can be persuaded more in simulated environments in which there are rewarding situations created to motive them for a targeted behavior suggested by Fogg [45]. For example, people can be influenced by the computer simulations that reward target behaviors in a virtual world, such as giving virtual rewards for exercising, and thus can perform the target behavior more frequently and effectively in the real world. To motivate people to achieve their goals, mobile health applications can leverage a wider range of influence strategies, from offering simulations that give insight to establishing a system of digital rewards to motivate users. The optimal strategy can make use of a number of proven approaches simultaneously which are based upon relevant methods and theories while targeting the individuals to promote physical activity and increase their participation aiming at chronic diseases prevention and intervention.

4 Research Approach

A design science research methodology [71] was used to determine requirements for a persuasive artificial intelligence voice-activated (AI VA) application, translate prescribed program recommendations for a physical activity (PA) program into the AI VA application, and design, build, and deploy the system in a small controlled pilot study. Four participants engaged in a 5-day pilot test who then were engaged in a mixed-method evaluation to assess user insight and validate the system model for future deployment and use.

4.1 Persuasive Design Approach

With the aim to encourage and promote PA, computing technologies can present data and graphics, rich audio and video, animation, simulation, or hyperlinked content. Persuasive technologies can create a significant impact by incorporating multimodal interactions, mainly voice, audio, video, and data, during an intervention. As suggested by Fogg [45], interactivity gives computing technology a strong advantage over other persuasive media. Persuasive technologies draw their strengths from being interactive. Additionally, as mentioned before the computers, technology tools and smart apps also have six distinct advantages over human beings as they can (1) be more persistent than human beings, (2) offer greater anonymity, (3) manage huge volumes of data, (4) use many modalities to influence, (5) scale easily, and (6) go where humans cannot go or may not be welcome. These are important features which aid during the course of promoting PA. There is a growing interest to investigate the capabilities of AI devices such as Alexa while promoting behavior change with the use of persuasive technology features. This study focused on the design of an AI PA coach based on persuasive technology principles. We expect that integrating real-time exercise data from a wearable activity tracker with AI VA will allow for effective and timely promotion of PA. Participants are encouraged to achieve their PA goal (i.e., steps) and use the AI VA to assist them with the effort.

4.2 AI VA System Design

We adapted a commercially available Artificial Intelligence Voice Assistant (AI VA) device (Echo Show/Alexa) paired with the Fitbit Charge 3 wearable physical activity (PA) monitoring device to incorporate persuasive technology tools and behavior change techniques. This AI VA device is programmed based on the Coventry, Aberdeen, and London–Refined (CALO-RE) taxonomy of behavior change techniques by Michie et al. (2011) and Fogg's (2003) persuasive technology model which is defined as "an interactive product designed to change attitudes or behaviors or both by making a desired outcome easier to achieve through persuasion and social influence, but not through coercion nor deception." The AI VA device includes some behavior change techniques defined in the CALO-RE taxonomy such as self-monitoring, feedback, positive reinforcement as rewards, social support (jokes, images, and music), coaching (Alexa itself is a virtual coach, embodied conversational agent), and tailored messages [55]. In addition to possessing the six distinct advantages over human beings, the device is in frequent interaction with the participants and adjusting itself based on user inputs, needs, and situations.

The AI VA was programmed to follow the user through voice-assisted statements for both event-based (user interacts with device) and non-event-based triggers (device interacts with user after specified period of no interaction) on the Echo Show. The Alexa is integrated with the Fitbit API to receive data from the Fitbit

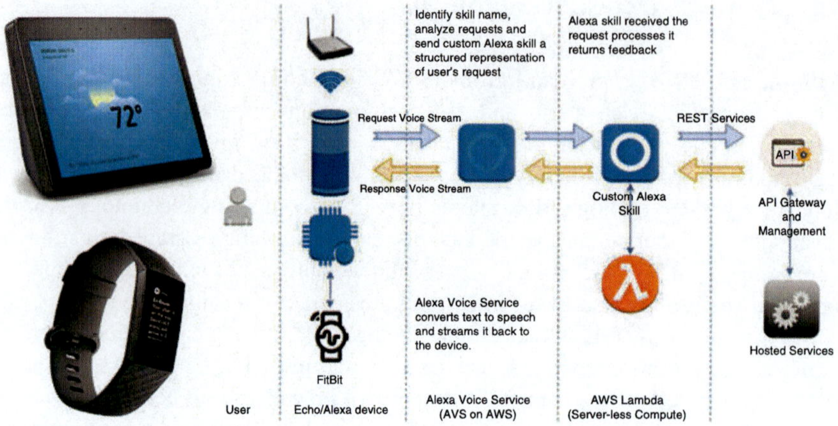

Fig. 2 Artificial intelligence voice-assisted (AI VA) system architecture

to monitor the subject's PA. The deployment allows for keeping statistics on the usage of the device. The design implementation can be seen in Fig. 2. The Alexa and Fitbit data are sent securely over the network using TLS v1.3 (Transport Layer Security) to the cloud-based Alexa Voice Service which acts as a gateway for the back-end programming on AWS Lambda.

The API gateway collects statistics of the usage of the system by the user and other user-related metadata (e.g., frequently used voice commands) essential for PA analysis and saves it on the hosted services securely under a VPC (Virtual Private Cloud) bound by security groups for further analysis. The depth of access to the back end is governed by an ACL (access control list) in compliance with HIPAA to protect the privacy of the user.

4.3 AI VA Physical Activity Coach

The PA motivation program incorporated into the AI VA system and designed for elderly patients (+65) was adapted based on literature review of in-person, phone-based, and computer-enhanced PA programs as found in the literature (see, e.g., [72–74]). The research and development team translated key motivational principles, PA coaching concepts, and goal-oriented designs into detailed interaction flowcharts across a two-week period of time. Decision modeling centered around meeting and increasing user step goals was incorporated into the system design. The logic for the functionality of the PA counseling system was then programmed in the AWS Lambda service primarily in Python (v3.7) using JSON-formatted guidance decision trees. Figure 3 illustrates a portion of voice logic that was created and implemented for one morning interaction at one day of the PA program starting with

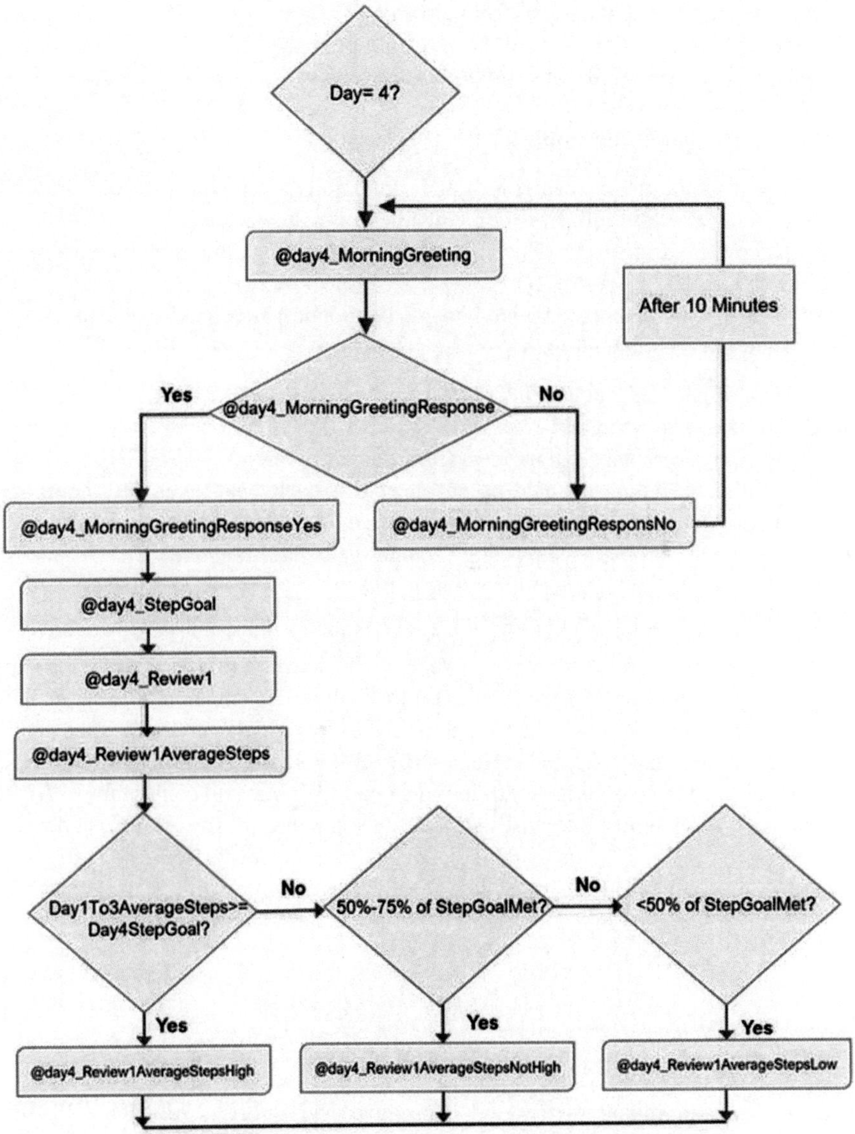

Fig. 3 Example of interaction logic

a personalized greeting and following with a review and an assessment of physical activity goals from the prior day.

The full logic for each day of the PA program consists of multiple persuasive interactive features, including:

- Personalized greeting

- Review physical activity goal from prior day
- Assess physical activity level achieved from prior day
- Feedback on low, moderate, and high achievement
- Motivational phrases
- Physical activity education:
  - Social support: How can your friends and family assist you with your activity?
  - Making exercise fun: How can you enjoy exercise each day?
  - Decrease sitting time: How to reduce your sitting time and increase your activity?
  - Gain self-confidence: How to become confident that you can exercise?
  - Injury prevention: How to exercise safely?
- Review of barriers and benefits to PA (optional)
- Check-in at afternoon and evening
- Daily goal assessment and review (afternoon and evening)
- Motivational content adapted based on goal achievement level (afternoon and evening)
- Review health problems/symptoms (standardized questionnaire)
- Referrals to health-care providers (based on responses to questionnaire)

Users are asked by the AI VA to choose three or more items such as social support, environmental resources, and/or activity barriers to ask Alexa each day. For example, if the participant is finding it difficult to identify a place to walk, they are instructed to ask Alexa: "Alexa, where is the closest park for me to walk within a 10-mile radius of my home?" Alexa will use the keyword "park" and "10-mile radius" to assist the participant with finding a park. We track all commands to Alexa related to PA to identify the most commonly used requests. The AI VA is adaptive according to the users' goals by taking goal achievement levels from each afternoon and evening into consideration. We tested this functionality with four older adults (65+) over a 5-day period. This is discussed in the next section.

4.4 Pilot Test

In this study, a mixed method of qualitative and quantitative data collection techniques was used. The AI VA application was pilot tested with the aim of conducting a proof of concept to refine the application and validate baseline assumptions about how the system would be utilized by a set of users. The goal was for users to increase light- to moderate-intensity PA by encouraging an increase in daily steps. Based on recommendations for step goals for older adults [75], participants were asked to establish a baseline step goal. The step goal is tailored to each participant and gradually increases based on a percentage change from baseline. The participants were provided an Echo Show and Fitbit Charge 3 for a period of 5 days, the users phone being paired with the home Echo device, where participant PA was tracked and reported. The Echo device receives the Fitbit tracker information (primarily steps) each day and alerts the participant if she/he have not reached her/his daily step goal. Participants received prompts at home at three daily intervals (morning, afternoon, and evening) where they were provided the opportunity to review benefits/barriers of exercise, watch walking videos, and receive feedback on their step goals from the previous day.

Utilization data was captured and analyzed for each user, and qualitative assessment was used to capture the end user's experience with the system as well as its perceived effects on behavior change outcomes relative to PA. At the end of the 5-day pilot period, in-depth interviews were conducted to elicit information about the technology usage and usability of the AI VA PA program. Interview data was collected, transcribed, and analyzed for themes as they relate to the Fogg and Michie et al. models [45, 55]. We also assessed the technology acceptance, perceived ease of use, and usefulness [76] in motivating PA to help determine the utility of these measure for a large-scale future study.

5 Findings and Discussion

Analysis of the qualitative interviews categorized participant responses across themes based on prevalent persuasive techniques. Table 1 below shows the persuasive techniques that were noted by participants during interviews in column one and the extent to which participants discussed the technique in column two. We assumed that the larger the number of participants to discuss a certain technique, the more influence it had. We found that *reducing complexity*, *positive reinforcement*, and *social support* as incorporated into the AI VA system had the most influence on participants at this phase of research. There are many other persuasive techniques that are not listed in the table below because they were not discussed by participants. We do not believe that this necessarily means that the techniques are not included in the system design or that participants did not experience them at any point in the beta test period. Additional techniques may have a stronger effect and be discussed by participants in the future when a more extensive study design is implemented, including a longer trial period and a larger number of research participants (Table 1).

User evidence of the three primary themes, reducing complexity, the use of positive reinforcement (conditioning), and social support, were viewed as most positive by the participants and were generally supported as useful and motivating. Reducing complexity activity to encourage users to continue with the PA program was a concept supported by several of the user comments as well as usability scale scores. For example, users noted that they were motivated "because the device made it so easy to want to exceed my challenge," and "the Fitbit and Alexa make it so easy." Participants indicated that the use of positive reinforcement techniques (conditioning, a method that uses positive reinforcements to increase the instances of a behavior) had a positive influence on the participants while using the AI VA

Table 1 Persuasive techniques from participant interviews

Persuasive techniques (Fogg and Michie et al.)	Level of participant agreement
Reducing complexity	+++
Positive reinforcement	+++
Social support	+++
Tailoring	+
Conditioning	+
Goal setting	++

+ low support, ++ mid-level support, +++ high support

device. For example, some of the participant responses received included "You're just so encouraged [by the device feedback]"; "Just her positive reinforcement. You're only so many steps away. One time I think she told me to have a blessed day, that was cute"; "[From daily conversations] I thought it was pretty encouraging from the afternoon session"; "I thought the introductory part was good, was very supportive"; "The prompt in the afternoon was always 'you've exceeded your goal, congratulations,'" and similar supportive comments like "It said congratulations [to me]." AI VA as a social actor uses voice, audio, and images to convey social presence and offers praise and congratulatory messages (i.e., positive reinforcement) via voice to motivate people during their PA. This social support aspect included audio feedback, jokes, positive images, and music that were perceived to be positive by the participants. For example, participants commented, "I liked if she [Alexa] always asked me if I was dying or not. The health questions"; "They [the jokes] were hilarious, I love a corny joke"; and "They [the jokes] were cute." Overall reaction from participants on whether the device helped them increase their PA was highly positive. One participant commented that even though she/he "... never made it to the 8,000 steps in the five days," she/he still found the system very helpful for increasing PA.

Participants were asked a series of standardized questions regarding their overall reactions to the system, extent to which the system was learnable, perspectives about system capabilities, usability, and satisfaction with the system. Users rated the usability and satisfaction features to be high. The lowest satisfaction score was relative to "learning the exercise topic (e.g., social support, making exercise fun)." As shown in Table 2, overall reactions were generally positive, with a moderate rating for flexibility. We believe this rating may have to do with the newness of the VA technology for the users and the prevalence of bugs and errors at this phase of work.

In Table 3 above, users generally felt the system to have high learnability with the highest rating being "learning to operate the system" and the lowest being in the case of "remembering names and use of commands." The low rating may be due to requiring users to learn a series of Alexa commands on their own with limited training and lack of quick reference sheets.

In Table 4 below, users rated the system speed and voice speed to be fast enough, while system reliability received only a moderate rating. We believe the moderate

Table 2 Participant perspectives about the system

Overall reactions to the system (0–9 scale)		
Terrible	7.75	Wonderful
Difficult	8.25	Easy
Frustrating	8	Satisfying
Dull	7	Stimulating
Rigid	5.5	Flexible
Hard to follow	8	Easy to follow
No help for my physical activity	8.5	Helpful to increase my physical activity

Table 3 Participant perspectives on system learnability

Learning (0–9 scale)			
Learning to operate the system	Difficult	8.25	Easy
Exploring new features (videos, skills)	Difficult	7.5	Easy
Remembering names and use of commands (e.g., Alexa, play me a walking video)	Difficult	5.75	Easy
Tasks can be performed in a straightforward manner	Never	7	Always
Visual aids on the screen	Unhelpful	7.75	Helpful
Ease of using the manual to problem solve	Confusing	8	Clear

Table 4 Participant perspectives on system capabilities

System capabilities (0–9 scale)			
System speed	Too slow	8.5	Fast enough
System reliability	Unreliable	5.5	Reliable
Voice speed	Too slow	9	Fast enough

rating was due to (1) the general immaturity of voice-activated technologies and (2) errors in our system logic that were repaired throughout the duration of the pilot test.

5.1 Conclusion

In this study, we constructed a conceptual model to motivate PA using an AI VA approach. The conceptual model was developed using persuasive technology theory and techniques and literature review of PA programs for older adults and people with chronic conditions. An AI VA functional system was designed and developed using the Echo Show/Alexa voice assistant device and cloud service, custom code and configuration of AI and VA components, and coupled with physical activity trackers (Fitbit). The conceptual model guided logical design, including VA workflow and interaction logic; user-specific algorithmic features obtained via literature review on PA programs; VA algorithmic features that control when, how, and what type of interactions will take place; VA algorithmic features based on user PA goals and activity tracking; and predetermined voice scripts delivered by the VA based on the algorithmic controls. The conceptual model was implemented, and preliminary testing results demonstrate a functional system with moderate to good usability, learnability, satisfaction, and performance. Users found key-persuasive techniques to be beneficial to their user experience and goal achievement, including the ability of the system to reduce complexity and provide positive reinforcement and social support. Challenges to date include low to moderate technology maturity for VA devices (e.g., some unnatural voice prompts and responses) and gaps to emotional acceptance of computerized voice interactions. The system model provides an evidence-based foundation for interacting with older (65+) participants with AI VA for the purpose of motivating PA and a tested model for capturing and analyzing PA and behavior change data, and providing feedback, education, and motivational guidance for goal achievement.

Study limitations include the small number of participants at this phase of work. Future research will refine the system model based on user feedback and conduct a 6-week trial with a larger number of users, tracking impacts on PA levels, goal achievement, and long-term system acceptance.

References

1. World Health Organization, Global action plan for the prevention and control of noncommunicable diseases 2013–2020 (2013). Available at https://apps.who.int/iris/bitstream/handle/10665/94384/9789241506236_eng.pdf. Accessed on 26 Mar 2020
2. The Centers for Disease Control and Prevention, About chronic diseases (October 23, 2019). Available at https://www.cdc.gov/chronicdisease/about/index.htm. Accessed on 26 Mar 2020
3. World Health Organization. Chronic diseases and health promotion. Available at https://www.who.int/chp/about/integrated_cd/en/. Accessed on 26 Mar 2020
4. The Centers for Disease Control and Prevention's National Center for Chronic Disease Prevention and Health Promotion, Chronic diseases in America (October 23, 2019). Available at https://www.cdc.gov/chronicdisease/resources/infographic/chronic-diseases.htm. Accessed on 26 Mar 2020
5. The Centers for Disease Control and Prevention, Lack of physical activity (September 25, 2019). Available at https://www.cdc.gov/chronicdisease/resources/publications/factsheets/physical-activity.htm. Accessed on 26 Mar 2020
6. P. Tuso, Strategies to increase physical activity. Perm. J. **19**(4), 84–88 (2015). https://doi.org/10.7812/TPP/14-24
7. H.W. Simons, J. Morreale, B. Gronbeck, *Persuasion in Society* (Sage Publications, Thousand Oaks, 2001)
8. W.D. Crano, R. Prislin, Attitudes and persuasion. Annu. Rev. Pschol. **57**, 13.1–13.30 (2005)
9. H. Oinas-Kukkonen, Discipline of information systems: A natural strategic alliance for web science, in *Proceedings of the Second International on Web Science Conference (WebSci 10)*, Raleigh, NC, USA, 26–27 Apr 2010
10. S. Chatterjee, A. Price, Healthy living with persuasive technologies: Framework, issues, and challenges. J. Am. Med. Inform. Assoc. **16**(2), 171–178 (2009). https://doi.org/10.1197/jamia.M2859
11. M. Cabrita, H. Op den Akker, M. Tabak, H.J. Hermens, M.M.R. Vollenbroek-Hutten, Persuasive technology to support active and healthy ageing: An exploration of past, present, and future. J. Biomed. Inform. **84**, 17–30 (2018). https://doi.org/10.1016/j.jbi.2018.06.010

12. The Centers for Disease Control and Prevention, Why should people be active? (April 10, 2020). Available at https://www.cdc.gov/physicalactivity/activepeoplehealthynation/why-should-people-be-active.html. Accessed on 13 Apr 2020
13. J.E. Fulton, D.M. Buchner, S.A. Carlson, D. Borbely, K.M. Rose, A.E. O'Connor, J.P. Gunn, R. Petersen, CDC's active people, healthy Nation^{SM}: Creating an active America, together. J. Phys. Act. Health **15**(7), 469–473 (2018). https://doi.org/10.1123/jpah.2018-0249
14. The U.S. Department of Health & Human Services (HHS), Importance of physical activity (January 26, 2017). Available at https://www.hhs.gov/fitness/be-active/importance-of-physical-activity/index.html. Accessed on 26 Mar 2020
15. The Centers for Disease Control and Prevention, Adult physical inactivity prevalence maps by race/ethnicity (January 2020). Available at https://www.cdc.gov/physicalactivity/data/inactivity-prevalence-maps/index.html. Accessed on 2 Apr 2020
16. The Centers for Disease Control and Prevention, Active people, healthy Nation^{SM} (April 10, 2020). Available at https://www.cdc.gov/physicalactivity/activepeoplehealthynation/index.html. Accessed on 26 Mar 2020
17. W.L. Haskell, S.N. Blair, J.O. Hill, Physical activity: Health outcomes and importance for public health policy. Prev. Med. **49**(4), 280–282 (2009)
18. M. Reiner, C. Niermann, D. Jekauc, A. Woll, R. Dishman, R. Washburn, et al., Long-term health benefits of physical activity – a systematic review of longitudinal studies. BMC Public Health **13**(1), 813 (2013). https://doi.org/10.1186/1471-2458-13-813
19. P. Kokkinos, Physical activity, health benefits, and mortality risk. ISRN Cardiol **2012**, 718789 (2012)
20. The Centers for Disease Control and Prevention, Overcoming barriers to physical activity (April 10, 2020). Available at https://www.cdc.gov/physicalactivity/basics/adding-pa/barriers.html. Accessed on 12 Apr 2020
21. P. Lally, B. Gardner, Promoting habit formation. Health Psychol. Rev. **7**, S137–S158 (2013). https://doi.org/10.1080/17437199.2011.603640
22. M.S. Hagger, Habit and physical activity: Theoretical advances, practical implications, and agenda for future research, in *Psychology of Sport & Exercise* (2018). https://doi.org/10.1016/j.psychsport.2018.12.007
23. N. Kaushal, R. Rhodes, J. Spence, J. Meldrum, Increasing physical activity through principles of habit formation in new gym members: A randomized controlled trial. Ann. Behav. Med. **51**, 578–586 (2017). https://doi.org/10.1007/s12160-017-9881-5
24. R. Orji, K. Moffatt, Persuasive technology for health and wellness: State-of-the-art and emerging trends. Health Informatics J. **1**, 7–9 (2016). https://doi.org/10.1177/1460458216650979
25. H. Oinas-Kukkonen, M. Harjumaa, Persuasive systems design: Key issues, process model, and system features. Commun. Assoc. Inf. Syst. **24**, 485–500 (2009)
26. E. Anderson, J.L. Durstine, Physical activity, exercise, and chronic diseases: A brief review. Sports Med. Health Sci. **1**, 3–10 (2019)
27. D. Nunan, K.R. Mahtani, N. Roberts, C. Heneghan, Physical activity for the prevention and treatment of major chronic disease: An overview of systematic reviews. Syst. Rev. **2**, 1–6 (2013)
28. J.L. Durstine, B. Gordon, Z. Wang, X. Luo, Chronic disease and the link to physical activity. J. Sport Health Sci. **2**, 3–11 (2013)
29. Global action plan on physical activity 2018–2030: More active people for a healthier world. Geneva: World Health Organization; 2018. Licence: CC BY-NC-SA 3.0 IGO
30. Mayo Clinic, Exercise and chronic disease: Get the facts (2018). Available at https://www.mayoclinic.org/healthy-lifestyle/fitness/in-depth/exercise-and-chronic-disease/art-20046049. Accessed on 26 Mar 2020
31. D.E. Warburton, C.W. Nicol, S.S. Bredin, Health benefits of physical activity: The evidence. CMAJ **174**(6), 801–809 (2006). https://doi.org/10.1503/cmaj.051351
32. F.W. Booth, C.K. Roberts, M.J. Laye, Lack of exercise is a major cause of chronic diseases. Compr. Physiol. **2**(2), 1143–1211 (2012). https://doi.org/10.1002/cphy.c110025

33. K. González, J. Fuentes, J.L. Márquez, Physical inactivity, sedentary behavior and chronic diseases. Korean J. Fam. Med. **38**(3), 111–115 (2017). https://doi.org/10.4082/kjfm.2017.38.3.111
34. World Health Organization. Physical activity. Available at https://www.who.int/health-topics/physical-activity. Accessed on 26 Mar 2020
35. J.A. Knight, Physical inactivity: Associated diseases and disorders. Ann. Clin. Lab. Sci. **42**, 320–337 (2012)
36. The U.S. Department of Health and Human Services, The physical activity guidelines for Americans (2018). Available at https://health.gov/sites/default/files/2019-09/Physical_Activity_Guidelines_2nd_edition.pdf. Accessed on 26 Mar 2020
37. D. Riebe et al. (eds.), *ACSM's Guidelines for Exercise Testing and Prescription*, 10th edn. (Wolters Kluwer Health Lippincott Williams & Wilkins, Philadelphia, 2018)
38. B.K. Pedersen, B. Saltin, Exercise as medicine - Evidence for prescribing exercise as therapy in 26 different chronic diseases. Scand. J. Med. Sci. Sports **25 Suppl 3**, 1–72 (2015). https://doi.org/10.1111/sms.12581
39. W. Ijsselsteijn, Y. De Kort, C. Midden, B. Eggen, E. van den Hoven, Persuasive technology for human well-being: Setting the scene (2006), pp. 1–5. https://doi.org/10.1007/11755494_1
40. D.E. Conroy, C.H. Yang, J.P. Maher, Behavior change techniques in top-ranked mobile apps for physical activity. Am. J. Prev. Med. **46**, 649–652 (2014). https://doi.org/10.1016/j.amepre.2014.01.010
41. K. Mercer, M. Li, L. Giangregorio, C. Burns, K. Grindrod, Behavior change techniques present in wearable activity trackers: A critical analysis. JMIR Mhealth Uhealth **4**(2), e40 (2016)
42. A. Direito, L.P. Dale, E. Shields, R. Dobson, R. Whittaker, R. Maddison, Do physical activity and dietary smartphone applications incorporate evidence-based behaviour change techniques? BMC Public Health **14**, 646 (2014). https://doi.org/10.1186/1471-2458-14-646
43. B.J. Fogg, Fogg behavior model (2009). Available at https://behaviordesign.stanford.edu/fogg-behavior-model. Accessed on 2 Apr 2020
44. B.J. Fogg, A behavior model for persuasive design, in *Persuasive '09. 2009 Presented at: 4th International Conference on Persuasive Technology* (April 26–29 2009), Claremont, CA, USA
45. B.J. Fogg, *Persuasive Technology: Using Computers to Change What We Think and Do* (Morgan Kauffman Publishing, Amsterdam/Boston, 2003)
46. H. Oinas-Kukkonen, M. Harjumaa, Towards deeper understanding of persuasion in software and information systems, in *Proceedings of the First International Conference on Advances in Human-Computer Interaction (ACHI 2008)* (2008). electronic publication. ISBN 978-0-7695-3086-4, pp. 200–205
47. K. Bosworth, D.H. Gustafson, R.P. Hawkins, B. Chewning, P.M. Day, BARNY: A computer based health information system for adolescents. J. Early Adolesc. **1**(3), 315–321 (1981)
48. H. Oinas-Kukkonen, A foundation for the study of behavior change support systems. Pers. Ubiquit. Comput. **17**, 1223–1235 (2013). https://doi.org/10.1007/s00779-012-0591-5
49. H. Oinas-Kukkonen, Behavior change support systems: A research model and agenda, in *Proceedings of the Persuasive Technology Conference* (2010), pp. 4–14
50. W.C. King, M.M. Dent, E.W. Miles, The persuasive effect of graphics in computer-mediated communication. Comput. Hum. Behav. **7**(4), 269–279 (1991)
51. H.C. Kelman, Compliance, identification, and internalization: Three processes of attitude change. J. Confl. Resolut. **2**(1), 51–60 (1958). https://doi.org/10.1177/002200275800200106
52. A. Bandura, *Self-Efficacy: The Exercise of Self-Control* (W.H. Freeman, New York, 1997)
53. A. Bandura, *Social Foundations of Thought and Action: A Social Cognitive Theory. Prentice Hall Series in Social Learning Theory* (Prentice Hall, Englewood Cliffs, 1986), p. 617
54. A. Bandura, Health promotion from the perspective of social cognitive theory. Psychol. Health **13**(4), 623–649 (1998). https://doi.org/10.1080/08870449808407422
55. S. Michie, S. Ashford, F.F. Sniehotta, S.U. Dombrowski, A. Bishop, D.P. French, A refined taxonomy of behaviour change techniques to help people change their physical activity and healthy eating behaviours: The CALO-RE taxonomy. Psychol. Health **26**(11), 1479–1498 (2011)

56. M.S. Hagger, D.A. Keatley, D.K.-C. Chan, CALO-RE taxonomy of behavior change techniques, in *Encyclopedia of Sport and Exercise Psychology*, ed. by R. C. Eklund, G. T. Tenenbaum, (SAGE, Thousand Oaks, 2014), pp. 100–105
57. A.N. Sullivan, M.E. Lachman, Behavior change with fitness technology in sedentary adults: A review of the evidence for increasing physical activity. Front. Public Health **4**, 289 (2016)
58. C.J. Greaves, K.E. Sheppard, C. Abraham, et al., Systematic review of reviews of intervention components associated with increased effectiveness in dietary and physical activity interventions. BMC Public Health **11**, 119 (2011). https://doi.org/10.1186/1471-2458-11-119
59. S. Consolvo, P. Klasnja, D. McDonald, J. Landay, Goal-setting considerations for persuasive technologies that encourage physical activity, in *Proceedings of the 4th International Conference on Persuasive Technology (Persuasive '09)* (2009). Association for Computing Machinery, New York, NY, USA, Article 8, 1–8. https://doi.org/10.1145/1541948.1541960
60. L. Lewis, A. Rowlands, P. Gardiner, M. Standage, C. English, T. Olds, Small steps: Preliminary effectiveness and feasibility of an incremental goal-setting intervention to reduce sitting time in older adults. Maturitas **85**, 64–70 (2016). https://doi.org/10.1016/j.maturitas.2015.12.014
61. H. op den Akker, V.M. Jones, H.J. Hermens, Tailoring real-time physical activity coaching systems: A literature survey and model user model. User-adapt. Interact. **24**(5), 351–392 (2014) https://doi.org/10.1007/s11257-014-9146-y
62. J. Fanning, S.P. Mullen, E. Mcauley, Increasing physical activity with mobile devices: A meta-analysis. J. Med. Internet Res. **14**(6), e161 (2012). https://doi.org/10.2196/jmir.2171
63. W.N. Wan Ahmad, N. Mohamad Ali, A study on persuasive technologies: The relationship between user emotions, trust and persuasion. Int. J. Interactive Multimed. Artif. Intell. **5**(1), 57–61 (2018). https://doi.org/10.9781/ijimai.2018.02.010
64. W.N. Wan Ahmad, N. Mohamad Ali, Engendering trust through emotion in designing persuasive application, in *Advances in Visual Informatics*, ed. by H. B. Zaman, P. Robinson, P. Olivier, T. K. Shih, S. Velastin, vol. 8237, (Springer International Publishing. Lecture Notes in Computer Sciences, Cham, 2013), pp. 707–717
65. S. Berkovsky, J. Freyne, H. Oinas-Kukkonen, Influencing individually: Fusing personalization and persuasion. ACM Trans. Interact. Intell. Syst. **2**(2), 9 (2012)
66. D.H. MacKenzie, Effects of various physical activities on the physical fitness of university men. Res. Q. Am. Phys. Educ. Assoc. **6**, 125–143 (1935)
67. Z. Ruttkay, J. Zwiers, H. van Welbergen, D. Reidsma, Towards a reactive virtual trainer, in *Intelligent Virtual Agents*. IVA 2006. Lecture Notes in Computer Science, ed. by J. Gratch, M. Young, R. Aylett, D. Ballin, P. Olivier, vol. 4133, (Springer, Berlin, Heidelberg, 2006)
68. H.B. Jimison, Patient specific interfaces to health and decision-making information, in *Health Promotion and Interactive Technology: Theoretical Applications and Future Directions*, ed. by R. L. Street, W. R. Gold, T. Manning, (Lawrence Erlbaum, New Jersey, 1997)
69. R.P. Hawkins, M. Kreuter, K. Resnicow, M. Fishbein, A. Dijkstra, Understanding tailoring in communicating about health. Health Educ. Res. **23**(3), 454–466 (2008). https://doi.org/10.1093/her/cyn004
70. M.W. Kreuter, V.J. Strecher, Do tailored behavior change messages enhance the effectiveness of health risk appraisal? Results from a randomized trial. Health Educ. Res. **11**(1), 97–105 (1996). https://doi.org/10.1093/her/11.1.97
71. K. Peffers, T. Tuunanen, M.A. Rothenberger, S. Chatterjee, A design science research methodology for information systems research. J. Manag. Inf. Syst. **24**(3), 45–77 (2008)
72. A. Albergoni, F.J. Hettinga, A. La Torre, M. Bonato, F. Sartor, The role of technology in adherence to physical activity programs in patients with chronic diseases experiencing fatigue: A systematic review. Sports Med Open. **5**(1), 41 (2019). https://doi.org/10.1186/s40798-019-0214-z

73. M. Friedrich, G. Gittler, Y. Halberstadt, T. Cermak, I. Heiller, Combined exercise and motivation program: Effect on the compliance and level of disability of patients with chronic low back pain: A randomized controlled trial. Arch. Phys. Med. Rehabil. **79**(5), 475–487 (1998)
74. A. Linden, S.W. Butterworth, J.O. Prochaska, Motivational interviewing-based health coaching as a chronic care intervention. J. Eval. Clin. Pract. **16**(1), 166–174 (2010). https://doi.org/10.1111/j.1365-2753.2009.01300.x
75. C. Tudor-Locke, C.L. Craig, Y. Aoyagi, R.C. Bell, K.A. Croteau, I. De Bourdeaudhuij, B. Ewald, A.W. Gardner, Y. Hatano, L.D. Lutes, S.M. Matsudo, How many steps/day are enough? For older adults and special populations. Int. J. Behav. Nutr. Phys. Act. **8**, 80 (2011). https://doi.org/10.1186/1479-5868-8-80
76. F. Davis, Perceived usefulness, perceived ease of use, and user acceptance of information technology. MIS Q. **13**(3), 319–340 (1989). https://doi.org/10.2307/249008

A Proactive Approach to Combating the Opioid Crisis Using Machine Learning Techniques

Ethel A. M. Mensah, Musarath J. Rahmathullah, Pooja Kumar, Roozbeh Sadeghian, and Siamak Aram

Abbreviations

EHR	Electronic Health Record
ML	Machine Learning
PDMP	Prescription Drug Monitoring Program

1 Introduction

Each year, an estimated 15 million people suffer from opioid addiction worldwide [1]. In the United States alone, prescription opioid abuse affects more than 2 million people and is the leading cause of death in adults under the age of 50 [1]. Opioid addiction is characterized by a powerful, compulsive urge to use opioid drugs even when no longer medically required. Overreliance on prescription opioids for the treatment and management of severe and chronic pain is a leading cause of opioid dependence and addiction. Commonly prescribed opioids include oxycodone, fentanyl, buprenorphine, methadone, oxymorphone, hydrocodone, codeine, and morphine. No unique cause of opioid addiction has been identified. The prevalence

E. A. M. Mensah · M. J. Rahmathullah · P. Kumar · R. Sadeghian
Department of Analytics, Harrisburg University of Science and Technology, Harrisburg, PA, USA
e-mail: emensah@my.harrisburgu.edu; mrahmathullah@my.harrisburgu.edu; pkumar@my.harrisburgu.edu; RSadeghian@harrisburgu.edu

S. Aram (✉)
Department of Information System and Engineering Management (ISEM), Harrisburg University of Science and Technology, Harrisburg, PA, USA
e-mail: SAaram@harrisburgu.edu

H. R. Arabnia et al. (eds.), *Advances in Computer Vision and Computational Biology*, Transactions on Computational Science and Computational Intelligence,
https://doi.org/10.1007/978-3-030-71051-4_30

of opioid use, misuse, and addiction is potentially increasing and facilitating other health problems such as increased risk of hepatitis B and C and HIV/AIDS. While variations exist in the choice of opiates, age range, and sex, overall, there is an increasing trend in opioid and substance abuse reported. Despite extensive research into the prevalence, scope, causes of use, and misuse of opioids, there are identified gaps in available data that significantly limit the understanding of the interrelated phenomena modeled in a system-dynamic approach which undermines policies and interventions aimed at easing the effects of the opioid crisis [2]. The application of big data analytics to the opioid crisis is a relatively new and emerging area. Multiple studies have been conducted using Machine Learning and big data analytics techniques in identifying and predicting opioid use disorder.

Addiction is a complex disease that affects an individual both physically and psychologically. The exact cause of opioid use and misuse is unknown, but many factors including the presence of mental health disorders, painful physical conditions, and socioeconomic and demographic factors play a major role [3]. The rate of drug overdose deaths in the United States has increased by 137% since 2000, with a 200% increase in deaths involving opioids (prescription drugs and heroin). Southern and Midwestern states have witnessed substantial increases in opioid-related mortality rates [4]. To effectively combat the opioid crisis, it is important to identify which groups are most affected by the health crisis and potential contributing factors. Research shows some populations are at a higher risk for opioid abuse than others including populations with low education levels, high rates of unemployment, and high poverty rates. As part of the effort to curb prescription opioid rates, states have initiated Prescription Drug Monitoring Program (PDMP). PDMPs are state-run electronic databases of prescription for controlled substances which provide useful information regarding a patient's prescription history and can be used to determine patients who are potentially at risk of abusing or are currently abusing controlled substances [5]. A review of prescription rates data reveals higher availability of opioids in rural communities. For example, OxyContin was aggressively marketed to Appalachia and surrounding communities. Over the past four decades, the restructuring of employment has led to the concentration of high-wage, high-skill, service, and technology jobs in urban areas while simultaneously moving livable-wage production jobs from rural areas [6]. This has resulted in the growing mismatch of skills and available jobs in most regions of the United States. According to the National Institute of Health (NIH), more than 50 million Americans suffer from chronic pain, of which 25 million lack effective, safe, non-opioid pain management solutions. Undertreatment of pain can result in many adverse effects and amounts to poor and unethical medical practice. Inadequate management of acute pain negatively impacts patients' health and well-being and may increase the risk of development of chronic pain [7]. Pain is a common and inordinately disabling condition in the US workforce. An estimated $61.2 billion per year is lost due to pain-related ailments and associated lost productivity [8]. Currently, opioids are the preferred treatment for most moderate to severe acute pain; however, the negative side effects impede their use and thus clinical effectiveness [7].

The socioeconomic impact of substance and opioid addiction cannot be underestimated. Currently, not many alternatives are available for the treatment of chronic pain because of the complex circuitry involved in pain. To effectively and efficiently treat pain management, it is important to identify "the nature and likely afferent source of pain," combining medication that act "synergistically" to minimize the dosage of any particular drug and thereby reduce any potential side effects [9].

Many strategies and policies have been proposed to address the opioid epidemic and some progress made. The application of big data analytics to the opioid crisis is a relatively new and emerging area. The social, infrastructural, and economic costs of opioid and substance abuse are enormous. Prescription opioid use, abuse, and resulting consequences is an epidemic that needs to be addressed in judicious, effective, and efficient manner. Many of the solutions and policies proposed to address prescription opioid use, abuse, and its consequences have largely been reactive.

Several different Machine Learning algorithms have been widely developed and discussed in literature to enable early intervention to reduce potential long-term opioid usage [10, 11]. Recently, to predict postoperative prolonged opioid prescription after anterior cervical discectomy [12] and surgery for lumbar disc herniation [13] and to increase the patient's surveillance after surgery to potentially reduce the long-term opioid use, Random Forest, ANN, SVM, elastic-net penalized Logistic Regression, and Stochastic Gradient Boosting algorithms have been studied [14]. SVM, ANN, Logistic Regression, and Decision Tree models were used to predict the prescription opioid misuse in patients, wherein SVM achieved 100% accuracy for classic training and testing sets [15].

In another study conducted to combat the opioid epidemic, various Machine Learning models were evaluated for predicting patients that were vulnerable to opioid use abuse and also for risk stratification, i.e., to help identify patients and provide physicians with real-time pre or post decision-making prescription alerts. The research suggested that the Gradient Boosting (XGBOOST) Forest had the lowest misclassification rate, highest sensitivity, highest accuracy, and highest RoC index [16].

In this research, a mixture of qualitative and quantitative methods was employed to understand the scope of previous research. This work is an experimental study that seeks to use predictive methodology/analysis as a proactive approach in addressing the opioid crisis.

2 Method

2.1 Data and Measures

Socioeconomic indicators such as household income vary geographically across US states and counties. The independent variables used in this study are education attainment, specifically percentage of adults with bachelor's degree or higher, unemployment rate, and poverty rate. States and counties unemployment data was retrieved from the USDA website for all states including Puerto Rico. The data source is US Department of Labor and Bureau of Labor Statistics (BLS) [17]. Unemployment data is collected through the Local Area Unemployment Statistics (LAUS) program [17]. Poverty and income data for 2013–2017 were retrieved from the USDA Census Bureau for all counties and states using information from the US Census Bureau and does not include data for Puerto Rico. State and county Supplemental Nutrition Assistance Program (SNAP) data, aggregate tax (IRS state-level data), and data from the American Community Survey (ACS) are inputs for the Small Area Income and Poverty Estimates. Income and poverty thresholds vary by income and family size and composition but do not vary geographically across the United States.

The 2018 income poverty threshold is $12,784 for an individual and $16,247 for two people [18]. Education attainment data was retrieved from the US Department of Agriculture (USDA). For the purposes of this research, the average of education data from 2013 to 2017 were used. Drug poisoning mortality rates for the years 1999–2017 in the United States were retrieved from Centers for Disease Control and Prevention and National Center for Health Statistics. The United States county-level Federal Information Processing Standard (FIPS) codes data was retrieved from the US Census Bureau. County-level FIPS codes are five-digit codes consisting of two-digit state identifier and three-digit county identifier assigned by the National Institute of Standards and Technology (NIST) that uniquely identify geographic areas of the United States [18]. The official list of FIPS codes for the year 2017, used in this research, identifies 3142 counties and county equivalents of the United States. The dependent variable in this study is risk level which has three categories, low (0), medium (1), and high (2), and is assigned based on a calculated relative risk score using unemployment rate, percent of adults with a bachelor's degree or higher, and poverty rate as inputs. This score is calculated using mean [19]. A county is assigned a "low" value if the combined related score calculated is less than or equal to 12, "medium" if the combined relative score is greater than 12 but less than 15, and "high" for all counties with a relative combined score of more than 15.

2.2 *Data Analysis*

The design of this study is experimental and examines the correlation between high poverty, high unemployment, low education rates, and opioid abuse disorder. Datasets were retrieved from the US Department of Agriculture (USDA) website compiled by the Economic Research Service. The data included county-level poverty, education (including median household income), and unemployment data for all 50 US states including Puerto Rico; however, data for Puerto Rico was removed for the purpose of this research. Opioid overdose death data was also derived from the Centers for Disease Control and Prevention (CDC) for all counties and states. Statistical data wrangling methods including imputing null values and formatting to standardize data for analysis using required packages and libraries were employed. Data visualization was used to describe the relationship between unemployment, poverty, and education on opioid abuse, dependence, and overdose. Machine Learning models including Support Vector Machine (SVM), Decision Tree, Logistic Regression, and more advanced models like Gradient Boosting (XGBOOST), AdaBoost, and MLP (Multiple Layer Perceptron) were created to predict opioid abuse, dependence, and overdose based on a relative combined score, considering unemployment, education, and poverty rates. The accuracy of the models was measured and compared to determine which model performed better at predicting opioid abuse and potential overdose. Counties were then classified as low, medium, or high risk for opioid abuse, dependence, and overdose. The dependent variable in this study is risk level, with three categories. A county is assigned a "low" value if the combined related score (of unemployment rate, percent of adults with a bachelor's degree or higher, and poverty rate) calculated is less than or equal to 12, "medium" if the combined relative score is greater than 12 but less than 15, and "high" for all counties with a relative combined score of more than 15. Research shows that both individual and community well-being is significantly impacted by labor-market conditions. Areas with low levels of educational attainment are generally clustered in areas of "high and persistent poverty." Education attainment is closely linked to labor-market outcomes as those who receive higher education generally receive higher earnings and are less likely to be unemployed. These factors tend to self-perpetuate, and the cycle of poverty can be hard to break.

In this study, data analysis was conducted in two phases—qualitative and quantitative. First, previous research was identified and evaluated to inform prevalence of opioid abuse disorder in the United States. Review of previous research identified trends in opioid use and abuse, prescription opioids prescribing patterns, and areas and/or groups impacted as well as current policies and programs implemented to address the health crisis. Quantitative analysis included using Excel formulae to calculate mean of average rates of opioid-related overdose deaths, unemployment, and poverty. Data wrangling and cleanup were performed using Python packages including pandas and NumPy. Poverty, unemployment, education, and drug overdose death rates datasets had varying number of observations. FIPS codes data from the US Census Bureau was used to standardize all the datasets for consistency, after which all the datasets were merged to obtain a single file and unneeded columns removed to avoid processing of a large file. The exploratory data analysis was carried out using visualization to describe the relationships between independent variables, with bar plots, line graphs, correlation plots, heatmaps, and box plots. In preprocessing step, the imbalanced dataset was balanced by up-sampling classes (i.e., classes 0 and 2) using resampling technique with replacement. Figures 1 and 2 show how data is distributed across three categories "before" and "after" data balancing. The dataset was split into train and test set along 75% and 25% margin, respectively, before training the Machine Learning models to predict opioid abuse disorder. Models were evaluated using cross-validation approach with kFold of 10 to overcome any problem due to high variance. The test accuracy of the models was

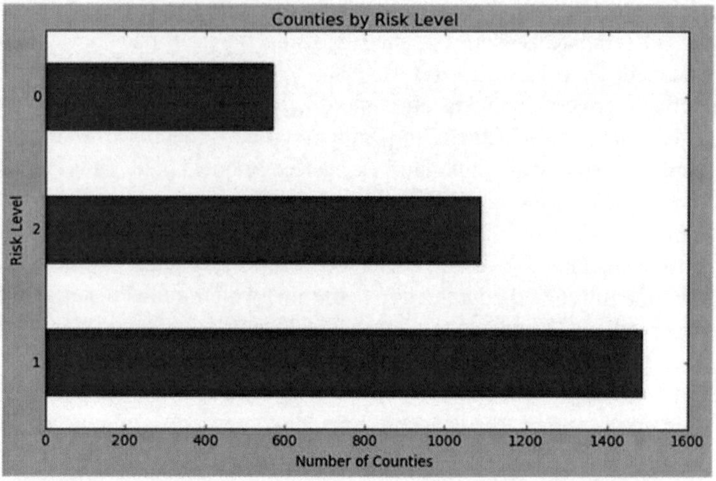

Fig. 1 Data distribution across three categories of risk level before data balancing

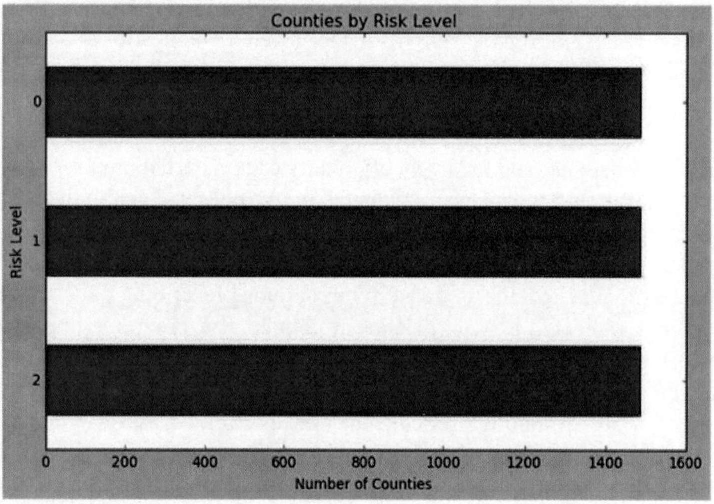

Fig. 2 Data distribution across three categories of risk level after data balancing

then compared to determine which model performed best at predicting county-level opioid abuse disorder based on unemployment, education, and poverty rates.

3 Results

Opioid abuse disorder and resulting consequences are growing, and this is an expensive problem in the United States. Federal agencies and states have implemented various policies and programs to combat the opioid crisis; however, these efforts

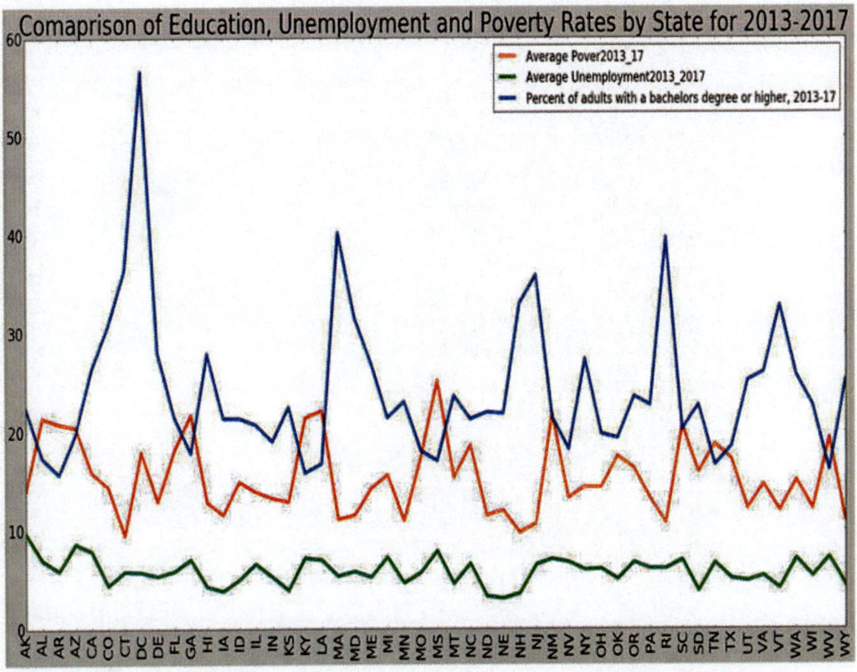

Fig. 3 Average rates of unemployment, education, and poverty levels from 2013 to 2017 period for each state in the United States

have largely been reactive instead of proactive including PDMPs. Socioeconomic indicators such as education, poverty, and unemployment rates are factors that contribute to the prevalence of opioid abuse disorder and vary widely across the United States. Figure 3 shows the distribution of average rate of unemployment, education, and poverty levels across all states of the United States for period 2013–2017.

Preliminary analysis explored the relationship between education, poverty, and unemployment, as shown in Fig. 4. Significant positive relationship was identified between unemployment and poverty. As unemployment increased, so did poverty and vice versa. However, negative relationship was found between education attainment (i.e., percent of adults with a bachelor's degree or higher) and poverty. Similarly, education attainment and unemployment were negatively correlated. An increase in educational attainment resulted in a decrease in poverty levels. An inverse relationship was observed between education level and poverty. Overall, there was a stronger positive relationship between unemployment and poverty.

It was hypothesized that states with higher unemployment rates, higher poverty rates, and lower percentage of higher education attainment are at higher risk for opioid use, abuse, and dependence. To identify which counties are at higher risk of opioid abuse disorder, a relative cumulative score was calculated for each county

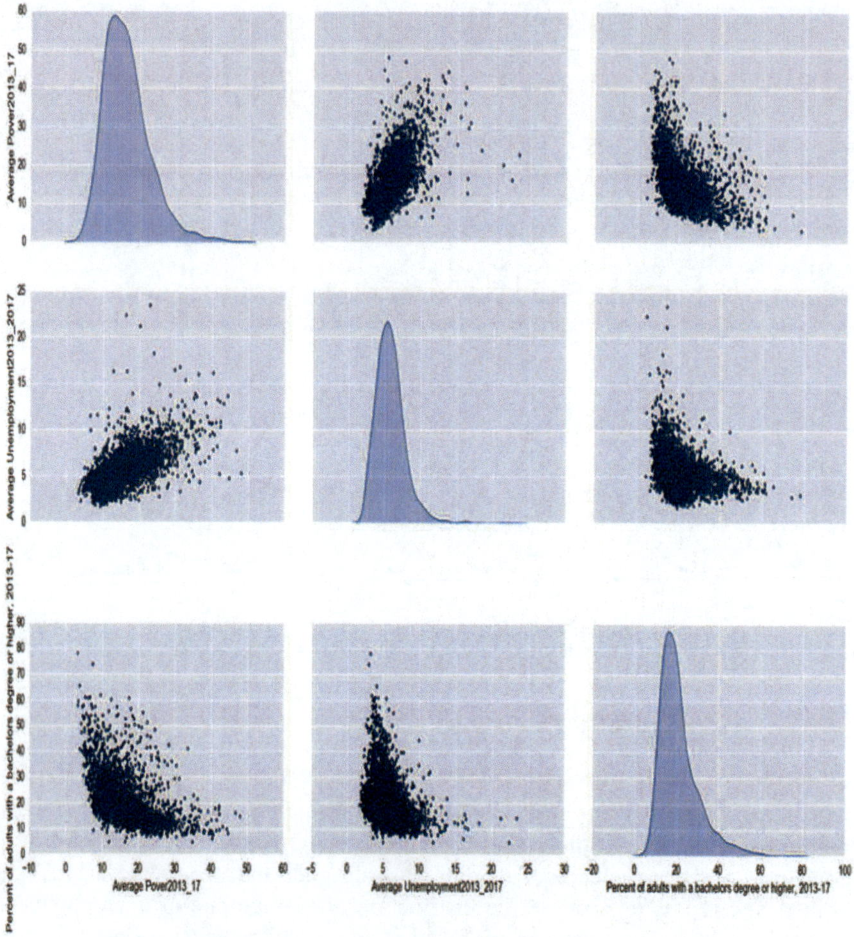

Fig. 4 Seaborn correlation plot showing relationship between poverty, education, and unemployment rates

using education attainment (i.e., percent of adults with a bachelor's degree or higher), poverty, and unemployment rates. The higher the score, the higher the risk and vice versa. Consistent with the present study's hypotheses as shown in Fig. 5, asserts with higher relative calculated scores had slightly higher average overdose rates.

A plotted US map of risk level at county level is shown in Fig. 6 with corresponding risk levels from 0 to 2, for low, medium, and high, respectively. For all 3142 counties tested, 1086 (35%) counties were identified to be at high risk, 1486 (47%) had medium risk, and only 569 (18%) had low risk of opioid abuse disorder.

Various Machine Learning models were trained to predict opioid use, abuse, and dependence based on available data as shown in Fig. 7.

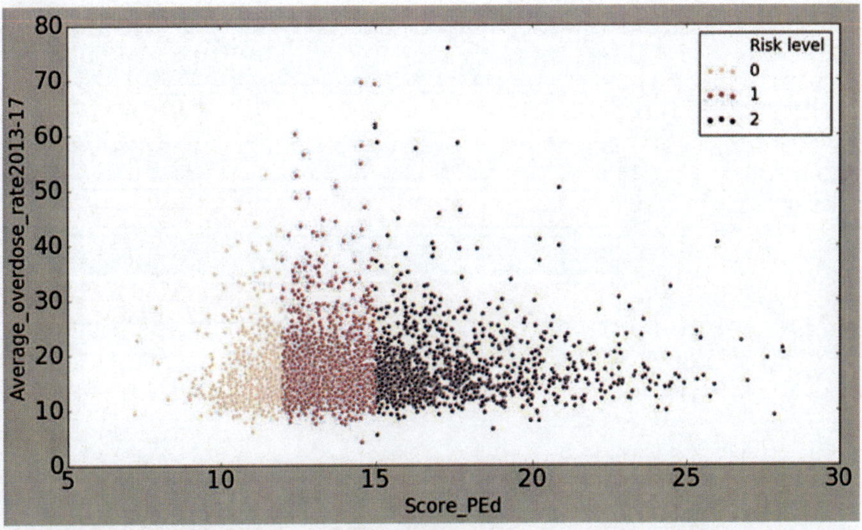

Fig. 5 Scatterplot distribution of average overdose rate for 2013–2017 based on relative calculated score using unemployment, poverty, and education rate data

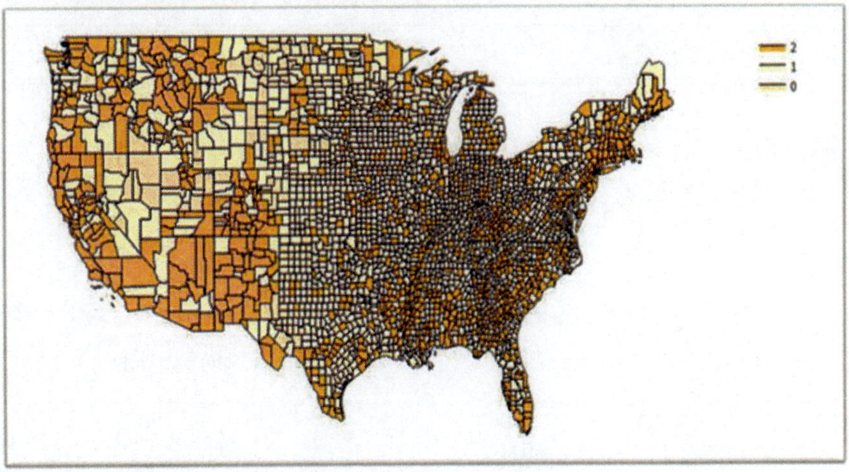

Fig. 6 County level map of United States showing predicted risk levels of opioid abuse disorder

Gradient Boosting (XGBOOST) performed the best with an accuracy score of 96.7% compared with Decision Tree and Support Vector Machine (SVM) which had 92% and 91%, respectively.

Figure 8 explains the mean accuracy and error across different applied algorithms. This can be attributed to the fact that XGBOOST is more robust and computationally more efficient and thus a better classification model for the given dataset.

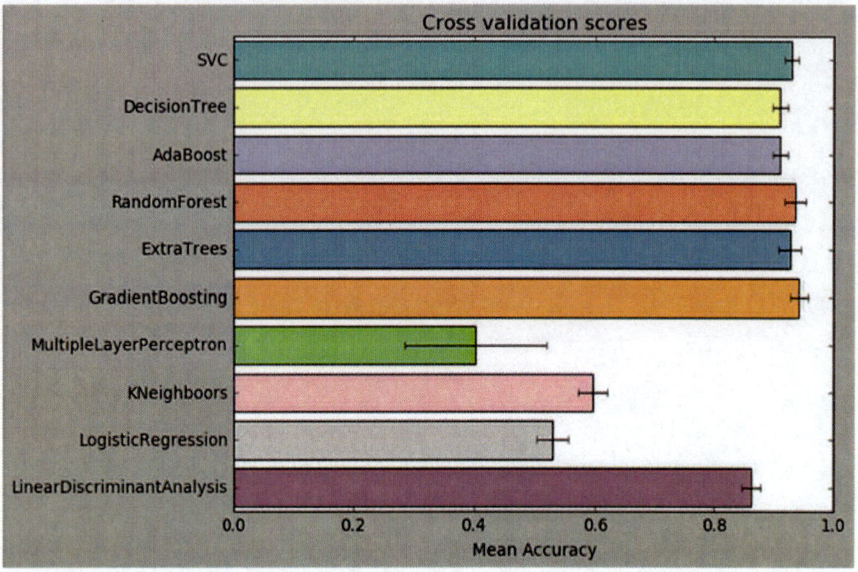

Fig. 7 Cross-validation scores for various applied algorithms

	CrossValAccuracy	*CrossValerrors*	*Algorithm*
0	92.95%	0.011955	SVC
1	91.09%	0.012370	DecisionTree
2	91.00%	0.013207	AdaBoost
3	93.59%	0.017715	RandomForest
4	92.75%	0.019052	ExtraTrees
5	94.31%	0.014239	GradientBoosting
6	40.17%	0.116548	MultipleLayerPerceptron
7	59.56%	0.024690	KNeighboors
8	52.89%	0.026011	LogisticRegression
9	86.17%	0.016278	LinearDiscriminantAnalysis

Fig. 8 Cross-validation scores of different algorithms

The average F1 score of all the three classes is 0.97, and the individual distribution of metrics of the final model used for prediction of opioid is as shown in Fig. 9.

Receiver Operating Characteristic (ROC) curve illustrates the trade-off between sensitivity (also known as true positive rate, TRP) and specificity (also known as

	precision	*recall*	*f1-score*	*support*
0	0.95	1.00	0.97	339
1	0.98	0.92	0.95	383
2	0.97	0.98	0.98	393
accuracy			0.97	1115
macro avg	0.97	0.97	0.97	1115
weighted avg	0.97	0.97	0.97	1115

Fig. 9 Precision, Recall, and F1 score of XGBOOST model

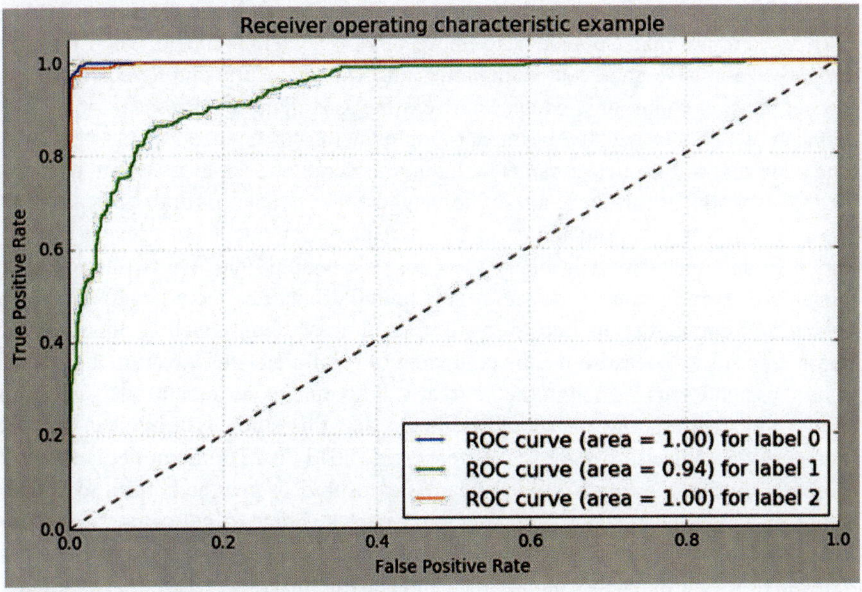

Fig. 10 Receiver Operating Characteristic curve

false positive rate, FPR) at various threshold settings for the XGBOOST model (as shown in Fig. 10). Any increase in sensitivity will be accompanied by a decrease in specificity. The area under the curve gives the measure of text accuracy. Here, area under ROC curve for classes 0 and 2 equals to 1 and class 1 equals to 0.94.

4 Discussion

The results of this study demonstrate a significant positive association between low education attainment, high poverty, and high unemployment. Additionally, the results show the risk of opioid use and abuse is more widespread geographically across the United States and is not peculiar to rural and/or low-income areas. It was hypothesized that areas plagued by a combination of low education levels and high unemployment and poverty are at risk of opioid abuse disorder. While the results of the study show this to be generally true, there is some evidence to suggest that metropolitan/urban areas are equally at risk of opioid abuse and dependence compared with their rural counterparts, if not greater. This is seen by the high concentration of high-risk areas in the western, southwest, and northeastern parts of the United States as shown in Fig. 6. This can be attributed to the fact that many people who abuse prescription opioids do so for recreational purposes, potentially as a way of relaxing or social "event." This phenomenon is very likely among the highly educated and professionals who may be seeking a "getaway" from their busy lives. Additionally, it is possible migration patterns influence how and where opioid-related overdose deaths are recorded and therefore impact data collection efforts.

For example, many people who abuse opioids generally begin when they are employed and have good socioeconomic status (i.e., gainfully employed and live in decent housing conditions). However, over time as addiction to prescription opioids worsens which can negatively impact employment and financial status, they may end up in less stable environments including rural and/or poor areas where potential overdose deaths occur. Previous studies suggest that people in rural areas are more likely to suffer from opioid addiction due to a lack of or inadequate access to medical facilities and services. It is likely the case that people who live in metropolitan areas have more resources to treat their opioid addiction, including therapy and addiction treatment compared to those in rural areas. Consequently, metropolitan areas record less overdose deaths compared to rural areas despite similar levels of opioid use and abuse. Though the internal validity and experimental realism of this study seem quite strong, it should be noted that this study is limited in that the amount of data used from the last 5 years (i.e., 2013–2017) may not be enough to properly understand trends in the variables measured. It may be helpful to include more data, as well as data from previous years in order to get a more complete picture of trends. Additionally, due to lack of data for multiple years, averages were computed for all independent variables and used in analyses. Also, the constructed measure calculated using educational level, unemployment, and poverty rates used to determine risk level is arbitrary and may not be an objectively accurate measure. For the purposes of this study, it was important to use a computed measure as a dependent variable for statistical analysis and prediction in the Machine Learning models. The model built in this research has greater accuracy in predicting risk level of opioid cases when compared to previous studies [16].

Intentional abuse of prescription opioids and over-the-counter (OTC) medicines has climbed steadily with sharp increases in the use of synthetic opioids such as heroin, fentanyl, and fentanyl analogs leading to marked increases of opioid-related overdose deaths. Data from the 2005 National Survey on Drug Use and Health showed that 6.4 million (2.6%) people in the United States aged 12 and older had used prescription drugs during the past month for nonmedical reasons [20]. This number is alarming, especially considering the rapidly rising rates of prescription opioids among young adults. Prescription opioid abuse has severe negative impacts on both individuals and communities. Among the many negative impacts include impact to family and society structures, loss of productivity, increased risk of health complications from prolonged use, incarceration, and, in some cases, premature death. Studies show that people who use prescription opioids generally progress to use of heroin and other synthetic opioid to achieve a bigger high as tolerance is built to prescription opioids, and users do not obtain the same level of euphoria that opioids produce from prescription drugs. Adverse effects of use of illicit drugs cannot be understated. According to the Centers for Disease Control and Prevention (CDC), unintentional deaths resulting from drug overdoses are the second leading cause of accidental death in the United States [21]. Future research should focus on including more patient-specific available data in order to build prediction models that more accurately represent the sample population. For example, data obtained from physician offices' Electronic Health Records (EHR) as well as from Prescription Drug Monitoring Program (PDMPs) can offer useful insights into individuals and communities or development of targeted solutions. In addition, data from PDMPs may provide a more accurate description of prescribing habits and better capture individual and communities' responses to the opioid epidemic.

5 Conclusions

Education, poverty, and unemployment are interrelated phenomena that impact opioid use, abuse, and dependence. The results of these studies found that advanced forest model, viz., Gradient Boosting (XGBOOST), was best compared to other traditional Machine Learning algorithms at predicting opioid abuse disorder. Previous studies showed that people who have lower socioeconomic status are at higher risk of opioid misuse. Understanding the role and impact of each one of these factors is critical to effectively tackle the opioid crisis. However, they may be deeper underlying issues not related to education, unemployment, and poverty that need to be examined in order to develop comprehensive solutions and programs to tackle the opioid epidemic. Also, we should note that there is not a general solution for all Opioid-related disorders. Individualized approaches that consider complete patient history and characteristics are likely to yield better and efficient results in efforts to tackle the opioid epidemic.

Acknowledgments Sincerest thanks to Mr. Arnie Miles who was instrumental in the creation of a quality manuscript.

Competing Interests The authors declare they have no competing interests.

Consent for Publication The authors consent to the publication of this manuscript.

Ethic Approval and Consent to Participate Not applicable

Availability of Data and Materials All datasets and software used for this study are open source and readily available at the resources listed in the data and measures section.

Funding Not applicable

References

1. Opioid Addiction (2020, March 3), Retrieved 12 Dec 2019, from https://pubmed.ncbi.nlm.nih.gov/28952972/. Misuse of prescription opioids, and addiction is rapidly increasing
2. T.D. Schmidt, J.D. Haddox, A.E. Nielsen, W. Wakeland, J. Fitzgerald, Key data gaps regarding the public health issues associated with opioid analgesics. J. Behav. Health Serv. Res. **42**(4), 540–553 (2015)
3. C. Katz, R. El-Gabalawy, K.M. Keyes, S.S. Martins, J. Sareen, Risk factors for incident nonmedical prescription opioid use and abuse and dependence: Results from a longitudinal nationally representative sample. Drug Alcohol Depend. **132**(1–2), 107–113 (2013)
4. G. Eigner, B. Henriksen, P. Huynh, D. Murphy, C. Brubaker, J. Sanders, D. McMahan, Who is overdosing? An updated picture of overdose deaths from 2008 to 2015. Health Serv. Res. Manag. Epidemiol. **4**, 2333392817727424 (2017)
5. K.M. Keyes, M. Cerdá, J.E. Brady, J.R. Havens, S. Galea, Understanding the rural–urban differences in nonmedical prescription opioid use and abuse in the United States. Am. J. Public Health **104**(2), e52–e59 (2014)
6. S.M. Monnat, K.K. Rigg, The opioid crisis in rural and small town America (2018)
7. R. Sinatra, Causes and consequences of inadequate management of acute pain. Pain Med. **11**(12), 1859–1871 (2010)
8. W.F. Stewart, J.A. Ricci, E. Chee, D. Morganstein, R. Lipton, Lost productive time and cost due to common pain conditions in the US workforce. JAMA **290**(18), 2443–2454 (2003)
9. M. Roe, A. Sehgal, Pharmacology in the management of chronic pain. Anaesth Intensive Care Med. **17**(11), 548–551 (2016)
10. A.S. Wadekar, Understanding Opioid Use Disorder (OUD) using tree-based classifiers. Drug Alcohol Depend. **208**, 107839 (2020)
11. Z. Che, J.S. Sauver, H. Liu, Y. Liu, Deep learning solutions for classifying patients on opioid use, in *AMIA Annual Symposium Proceedings*, vol. 2017, (American Medical Informatics Association, 2017), p. 525
12. Local Area Unemployment Statistics (n.d.), Retrieved 7 Dec 2019, from https://www.bls.gov/lau/#tables
13. U.C. Bureau, Small area income and poverty estimates (saipe) program (2018, October). The United States Census Bureau. Retrieved from https://census.gov/programs-surveys/saipe.html
14. A.V. Karhade, P.T. Ogink, Q.C. Thio, T.D. Cha, W.B. Gormley, S.H. Hershman, et al., Development of machine learning algorithms for prediction of prolonged opioid prescription after surgery for lumbar disc herniation. Spine J. **19**(11), 1764–1771 (2019)
15. G. van Rossum, *Python tutorial (No. CS-R9526)* (Centrum voor Wiskunde en Informatica (CWI), Amsterdam, 1995)
16. J.E. Lessenger, S.D. Feinberg, Abuse of prescription and over-the-counter medications. J. Am. Board Fam. Med. **21**(1), 45–54 (2008)
17. S. Okie, A flood of opioids, a rising tide of deaths. N. Engl. J. Med. **363**(21), 1981–1985 (2010)
18. A.V. Karhade, P.T. Ogink, Q.C.B.S. Thio, M.L.D. Broekman, T.D. Cha, S.H. Hershman, J. Mao, W.C. Peul, A.J. Schoenfeld, C.M. Bono, et al., Machine learning for prediction of sustained opioid prescription after anterior cervical discectomy and fusion. Spine J. **19**(6), 976–983 (2019)
19. A.V. Karhade, P.T. Ogink, Q.C.B.S. Thio, T.D. Cha, W.B. Gormley, S.H. Hershman, T.R. Smith, J. Mao, A.J. Schoenfeld, C.M. Bono, et al., Development of machine learning algorithms for prediction of prolonged opioid prescription after surgery for lumbar disc herniation. Spine J. **19**(11), 1764–1771 (2019)
20. J. Huinker, Using machine learning to predict prescription opioid misuse in patients (2019)
21. N. Kaur, G. Chakraborty, M. Mcgaugh, Machine learning approach to combat the opioid epidemic (2020)

Security and Usability Considerations for an mHealth Application for Emergency Medical Services

Abdullah Murad, Benjamin Schooley, and Thomas Horan

1 Introduction

Mobile devices are being used increasingly to collect, share, and manage patient data across interorganizational networks of cooperating healthcare providers in order to facilitate healthcare delivery [1, 2]. A major motivation for this phenomenon is the growing demand for organizations to collect, transmit, access, and modify electronic patient health information (PHI) efficiently while satisfying both healthcare patients and providers. Many believe that these devices and applications hold significant potential to improve healthcare [1, 2], but concerns continue to surface about information security and privacy [3]. Designing and developing mobile health (mHealth) applications in a manner that (1) adheres to PHI privacy and security rules and regulations, (2) has an acceptable level of usability, and (3) facilitates improvements to healthcare delivery poses significant challenges [4–7].

Few studies have directly referenced the commonly accepted security practices and methodologies involved in designing and implementing interorganizational healthcare enterprise mHealth applications. This may be due to the relative "newness" of interorganizational information sharing during the process of care, as most information sharing of patient records occurs in non-time-critical circumstances. While health information exchange (HIE) for more real-time information sharing

A. Murad
Umm Al-Qura University, Mecca, Saudi Arabia

B. Schooley (✉)
University of South Carolina, Columbia, SC, USA
e-mail: bschooley@cec.sc.edu

T. Horan
University of Redlands, Redlands, CA, USA

H. R. Arabnia et al. (eds.), *Advances in Computer Vision and Computational Biology*, Transactions on Computational Science and Computational Intelligence,
https://doi.org/10.1007/978-3-030-71051-4_31

has increased, it is most often not conducted in mobile environments. We have found a scarcity of comprehensive and generalizable frameworks and examples of secure mHealth applications that can facilitate healthcare provision across health provider organizations for the purpose of continuity of care.

This chapter discusses a case in which a research team designed and implemented security principles for an mHealth application to secure PHI. This chapter describes the standards applied, how they were applied, and the process used regarding physical and technical guidelines specified by the Health Insurance Portability and Accountability Act (HIPAA). We describe a practitioner-oriented system aimed at sharing multimedia patient information between emergency medical services (EMS) paramedics in the field and charge nurses in an emergency department using service-oriented architecture (SOA).

The study applied a design science research methodology (DSRM) to design, demonstrate the use, and evaluate the aforementioned mHealth application in terms of its security and usability. The application incorporates 11 security principles that have been presented by the Office of the National Coordinator (ONC) for health IT, U.S. Department of Health and Human Services, to help guide the development of mHealth applications. Taken together, the application and the design process provide a normative architecture – a heuristic for applying security to future interorganizational enterprise mHealth systems. We examine the heuristic in relation to security and usability goals within the context of a case example, providing an illustration of its application and testing.

2 mHealth Security Challenges

The challenges of achieving information privacy and security in healthcare organizations is a common topic for discussion [4, 6]. Some of the barriers to adopting electronic health records (EHRs) on Internet and mobile platforms include increased concerns about the security, confidentiality, and privacy of patient health data [8]. Specific to mHealth, the evolution of modern technology platforms, enhanced communication capabilities, hardware portability, user and data mobility, and changing user patterns have increased the complexity of information security design and implementation [4]. These developments require that data be protected, in response to a wide range of security threats including malware, phishing and social engineering, direct attack by hackers, data communication interception and spoofing, loss and theft of devices, malicious insider actions, and user policy violations [3, 9].

For risk-sensitive systems such as homeland security, defense, critical infrastructures, and healthcare, mobile device and application security must be considered together. Common security attributes that should be present in these information-sensitive applications include authentication, authorization, accountability, availability, confidentiality, integrity, device and user management, and physical security [10].

While data security standards for HIPAA compliance have been discussed extensively, a lack of security standardization has been identified as a significant barrier to assuring privacy and interoperability and achieving healthcare improvements from mHealth technologies [4]. What is needed is a standardized framework to implement HIPAA standards and ensure they are enforced. This chapter aims to contribute in this regard by providing a framework for securing PHI across mHealth applications and devices, without sacrificing usability for time-critical interorganizational contexts.

2.1 *Usability and Security in mHealth*

Usability has been defined by a variety of standards. Simply, a usable system is one that performs effectively, efficiently, and to the satisfaction of users [11]. Of the many standards defining usability, some also indicate the importance of security for critical systems [12]. The design of usable yet secure systems raises important considerations of how to solve perceived conflicts between these two goals [13]. Many believe usability to be an important component of security. Yet the fundamental question remains for designers: how to ensure usability without compromising security and vice versa [13, 14]? One descriptive model, depicting the use of compromise in resolving this challenge, is shown in Fig. 1.

The literature has identified some of the factors underlying this challenge: system implementers treating security or usability as an add-on to a finished product [15] and conflicts of interest existing between the system owner and its users [16]. These factors should be taken into account when developing usable and secure systems.

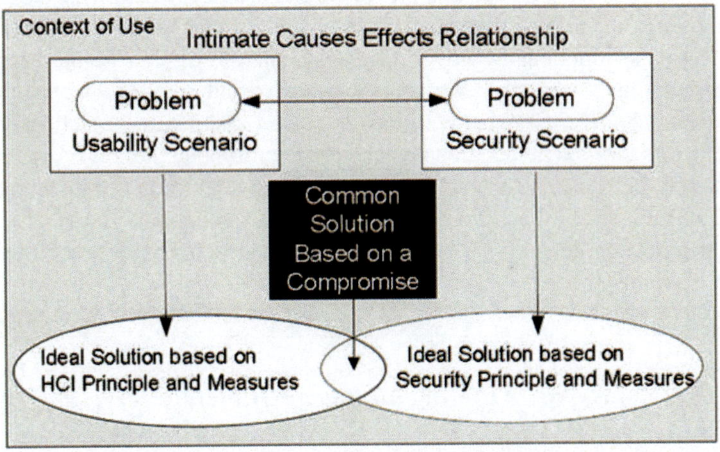

Fig. 1 Usability and security trade-off: a common solution based on a compromise [13]

Healthcare software applications continue to face these usability and security challenges [6]. In the application presented in this paper, paramedics required a highly usable application in order to interfere as little as possible in emergency patient care. Yet, at the same time, hospitals required protection of PHI that occurred during EMS communications with the ER while in the field and during patient handoff in the ER. All organizations had to agree on the security and usability framework in order to proceed. Required PHI protections may be difficult to achieve in these mobile, time-critical, real-time information exchanges. For example, the HIPAA requirement for data encryption/decryption can consume significant processing and bandwidth resources, causing application inefficiency. Further, each participating organization in an interorganizational network may have different encryption/decryption requirements – some that may be overly restrictive and impede usability. Researchers have recently begun to propose mHealth architectures and frameworks that strike a balance between security and privacy with metrics representing usability for secure, mobile, wearable, and easy-to-use mHealth applications that may apply to interorganizational contexts [17].

Other researchers [7, 18] developed and tested a framework to support policy enforcement on the security and privacy needs of health data, including the mechanisms required to support such policies on mHealth applications. Kainda and associates proposed a security and usability threat model detailing the various factors pertinent to the security and usability of secure systems [16]. And Josang and colleagues proposed a way to incorporate a set of security and usability principles into existing and future security solutions [19]. Standard-setting bodies, including the National Institute of Standards and Technology (NIST), the Federal Information Processing Standards (FIPS), and the International Organization for Standardization (ISO), provide specific definitions and guidance on applying technical standards in collecting, storing, and transmitting sensitive data. However, guidelines are lacking on HIPAA implementation for secure and usable mHealth systems. Previous research has emphasized the importance of using behavioral science theories to create exercise programs to aid in the transformation of short-term changes into long-term habits. Habitual behaviors, such as physical activity, are represented in associative memory and experienced as low effort and automatic actions independent of goals and intentions. People can easily build habits by repeating an action consistently in the same context [21, 22]. Several studies demonstrate the pervasive impact of habit and past behavior on physical activity adherence. In order to promote long-term and continuous participation in physical activity, interventions should seek to tap into processes linked to habit formation [23].

2.2 *HIPAA Security and Healthcare Efficiency*

The Health Insurance Portability and Accountability Act (HIPAA) and the Health Information Technology for Economic and Clinical Health (HITECH) Act address privacy and security of health information when it is accessed by entities engaged in healthcare-related activities. Title II of HIPAA includes a section (Administrative Simplification) on requiring improved efficiency in healthcare delivery by standardizing electronic data interchange (EDI) and on protecting confidentiality and security of health data through setting and enforcing standards. Thus, HIPAA presents efficiency and security as integrated requirements.

The HIPAA security rule is presented as a set of security safeguards divided into three categories – administrative, physical, and technical – for the purpose of guarding data integrity, confidentiality, and availability. The standards were designed for implementation by organizations of all sizes to help promote advances in technology and enable organizations to choose how to implement solutions. While the standards can be met in a variety of ways that are considered reasonable and appropriate to each specific organization, organizations are required to meet the standards. An implementation specification is an additional requirement, within a standard, that provides specific direction to the implementation. This chapter focuses on providing a set of implementation specifications for enterprise mHealth applications. While HIPAA is considered to provide broad guidance, it has also been compared with other security frameworks. For example, one assessment found HIPAA to be more stringent in seven categories than the international security framework ISO 17799:2005 [5]. These frameworks do not, however, provide a "how to" implementation guide to healthcare providers, though significant demand exists for such frameworks.

2.3 *mHealth Security Guidance from the Office of the National Coordinator*

The Office of the National Coordinator (ONC) for Health Information Technology, U.S. Department of Health and Human Services, conducted a multiagency workshop on March 16, 2012, followed by 30 days of public comment for the purpose of "gather[ing] tips and information that would be most useful to healthcare providers and professionals using mobile devices in their work" [20]. The result was a set of guidelines released on the ONC website to help healthcare providers protect and secure patient health information when using mobile devices [21]. While the content is "provided for informational purposes only and does not guarantee compliance with federal or state laws," it does provide a high-level practical guide, which is in high demand due to the confusion surrounding privacy and security compliance in the realm of designing mHealth systems. The research described in this chapter used this high-level guidance as a starting place and added the requirements across interorganizational participants to illustrate how one multi-organizational, enterprise-level, mobile system applied these principles and how these principles map to high-level federal guidance (i.e., HIPAA). Thus, this study aims to substantiate the principles presented herein and to formulate a normative architecture and heuristic for the design and implementation of future mHealth systems.

3 Research and Design Methods

Design science research (DSR) has been known for its practicality in creating and evaluating information technology (IT) artifacts that address an organizational problem [22]. The design science methodology includes conceptual principles, practice rules (guidelines), and a procedure for carrying out the research [22, 23]. The primary design, development, and evaluation of the artifact component of this study are based on the DSRM process model and include problem identification, defining the objective of a solution, design and development, artifact demonstration, evaluation, and communication [23].

3.1 Solution Objective

The objective of the research team was to develop a secure yet usable mHealth application to support interorganizational emergency medical services (EMS). Paramedics used the mobile application to collect on-scene pre-hospital information, including multimedia data, and submit it to a receiving hospital prior to the patient's arrival. We have noted that HIPAA Section 164.312(a)(1) provides for an emergency access procedure to bypass some security safeguards in order to more efficiently obtain the necessary PHI during an emergency. Nevertheless, the law maintains that security should not disappear completely in cases of emergency. In addition, the law does not specify that collecting and transmitting PHI during an emergency is equivalent to accessing PHI during an emergency. Thus, for the purposes of this application, we have assumed that HIPAA applies to the collection, storage, and transmission of PHI during a medical emergency.

3.2 Security Requirements

Emergency practitioners requested a unique set of characteristics in the design of a mobile application. First, the application must be available to users with or without an available data network connection, and a record must be sent immediately when data network connectivity is detected. This is particularly important in rural and remote areas with intermittent network connectivity. Second, users must be able to record and send an audio report to a receiving emergency department, as audio communication between medics and emergency department staff is expected. Third, the system must be able to collect images and video. Fourth, the system must be simple to use, interfering at little as possible with patient care. And fifth, the system must be able to send patient data efficiently and with high reliability.

3.3 Security Risks and Practices

Several security risk scenarios have been associated with mHealth applications, including lost or stolen mobile devices, unintentional downloads of viruses or other malware, or use of an unsecured Wi-Fi network. To mitigate these risks, as well as a myriad of others, 11 security practices were proposed for the design and implementation of mHealth applications. These practices, adopted and published on the ONC website (www.healthIT.gov), appear in Table 1. Additional security requirements from case study participants included deleting all encrypted patient information from the device at the conclusion of patient handover; simple multi-factor authentication; same device used for each crew number (associated with an ambulance); >99% reliability to send patient records to the ER; and more specific implementation requirements described further below. These security practices were incorporated into the application design, and performance metrics were used to evaluate usability as indicated by average use time, average time to encrypt, average response time, and the value perceived by users.

Table 1 Security threats vs. security guidance

Security threat	ONC mHealth security guidance	HIPAA compliance
Loss, theft of devices, malicious insider actions, and data-communication interception	1. The use of user-authentication mechanism 2. The use of encryption 3. The use of remote device activation and data wiping mechanisms 4. The use of a policy to maintain physical control of mobile devices 5. The ability to delete all stored health information before discarding or reusing the mobile device	164.312(a)(1) Access Control 164.312(d) Authentication 164.312(c)(1) Integrity 164.310(d) Physical Control
Malware, phishing, social engineering, direct attack by hackers and spoofing	6. The use of a policy to disable and to not install file-sharing applications 7. The use of a firewall 8. The use of security software 9. The use of a mechanism/policy to keep security software up-to-date 10. The use of a policy to enforce researching mobile applications (apps) before downloading	164.312(a)(1) Access Control
Data communication interception	11. The ability to maintain adequate security to send or receive health information over public Wi-Fi networks	164.312(e)(1) Transmission Security

3.4 Design and Development

The artifact is the mHealth application, which consists of a mobile application used to collect pre-hospital patient information in emergency medical settings via an Android smartphone. Digital voice recordings (i.e., the paramedic's verbal patient report), pictures, video, and patient data (e.g., age, gender, date of birth, name, patient indicators, patient interventions) are then sent to the receiving hospital's emergency department prior to patient arrival. Researchers engaged paramedics, nurses, and emergency physicians to determine user requirements and to design, develop, and test the application in multiple iterations. The resulting application was field-tested in 20 ambulances and seven hospital emergency departments transmitting live patient information.

3.5 System Overview

As shown in Fig. 2, the system consists of a mobile smartphone equipped with an application by which paramedics/emergency medical technicians (EMTs) can securely capture pictures, digital audio recordings, video, patient indicators, and incident information and send it securely to the ER (via phone call, text, email, or iPad application).

The information collected at the scene can be viewed through a secure web-based interface, via an iPad application for practitioners on demand, or via phone calls to registered phone numbers. To address the system's security and privacy dimensions, the ONC and HIPAA guidance, along with participant requirements, was applied and incorporated into the mHealth system design.

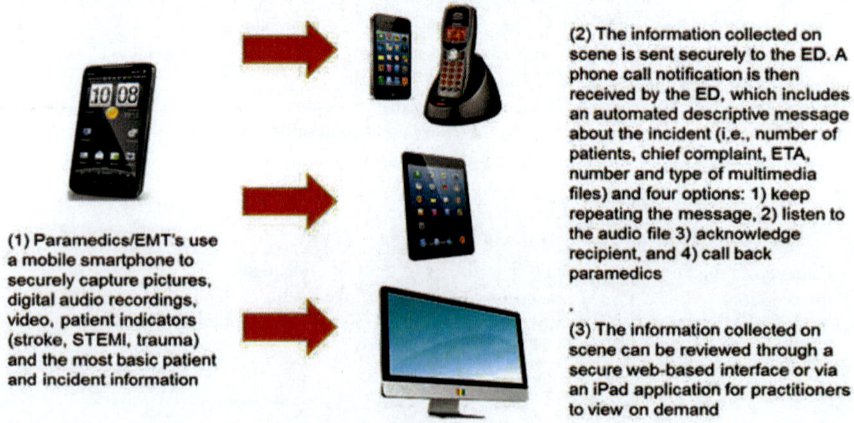

Fig. 2 CrashHelp information exchange process

3.6 Usability for Time-Critical Emergency Care

Critical to the application were end-user requirements that the mobile application be useful across a time-critical workflow. Users wanted the application to be just as easy to use as their existing two-way radios yet have more utility. For example, users wanted to be able to record data when they wanted, as opposed to requiring someone on the other end of the radio to "pick up" before communicating. Asynchronous communications; easy to enter data elements; single touch capability to take pictures, add video, and record dictation notes to be sent to the ER; and quick selection of final hospital destination were paramount features for the app not getting in the way of patient care. These features were considered along with the security features detailed below.

3.7 Usability and User Authentication

To send a patient record, a unique personal identification number (PIN) must be entered that is associated with each mobile user (paramedic) and his/her organization. In order to balance usability with security, the mHealth application implemented PINs instead of usernames and passwords. Entering long passwords was considered too time-consuming for paramedics involved in emergency incidents. Even though HIPAA does not explicitly define the required level of authentication, Luxton and colleagues propose that two-factor authentication be considered and discussed within the field [4]. In our system, we authenticate the device ID together with the user-entered PIN and digital certificate residing within the app. This system authenticates paramedics and mobile devices to specific organizations; thus, the server checks the mobile user's password, the mobile device's serial number, and the organization to which the user belongs to enhance user efficiency in emergency situations. The device screen lock-out mechanism is also used and is set to time out after a period of inactivity (duration can be configured). The screen unlocks using a unique PIN separate from the app PIN.

3.8 Encryption

Encryption can be defined as the process of encoding data in a way that only authorized personnel can read it. Encryption may not eliminate the risk of reading the data by hackers, but it definitely reduces that risk to a low percentage depending on the encryption's strength and hackers' knowledge of cryptography. In subsequent sections, we discuss encrypting data as it is (1) stored temporarily in the mobile device and (2) transferred securely to the system server. We control this process as opposed to allowing the device and/or Android system defaults in order to maintain process control.

Patient information collected by paramedics is saved in hidden files on the device and encrypted periodically or prior to transmitting data, whichever occurs first. The requirement is to ensure efficient encryption to avoid delaying emergency data transmission to an emergency department. The file encryption applied is an integrated cryptosystem, also called "hybrid mode." This hybrid mode encryption uses a symmetric key encryption to encrypt the message while using an asymmetric key encryption to encrypt the symmetric key used to encrypt the message [24]. Therefore, the message representing the largest amount of data is encrypted using a light encryption (the symmetric encryption) [25]; the key to decrypt it, which is small in size, is encrypted using a strong technique (the asymmetric encryption), as shown in Fig. 4. The integrated symmetric and asymmetric key cryptosystem enables safe key distribution and fast performance by combining the convenience of a public-key cryptosystem with the efficiency of a symmetric-key cryptosystem.

All data communication and transmission between the mobile device and the system server is accomplished over an encrypted channel using Secure Socket Layer/Transport Layer Security (SSL/TLS).

3.9 Remote Device Activation and Data Wiping

The mHealth app can only be installed, reinstalled, updated, activated, and deactivated by a system administrator. The app cannot be downloaded from an online marketplace. This is managed using mobile device management (MDM) functionality internal to the server-side application, as opposed to using a third-party vendor. This is to maintain organizational control over the app distribution and utilization itself. The system administrator sends a download link to a specific device, downloads and installs the app to the device, and then enters a unique activation code to open and enable its use. Only system administrators and representatives of authorized organizations (i.e., hospital, ambulance provider) can initiate the activation by using the server-side MDM Administrator Portal.

As noted in Sect. 3.7, after a paramedic creates a patient record in the mobile application, all data is encrypted periodically to the device. Once the record is sent, all encrypted files are wiped from the device. In the case of a "send" failure, the encrypted records are purged automatically after 24 hours (or other configurable time frame). This purging mechanism may provide an alternative to having a remote mechanism wipe data off the phone if the device is lost or stolen. When necessary, the system administrator can wipe data off the phone manually via the mandated third-party security suite installed on all phones. More details are provided below.

3.10 *Policy to Disable and/or Not Install File-Sharing Applications*

Each separate organization that uses the application determines its own practice for users to install applications, which can pose a significant security risk. Instead, we recommend an MDM policy that does not allow users to download any apps. This policy could be enforced through configuring user profiles on mobile devices to restrict installation of any file-sharing applications. A second mechanism for enforcing such restrictions is peer review: Each device is assigned to a paramedic ambulance unit (team), in which each unit works on one ambulance per work shift. The device is passed from one medic unit to the next, which can review if any apps have been downloaded.

3.11 *Firewall and Security Software*

We have enforced the policy that all mobile devices have a third-party security suite installed. This is to enable protection to stop unwanted intrusions from hacking into the mobile device. As noted in Sect. 3.8, a comprehensive third-party security suite is installed on all smartphones. The comprehensive third-party security suite is configured to receive daily automatic updates to keep current with known threats. Although we have enforced a "no downloading" policy, the security software suite is equipped with a "security advisor" feature. This feature helps users avoid risky behavior, such as downloading malicious applications.

3.12 *Physical Control of Mobile Devices*

While bring-your-own-device (BYOD) initiatives have been gaining traction in the business world with enhanced security due to MDM and device virtualization, we have enforced a policy that prohibits the use of personal mobile devices. The mHealth application described here is only installed on EMS agency-owned mobile devices, checked out by on-duty medic units, and managed by the aforementioned MDM software and system administrator. This is because of well-documented hacks to MDM software on personal phones. To maintain adequate security for sending or receiving health information over public Wi-Fi networks, data files must be encrypted locally on the device, and all data communication and transmission with the server must be communicated over an encrypted channel using SSL-TLS.

3.13 Deletion of All Stored Health Information Before Discarding or Reusing the Mobile Device

As noted in Sect. 3.8, all data are wiped after the completion of each record transmission. The only remaining data are log file data that contain no personal health information – just information about the use of the application. Devices are destroyed when they will no longer be used for collecting patient information. Some security practices described above overlap to prevent one type (dimension) of security threats, but some do not. Table 2 summarizes the security dimensions and their associated interventions.

4 Demonstration

The mHealth application was developed, tested, refined, and then field-tested with paramedics. A 10-month pilot test conducted in the Boise, Idaho, region included the following participating organizations: Ada County Paramedics, Canyon County Paramedics, St. Alphonsus Boise Hospital, St. Alphonsus Nampa Hospital, St. Alphonsus Eagle Hospital, St. Luke's Boise Hospital, St. Luke's Meridian Hospital, and West Valley Medical Center. Twenty ambulances across two agencies were each provided with a mobile smartphone for the duration of the pilot test, through sponsorship of the Idaho EMS Bureau. The system was used for transmitting and receiving 1513 patient records and over 300 pictures and 1000 voice-recorded patient descriptions during the pilot test. The application demonstrated the use

Table 2 Summary of security dimensions and interventions

	SAD	SAC	SDD	SDC
App activation/deactivation	X			
PIN number		X		
Device lock password		X		
File encryption			X	
Delete data after record is sent			X	
Remote data wipe			X	
Disable download outside the market			X	
Disable install file-sharing apps			X	
Anti-virus software		X	X	
Update anti-virus software		X	X	
Firewall		X		
No use of personal devices		X	X	
TLS/SSL communication encryption				X

SAD Secure application distribution, *SAC* Secure access to devices, *SDD* Secure on-device data, *SDC* Secure data communication

Table 3 Summary of usability evaluation metrics

Factor	Metric	Description	Section
Efficiency	Encryption time Use time Response time	The time to: Encrypt incident's files Create an incident Transmit an incident	Efficiency
Effectiveness	Task/record completion	The number of times task was accomplished	Effectiveness
Accuracy	Incidents transmittal success rate	Percentage of successfully transmitted incidents	Reliability
Satisfaction	Qualitative analysis of users' experience	Asked users to comment on value of using the system	User Perceived Value (Satisfaction)

and value of integrating multimedia information into the pre-hospital to hospital communication process. Approximately 46% of all paramedics ($n = 81$) used the application at least once, and more than 15% of paramedics used the system at least ten times. Although paramedics were not required to use the system at any time, the consistency and frequency of their use provided a solid base of experience to draw from and enhanced the validity of research evaluation findings. A summary of findings from the pilot evaluation is presented below, in Sect. 5.

5 Evaluation

The goal of this study was to provide researchers and practitioners with an example and heuristic for designing practitioner-oriented mHealth applications that achieve both security and usability goals. As noted in Table 3, this study breaks usability into the following components: (1) efficiency measured by encryption time, transmission time, and use time; (2) effectiveness measured by completion of record transmittals (also called total number of task successes); (3) accuracy measured by success rate of incident transmittals; (4) satisfaction measured by qualitative feedback on users' perceived value of the system; and (5) learnability (ease of use) measured by qualitative feedback from users on system's ease of use.

5.1 Data Analysis

For the first three measures (efficiency, effectiveness, and accuracy), the research team analyzed log files collected from mobile devices. Each phone collected multiple log files, with each log file representing one incident record. Data were collected from each of the 16 mobile devices used by paramedics, with each phone having between 400 and 480 log files. The log files capture the paramedic's experience with using the mobile device and were designed to capture predefined

Table 4 An example of actions captured inside a log file

2013-05-20 13:53:52 MDT	Click	Start incident
2013-05-20 13:53:52 MDT	Incident	New incident created
2013-05-20 13:53:52 MDT	Application	Camera tab displayed
2013-05-20 13:53:57 MDT	Application	Audio tab displayed
2013-05-20 13:53:57 MDT	Click	Audio tab clicked
2013-05-20 13:53:58 MDT	Click	Audio recording start

actions for the measurement of specified tasks. In other words, log files capture every click or navigation (also called an action) that occurs while using the mobile app. Table 4 presents a sample of six actions inside a log file. For our analysis, we used a random sample chosen by selecting one of the phones at random. This sample included 460 log files, from which we excluded 121 log files that were either (1) the output of application testing and not the result of real usage or (2) statistical outliers, due to starting but not completing a record (>10 minutes elapsed usage time). As the average transport time from the emergency scene to the hospital is 7–13 minutes, participants indicated that use times longer than 10 minutes would not be representative of normal use. Average use time of the excluded records is 1 hour and 51 minutes and 12 seconds (1:51:12); thus, they were eliminated from examination. Details on calculating the average use time are provided in section "Use Time".

Table 4 comprises three columns and six rows, with the three columns capturing the date/time when an action occurred, the type of user action, and a brief task description. Each row represents one action, and this sample illustrates a short list of only six actions. On average, log files contain 20–40 rows, depending on the user's engagement with the app for a particular incident.

Efficiency

This study measures efficiency in terms of (1) practitioner usage time; (2) encryption time of an average-size patient record, compared to the times for other encryption algorithms found in the literature; and (3) record transmission response time over a cellular network. Details about each measure are provided in sections below.

Use Time

Use time is the time a paramedic spends completing a set of tasks that result in sending one patient record – the time from record initiation until clicking "Send." This may include the time a user spends on each of the mobile app's four screens, also called tabs. The four tabs, illustrated in Fig. 3, are Camera (to take a picture or record a video), Audio (to record an audio), Patient (to enter the patient's information such as name, gender, date of birth, incident type, and interventions

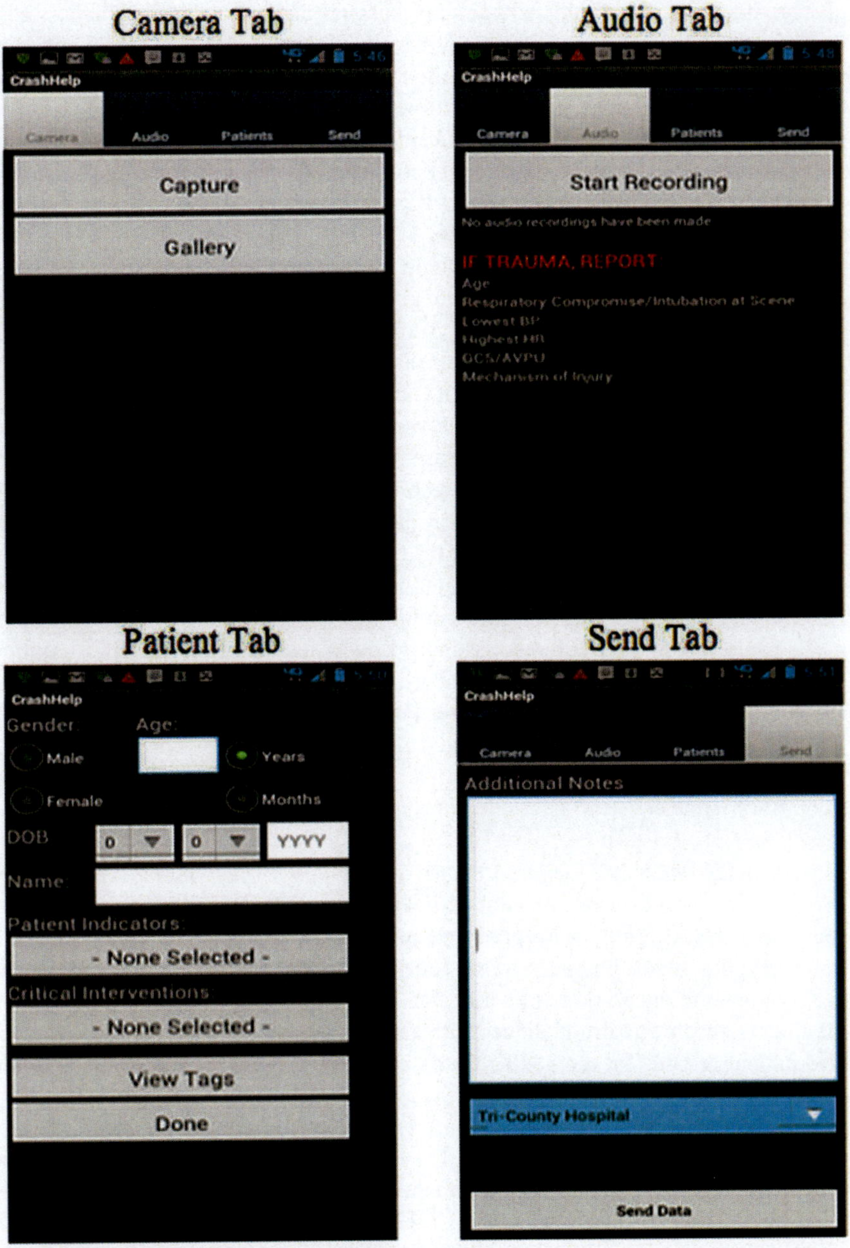

Fig. 3 The four tabs (screens) of the mHealth app

given), and Send (to select the receiving hospital and enter the paramedic's PIN number to send an incident). Paramedics were allowed to use the mobile app with no restrictions. The users' varying skill levels with using smartphones may have been an important factor in their use time. This justifies the reason we used the average use time as a metric instead of using one random use time record.

Analysis of the log files showed that paramedics spend an average of 31 seconds at the Camera tab, 45 seconds using the Audio tab, 63 seconds (~1 minute) at the Patient tab, and 27 seconds at the Send tab. If all four tabs were used for each incident, the average use time would be the sum of the individual averages: 166 seconds (~2.8 minutes). However, our records showed that paramedics used the Camera tab in 22% of incidents, the Audio tab in 78% of incidents, the Patient tab in 46% of incidents, and the Send tab in 100% of incidents. Therefore, the weighted average use time is the sum of Camera tab use (31 seconds * 0.22), Audio tab use (45 seconds * 0.78), Patient tab use (63 seconds * 0.46), and Send tab use (27 seconds * 1.0), yielding an average use time for the mHealth app of 97.7 seconds (~1.6 minutes). Although researchers recorded the amount of time users expended to successfully capture and send patient data, it is not known whether users were continually using the application during that time period. Participant interviews noted that typical use of the app included intermittent use when not caring for the patient. Thus, the app was not used continuously. Other responses indicated that participants did not feel the use of the app was less efficient than the required two-way radios that have a gold standard 30-second use time. Analysis of user satisfaction is described in section "User Perceived Value (Satisfaction)".

Encryption Time

Silva et al. [26] evaluated the performance of four types of encryptions (AES, 3DES, RC4, and Blowfish) on seven mobile devices using an mHealth application and found that the AES algorithm produced better results. As mentioned in Sect. 3.8, our encryption algorithm is a hybrid mode encryption that utilizes both symmetric and asymmetric encryptions (see Fig. 4). The phones used by paramedics during the field test were Motorola phones with a processor speed of 1 GHz. The average-size patient record (for the 1513 records sent during the pilot test) contained one 27-second long audio file (28 KB), one picture image (451 KB), and basic text information (4 KB). Taken together, the average size of a patient record was 483 KB. AES takes 0.0045 seconds to encrypt that same amount of data (483 KB) using the same phone; by comparison, we found that our application encrypted the data in an average of 0.0028 seconds, which was acceptable to study participants as they did not find this to be a barrier to efficient use.

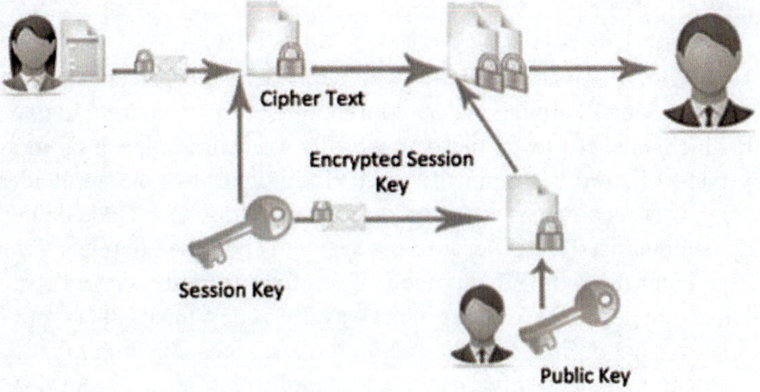

Fig. 4 Integrated symmetric and asymmetric key cryptosystem (hybrid mode)

Response Time Over Cellular Networks

Our definition of response time is similar to round-trip time (RTT) used in telecommunications. In this study, response time is the time interval between the app sending a patient record to the server over a cellular network and receiving a message from the server indicating that all information has been received. Patient records vary in size depending on the number of images sent, the length of the audio and video files, and the size of the text recording basic patient information such as name, gender, age, mechanism of injury, and intervention, as input by paramedics at the emergency scene. For more than 1500 patient records sent by paramedics, the average recorded response time across all records was 11.42 seconds. However, the response time for sending one average-size patient record (483 KB), is 7.4 seconds. The longer response time calculated over 1500 patient records was due to several large outlier response time records that resulted from user errors (e.g., forgetting to stop the audio or video recordings). This was considered an acceptable response time by study participants.

Effectiveness

The international standard ISO 9241-11 presents effectiveness in terms of the extent to which users can complete tasks and achieve desirable goals. In our study, effectiveness is measured by the total number of tasks completed by paramedics – including number of completed reports sent, recorded audio files, captured images, and videos – and made available to emergency departments. Across all 1513 records, there were 1121 completed audio files, 306 images captured with the camera, and five captured videos. The qualitative analysis discussed in Sect. 5.2 describes the utility of these completed tasks.

Reliability

In the context of this study, reliability is defined as the percent of successfully transmitted incidents. Through our random sample of log files, we found nine errors out of 460 incidents. However, these nine errors were all of type "user input error," meaning that users did not input the right PIN number to send an incident. Even though they were recorded as errors in log files, we chose to exclude them from our reliability calculation. This is because the system is designed to reject access when users fail to enter the right PIN numbers. Therefore, from the system's standpoint, the system responded to these errors in the way it was designed. Other types of errors we searched for but did not find are "server errors," meaning either that the server was down or the connection was lost, and "application errors," meaning that the phone app did not function properly or crashed. Therefore, according to our random sample, the system's reliability is at 100%, greater than the required reliability of >99%.

A more complete reliability assessment should inherit the reliability of the other systems for which our application depends on. For example, we are hosting our data and server application on Amazon Cloud instances. According to Amazon, the server up time is 99.99%. Another factor is the cell phone coverage ratio for the geographic area where the application was used. We did not experience failures in this regard, and we believe this was partially the result of our algorithm to continue resending a record if/when cell coverage is not detected. Even so, it is still conceivable that a cell connection could be unavailable for a long period of time, which could result in a transmission error. Hence, it is expected that the reliability percentage could decrease below 99.99% in areas with limited cell phone coverage, such as rural areas. We were not able to determine the reliability of these dependencies and thus report only that which we were able to measure.

5.2 *Qualitative Analysis*

User Perceived Value (Satisfaction)

Researchers sought to understand whether the application response times and use times were acceptable to users, the general attitudes of users toward the system, and whether security features previously described were perceived as barriers to efficient data collection and transmission. At the conclusion of the pilot test, field visits were made to each participating organization. Qualitative data were collected via a series of focus groups and semi-structured interviews with 22 paramedics who had used the system at least once during the pilot test. All interviewees signed a consent form to voluntarily participate in this research. A series of questions were asked to understand perceptions about the system's utilization, usability, and efficiency (see Appendix A). Despite the mobile application being designed to comply with the security practices, none of the paramedics perceived performance degradation or use complexity. Instead, paramedics described how using the smartphone application did not seem to interfere with current on-scene medical care practices and, in some cases, assisted current processes more effectively than using traditional two-way radios to communicate with emergency departments.

More generally, paramedics found the system valuable for augmenting current practices. For example, the system permitted the audio recordings to be retained and accessed by downstream medical practitioners in the hospital. One paramedic explained:

> Like a radio report sent, they [the hospitals] need this report.

Paramedic participants also described how the design of the mobile health application aided efficient data entry and on-scene multitasking. For example, one participant noted:

> I take pictures or do the audio while I'm walking to the rig. Maybe it's a generational thing, but I use it while I'm doing other things, so you know it doesn't really get in the way more than what we already do.

Other paramedics thought the system was most valuable with severe incidents, especially when using pictures to describe the intensity of crash accidents or trauma situations. Asked when the system is most valuable, one paramedic replied:

> Well, like I said, the scene of an MVC, just to understand it a little bit better, would be helpful for us; trauma situations where the presentation would certainly affect the initial interventional process, meaning like an open fracture or something that was very deformed or a foreign body that is like, 'Wow, that shouldn't be there,' not just your ordinary things.

To our surprise, some paramedics saw value in using the system to validate a patient's medical condition, especially for patients who recover by the time they reach the hospital. When asked for examples, two paramedics responded:

> We had an elderly man that was having a stroke. We took a picture of him sitting up, and you could definitely see the whole side was down and he was looking bad. Then you saw the next picture when he's lying on the stretcher. Then on the next one, he's sitting up smiling, everything has resolved, and he's back. When you come in and tell the doctor what you saw in the field and they're like 'okay!' [a skeptical expression] ... it's not the same as seeing it as a picture.

Preregistration is another use of the system that was previously not possible. Before introduction of our secure system, paramedics were not allowed to send identifying patient information (e.g., name and date of birth) over the radio due to concerns about patient security. Because radio devices use the air medium for communication, intruders could easily tune to these communication frequencies and listen to the information. Preregistration also helps expedite patients' treatments. In addition, over 70% of patients who come to the emergency rooms are return patients, meaning that their name and date of birth could be used to pull up their medical history, if needed. One charge nurse shared a real example, in which a patient had to be transported to the hospital by air transport. Within the 20-minute transport time, the emergency department personnel were able to use the patient's name and date of birth to review the medical history and also contacted the primary physician with quick questions. By the time the patient arrived at the hospital, the room had been assigned, and the necessary medical personnel had assembled to start immediate interventions. Such high-quality information requires a sophisticated system to facilitate the communication, and this leads to an important question: "How hard is it to learn to use the system?" Section "Learnability (Ease of Use)" will address this question.

Learnability (Ease of Use)

This study defines learnability as the degree of difficulty experienced by users while learning to use the system efficiently. One of the major design goals of our system is to build a sophisticated but easy-to-use system to facilitate the information exchange between paramedics and ED personnel. Due to the nature of EMS personnel's busy work schedules, it should be possible to learn to use the system with minimal training. To this end, both in-person and web-based training sessions were conducted in September and October 2012 for each participating organization. The hands-on training sessions lasted approximately 1 hour. For participants who could not attend live sessions, a video-recorded training session was distributed via a web-based education and training system. Training materials, including user guides, quick reference guides, and log-in information, were distributed to participants. Technical implementation guides and documentation were distributed to information technology (IT) staff at each participating organization. Asked to comment on ease of use, users had a range of responses. In general, more positive comments have been received from the younger EMS personnel. One paramedic said:

> I actually found it (the system) to be faster and more user-friendly than actually calling in to the hospital. And I think probably a lot of that is generational things.

On the other hand, one paramedic thought the buttons on the mobile device were too small for his "fat thumbs," which made patient information entry very time-consuming. Suggested interventions would minimize interacting with the mobile device by hand and might include the use of wearable devices.

6 Discussion

6.1 A Heuristic for Security Implementation

Analysis demonstrates that the ONC guidelines for mHealth application security may be useful as a heuristic, or guide, for developing future mHealth applications. Further, the case example described in this chapter demonstrates that the guidelines can be implemented while balancing usability goals. However, the degree to which the ONC guidelines can be followed may depend on the case context in which the application is used. The password is a clear example of how the context may play a role in the degree of usability required. According to ONC guidelines, the password should be a strong password that is at least six characters long and combines letters (uppercase and lowercase) and numbers. Yet such passwords might not be appropriate for mHealth apps for EMS due to the time-critical nature of their work. Our initial feedback from paramedics who tested the app was that passwords should be as short and simple as possible. One way to avoid strong password complaints from health practitioners would be to use biometric fingerprints (or another marker) associated with each user. At the time of our study, the Android phones limited the number of fingerprint profiles allowed, thus limiting the number of paramedics that could use the phone. As such, this limitation did not fit with the chosen workflow model to pass the phone along to multiple shifts of paramedic crews. Another solution would be to separate the device's password from the app's password. Making the device password in compliance with security guidelines was acceptable to the affected healthcare organizations because paramedics could enter the password on their way to an emergency scene. However, the app's password, which must be entered when sending patient information from the scene to the hospital, could be as simple as a four-digit PIN. It is clear that the context of the case created this trade-off between security and usability and is critical to consider when designing security guidelines for mHealth applications.

Another factor to highlight regarding security guidelines is the lack of specificity for most interorganizational mHealth security systems. Guidelines have not been designed to be specific but addressed on a case-by-case basis. They also generally do not address which security components can be fulfilled using third-party software applications vs. built-in hardware functionality. In today's mobile computing environment, designers of mHealth can adhere to more than 35% of security guidelines noted herein using third-party software default configurations. In sum, the heuristic for practitioner-oriented interorganizational mHealth security implementation includes the following considerations: ONC mHealth guidelines, specific end-user (health practitioner) usability goals for the specified health context, and interorganizational security requirements (agreed upon by participating organizations).

6.2 Security Context: Extending the Security Heuristic for Time- and Information-Critical Systems

In a fast-paced and time-critical working environment such as EMS, mHealth applications must perform efficiently to achieve improvement in emergency health services. At the same time, healthcare organizations cannot allow security to be compromised in the interests of urgency. As shown in Sect. 5 of this chapter, both quantitative and qualitative analysis supported the efficiency of the mHealth application and its value in improving communication between ambulance providers and hospital emergency departments. However, for emergency care, none of the security or usability measures evaluated in this chapter matter if patient care is inhibited. Thus, an important heuristic is patient centeredness, or the ability of the app to facilitate patient-centered care. Among its strong points is the capacity of mHealth apps to provide HIPAA-compliant patient information capture, storage, and transmission capabilities without (1) harming the patient (due to delayed care and/or PHI breaches) and (2) delaying the practitioner on both ends of the communication (paramedics and ER staff) to accomplish their patient care duties. Rather, the system should provide value to enhance care as was perceived by the participants of this study (in the form of enabling patient decisions sooner in the interorganizational care process). Table 1 presented potential security threats when using a mobile technology in healthcare. These can and must be addressed but can be accomplished while also considering patient safety and practitioner efficiency as was demonstrated in this research study.

7 Conclusion

This study demonstrated and tested comprehensive mHealth security practices along with accomplishment of usability goals through a live implementation. The emergency medical services application described herein was pilot tested in a live field-test environment to observe its combined utility, usability, and security. The application was designed using frameworks from literature, ONC guidance, and stakeholder requirements. This research makes several contributions. In this article, we illustrate an integrated approach to securing PHI and suggest an approach for designing and implementing security practices for practitioner-oriented mHealth applications. Further, the interorganizational EMS context may be applicable to other interorganizational, time-critical patient care settings where continuity of care is critical to achieving positive outcomes. It provides a set of illustrations and heuristics for addressing mHealth security and usability together in contexts where information must be shared across multiple healthcare providers. In addition, the study helps substantiate and elaborate on the mHealth security design principles proposed by ONC.

While this study focused on the security of mobile devices issued by a healthcare organization to practitioners for intermittent and temporary use, future studies should investigate personal device models for securing mHealth applications (e.g., BYOD). Further, continued research bridging usability and security trade-offs in a mobile healthcare environment should consider the growing wearable device market (e.g., smartwatches, glasses, etc.). These studies should be undertaken with emphasis on patient-centered care workflows and practitioner needs for high efficiency, effectiveness, and safety. The study of design trade-offs in an integrated, complex, dynamic, and "live" test environment, such as the one presented herein, also provides valuable insights for practice to enhance planning and implementation of interorganizational mHealth systems.

The findings presented in this chapter are not meant to be a one-size-fits-all model. Rather, the goal is to provide an example of an implementation and live field test that may help to validate a set of guiding principles that can and should be developed and improved over time.

Acknowledgments This work was funded by the Federal Highway Administration, U.S. Department of Transportation. The authors would like to thank Yousef Abed for his excellent contributions to the system's design and implementation. A prior version of this manuscript has been published as a portion of Dr. Murad's dissertation by ProQuest Dissertations Publishing.

References

1. L. Washington, Managing health information in mobile devices. J. AHIMA **83**(7), 58 (2012)
2. World Health Organization, *mHealth: New Horizons for Health through Mobile Technologies: Second Global Survey on eHealth* (World Health Organization, Geneva, 2011)
3. D. Dagon, T. Martin, T. Starner, Mobile phones as computing devices: The viruses are coming! IEEE Pervasive Comput. **3**(4), 11–15 (2004)
4. D.D. Luxton, R.A. Kayl, M.C. Mishkind, mHealth data security: The need for HIPAA-compliant standardization. Telemed. e-Health **18**(4), 284–288 (2012)
5. G. Thomas, R.A. Botha, Secure mobile device use in healthcare guidance from HIPAA and ISO17799. Inf. Syst. Manag. **24**(4), 333–342 (2007)
6. V. Stanford, Pervasive health care applications face tough security challenges. IEEE Pervasive Computing **1**(2), 8–12 (2002)
7. M. Ahmed, M. Ahamad, Protecting health information on mobile devices, in *Proceedings of the Second ACM Conference on Data and Application Security and Privacy*, (ACM, New York, 2012), pp. 229–240
8. K. Patrick, W.G. Griswold, F. Raab, S.S. Intille, Health and the mobile phone. Am. J. Prev. Med. **35**(2), 177–181 (2008)
9. J. Friedman, D.V. Hoffman, Protecting data on mobile devices: A taxonomy of security threats to mobile computing and review of applicable defenses. Inf. Knowl. Syst. Manag. **7**(1), 159–180 (2008)
10. J. Sathyan, M. Sadasivan, Multi-layered collaborative approach to address enterprise mobile security challenges, in *2010 IEEE 2nd Workshop on Collaborative Security Technologies*, (2010), pp. 1–6
11. N. Bevan, Human-computer interaction standards. in *Advances in Human Factors/Ergonomics*, vol. 20, (Elsevier, 1995), pp. 885–890
12. A. Abran, A. Khelifi, W. Suryn, A. Seffah, Usability meanings and interpretations in ISO standards. Softw. Qual. J. **11**(4), 325–338 (2003)
13. C. Braz, A. Seffah, D. M'Raihi, *Designing a Trade-off Between Usability and Security: A Metrics Based-Model* (Springer, New York, 2007)
14. P. Gutmann, I. Grigg, Security usability. IEEE Secur. Priv **3**(4), 56–58 (2005)
15. K.-P. Yee, Aligning security and usability. IEEE Security & Privacy **2**(5), 48–55 (2004)
16. R. Kainda, I. Flechais, A. Roscoe (2010), Security and usability: Analysis and evaluation, in *2010 International Conference on Availability, Reliability and Security*, pp. 275–282. IEEE
17. J. Sorber, M. Shin, R. Peterson, C. Cornelius, S. Mare, A. Prasad, Z. Marois, E. Smithayer, D. Kotz (2012), An amulet for trustworthy wearable mHealth, in *Proceedings of the Twelfth Workshop on Mobile Computing Systems & Applications*, pp. 1–6. ACM
18. R. Gardner, S. Garera, M. Pagano, M. Green, A. Rubin, Securing medical records on smart phones, in *Proceedings of the First ACM Workshop on Security and Privacy in Medical and Home-Care Systems*, (ACM, New York, 2009), pp. 31–40

19. A. Josang, B. AlFayyadh, T. Grandison, M. AlZomai, J. McNamara (2007), Security usability principles for vulnerability analysis and risk assessment, in *Twenty-Third Annual Computer Security Applications Conference (ACSAC 2007)*, pp. 269–278. IEEE
20. L. Washington, Managing health information in mobile devices. J. AHIMA **83**(7), 58–60 (2012)
21. Office of the National Coordinator for Health IT (2013), Your mobile device and health information privacy and security. Washington, DC
22. A.R. Hevner, S.T. March, J. Park, S. Ram, Design science in information systems research. MIS Q. **28**(1), 75–105 (2004)
23. K. Peffers, T. Tuunanen, M.A. Rothenberger, S. Chatterjee, A design science research methodology for information systems research. J. Manag. Inf. Syst. **24**(3), 45–77 (2007)
24. E. Fujisaki, T. Okamoto, *Secure Integration of Asymmetric and Symmetric Encryption Schemes Advances in Cryptology — CRYPTO' 99* (Springer, Berlin/Heidelberg, 1999)
25. Z. Liu, X. Li, Z. Dong, *A Lightweight Encryption Algorithm for Mobile Online Multimedia Devices Web Information Systems – WISE 2004* (Springer Berlin, Heidelberg, 2004)
26. B.M. Silva, J.J. Rodrigues, F. Canelo, I.C. Lopes, L. Zhou, A data encryption solution for mobile health apps in cooperation environments. J. Med. Internet Res. **15**(4), e66 (2013). https://doi.org/10.2196/jmir.2498

Semantic Tree Driven Thyroid Ultrasound Report Generation by Voice Input

Lihao Liu, Mei Wang, Yijie Dong, Weiliang Zhao, Jian Yang, and Jianwen Su

1 Introduction

Ultrasound and other medical imaging are widely used in clinical practice for diagnosis and treatment [1–4]. For ultrasound, radiologists need to operate machines, examine images, provide professional interpretations of images, and write the explicit reports. It is challenging for radiologists to complete these tasks in a short time. Currently, ultrasound examinations normally require two medical staff in China, one for ultrasound checking and diagnosis, another one for data recording and report typing. This process causes a waste of human resources and the report writing is error-prone.

Currently, automatic speech recognition techniques [5–8] have become quite mature. Automatic speech recognition in the medical domain is gaining increasing interest in both academic and research areas. The recent study [9] demonstrates that

L. Liu · M. Wang · W. Zhao (✉)
School of Computer Science and Technology, Donghua University, Shanghai, China
e-mail: 2181757@mail.dhu.edu.cn; wangmei@dhu.edu.cn

Y. Dong
Department of Ultrasound, Ruijin Hospital, School of Medicine Shanghai Jiao Tong University, Shanghai, China
e-mail: dyj11584@rjh.com.cn

J. Yang
School of Computer Science and Technology, Donghua University, Shanghai, China

Computing Department, Macquarie University, Sydney, NSW, Australia
e-mail: jian.yang@dhu.edu.cn

J. Su
Department of Computer Science, University of California, Santa Barbara, CA, USA
e-mail: jianwen_su@ucsb.edu

H. R. Arabnia et al. (eds.), *Advances in Computer Vision and Computational Biology*, Transactions on Computational Science and Computational Intelligence,
https://doi.org/10.1007/978-3-030-71051-4_32

the accuracy rate of medical speech recognition is over 95%. The speech recognition tool Nuance [10] has an accuracy rate of 99% and is 3 times faster than typing. However, most of the current automatic speech recognition solutions in the medical domain focus on fast, accurate, and responsive clinical speech recognition [11–14]. There is still a gap from the simple speech recognition to generate comprehensive reports. A few applications [15–18] have been proposed for report generation via voice input. One existing way is to capture the voices of radiologists and translate them to text [15, 17]. The translation results are used as reports. As shown in Fig. 1, a medical report consists of several sections describing medical observations in detail. The translating voice-to-text method needs radiologists to speak out the whole ultrasound report, which slows down the ultrasound examination process. It is obviously an inefficient solution. Another popular way is to pre-define a set of templates in the system and select a template to generate a report [16, 18]. In this solution, the proper template is invoked at first. Then the radiologist speaks out the normal and abnormal observations which will be fed in the template. The application recognizes the voice and embeds the recognized text into the template. In such a way, the reports are generated according to templates. How to define, choose, and manage the templates is often quite challenging. If the observations show a big variance with the invoked template, it is difficult for the radiologist to modify the template by voice. So they need to return to typing it, resulting in additional workload. Normally, the pure templates-based solutions are lacking of the flexibility to deal with rich situations.

The aim of this work is to develop an automatic ultrasound report generation system with less voice input and more flexibility. It can be observed that radiologists follow certain patterns with semantic structures when they write ultrasound reports. Motivated by this idea, we construct the semantic structure by mining more than 40,000 real world thyroid ultrasound reports and getting the opinions of radiologist experts. Then we model the report generation process as a semantic tree driven sample generation process. Specifically, the report generation is decomposed into two stages. In the first stage, the radiologist only needs to input a few key descriptions by voice. The system can automatically generate the ultrasound semantic tree instance by analyzing the semantic relations between the inputs and the tree structure. A tree-to-text algorithm is employed in the second stage to generate the smooth and clear natural language text report. This solution can significantly save labor cost and improve the work efficiency. An example of an ultrasound report and the description input is shown in Fig. 1. The number of speech input characters is only 23.88% (16/67) of the characters in the report. This significantly reduces the radiologist's burden.

The main contributions of this work are:

- We design a system to automatically generate ultrasound reports via voice input. By incorporating the semantic tree structure, the radiologists do not need to follow the fixed templates. They just need to speak out their specific observations for individual patients. Our method generates the complete report automatically.

Ultrasound report	Individual description
术后，右叶：前后径：10mm，左右径： 1 2 3 4 5 6 7 8 9 10 11 12 13 9mm；左叶：前后径：9mm，左右径： 8mm；峡部已切除。残余甲状腺内部呈 密集中等回声，回声分布欠均匀。CDFI： 未见明显异常血流信号。 58 59 60 61 62 63 64 65 66 67	右叶，10，9，左叶，9， 1 2 3 4 5 6 7 8，峡部已切除，不均匀 8 9 10 11 12 13 14 15 16

Fig. 1 An example of an ultrasound report and the description input

- We develop algorithms to automatically generating long and semantic-coherent ultrasound reports based on the minimum inputs. The tree instance generation (TIG) algorithm is proposed to generate the semantic tree with keyword inputs. The tree-to-text (TTT) algorithm is proposed to generate text from a tree structure to ensure that the text has no redundant information and is fluent.
- We randomly selected practical ultrasound texts from the thyroid ultrasound examination data of a prestigious hospital in China to test the proposed system. The experimental results show that the proposed solution can generate accurate reports.

The rest of the paper is organized as follows. Section 2 presents the methodology for generating reports automatically, including the detailed process structure, the specification of the semantic tree, and the proposed algorithms. Section 3 provides the experimental results and analysis. Section 4 discusses the related work.

2 Methodology

In this section, we first provide an overview of the proposed method. Then, we present the structure of the semantic tree. Finally, we provide the details of two core algorithms as the tree instance generation (TIG) algorithm and the tree-to-text (TTT) algorithm.

2.1 Overview

Figure 2 shows an overview of our proposed solution. The system input is the description for an individual patient. The embedded speech recognition interface parses and translates the voice into text. After that, the ultrasound semantic tree instance generation module (TIG algorithm) is invoked to generate the semantic tree instance and the text generation module (TTT algorithm) is invoked to generate the report. Exception management module automatically updates the ultrasound semantic tree based on the execution log as adding the missing attributes in the

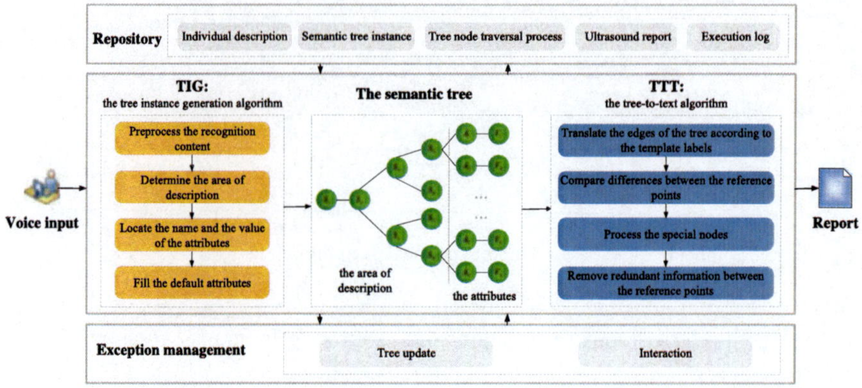

Fig. 2 Overview of the proposed solution

semantic tree. When encountering problems such as semantic logic conflict, the system will interact with radiologists to solve these problems and generate the proper semantic tree instance. The ultrasound information repository holds both the intermediate results and the final results including the individual descriptions, generated semantic tree instances, tree node traversal process records, execution logs, and the ultrasound reports.

It should be noticed that all the examples of report generation in this paper are in Chinese. Actually the report generation process in other languages will be the same. Although this work focuses on the thyroid ultrasound report generation, the method has the generality which can be easily modified to satisfy the requirements of other types of ultrasound report generation.

2.2 *Semantic Tree*

By analyzing the structures and contents of more than 40,000 thyroid ultrasound reports and discussing with the thyroid ultrasound experts, we specify the semantic tree $\mathcal{T}$ as the hierarchical representation of the thyroid ultrasound report. The nodes of $\mathcal{T}$ are labeled with organs/regions (area examined), the attribute names (what are examined), and the attribute values (what are observed). The edges of $\mathcal{T}$ denote the "is a part of" relationship, region-attribute, and attribute value relationship. The thyroid ultrasound semantic tree has three subtrees, which are thyroid subtree, parathyroid subtree, and cervical lymph node subtree, respectively. Each subtree includes the area layers, the attribute name layer, and the attribute value layer. The tree instance generated based on semantic tree T is illustrated in Fig. 3.

We further calculate the probability of each attribute and attribute value in different description ranges under abnormal and normal conditions, and then divide the attributes in the ultrasound semantic tree into three categories: (1) the normal

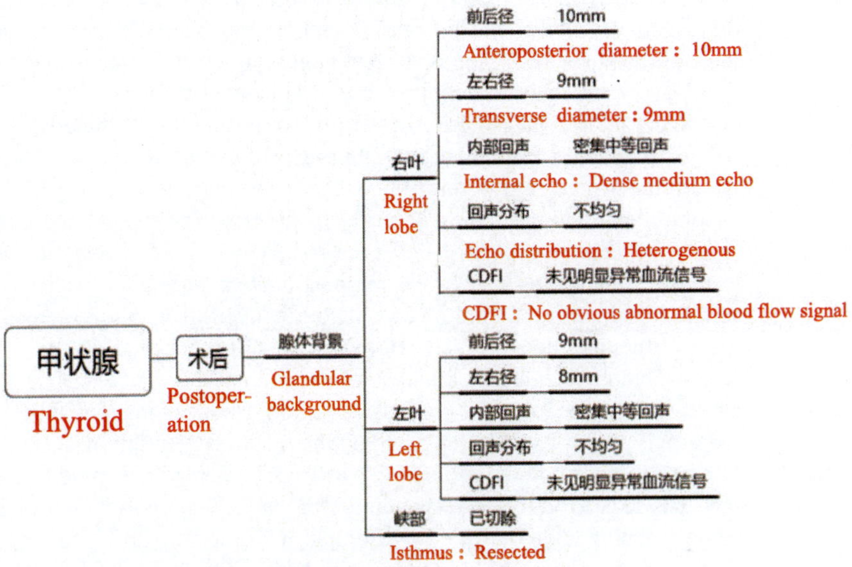

Fig. 3 The semantic tree instance of the example

attribute set; (2) the required attribute set, including attributes that must be abnormal when the lesion is present and is intended to alert the radiologist if there is any omission of ultrasound information; (3) the supplementary attribute set, including attributes that the radiologist can optionally describe, which may not be displayed in the ultrasound report when the attributes are normal. There is no intersection between/among these three attribute sets.

2.3 *Algorithms*

TIG

TIG is used to generate semantic tree instance according to the voice input. The instance of the semantic tree $\mathcal{T}$ is denoted as T, for which the nodes and the edges are the subset of $\mathcal{T}$. Given the individual description voice input $I = \{s_1, s_2, \ldots, s_n\}$, where s_i is the string to describe the key information of the individual observations. By analyzing the relationships between s_i and the nodes in $\mathcal{T}$, also the logical order of s_i with other s_j, $j \in \{1, 2, \ldots, i-1, i+1, \ldots, n\}$, we design a series of rules to locate the nodes, establish the edges, and fill the default nodes to generate the semantic tree instance according to the input. We use thyroid subtree as an example to illustrate the process. The steps are as follows:

Step 1: Voice recognition and preprocessing. The radiologist inputs the necessary description by voice, and the speech recognition interface converts the voice into characters. The speech recognition results cannot achieve 100% accuracy, so the system preprocesses the recognition content (ln:2), correcting the recognized error keywords, separating the attribute values, parsing the input according to the Chinese punctuation.

Step 2: Determine the area of the description (ln:5). Specifically, it is the process of identifying and generating branches of the tree. The second and third layers are mainly expanded based on the keywords of the input. For example, if s contains keywords corresponding to nodules, the focal lesion should be added to the third layer. The fourth layer involves more precise areas (parts and nodules). Therefore, the default input order of the area (e.g., right lobe, left lobe, isthmus) also needs to be specified to ensure the correctness of the location. Furthermore, the system can interact with the radiologist and judge the area based on the previous description.

Step 3: Locate the name and the value of the attribute. When no exit condition is met, s is located to the corresponding attribute according to the attribute value mapping table (ln:6.1). For example, s would be mapped to shape, when including keyword like "plump." But some attribute value keywords are the same, the default input order of attribute values (e.g., antero-posterior diameter transverse diameter) is designed to assist attribute locating. Considering that some attributes are unavoidably missed in the semantic tree, the system would analyze the input logic and interact with the radiologist to find the missed content. The process is marked as an execution log. If locating the attribute is successful, the attribute name node and the attribute value node are added in the tree. The exit condition (ln:6) is: (1) I has been completely processed; or (2) s involves keywords corresponding to another part or nodule; or (3) s is conformed to the default input orders for describing another part or nodule.

Step 4: Check the required attributes (ln:8). After each round of text processing, the attribute set of the generated semantic tree instance (T) is compared with the required attribute set (RA). Required but unmentioned attributes are marked in T to remind the radiologist if some necessary attributes are missed. This can reduce the error rate of the reports.

Step 5: Fill the default attributes (ln:9). When the radiologist states that the input of the ultrasound report has finished, T is compared with the normal attribute set (NA). Then the missed attribute names and the corresponding normal attribute values are added to T. This operation avoids repeating a large number of default attributes, which will significantly reduce the burden on radiologists.

TIG is a recursive algorithm which inputs a clause recognized by the speech recognition software (I), the normal attribute set (NA), and the required attribute set (RA). It also takes the semantic tree instance (T) as its input and output (when its termination condition is satisfied).

Algorithm TIG

Input: clause I, attribute sets NA and RA, tree T
Output: tree T
0. $Array\_clause = \emptyset$; Initialize $T = \emptyset$;
1. **If** $T = \emptyset$ **Then** $T.1F \longleftarrow Thyroid$; **End If**
2. $Array\_clause \longleftarrow$ preprocesse I;
3. **While** $Array\_clause \neq \emptyset$ **Then**
4. $s \longleftarrow Array\_clause.pop()$;
5. Determine the area based on keywords and the default input orders;
5.1 $T.2F \longleftarrow Postoperation/Preoperation$;
5.2 $T.3F \longleftarrow Glandular\ background/Lesion$;
5.3 $T.4F \longleftarrow parts\ and\ nodules$;
6. **While** s *does not conform to the exit condition* **Then**
6.1 s is located to the corresponding attribute according to the mapping table and the default input orders;
6.2 $T.5F \longleftarrow Attribute\_name$;
6.3 $T.6F \longleftarrow Attribute\_value$;
6.4 $s \longleftarrow Array\_clause.pop()$;
6.5 **End While**
7. **End While**
8. Compare T with RA. Required but unmentioned attributes are marked;
9. Compare T with NA. T is filled with the default attributes;
10. return T;

The semantic tree instance generated by the example in Fig. 1 is shown in Fig. 3. The process is as follows. Firstly, the tree is initialized, $T.1F \longleftarrow Thyroid$. Then the input is preprocessed to obtain $Array\_clause$ = {right lobe, 10, 9, left lobe, 9, 8, the isthmus has been resected, heterogenous}. Since $Array\_clause$ contains "resected," $T.2F \longleftarrow postoperation$. After that, let s = "right lobe," which belongs to the glandular background, $T.3F \longleftarrow glandular\ background$, $T.4F \longleftarrow right\ lobe$. Let s = "10," which is positioned to the anteroposterior diameter according to the attribute value mapping table and the default input order, $T.5F \longleftarrow anteroposterior\ diameter$, $T.6F \longleftarrow 10mm$. Let s = "9," which does not meet the exit condition, step 3 should be repeated. When the exit condition is encountered, step 2 and step 3 are repeated until $Array\_clause = \emptyset$. Finally, default attributes are filled and a semantic tree instance is generated.

TTT

Although the semantic tree is understandable, it is still necessary to provide the natural language based reports in real applications.

Template labels ($l(x, y)$)	Examples		
	Parent nodes(x)	Child nodes(y)	Description
$x +$ "：" $+y$	前后径 (Anteroposterior diameter)	10mm	前后径：10mm (Anteroposterior diameter: 10mm)
$x + y$	回声分布 (Echo distribution)	不均匀 (Heterogenous)	回声分布不均匀 (Echo distribution is heterogenous.)
y	部位 (Position)	左侧 (Left side)	左侧 (Left side)

Fig. 4 The examples of the template labels

In this section, we present our proposed tree-to-text (TTT) algorithm. At first, we define template labels, reference points, and special points for the tree nodes. Template labels are used to get the fluent text. Reference points are used to eliminate redundant information to obtain a concise text. Special nodes are used to make the text structure more clear. Then we design the TTT algorithm on the foundation of these definitions.

Template Label There are specific correlations between parent nodes and child nodes in the tree. For producing smooth text, we define template labels to connect two nodes. A template label is defined as $l(x, y)$, where x is the parent node and y is the child node. Several template labels are shown in Fig. 4.

Reference Point (*rp*) The child nodes with the same parent node are called sibling nodes. If there are multiple sibling nodes with the same name, these sibling nodes are recorded as reference points. In the thyroid subtree, right lobe, left lobe, and isthmus of the glandular background are marked as reference points.

Special Point (*sp*) Since some child nodes between rps have different contents in most cases, these nodes are defined as special points. When generating text, special points are handled according to the text structure. This ensures that the generated text conforms to general description habits. For example, the attribute values of the anteroposterior diameter between right lobe and left lobe are mostly different, so the anteroposterior diameter is the special point.

Deduplication of rps is a key step in keeping the text concise. The reference points comparison algorithm (RPC) is developed for this task. The input is the parent node of rps and the name set of the child nodes of rps. The output is the set of different child nodes between rps (M). The process has two steps. Firstly, rps and the child nodes are obtained according to the parent node of rps. Secondly, the different child nodes (excluding sps) between rps are recorded and stored in M. The recorded nodes have one of the following properties: (1) the child node names only appear in some rps, or (2) the child node names are same, but the content behind the child nodes is different.

The process of TTT is as follows: (1) the traversal starts at the root node ($RNode$), and then the edges of the tree are translated according to the template labels (ln:2.3) until rp is found (ln:2); (2) RPC is used to obtain the set of different child nodes (M) (ln:3.1); (3) the child nodes ($CNodes$) of rps are processed in the order of sps, the same nodes (not included in M), and the different nodes (included in M) according to the template labels (ln:3.2–3.4); (4) the parent node ($PNode$) of rps is obtained to find the unprocessed nodes (ln:4.1–4.4). The complete natural language text is obtained when all leaf nodes are processed.

The process of generating text from the example semantic tree instance in Fig. 3 is as follows: (1) when traversing to the rps (right lobe, left lobe, isthmus), $Cstr$ = "Postoperation,"; (2) there is no different child node between rps, $M = \emptyset$; (3) after processing sps (anteroposterior diameter, transverse diameter, resected), $Cstr$ = "Postoperation, right lobe: anteroposterior diameter: 10 mm, transverse diameter: 9 mm; left lobe: anteroposterior diameter: 9 mm, transverse diameter: 8 mm; isthmus: resected.", and the remaining child nodes are processed according to M; (4) all leaf nodes have been processed in the previous step, so the traversal has ended. The generated ultrasound report is shown in Fig. 5.

Algorithm TTT

Input: tree T

Output: clause $Cstr$

```
0.    TNode = T.RNode;
1.    While there are leaf nodes that are not translated Then
2.        While TNode is not the rp && TNode != NULL Then
2.1           /*Get TNode's first unprocessed CNode from left to right*/
2.2           TNode = TNode → CNode;
2.3           Cst += Translate edge(TNode, TNode → PNode);
2.4       End While
3.        If TNode is rp Then
3.1           M = RPC(TNode → PNode, Name);
3.2           Cstr += Process sps;
3.3           Cstr += Process the nodes that don't belong to M;
3.4           Cstr += Process the nodes that belong to M;
3.5       End If
4.        /*Return to PNode to find untraversed nodes*/
4.1       TNode = TNode → PNode;
4.2       While All CNodes of TNode are traversed && TNode isn't RNode Then
4.3           TNode = TNode → PNode;
4.4       End While
5.    End While
6.    return Cstr;
```

术后，右叶：前后径：10mm，左右径：9mm；左叶：前后径：9mm，左右径：8mm；峡部：已切除。残余甲状腺内部回声呈密集中等回声，回声分布不均匀，CDFI：未见明显异常血流信号。

Postoperation, right lobe: anteroposterior diameter: 10mm, transverse diameter: 9mm; left lobe: anteroposterior diameter: 9mm, transverse diameter: 8mm; isthmus: resected. In the residual thyroid, internal echo is a dense medium echo, and echo distribution is heterogenous. CDFI : no obvious abnormal blood flow signal.

Fig. 5 The ultrasound report of the example

3 Experimental Results and Analysis

3.1 Experimental Setup

The experimental data were obtained based on the ultrasound examination data of thyroid from the ultrasonic department of a hospital in Shanghai, China. The total number of reports was 464,681. We selected 4 testers who were familiar with the thyroid ultrasound report for voice input. Each of them randomly selected 100 data for testing. Moreover, the glandular background should be described first, followed by the focal lesion. The following experiments are conducted:

- Calculate the ratio of the input characters and the number of the characters of the original report to verify the effectiveness of TIG in reducing input characters.
- Calculate the accuracy of the semantic tree instance to illustrate the feasibility of obtaining the complete information only by inputting individual descriptions.
- Calculate the BLEU (Bilingual Evaluation Understudy) scores to objectively evaluate the similarity between the generated text and the original ultrasound report.
- Carry out the subjective evaluation to evaluate the accuracy, simplicity, fluency, and unambiguity of generated reports.

3.2 Experimental Results

The Character Ratio

We made statistics on the number of the input characters (IC) and the number of the characters of the original report (TC), and then calculated the character ratio (CR) as follows:

$$CR = \frac{IC}{TC} \tag{1}$$

Table 1 The statistics of the character ratio

	Range				
	[0,0.2)	[0.2,0.4)	[0.4,0.6)	[0.6,0.8)	[0.8,1]
n	49	235	68	41	7
SR	12.25%	58.75%	17%	10.25%	1.75%
Avg	0.1147	0.3060	0.4603	0.6618	1
CR_{min}	0.0492	0.2000	0.4000	0.6000	\
CR_{max}	0.1967	0.3974	0.5952	0.7692	\
$TAvg$	0.3574				

We divided the value of the ratio CR into 5 ranges [0,0.2), [0.2,0.4), [0.4,0.6), [0.4,0.6), and [0.8,1] for analysis, as shown in Table 1. In order to interpret the results, we have the following notations: N (400): the total number of the samples. n: the number of the samples in each range. SR: The proportion of n in N. Avg: the average of the ratios in each range. $TAvg$: the average of the ratios of all samples. CR_{min}: the minimum value of CR. CR_{max}: the maximum value of CR. During analysis, we removed the special cases (0 and 1) to count CR_{min} and CR_{max}.

Table 1 shows that the number of samples in [0.2, 0.4) is the largest, with a total of 235, accounting for 58.75%. In other words, more than half of ultrasound reports require less than half of the characters of the report as the input to generate a complete report. In particular, CR_{min} in the whole sample is 0.0492. The total number of characters in this sample is 61, while the number of individual description characters is only 3. Although CR_{max} in the whole sample is 0.7629. Compared with the complete ultrasonic report by voice input, it can still significantly reduce the workload of radiologists. Moreover, $TAvg$ is 0.3574. It indicates that the proposed TIG algorithm can effectively reduce the number of characters required to generate an ultrasound report, which can accelerate the speed of ultrasound examination and greatly reduce the burden of radiologists.

The Accuracy of the Semantic Tree Instance

This experiment testifies the effectiveness of semantic tree instance generation. The main reasons that may cause errors in the semantic tree instance generation include the speech recognition problem (SRP), special text problem (STP), and tree structure problem (TSP). SRP is due to noise, speech speed, accent, and other reasons. The results of speech recognition inevitably contain error messages. STP is due to special description habits of the testers. All of these problems may cause the incorrect location of an attribute value or the failed location of the attribute. In the proposed method, the preprocessing step is designed to deal with SRP, the tree update function in exception management module will be triggered according to the execution log to update the semantic tree structure at the end of each test round.

Table 2 The result statistics of the semantic tree

	The first round				The second round			
		Incorrect				Incorrect		
Tester	Correct	SRP	STP	TSP	Correct	SRP	STP	TSP
1	93	1	2	4	99	0	1	0
2	89	1	4	6	97	0	3	0
3	92	2	3	3	97	0	3	0
4	96	0	2	2	98	0	2	0
Total	370	4	11	15	391	0	9	0
Accuracy	92.5%				97.75%			

Table 3 The BLEU scores

	BLEU-1	BLEU-2	BLEU-3	BLEU-4
Average	0.8059	0.7561	0.7108	0.6714
Maximum	0.9577	0.9577	0.9470	0.9360
Minimum	0.5806	0.5652	0.5054	0.4481

The number of correct and incorrect semantic tree instances generated in the first test round and the second round is illustrated in Table 2. According to the table, the overall accuracy is 97.75%, which demonstrates the effectiveness of the proposed semantic tree instance generation algorithm. The detailed information about the error caused by different reasons in each round is also listed in the table. From the table, we can see that SRP and TSP are well resolved in the second test round. Most of the wrong results are corrected by exception management module. The number of incorrect tree instances caused by SRP and TSP is reduced from 4 and 15 to 0 and 0. STP is difficult to be resolved. After each round of the test, testers are trained to avoid inputting special text. The number of incorrect tree instance is reduced from 30 to 9.

BLEU

BLEU is mainly used for automatic machine translation evaluation by calculating the similarity between sentences in machine translation and standard translation [19]. BLEU-1, BLEU-2, BLEU-3, and BLEU-4 are used in this paper to evaluate the similarity of the generated reports and the original ones. We randomly select 60 samples from the correct semantic tree instances for evaluation. The BLEU scores are shown in Table 3.

From the table, we can see that the highest scores of BLEU-1,2,3,4 are all above 0.9 and the average scores of BLUE-2,3,4 are not so high. That is because the different lengths and word orders of the texts will affect their values. In the proposed method, the redundant information in the semantic tree is merged, so fewer sentences are generated than that of the original report. The second reason is that the semantic tree contains the default information unmentioned in the original report,

Table 4 The result of subjective evaluation

	Ratio					
Criteria	1	2	3	4	5	Overall score
Accuracy	0/4	0/4	0/4	0/4	4/4	5
Simplicity	0/4	0/4	0/4	0/4	4/4	5
Fluency	0/4	0/4	0/4	1/4	3/4	4.75
Unambiguity	0/4	0/4	0/4	0/4	4/4	5

so the generated text may have more content. In other words, a lower BLEU score does not affect the accuracy of the report. Instead, it is more concise than the original report.

Subjective Evaluation

BLEU-1,2,3,4 can objectively evaluate the similarity between the generated reports and the original ones. To further verify the effectiveness of the generated report, each generated text is evaluated according to the following four criteria: (1) accuracy, which means the text has the same semantics as the original text and no information is missed; (2) simplicity, which means the generated report is concise and has no redundant information; (3) fluency, which means the sentences are smooth and fluent; (4) unambiguity, which means the text is logic clear and has no ambiguity. The tester scores each criterion based on the output text report, with a maximum of 5 points and a minimum of 1 point. For each score, the ratio of the actual number of scorers to the total number of testers is listed in Table 4.

According to Table 4, the overall assessments of accuracy, simplicity, and unambiguity are 5. As for fluency, one tester rated it as 4. The overall evaluation of fluency is 4.75. The subjective evaluation results show that Algorithm TTT can effectively translate the tree into the text, which has complete information, concise sentences, unambiguous meaning, and is relatively fluent. The description logic of the generated text is consistent with that of the real report.

4 Conclusion and Future Work

In this paper, a system for automatically generating ultrasound reports via voice input has been proposed. By specifying the semantic tree and using it as an intermediary, we propose two algorithms for semantic tree instance generation and tree-to-text generation. The experimental results show that the overall accuracy of the semantic tree is high and the output text is concise and unambiguous. In the future, we plan to cover more interactions and extend the proposed method to generate ultrasound reports about other body parts.

Acknowledgement This work was supported by the National Key R&D Program of China under Grant 2019YFE0190500.

References

1. V.Y. Park, K. Han, Y.K. Seong, M.H. Park, E. Kim, Moon, H.J. et al., Diagnosis of Thyroid nodules: performance of a deep learning convolutional neural network model vs. radiologists. Sci. Rep. 9, 17843 (2019). https://doi.org/10.1038/s41598-019-54434-1
2. X. Mei, H. Lee, K. Diao, M. Huang, B. Lin, C. Liu, et al., Artificial intelligence–enabled rapid diagnosis of patients with COVID-19. Nat. Med. **26**, 1224–1228 (2020). https://doi.org/10.1038/s41591-020-0931-3
3. X. Wang, Y. Peng, L. Lu, Z. Lu, R.M. Summers, TieNet: Text-image embedding network for common thorax disease classification and reporting in chest X-rays, in *The IEEE Conference on Computer Vision and Pattern Recognition* (2018), pp. 9049–9058
4. P. Kisilev, E. Walach, E. Barkan, B. Ophir, S. Alpert, S.Y. Hashoul, From medical image to automatic medical report generation. IBM J. Res. Develop. **59**(2/3), 2:1–2:7 (2015)
5. A. Graves, N. Jaitly, Towards end-to-end speech recognition with recurrent neural networks, in *International Conference on Machine Learning* (2014), pp. 1764–1772
6. Y. He, T.N. Sainath, R. Prabhavalkar, I. McGraw, R. Alvarez, D. Zhao, et al., Streaming end-to-end speech recognition for mobile devices, in *2019 IEEE International Conference on Acoustics, Speech and Signal Processing* (2019), pp. 6381–6385
7. D. Amodei, S. Ananthanarayanan, R. Anubhai, J. Bai, E. Battenberg, Deep speech 2: End-to-end speech recognition in English and mandarin, in *Proceedings of the 33rd International Conference on Machine Learning* (2016), pp. 173–182
8. L.E. Shafey, H. Soltau, I. Shafran, Joint speech recognition and speaker diarization via sequence transduction, in *Conference of the International Speech Communication Association* (2019), pp. 396–400
9. L. Zhou, S.V. Blackley, L. Kowalski, B. Adam, E. Kontrient, D. Mack, et al., Analysis of errors in dictated clinical documents assisted by speech recognition software and professional transcriptionists. JAMA Netw. Open. **1**(3), e180530 (2018)
10. Nuance Communications, Control your computer by voice with speed and accuracy. https://www.nuance.com/en-gb/dragon.html#standardpage-mainpar_backgroundimage_copy. Accessed 18 Decemebr 2019
11. Nuance Communications, Dragon Medical One: Secure, cloud-based clinical speech recognition. https://www.nuance.com/en-au/healthcare/provider-solutions/speech-recognition/dragon-medical-one.html. Accessed 18 Decemebr 2019
12. Amazon Web Service, Amazon Transcribe Medical. https://aws.amazon.com/cn/transcribe/medical/. Accessed 16 January 2020
13. WebChartMD, Healthcare's leading dictation and medical transcription software. https://www.webchartmd.org/. Accessed 27 May 2020
14. VoiceboxMD, Medical Dictation for Physicians and Nurse Practitioners. https://voiceboxmd.com/medical-dictation/. Accessed 27 May 2020
15. A. Paats, T. Alumäe, E. Meister, I. Fridolin, Retrospective analysis of clinical performance of an Estonian speech recognition system for radiology: effects of different acoustic and language models. J. Digit. Imaging. **31**(5), 615–621 (2018)

16. T. Takao, R. Masumura, S. Sakauchi, Y. Ohara, E. Bilgic, E. Umegaki, et al., New report preparation system for endoscopic procedures using speech recognition technology. Endoscopy Int. Open **6**(6), E676–E687 (2018)
17. A. Trujillo, M. Orellana, M.I. Acosta, Design of emergency call record support system applying natural language processing techniques, in *Conference on Information Technologies and Communication of Ecuador* (2019), pp. 53–65
18. T.N. Hanna, H. Shekhani, K. Maddu, C. Zhang, Z. Chen, J. Johnson, Structured report compliance: Effect on audio dictation time, report length, and total radiologist study time. Emerg Radiol. **23**(5), 449–453 (2016)
19. K. Papineni, S. Roukos, T. Ward, W. Zhu, BLEU: A method for automatic evaluation of machine translation, in *Proceedings of the 56th Annual Meeting of the Association for Computational Linguistics* (2002), pp. 311–318

Internet-of-Things Management of Hospital Beds for Bed-Rest Patients

Kyle Yeh, Chelsea Yeh, and Karin Li

1 Introduction

In a hospital environment, one of the roles of the medical staff is to enforce the medical instructions that patients have received, as this directly affects the safety and recovery time of patients. Internet of things (IoT) allows for real-time remote collection and interpretation of data, and immediate feedback of monitored status based on the collected data. In medical applications, IoT enables the collection of medical data of patients in a hospital and the dissemination of the patients' status to the medical staff immediately. This allows the medical staff to assess the condition of those in their care and take appropriate actions to prevent or mitigate worsening medical conditions or additional complications and injuries.

In this research, we developed a real-time bed-rest monitoring system based on IoT-connected pressure sensors. Hospital beds are equipped with IoT pressure sensors that detect whether or not the patient has vacated their prescribed bed rest. The devices transmit the data immediately upon vacancy to a central server, and they also transmit periodically to update the status of the patient. The server processes and interprets the data and then updates to a mobile application running on the nurses' mobile devices, alerting them if a patient ordered by a physician to bed rest has vacated the bed. It can also alert the staff in the nurses' station via a dedicated console or can be integrated into the hospital's in-patient management system.

Further work includes the management of comatose and immobile patients who need frequent movement by the medical staff. Using the IoT pressure and motion

K. Yeh (✉) · C. Yeh
Walnut Valley Research Institute, Walnut, CA, USA

K. Li
UC Riverside School of Medicine, Riverside, CA, USA

H. R. Arabnia et al. (eds.), *Advances in Computer Vision and Computational Biology*, Transactions on Computational Science and Computational Intelligence,
https://doi.org/10.1007/978-3-030-71051-4_33

sensing devices embedded into the hospital beds, the server can automatically sense when the patient has been moved [2]. It can keep track of when each patient has been moved and inform the medical staff if it is time to move a particular patient according to schedule. Also, the server can alert the medical staff if a patient is overdue for a move [3, 4].

2 Bed-Rest Management

Bed rest is a commonly prescribed medical treatment used to treat a wide array of illnesses. However, when patients vacate their beds during their prescribed bed rest, the probability of further injury from falling increases dramatically. Our project aims to solve this issue by introducing a monitoring system designed to supervise the movement of those patients and allow the hospital staff the ability to react promptly and escort the patients back to bed. The idea of putting bed alarms to alert nurses and care staff of patient movement has already been implemented before in existing products. In previous works, bed alarms have been employed to signal bed absence. These bed alarms consist of a pressure sensor with a co-located, integrated alarm. If a bed-rest patient vacates their bed, the pressure sensor will detect the reduction in pressure and, with an audible alarm, alert the caregivers of the situation. In this particular study, 77% of nurses found this method useful for fall prevention, and 83% found this method useful for fall detection [1].

However, in a clinical situation, this is likely to disturb the other patients in the vicinity of the alarm. For our project, we aim to remove the audio aspect of these alarms. By enabling the sensors to send notifications to the medical staff via an IoT network consisting of a server and interconnected pressure devices integrated into hospital beds, thereby eliminating the disturbance created by the alarm. The medical staff must be alerted in case of an alarm whenever they are on duty. Therefore, this system sends alerts directly to mobile phones of the medical staff, which are on their persons during their shift.

3 Components

The embedded IoT medical system consists of the following elements:

1. Bed absence sensors suitable for hospital bed use
2. Internet-capable processing devices co-located and connected to the bed absence sensors, which collect, interpret, and transmit the sensor data
3. A Wi-Fi, 5G, or other suitable and secure network accessible from inside the hospital environment
4. A data collection server that receives the bed absence data for the hospital or the sector of the hospital which it is monitoring

5. Mobile devices or cellular phones that are normally carried by the attending nurses during their shift, running the mobile application that displays the status of the beds that the nurse is attending

3.1 Sensors

Pressure sensors such as pressure pads are commercially available and easy to obtain. These devices sense pressure through the distribution of the patient weight among the pad and sensors. In this system, the pressure pad is connected to a Wi-Fi module. The purpose of the module is to read real-time patient data from the sensors and relay the information to the data analysis server.

In addition to pressure sensors, it is also possible to utilize other sensing technology to assist in the monitoring of bed-rest-prescribed patients. Accelerometers are readily available to measure the movement on the bed. Here, patient motion can be monitored to further determine if a vacating event is occurring. In addition, the accelerometer may be able to determine the quality of sleep that the patient is experiencing, whether the patient is undergoing convulsions or epileptic events, or if the patient needs to be moved to prevent pressure ulcers. We would like to emphasize that the accelerometer is to be mounted on the bed and not worn on the wrist of the patient/user. This minimizes the workload on the hospital staff by reducing bodily attachments, as the patient may already have various monitoring devices and intravenous tubes attached to their bodies.

Heat sensors can also be deployed on the hospital bed to monitor the temperature of the bed as the patient is lying on the bed. This temperature will not be an accurate reading of the patient's body temperature due to the lack of direct contact between the sensor and the patient's body (shielded by gown, sheets, etc.). However, it does provide a relative difference in temperature when the patient is on the bed versus not on the bed. An additional temperature sensor can be mounted on the bed away from the patient that measures the ambient temperature of the bed. This second sensor will provide a baseline temperature reading of the bed without the patient, and its reading compared to the temperature sensor under the patient.

3.2 Microcontroller

The sensors will be connected via a suitable interface to a computing device (microcontroller). If the absence determination algorithm is simple enough for the sensing modality, the microcontroller would be able to directly determine if a vacating event has occurred. For more complicated algorithms, the microcontroller will simply transmit the received data.

For example, with a pressure pad, the algorithm to determine if the patient has vacated the bed is relatively simple. Either a lower threshold pressure level has been crossed, or a sudden decrease in pressure level can be used to trigger an alert for a vacating event.

The microcontroller must be equipped with networking capabilities, preferably wireless, which will be used to transmit the collected data to a server. Ideally, the microcontroller will be powered via an AC power adaptor. This provides a constant source of power delivered by the hospital. Since hospital beds are typically already powered, using AC power should be an option in a hospital environment. However, if such power is unavailable, rechargeable batteries can be deployed. Even if AC power is available, rechargeable batteries may be advantageous to provide backup power to the microcontroller and sensing devices in case of a power failure.

3.3 Network

The hospital must provide a network that the microcontrollers deployed on the hospital beds can connect to. Wi-Fi is probably the most prevalent wireless networking system deployed in a hospital (or most other modern environments). The network must provide adequate security against data interception and data breaches, and Wi-Fi provides this capability. It must be highly reliable (transmitted data is not lost or corrupted) and have low latency (transmitted data is received immediately). Bandwidth requirements are low for the hospital bed, as only a small amount of data is transmitted per second per bed.

Other data networking systems may be used, provided that the hospital possesses such a system or is willing to invest in such a system, and the system provides the necessary security. Wireless systems include 5G cellular networks. Wired systems that can be considered are Ethernet, powerline communication, coaxial, or telephone networking.

3.4 Server

The role of the central server is to receive the data sent by the microcontroller from sensors attached to the hospital beds. When a vacating event occurs, as determined by the microcontroller or by the algorithm running in the server, it will send an alert to the mobile device or cell phone carried by the responsible nurse and/or the console at the nurses' station.

It is often the case that there are multiple nurses on each hospital floor, each attending to a set of beds, some with bedrest order and some without.

The configuration of the assignment of the beds to each nurse must be simple and straightforward. Also, the bed-rest alert must be able to be turned on or off (permanently or temporarily) for each bed depending on whether a bed rest has been ordered for that patient and if the patient has been removed from the bed (by the hospital staff) for reasons such as imaging, diagnostic, or treatment sessions.

3.5 *Mobile Devices and Mobile Application*

The mobile application that notifies and alerts the responsible nurses of bed-rest violation will run on a mobile device that the nurses carry. For nurses with hospital-issued mobile phones that they carry on their persons during their shift, the mobile application can be installed and provisioned on these devices by the hospital IT staff. Dedicated devices can also be developed that connect to the hospital network and alert the nurse of bed-rest violations.

The hospital management or IT staff will be able to configure from the central server, or on the mobile devices, the assignment of the set of beds that are assigned to each particular mobile device/nurse. Also, the configuration will determine which assigned beds have their alerts disabled on a permanent (no bed-rest order) or temporary (patient in imaging, diagnostics, or treatment) basis.

The alert on the mobile device can provide (1) visible notification on the screen, (2) vibration of the device, and/or (3) one-time or periodic audible beep or alarm.

4 Initial System

For the initial presence sensing system development, we created a test system from the following components.

The ESP32 was chosen as the microcontroller because it is powerful and low cost and, most importantly, has integrated Wi-Fi capabilities [5]. The ESP32 is compatible with the Arduino Integrated Development Environment, a widely used open-source development system that uses the C++ coding language, making it simple for programming and updating. This platform features a built-in dual-core CPU with Wi-Fi connectivity and a wide operating temperature range from −40 °C to 125 °C. This development board is low cost and usually operates at 160 MHz with 4 MB of flash memory and 8 MB of PSRAM.

Wi-Fi networks are ubiquitous and secure with WPA2 [6]. The IoT servers will be connected over a 2.4-GHz Wi-Fi band. This is because ESP32 only supports the 2.4-GHz band, and the lower band is also more secure and has a longer range than the 5.0-GHz band [6].

For this initial development, we chose the Blynk cloud-based server. Blynk runs on the HTTPS API and is an IoT platform that allows machine learning and data analytics on mobile apps. Blynk [7] runs with the concept of a virtual pin, which enables data to be exchanged from a device to the server easily from the cloud.

Similarly, for the mobile application, we used the commercially available Blynk application. It is operational on both iOS and Android. The Blynk mobile application uses a drag-and-drop interface, allowing for a simple and user-friendly design.

For future development, we plan to migrate to more secure and robust servers and mobile devices. Cloud-based servers include Amazon Web Services [8], Google

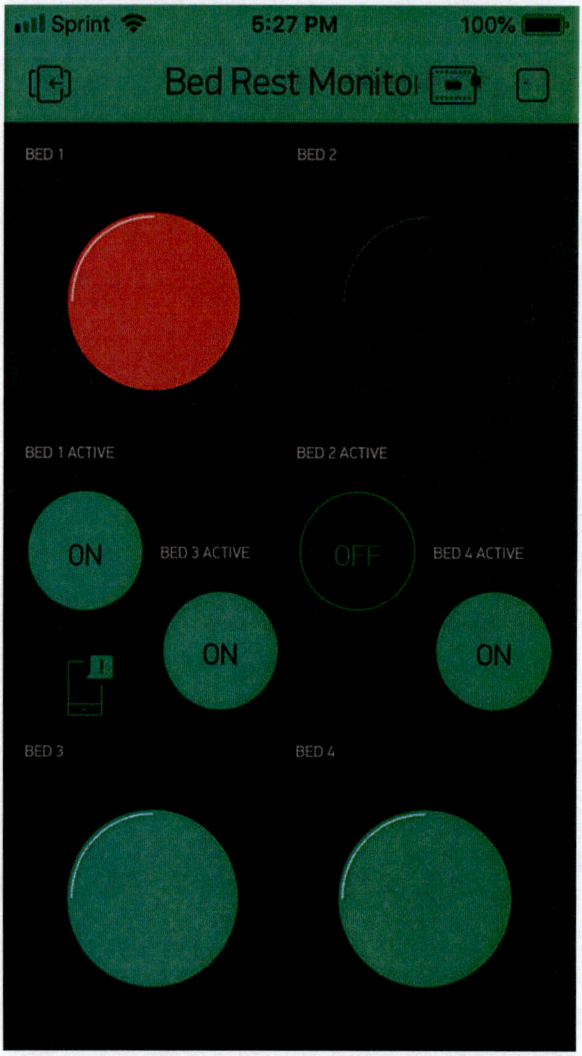

Fig. 1 Alarms, configuration to turn on/off

Cloud [9], and Microsoft Azure [10]; a variety of software exists if the hospital plans to host the servers in house.

For the mobile application, we plan to migrate to a more flexible React Native environment. React Native [11] runs on JavaScript while rendering in the platform's native user interface, enabling cross-platform sharing of code from a single codebase. React Native also supports both the Android and iOS operating systems.

Figure 1 shows the screenshot of the bed-rest management mobile application on the iOS environment. Here, bed occupancy status of Bed 1, Bed 3, and Bed 4 are

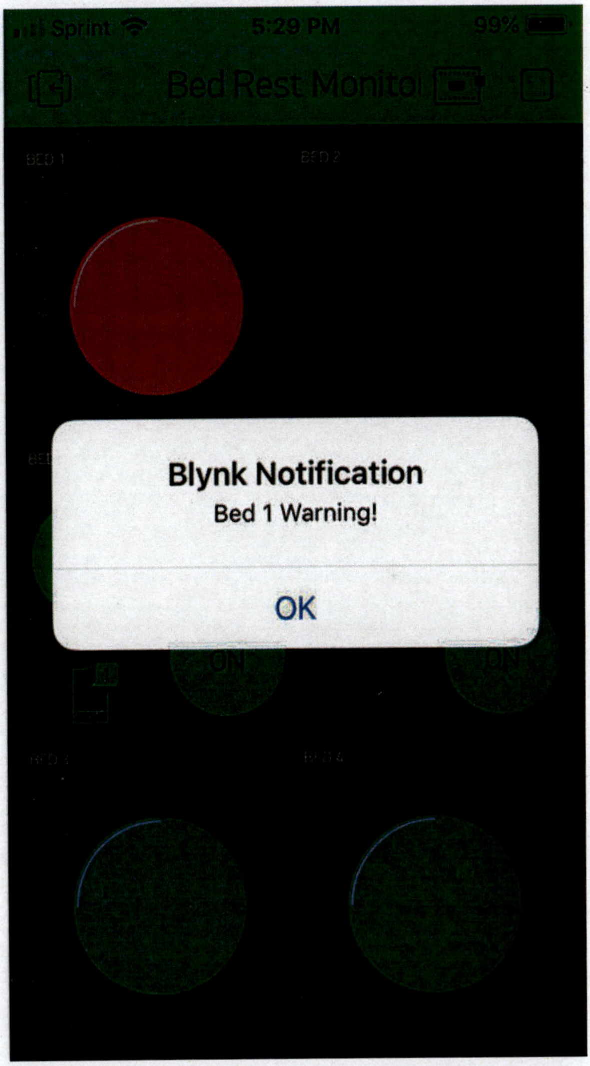

Fig. 2 Notifications

active. Bed 2 is turned off temporarily due to the patient being in treatment. Bed 1 is showing vacancy alert, while Bed 3 and Bed 4 are occupied as measured by the pressure sensor.

Figure 2 shows the screenshot of the mobile notification alert in real time as Bed 2 is vacated by the patient.

Figure 3 shows the screenshot of the mobile notification alert in real time as Bed 3 is vacated by the patient on the lock screen of the iOS device.

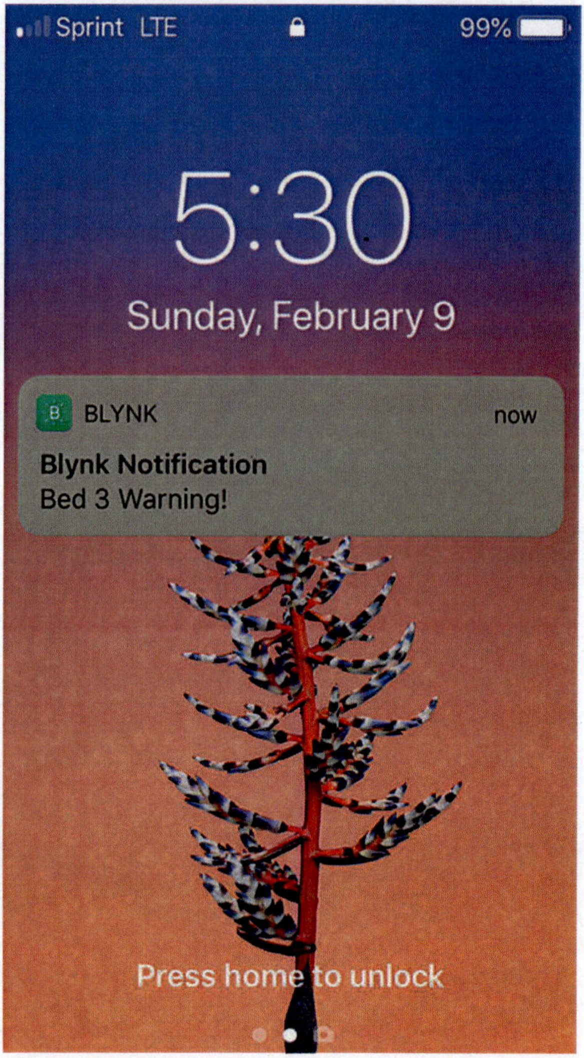

Fig. 3 Notification locked screen or home screens

Figure 4 shows a commercially available pressure sensing pad used to monitor patient presence on the bed.

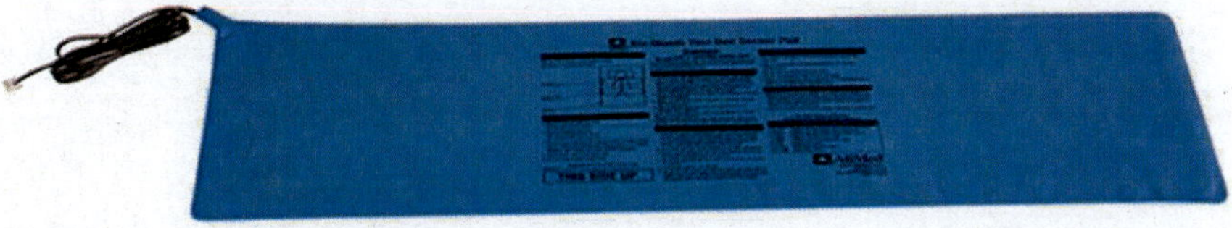

Fig. 4 Pressure sensing pad [12]

5 Conclusion and Future Work

We have created a novel IoT-based hospital bed-rest management system that uses integrated sensors (pressure sensors), Wi-Fi-connected microcontroller, cloud-based servers, and mobile applications. This alerts the hospital staff immediately of bed vacancy events that may lead to serious injuries and complications to patients ordered to bed rest in hospitals and to take mitigating actions to prevent such injuries and complications.

We propose the integration of additional sensors (accelerometer and thermal sensor) to the hospital beds that enable the noninvasive sensing of patient temperature and movement. These can be useful in monitoring patient relative temperature and the management of comatose patients for pressure ulcers (bed sores).

References

1. K. Subermaniam, R. Welfred, P. Subramanian, et al., The effectiveness of a wireless modular bed absence sensor device for fall prevention among older inpatients. Front Public Health **4**, 292. Published 2017 Jan 9. (2017). https://doi.org/10.3389/fpubh.2016.00292
2. S. Bhattacharya, R.K. Mishra, Pressure ulcers: Current understanding and newer modalities of treatment. Indian J Plast Surg. **48**(1), 4–16 (2015). https://doi.org/10.4103/0970-0358.155260
3. J.E. Mahoney, Immobility and falls. Clin. Geriatr. Med **14**(4), 699–726 (1998)
4. R.I. Shorr, A.M. Chandler, L.C. Mion, et al., Effects of an intervention to increase bed alarm use to prevent falls in hospitalized patients: A cluster randomized trial. Ann Intern Med **157**(10), 692–699 (2012). https://doi.org/10.7326/0003-4819-157-10-201211200-00005
5. https://www.espressif.com/en/products/hardware/esp32/overview
6. IEEE Standard for Information technology—Telecommunications and information exchange between systems Local and metropolitan area networks—Specific requirements - Part 11: Wireless LAN Medium Access Control (MAC) and Physical Layer (PHY) Specifications, in *IEEE Std 802.11-2016* (Revision of IEEE Std 802.11-2012), pp.1–3534 (14 Dec 2016)
7. https://blynk.io/
8. F.P. Miller, A.F. Vandome, J. McBrewster, Amazon web services (2010)
9. S.P.T. Krishnan, J.U. Gonzalez, Building your next big thing with google cloud platform: A guide for developers and enterprise architects (2015)

10. M. Copeland, J. Soh, A. Puca, M. Manning, D. Gollob, Microsoft azure: Planning, deploying, and managing your data center in the cloud (2015)
11. https://facebook.github.io/react-native/
12. https://www.alimed.com/alimed-sensor-pads.html

Predicting Length of Stay for COPD Patients with Generalized Linear Models and Random Forests

Anna Romanova

1 Introduction

In the current fast-changing environment, healthcare systems require extra flexibility and adaptability to high variation in hospital volumes and flow segmenting by patient types. Having analytical tools for predicting the length of stay (LOS) along with predictive models for patient demand can help our society respond to public health challenges more efficiently. Accurate predictive models for the LOS are instrumental in finding the right balance between patient demand and hospital capacity in terms of beds, nurses, mid-level providers, and physicians and are particularly important when addressing changes in demand for seasonal patients (e.g., flu and Covid-19 patients).

This study focuses on predicting the LOS for chronic obstructive pulmonary disease (COPD) patients using administrative, clinical, and operational data from a large teaching hospital in the southeastern United States. We investigate the performance of several predictive models including generalized linear models (GLM) and random forest methods and assess models' predictive ability by comparing their generalization errors.

A. Romanova (✉)
Department of Computer Science and Quantitative Methods, College of Business Administration, Winthrop University, Rock Hull, SC, USA
e-mail: romanovaa@winthrop.edu

H. R. Arabnia et al. (eds.), *Advances in Computer Vision and Computational Biology*, Transactions on Computational Science and Computational Intelligence,
https://doi.org/10.1007/978-3-030-71051-4_34

2 Data Processing and Methodology

2.1 Data Set

The data set for the analysis includes COPD patients admitted to the University of Tennessee Medical Center during the period of 2011–2018 with discharge dates between January 1, 2012, and December 31, 2018. Since misclassification of the COPD diagnosis is likely on admission [13], only patients with the principal diagnosis of COPD at discharge were included in this study. As such, the data set includes a total of 3696 COPD patients.

The data collected for this study comes from both the clinical and the administrative databases of the hospital and includes patient demographic characteristics (age, gender, race, and insurance type), clinical characteristics (vital signs on admission, classical COPD risk factors, procedures, and secondary diagnoses), and operational data (number of beds available and patient days).

The LOS, reported in days, was recalculated to be measured in hours based on the exact admission and discharge time in the clinical risk reports for each patient. The LOS measured in hours was used as the outcome variable in the analysis. The median LOS for the entire sample of the COPD patients during the study period was 4 days, or 96 hours. One day was reported as the shortest LOS, and an LOS of 52 days was the longest in the sample. Since a LOS of more than 9 days is considered unusual for most DRGs (diagnosis-related group), we performed the outlier diagnostics for the LOS variable and removed 74 observations where the LOS exceeded 18 days ($\geq$Q3 + 3IQR).

The distributions of *Age*, *Temp*, *HRate*, *SysBP*, and *DiasBP* appear to be normal, while *Oxygen*, *BMI*, glomerular filtration rate, *eGFR* (a measure of renal function,), and Braden score exhibit sample distributions that are highly skewed and might result in leverage points which have a detrimental impact on the estimation.

A vast majority of medical studies emphasize the importance of adjusting for comorbidities when modeling clinical outcomes [1]. Comorbidities may delay diagnosis, influence treatment choices, affect treatment progress, and impact the LOS. While several general comorbidity indices are available for measuring the impact of comorbidities, the Charlson Comorbidity Index (CCI) is the only index designed using statistical methodology [3]. Another advantage of the CCI is that it creates a continuous variable for scoring.

The CCI in this study, *Charlson_w*, was calculated using ICD-9 and ICD-10 codes for secondary diagnoses for COPD patients with comorbidity package in R [6]. We used the current version of the weighted Charlson score with 17 comorbidities [4]. COPD was excluded from the comorbidities list in our calculations since all patients had COPD as their primary diagnosis. The CCI is expected to have a right skewed distribution with a low mean [7], and the observed distribution of the *Charlson_w* for the COPD patients in the sample was consistent with the theory.

Tobacco use is a behavioral risk factor for COPD and must be controlled for when modeling clinical outcomes such as LOS and readmission rate. The *Tobacco.Use* variable is constructed from the clinical data reports and has three categories that denote patient use of tobacco: never a smoker, a former smoker, and a current smoker. Eighty-four percent of the recorded responses for COPD patients in the data set were either former or current smokers; more than two-thirds of patients have missing values for tobacco use.

Many studies suggest using a severity of illness indicator as an important covariate for the estimation of clinical outcomes. Mechanical ventilation is a commonly used indicator for the severity of illness in COPD patients [2], and an indicator variable for the use of invasive mechanical ventilation, *IMV*, is included in this study. We constructed the *IMV* variable from the primary and secondary procedures for COPD patients where the ventilator use was recorded.

The measures of hospital congestion on admission (*HCa*) and at discharge (*HCd*) were calculated as a daily ratio of patient days and observation days to beds available. Higher values for *HCa* and *HCd* denote higher daily hospital congestion. On average, the hospital was operating at a 77% capacity level over the study period, with some days reaching as high as 94% of total capacity.

2.2 Preliminary Selection of Predictor Variables and Missing Values Analysis

The *Race* variable was excluded from the analysis after finding that *Race* and *Insurance* variables were not independent ($\chi^2 = 15.9, df = 3, p\text{-value} = 0.001$). For *Race* and *Tobacco.Use*, the χ^2 test statistic was also significant (p-value $= 0.054$). Including *Race* together with other categorical predictors resulted in a singular matrix error with Amelia package, likely due to the dependencies discussed above.

Systolic and diastolic blood pressures were highly correlated ($r = 0.67043$, p-value <0.000). Only systolic blood pressure was retained as a potential predictor for the LOS based on the findings from the study by Palaniappan et al. [11]. According to Palaniappan et al., clinicians are more familiar with systolic blood pressure as a risk factor, and the use of other existing blood pressure measurements does not provide a clear advantage.

Temp variable values ranging between 34 and 49 degrees were assumed to be recorded in Celsius and converted to Fahrenheit. Temperatures outside reasonable ranges were assigned *NA*s.

BMI variable had a high percentage of missing values (around 30%). While patient height and weight were reported in the clinical data set, calculating BMI from the recorded values for height and weight was not plausible due to apparent inconsistences in the scales of measurement for the *Height* and *Weight* variables.

The clinical data set that contained patient vital signs and clinical risk factors had a large number of missing values for several fields. Figure 1 shows the missingness map for all predictor variables in our sample.

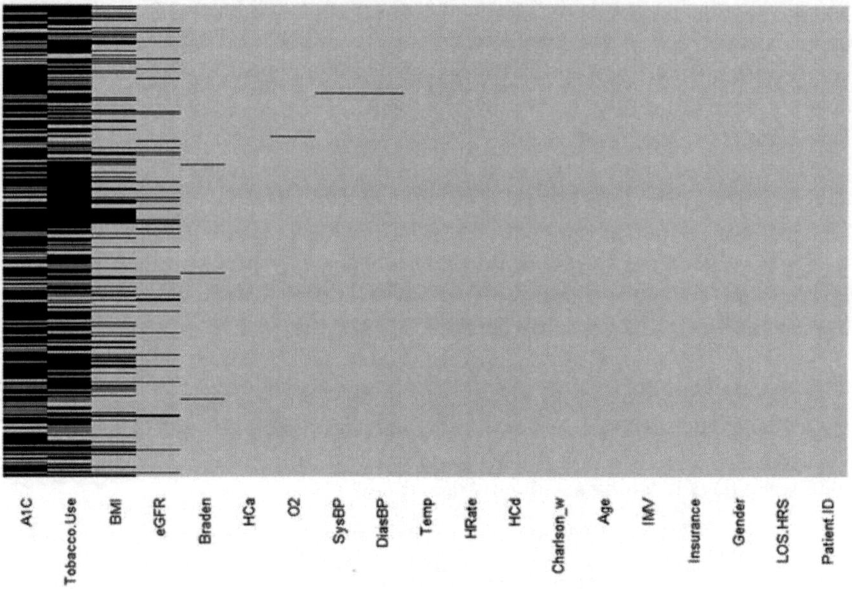

Fig. 1 Missingness map

The top four variables in terms of missingness were *A1C*, *Tobacco.Use*, *BMI*, and *eGFR*. Percent of missing values in the *A1C* variable was 78.7%; in *Tobaco.Use*, 70.6%; in *BMI*, 30.5%; and in *eGFR*, 8.2%. Keeping these four variables in the model would result in the loss of 3512 observations (about 95% of the entire sample). For the baseline model, we removed the three variables with the highest number of missing values from the analysis and continued working with the resulting sample of 2491 complete observations. To address the issue of the missing values, we performed multiple imputations of the missing values using Amelia package in R [8]. We generated 25 data sets with imputed missing values and used them for modeling the LOS with a full set of predictors.

2.3 Variable Selection and Model Development

The commonly used statistical modelling method for count data is the generalized linear model (GLM). The two specific models that can be used to predict the LOS are the Poisson and the negative binomial regression models.

While both Poisson and negative binomial regression models are designed to analyze count data, the two regression models have different assumptions about the conditional mean and variance of the dependent variable. Poisson models assume that the conditional mean and variance of the distribution are equal. Negative binomial regression models do not make the same assumption and correct for

Table 1 Baseline negative binomial regression model

	Estimate	Std. error	z Value	Pr(>|z|)	Significance
(Intercept)	3.67	1.4682	2.502	0.0124	*
Age	0.00	0.0016	2.959	0.0031	**
HCa	0.27	0.2701	0.981	0.3265	
HCd	0.51	0.2633	1.953	0.0508	.
Temp	0.01	0.0146	0.605	0.5449	
HRate	0.00	0.0007	−0.514	0.6069	
SysBP	0.00	0.0005	−1.097	0.2725	
O2	0.00	0.0019	0.389	0.6972	
eGFR	0.00	0.0005	1.074	0.2828	
Braden	−0.03	0.0052	−5.17	0.0000	***
Charlson_w	0.02	0.0087	2.509	0.0121	*
IMV1	0.36	0.1025	3.493	0.0005	***
GenderMale	−0.06	0.0289	−2.058	0.0396	*
InsuranceMedicare	−0.12	0.0431	−2.826	0.0047	**
InsurancePrivate	−0.25	0.0564	−4.441	0.0000	***
InsuranceUninsured	−0.24	0.0734	−3.202	0.0014	**

overdispersion in the data [5, 12]. The negative binomial regression produces a better fit for the LOS and is, therefore, a better modeling choice.

The probability distribution for a negative binomial variable that allows for different means μ_i for each y_i can be expressed as follows:

$$f\left(y_i;\mu_i,\upsilon\right)=\frac{\Gamma\left(y_i+\upsilon\right)}{y_i!\Gamma\left(\upsilon\right)}\left(\frac{\upsilon}{\upsilon+\mu_i}\right)^{\upsilon}\left(\frac{\mu_i}{\upsilon+\mu_i}\right)^{y_i}. \tag{1}$$

The means are based on the logarithmic link, $\boldsymbol{\mu} = \exp\left(\boldsymbol{X\beta}\right)$. The negative binomial parameters $\boldsymbol{\beta}$ and $\boldsymbol{\alpha}$, where $\alpha = \frac{1}{\upsilon}$, can be estimated using maximum likelihood. The asymptotic variance of $\hat{\boldsymbol{\beta}}$ can be estimated using

$$\hat{V}\left(\hat{\boldsymbol{\beta}}\right)=\left(X'\,\mathrm{diag}\left[\frac{\hat{\mu}_i}{1+\hat{\alpha}\hat{\mu}_i}\right]X\right)^{-1} \tag{2}$$

The list of potential covariates for the baseline negative binomial regression model for the LOS includes *Age*, *Gender*, *Temp*, *HRate*, *SysBP*, *O2*, *eGFR*, *Braden*, *Charlson_w*, *Insurance*, *IMV*, *HCa*, and *HCd*. The estimation results are shown in Table 1.

The baseline model identifies Age, Braden score, and use of a ventilator as highly significant predictors for the LOS. Insurance was significant as well, with private insurance, Medicare, and Uninsured categories contributing to a reduction in the LOS in comparison to the Medicaid category. Charlson Comorbidity Index and

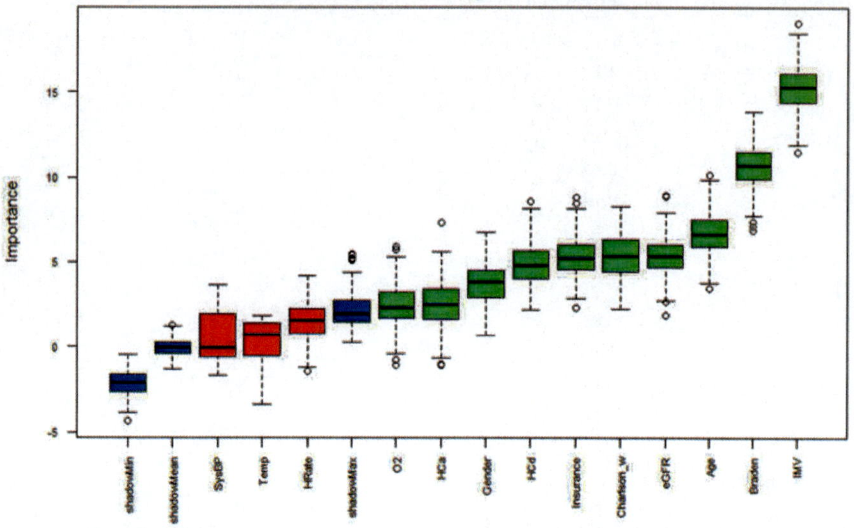

Fig. 2 Boruta variable selection results

gender were significant at a 5% level. The sign of the coefficient for the hospital congestion at discharge was positive, suggesting that it increases the LOS.

Variable selection plays an important role in predictive modeling. Selecting only those predictor variables that are uncorrelated and nonredundant can help reduce noise, train the model faster, and reduce model complexity. Boruta variable selection algorithm is a wrapper method built around the random forest classification algorithm. Its heuristic procedure provides stable and unbiased selection of important attributes [9]. We employed the Boruta variable selection algorithm for the baseline model, and Fig. 2 shows variable importance for the baseline predictors.

The Boruta algorithm agreed with the baseline regression model on *Temp*, *HRate*, and *SysBP* and classified them as unimportant predictors. It added oxygen (*O2*) and hospital congestion on admission (*HCa*) to the list of important predictors. *Age*, *HCd*, *Braden*, *Charlson_w*, *IMV*, *and Gender* were selected as important predictors by both the baseline regression and the Boruta algorithm.

We fitted a negative binomial regression model to the set of important predictors identified by the Boruta algorithm and compared its performance to the baseline model. The new model produced very similar generalization error, since the two sets of predictors did not differ greatly. The estimation results are shown in Table 2.

Random forest models have demonstrated high predictive accuracy in data mining and other disciplines, but they have not been used extensively with count data. We trained a random forest model on a baseline set of predictors using randomForest package in R [10]. The default values of mtry, ntree, and nodesize are often good options [10]; therefore, we used the default values in our analysis (ntree = 500, mtry = 4). The features were selected based on variable importance

Table 2 Baseline negative binomial regression model with Boruta predictors

	Estimate	Std. error	z Value	Pr(>|z|)	Significance
(Intercept)	4.439	0.3266	13.593	< 2e-16	***
Age	0.005	0.0016	3.018	0.0025	**
HCa	0.279	0.2698	1.035	0.3007	
HCd	0.516	0.2633	1.962	0.0498	*
O2	0.001	0.0019	0.291	0.7707	
eGFR	0.001	0.0005	1.086	0.2777	
Braden	−0.027	0.0052	−5.243	0.0000	***
Charlson_w	0.021	0.0087	2.462	0.0138	*
IMV1	0.347	0.1019	3.405	0.0007	***
GenderMale	−0.059	0.0288	−2.035	0.0419	*
InsuranceMedicare	−0.121	0.0431	−2.806	0.0050	**
InsurancePrivate	−0.249	0.0563	−4.415	0.0000	***
InsuranceUninsured	−0.235	0.0734	−3.195	0.0014	**

Table 3 Variable selection from the random forest model

	VarImp
Braden	207.169168
Age	118.380896
Insurance	92.356124
IMV	80.528444
HCd	70.813271
Charlson_w	61.29239
eGFR	58.860783
Gender	47.056827
O2	26.204149
HRate	15.7401
HCa	−8.253697
Temp	−21.610288
SysBP	−42.30066

and on the accuracy of the resulting predictive model. In the final selection, only those predictors that could improve the predictive accuracy were selected. Table 3 shows the results of the variable selection from the RF model.

We also estimated the LOS using the imputed missing values from Amelia package and a full list of available predictors. The regression coefficients were obtained by averaging the model coefficients from each of the imputed data sets. The RMSE and RMSE_holdout for the random forest model on imputed data were calculated as an average from each estimation run.

The negative binomial regression and random forest models on imputed data produced similar estimation results in terms of model accuracy and predictive ability. *Tobacco.Use*, *A1C*, and *BMI* that were omitted from the baseline model due to a large number of missing values were selected as important variables by the Boruta algorithm (Fig. 3).

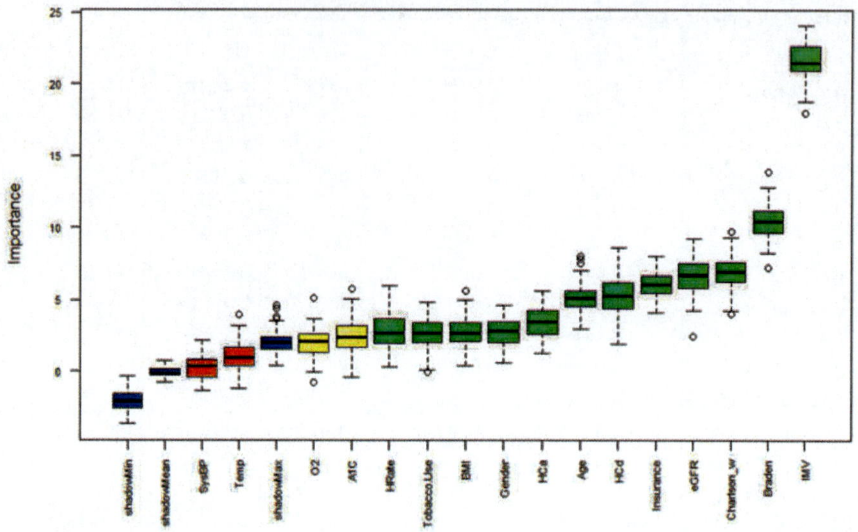

Fig. 3 The Boruta variable selection results for imputed data

Table 4 Model comparison

Model	RMSE	RMSE_holdout
NB_Baseline	69.65	70.92
NB_Baseline_Boruta	69.70	70.84
RF_Baseline	71.09	70.72
NB_Imputed	69.75	72.90
NB_Imputed_Boruta	69.77	72.92
RF_Imputed	69.93	72.75

3 Results and Discussion

In this study, we used the negative binomial regression and random forest methods to develop an optimal predictive model for the LOS of COPD patients. The models' predictive ability was assessed by calculating their generalization errors (RMSE_holdout) and is summarized in Table 4.

The Boruta feature selection algorithm and the random forest models did not outperform the baseline negative binomial regression model, confirming the idea that GLM is a better candidate for count data and for application where the number of predictor variables is not overly large. Using a regression model for predicting the LOS also has the advantage of interpretability as opposed to a black box machine learning model and is often a preferred method in many applications.

All models identified largely similar sets of important predictor variables. While some of those predictor variables, such as age, comorbidity score, and use of a ventilator, were expected to make the selection list, several others require special consideration, and the Braden score is one them. While usually not included in the studies of COPD patients, it was a significant predictor in the regression models, and it was given high importance by the Boruta algorithm and the random forest models as well.

Hospital congestion indices had positive signs of estimated coefficients, showing that shortage of hospital resources contributes to the extended LOS. Insurance variable was highly significant and requires further investigation. Tobacco use, eGFR, and oxygen were selected as important predictors for the COPD patients as well and should be included in future studies.

References

1. S. Austin, Y. Wong, R. Uzzo, J. Beck, B. Egleston, Why summary comorbidity measures such as the Charlson Comorbidity Index and Elixhauser score work. Med. Care **53**(9), e65–e72 (2015). https://doi.org/10.1097/MLR.0b013e318297429c
2. G. Brattebø, D. Hofoss, H. Flaatten, A.K. Muri, S. Gjerde, P.E. Plsek, Quality improvement report: Effect of a scoring system and protocol for sedation on duration of patients' need for ventilator support in a surgical intensive care unit. BMJ Br. Med. J. **324**(7350), 1386 (2002)
3. M. Charlson, P. Pompei, K. Ales, C. MacKenzie, A new method of classifying prognostic comorbidity in longitudinal studies: Development and validation. J. Chronic Dis. **40**(5), 373–383 (1987)
4. Y.-T. Chu, Y.-Y. Ng, S.-C. Wu, Comparison of different comorbidity measures for use with administrative data in predicting short-and long-term mortality. BMC Health Serv. Res. **10**(1), 140 (2010)
5. J.J. Faraway, *Extending the Linear Model with R: Generalized Linear, Mixed Effects and Nonparametric Regression Models* (CRC Press, New York, 2005)
6. A. Gasparini, Comorbidity: An R package for computing comorbidity scores. J. Open Source Softw. **3**(23), 648 (2018). https://doi.org/10.21105/joss.00648
7. S.F. Hall, A user's guide to selecting a comorbidity index for clinical research. J. Clin. Epidemiol. **59**(8), 849–855 (2006)
8. J. Honaker, G. King, M. Blackwell, Amelia II: A program for missing data. J. Stat. Softw. **45**(7), 1–47 (2011)
9. M. Kursa, W. Rudnicki, Feature selection with the Boruta package. J. Stat. Softw. **36**(11), 1–13 (2010)
10. A. Liaw, M. Wiener, Classification and regression by randomForest. R. News **2**(3), 18–22 (2002)
11. L. Palaniappan, L. Simons, J. Simons, Y. Friedlander, J. McCallum, Comparison of usefulness of systolic, diastolic, and mean blood pressure and pulse pressure as predictors of cardiovascular death in patients $\geq$60 years of age (the Dubbo study). Am. J. Cardiol. **90**(12), 1398–1401 (2002)
12. J.S. Simonoff, *Analyzing Categorical Data* (Springer Science & Business Media, New York, 2013)
13. B. Smith, F. Cheok, A. Heard, A. Esterman, A. Southcott, R. Antic, et al., Impact on readmission rates and mortality of a chronic obstructive pulmonary disease inpatient management guideline. Chron. Respir. Dis. **1**(1), 17–28 (2004)

Predicting Seizure-Like Activity Using Sensors from Smart Glasses

Sarah Hadipour, Ala Tokhmpash, Bahram Shafai, and Carey Rappaport

1 Introduction

The availability of a system capable of automatically classifying the physical activity performed by a human subject is extremely attractive for many applications in the field of healthcare monitoring and in developing advanced human–machine interfaces [3]. By the term physical activity, we mean any background activity that excludes the period of seizure happening. Wearable accelerometers are a novel tool that can detect and objectively characterize these movement abnormalities in both the clinical setting and the patient's home environment. Although accelerometry has yet to make it into the mainstream clinic, there is great promise for this technology in monitoring epileptic patients [4, 5].

2 Smart Glasses and Data Collection

Bose AR devices combine data from embedded motion sensors with GPS information from your phone, which they connect with via Bluetooth. GPS detects where a user is, and the nine-axis sensor can determine which direction they are looking and moving.

S. Hadipour (✉) · A. Tokhmpash · B. Shafai · C. Rappaport
Department of Electrical and Computer Engineering, Northeastern University, Boston, MA, USA
e-mail: hadipour.s@northeastern.edu; tokhmpash.a@northeastern.edu; shafai@ece.neu.edu; rappaport@ece.neu.edu
https://ece.northeastern.edu/; https://coe.northeastern.edu/people/shafai-bahram/; https://coe.northeastern.edu/people/rappaport-carey/

H. R. Arabnia et al. (eds.), *Advances in Computer Vision and Computational Biology*, Transactions on Computational Science and Computational Intelligence,
https://doi.org/10.1007/978-3-030-71051-4_35

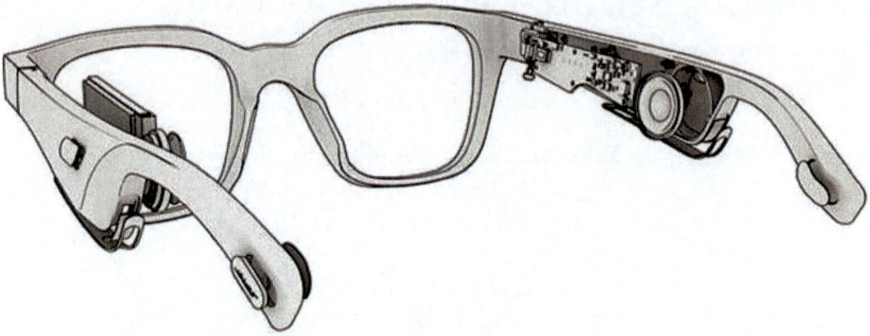

Fig. 1 The wearable sensor used in this study to perform activity detection. Picture courtesy of Bose

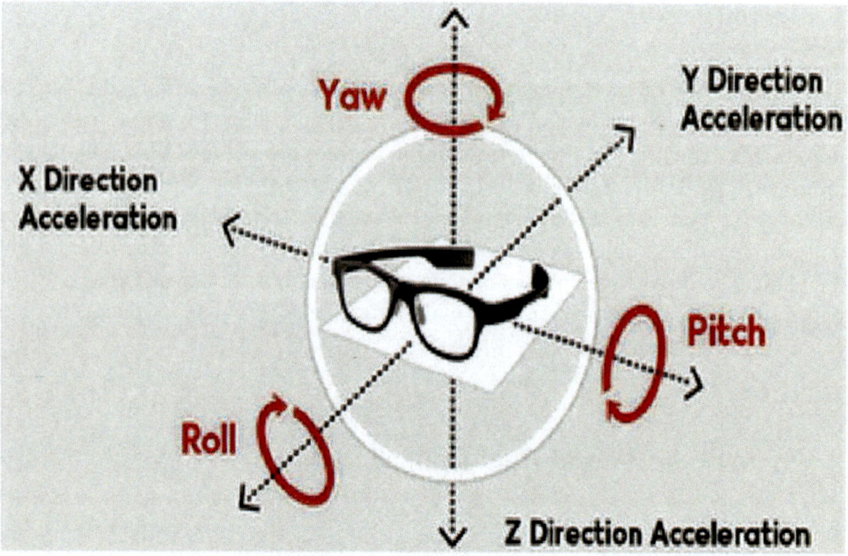

Fig. 2 The wearable sensor orientation used in this study

Figure 1 shows the structure of the wearable device used in this study which is a Bose AR frame.

An IMU used here is a specific type of sensor that measures angular rate, force, and sometimes magnetic field [6]. IMUs are composed of a 3-axis accelerometer and a 3-axis gyroscope, which would be considered a 6-axis IMU [7].

Figure 2 shows how the orientation of the data collected is and the corresponding time series plots would reflect this orientation.

3 Deep Neural Network (DNN)

In this study we show how to forecast time series data using a long short-term memory (LSTM) network. DNN have been studied in other works [8].

To forecast the values of future time steps of a sequence, we then train a sequence-to-sequence regression LSTM network, where the responses are the training sequences with values shifted by one time step. That is, at each time step of the input sequence, the LSTM network learns to predict the value of the next time step.

In our study we used the data set downloaded from the Bose portal that is designed for data collection. The example trains an LSTM network to classify the next activity as a seizure or not.

Figure 3 shows the time domain representation of the X, Y, and Z acceleration in the simulated seizure event.

And Fig. 4 shows the frequency domain representation of the X, Y, and Z acceleration in the simulated seizure event.

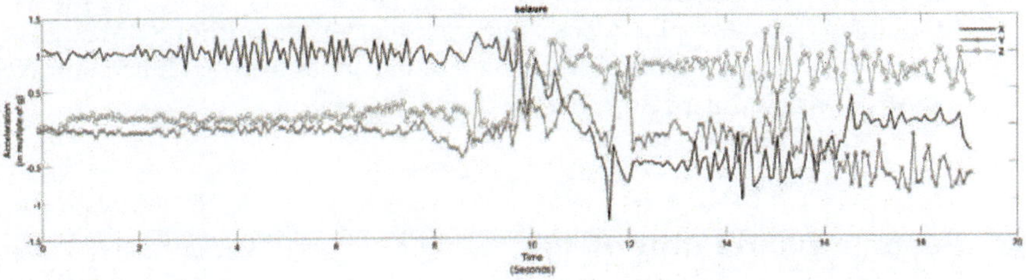

Fig. 3 Time series representation of a seizure like X, Y, and Z acceleration signals

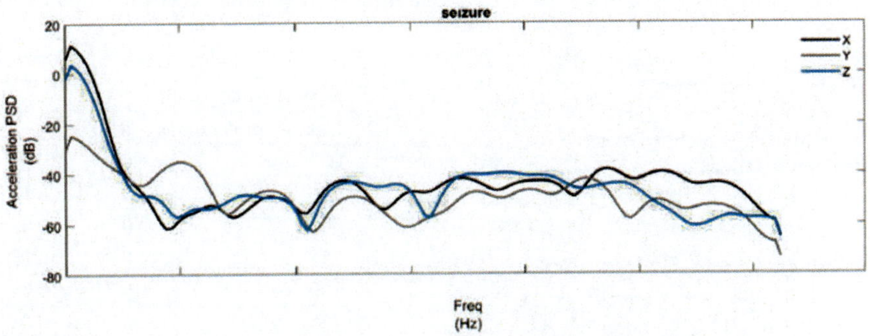

Fig. 4 Frequency representation [2] of a seizure like X, Y, and Z acceleration signals

4 Training Results

Long short-term memory (LSTM) is an artificial recurrent neural network (RNN) architecture [1] used in the field of deep learning. Unlike standard feedforward neural networks, LSTM has feedback connections. It can not only process single data points (such as images), but also entire sequences of data (such as speech or video).

For a better fit and to prevent the training from diverging, it is important to standardize the training data to have zero mean and unit variance. At prediction time, it is also important to standardize the test data using the same parameters as the training data.

For forecasting the values of future time steps of a sequence, we specified the responses to be the training sequences with values shifted by one time step. That is, at each time step of the input sequence, the LSTM network learns to predict the value of the next time step. The predictors are the training sequences without the final time step.

Finally we created an LSTM regression network. To prevent the gradients from exploding, we set the gradient threshold to 1 [9].

The training progress plot reports the root-mean-square error (RMSE) [10] calculated from the standardized data. Table 1 summarizes the Loss function values [11] and Root-Mean-Square Error over multiple iterations:

5 Summary and Future Work

We presented and analyzed a method to classify and distinguish between a simulated seizure and a non-seizure activity. To visualize the performance of the model we

Table 1 Loss function values and Root-Mean-Square Error over multiple iterations

Sample model results		
Number of iterations	RMSE	Loss
0	0.98	0.49
25	0.38	0.12
50	0.36	0.09
75	0.37	0.05
100	0.31	0.04
125	0.35	0.03
150	0.19	0.02
175	0.17	0.01
200	0.16	0.0
225	0.15	0.0
250	0.14	0.0

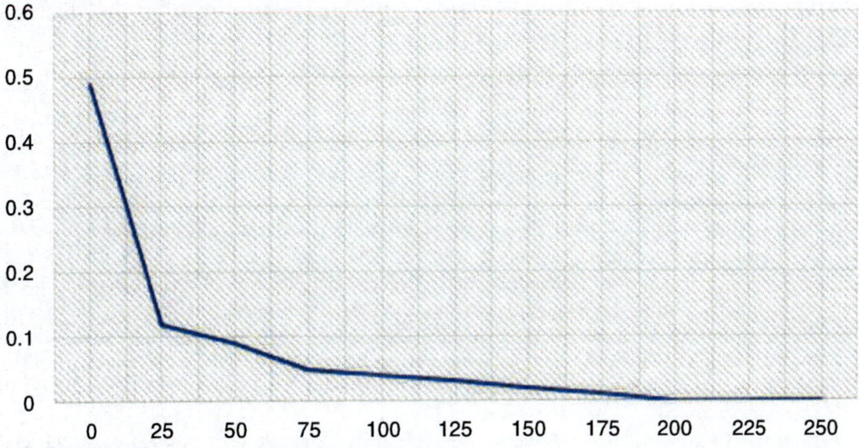

Fig. 5 Loss function values over multiple iterations

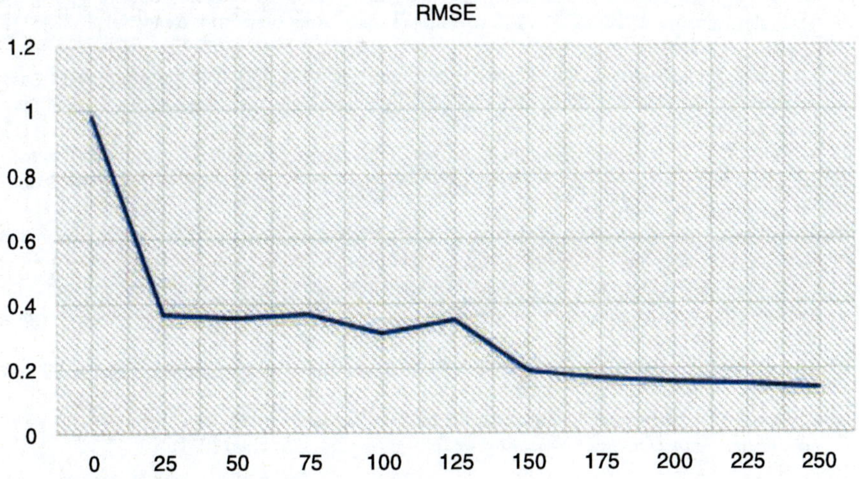

Fig. 6 Root-Mean-Square Error over multiple iterations

plotted the loss function as well as the Root-Mean-Square Error over multiple iterations.

Figure 5 shows a significant decline in the loss value and settling after 200 iterations.

Figure 6 shows a significant decline in the RMSE value and settling after 250 iterations.

This detector simplifies the implementation of the seizure prediction system into a wearable device. This system can be potentially coupled with a closed loop control system to suppress the seizure intensity and mitigate the consequences of the drug-resistant seizures.

For future work we are planning on using the non-patient specific classifier and compare it with the one designed in this study.

References

1. U. Orhan, M. Hekim, M. Ozer, EEG signals classification using the K-means clustering and a multilayer perceptron neural network model. Exp. Syst. Appl. **38**, 13475–13481 (2011)
2. K. Samiee, P. Kovács, M. Gabbouj, Epileptic seizure classification of EEG time-series using rational discrete short-time Fourier transform. IEEE Trans. Biomed. Eng. 62, 541–552 (2015)
3. T. Kangarloo, F. Hameed, C. Demanuele, D. Psaltos, H. Zhang, R. Lopez, et al. An observational study using multimodal wearable sensors and environmental monitors in healthy volunteers to characterize activities pertaining to health, wellbeing, and daily living, in *Movement Disorders* (Wiley, New York, 2018)
4. Aliverti2017,Munos2016 A. Aliverti, Wearable technology: Role in respiratory health and disease. Breathe **13**, e27–e36 (2017)
5. B. Munos, P.C. Baker, B.M. Bot, M. Crouthamel, G. de Vries, I. Ferguson, J.D. Hixson, L.A. Malek, J.J. Mastrototaro, V. Misra, A. Ozcan, L. Sacks, P. Wang, Mobile health: the power of wearables, sensors, and apps to transform clinical trials. Ann. New York Acad. Sci. **1375**, 3–18 (2016)
6. T.T. Um, V. Babakeshizadeh, D. Kulic, Exercise motion classification from large-scale wearable sensor data using convolutional neural networks, in *IEEE International Conference on Intelligent Robots and Systems* (2017)
7. B. Wagstaff, V. Peretroukjin, J. Kelly, Improving foot-mounted inertial navigation through real-time motion classification, in *2017 International Conference on Indoor Positioning and Indoor Navigation, IPIN 2017* (2017)
8. S. Hadipour, A. Tokhmpash, B. Shafai, A comparative study on epileptic seizure detection methods, in *International Conference on Applied Human Factors and Ergonomics* (2020)
9. C.M. Vastrad, Performance analysis of neural network models for oxazolines and oxazoles derivatives descriptor dataset, in *International Journal of Information Sciences and Techniques* (2013)
10. R.O. Duda, P.E. Hart, D.G. Stork, Pattern Classification, 2nd edn. Computational Complexity (1998)
11. Z. Zhang, M.R. Sabuncu, Generalized cross entropy loss for training deep neural networks with noisy labels, in *Advances in Neural Information Processing Systems* (2018)

Epileptic iEEG Signal Classification Using Pre-trained Networks

Sarah Hadipour, Ala Tokhmpash, Bahram Shafai, and Carey Rappaport

1 Introduction

In the past, seizure classification methods were applied by extracting features from the time series signals. This work describes how pre-trained sophisticated models can now be used in classification of naturally occurring seizure signals in drug-resistant epileptic patients.

These pre-trained models are Neural Network models trained on large benchmark datasets. These open-source models have greatly benefited The Deep Learning community and played a major role in the rapid advances in Computer Vision research [1–3].

It is possible that other researchers and practitioners may use these state-of-the-art models instead of re-inventing everything from scratch. The word pre-trained here means that the deep learning architectures have been already trained on some huge dataset and thus carry the resultant weights and biases with them [4, 5].

Recently some research discoveries say that pre-trained models may have very limited help for some tasks [6]. However, such pre-trained models are mainly trained using natural images. There is a difference between natural images and medical images, where in the latter, networks may be fine-tuned using a technique known as transfer learning. It has been argued that transfer learning may have a very limited effect when switching data content from one type to another. If so, transfer learning in this case may be no better than training with randomly initialized weights (from

S. Hadipour (✉) · A. Tokhmpash · B. Shafai · C. Rappaport
Department of Electrical and Computer Engineering, Northeastern University, Boston, MA, USA
e-mail: hadipour.s@northeastern.edu; tokhmpash.a@northeastern.edu; shafai@ece.neu.edu; rappaport@ece.neu.edu
https://ece.northeastern.edu/; https://coe.northeastern.edu/people/shafai-bahram/; https://coe.northeastern.edu/people/rappaport-carey/

H. R. Arabnia et al. (eds.), *Advances in Computer Vision and Computational Biology*, Transactions on Computational Science and Computational Intelligence,
https://doi.org/10.1007/978-3-030-71051-4_36

scratch), since the networks learn very different high-level features in the two tasks. Certainly, we know if we have enough data, training from scratch is a feasible approach. However, in the health care field that may not be always possible.

We have put this hypothesis to test and used one of the common pre-trained models to see how our results compare.

2 Spectrogram of Medical Signals and Convolutional Neural Network

In our experiment we used transfer learning to retrain a convolutional neural network to classify a new set of images [7].

Pre-trained image classification networks have been trained on over a million images and can classify images into hundreds of categories [8–10]. The networks have learned many feature representations for a variety of images. The network takes an image as input, and then outputs a label for the image.

Transfer learning is commonly used in deep learning applications [11]. We take a pre-trained network and use it as a starting point to learn a new task. Fine-tuning a network with transfer learning is usually much faster and easier than training a network from scratch with randomly initialized weights. We then quickly transfer the learned features to a new task using a smaller number of training images.

Figure 1 shows our approach and summarizes the high-level tasks:

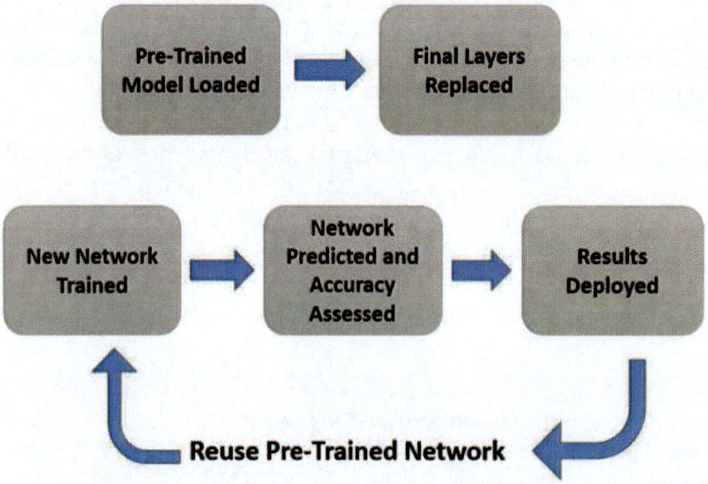

Fig. 1 Pre-training block diagram

In order to obtain the iEEG images of the brain signals we used the spectrogram technique. This technique has been used for medical purposes in the past such as phonocardiogram [12], electromyography [13], electrocardiogram [14].

The spectrogram uses the short-time Fourier transform of the input signal and outputs an image in which each column contains an estimate of the short-term, time-localized frequency content of the iEEG signal.

The following Figs. 2 and 3 plot the spectrogram image of the preictal and interictal iEEGs collected from a patient with naturally occurring epileptic seizures.

The interictal period is often used by neurologists when diagnosing epilepsy since an iEEG trace will often show small interictal spiking and other abnormalities known by neurologists as subclinical seizures.

Preictal refers to the state immediately before the actual seizure.

Visually inspecting there is a clear distinction between the two states so we anticipate a good classification result.

Additionally training neural networks is easiest when the inputs to the network have a reasonably smooth distribution and are normalized which has been accomplished here.

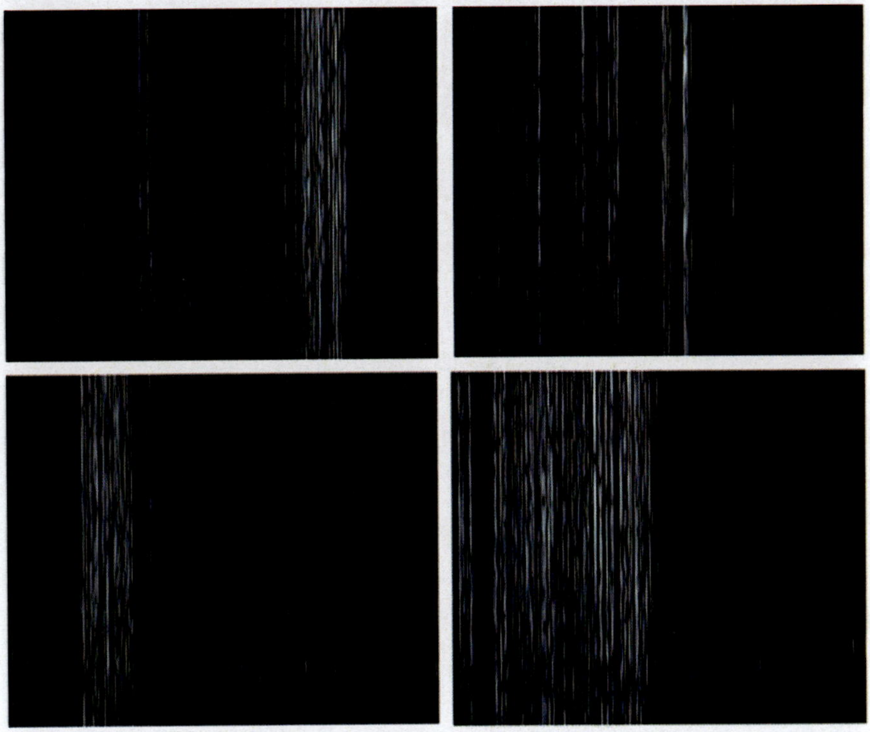

Fig. 2 Spectrogram of interictal iEEG signals

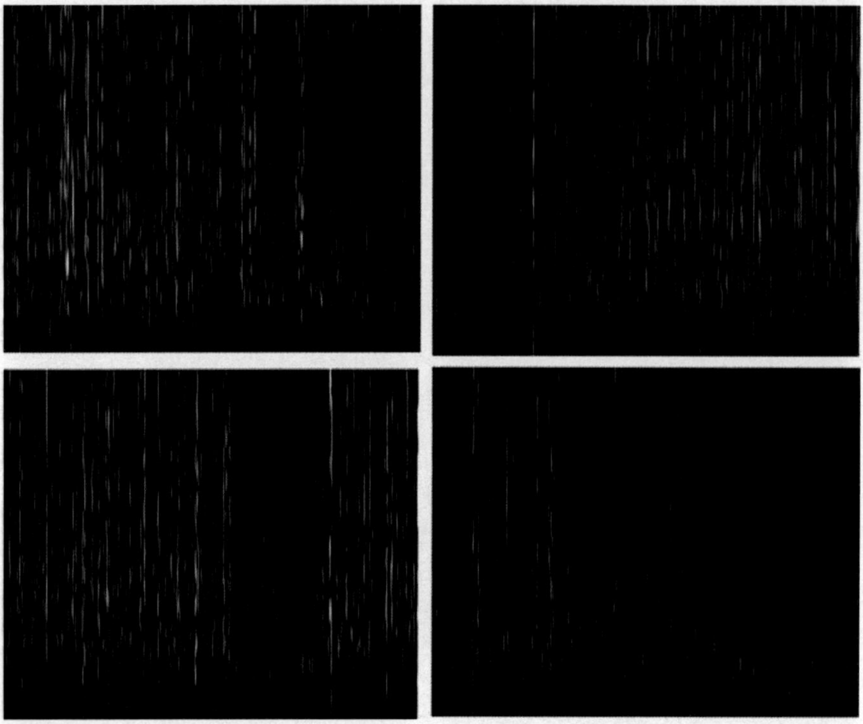

Fig. 3 Spectrogram of preictal iEEG signals

3 Performance Results

In order to find out how our CNN is performing we used accuracy and the loss as the performance metrics. Accuracy is one of the most common metric for evaluating classification models. Informally, accuracy is the fraction of predictions our model got right. Formally, accuracy has the following definition [15]:

$$Accuracy = \frac{Numberofcorrectpredictions}{Totalnumberofpredictions}$$

Figure 4 shows the accuracy achieved over multiple iteration and batches. The overall accuracy improves as we train the model over and over.

For the second performance metrics we used the loss values. In most cases CNNs use a cross-entropy loss [16] . For a single image the cross-entropy loss looks like this:

$$-\sum_{c=1}^{M}(y_c . \log \hat{y_c})$$

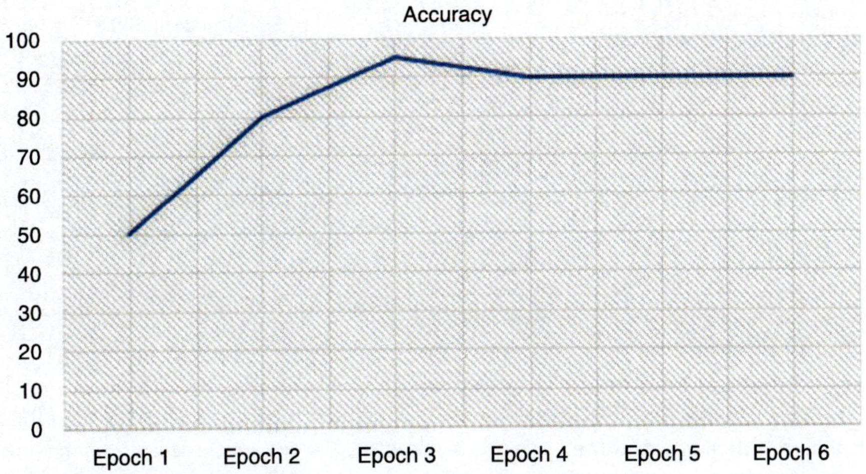

Fig. 4 Accuracy settling after four epochs

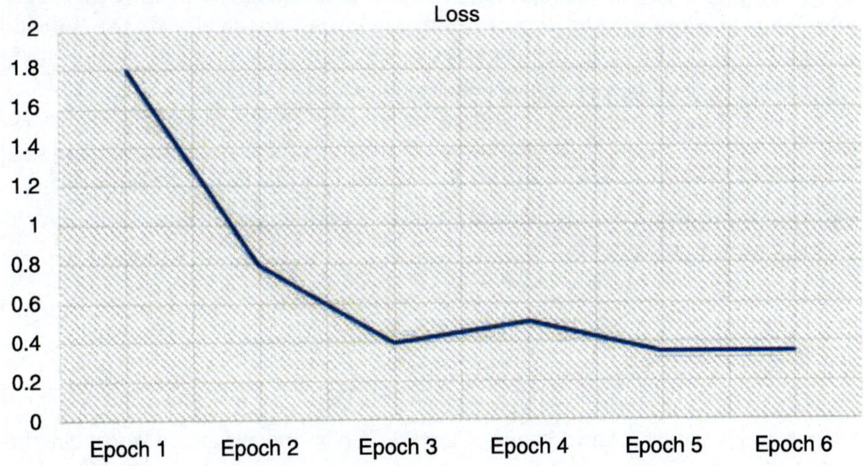

Fig. 5 Loss function converging after five epochs

where M is the number of classes and y_c is the model's prediction for that class (i.e. the output of class c).

Figure 5 shows the loss function values over multiple batches and iterations. The loss function value declines from the first to the last epoch.

Table 1 Accuracy and Loss performance measure for our classifier network

Sample model results		
Parameters	Loss	Accuracy
Epoch 1	1.8	50.1%
Epoch 2	0.8	80.4%
Epoch 3	0.4	95.6%
Epoch 4	0.5	90.8%
Epoch 5	0.35	90.9%
Epoch 6	0.35	91%

4 Summary

Transfer learning has been recommended in research works as one of the solutions to the insufficiency of training data in healthcare. While transfer learning helps our training process in terms of reducing size of required training dataset and saving training time, it is also important to understand and study the nature of the data. Using pre-processing techniques that are specific to the nature of the data should be applicable to our specific area of healthcare images first to classify the epileptic seizures.

The summary of the performance measures is shown in Table 1:

As we increase the number of epochs we achieve a high accuracy rate. The loss function also shows a good drop from epoch 1 to 6. An epoch is one complete presentation of the dataset to be learned to our learning machine. Learning machines like feed-forward neural nets that use iterative algorithms often need many epochs during their learning phase.

5 Future Work

Deep learning Convolutional Neural Network (CNN) models are powerful classification models but require a large amount of training data. In niche domains such as epilepsy and seizure detection, it is expensive and difficult to obtain a large number of training samples. One method of classifying data with a limited number of training samples is to employ transfer learning. In this research, we evaluated the effectiveness of intracranial EEG signal classification using transfer learning from a larger base dataset to a smaller target dataset using the pre-trained CNN. We obtained 82.4% average validation accuracy on the target dataset in fivefold cross-validation. The methodology of transfer learning from a pre-trained CNN to a project-specific and a much smaller set of classes and images was extended to the domain of spectrogram images.

Transfer learning works fairly well in medical images. Most published deep learning models for healthcare data analysis are pre-trained on popular models. Pre-training most times does not necessarily need to be done on dataset of similar domain but just to give a model a general context about objects. This has been proven to help deep models converge faster compared to when they are trained from scratch.

References

1. D. Marmanis, M. Datcu, T. Esch, U. Stilla, Deep learning earth observation classification using ImageNet pretrained networks.IEEE Geosci. Remote Sensing Lett. **13**, 105–109 (2016)
2. G. Carneiro, J. Nascimento, A.P. Bradley, Unregistered multiview mammogram analysis with pre-trained deep learning models, in *Lecture Notes in Computer Science (Including Subseries Lecture Notes in Artificial Intelligence and Lecture Notes in Bioinformatics)* (2015)
3. A. Singla, L. Yuan, T. Ebrahimi, Food/non-food image classification and food categorization using pre-trained GoogLeNet model, in *MADiMa 2016 - Proceedings of the 2nd International Workshop on Multimedia Assisted Dietary Management, Co-located with ACM Multimedia 2016* (2016)
4. K. Samiee, P. Kovács, M. Gabbouj, Epileptic seizure classification of EEG time-series using rational discrete short-time Fourier transform. IEEE Trans. Biomed. Eng. **62**, 541–552 (2015)
5. U. Orhan, M. Hekim, M. Ozer, EEG signals classification using the K-means clustering and a multilayer perceptron neural network model. Expert Syst. Appl. **38**, 13475–13481 (2011)
6. R.B. Models, Rethinking business models for innovation. *Grenoble Ecole de Management PostPrint* (2011)
7. A. Verikas, M. Bacauskiene, Feature selection with neural networks. Pattern Recogn. Lett. **23**, 1323–1335 (2002)
8. T. Xiao, Y. Xu, K. Yang, J. Zhang, Y. Peng, Z. Zhang, The application of two-level attention models in deep convolutional neural network for fine-grained image classification, in *Proceedings of the IEEE Computer Society Conference on Computer Vision and Pattern Recognition* (2015)
9. W. Rawat, Z. Wang, Deep convolutional neural networks for image classification: A comprehensive review. Neural Comput. **29**, 2352–2449 (2017)
10. J. Deng, W. Dong, R. Socher, L.-J. Li, K. Li, L. Fei-Fei, ImageNet: A large-scale hierarchical image database, in *2009 IEEE Conference on Computer Vision and Pattern Recognition* (2009)
11. J. Behncke, R.T. Schirrmeister, M. Völker, J. Hammer, P. Marusič, A. Schulze-Bonhage, W. Burgard, T. Ball, Cross-paradigm pretraining of convolutional networks improves intracranial EEG decoding, in *Proceedings - 2018 IEEE International Conference on Systems, Man, and Cybernetics, SMC 2018* (2019)
12. A. Djebbari, F.B. Reguig, Short-time Fourier transform analysis of the phonocardiogram signal, in *Proceedings of the IEEE International Conference on Electronics, Circuits, and Systems* (2000)
13. T.N. Zawawi, A.R. Abdullah, E.F. Shair, I. Halim, O. Rawaida, Electromyography signal analysis using spectrogram, in *Proceeding - 2013 IEEE Student Conference on Research and Development, SCOReD 2013* (2015)
14. J.N. McNames, A.M. Fraser, Obstructive sleep apnea classification based on spectrogram patterns in the electrocardiogram, in *Computers in Cardiology* (IEEE, Piscataway, 2000)
15. R.O. Duda, P.E. Hart, D.G. Stork, *Pattern Classification*, 2nd edn. Computational Complexity (Wiley, New York, 1998)
16. Z. Zhang, M.R. Sabuncu, Generalized cross entropy loss for training deep neural networks with noisy labels, in *Advances in Neural Information Processing Systems* (2018)

Seizure Prediction and Heart Rate Oscillations Classification in Partial Epilepsy

Sarah Hadipour, Ala Tokhmpash, Bahram Shafai, and Carey Rappaport

1 Introduction

Epileptic seizures can be controlled with medication in 70% of the cases [1] and the remaining 30% can lead to serious physical injuries. Since approximately 1% of the world population is affected by epilepsy, creating a wearable technology able to predict epileptic seizures and warn the patient before they happen would be significantly helpful. Most of the existing studies are focused on epileptic seizure prediction [2] that uses the recordings of electroencephalogram (EEG) that practically speaking cannot be easily used in daily life and if they do the cost of such devices is still too high for some patients. On the other hand, electrocardiography (ECG) signal represents the electrical activities of the heart and have been used in detection and classification of cardiac disease. This means they could be useful in detecting other diseases such as epilepsy. From the previous studies done in this field [3] and [4], statistical correlation exists between heart rate variability features and epileptic pre-ictal and post-ictal states. These findings of underlying physiological mechanisms epileptic seizure detection can be done using the ECG signals. The portable nature of the ECG signals [5] makes them very good candidate for wearable device predictors.

In this chapter, we investigate a methodology to reliably predict epileptic seizures from the data provided by portable ECG recorders.

S. Hadipour (✉) · A. Tokhmpash · B. Shafai · C. Rappaport
Department of Electrical and Computer Engineering, Northeastern University, Boston, MA, USA
e-mail: hadipour.s@northeastern.edu; tokhmpash.a@northeastern.edu; shafai@ece.neu.edu; rappaport@ece.neu.edu
https://ece.northeastern.edu/; https://coe.northeastern.edu/people/shafai-bahram/; https://coe.northeastern.edu/people/rappaport-carey/

H. R. Arabnia et al. (eds.), *Advances in Computer Vision and Computational Biology*, Transactions on Computational Science and Computational Intelligence,
https://doi.org/10.1007/978-3-030-71051-4_37

In this chapter, we use a supervised classification method to detect pre-ictal heart rate variability patterns and predict epileptic seizures. We first take the ECG data and deal with the noise during the recording process and also the seizure onset. The next step would be to extract features to perform the prediction. These features are subsequently used to train a recurrent neural network (RNN) to achieve seizure prediction. At the end, we present the training result conducted using real ECG data gathered before, during, and after epileptic seizure episodes.

2 ECG Data Description and Visualization

In our study, we used the SZDB database from [3].

This database, composed of 7 records, contains more than 16 h of ECG sampled at 200 Hz. The data corresponds to heterogeneous group of patients with partial epilepsy during continuous EEG, ECG, and video monitoring. The recording involves 11 epileptic seizures lasting from 15 to 110 s. The EEG and video records were used by expert neurologists to tag the epileptic seizures. Thus, the ground truth is available and perfectly defined within this database: Figure 1 shows the seven recordings that include pre- and post-seizure ECGs.

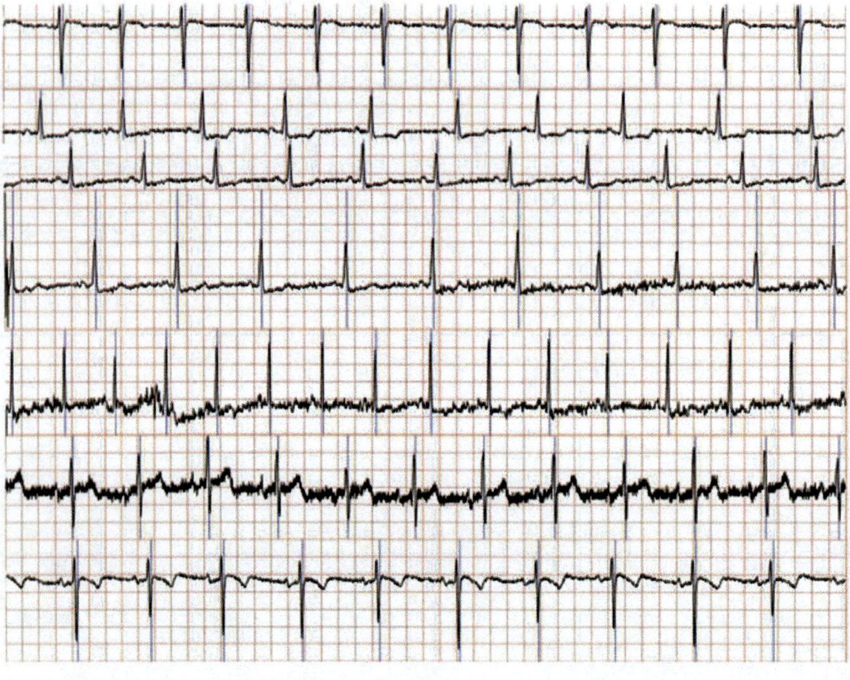

Fig. 1 ECG recording of pre- and post-seizure states

3 Methodology and Feature Extraction

One obvious way to go about feature selection is to start with morphological features and classical signal processing techniques [6–17]. But such features are not sufficient for accurately distinguishing among different types of patients [18, 19], which is because of ECG waveform and its morphological characteristics, for example, shapes of QRS complex and P waves significantly vary under different circumstances and for different patients. To extract the features automatically and increase the ECG based seizure detection accuracy, a deep learning based algorithm including deep recurrent neural networks is proposed, similar to other studies in [19]. Specifically, our approach is to use an ECG classification algorithm based on LSTM recurrent neural networks (RNNs). The classifiers will be discussed in the next sections.

Because of the nature of the electrical conduction system of the heart, ECG waveform is a good fit to be processed by RNNs. The conduction slows through the atrioventricular node that causes a time delay. This means temporal dependencies naturally exist in this waveform. Among all deep learning methods, RNNs capture such temporal dependencies in sequential data most efficiently.

The features we extracted for be to fed the RNN are in two main categories. First, the features that are extracted from the signal in between two heartbeats or precisely between the two R-peaks. And the second are the features that are centered more around the onset of each heartbeat. The following sections explain each category in detail.

3.1 *Inter-Beat Intervals Features*

In order to calculate the inter-beat features, we need to first estimate the inter-beat intervals that are defined as the time between consecutive heartbeats. A common approach to obtain them is to measure the time between consecutive R-peaks in an ECG that is called the R-R intervals or RRI. To do so, we need to perform two main steps: the first step is to process the raw ECG and detect the existing R-peaks and secondly to robustly estimate the RRI.

RRI Detection and Heart Rate Variability Features The RRI can be computed by subtracting the time steps of consecutive heartbeats. However, intervals of extreme noise may appear due to the epileptic seizures. During these intervals, it is difficult to detect the R-peaks. Knowing there is a correlation between heart rate variability features and pre-ictal states, we can find a significant correlation with a set of four time domain features and three frequency domain features. The time domain features are:

1. mean;
2. standard deviation;

3. root mean square of differences between adjacent values (RMS);
4. total power.

The frequency domain features are:

1. power of the power spectrum density (PSD) band 0.04–0.15 Hz;
2. power of the PSD band 0.15–0.4 Hz;
3. ratio between these two frequency features.

All these features are computed within a sliding window over the RRI estimates whose size will be experimentally assessed. Even though these features are a good representation of the inter-beat signals, they are not sufficient to distinguish between pre-seizure and normal states. To achieve more correlation and more features, we will look into the heartbeat features in the next section.

3.2 Segmentation and RR Interval Features

Using the same windowing technique, we digitized ECG samples and segmented them into a sequence of heartbeats. Once again, the segmentation is performed based on detecting the R-peaks. Every segment (heartbeat) is defined as a fixed length signal that contains a half second of the input ECG signal before the detected R-peak and a half second after. Based on this information, we also extract the following four features for heartbeat :

1. the past RR interval;
2. the next RR interval;
3. the sum of the ten consecutive intervals centering around the current heartbeat as the local average of the five past and the five next RR intervals;
4. the average duration of the RR intervals in each person's train data.

The fourth feature is the average RR in every individual's train data recording. This feature varies among people with different average heart rates as it can be quite larger in athletes because they have slower heart rates. We have decided not to employ other handcrafted morphological features such as those that are based on Q, S, or T since such features are not optimal in representing the characteristics of the underlying signal. They are also non-patient specific and therefore do not efficiently represent the differences among the ECG classes [18, 19]. Our algorithm automatically extracts features using wavelet and recurrent neural networks.

3.3 Wavelet Features and Background on Wavelet Transform

ECG signals are frequently non-stationary meaning that their frequency content changes over time. Therefore, traditional signal processing techniques would not

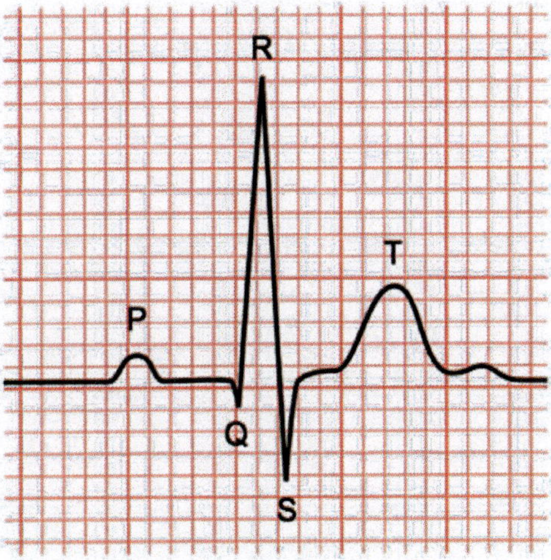

Fig. 2 QRS complex of an ECG recording

suffice. Wavelet transform decomposes signals into time-varying frequency (scale) components. Because signal features are often localized in time and frequency, analysis and estimation are easier when working with sparser signals like ECGs. The QRS complex consists of three deflections in the ECG waveform. The QRS complex reflects the depolarization of the right and left ventricles and is the most prominent feature of the human ECG.

Figure 2 shows an ECG waveform where the R-peaks of the QRS complex have been annotated.

We use wavelets to build an automatic QRS detector and estimate the R-R interval. The wavelet transform separates signal components into different frequency bands enabling a sparser representation of the signal. We found a wavelet that resembles the feature we are trying to detect.

The "sym4" wavelet resembles the QRS complex, which makes it a good choice for QRS detection. Figure 3 illustrates this more clearly, as an example of an extracted QRS complex, and plots the result with a dilated and translated "sym4" wavelet for comparison.

The ECG waveform is decomposed down to level 5 using the default "sym4" wavelet. A frequency-localized version of the ECG waveform is reconstructed using only the wavelet coefficients at scales 4 and 5 that will cover the passband shown to maximize QRS energy. The scales correspond to the following approximate frequency bands:

- Scale 4—[11.25, 22.5) Hz;
- Scale 5—[5.625, 11.25) Hz.

Another technique is to square the magnitudes of the original data. This makes it a lot easier to find the wavelet transform to isolate the R-peaks. Figure 4 shows the raw, squared raw data and the wavelet reconstruction of the ECG recordings.

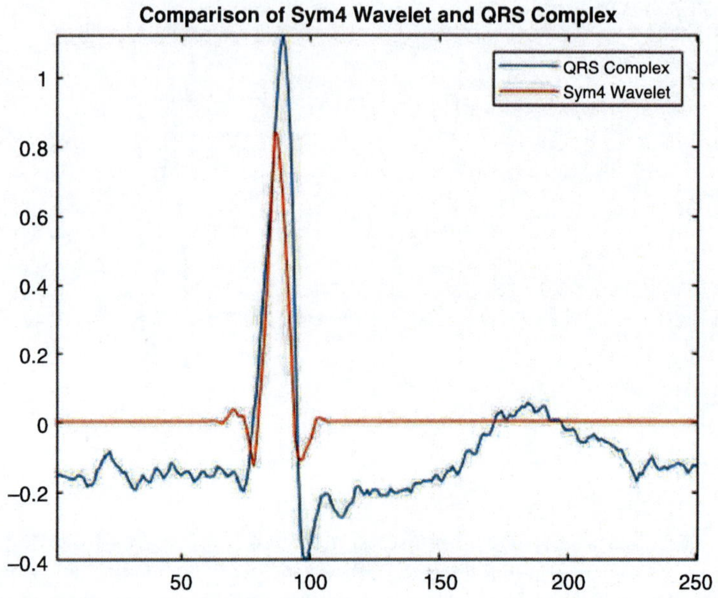

Fig. 3 Comparison of Sym4 wavelet and QRS complex

This shows how a wavelet QRS detector based on a signal approximation and proves that the wavelet transform can isolate signal components and provide a multiscale analysis of the signal to enhance peak detection. By applying a type of wavelets called low-order Daubechies [20] that have somewhat of good time resolution and frequency resolution, we will get (A4, D4, D3, D2, D1) coefficients. These coefficients will be the last five to join the rest of the features extracted in the previous sections.

4 Recurrent Neural Network (RNN)

Figure 5 shows a simple RNN cell. x_t is the input vector at time t. h_t and c_t are state vectors that are carried from time $t1$ to time t and, hence, act as memory by encoding previous information. h_t is also considered as the cell output. Size of vectors h and c is denoted by N_h and is known as the number of hidden units. The cell works based on the following equations:

$$\begin{aligned} &m_t[j] = \\ &\tanh\left(\sum\nolimits_{k\in[1,N_x]} w[j,k]x_t[k] + \sum\nolimits_{k\in[1,N_h]} u[j,k]h_{t-1}[k] + b[j]\right) \\ &c_t[j] = c_{t-1}[j] + m_t[j] \\ &h_t[j] = \tanh\left(c_t[j]\right). \end{aligned} \tag{1}$$

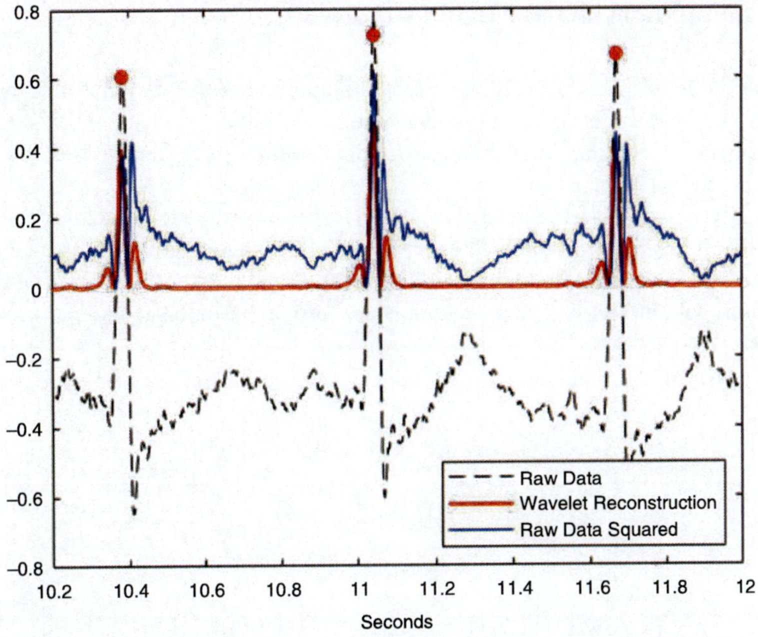

Fig. 4 Comparison of raw, squared raw data and the wavelet reconstruction of the ECG recordings

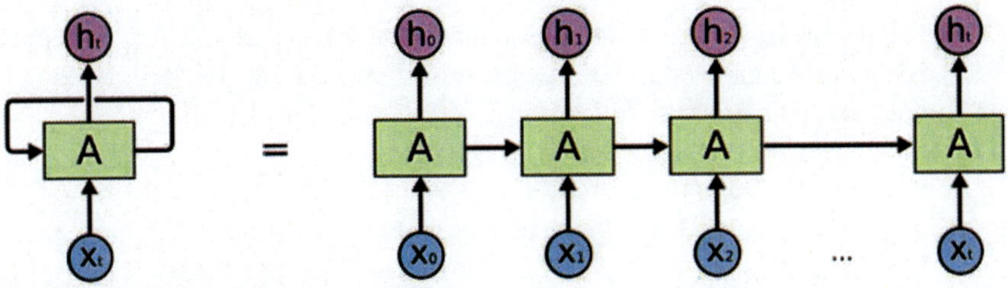

Fig. 5 A simple recurrent neural network (RNN)

An intermediate vector m_t is formed by applying *tanh* activation function on a linear combination of x_t and $ht1$, i.e., current input and previous output, respectively, $j[1, N_h]$. Weight matrices w and u and bias vector b are determined during the training phase. The state vector c_t is formed by accumulating m_t over time. The output vector ht is formed by applying *tanh* activation function on c_t. It can be seen that the output is related to all previous inputs.

5 Long Short-Term Memory (LSTM)

In the above simple RNN cell, the effect of all previous information is accumulated in the internal state vector. Gradient-based algorithms may fail when temporal dependencies get too long because gradient values may increase or decrease exponentially [21].

LSTM solves this issue by allowing us to forget according to the actual dependencies that exist in the problem. The dependencies are automatically extracted based on the data. This is achieved through forget, input, and output gates [21]. The LSTM cell is shown in Fig. 6. The gate signals are formed based on x_t and h_{t1} as shown below:

$$
\begin{aligned}
&f_t[j] = \\
&\sigma\left(\sum_{k\in[1,N_x]} w_f[j,k]x_t[k] + \sum_{k\in[1,N_h]} u_f[j,k]h_{t-1}[k] + b_f[j]\right)\\
&i_t[j] = \\
&\sigma\left(\textstyle\sum_{k\in[1,N_x]} w_i[j,k]x_t[k] + \sum_{k\in[1,N_h]} u_i[j,k]h_{t-1}[k] + b_i[j]\right)\\
&o_t[j] = \\
&\sigma\left(\textstyle\sum_{k\in[1,N_x]} w_o[j,k]x_t[k] + \sum_{k\in[1,N_h]} u_o[j,k]h_{t-1}[k] + b_o[j]\right).
\end{aligned}
\tag{2}
$$

The above equations denote the sigmoid activation function and $j[1, N_h]$. In the LSTM cell, m_t is computed as before, i.e., it is modified based on the forget, input, and output gate signals as the following:

$$
\begin{aligned}
c_t[j] &= f_t[j] \times c_{t-1}[j] + i_t[j] \times m_t[j]\\
h_t[j] &= o_t[j] \times \tanh\left(c_t[j]\right).
\end{aligned}
\tag{3}
$$

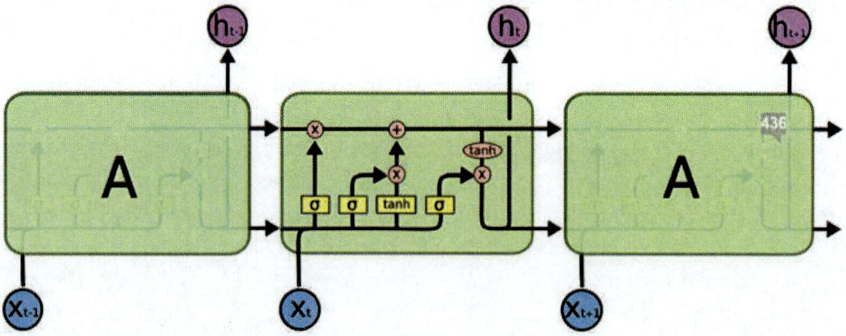

Fig. 6 A long short-term memory (LSTM) network model

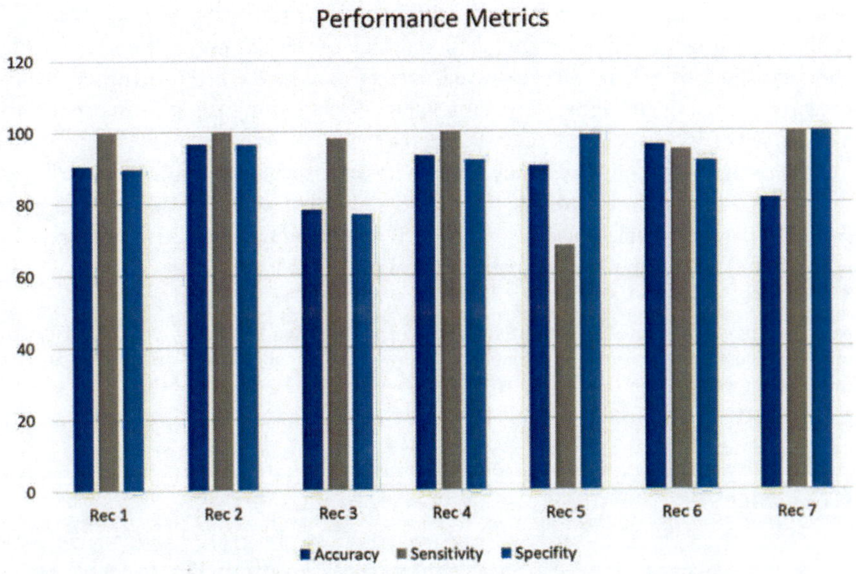

Fig. 7 Performance metrics in three categories: accuracy, sensitivity, and specificity

The forget gate f_t controls carrying of state vector c from time $t1$ to time t. The input gate adjusts the accumulation of mt in ct. As shown in (9), the output h_t is formed by applying $tanh$ activation function on c_t and is then adjusted by the output gate o_t. As the above equations show, the LSTM output still depends on all previous inputs. Previous information is neither completely discarded nor completely carried over to the current state. Instead, influence of the previous information on the current state is carefully controlled through the gate signals [21].

6 Performance results

The results were assessed in terms of sensitivity, specificity, accuracy, sensitivity (Sens), and specificity (Spec), which reflect the performance of imbalanced classification. An overview of how these parameters are obtained for each recording can be found in Fig. 7.

7 Conclusion

This chapter constitutes a first step toward a wearable epileptic seizure prediction device. Compared to most common approaches of using EEG signals in our study, we use input data obtained from ECG. In this chapter, we processed the ECG explicitly and dealt with the intervals of extreme noise that may appear during the epileptic seizures. Then, the processed data is used to train the recurrent neural network precisely the long short-term memory variation that will subsequently classify new ECG data as pre-ictal or normal.

The results show high accuracy, sensitivity, and specificity have been achieved for most of the ECG recordings. They also show that a LSTM trained with data from one patient is almost useless with a different patient. Thus, the system must be properly trained for the specific patient who is going to use it.

Acknowledgments The ECG data used in this chapter is taken from MIT and BIH database. Figures 3 and 4 are taken from an example on mathworks.com, and the network pictures are also from C.Olah weblog.

References

1. M.J. Eadie, Shortcomings in the current treatment of epilepsy. Expert Rev. Neurother. **12**(12), 1419–1427 (2012)
2. K. Gadhoumi, J.M. Lina, F. Mormann, J. Gotman, Seizure prediction for therapeutic devices: a review. J. Neurosci. Methods **260**, 270–282 (2016)
3. I.C. Al-Aweel, K.B. Krishnamurthy, J.M. Hausdorff, J.E. Mietus, J.R. Ives, A.S. Blum, D.L. Schomer, A.L. Goldberger, Postictal heart rate oscillations in partial epilepsy. Neurology **53**(7), 1590–1590 (1999)
4. K. Fujiwara, M. Miyajima, T. Yamakawa, E. Abe, Y. Suzuki, Y. Sawada, M. Kano, T. Maehara, K. Ohta, T. Sasai-Sakuma, T. Sasano, M. Matsuura, E. Matsushima, Epileptic seizure prediction based on multivariate statistical process control of heart rate variability features. IEEE Trans. Biomed. Eng. **63**(6), 1321–1332 (2016)
5. M.M. Baig, H. Gholamhosseini, M.J. Connolly, A comprehensive survey of wearable and wireless ECG monitoring systems for older adults. Med. Biol. Eng. Comput. **51**(5), 485–495 (2013)
6. T. Teijeiro, P. Felix, J. Presedo, D. Castro, Heartbeat classification using abstract features from the abductive interpretation of the ECG. IEEE J. Biomed. Health Inform. **22**(2), 409–420 (2018)
7. P. De Chazal, M. O'Dwyer, R.B. Reilly, Automatic classification of heartbeats using ECG morphology and heartbeat interval features. IEEE Trans. Biomed. Eng. **51**(7), 1196–1206 (2004)
8. K.I. Minami, H. Nakajima, T. Toyoshima, Real-time discrimination of ventricular tachyarrhythmia with Fourier-transform neural network. IEEE Trans. Biomed. Eng. **46**(2), 179–185 (1999)
9. M. Lagerholm, G. Peterson, Clustering ECG complexes using Hermite functions and self-organizing maps. IEEE Trans. Biomed. Eng. **47**(7), 838–848 (2000)
10. L.Y. Shyu, Y.H. Wu, W. Hu, Using wavelet transform and fuzzy neural network for VPC detection from the Holter ECG. IEEE Trans. Biomed. Eng. **51**(7), 1269–1273 (2004)
11. O.T. Inan, L. Giovangrandi, G.T. Kovacs, Robust neural-network-based classification of premature ventricular contractions using wavelet transform and timing interval features. IEEE Trans. Biomed. Eng. **53**(12), 2507–2515 (2006)
12. F. Melgani, Y. Bazi, Classification of electrocardiogram signals with support vector machines and particle swarm optimization. IEEE Trans. Inf. Technol. Biomed. **12**(5), 667–677 (2008)

13. D.A. Coast, R.M. Stern, G.G. Cano, S.A. Briller, An approach to cardiac arrhythmia analysis using hidden Markov models. IEEE Trans. Biomed. Eng. **37**(9), 826–836 (1990)
14. Y.H. Hu, S. Palreddy, W.J. Tompkins, A patient-adaptable ECG beat classifier using a mixture of experts approach. IEEE Trans. Biomed. Eng. **44**(9), 891–900 (1997)
15. P. De Chazal, R.B. Reilly, A patient-adapting heartbeat classifier using ECG morphology and heartbeat interval features. IEEE Trans. Biomed. Eng. **53**(12), 2535–2543 (2006)
16. W. Jiang, S.G. Kong, Block-based neural networks for personalized ECG signal classification. IEEE Trans. Neural Netw. **18**(6), 1750–1761 (2007)
17. T. Ince, S. Kiranyaz, M. Gabbou, A generic and robust system for automated patient-specific classification of ECG signals. IEEE Trans. Biomed. Eng. **56**(5), 1415–1426 (2009)
18. R. Hoekema, G.J. Uijen, A. Van Oosterom, Geometrical aspects of the interindividual variability of multilead ECG recordings. IEEE Trans. Biomed. Eng. **48**(5), 551–559 (2001)
19. S. Kiranyaz, T. Ince, M. Gabbouj, Real-time patient-specific ECG classification by 1-D convolutional neural networks. IEEE Trans. Biomed. Eng. **63**(3), 664–675 (2016)
20. P. De Chazal, B.G. Celler, R.B. Reilly, Using wavelet coefficients for the classification of the electrocardiogram, in *Annual International Conference of the IEEE Engineering in Medicine and Biology - Proceedings* (2000)
21. S. Hochreiter, J. Schmidhuber, Long short-term memory. Neural Comput. **9**(8), 1735–1780 (1997)

A Comparative Study of Machine Learning Models for Tabular Data Through Challenge of Monitoring Parkinson's Disease Progression Using Voice Recordings

Mohammadreza Iman, Amy Giuntini, Hamid Reza Arabnia, and Khaled Rasheed

1 Introduction

Parkinson's disease is a neurodegenerative disorder, affecting the neurons in the brain that produce dopamine. Parkinson's disease can cause a range of symptoms, particularly the progressive deterioration of motor function [1–3]. When diagnosed with Parkinson's disease, a person's health may deteriorate rapidly, or they may experience comparatively milder symptoms if the disease progresses more slowly. In our research, we are mainly concerned with how Parkinson's disease can affect speech characteristics. People with Parkinson's may display dysarthria or problems with articulation, and they may also be affected by dysphonia, an impaired ability to produce vocal sounds normally. Dysphonia may be exhibited by soft speech, breathy voice, or vocal tremor [1–3].

The authors Mohammadreza Iman and Amy Giuntini contributed equally to this work.

M. Iman (✉) · H. R. Arabnia
Department of Computer Science, Franklin College of Arts and Sciences, University of Georgia, Athens, GA, USA
e-mail: hra@uga.edu

A. Giuntini · K. Rasheed
Institute for Artificial Intelligence, Franklin College of Arts and Sciences, University of Georgia, Athens, GA, USA
e-mail: khaled@uga.edu

H. R. Arabnia et al. (eds.), *Advances in Computer Vision and Computational Biology*, Transactions on Computational Science and Computational Intelligence,
https://doi.org/10.1007/978-3-030-71051-4_38

People with Parkinson's disease do not always experience noticeable symptoms at the earliest stages, and therefore, the disease is often diagnosed at a later stage. As there is not currently a cure, people diagnosed with Parkinson's must rely on treatments to alleviate symptoms, which is most effective with early treatment. Once a diagnosis is made, the patient must regularly visit their physician to monitor the disease and the effectiveness of treatment. Monitoring the progression of the disease through a voice recording captured by the patient at their own home can make the process faster and less stressful for the patient. The possibility of lessening the frequency of doctor visits can be cost-effective and allow the patient to follow a more flexible schedule [1–3].

One of the most prominent methods of quantifying the symptoms of Parkinson's disease is the Unified Parkinson's Disease Rating Scale (UPDRS) that was first developed in the 1980s. The scale consists of four parts: intellectual function and behavior, ability to carry out daily activities, motor function examination, and motor complications. Each part is composed of questions or tests where either the patient or clinician will give a score with 0 denoting normal function and the maximum number denoting severe impairment. The clinician calculates a UPDRS score for each section as well as a total UPDRS score that can range from 0 to 176. In this chapter, we are concerned with the motor UPDRS that can range from 0 to 108.

All the machine learning techniques and data analysis in this project have been done using the Waikato Environment for Knowledge Analysis (Weka), free software developed at the University of Waikato [4]. Weka is a compilation of machine learning algorithms written in Java. All the applied methods in this study are based on 10-fold cross-validation.

1.1 Dataset

We obtained the data from UC Irvine's machine learning repository. The data consists of a total of 5875 voice recordings from 42 patients with early-stage Parkinson's disease over the course of 6 months. Voice recordings were taken for each subject weekly, and a clinician determined the subject's UPDRS scores at the onset of the trial, at 3 months, and at 6 months. The scores were then linearly interpolated for the remaining voice recordings [2].

The raw data from the original paper had 132 attributes, but the publicly available data contains 22 features, including the test time, sex, and age. Table 1 categorizes these features. The remaining features are the data related to the voice recordings. While abnormalities in any of these features could be symptomatic of many causes, they also provide measurements for several symptoms of Parkinson's disease.

The data contains four features that measure jitter and six that measure shimmer. Jitter measures the fluctuations in pitch, while shimmer indicates fluctuations in amplitude. Common symptoms of Parkinson's disease include difficulty in maintaining pitch as well as speaking softly. Therefore, measurements of both jitter

Table 1 Dataset attributes

Attribute	Brief description
Subject	Integer that uniquely identifies each subject (not used in training/test)
Age	Subject age
Sex	Subject gender '0'—male, '1'—female
Test time	Time since recruitment into the trial. The integer part is the number of days since recruitment.
Motor UPDRS	Clinician's motor UPDRS score, linearly interpolated
Total UPDRS	Clinician's total UPDRS score, linearly interpolated (not used)
Jitter (%), Jitter(Abs), Jitter:RAP, Jitter:PPQ5, Jitter:DDP	Several measures of variation in fundamental frequency
Shimmer, Shimmer(dB), Shimmer:APQ3, Shimmer:APQ5, Shimmer:APQ11, Shimmer:DDA	Several measures of variation in amplitude
NHR,HNR	Two measures of ratio of noise to total components in the voice
RPDE	A nonlinear dynamical complexity measure
DFA	Signal fractal scaling exponent
PPE	A nonlinear measure of fundamental frequency variation

and shimmer can be used to detect and measure these symptoms and can be useful to map the voice data to a UPDRS score.

The recurrence period density entropy (RPDE) measures deviations in the periods of time-delay embedding of the phase space. When a signal recurs to the same point in the phase space at a certain time, it has a recurrence period of that time. Deviations in periodicity can indicate voice disorders, which may occur as a result of Parkinson's disease [1].

Noise-to-harmonics and harmonics-to-noise ratios are derived from estimates of signal-to-noise ratio from the voice recording. Detrended fluctuation analysis (DFA) measures the stochastic self-similarity of the noise in the speech sample. Most of this noise is from turbulent airflow through the vocal cords [1]. Each of these measures can capture the breathiness in speech that can be a symptom of Parkinson's disease.

A common symptom of Parkinson's disease is an impaired ability to maintain pitch during a sustained phonation. While jitter detects these changes in pitch, it also measures the natural variations in pitch that all healthy people exhibit. It can be difficult for jitter measurements to distinguish between these two types of pitch variations. Pitch period entropy (PPE) is based on a logarithmic scale rather than a frequency scale, and it disregards smooth variations [1]. Therefore, it is better suited to detect dysphonia-related changes of pitch.

1.2 Document Organization

The next section gives an overview regarding the previous research that has been done on this dataset and a similar dataset. Then in the section titled Machine Learning Strategies and Our Research Road Map, you can find the details about feature analysis and selection, a brief description of the methods that we applied, followed by the different approaches and their results. The last section, discussion and conclusion, is about future works and summarization of our study on this dataset.

2 Related Work

Approximately 60,000 Americans are diagnosed with Parkinson's disease each year, but only 4% of patients are diagnosed before the age of 50 [1–3]. In order to diagnose Parkinson's disease earlier, there have been several works, based on a dataset of voice recordings of patients with Parkinson's disease and healthy patients. First, work by Max Little on this initial dataset predicts whether a subject is healthy or has Parkinson's disease using phonetic analysis of voice recordings to measure dysphonia [1]. Much similar work has been done to create models that can accurately predict whether a person has Parkinson's disease or is healthy based on the phonetic analysis of voice recordings. Max Little et al. introduced the dataset and found success with SVM (support vector machine) that indicated that voice measurements can be a suitable way to diagnose Parkinson's disease [1]. Further research has contributed methods to solve this problem with various machine learning techniques [5] that successfully used artificial neural networks as well as a neuro-fuzzy classifier. The neuro-fuzzy classifier achieved a high accuracy on the testing set for this binary classification problem. The work to classify people as healthy or having Parkinson's disease has favorable results, but due to unbalanced data available, we cannot know whether a model is reliable. The subsequent work was on a more complex dataset, to monitor patients with early-stage Parkinson's disease [2], which is the basis for this chapter. Age, sex, and voice are all important factors to identify Parkinson's disease or, in other words, are used by clinicians to calculate a UPDRS score. Therefore, both the above ideas seem promising for identification and monitoring of people with Parkinson's disease. As for this chapter, we are more concerned with the more recent data and work [2], which attempts to map data from voice recordings to UPDRS scores. The original authors have tackled this problem as a regression problem, by using logistic regression and CART (classification and regression tree). In their work, they have mentioned that by using the CART method, they could reduce the mean absolute error to 4.5 on the training set and 5.8 on the testing set. However, in this chapter, even with 10-fold cross-validation, we achieved a mean absolute error even lower than 1.9.

3 Machine Learning Strategies and Our Research Road Map

In this section, we examine at first the correlation of the features to the class and discuss feature selection. Next, we describe the machine learning techniques that we applied to this dataset in different manners. We applied regression methods to the data with a continuous class in an attempt to map the phonetic features to the severity of the symptoms from Parkinson's disease. We also undertook this as a classification problem and tried various classification techniques.

3.1 Feature Selection

The 22 features accessible in the dataset had already been selected from 132 attributes of the raw data, which is not available to the public [2]. We selected 18 features for this chapter after excluding the subject, test time, and total UPDRS features from the 22 available ones. We selected the motor UPDRS as the target attribute. Also, motor UPDRS has a high correlation with total UPDRS, so we used motor UPDRS as our sole class. Table 2 shows the correlation between each of those 18 features with motor UPDRS, ordered by correlation.

Table 2 Features correlation with motor UPDRS

Rank	Correlation	Attribute
1	0.2737	Age
2	0.1624	PPE
3	0.1366	Shimmer:APQ11
4	0.1286	RPDE
5	0.1101	Shimmer:dB
6	0.1023	Shimmer
7	0.0921	Shimmer:APQ5
8	0.0848	Jitter
9	0.0843	Shimmer:APQ3
10	0.0843	Shimmer:DDA
11	0.0763	Jitter:PPQ5
12	0.075	NHR
13	0.0727	Jitter:DDP
14	0.0727	Jitter:RAP
15	0.0509	Jitter:Abs
16	0.0312	Sex
17	-0.1162	DFA
18	-0.157	HNR

3.2 Regression-Based Methods

We created regression models to determine a relationship between the features and the continuous class (motor UPDRS). We tried many different techniques in different categories of machine learning methods, including trees, functions, multi-layer perceptron, and instance-based learning. Table 3 shows the correlation coefficient and mean absolute error for the top performing regression models. We omitted results that did not compare well to the top models.

Overall, the tree-based regression models performed the best. The previous work on this data measured their results by using the mean absolute error. For this reason, we also observed the mean absolute error for each method, so we could meaningfully compare our results to the previous works. For more insight into the results, we also noted the correlation coefficient.

Table 3 Regression-based methods' results

Method	Correlation coefficient	Mean absolute error
M5P tree	0.9463	1.9285
SVM (nu-SVR)	0.9335	2.0612
REPTree	0.9282	2.0157
k-NN	0.8619	2.8239

M5 model tree [6] combines decision and regression trees. M5 model (M5P) first constructs a decision tree, and each leaf of that tree is a regression model. Therefore, the output we get out of the M5 model are real values instead of classes. As our dataset's dependent variable has continuous values, we chose this method. It is different from a classification and regression tree (CART) method as CART generates either a decision or regression tree based on the type of dependent variable and M5 model tree uses both techniques together. This method is one of the best performers.

Support vector machines (SVMs) [7] are another popular machine learning algorithm that can handle both classification and regression with the detection of outliers. SVM tries to find an optimal hyperplane that categorizes the new inputs. We attempted two methods: epsilon-SVR and nu-SVR. There are multiple kernels to find the optimal hyperplane, including linear, radial, sigmoidal, and polynomial. Since the data was complex and has a high dimensionality, radial kernel tends to work faster and better than any other kernel type. We found that nu-SVR performed better than epsilon-SVR for this data. The nu-SVR method got 0.9335 as the highest correlation coefficient, only marginally higher than epsilon-SVR, which achieved 0.9301 for the correlation coefficient. However, the mean absolute error of 2.06 was also slightly higher compared to that of epsilon-SVR, 2.02.

Reduced error pruning tree [8], or REPTree, is Weka's implementation of a fast decision tree learner. The REPTree is sometimes preferred over other trees because it prevents the tree from growing linearly with the sample size when growth will not improve the accuracy [9]. It uses information gain to build a regression tree and prunes it with reduced error pruning. The REPTree for classification yielded a correlation coefficient of 0.92 and a mean absolute error of 2.02.

3.3 *Instance-Based Learning*

Instance-based learning, such as k-nearest neighbors (k-NN) [10], uses a function that is locally approximated and defers computation to the classification or value assignment. Instead of generalizing the data, new instances are assigned values based directly on the training data. As a regression method, k-NN outputs the average of the values of the instance's nearest neighbors. We applied the k-NN algorithm to the discretized data and classified instances based on the seven nearest neighbors. We used Manhattan distance and weighted the distance with one divided by the distance. This method yielded a correlation coefficient of 0.86 and 2.83 as the mean absolute error.

3.4 *Ensemble Methods*

Using ensemble methods, we combined several regression techniques with other methods in an attempt to improve upon the best results we achieved. Some of these methods include bagging, boosting, stacking, voting, and iterative absolute error regression in conjunction with other regression methods.

Bagging [11], or bootstrap aggregation, uses multiple predictions of a method with high variance. Many subsamples of the data are made with replacement, and a prediction is made with a machine learning method for each subsample. The result from bagging is the average of the result of all of these predictions.

Stacking [12] makes use of several machine learning models. We applied multiple methods to the original dataset. There is a metalayer that uses another model that uses the individual results as its input and creates a prediction. Our best stacking result stacked M5P tree and REPTree, and we used M5PTree as the model for the metalayer.

Voting [13], or simple averaging for this regression problem, used multiple machine learning methods. The average of their results was the output for the voting algorithm. Our best model with this ensemble method was once again the M5P tree and the REPTree.

Random forest [14] is a tree-based ensemble learning method that can be used for both classification and regression. It operates by constructing a multitude of decision trees at training time and outputting class that is the mode of classes (classification) or mean prediction (regression) of the individual trees. These trees are generally fast and accurate but sometimes suffer from over-fitting.

Table 4 Regression-based ensemble methods' results

Ensemble method	Correlation coefficient	Mean absolute error
Bagging M5P tree	0.9529	1.8674
Stacking M5P tree with REPTree by M5P tree	0.9502	1.8563
Vote M5P tree and REPTree	0.9465	1.9163
Random forest	0.9167	2.7372

Tree-based methods did provide the best results and tend to work well in ensemble methods due to their high variance. The best performing model was bagging with the M5P tree as the base method. This yielded a correlation coefficient of 0.95 and a mean absolute error of 1.87. Table 4 features some of the best ensemble methods for regression.

3.5 *Verification*

In order to confirm that our results are consistent with real values for the motor UPDRS scores and not just fitting to the linear interpolation, we also tried the regression techniques on a subset of the data. In this subset, we used only instances in which the value for the motor UPDRS was a whole number. While some interpolated instances may coincidentally have a whole number for the motor UPDRS, this method ensured that much of the subset was the data where a clinician examined the patient and calculated a UPDRS score.

The results we achieved with this subset of the data surpassed those of the whole dataset. In particular, the M5P model has a correlation coefficient of 0.95 and a mean absolute error of 1.87. These results indicate that our findings from regression methods are reliable and are not simply fitting to the linearly interpolated data.

3.6 *Classification by Discretization*

In addition to the regression models, we also attempted other methods of modeling the data. Below we briefly summarize these different approaches to this problem since the results were not promising.

To classify the instances into meaningful intervals, we discretized the data. According to the work of Pablo Martinez-Martin et al. [15], UPDRS scores can be used to indicate the severity of the disease. These authors classified motor UPDRS scores from 1 to 32 as mild, 33 to 58 as moderate, and 59 and above as severe. Using these intervals, the data we used had 5254 instances with mild Parkinson's disease and only 621 instances that were moderate, and no severe cases.

We used multiple tree-based methods, including C4.5, classification and regression tree, and LogitBoost alternating decision tree. Weka's J48 algorithm [16] is essentially an implementation of the C4.5 algorithm (a type of decision tree methods). C4.5 is an improvement over the ID3 algorithm. J48 is capable of handling discrete as well as continuous values. It also has an added advantage of allowing a pruned tree. Our data has attributes with continuous values, so we chose the J48 classifier as one of the methods and tried multiple configurations.

SimpleCART [17] is a type of classification and regression tree. The classification tree predicts the class of the dependent variables, while the regression tree outputs a real number. The SimpleCART technique produces either a classification or regression tree based on whether the dependent variable is categorical or numeric, respectively. The class attribute of our dataset is of numeric type, but after discretizing the class label into bins, we converted it into a categorical type, so the SimpleCART algorithm treated our discretized dataset as a classification problem.

LADTree (LogitBoost alternating decision tree) [18] is a type of alternating decision tree for multi-class classification. Alternating decision tree was designed for binary classification. ADTrees can be merged into a single tree; therefore, a multi-class model can be derived by merging several binary class trees using some voting model. LADTree uses LogitBoost strategy for boosting. In simple terms, boosting gives relatively more weight to misclassified instances compared to correctly classified instances for the next iteration of boosting. Generally, the boosting iteration is directly proportional to the number of iterations.

Bayes Net [19] is a probabilistic directed acyclic graphical model. This model represents a set of variables and their conditional dependencies through a direct acyclic graph. Each node's output depends on the particular set of values of its parent nodes. The nodes that are not connected to each other are considered as conditionally independent nodes from each other. Unlike the Naïve Bayes [20] assumption of conditional independence, Bayesian belief networks describe conditional independence among a subset of variables.

K-nearest neighbors (K-NN) [10] can also be used for both classification and regression problems. When used for classification, k-NN classifies a new instance with the class held by the majority of its nearest neighbors. We applied the K-NN algorithm [10] to the discretized data and classified the motor UPDRS values for instances based on the six nearest neighbors and measuring using Manhattan distance.

The multi-layer perceptron (MLP) is a type of artificial neural network [21, 22]. An MLP consists of one or more layers with a different number of nodes in each, called the network architecture. Using some activation function such as sigmoid in each node combined with the backpropagation technique makes such networks useful for machine learning classification and regression tasks. For this dataset, we applied variant network architectures, single-layer to five-layer networks with a range of 1–10 nodes in each.

The state of the art, known as deep learning, is the developed MLP into more layers containing more nodes with more options of activation functions and training algorithms [23]. We tried several different architectures of deep neural network

(DNNs) using Keras [24] and Tensorflow [25]. The results were not promising in comparison to listed models.

After all, the classification results did not compare well to the regression-based methods. We speculate that this is because of the unbalanced data.

3.7 *Multi-Instance Learning*

We also used multi-instance learning [26]. For each subject in this dataset, there are approximately six voice recordings for each time step. Rather than considering each of these recordings by itself, multi-instance learning collects these instances into bags. Each bag holds one person's voice recording data that was taken at the same time step, and every instance in the bag is assigned to the same class. We have 995 bags for the 42 subjects, amounting to about 24 per subject, or one per week.

We propositionalized the bags, creating one instance for each bag with the mean of the values of the aggregated instances. This creates 995 instances, one for each person at every time interval. We then were able to apply single-instance classifiers, including Bayesian methods, decision trees, SVMs, and multi-layer perceptron. These methods yielded similar results to those that we achieved with classification using the data with all 5875 instances.

The results of this approach were similar to those of the classification models and not significant compared to the regression results.

4 Discussion and Conclusion

Our results from the classification problem indicate that these measures of dysphonia may be used to determine the severity of the symptoms of Parkinson's disease. Results with higher accuracy as well as a better ability to predict the minority class suggest a higher likelihood that model can be accurately used with more diverse data. However, we found the regression results to be even more promising. We favored regression over classification with this data because, in order to classify, we must discretize into bins. Meanwhile, regression techniques can map the UPDRS score to a more precise value. It is more meaningful for a model to output a motor UPDRS score of 15 than to say it is in the range of 0–16. Our best performing regression method was bagging using the M5P model tree as the base method, which achieved a correlation coefficient of 0.95 and a mean absolute error of 1.86.

To our knowledge, the only existing work on this data belongs to the same authors who created this dataset [2]. We tried many regression methods and compared them to the findings of these authors. We only compiled our significant findings in this report. Our regression methods resulted in high correlation coefficients. However, the previous work made no mention of the correlation coefficient, so we used the mean absolute error to compare our results. The best results from this earlier work had mean absolute errors of 4.5 on the training set and 5.8 on the testing set. We were able to lower the mean absolute error to 1.9, a significant decrease from the earlier work's mean absolute errors. We attained the lower mean absolute error despite using 10-fold cross-validation, which makes our results more reliable. These models indicate that motor UPDRS can be calculated using these voice measurements in the early stages of the disease with even more precision than previously thought. These results suggest that voice recordings may be a reliable approach to monitoring Parkinson's disease from the comfort of the patient's home, potentially reducing the frequency of doctor visits and giving patients more freedom with their time.

There are many possibilities of future work on this type of data. Researchers are currently collecting more data of this type. If more data is collected from patients at all stages of Parkinson's, similar techniques could be applied to determine whether vocal parameters can still be mapped to UPDRS scores at a later stage of the disease. Additionally, data from the later stages of Parkinson's could be used to attempt to predict the progression of the disease.

As a result of our comparative study of machine learning methods, we discovered that the new methods of deep learning are not as efficient and competitive as trees for many tabular data. A data scientist needs to know about all machine learning methods and different types of datasets to achieve the best accuracy and efficiency. The results of our comparative study of variant machine learning models support the same claim of [27–29] that for many tabular data, the older models (e.g., decision trees) outperform cutting edge deep learning models. Also, we should consider that some machine learning models such as decision trees are much faster than DNNs and could be run in very simple machines like on edge devices (e.g., cell phones).

Acknowledgment Here we want to appreciate the help of Pawan Yadav and Ankit Joshi for part of the early implementation of the experiments.

References

1. M.A. Little, P.E. McSharry, E.J. Hunter, J. Spielman, L.O. Ramig, Suitability of dysphonia measurements for telemonitoring of Parkinson's disease. IEEE Trans. Biomed. Eng. **56**(4), 1015–1022 (2009)
2. A. Tsanas, M.A. Little, P.E. McSharry, L.O. Ramig, Accurate telemonitoring of Parkinson's disease progression by noninvasive speech tests. IEEE Trans. Biomed. Eng. **57**(4), 884–893 (2010)
3. A. Tsanas, M.A. Little, P.E. McSharry, L.O. Ramig, Using the cellular mobile telephone network to remotely monitor Parkinson's disease symptom severity. IEEE Trans. Biomed. Eng. (2012)
4. E. Frank, M.A. Hall, I.H. Witten, *The WEKA Workbench. Online Appendix for "Data Mining: Practical Machine Learning Tools and Techniques"*, 4th edn. (Morgan Kaufmann, Burlington, 2016)
5. M.F. Çağlar, B. Çetışh, İ.B. Toprak, Automatic recognition of Parkinson's disease from sustained phonation tests using ANN and adaptive neuro-fuzzy classifier. Mühendislik Bilimleri ve Tasarım Dergisi **1**(2), 59–64 (2010)

6. A. Etemad-Shahidi, J. Mahjoobi, Comparison between M5' model tree and neural networks for prediction of significant wave height in Lake Superior. Ocean Eng. **36**(15–16), 1175–1181 (2009)
7. I. Steinwart, A. Christmann, *Support Vector Machines* (Springer Science & Business Media, New York, 2008)
8. W.N.H.W. Mohamed, M.N. Salleh, A.H. Omar, A comparative study of reduced error pruning method in decision tree algorithms, in *2012 IEEE International Conference on Control System, Computing and Engineering* (IEEE, Piscataway, 2012), pp. 392–397
9. T. Elomaa, M. Kaariainen, An analysis of reduced error pruning. J. Artif. Intell. Res. **15**, 163–187 (2001)
10. Y. Liao, V. Vemuri, Use of k-nearest neighbor classifier for intrusion detection. Comput. Secur. **21**(5), 439–448 (2002)
11. L. Breiman, Bagging predictors. Mach. Learn. **24**(2), 123–140 (1996)
12. S. Džeroski, B. Ženko, Is combining classifiers with stacking better than selecting the best one? Mach. Learn. **54**(3), 255–273 (2004)
13. J. Kittler, M. Hatef, R.P.W. Duin, J. Matas, On combining classifiers. Trans. Pattern Anal. Mach. Intell. **20**(3), 226–239 (1998)
14. A. Liaw, M. Wiener, Classification and regression by random Forest. R News **2**(3), 18–22 (2002)
15. P. Martí-nez-Martín, C. Rodríguez-Blázquez, M. Alvarez, T. Arakaki, V. Campos Arillo, P. Chaná, W. Fernández et al., Parkinson's disease severity levels and MDS-Unified Parkinson's Disease Rating Scale. Parkinsonism Relat. Disord. **21**(1), 50–54 (2015)
16. J. R. Quinlan, *C4. 5: Programs for Machine Learning* (Elsevier, Amsterdam, 2014)
17. S. Kalmegh, Analysis of Weka data mining algorithm REPTree, simple cart and random tree for classification of Indian news. Int. J. Innov. Sci. Eng. Technol. **2**(2), 438–446 (2015)
18. G. Holmes, B. Pfahringer, R. Kirkby, E. Frank, M. Hall, Multiclass alternating decision trees, in *Proceedings of ECML* (2001), pp. 161–172
19. I. Ben Gal, Bayesian networks, in *Encyclopedia of Statistics in Quality and Reliability*, ed. by F. Ruggeri, R.S. Kennett, F.W. Faltin (Wiley, New York, 2007)
20. H. Langseth, T.D. Nielsen, Classification using hierarchical Naive Bayes models. Mach. Learn. **63**(2), 135–159 (2006)
21. S. Haykin, *Neural Networks: A Comprehensive Foundation*, 2nd edn. (Prentice Hall, Upper Saddle River, 1998). ISBN 0-13-273350-1
22. H. Ramchoun, M.A.J. Idrissi, Y. Ghanou, M. Ettaouil, Multilayer perceptron: architecture optimization and training. Int. J. Interact. Multimedia Artif. Intell. **4**(1), 26–30 (2016)
23. I. Goodfellow, Y. Bengio, A. Courville, *Deep Learning* (MIT Press, Cambridge, 2016)
24. A. Gulli, S. Pal, *Deep Learning with Keras* (Packt Publishing Ltd, Birmingham, 2017)
25. A. Sergeev, M. Del Balso, Horovod: fast and easy distributed deep learning in TensorFlow (2018). Preprint, arXiv:1802.05799
26. E. Frank, B. Pfahringer, Propositionalisation of multi-instance data using random forests, in *AI 2013: Advances in Artificial Intelligence*, ed. by S. Cranefield, A. Nayak (Springer, Cham, 2013)
27. I. Shavitt, E. Segal, Regularization learning networks: deep learning for tabular datasets, in *Advances in Neural Information Processing Systems* (2018), pp. 1379–1389
28. K.B.A. Omar, XGBoost and LGBM for Porto Seguro's Kaggle challenge: a comparison. Preprint Semester Project (2018)
29. K. Khosravi, B.T. Pham, K. Chapi, A. Shirzadi, H. Shahabi, I. Revhaug, I. Prakash, D.T. Bui, A comparative assessment of decision trees algorithms for flash flood susceptibility modeling at Haraz watershed, Northern Iran. Sci. Total Environ. **627**, 744–755 (2018)

ICT and the Environment: Strategies to Tackle Environmental Challenges in Nigeria

Tochukwu Ikwunne and Lucy Hederman

1 Introduction

Information and communications technology (ICT) encompasses all technologies that facilitate the processing, transfer and exchange of information and communication services [1], including the technology used to store, manipulate, distribute and create information [2]. Marzelle (quoted in UNDP [3]) suggests that ICTs are both traditional (such as radio, television, dance, drama folklore, print and fax) and new devices (such as the Internet, the World Wide Web, electronic mail, teleconferencing and distance learning tools including CD-ROMs, hypertext and the virtual classroom). ICT has continued to improve the way we live, work, interact with our environment and perceive our lives [4]. In addition, the proliferation of ICTs has played a key role in changing the lifestyle of many people, including older adults in recent times [5]. Further, it has shown[1] to have considerable potential to boost economic growth and promote international development [6, 7]. ICTs[2] are the main drivers of economic growth in African countries over the recent period 2007–2016 [8]. It is also suggested that technology plays an important role in driving the development of the information society and economy in developing countries, with many countries in Africa equally placed to take advantage of technology to facilitate socioeconomic development [9]. Technology is also widely recognized as having the potential to improve environmental performance and tackle climate change [10].

[1] http://www.smart2020.org/.

[2] www.climateactionprogramme.org.

T. Ikwunne (✉) · L. Hederman
ADAPT Centre, Trinity College Dublin, Dublin, Ireland
e-mail: ikwunnet@tcd.ie

H. R. Arabnia et al. (eds.), *Advances in Computer Vision and Computational Biology*, Transactions on Computational Science and Computational Intelligence,
https://doi.org/10.1007/978-3-030-71051-4_39

Moreover, it is claimed that ICT provides the bedrock for survival and development in a rapidly changing global environment [11]. However, climate change and global warming represent a complex set of challenges and long-term problems [12] that require collaborative solutions and the engagement of all countries on the planet. It is for this reason that a cohesive and coordinated international ICT policy between countries is required to respond to this emerging global reality and avert this continuous environmental degradation [4].

A developing nation like Nigeria that aspires to participate effectively and become a key player in the information age needs to have a robust ICT ecosystem driven by a vibrant national ICT policy. Many countries across the world face a challenge to efficiently address the quality of air, soil, wildlife, water, food and energy they provide to their citizens. The Smart 2020 Report written by the International Climate Group[1] recommends that ICT be intensively deployed both for enhancing the monitoring of environmental and human activities (industry, building, transport) and for distributed smart ICT systems to mitigate the pollution, waste and food quality and tackle supply and energy constraints. In the same vein, the Vision 2020 ICT and climate change in Nigeria written by the Eco Nigeria climate group[2] recommends that ICT play a major role in climate change mitigation and adaptation. Also, according to the World Development Report 2010,[3] the use of ICT is predicted to reduce total greenhouse gases by 15% by 2020. Beyond climate change mitigation, ICT has a prominent role to play in realizing Nigeria's Vision 2020 mandate of building a large, diversified, sustainable and competitive economy that harnesses the energies and talents of its people and guarantees a high standard of living and quality of life for its citizens. This proposed convergence between climate change mitigation and meeting growth targets is particularly important to Nigeria. At the same time, ICTs are instrumental to greenhouse gas mitigation; on the other hand, it is also said that the ICT sector and ICT products are currently responsible for about 2% of global greenhouse gas emissions. Unfortunately, the high rate of growth in ICT penetration and increases in processing power means that without mitigation, the harmful contributions of ICT are likely to grow quickly. Thus, it is fair to say that ICT is part of the problem. ICT not only requires energy resources but also offers several opportunities to move global environment research, planning and implementation forward. Developed countries in the Global North such as the United States, the United Kingdom, France, Switzerland and Germany have adopted the use of ICTs to significantly reduce greenhouse gas emissions while increasing energy efficiency and reducing the use of natural resources. This is achieved by using ICTs for travel replacement, dematerialization and reduced energy consumption and many more different aspects of work on the environment, including environmental observation, analysis, planning, management and protection, mitigation and capacity building [13]. But not all countries have the capacity to take advantage of these technologies in order to use the full potential of ICTs for environmental action. There is a need to strengthen the capacity of

[3]https://greennigeria.wordpress.com/tag/ict-climate-change-nigeria/.

developing countries, particularly Nigeria, to benefit from the use of ICTs for managing the environment in meeting the targets of the Vision 2020.

2 ICT and Economy Growth in Nigeria

Nigeria possesses one of the fastest growing telecommunications industries in the world [14]. Nigeria's telecommunications industry was liberated with the return of democracy in 1999. This led to the granting of mobile telecommunication licenses by the Nigerian Communications Commission (NCC) to three providers: Econet, Mobile Telephone Network (MTN) and M-tel. This was followed by the licensing of the Second National Operator (SNO) in 2003, that is, Globacom and Universal Access Service licenses of 2006 which include fixed telephony, very small aperture terminal (VSAT) and Internet service providers. Also, in March 2008, the NCC gave license to another Global System for Mobile (GSM) operator known as Etisalat [15]. In 2000, the Federal Government of Nigeria through its privatization and deregulation policies embarked on an aggressive drive toward the provision of more efficient ICT services in the nation and investment in ICT. The policy success led to the establishment of National Telecommunication Policy in December 2001. The policy recognized the need for the establishment of an enabling environment for deregulation, rapid investment in ICT and rapid expansion of the telecommunication services in the country. Since then, there has been a progressive impact on economic growth in terms of empowerment of women, organizational growth and employment generation in the banking sector and the construction industry [16].

Figure 1 shows that Nigeria had approximately 92.3 million Internet users in 2018. This figure is projected to grow to 187.8 million Internet users in 2023. The Internet penetration amounted to 47.1% of the population in 2018 and is set to reach 84.5% in 2023 [17].

The number of smartphone users in Nigeria is forecast to grow to more than 140 million by 2025 [18]. Currently, estimates from different sources put the number of smartphone users in Nigeria at roughly 25 and 40 million. The exact number of users is hard to pin down; however, the data shows a strong growth outlook for the Nigerian smartphone market with user numbers to at least triple within the next 5–

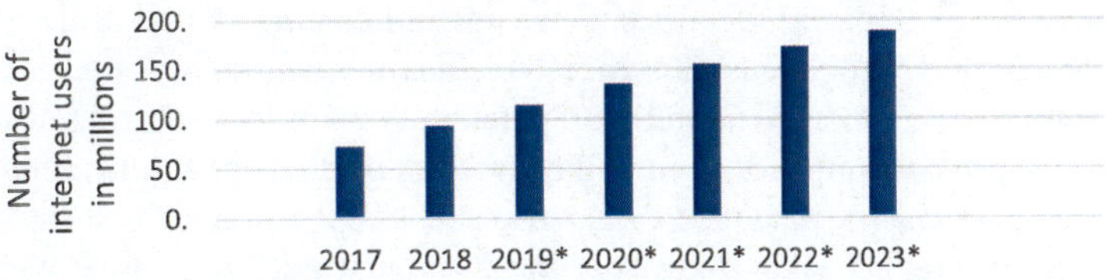

Fig. 1 Number of Internet users in Nigeria from 2017 to 2023. (Source: Nigeria; Statista Digital Market Outlook)

Table 1 Number of smartphone users in Nigeria from 2014 to 2025 (in millions). (Source: Nigeria; Statista Digital Market Outlook)

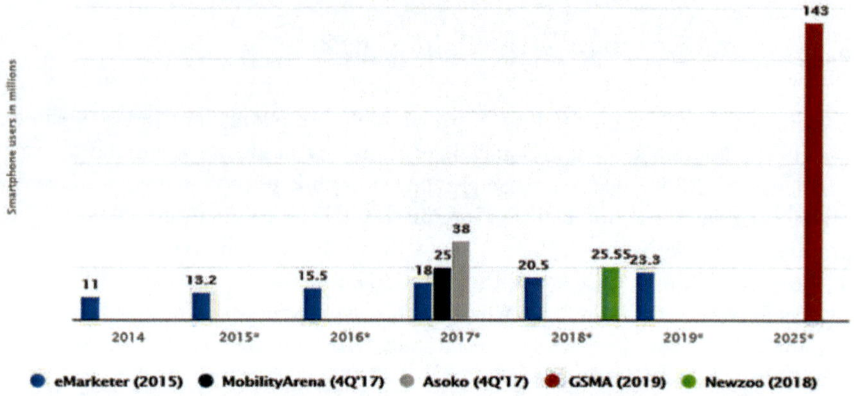

6 years [18] as shown in Table 1. According to Akwani [19], the fastest growing employer of labour in Nigeria today is the telecommunications industry.

3 Types of Pollution and Environmental Issues in Nigeria

This section discusses the various types of environmental pollution that occurs in Nigeria.

3.1 Water Pollution

Water quality issues are a major challenge that humanity is facing in the twenty-first century and cover any chemical, physical, or biological change in the quality of water that has a harmful effect on any living thing that drinks or uses or lives in it [20]. Waste from industries such as breweries, textiles, bottling, paper, pharmaceutics, meatpacking, dairies, paint, metal finishing and oil drilling contain carbonaceous and nitrogenous substances, organic/inorganic matter, toxic chemicals and heavy metals. If such harmful or potentially harmful industrial wastes are dumped in surface dumpsites or in gullies, valleys or drainage basins, liquids from dissolved solid wastes percolate freely and are swept by rain flood into surface water such as streams, lakes and rivers and also burst into water pipes and nearby underground water system. The result is extensive chemical pollution of water. An example is River Kaduna which plays a very important role as the major source of water supply and common sink of all waterborne wastes produced by the industries.

Another example is the stream serving as waste sink to NICHEMTEX, a textile company in Ikorodu at Lagos State. Most other industries along Ikeja, Ijora and Apapa rivers, to mention but a few, discharge their effluents and untreated wastes directly into open public drains.

3.2 Air Pollution

Air pollution refers to all combustion gases and particles released into the air that include sulphur and nitrogen oxides, carbon monoxide and soot particles, as well as smaller quantities of toxic metals, organic molecules and radioactive isotopes [21]. The atmosphere is a complex natural gaseous system that is essential to support life on planet Earth. Stratospheric ozone depletion due to air pollution has long been recognized as a threat to human health as well as to the Earth's ecosystems. The quality of air is affected by smoke, dust, automobile exhausts and gaseous waste from factories. The important list of gaseous emulsions from Nigerian industries includes sulphur dioxide, carbon monoxide and oxides of nitrogen particulate matter and heavy metal dust. These gaseous substances irritate the lungs and pose a serious threat to the health of people, especially older people and children. The two biggest sources of air pollution in Nigeria are vehicular emissions and industrial plants [22].

3.3 Land Pollution and Heavy Metals

Land pollution includes all the natural resources used in the production of the minerals in the ground, forests, waterfalls, fertile soil and so on. Disposal of solid and hazardous waste on land is dangerous when not dealt with in an environmentally friendly way. The danger is that these wastes may pollute groundwater used for drinking and soils used for grazing and farming. Unwanted health and environmental impacts such as contamination of soil and possibly of food products grown thereon are potential consequences of improper disposal of hazardous wastes on the land which are found in most communities in Nigeria. In the oil-producing areas of the country, oil spillage of differing intensity resulting from burst pipelines, tanks, tankers, drilling operations, etc., is a common phenomenon [15].

Heavy metals occur as natural constituents of the Earth's crust and are persistent environmental contaminants since they cannot be destroyed. Mercury and lead are examples of heavy metals. They are widely used in technology but are so toxic that minute quantities can destroy life. In Nigeria today, numerous studies have shown that industrial activities release heavy metals either as solid, gas or liquid in the form of wastewater or effluents that are released into water ways or bodies [15]. Cadmium is a heavy metal of considerable environmental and occupational concern, and it is frequently used in various industrial activities [23]. Cadmium is also present in trace amounts in certain wraps of foods and foods such as leafy vegetables, potatoes, grains and seeds, liver and kidney, and crustaceans and molluscs [24]. Also, a common thing seen on the streets in Nigeria is the wrap of some food items such as kola nuts, eba, moi-moi, agidi, maize and so on. In most cases, the leaves on the streets find their way to gutters, and when there is a heavy rainfall, lakes, dams, streams and other water bodies used by local communities for drinking and other household activities may be contaminated. The toxicities of these heavy metals can range from severe illness to death of both plants and animals.

4 Potential Roles of ICT in Tackling Environmental Challenges

As stated earlier, the impacts of human activities on the environment are critical issues of concern confronting general life on Earth. It is clear that ICT requires energy resources, but they also offer several opportunities to move the global environment research, planning and implementation forward [4]. This section provides an overview of ICT's role in engaging mankind to mitigate against environmental degradation. It is suggested that there is a need to partner with the more developed countries to ensure the transfer and localization of software technologies which can promote climate action and greenhouse gas emission mitigation in Nigeria and in developing countries in general. This is because encouraging ICT development in Nigeria will ultimately inspire local innovations and will promote the use of sustainable sources of energy. It is the long-term potential of ICT to completely transform existing operating systems and business models that will have the biggest impact on emission reductions and environmental degradation [25]. In a report on the use of ICT for e-environment, Labelle [26] identified six categories of application of ICTs for the environment. These are ICT for environmental observations, analysis, planning, management and protection, mitigation and capacity building.

4.1 ICT Services for Environmental Observations: Satellite Observations and Direct Sensors

ICT Services for Environmental Observations are tools that are used to acquire environmental information, monitoring, data recording and storing them in a standardized format. This category includes making a detailed observation and presentation of data on Earth resources and environment. A typical example is the variety of remote sensing observations, which are used to help researchers gather large information about environmental systems. Sensors generate large amount of data in digital form which poses a challenge to the researchers and decision makers, particularly in developed worlds where the researchers could help interpret environmental information for government. Advances in the use of remote sensing technologies have allowed much more detailed observation and analysis of the Earth and are applied in agriculture, forestry and range, biophysical-spectral models, ecology, Earth and environmental science, geography and land information, geology and geosciences, hydrology and water resources, image processing and analysis, and atmospheric science and meteorology. Generally, remote sensing refers to the activities of recording, observing, or sensing objects at faraway or isolated or remote places. We have different types of remote sensor such as satellite remote sensing, optical and infrared remote sensing, macrowave remote sensing and remote sensing images, all with different functions. Thus, there is need for a robust system and well-maintained satellite-based remote sensing and for satellite meteorology to study atmospheric and weather sciences using satellite data to facilitate the effective management of our environment in Nigeria. Information from the observations should be provided to the policymakers, disaster management organizations, commercial interests and the general public. This is because several countries, including Argentina, Canada, China, France, India, Indonesia, Mexico, Saudi Arabia, Thailand and the United States, have implemented satellite-based multi-point telecommunication systems for their National Meteorological Telecommunication Networks. The World Meteorological Organization (WMO) provides the backbone of the Global Observing System (GOS) which is comprised of observation stations located on land, at sea, on aircraft and on meteorological satellites. GOS is a composite system of complex methods, techniques and facilities for measuring meteorological and environmental parameters. It provides observations of the atmosphere and the Earth's surface (including ocean surface) from all parts of the globe and from outer space. The system ensures that critical information is available to every country to generate weather analyses, forecasts and warnings on a day-to-day basis.[4]

4.2 *ICT Services for Environmental Analysis: Grid Computing and GIS Systems*

Environmental analysis must deal with the use of various computational and processing tools to perform analysis on the environment, focusing on the interaction between human and nonhuman components of the biosphere. Once environmental data has been collected and stored, various computational and processing tools are required to perform the analysis and comparison of data available. Recent development of information and communication technologies provides very powerful platforms for effective processing of multiple data sources, particularly web searches, database systems and data mining tools oriented on key environmental components and their descriptors, regionally specific data aggregation, mapping of

[4] https://www.britannica.com/science/Cenozoic-Era.

segmentation of the regions using geographic information system (GIS) technology, automated processing of laboratory tests, algorithms and statistical packages, energy-efficient programmes in CPU design and grid computing. GIS is a new way of thinking that integrates geographic information into how we understand and manage our planet. Grid computing enhances access to environmental data and encourages networking and virtual collaboration. It collects computer resources from multiple locations to reach a common goal by setting up grid networks for computation analysis. Applying these two ICT services for environmental analysis, Worthington [27] suggested that the potential total emission avoidance from the implementation of smart building solutions, for example, is estimated to be as high as 1.68 Gt carbon IV oxide emission (C02e) by 2020.

4.3 *ICT for Environment Planning, Management and Protection, Mitigation and Capacity Building for Environmental Sustainability*

Environmental planning involves decision-making to carry out development considering the natural environmental, social, political, economic factors and providing a holistic framework to achieve sustainable outcomes. It starts with a study and evaluation that are based on the outcome information of the environmental observation and analysis, which is then used to develop environmental policies and strategies.

It might be reasonable to assume that the implementation and enforcement goal is to maximize the environmental benefits of compliance. Several governments have recommended ambitious policy goals, both to enable ICTs to address issues related to climate change and to encourage the sector to remediate its own carbon footprint. For instance, in 2008, the European Union (EU) Heads of State and Government set a policy to reduce EU greenhouse gas emissions by at least 20% below 1990 levels, to allow 20% of EU energy consumption to come from renewable resources, and recommended that the ICT sector fulfil its EU 2020 goals by 2015.[5]

There is no doubt that ICTs impose their challenges on the environment. These challenges come as a result of their use and disposal and can be mitigated using innovative or novel ICT tools in a more environmentally friendly way and by modifying human behaviour resulting in action that reduces or eliminates negative impact on the environment. The potential mitigation benefits of ICT should centre on social media applications that promote ecological behaviour and the use of smart grid applications for automatic calculation of carbon footprint, that is, the amount of carbon dioxide produced through vehicle emissions, electricity use and fuel consumption. ICT tools that support sustainable consumption must simplify complex information and present it in a more personal and motivating manner. For

[5] https://ec.europa.eu/clima/policies/strategies/2020_en.

example, it is estimated that the amount of fuel wasted by congestion in US urban areas alone has increased to 480%, from 500 million gallons to 2.9 billion gallons from 1982 to 2005 [27]. In this era of heightened concern regarding climate change, how we organize traffic and travel has become a critical concern, particularly for urban environments. Logically, if there is less traffic, there is less CO_2. ICT services and solutions can help to optimize traffic congestion and avoid them completely, where possible. For instance, improvements in supply chain logistics can minimize travel among distribution networks. The use of vehicle telematics solutions can optimize loading and route management for goods transport vehicles, taking more traffic off the road and lowering company logistics costs.

There is a need for capacity building which involves the integration of environmental awareness and content into formal education. Environmental public awareness simply means the ability to understand our surroundings, including the laws of the natural environment, sensitivity to all the changes occurring in the environment, understanding of cause-and-effect relationships between the quality of the environment and human behaviour and a sense of responsibility for the natural resources, with the aim of preserving and conserving them for future generations. To improve environmental condition, action can be taken in a variety of areas to increase environmental awareness and education. Some of these categories are implementation of environmental legal rights and responsibilities and associated consequences, use of the media, awareness raising campaigns, incorporation of environmental issues in mainstream education from primary to tertiary, increasing awareness and education in target groups and encouragement of public participation in environmental matters. The main goal of any environmental conscious individuals or groups is to increase awareness because that is the only way to attain a more sustainable environment. In practice, this will mean purchasing eco-labelled cleaning products (such as multi-purpose cleaner and window cleaner), making sure staff are trained on the use of the correct dosage, employing chemical-saving techniques (such as using micro-fibre cloths) and ensuring that an appropriate cleaning needs analysis is carried out so that areas are not "over-cleaned" [28].

5 Conclusions and Recommendations

ICT has the potential to give better insight into the complex interaction between natural resources and environmental dynamics for sustainable use. Poor analytical assessment and inadequate monitoring of natural resources have been a big challenge resulting in degradation and constitute a major risk to environmental security in Nigeria. There is a need to raise awareness of the importance of collecting, measuring and analysing scientific data from the environment and the need to share these data to the public with the help of ICT. Much of this data is or can be georeferenced and could add significant value to the historical record of life, ecosystems and other natural systems, including past events of environmental significance and how these have changed over time. Priority should be given to deployment of ICTs by governments for the purpose of environmental management. Agencies in Nigeria such as the National Information Technology Development Agency (NITDA), Ministry of Science and Technology, Ministry of Information Communication and Nigerian Communications Commission exist specifically to address this situation and initiate e-Government Interoperability Framework. The Nigerian ICT industry should also recognize the ever-increasing importance of systems and software interoperability to enable the integration of systems and business/government processes.

Establishment of human and institutional capacity to undertake environmental planning activities on their own and collaborate with the international development community is also essential. Moreover, there is an urgent need to assign the environment a more important and higher profile in ICT strategic planning initiatives at both local and national levels so that the use of ICTs for the environment is integrated into planning processes from the beginning along with other national priorities and initiatives.

Acknowledgement This publication has emanated from research supported in part by a grant from Science Foundation Ireland under grant number 18/CRT/6222.

References

1. A. Osterwalder, ICT in developing countries (2002). Lausanne, Switzerland, University of Lausanne, pp. 1–13
2. B. Meadowcroft, The impact of information technology on work and society (2006). Retrieved from the internet. Available at: www.m-w.com/cgi-bin/netdict?society
3. United Nations Development Program (UNDP). Information, communication and knowledge-sharing, gender in development, learning and information pack (2002). UNDP, New York. Available at: http://www.undp.org/gender/infopack.htm
4. T.A. Ikwunne, *ICT for Greener Environment: A Case for Nigeria* (Great AP Express Publications LTD, Nigeria, 2014)
5. K.R. Acharya, J.R. Bautista, J.R. Wilson, J. Nahachewsky, J.L. Briere, S. Flanagan, J. Pilgrim, Aging, E-literacy, and technology: Participatory user-centered design for older adults' digital engagement. J. Literacy Technol. **16**(2), 3–32 (2015)
6. E.M. Ahmed, R. Ridzuan, The impact of ICT on East Asian economic growth: Panel estimation approach. J. Knowl. Econ. **4**(4), 540–555 (2013)
7. A. Yousefi, The impact of information and communication technology on economic growth: Evidence from developed and developing countries. Econ. Innov. New Technol. **20**(6), 581–596 (2011)
8. E.A. Cortés, J.L.A. Navarro, Do ICT influence economic growth and human development in European Union countries? Int. Adv. Econ. Res. **17**(1), 28–44 (2011)
9. C. Dzidonu, *A Blueprint for Developing National ICT Policy in Africa* (African Technology Policy Studies Network, Nairobi, 2002)
10. J. Houghton. ICTs and the environment in developing countries: Opportunities and developments. The development dimension ICTs for development improving policy coherence: improving policy coherence (2010), p. 149
11. D.O. Odedele, O.A. Ogbolumani, Deployment of sustainable ICT infrastructure in Nigeria Vis a Vis the nation building. Am. J. Eng. Technol. Soc. **2**(3), 60 (2015)

12. G.R. Shaver, J. Canadell, F.S. Chapin, J. Gurevitch, J. Harte, G. Henry, et al., Global warming and terrestrial ecosystems: A conceptual framework for analysis: Ecosystem responses to global warming will be complex and varied. Ecosystem warming experiments hold great potential for providing insights on ways terrestrial ecosystems will respond to upcoming decades of climate change. Documentation of initial conditions provides the context for understanding and predicting ecosystem responses. Bioscience **50**(10), 871–882 (2000)
13. International Telecommunication Union, ICTs for e-Environment: Guidelines for developing countries, with a focus on climate change, (ITU, Geneva, 2008), p. 25
14. F.O. Asogwa, K.K. Ohaleme, R.O. Ugwuanyi, The impact of telecommunication expenditure on economic growth in Nigeria. J. Econ. Sustain. Dev. **4**(13), 40–44 (2013)
15. I. Aigbedion, S.E. Iyayi, Environmental effect of mineral exploitation in Nigeria. Int. J. Phys. Sci. **2**(2), 33–38 (2007)
16. O.A. Okogun, O.M. Awoleye, W.O. Siyanbola, Economic value of ICT investment in Nigeria: Is it commensurate. Int. J. Econ. Manag. Sci. **1**(10), 22–30 (2012)
17. J. Clement, Number of internet users in Nigeria from 2017 to 2023 (2019), https://www.statista.com/statistics/183849/internet-users-nigeria/
18. E. Ndukwe, The role of telecommunications in national development. Nigerian Tribune, No. 13, 467, Tuesday 21 September (2004)
19. O. Akwani. Telecom operators creating new employment in Nigeria (2005), https://imdiversity.com/villages/global/travel-diaries/
20. R.P. Schwarzenbach, T. Egli, T.B. Hofstetter, U. Von Gunten, B. Wehrli, Global water pollution and human health. Annu. Rev. Env. Resour. **35**, 109–136 (2010)
21. P.O. Agbaire, E. Esiefarienrhe, Air pollution tolerance indices (apti) of some plants around Otorogun Gas Plant in Delta State, Nigeria. J. Appl. Sci. Environ. Manag. **13**(1), 11–14 (2009)
22. C.A. Odilara, P.A. Egwaikhide, A. Esekheigbe, S.A. Emua, Air pollution tolerance indices (APTI) of some plant species around llupeju industrial area, Lagos. J. Eng. Sci. Appl. **4**(2), 97–101 (2006)
23. P.B. Tchounwou, C.G. Yedjou, A.K. Patlolla, D.J. Sutton, Heavy metals toxicity and the environment. Published in final edited form as: EXS **3**, 133–164 (2012)
24. S. Satarug, J.R. Baker, S. Urbenjapol, M. Haswell-Elkins, P.E. Reilly, D.J. Williams, et al., A global perspective on cadmium pollution and toxicity in non-occupationally exposed population. Toxicol. Lett. **137**, 65–83 (2003)
25. M. Webb, Smart 2020: Enabling the low carbon economy in the information age (The Climate Group, London), **1**(1), 1 (2008)
26. R. Labelle, ICTs for e-Environment guidelines for developing countries, with a focus on climate change. International Telecommunications report (2008), http://www.itu.int/ITU-D/cyb/app/docs/itu-icts-for-e-environment. pdf
27. T. Worthington, *Green Technology Strategies* (Tomw Communications Pty Ltd, Belconnen, 2009)
28. ICLEI. Local sustainability 2012: Showcasing progress. Case studies, ICLEI Global Report · Analysis · Sustainability · ICLEI - Local Governments for Sustainability World Secretariat Kaiser-Friedrich-Str.7, 53113 Bonn, Germany (2012). Avaliable at: www.iclei.org

Conceptual Design and Prototyping for a Primate Health History Knowledge Model

Martin Q. Zhao, Elizabeth Maldonado, Terry B. Kensler, Luci A. P. Kohn, Debbie Guatelli-Steinberg, and Qian Wang

1 Introduction

In 1938, a group of rhesus macaques (*Macaca mulatta*) from India were introduced to Cayo Santiago (CS), Puerto Rico, to ensure a steady supply for research and vaccine development in the continental USA during WWII [1, 4–7, 10–12, 14–19].

Systematic daily tracking of all rhesus monkeys on the island began in 1956 under the National Institutes of Health's (NIH) Laboratory of Perinatal Physiology (LPP) in San Juan. The LPP closed in 1970, and the Caribbean Primate Research Center (CPRC) was established under the University of Puerto Rico (UPR) School of Medicine with base support coming from NIH. The daily census, which began in 1956, has continued uninterrupted to the present day. The colony has been naturally divided into more than 26 matrilineal families. The data collected during

M. Q. Zhao (✉)
Department of Computer Science, Mercer University, Macon, GA, USA
e-mail: zhao_mq@mercer.edu

E. Maldonado · T. B. Kensler
Caribbean Primate Research Center, University of Puerto Rico Medical Sciences Campus, San Juan, Puerto Rico

L. A. P. Kohn
Department of Biological Sciences, Southern Illinois University Edwardsville, Edwardsville, IL, USA

D. Guatelli-Steinberg
Department of Anthropology, The Ohio State University, Columbus, OH, USA

Q. Wang (✉)
Department of Biomedical Sciences, Texas A&M University College of Dentistry, Dallas, TX, USA
e-mail: qian.wang@tamu.edu

H. R. Arabnia et al. (eds.), *Advances in Computer Vision and Computational Biology*, Transactions on Computational Science and Computational Intelligence,
https://doi.org/10.1007/978-3-030-71051-4_40

the past 64 years for over ten generations of monkeys makes the rhesus colony at Cayo Santiago one of the most useful primate databases in biomedical and anthropological research. In addition, in 1971, the CPRC rhesus monkey skeletal collection was established, and at present, up to eight generations are in the collection. This is a unique translational resource for genetic and age-related studies: ancestors of nonhuman primates available in a skeletal collection plus their descendants living in similar conditions [1, 5, 14]. However, there is no integrated database on the Cayo rhesus colony and the derived skeletal collection, limiting the use of this rhesus resource for the reconstruction of the health history of the colony for the purpose of biomedical and anthropological studies. The need to integrate data warrants the construction of a complete demographic profile of the colony at Cayo Santiago.

We have started a collaborative research project with a group of scientists in four universities in the USA involved to carry out the studies. In our long-term project, there are three aims toward building a searchable database of Cayo Santiago monkey health history for anthropological and biomedical/translational studies of the effects of environment and genetics on bone development, aging, and pathologies.

1. Document morphological and pathological conditions of the Cayo Santiago skeletal collection.
2. Build a Cayo Santiago rhesus health database.
3. Test hypotheses about secular trends and familial disparities in health and other features using the Cayo Santiago rhesus health database.

This chapter discusses the conceptual design and prototyping of this database (DB) and related graphical user interfaces (GUI) to include all necessary information and facilitate searchable outputs while allowing the continuing input of information in the future, similar to a knowledge model [20, 21]. Meanwhile, it must be pointed out that *like any database of human subjects and following regulations and requirements set by the Caribbean Primate Research Center, this project treats every monkey as a patient and thus protects its privacy as we practice with human patients.*

2 Data Needs and Conceptual Data Models

Building the proposed database and related GUIs needs to have thorough plans that address all phases of the application development life cycle [22], as illustrated in Fig. 1. In this early stage of the development process, the key activity is to collect and analyze requirements for the proposed system and come up with conceptual design models. In this section, we will discuss data needs and conceptual data models. Functional requirements in terms of use cases and GUI design concepts will be discussed in the next section.

In our planned project, individual skeletal remains will be screened and measured for documenting morphological and pathological conditions for a wide spectrum of

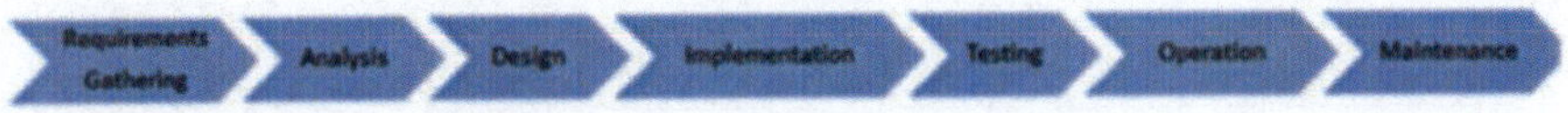

Fig. 1 Illustration of the application development life cycle (ADLC)

bone and tooth health and pathology. Five sets of data will be collected for each skeleton:

1. The demographic and genealogical information of all specimens and body mass and sitting height when available.
2. The bone conditions of all available skeletal parts, including age-related and pathological features (such as abnormalities, diseases, and trauma) and non-metric harmless bone features (such as supernumerary teeth, suture type at the pterion, and hyperostosis). Color images of morphological and pathological features of interest will be generated using a high-quality camera, Cannon EOS 50D.
3. Bone density will be measured by a portable Omnisense 8000S Mobile Sonometer Bone Densitometry System. Specimens of special interest will be further examined using X-ray or quantitative CT scanning facilities.
4. Measurements of skeletal size of both cranial and postcranial skeletons [2, 15].
5. Linear enamel hypoplasia (developmental defects of enamel) from dental replicas under a Leica DMS1000 digital monocular microscope and then a measuring microscope (Spectra Services) and VisionGauge software to measure perikymata (growth increment) spacing.

For data collection, an interactive bone survey program will be generated using Qualtrics, a web-based data collection tool that is secure, and Texas A&M University has a license for all faculty and staff to use.

The proposed integrative database will incorporate health data obtained in this project (scans, measurements, and observation data) with subject genealogy information of the rhesus families maintained by the CPRC. A standard relational data model will be used to provide a normalize the database (Fig. 2).

Originally, the genealogical data are recorded using Excel files, each for a different family. In these files, each row keeps track of a leaf node (i.e., a subject with no descendant) in the respective family tree, including information of its own (gender, birth, and death dates) and information about its female ancestors all the way back to the family founder.

To remove the redundancy in the original dataset is to split it into two tables, one for family and the other for subjects. Each row of the Subject table records a distinct animal subject, which is related to the corresponding family through a foreign key (FK) FamilyID to the primary key (PK) in the Family table. Each subject entry is related to its mother through another foreign key MotherID, which is the mother's SubjectID, to keep mother-child mapping.

Additional tables will be used to store subject morphology and pathology information (such as bone density, disease, and image) when they become available.

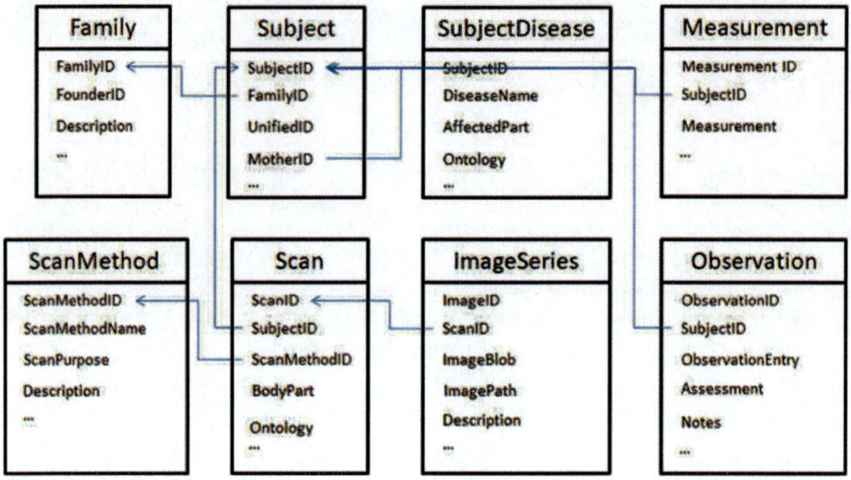

Fig. 2 Conceptual data model for the Cayo Santiago Rhesus Health Database. Per regulations and requirements set by the Caribbean Primate Research Center, this project treats every monkey as a patient and thus protects its privacy as we practice with human patients. All assigned IDs will be a coded ID, not original tattoos

Similar relational design has been used [13] and shows great extensibility. More tables may be added as needed to demonstrate a high-level abstraction of the database schema that captures the major data sets (i.e., database tables) and the relationships among them (Fig. 3). As will be discussed in the following section, other kinds of information need to be stored to keep track of valid users, access control, user activities, etc. Additional tables will be added to in later stages (such as detailed design phase) to store those kinds of information.

2.1 Unified Coding Scheme

The unified code includes all the information regarding the subject with a FI-GE-MSEQ-SS-G-BY-DY-SSEQ pattern, which is detailed in the unified coding scheme. When used in various lengths (including certain parts in the multi-part pattern), it can present data needed in various scenarios. For instance, FI (family ID) and SSEQ (subject sequence number within the family) can uniquely identify a subject; FI, MSEQ (mother sequence number), and SS (sibling sequence number) can also identify a subject and focus on a subject's social status.

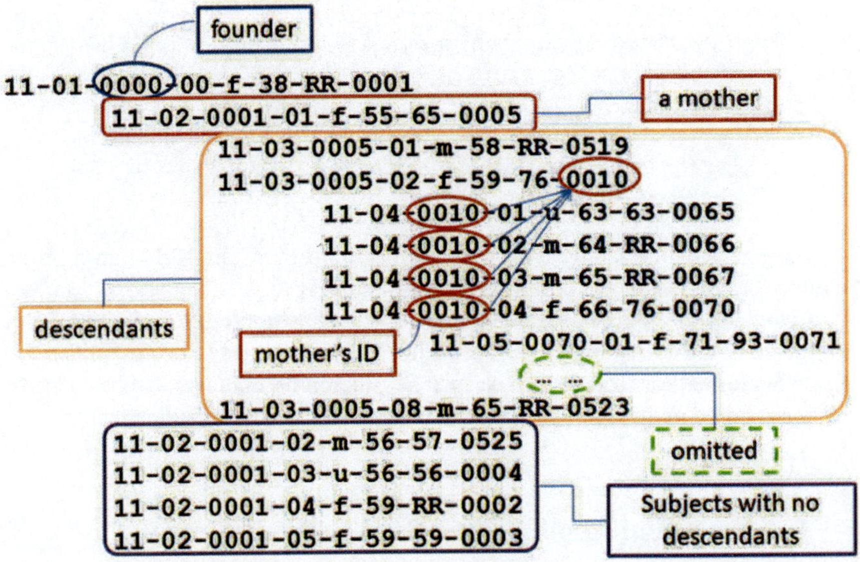

Fig. 3 A partial family tree with subjects represented in the FI-GE-MSEQ-SS-G-BY-DY-SSEQ pattern

The FI-GE-MSEQ-SS-G-BY-DY-SSEQ pattern consists of the following parts:

- FI: two-digit family ID.
- GE: two-digit generation number within a family, with 01 for the family founder.
- MSEQ: four-digit subject sequence number within a family for the mother of this subject; 0000 is used for family founder, whose mother is not in this database.
- SS: sibling sequence number for direct children from the same mother subject.
- G: one-character code for individual's sex, with valid values "f," "m," and "u."
- BY: Exact birth date with four-digit birth year, two-digit birth month, and two-digit birth day.
- DY: Exact death date with four-digit death year, two-digit death month, and two-digit death day.
- "RR" and ".." used for subjects that are removed and still alive, respectively, with exact date of removal.

(continued)

- CPRC-LPM-CM: Current CPRC LPM's skeletal catalog number assigned to each skeleton.
- SSEQ: four-digit subject sequence number within family.

A segment of the family tree representing subjects in family 11 (an arbitrary number for now) using the unified code is given in Fig. 3.

A UnifiedCode column is added to the Subject table to protect subject's privacy. On the other hand, ontology links are added in certain tables to be compliant with medical informatics standards. To be specific, Uberon [9] numbers will be added for diseases (stored in the SubjectDisease table) and body part (in the Scan table).

3 Use Cases and Application Design Concepts

Convenient user interfaces need to be developed to support various kinds of users to use the database we are building. Users can be categorized into the following types: (1) staff in charge of collecting and entering data, (2) researchers involved in this project using the data to "test hypotheses on secular trends and familial disparities," and (3) general public in research communities searching for related information to support their research.

While the three groups may overlap with one another, the first two groups of users are closely related to the collaborative research project. It is appropriate to develop two sets of interfaces: a window-based GUI app for staff operators/researchers to use, such as for loading and editing data and for data visualization and manipulation, and a web-based application for general research communities to access data and use in their studies.

The web-based application is designed to be a searchable and computer-interoperable knowledge model to discover previously unknown associations from the rhesus family data. It will be developed in the last stage of the multi-year project when the database is constructed and loaded with newly collected data. In this chapter, our focus will be on the window-based interfaces for staff and project researchers.

Like many information systems, this proposed system will need to support the following use cases:

- User authentication and role-based accessibility control: Only authorized users will be able to log into the system with valid credentials. Based on their job functions (or roles), they will be able to access (search only or manipulate) the right types of data (e.g., family and/or pathology).

- Data entry and editing: The system will provide support in several different approaches.
  - Converting existing datasets (Excel spreadsheets) used to track subject and family information and automatically loading them into the new relational database
  - Providing convenient forms and/or dialog boxes to allow for manual data entry and editing, as well as data quality checking
  - Integrating with other specialized data collection tools such as Qualtrics to load data into targeted tables
- Provide a comprehensive window (Fig. 4) with multiple panels or tabs to support various kinds of data visualization and analytics tasks. This window will include:
  - A main panel that displays an interactive family tree with all subjects from the selected family displayed, and with indications, e.g., as a mother, a male, a female, or an unknown gender subject with no descendant.
  - A side panel displaying morphological and pathological data in tabular form for an individual selected in the family tree.
  - Separate panels will display scan images for the selected subject when available.
  - Other panels displaying additional notes/descriptions.
- The comprehensive window will anchor menus or tabs to allow insider researchers to conduct searching, filtering, and analytical tasks, such as:
  - Displaying distribution and trends with common charts (e.g., histogram, scatter plots)
  - Partial family tree with filtering criteria in place and/or with father information available from DNA to be conducted in this project

4 Database and Application Prototyping

Efforts to parse subject information have been tested in three families stored in Excel spreadsheets, which was prepared by E.M. and released by CPRC to Q.W. at the early stage of preparing for this project. Original data for each subject includes a unique code (or ID), sex, years born and died, and the mother's code. Additional data derived from the dataset include generation within the family, family number, sibling sequence number, and each subject's life span. As mentioned above, a unified coding scheme is proposed to provide a unique identifier for each subject. Some pilot studies have been conducted to test the effectiveness of the conceptual data models and provide a prototype that implements the design concepts. Before a detailed plan for new data collection contents and procedures is established, a *simplified database schema* is developed in these proof-of-concept efforts. It can

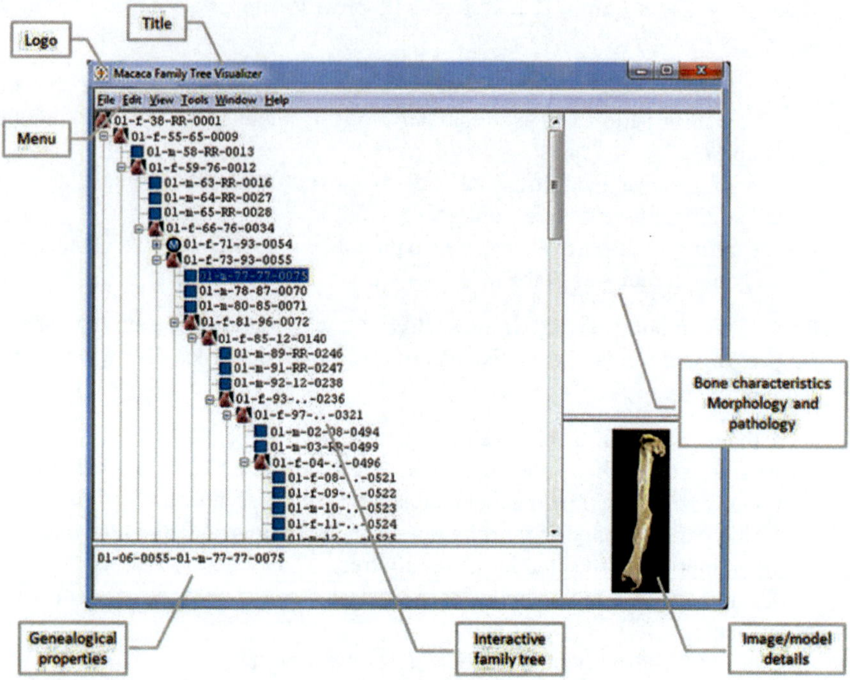

Fig. 4 Illustration of the layout of the window-based user interface

manage the existing subject data and can associate various kinds of scan imagery and conventional physical measuring data related to the subjects. With detailed data management needs provided, this simplified schema can be extended to store all collected data as proposed.

A simplified implementation was prototyped in the fall of 2019 using SQL Server on a virtual machine at Mercer University's Computer Science Department (Fig. 5). The Family and Subject tables are populated with data originally from CPRC, with derived values like generation, life span, and a unified subject ID. Dummy data collected from online sources are used to populate other tables (such as Scan and ImageSeries) to provide test data necessary for the graphical interface development efforts. To be compliant with standard bioinformatics ontologies (such as Uberon) for interoperability with other data sources and search tools, Uberon IDs for body parts (bones or teeth) and diseases will be included in related tables.

Framework of the GUI design for the window-based application was developed in the spring of 2020. It includes a comprehensive window that can anchor components for displaying a family tree, series of scan images, tabular presentation of basic body measures, dialog boxes that support data entry and update, as well as some data analytics tasks.

Interactive family tree (shown in Fig. 6) can be used to display all subjects in the same family. The Search menu can facilitate selecting a family by family ID, and a

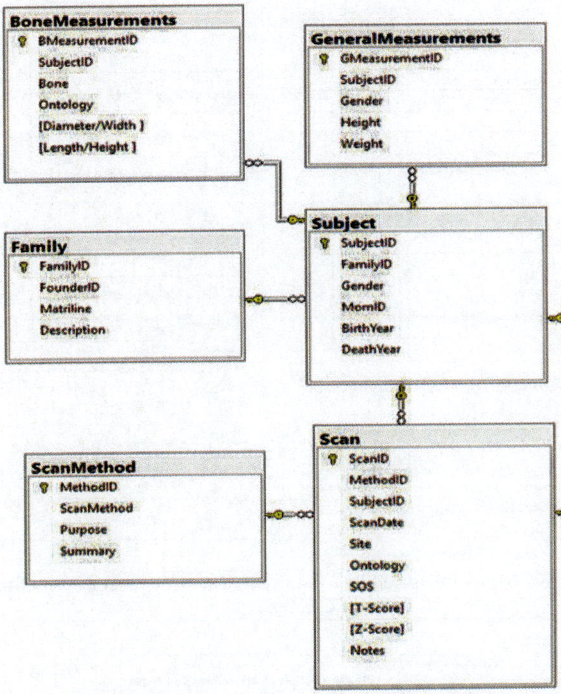

Fig. 5 Relational schema of a prototype database for testing purpose. Note: Though this looks similar in the flowchart, Fig. 2 presents a "conceptual" data model, developed in "analysis" phase of the ADLC, with certain details omitted intentionally to deal with layers of complexity. Figure 5 is a design model or DB schema that is specialized for this simplified prototype implementation of the more abstract analysis model. Again, per regulations and requirements set by the Caribbean Primate Research Center, this project treats every monkey as a patient and thus protects its privacy as we practice with human patients. All assigned IDs will be a coded ID, not original tattoos

matriline family tree starting from the founder can be generated using data from the DB and displayed in the panel. Various icons are used to indicate mother, female or male descendants, as well as subjects whose gender is labeled as U (for unknown). Subtrees starting from each mother node can be expanded or collapsed to show or hide details. When a subject node is selected, related imagery and measurement data will be displayed in corresponding panels as illustrated in Fig. 4.

Certain GUIs that can be used to support data entry/editing and data analytics tasks have also been developed in the prototype system. Dialog boxes for manipulating data in a table are provided to support operational staff to view and edit data in the DB. These dialog boxes can pop up from the menus. A screenshot of a dialog box used for manipulating entries in the ImageSeries table is shown in Fig. 7a. Operation staff can use this interface to edit data collected from the scan, add a new image, or delete an image, as necessary. Values in primary key and/or foreign key fields are not changeable in this interface.

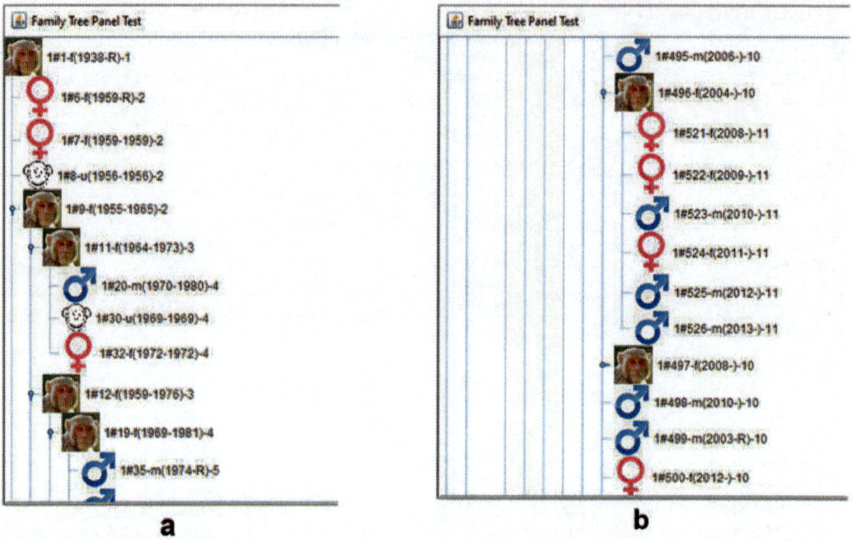

Fig. 6 Illustrations of the interactive family tree panel. (**a**). Family tree starting from the founder. (**b**). Tree expanded to 11th generation (with M, F, U, and Mom icons)

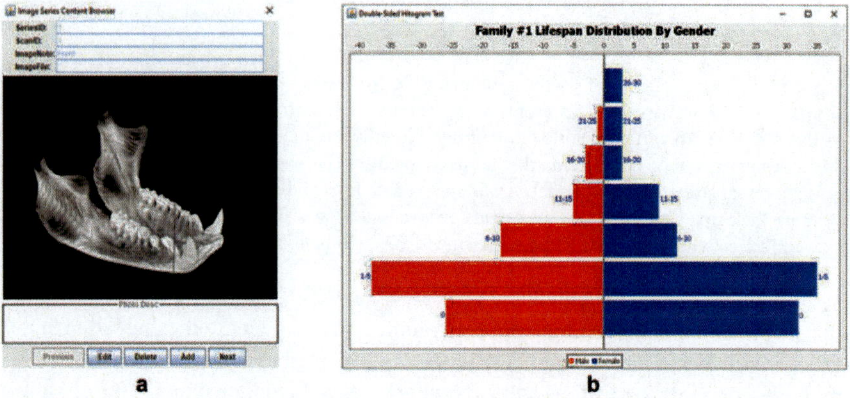

Fig. 7 Screenshots of additional user interfaces. (**a**). Dialog box for manipulating entries in the ImageSeries table. (**b**). Additional window for showing data analytics results

Figure 7b shows a screenshot of a separate window showing a dual histogram of subject count by gender using data from one rhesus family. Only subjects with a known death year value (i.e., not removed or still alive) and whose gender is not labelled as unknown (U) are included. Life span values are calculated using the difference between death year and birth year data and categorized in bins for 0, 1–5, 6–10, and so on. An open source Java charting API JFreeChart [3] is used in generating the two-sided bar chart.

An SQL Server [8] instance has been set up on Amazon Web Services (AWS) cloud-based facility to build the simplified database to concept-prove the possibility of exposing the proposed database to the research community after it is built. Other cloud-based technologies to make the data accessible will be explored for the web-based application to be developed later. Integrated data and information could be extracted in Excel, comma-separated values (CSV), or other forms for easy data mining.

5 Conclusions and Future Work

With careful design and data collection, we will build a web-based interface and make it useful for future scientific queries and studies with proper privacy protection mechanisms. Hypotheses regarding sex-based difference, aging, geographic adaptations, and impacts of natural disasters such as hurricanes could be tested to examine the correlation between natural and/or independent factors and anato-physiological features for developmental, evolutionary, and biomedical studies.

Acknowledgments The CPRC Skeletal Collection has been supported by National Institutes of Health (NIH) contracts NIH 5 P40 OD012217. This project is supported by NSF grants to M.Q.Z., L.K., D.G.S., and Q.W. (NSF #1926402, 1926481, 1926528, 1926601). We thank Dr. Melween I. Martinez Rodriguez (current CPRC director), Mr. Bonn V Aure Liong, Dr. Angelina Ruiz-Lambides, and other CPRC staff members for their support and help. Coauthor Terry B. Kensler, who currently manages the collection, is thanked for her excellent curatorial skills. Dr. Li Sun is thanked for her help, support, and patience. Special thanks go to Mr. Jesse Sowell for setting up the database servers and the students at the Mercer University's Computer Science Department for their contributions. We also thank the editor and reviewers for their very constructive comments.

References

1. D.C. Dunbar, Physical anthropology at the Caribbean Primate Research Center: Past, present, and future, in *Bones, Genetics, and Behavior of Rhesus Macaques: Macaca mulatta of Cayo Santiago and Beyond*, ed. by Q. Wang, (Springer, New York, 2012), pp. 1–35
2. L.A.P. Kohn, Z. Bledsoe, Genetic and group influences on postcranial morphology in rhesus macaques (*Macaca mulatta*) of Cayo Santiago, in *Bones, Genetics, and Behavior of Rhesus Macaques: Macaca mulatta of Cayo Santiago and Beyond*, ed. by Q. Wang, (Springer Verlag, New York, 2012), pp. 117–129
3. JFree.org, The most widely used chart library for Java (2020). Accessed on 10 May 2020
4. M. J. Kessler (ed.), Proceedings of the meeting to celebrate the 50th anniversary of the Cayo Santiago Rhesus Monkey Colony. P. R. Health. Sci. J. **8**(1), 1–200 (1989)
5. M.J. Kessler, R.G. Rawlins, A 75-year pictorial history of the Cayo Santiago rhesus monkey colony. Am. J. Primatol. **78**, 6–43 (2016)
6. M.J. Kessler, Q. Wang, A.M. Cerroni, M.D. Grynpas, O.D.G. Velez, R.G. Rawlins, K.F. Ethun, J.H. Wimsatt, T.B. Kensler, K.P.H. Pritzker, Long-term effects of castration on the skeleton of male rhesus monkeys (*Macaca mulatta*). Am. J. Primatol. **78**, 152–166 (2016)

7. H. Li, W. Luo, A. Feng, M.L. Tang, T.B. Kensler, E. Maldonado, O.A. Gonzalez, M.K. Kessler, P.C. Dechow, J.L. Ebersole, Q. Wang, The odontogenic abscess in rhesus macaques (*Macaca mulatta*) from Cayo Santiago. Am. J. Phys. Anthropol. **167**, 441–457 (2018)
8. Microsoft Corp, SQL server technical documentation (2020), https://docs.microsoft.com/en-us/sql/sql-server/?view=sql-server-ver15. Accessed on 10 May 2020
9. C.J. Mungall, C. Torniai, G.V. Gkoutos, S.E. Lewis, M.A. Haendel, Uberon, an integrative multi-species anatomy ontology. Genome Biol. **13**(1), R5 (2012)
10. J.E. Turnquist, N. Hong, Current status of the Caribbean Primate Research Center Museum. P R Health Sci. J. **8**, 187–189 (1989)
11. R. G. Rawlins, M. J. Kessler (eds.), *The Cayo Santiago Macaques* (State University of New York Press, Albany, 1986)
12. D.S. Sade, B. Chepko-Sade, J. Schneider, S.S. Roberts, J.T. Richtsmeier, *Basic Demographic Observations on Free-Ranging Rhesus Monkeys* (New Haven, Human Relations Area Files Press, 1985), pp. 1–98
13. D. Seo, S. Lee, S. Lee, H. Jung, W.K. Sung. Construction of Korean spine database with degenerative spinal diseases for realizing e-spine, KSII. The 8th Asian Pacific international conference on information science and technology (APIC-IST) 2013, Jeju, Republic of Korea (2013)
14. Q. Wang (ed.), *Bones, Genetics, and Behavior of Rhesus Macaques: Macaca mulatta of Cayo Santiago and Beyond* (Springer, New York, 2012)
15. Q. Wang, P.C. Dechow, S.M. Hens, Ontogeny and diachronic changes in sexual dimorphism in the craniofacial skeleton of rhesus macaques from Cayo Santiago, Puerto Rico. J. Hum. Evol. **53**, 350–361 (2007)
16. Q. Wang, M.J. Kessler, T.B. Kensler, P.C. Dechow, The mandibles of castrated male rhesus macaques (*Macaca mulatta*): The effects of orchidectomy on bone and teeth. Am. J. Phys. Anthropol. **159**, 31–51 (2016)
17. Q. Wang, L.A. Opperman, L.M. Havill, D.S. Carlson, P.C. Dechow, Inheritance of sutural pattern at the pterion in rhesus monkey skulls. Anat. Rec. **288A**, 1042–1049 (2006)
18. Q. Wang, D.S. Strait, P.C. Dechow, Fusion patterns of craniofacial sutures in rhesus monkey skulls of known age and sex from Cayo Santiago. Am. J. Phys. Anthropol. **131**, 469–485 (2006)
19. Q. Wang, J.E. Turnquist, M.J. Kessler, Free-ranging Cayo Santiago rhesus monkeys (*Macaca mulatta*): III. Dental eruption Patterns and dental pathology. Am. J. Primatol. **78**, 127–142 (2016)
20. M.Q. Zhao, Knowledge representation and reasoning for impact/threat assessment in cyber situation awareness systems. Final Report to AFRL/RI, Rome, NY, June 2010 (2010)
21. M.Q. Zhao, Analysis tool development for quantifying the SITA system. Technical Report to AFRL/RI, Rome, NY, August 2012 (2012)
22. M.Q. Zhao, A first course in database systems using SQL server. Published by Linus Learning, Ronkonkoma, NY, 2018 (2018)

Implementation of a Medical Data Warehouse Framework to Support Decisions

Nedra Amara, Olfa Lamouchi, and Said Gattoufi

1 Introduction

2600 new instances of breast cancer growth are enlisted each year in Tunisia, which could arrive at 3800 cases by 2024, as indicated by the leader of the Tunisian association for breast cancer disease [1]. The most widely recognized cancer growth in ladies is breast cancer diseases. Breast cancer disease rate expanded from 17/100 000 out of 2000 to 32.9/100 000 out of 2015 [1]. The occurrence pace of breast disease is on the ascent, and analyses frequently happen at a late stage (35% at the limited stage; 45% at the local stage; 20% at the metastatic stage) [2]. Breast malignancy screening is regulated by the National Office of Family and Populace (NOFP) and the Directorate of Basic Health Care (DBHC), while breast cancer disease cannot be forestalled yet can be controlled through early discovery and suitable treatment. The early detection of breast malignant growth expands the endurance rate in a patient [3]. Whenever identified in the beginning periods, breast cancer disease is exceptionally treatable by a medical procedure, radiation treatment, chemotherapy, and hormonal treatment. In this manner, mammography is a critical imaging methodology for the early detection of breast cancer growth [4].

As standard screening assessment turns out to be progressively popular, a gigantic measure of breast imaging information has been aggregated [3]. To analyze breast anomalies successfully, radiologists anticipate that helpful access should efficiently breast imaging-related data. Most breast malignant growth-related infor-

N. Amara (✉) · S. Gattoufi
Institute of Management, University of Tunis, Bardo, Tunisia
e-mail: said.gattoufi@isg.rnu.tn

O. Lamouchi
LR-RISC-ENIT (LR-16-ES07), Tunis, Tunisia

H. R. Arabnia et al. (eds.), *Advances in Computer Vision and Computational Biology*, Transactions on Computational Science and Computational Intelligence,
https://doi.org/10.1007/978-3-030-71051-4_41

mation, be that as it may, spread across various sources, making them difficult to get to. Besides, clinical data systems, for example, hospital information system (HIS), radiological information system (RIS), and picture archiving and communication system (PACS), as a rule, have activity execution prerequisites furthermore high reliable use. Conversely, decision support systems regularly have shifting execution necessities [5].

These distinctions can make it hard to join medical operational help and decision support prepared inside a unique data system, particularly concerning capacity planning, store management, and system execution tuning. Therefore, system administrators are typically hesitant to permit decision help exercises performed on their medical systems. Decision help information normally needs to be gathered from an assortment of working (regularly unique systems) and kept in an incorporated data store dwelled on a different platform. The ascent of customized medication and the accessibility of high-throughput clinical investigations with regards to clinical treatment have expanded the requirement for satisfactory tools for translational scientists to oversee and investigate this information. We checked on biomedical writing for translational platforms permitting the administration and investigation of medical data and identified a few openly accessible platforms: BRISK, caTRIP, cBio Cancer Portal, G-DOC, iCOD, iDASH, tranSMART, and Extensible Neuroimaging Archive Toolkit (XNAT). An enormous heterogeneity was seen with respect to the ability to oversee medical data, their security, and interoperability highlights. The expository and representation includes emphatically rely upon the thought about platforms [6]. Thus, the accessibility of the systems is variable. Li et al. [7] give an associate framework to client self-social insurance just as an integral framework for doctors' diagnosis of their day by day work. These platforms are proprietary and do not have the essential consistency with principles that would take into account cross-institutional information trade.

The mammography information data warehouse (MDW) is a significant apparatus for such a setting since it is characterized as a far-reaching database intended to help on decision making in business administration. DW has the properties of being coordinated, subject-situated, non-volatile, and time-variation [8]. Data warehousing is a wide domain focused on a MDW. Its application needs the integration of data originating from a few interior and outer sources (breast imaging, textual report, and excel and CSV files) to a more extensive specific database. This condition gives a far-reaching perspective on the whole association by the entrance to verifiable and solid data to aid the decision making, with the base conceivable over-burden on the value-based frameworks [9]. A few investigations have been led with various objectives, concerning medical data warehousing conditions. Einbinder et al. [10] introduced an investigation and development of an information store that comprises a DW for supporting the exploration and instruction in a scholarly clinical center and furthermore with the capacity of giving information to directors and managers. Evans et al. [11] depicted a contextual analysis about an endeavor DW applied to clinical registers, in this way, permitting association information with various records from inpatients and outpatient units to be incorporated and further broke down. Kerkri et al. [12] introduced a medical data warehousing platform that refocuses on patient clinical data from various medical information sources at a local level and incorporates them into a unique and more extensive information system. The incorporated data put away in the DW archive give significant information about the patients. Accordingly, it offers enhancements for finding and clinical decisions, giving experts solid, protected, and controlled data. Sebaa et al. [13] presented a data warehouse employed as the capacity of a lot of medical data, satisfying in as a principal part of a system that holds proof-based treatment. This examination additionally remarked on the principle moves identified with a mix of low-grained and time-segregated information into a DW.

The Tunisian general health system, just as that of a few different nations, presents genuine problems in data the board and an absence of getting ready for managing its requests and the controlling of its assets considering a confined time extend [14]. Among these problems, we can make reference to the complexity in managing human resources (HR) [15], just like materials, advances, and assets. The sending of normalized joint activities is fundamental to limit such issues. In Tunisia, an initial step was taken toward taking care of these issues. Worried about the open social insurance assets circulation, the Health Ministry of the Tunisian Government has built up laws and processes with respect to the public system medicinal services arranging and association. One of these processes is the star schema—presented for medical data warehouse entails a exhaustive description of resources, facilities, and activities related to the public healthcare system [14]. The proposal mammography data warehouses emerged for two reasons: first, the need to give a single, perfect, steady wellspring of data for decision support purposes; second, the need to do as such without affecting operational systems. An incorporated advanced mammography data warehouse can encourage analysis, instruction, and research in the territory of breast cancer disease. Having the option to solidify clinical data and arrange persistent records by their medical pictures, family history, and pathologies can give valuable data to both a clinician and a scientist to analyze, learn, and study different parts of breast malignant growth. A lot of analytic tools can make this fixed data open with adaptability, accommodation, and speed. This condition means to empower manager, regional, and local levels to construct complex specially appointed inquiries in a powerful manner, getting a wide assortment of perspectives with respect to the total and refining of medical data. Along these lines, we proposed to develop an advanced mammography data warehouse that can give significant data to the two clinicians and analysts at Salah Aziaz Hospital.

In this chapter, we built up a data warehousing condition, called the medical analytical framework (MAF). This condition comprises a mammography data warehouse, got to by a lot of analytic tools. The MAF supplies information incorporation from heritage databases and from records created by territorial health centers. The MAF analytics tools permit administrators to construct diagnosis reports and produce complex impromptu queries upon health measures.

2 Material and Method

2.1 Data Warehouse System

A classic data warehousing design includes a blend of components that make it a rich situation for information stockpiling, in particular: operational source systems, staging zone, visualization zone, and data access tools [16].

The primary component of the data warehousing architecture is the operational source systems that incorporate different heterogeneous information sources with various structures and arrangements, for example, relational databases, level documents, spreadsheets, and others [13].

For the proposed study, the scientist researcher will gather data from different existing medical operational data systems over the medical center. The breast imaging information, including persistent demographics, related patient history, textual reports, advanced mammography, ultrasound picture, MRI, pathology, and cytology information, will be gained from HIS, RIS, PACS, and operational databases.

1. Textual data source: Patient demographics from Salah Azaiz Hospital Information System. Symptomatic mamograms imaging reports from the Salah Azaiz RIS system, which will be a significant source of radiological discoveries. Related patient history information gathered from the paper-based clinical records at the Breast Imaging Section of the hospital radiology department. Pathology and cytology report for each center biopsy from the hospital radiology department.
2. Imaging information: Selected mammogram films chronicled in the Breast Imaging Section will be filtered utilizing Lumisys Laser Scanner and put away into the proposed data warehouse. Mammogram imaging is a critical data source for medical decisions [17]. As of now accessible data recovery and decision support systems depend fundamentally on the extracted content. We will probably discover promising methodologies for giving clinical proof at the purpose of service, utilizing data contained in the medical text, and mammogram imaging. We examined two ways to deal with finding illustrative proof: a supervised machine learning approach, in which mammogram imaging is delegated being applicable to a data need or not, and a pipeline data recovery approach, in which pictures were recovered utilizing related text and afterward re-ranked utilizing content-based image retrieval (CBIR) methods. In this chapter, Rahman [18] presents an incorporated order and retrieval based diagnostic guide for tumor cancer recognition by removing and consolidating a few profound highlights by utilizing move learning and a multi-reaction straight relapse (MLR)-based meta-learning approach.

The second component is the data staging zone, which includes a few information preprocessing assignments, for example, management of cleaning, joining and normalizing; data storing; and arranging and consecutive preparing.

The third component is the introduction zone wherein the information is organized in data marts in view of a unique business process; in addition, the data marts are adjusted in a normalized manner to be additionally incorporated.

The last component introduces the data access tools that incorporate: ad hoc query outfits, textual report, analytical applications, data mining, and others. Among the first, second, and third components, the extract, transform, and load (ETL) process extract implies that medical data gotten by different data sources and duplicated to another incorporated database for additional readiness.

1. Medical data extraction is the way toward catching information from operational databases and different sources. Numerous devices are accessible to help in this process, including framework gave utilities, custom concentrates on projects, and business extricates items. Specially appointed program utilities will be created in house to remove clinical data such as machine learning algorithms and content-based image retrieval (CBIR) methods.
2. Few medical data sources control information quality satisfactorily. This, information frequently requires cleaning before it tends to be gone into the decision support database. Cleansing of medical information, for example, tolerant demographics, will remember filling for missing qualities, family history, rectifying typographical and other information errors, setting up standard truncations and configurations, supplanting equivalent words by standard identifiers, etc. Information that is known to be in error and cannot be cleansed down will be dismissed.
3. After the cleaning task, the information will presumably still not be in the structure of the decision support system needs; thus it should be changed properly. For the most part, the necessary structure will be a lot of documents, one for each table recognized in the physical schema; thus, changing, the information may include parting and additionally joining source archives alongside the lines.
4. Consolidation is especially significant when a few data sources should be combined. In such a case, any understood connections among data from several sources should be made explicit.
5. After completing all the above data arrangement forms, data ought to be loaded, which incorporates (a) moving the changed and solidified data into the decision support database, (b) checking it for consistency, and (c) construct any vital index.

The extraction of radiological discoveries will be performed on radiological reports, as a rule in a free-content structure. This information is then cleaned, transformed, and loaded into the DW. Mammography images, either scanner or initially advanced, will be investigated to extract significant picture substance. The substance descriptors are put away in the textual database, while the medical images themselves are stored in the advanced image database.

Another significant component of a data warehousing condition is the ODS (operational data store) that is an extension of the data warehouse engineering, and it contains operational information that is incorporated from heritage data source systems. In contrast to the DW storehouse, the ODS has the particularity of being modified.

The typical methodology for a data warehouse configuration is dimensional modeling that incorporates the star model, dimension tables, and fact tables. This modelization is frequently applied to data marts that are a subset of a data warehouse and are molded by handling necessities. The star diagram involves a focal table (fact table) containing the measures. Contextual properties in the fact table are standardized by the dimension tables, which contain verbose depictions, for example, textual attributes and discrete numbers, and a unique primary key field called a substitute key. The primary keys in each dimension are combined with foreign keys in the fact table. In addition, complex dimension tables can introduce more than one implanted hierarchical constitutions. At that point, if a dimension is standardized, the hierarchies produce a structure known as the snowflake model [19]. To get to data in the data warehouse, we, for the most part, utilize an OLAP server. OLAP (online analytical processing) includes complex queries over enormous quantities of records. OLAP servers can be relational or multidimensional systems. A relational OLAP is an all-encompassing relational system that maps procedure on dimensional information to standard relational activity (SQL) [20, 21]. Ordinarily, the OLAP data are spoken to as a multidimensional data cube [22].

2.2 *Implementation Tools*

To realize all the components of the MAF, we received the accompanying arrangement of tools so as to aid the execution procedure steps: Microsoft SQL server for modeling the entity-relationship diagram of the MAF's databases and star model; SQL Server Integration Services to execute the ETL procedure among the information sources, the MAF's databases; SQL Server Analysis Services and SQL Server Reporting Services for the creation and trial of the OLAP cube schema; blueprints; and gives the center interface to analyze and visualize the DW's data by methods for cutting advanced inquiry devices and fundamental reports.

2.3 *Medical Analytical Framework*

The MAF comprises components that are flexibly the necessary functions to get, get ready, and integrate data into a DW store. Besides, it gives to get to instruments to create complex analysis over this data. Figure 1 illustrates the MAF, wherein we can perceive how the components are composed, how data are moved from data sources to the DW system, and how doctors can get to data.

The primary component in our framework speaks to the general medical system data sources, for example, the source of breast imaging and textual reports. Every one of these sources gives information in various arrangements and structures (for

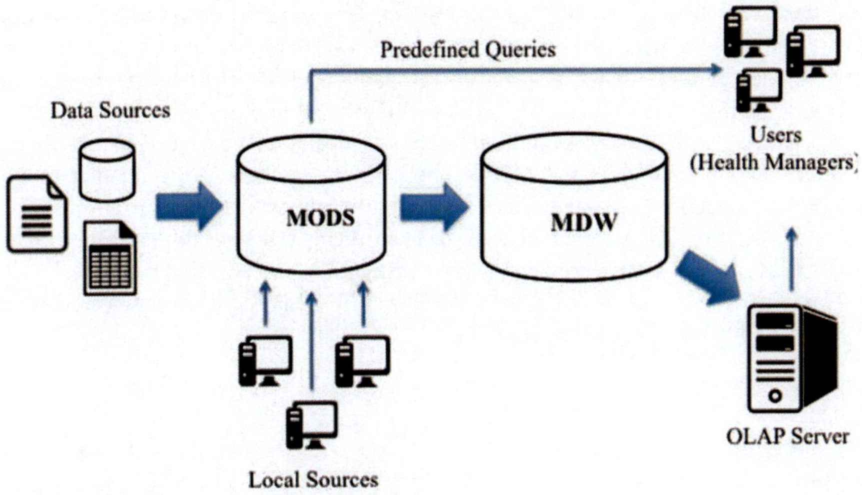

Fig. 1 Medical analytical framework environment

instance: spreadsheets, semi-structured records, and relational databases, and so forth).

The second component is the medical operational data store (MODS), where the information is integrated through a typical and structured format. The MODS displayed utilizing entity-relationship concepts and presented the qualities of an ODS. Thus, by methods for this database, we can amass the data given by the various sources. Also, it empowers us to make accessible predefined inquiries to the users.

The third component is the mammography data warehouse (MDW) that was structured utilizing the dimensional displaying techniques, in this manner star diagrams were executed through the meaning of dimension and fact tables, with their separate measures.

The last component is the OLAP server that permits doctors to get to the dimensional data put away in the MDW. This access is given by methods for OLAP devices, so doctors perform tasks including drill down, roll up, slice and dice, pivot, and drill over.

To execute the data warehousing condition, we followed a lot of steps that guided us to develop all the necessary segments: MODS creation; MDW dimensional modeling; ETL usage; OLAP Server's setting; investigation building; and approval.

In the first place, we analyzed how health data have been sorted out and organized in their data sources. At that point, we modeled and built up the MODS that incorporates data originating from numerous open data sources, for example, excel files accessible on database records and image databases accessible on Salah Azaiz Hospital. In the third step, we demonstrated the DW storehouse, by deciding the preparing necessities and building all the star diagrams. At that point, we actualized the extract, transform, and load process for information loading of both MODS and MDW databases. MODS got information extricated from open data sources, and HMDW got data from HMODS. In addition, before information extraction, we applied changes to set it up for every database of the HMAF. In this manner, to arrange the OLAP server, we developed the data cube of the medical handling necessities. In the analysis building step, we designed interfaces to get to the information put away in the MDW. These interfaces permit the doctors to run complex specially appointed queries over multidimensional data in an amicable manner. At long last, we applied a survey to medical staff so as to assess the ease of use of MAF. The survey utilized in our investigation was adjusted from the CSUQ (Computer System Usability Questionnaire) [23]. This method empowered us to survey and validate our framework.

3 Results

3.1 Medical Operational Data Store

As a case study, we applied MAF to the Tunisian healthcare system, more specifically with data concerning breast cancer. We structured this incorporated database dependent on the indicators introduced in the health records. MODS has 5 tables with an aggregate of 102 properties. Examples of MODS' tables are: "Hospital," "Doctors," "Patient," "image_Group," and "Images."

3.2 Star Schemas

The itemized star diagram, as appeared in Fig. 2, shows the data layer design of the MDW. The designed MDW utilizes a denormalized diagram, as appeared in the star diagram, and the dimensional tables, such as DIM_PATIENT, DIM_DATE, DIM_HOSPITAL, DIM_IMAGE DETAILS, DIM_IMAGE, contain denormalized or repetitive data. Such de-normalization may expedite data mining and business intelligence procedures. The fact tables have the same dimensions but at different levels of granularity. Each fact table gets its own measure group. Fact tables below demonstrate the fact and dimension tables of the medical data warehouse in detail: two fact tables. The fact tables that describe the subject matter are named FACT_DIAGNOSTICS and FACT_FORECAST. The tables consist of the case ID, Id_patient, Id_hospital, Id_date, and id_image. The FACT_DIAGNOSTICS consists of two measurements, the diagnosed_status and the treatment_results. The FACT_FORECAST table consists of the measurement RiskFactors.

Dimension Tables
Figure 3 underneath lists the 5 dimension tables that detail every element in the fact tables.

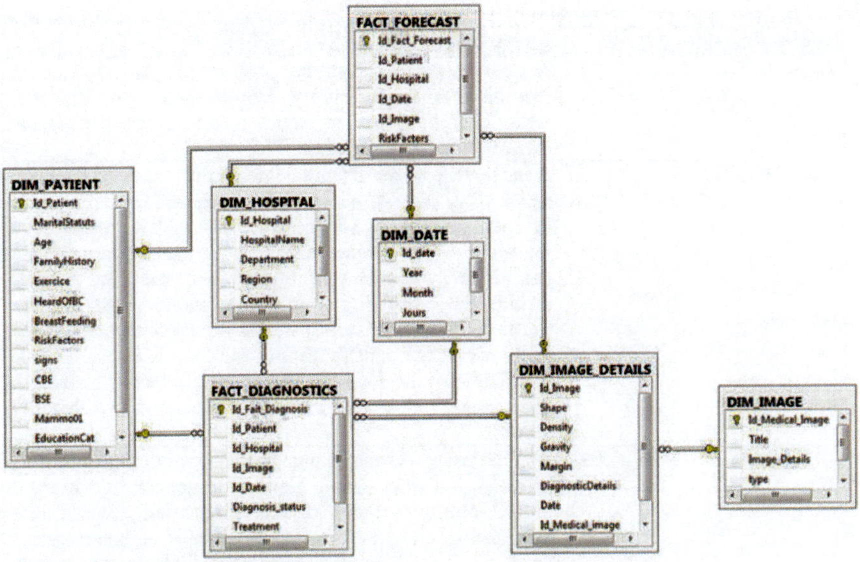

Fig. 2 Medical data warehouse star diagram

3.3 *ETL Tools*

We made changes to enhance all the undertakings of information readiness and loading from MODS to MDW databases. Figure 4 presents the transformation of the "DIM_DATE" for instance of the ETL procedure. This transformation has a progression of steps, where the first produces 100 lines and 2 fields, one field as the table identifier and the other field speaking to the years. The accompanying advances play out the arrangement of the fields, checking the identifier field from 0 to 99 and tallying the year field from 2012 to 2019. The "month range" and "day run" steps play out the mix between year, month, and day. Ultimately, the Insert and/or Update Year step executes the loading of data to the dimension table.

3.4 *OLAP Server*

A cube is developed dependent on dimensions of a medical data warehouse so as to perform OLAP activities. It is structured and actualized by utilizing SQL Server Analytical Service [24]. The dimensions and pecking orders are actualized to permit applying OLAP activities (slice, dice, drill through, drill up, and drill down).Two powerful hierarchies are actualized, which are date and address hierarchy.

All dimensions are picked to construct the cube. After the cube execution finished, it very well may be seen straightforwardly by dropping dimensions of

Dimension tables	Dimension description
DIM_PATIENT	A table that stores patient information, such as patient name, date of birth, family history, Marital status, sport exercise, signs, Education etc. The data is used to show demographic data for breast cancer disease.
DIM_HOSPITAL	A table that stores Hospital information, such as Hospital name, City, address, phone Number, zip code, building date, specialty, emergency Services. The data is used to show data for breast cancer disease. Hospitals are the most significant part of our lives, attempting to give the best medical supports to individuals suffering from breast cancer disease, for our situation. It is particularly hard for the medical staff to keep up its everyday hospital's features and records manually. That is the reason the hospital dimension is required to track a wide range of characteristics options of an emergency hospital.
DIM_IMAGES_DETAILS	A table that stores mammography images information , such as categorical mass shape, gravity, categorical mass margin, ordinal density, Gravity, date of diagnostics, a breast self-examination, a clinical breast exam, number of mammograms per year. The data is used to show the digital mammography images storage for diagnosis. An essential for a fruitful screening task is that the mammograms contain adequate diagnostic data to have the option to detect breast cancer disease.
DIM_IMAGE	A table that stores Image information, such as image title, type, suspect, equipment, and textual description of the Physical and Technical Aspects of mammography images. The data is used to show general image properties.
DIM_DATE	In the dimension table "DIM_ DATE" we can see that there are hierarchies of attributes among their traits, for example, in the dimension table "DIM_ DATE" there is an implicit hierarchy among the dates "year", "month" and "day".

Fig. 3 Dimension tables of the medical data warehouse

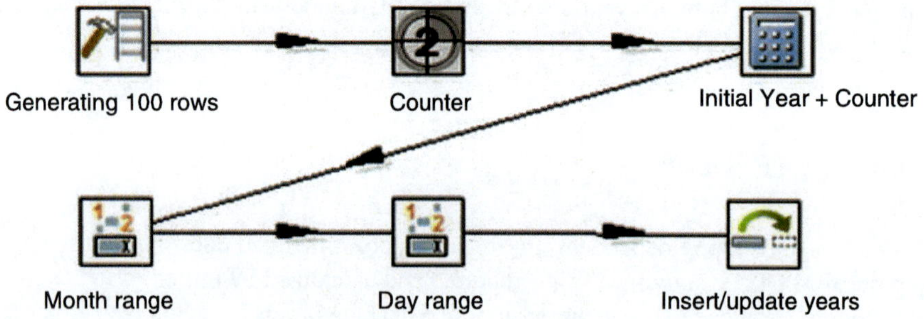

Fig. 4 Transformation of dimension Dim_Date

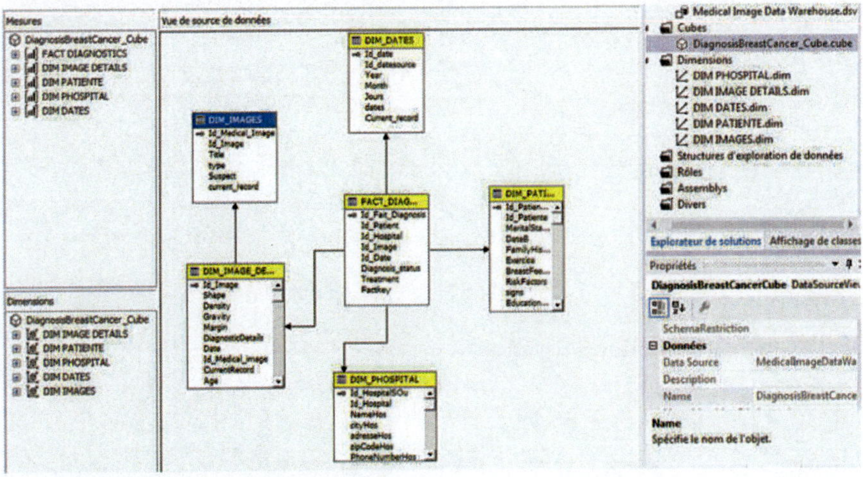

Fig. 5 Diagnosis breast cancer cube

individuals and measurement. The unique cube can be built to analyze information dependent on explicit dimensions and measurements. This product executes MDX (multidimensional expressions) demands that are a language deciphered by Mondrian and are utilized to perform inquiries on OLAP schema. These schemas comprise XML metadata models that are made in a cube structure. Figure 5 illustrates the cube in the interface of visual studio, business intelligence environment, and SSAS package. We can see our star diagram with the fact tables, the dimension tables, and the measures.

3.5 Analyses

In the implementation of actualizing the SSAS package, the following stage is to see the cube utilizing SSMS. SSMS permits the experts to see the subsequent cube by dropping each dimension part without any problem. It additionally gives filtering conditions to bar a few values or add more values to get accurate outcomes [25].

Figure 6 shows the number of explicit diseases (breast cancer tumors) characterized by a fourth of the year for a particular gender (female). The analysts can likewise be gathering numerous diseases for some areas and sexes.

The output file additionally developed with an entrance database that held more than one a huge number of the clinical record. A significant number of determining attributes are included based on the first properties, for example, (Age Class from Age), (Day, Month, Year, Quarter, and Season from date of finding). Some change forms are applied, for example, evacuating spaces inside the trait's qualities and

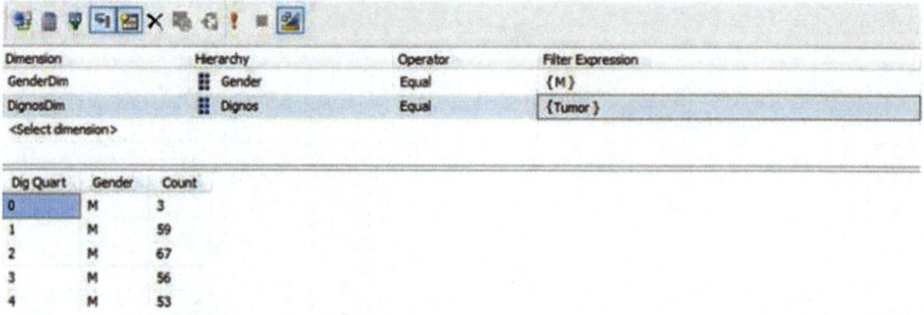

Fig. 6 Analysis result of filters applied on breast cube

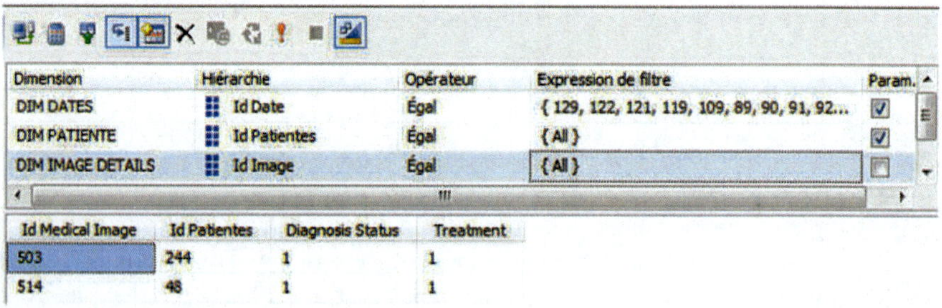

Fig. 7 Analysis result of filters applied on breast cube

changing over sexual gender into a unique character (Male into M, Female into F, and others into U).

Excel table gives the device to interface with SQL Server Analysis Server and views cube in an adaptable manner. When the association built up to cube, the expert can pick the dimension individuals and measurements without any problem. Next, we apply filters on the dimensions tables so that the results are restricted to the analysis status. In our example, we chose as a filter: date equal to a set of dates, id patient equal to all patients, and id image equal to all images. Figure 7 illustrates the concluding result of the filters applied to the analysis example.

The output file additionally developed with an entrance database that held more than one a huge number of the clinical record. A significant number of determining attributes are included based on the first properties, for example, (Age Class from Age), (Day, Month, Year, Quarter, and Season from date of finding). Some change forms are applied, for example, evacuating spaces inside the trait's qualities and changing over sexual gender into a unique character (Male into M, Female into F, and others into U).

Figure 8 shows the breast tumor disease characterized by gender and age class. Each shading speaks to the age class and shows the exact number of contaminations. Clearly, age class 5 (40–65 years) is tainted with high rate numbers among the other age classes.

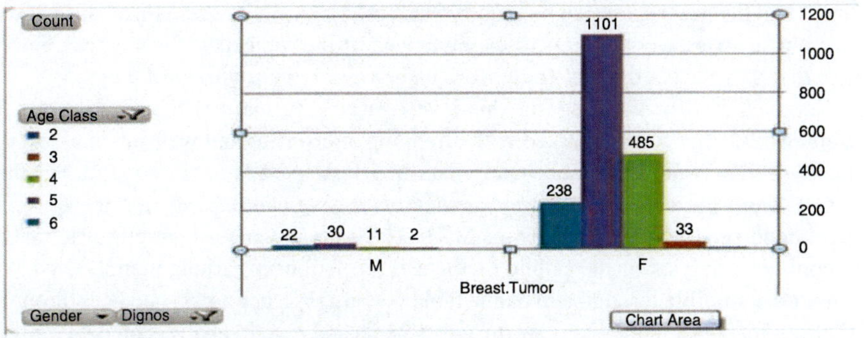

Fig. 8 Breast cancer tumor using age group and gender

Right off the bat, to execute this analysis we have to open our cube in the OLAP server. The OLAP table begins with the aggregate sum of the measures alongside the columns (dimensions) as should be obvious in Fig. 6.

In this manner, we apply filters on the table with the objective that the results are constrained to the analysis condition. In dimension "City," we picked just the "cities" as for the prosperity locale part of Salah Azaiz. Figure 6 presents the decisive result of the filters applied to the analysis model.

3.6 Validation of the MAF

Among them, there were three directors of healthcare planning, three healthcare secretaries, one doctor responsible for healthcare planning, one specialist on healthcare management and planning, one technical assistant of healthcare planning, and one technical coordinator of an informed healthcare center. All of them were not familiar with the software; therefore, we gave them a short demonstration of how the platform works, and then we let them play and test freely. After that we requested them that to answer a survey. This survey, adjusted from the Computer System Usability Questionnaire (CSUQ), is made out of 10 inquiries, in particular: (1) It was easy to utilize this framework; (2) I am ready to proficiently finish my work utilizing this framework; (3) I feel great utilizing this framework; (4) It was anything but difficult to figure out how to utilize this framework; (5) Whenever I commit an error utilizing this framework, I recoup effectively and rapidly; (6) It is anything but difficult to track down the data I need; (7) The data is successful in helping me complete the assignments and situations; (8) The association of data on the framework is clear; (9) The interface of this framework is amiable; (10) Generally, I am satisfied with this framework. Each question is compared to an affirmation and a rating scale between 1 ("emphatically dissent") and 7 ("firmly concur"). The general normal, thinking about all inquiries, was 6.02. Questions 4 and 7 had the best scores and no inquiry was under 5.7. Along these lines, this shows that our structure was very much acknowledged by the subjects of the medical region and that they accept that our framework can turn into their work profitable.

By methods for the usage of this investigation, we can say that our proposed framework helps users occupied with arranging and sorting out well-being assets to make decisions dependent on steady data in a fast and adaptable way. As per the results from the evaluation led by medical users, we can express that these users have endorsed the tools given by the MAF. The tools of the MAF empower to make a complex analysis of the public medical information in various manners, which should be possible through a dynamic table that alters as per users' needs or through outlines that permit users to perform assessments and pattern analysis on data for the duration of the time. Furthermore, these devices additionally permit users to spare their inquiries in the OLAP server such that a modified arrangement of questions can be made for various classes of users, objectives, and contexts.

Our study additionally indicated genuine trouble in regard to the information acquisition for loading on the framework, because of the way that data is disseminated in a non-normalized way, in various formats, and on several sources of the medical system. Hence, our framework fills in as an underlying example to build up an organization on this medical data.

4 Conclusions

In this chapter, we proposed the execution of a medical analytical data warehousing framework, which we named MAF, so as to help users of the public healthcare system giving information and a tool set containing process, to perform complex analysis. We can presume that the objective of our investigation in developing a framework to help analyze and improve the decision-making process was practiced by a successful and agreeable way, since MAF advances data integration and encourages and makes as adaptable as conceivable the data analysis movement, on the medical management condition.

As future work, this framework requests enhancements with respect to information insertion and updation in MODS. The flexibility of information by the cities is fundamental for the data maintenance of MAF. With refreshed information on MODS, therefore, when another load is acted in MDW, it is conceivable to fabricate an analysis of current information just as on prior historical information.

References

1. R. Sharma, Breast cancer incidence, mortality and mortality-to-incidence ratio (MIR) are associated with human development, 1990–2016: evidence from global burden of disease study 2016. Breast Cancer **26**(4), 428–445 (2019)

2. F. Belaiba, I. Medimegh, M. Ammar, F. Jemni, A. Mezlini, K.B. Romdhane, L. Cherni, A. Benammar Elgaaïed, Expression and polymorphism of micro-RNA according to body mass index and breast cancer presentation in Tunisian patients. J. Leukoc. Biol. **105**(2), 317–327 (2019). https://jlb.onlinelibrary.wiley.com/doi/abs/10.1002/JLB.3VMA0618-218R
3. R.T. Chlebowski, E. Aiello, A. McTiernan, Weight loss in breast cancer patient management. J. Clin. Oncol. **20**(4), 1128–1143 (2002)
4. Y. Feng, M. Spezia, S. Huang, C. Yuan, Z. Zeng, L. Zhang, X. Ji, W. Liu, B. Huang, W. Luo, B. Liu, Y. Lei, S. Du, A. Vuppalapati, H. Luu, R. Haydon, T.-C. He, G. Ren, Breast cancer development and progression: risk factors, cancer stem cells, signaling pathways, genomics, and molecular pathogenesis. Genes Dis. **5**, 05 (2018)
5. D.B. Larson, J.B. Kruskal, K.N. Krecke, L.F. Donnelly, Key concepts of patient safety in radiology. Radiographics **35**(6), 1677–1693 (2015)
6. S. Timón, M. Rincón, R. Martínez-Tomás, Extending xnat platform with an incremental semantic framework. Front. Neuroinform. **11**, 57 (2017)
7. D. Li, H.W. Park, E. Batbaatar, Y. Piao, K.H. Ryu, Design of health care system for disease detection and prediction on Hadoop using DM techniques, in *Conference on Health Informatics and Medical Systems* (2016)
8. R. Kimball, J. Caserta, *The Data Warehouse ETL Toolkit* (Wiley, Indianapolis, 2004)
9. S. Gao, S.P. Low, From lean production to lean construction, in *Lean Construction Management* (Springer, Singapore, 2014), pp. 27–48
10. J.S. Einbinder, K.W. Scully, R.D. Pates, J.R. Schubart, R.E. Reynolds, Case study: a data warehouse for an academic medical center. J. Healthc. Inf. Manag. **15**(2), 165–176 (2001)
11. R.S. Evans, J.F. Lloyd, L.A. Pierce, Clinical use of an enterprise data warehouse, in *AMIA Annual Symposium Proceedings*, vol. 2012 (American Medical Informatics Association, Bethesda, 2012), p. 189
12. E. Kerkri, C. Quantin, F. Allaert, Y. Cottin, P. Charve, F. Jouanot, K. Yétongnon, An approach for integrating heterogeneous information sources in a medical data warehouse. J. Med. Syst. **25**(3), 167–176 (2001)
13. A. Sebaa, F. Chikh, A. Nouicer, A. Tari, Medical big data warehouse: architecture and system design, a case study: improving healthcare resources distribution. J. Med. Syst. **42**(4), 59 (2018)
14. P. Vallejo-Gutiérrez, J. Bañeres-Amella, E. Sierra, J. Casal, Y. Agra, Lessons learnt from the development of the patient safety incidents reporting and learning system for the Spanish national health system: Sinasp. Rev. Calid. Asist. **29**(2), 69–77 (2014)
15. S. Khan, A. Vandermorris, J. Shepherd, J.W. Begun, H.J. Lanham, M. Uhl-Bien, W. Berta, Embracing uncertainty, managing complexity: applying complexity thinking principles to transformation efforts in healthcare systems. BMC Health Serv. Res. **18**(1), 192 (2018)
16. U. Dayal, M. Castellanos, A. Simitsis, K. Wilkinson, Data integration flows for business intelligence, in *Proceedings of the 12th International Conference on Extending Database Technology: Advances in Database Technology* (2009), pp. 1–11
17. S. Krishnan, R.B. Rao, M. Dundar, G. Fung, Systems and methods for automated diagnosis and decision support for breast imaging. US Patent 7,640,051, 29 Dec 2009
18. M.M. Rahman, A decision support system for skin cancer recognition with deep feature extraction and multi response linear regression (MLR)-based meta learning (2019)
19. R. Kimball, M. Ross, W. Thornthwaite, J. Mundy, B. Becker, *The Data Warehouse Lifecycle Toolkit* (Wiley, Indianapolis, 2008)
20. C. Coronel, S. Morris, *Database Systems: Design, Implementation, & Management* (Cengage Learning, Boston, 2016)
21. W.H. Inmon, D. Strauss, G. Neushloss, *DW 2.0: The Architecture for the Next Generation of Data Warehousing* (Elsevier, Amsterdam, 2010)
22. A. Nanda, S. Gupta, M. Vijrania, A comprehensive survey of OLAP: recent trends, in *2019 3rd International Conference on Electronics, Communication and Aerospace Technology (ICECA)* (IEEE, Piscataway, 2019), pp. 425–430
23. J.R. Lewis, Measuring perceived usability: SUS, UMUX, and CSUQ ratings for four everyday products. Int. J. Hum. Comput. Interact. **35**(15), 1404–1419 (2019)

24. B. Benatallah, S. Sakr, D. Grigori, H.R. Motahari-Nezhad, M.C. Barukh, A. Gater, S.H. Ryu et al., *Process Analytics: Concepts and Techniques for Querying and Analyzing Process Data* (Springer, Berlin, 2016)
25. P.J. Potts, *A Handbook of Silicate Rock Analysis* (Springer Science & Business Media, New York, 2012)

Personalization of Proposed Services in a Sensor-Based Remote Care Application

Mirvat Makssoud

1 Introduction

Nowadays, the proliferation of Internet of things (IoT) devices such as sensors is offering promising solutions for e-health domain [1]. In this context, remote patient monitoring (RPM) at home represents a great opportunity to reduce medical costs and to improve the quality of life of both patients and their families [2]. It allows patients to be monitored remotely in their homes at any time by means of sensing devices in order to be able to offer services tailored to the needs and daily situations of the patients and detect earlier any critical health condition and actuate different actions in the form of services according to the detected situation consequently [3].

Based on this context, we propose a home-based care system capable of collecting massive data flows from the sensors located at patient's home and analyzing and filtering them in order to offer services adapted to the needs and daily situations of the patients. It provides an extensible and efficient prototype for monitoring and handling the patient's chronic conditions.

To test our application, we set up the OM2M platform to be able to collect data flows from the sensors deployed in the patient's environment [4]. Indeed, OM2M is an open source service platform based on the oneM2M standard, and it follows a RESTFUL approach with open interfaces to enable developing services and applications independent of the underlying network.

The chapter is organized as follows: Section 2 discusses related works. Section 3 presents the architecture of the system. Section 4 shows the services personalization steps. Section 5 discusses the exploitation of services. We will end this chapter with a conclusion and future works.

M. Makssoud (✉)
Lebanese University, Tripoli, Lebanon

H. R. Arabnia et al. (eds.), *Advances in Computer Vision and Computational Biology*, Transactions on Computational Science and Computational Intelligence,
https://doi.org/10.1007/978-3-030-71051-4_42

2 Related Works

Nowadays, the proliferation of new technologies such as IOT and smart devices is revolutionizing the development of healthcare systems [5]. It places the patient in the center of the treatment process [6]. Many healthcare initiatives have been presented in the literature. A holistic approach to design and implementation of a medical teleconsultation workspace is proposed in [7]. This system presents a system architecture implementation called TeleDICOM II based on service-oriented architecture (SOA) and virtual organization (VO) concepts. A cloud-based mobile system to improve respiratory therapy services at home is also proposed in [8]. The platform uses vital signs monitoring as a way of sharing data between hospitals, caregivers, and patients. Using an iterative research approach and the user's direct feedback, they show how mobile technologies can improve a respiratory therapy and a family's quality of life. [9] presented a software agent approach for telemonitoring of patients at home. In particular, it is considered as an alarm raising system that addresses the issue of the increasing medical needs of maintaining people at home in loss of autonomy.

A common feature of systems using sensing devices is that they collect a large amount of data in real time which need to be processed quickly to make real-time decisions. Most of existing researches have been conceived as stand-alone by offering very specific services to particular needs such as detecting alarm situations. However, with the appearance of cloud computing technology, it is time to take advantage of services proposed by patient remote care systems in the developed countries to be offered to patients located anywhere in the world and, in particular, in the developing countries which suffer from lack of care [10]. In this context, we propose an extensible and adaptive prototype which models and defines medical services located in the cloud in order to offer them to patients in terms of their needs and daily situations.

3 Functional Architecture of the System

The general architecture of the system, as shown in Fig. 1, is composed of two modules: (1) services personalization and (2) services exploitation. The first module, services personalization, is based on assigning services to patients according to their needs defined in profiles. The second module, services exploitation, consists of collecting data flows from patient's home in order to analyze them, filter them, and extract the services that correspond to the patient's needs.

In the following sections, we will describe each of these modules. We will start with the personalization of services.

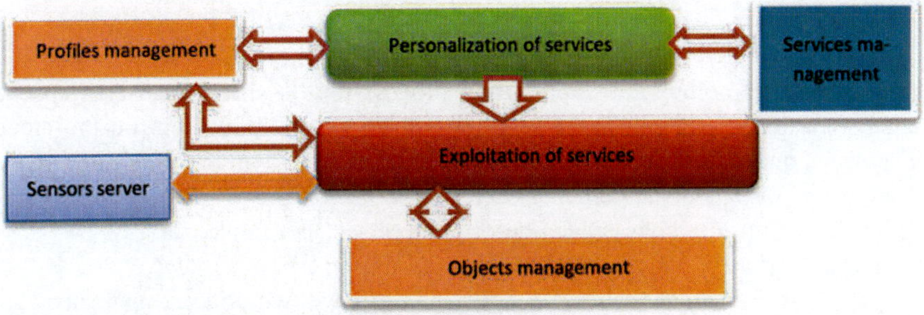

Fig. 1 Functional architecture of the system

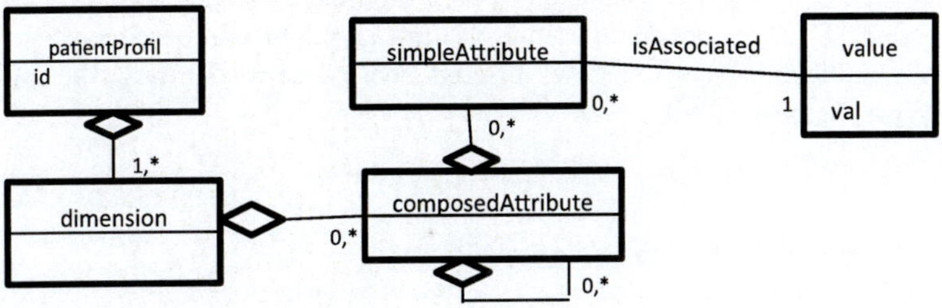

Fig. 2 Meta-description of profile model

4 Services Personalization

This module focuses on the use of profiles and services in order to offer to a patient services related to the elements defined in his profile. Before describing services personalization process, we will give an idea on how a patient's profile and a services model are described. We will start with the patient's profile.

4.1 Patient's Profile

The patient's profile is defined as a collection of knowledge characterizing a patient in its daily environment. a generic model must be proposed to cover all characteristics that differentiate between patients.

Figure 2 represents a meta-description of the model that provides a high level abstraction of the profile elements.

4.2 Services Model

A service is an autonomous application process that is able to satisfy a specific need for a given patient. These services can be located anywhere on the cloud. Therefore, our system must be able to access and exploit them in the monitoring and remote care of patients at home. A generic model is proposed to cover all services' diversities. Figure 3 shows a meta-description of services model.

The class *data* contains data used to identify a service.

The class *criteria* describes that a service can have two criteria: mandatory and optional.

A service has the objective to satisfy a given need. This need may involve several patients. So a service is associated with a profile element in general and not with any patient. This element could be either a dimension or a composed attribute in the case where the dimension expresses different needs described through the definition of several composed attributes.

4.3 Personalization of Services

Ce scenario consists of searching for correspondence between patients' profiles and services' profiles. The matching search is generally performed by a matching program that compares the service's structure ("profile" node in the services model) to the patient profile structure and especially to the dimension part with the descending nodes (composed attributes and simple attributes).

This scenario occurs in two different cases:

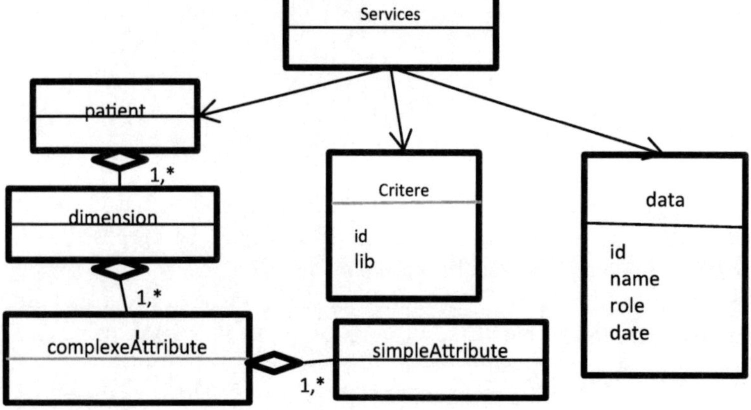

Fig. 3 Meta-description of services model

- The creation of a new service: Once a service has been created, it is proposed to all patients to look for a correspondence between this service (matching from the node "profile") and the structure of each patient profile. If a match is found, then it will be offered to each patient concerned.
- Adding a simple attribute to a patient's profile structure: a notification with attribute ID and profile ID is received when a new element is added in the patient profile, and the matching program is triggered to review the patient services list.
  - If the notification = 1, the profile attribute ID and the simple attribute ID for every service are matched. If a match is found, the service is offered to the concerned patient.
  - If the notification = 2, the correspondence search module sends a notification to the services module to notify the services administrator to perform a correspondence search between the new attribute and all services.

5 Exploitation of Services

5.1 *Object Management*

This module allows defining sensors that are deployed in the patient's platform.

Object Model Figure 4 represents an abstract description of an object model describing a sensor and collected data.

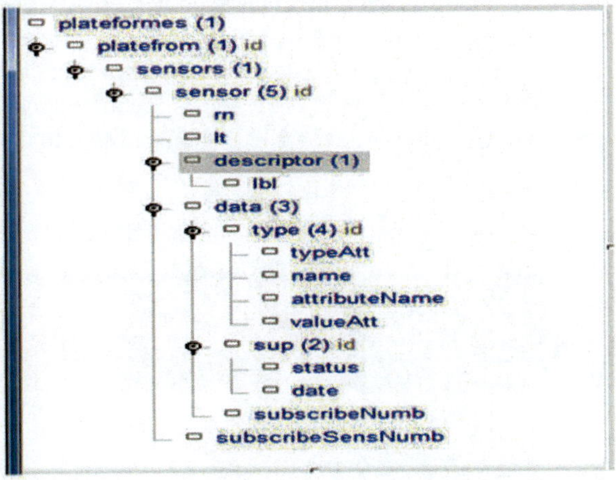

Fig. 4 Object model

When a new sensor is added, our application receives a data stream sent by the OM2M server including the sensor identifier (**ri**) which is represented in our model by the **id** attribute, its name (**rn**), its commissioning date (**lt**), a general description (**lbl**), and the platform identifier (**pi**) which is represented in our model by the **id** attribute.

The *descriptor* element is dedicated to providing a general description of the sensor such as its location and type, and the *data* element contains the data format as it is received from the OM2M server. These two steps are described in detail in the following section. Each element must be assigned a subscription number in order to ensure that it receives data flows and is informed of any changes by the OM2M server.

5.2 Services Exploitation Scenario

The exploitation of services as illustrated in Fig. 5 is organized into three modules: (1) data flow extraction and analysis module, (2) data filtering module, and (3) services processing module.

The first module consists of receiving data flows from the OM2M server in real time and extracting some information important for the filtering process.

The second module, data filtering, consists of selecting services according to the data extracted from the sensors.

The last module, processing services, mainly deals with the steps of triggering services whatever their location.

Flow Extraction and Analysis Module This module consists of processing the data flows in order to extract the data required for the filtering module and the object model. Indeed, during the analysis, some data extracted from the flows can be used to feed the object model. Other data such as the sensor identifier (sensorId), attribute name (attributeName), and value (value) are extracted and sent to the filter module.

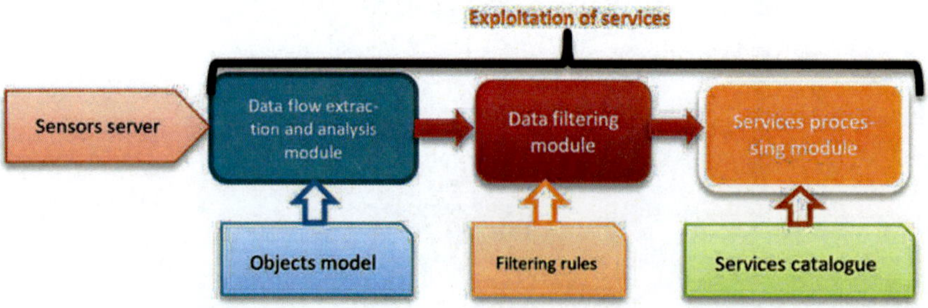

Fig. 5 Exploitation of services

When the system starts receiving data flows from the OM2M server in the form of messages in XML format, each message is processed to extract the type (**ty**), node name (**rn**), node identifier (**ri**), and parent node identifier (**pi**). The value of **ty** will be analyzed. Here, we distinguish three cases:

- If ty =2, it is about creating a new sensor (newSensAE).
- If ty = 3, it is about creating a new container (newSensCnt) in the sensor whose name is designated in pi.
- If ty =4, the value of **rn** is analyzed:
  - If rn = « data », it is data collected from sensors (newDataContent).
  - Otherwise, it is data about the description of the sensors (newInstDesc).

As shown in Fig. 6, the "streamingReception" process receives data streams and sends XML messages to the "messageParsing" process. The latter communicates in parallel with the four processes—newSensorAE, NewSensCnt, newInstDesc, and newDataContent—depending on the value of the node **ty**.

This process generates two XML documents, "ObjectXMLFile" and "XMLtmp," as a result. The first document concerns the final description of the sensors in their platforms. The second file stores the temporary data extracted from the collected flows for analysis to extract the nodes to be inserted in the "ObjectXMLFile" document. Indeed, extracted flows can include data about a sensor's description. This data can be redundant. Only relevant data are taken into consideration. For this reason, this data is stored in a temporary document and processed via an interface to select the instances necessary for the system.

When it is a new sensor (**ty** = **2**), the process "newSensAE" is executed. It takes as input the variables **ri** (sensor ID), **rn** (sensor name), **pi** (sensor parent ID), **lbl** (sensor description), and **lt** (commissioning). It retrieves in the document ObjectXMLFile.xml the platform that has an identifier = **pi** to insert in this platform a sensor with an identifier = **ri**, a name = **rn**, and **lt** in a node of the same name.

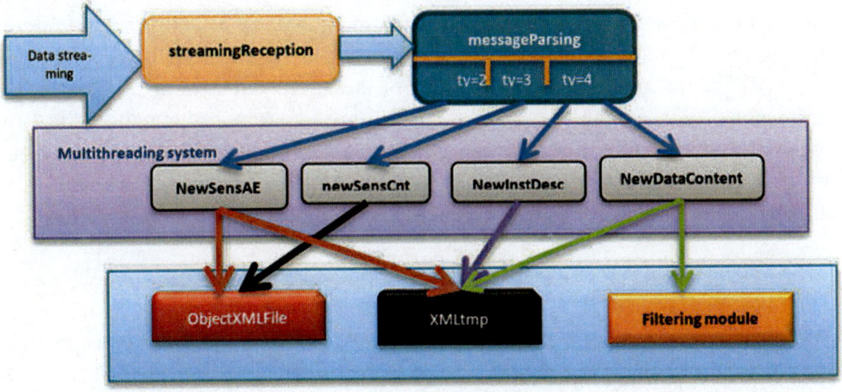

Fig. 6 Data flows analysis steps

A descriptor element is created to insert the variable **lbl** into a node with the same name.

<plateforme id = pi> <sensor id = ri>

<rn> rn </rn> <lt> lt </lt>

<descriptor> <lbl> lbl </lbl> </descriptor> <sensor> . . . .

</plateforme>

When it is a new container in a given sensor (**ty** = **3**), we look in the document ObjectXMLFile for the sensor that has an identifier corresponding to **pi** knowing that the **pi** refers to the identifier of a sensor. If found, a new **rn** node is inserted as a child node in the parent node "sensor" with an identifier **id** that corresponds to the **ri** retrieved as follows:

<sensor id = pi> . . . . *<rn id = ri> </rn> </sensor>*

When **ty** = **4** and the received data concerns a container different from "data," this signifies that the data collected in the node "con" concerns the description of the sensor. In this case, the node "con" will be inserted in the XMLtmp document of this form:

<container id =ri> <con> . . . . . . *</con> </container>*

ri represents the identifier of the container already inserted. This part of the XML code will then be displayed in a graphical interface. Thus, the user chooses the instances with the values they find relevant so that they are inserted in the final XML document as child nodes of the node « **descriptor** ».

In the case where the received data (**ty** = **4**) concerns a "data" container (**rn** = **data**) with a **pi** corresponding to the sensor identifier, we search in an already created map if idSensor exists. Here, we have two possibilities:

- **idSensor** does not exist in the map. Received data will be inserted into the XMLtmp file.

  <data id=pi> <con> . . . . *</con> </data>*

  The sensor ID (the **pi** instance in the received data) and the type that takes the value −1 will also be added to the map. Thus, the user chooses via a graphical interface the instances that are likely to contain the data to be analyzed and filtered. Once these instances are chosen, they are inserted into the final XML file in the **data** node with the instance **type** that takes one of these two values (1 or 2). 1 means that the received data contains four instances, among which we distinguish the name of the attribute that contains the desired information. 2 means that we only have one instance which is the name of the attribute. The sensor identity as well as the attribute name and type with its value will also be added to the map.

- In case *idSensor* exists. We extract the attribute name as well as the type. We are faced with two alternatives:

  - The type = −1; then the data received will be ignored until the instances are selected as explained above.
  - The type! = −1; then we extract the attribute name and search in the received data for the attribute value that corresponds to the one found in the map.

Then the three instances will be sent to the filtering process in this form: <idSensor,attributeName,value>.

Since data flows arrive massively in real time, the system must process them quickly. For this reason, the multithreading technique is adopted. Indeed, when a new data stream is received and after extraction of **ty**, the system creates a thread to support the processing of the flow data in the "data extraction and analysis" module.

Data Filtering This module consists of selecting services according to the data extracted from the sensors. This selection will be performed according to filtering rules previously defined. So the first step of this module is to define the model of the filtering rules, and then the second step is to use these rules to filter received data

Filtering Rules As shown in Fig. 7, filtering rules are defined to be applied to data collected from the sensors. Thus, for a given sensor, several rules can be defined. Each rule can be linked to one or more services. It can also contain one or more conditions of the form <subject, conditionOp, value>. The term conditionOp may correspond to "==, <>, >, >=, <, <=".

If there are several conditions that are linked by "AND" or "OR" connection operations such as "C1 and C2 or C3" with C1, C2, and C3 three conditions, two cases are possible:

- Both conditions C1 and C2 which are linked by the AND connection operation are combined as follows:

<connection> <connectionOp>AND</connectionOp>
<condition id=C1> ———— </condition>
<condition id=C2> ———— </condition> </connection>

- Condition C3 is represented independently in the <connection> tag as follows:

<connection> <condition> .... </condition> </connection>

The filter rule model also contains a "query" element in order to accelerate the filtering. For this purpose, once the rules are defined for a given sensor, the system forms a query from these rules and saves it in the rule model. Thus, each time data

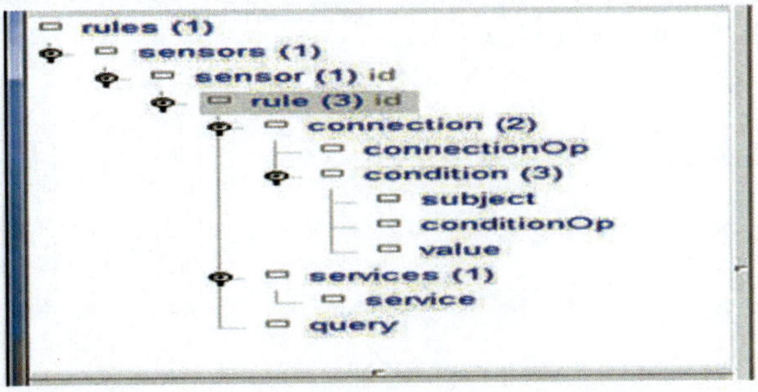

Fig. 7 Filtering rules model

occurs in the filtering module, instead of searching for all conditions for a given sensor and making a query, the system searches directly for the query.

Data Filtering Process When the data <sensorId, attributeName, value> are received, the system searches in the filter rules for a sensor whose identifier corresponds to sensorId. When it is found, the system extracts the queries located in the *query* nodes as well as the services for each query. Then the system executes each request consecutively on the instances data <attributeName ,value>. If a query returns true, then the services related to this query are sent to the trigger module. Otherwise, we move on to the next request and so on. If no query returns true, the data is ignored.

Services processing module This module is under development. We are working on two points: (1) the definition of the frequency of a service between the last triggering and the new one and (2) the preparation of input data if required for a service.

6 Conclusion

Nowadays, we are facing a proliferation of new technologies such as IOT and sensing devices. This major step in technological progress has led researchers to exploit it for the benefit of the medical sector.

This article has presented an approach that aims to leverage services in the cloud for the benefit of patients at home wherever their location in the world. This approach is divided into two steps. First, it must be able to identify services, define them in a generic model, and associate them with patients according to their needs and medical situations. The second step of the system is to collect data from sensors located at the patient' home, filter them, and extract the adequate services that match the situation of the patient concerned.

Presently, we are working on the second step. The processes of data collecting and filtering are under test. Currently, we are developing how to trigger services. This step is facing a set of challenges such as the trigger frequency, the definition of input data required by a service before triggering, and the determination of output data generated by an executed service.

References

1. A. Zanella, N. Bui, A. Castellani, L. Vangelista, M. Zorzi, Internet of things for smart cities. IEEE Internet Things J. **1**(1), 22–32 (2014). (Cited in pages viii, 2, 19, 20, 23 and 110)
2. S. Sotiriadis, L. Vakanas, E. Petrakis, P. Zampognaro, N. Bessis. Automatic Migration and Deployment of Cloud services for healthcare application development in FIWARE, in *Proceedings of the 2016 30th International Conference on Advanced Information Networking and ApplicationsWorkshops (WAINA)*, Crans-Montana, Switzerland (March 2016), pp. 416–419, 23–25
3. R. Kumar, M.P. Rajasekaran, An IoT based patient monitoring system using raspberry pi, International Conference on Computing Technologies and Intelligent Data Engineering (ICCTIDE'16) (2016)
4. M. Ben-Alaya, S. Medjiah, T. Monteil, K. Drira, Toward semantic interoperability in oneM2M architecture. IEEE Commun. Mag. **53**(12), 35–41 (2015). (Cited in pages viii, 18, 19, 20, 23, 33, 39, 45, 80, 85 and 110)
5. Z. Pang, L. Zheng, J. Tian, S. Kao-Walter, E. Dubrova, Q. Chen, Design of a terminal solution for integration of in-home health care devices and services towards the Internet-of-Things. Enterp. Inform. Syst. **9**(1), 86–116 (2015)
6. FI-WARE cost-effective creation and delivery of future internet applications. Available online: http://www.fi-ware.eu/. Accessed on 1 Oct 2014
7. A. Pouryazdan, R.J. Prance, H. Prance, D. Roggen, Wearable electric potential sensing: A new modality sensing hair touch and restless leg movement, in *Proc. ACM Int Joint Conf on Pervasive and Ubiquitous Computing: Adjunct* (2016), pp. 846–850
8. C. Łukasz, F. Malawski, P. Wyszkowski, Holistic approach to design and implementation of a medical teleconsultation workspace. J. Biomed. Inform. **57**, 225–244 (2015)
9. N.A. Risso, A. Neyem, J.I. Benedetto, M.J. Carrillo, A. Farías, M.J. Gajardo, O.A. Loyola, Cloud-based mobile system to improve respiratory therapy services at home. J. Biomed. Inform. **63**, 45–53 (2016)
10. A. Bagula, M. Mandava, H. Bagula, A framework for healthcare support in the rural and low income areas of the developing world. J. Netw. Comput. Appl. **120**, 17–29 (2018)

A Cross-Blockchain Approach to Emergency Medical Information

Shirin Hasavari, Kofi Osei-Tutu, and Yeong-Tae Song

1 Introduction

Emergency medical services (EMS) are the practice of medicine involving the evaluation and management of patients with acute traumatic and medical conditions in an environment outside the hospital [2]. Therefore, in a medical emergency, accessing a patient's clinical and medical record can make a difference especially in life or death situation. Thus, any effort to enable this carries a high value. Accessing a patient's health information across a disparate network of healthcare settings and providers involves some or all of the following requirements [3–6].

- Shared vision and motivation
- Technical infrastructure
- Healthcare information technology standards
- Compliance with HIPAA privacy law
- Data security and reliability
- Effective patient identification management and matching processes
- Patient consent management
- Funding grants
- Data governance and authority decisions
- Connecting systems performance and scalability
- Consistent view of a patient data
- IT vendors and state and federal regulations
- Innovative solutions
- Auditability and more

S. Hasavari · K. Osei-Tutu · Y.-T. Song (✉)
Department of Computer & Information Sciences, Towson University, Towson, MD, USA
e-mail: shasavari@towson.edu; koseitutu@towon.edu; ysong@towson.edu

H. R. Arabnia et al. (eds.), *Advances in Computer Vision and Computational Biology*, Transactions on Computational Science and Computational Intelligence,
https://doi.org/10.1007/978-3-030-71051-4_43

The list indicates that coordination and ongoing maintenance of such an ecosystem are very challenging due to its scope and changing and evolving nature. If one index is changed, it can affect the others. That is why currently available solutions and even proposed new technologies are not capable of meeting all the necessary requirements. A realistic vision is that there is always a trade-off between the requirements. Our proposed system is not an exception as well.

This chapter is organized as follows:

Section 2 describes the permissioned blockchain technology to build a peer-to-peer network of sharing and searching healthcare information.
Section 3 discusses current approaches that provide a patient's data lookup service in either regional or statewide level and their benefits and challenges.
Section 4 describes our architecture consisting of a client application that is going to connect dynamically to different permissioned blockchain networks providing emergency staff with the patient's emergency relevant data like current problems, allergies, medications, and demographic information and allowing them to send a patient's care report to record and update on the distributed ledgers.
Section 5 discusses our challenges.
Section 6 presents our conclusion.

2 A Permissioned Blockchain Technology (HLF)

Current electronic health record systems are not interoperable, and patients' medical records are distributed [7, 8]. Thus, to have a consistent view of a patient's clinical and medical data while a patient walks from a medical facility to another, a technical infrastructure is required. During a patient's visit to one facility, a copy of part or all data gathered from that visit needs to be sent to others based on previously agreed-upon business logic and policy without relying on a third party that oversees and validates the exchanging or sharing of data. This way, these healthcare facilities create a peer-to-peer network among themselves, and a node will represent each participant on the network. Figure 1 illustrates this mechanism.

These healthcare facilities are able to share patient's data such that once the data is born in any of the healthcare setting, then it will be distributed among the members synchronously (distributed ledger) based on the agreed-upon consensus mechanism. The ordering node will perform the data distribution task. There is a good number of articles and websites about the Hyperledger Fabric network platform [9].

Each hospital or healthcare facility needs to install and create the following Hyperledger Fabric components.

Peer node: organizations can join the network using their peer nodes. Peer node is a network entity that calls a chaincode program (smart contract) to perform read/write tasks against the ledger. It represents an organization or a healthcare facility that performs a transaction. Once the request of recording a patient data on the ledger from client application is received, it calls the chaincode to read

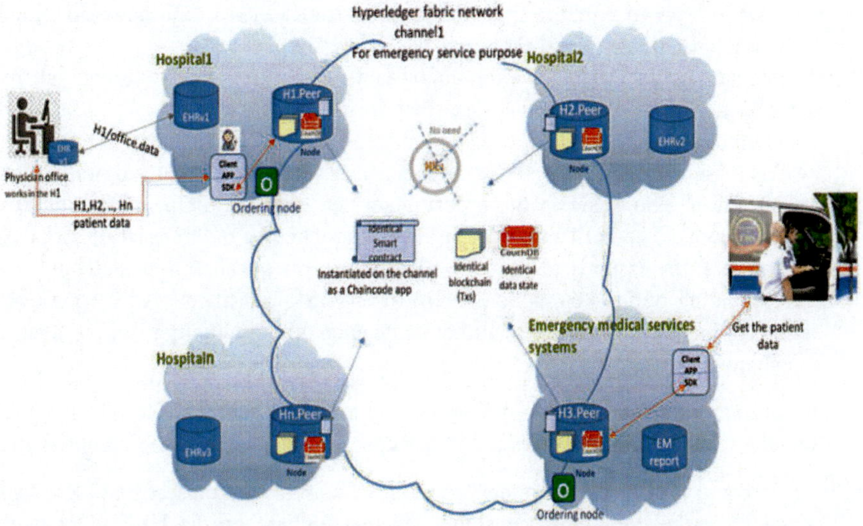

Fig. 1 A Hyperledger Fabric subnetwork (channel) among decentralized healthcare settings

the data from the state database to build a read set indicating the latest state of the patient's data. A specified number of peer nodes representing other members on the channel perform the same task simultaneously, based on the agreed-upon endorsement policy, and create read sets from their own state databases ensuring that all data states are identical. In this stage, no data is recorded on the ledger. It is only for initial data state validation. The nodes create write sets as well, which to be added to the blockchain and update the state database in the next steps.

Channel: A private Hyperledger Fabric subnetwork of members, consisting of member peers, the shared ledger, chaincode application, and the ordering service node for the purpose of conducting private and confidential transactions.

Smart contract or chaincode: an application instantiated on the channel and called by the peer command sitting on the peer node that reads/writes the data against the ledger.

Ledger: A blockchain and a state database.

Blockchain: A chain of blocks linked to one another; it keeps all transaction history in an immutable manner. Each block holds the hash value of the previous block so that if one block is changed, it affects all blocks after itself to make it impossible or very difficult to alter.

State database (Couchdb or Leveldb): A non-SQL database that keeps the latest state of the data.

Ordering node: A messaging queue and broadcasting service, which gets the data from client application that performs and verifies the endorsement policy. It builds the blocks of data and then broadcasts copies of the data to the other members' peers to commit/append it to their blockchains as a new block and then update their state databases.

Certificate authority: An HLF component that issues identities for members by generating a public and private key that forms a key pair that can be used to prove identity.

Membership service provider (MSP): a peer uses its private key to digitally sign a transaction. The MSP on the ordering service contains the peer's public key that is then used to verify that the signature attached to the transaction is valid. The private key is used to produce a signature on a transaction that only the corresponding public key, which is part of an MSP, can match. All components of an HLF network use MSP to authenticate each other mutually to communicate and share resources.

To interact with the network and connect to a peer to submit a request or transaction, we need a client application that includes one of the following components:

CLI, SDK, and API: used to connect to peers to submit the transaction (TX). This concept can be confusing for some new researchers on the HLF blockchain technology. Actually, an organization uses peers to record/read data to/from ledger. Therefore, to connect to a peer, other components of Hyperledger Fabric are required like CLI peer or SDK component; otherwise, the existing applications or a web/mobile application which organizations use to submit transactions is not capable of connecting to their peer nodes directly. Therefore, these applications need to import SDK component in their code. An application providing command line environment like Ubuntu terminal uses CLI peer component to connect to peers to submit the transactions from terminal. The application imports SDK into its code.

3 Related Work

The term "HIE" does not have a consistent term in health information technology. It is used both as a verb indicating exchanging of healthcare data and a noun as healthcare information exchange service provider. Effective October 1, 2018, Maryland law defines an HIE as an entity that provides or governs organizational and technical processes for the maintenance, transmittal, access, or disclosure of electronic healthcare information between or among healthcare providers or entities through an interoperable system [10]. Healthcare providers and entities like hospitals, clinics, image centers, labs, and pharmacies need to exchange and share patients' data among themselves for quality patient care, hence reducing mortality rate [11]. HIEs connect these healthcare entities, oversee, and govern the data exchange among them. Figure 2 shows an architecture of regional HIE networks (RHIOs) (Fig. 3).

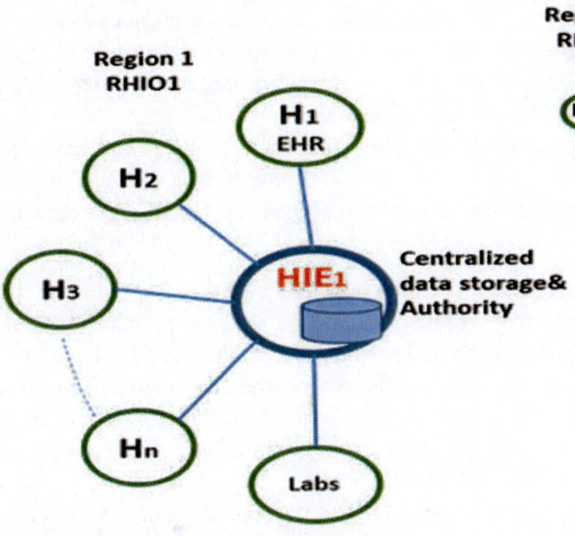

Fig. 2 Regional HIE networks (RHIOs)

Fig. 3 Healthcare facilities and entities exchanging data with RHIOs using their EHR interfaces

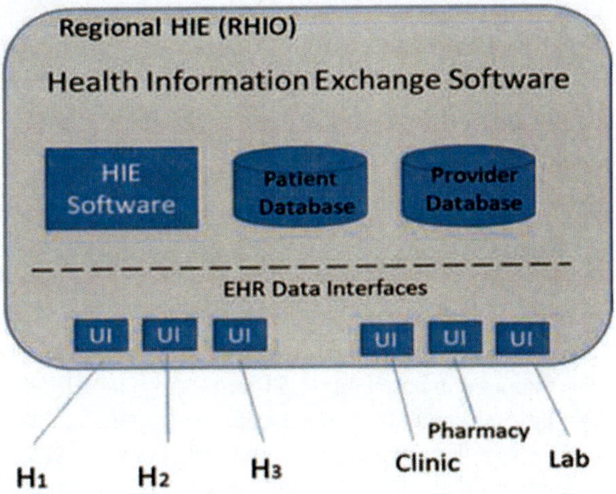

Centralized Data Storage and Governance Problem

All healthcare settings and entities must send their agreed-upon data to the HIE's document repository through an Electronic Health Record interface, and then a document registry database provides a pointer to the document repository. All healthcare settings need to feed patients' demographics and clinical and medical information to the HIE, and the data is updated when it is updated in the original healthcare setting [12]. An HIE organization is a centralized site which governs and oversees all data exchanged and shared among the participants. It also decides on the data validation. Real-world experience shows that a centralized data storage and authority is an attractive target for the cyber-criminals that leads to data privacy and security problem [1]. On the other hand, the data governance and authority shifts away from healthcare settings, which are the original producer of patient's data, to a third party. Once hospitals create a secure HLF channel among themselves, every member has the same identical data, which they have produced and validated, and they do not need to move the data they have produced to a third centralized data authority and governance to hold, validate, aggregate, exchange, and share data among members.

Fund-Bound Financial Sustainability and Viability Problem
RHIOs must continue to rely on government funding or receive grants from other stakeholders to ensure continuity. There is a substantial risk that many current efforts to promote health information exchange will fail when public funds supporting these initiatives are depleted [13]. Since RHIOs are often created through and operate from a grant, they are frequently working against a ticking clock. The sunset dates on these grants are typically only 2–3 years, and given the enormity of the task at hand, this is often not enough time for an RHIO to become financially sustainable on its own. This is a key obstacle in achieving health information exchange today [14].

Consistent View of a Patient's Data Problem
Once data is produced from a patient's visit, it is submitted to the HIE which aggregates the data with other data coming from other entities before sending it to the requesting service, so producing a real-time and consistent view of a patient's data is not always available.

3.1 Fast Healthcare Interoperability Resource (FHIR)

FHIR is a specification for exchanging clinical and administrative healthcare data. The standard is based on REST and OAuth developed by the HL7 organization that can be used as a stand-alone data exchange standard but can and will be used in partnership with existing widely used standards [15]. FHIR resources, as key core components, are used to build data exchange capabilities that become a popular approach among developers and providers. A patient's administrative, clinical, and medical data is categorized and defined as resources stored in an FHIR server from which apps and services will draw health data. It is a standard developed for electronic health record interoperability, so the standard apparently can be adopted by any technology used to exchange and share data like HIEs. The reality is that there are different versions of FHIR and it has its own challenges.

Challenges with FHIR

Semantic Interoperability FHIR may not help healthcare facilities/entities achieve semantic interoperability. Healthcare organizations seeking semantic interoperability are still challenged by variations in FHIR that prevent them from smoothly exchanging information [16].

Consistent View of a Patient's Data and Availability of All Resources Pertaining to a Patient A user application searching for a patient's data needs to connect to different servers holding resources and then aggregate them to have a consistent view of a patient's data. Here, the problem is that a healthcare facility needs to support a third-party application such as Apple's Health app to allow data storage or a user to look up through resources held by the facilities or a cloud storage on behalf of the facility. Therefore, the providers and consumers are forced to select vendors that they choose to use [17]. This way, the application supported to look up a patient's data may not be supported by facilities holding the same patient's resources. Thus, there is no consistent and holistic view of a patient's data available to consumers. Another problem is: how many resources are going to be collected and aggregated to produce the optimal result? The question coming to mind is whether it is real time accessing a patient's data scattered as resources on many FHIR servers.

Security FHIR depends on external encryption to secure data, but blockchain is inherently secure because of the way the data is passed through the platform, making security breaches of patient data less likely.

3.2 *Inter-blockchain Communication*

This is a survey of all proposed solutions on how to leverage the permissioned blockchain network technologies to exchange data between one another. The approaches do not address the problem of how a patient's data can be searched across all networks at a time [18].

4 Our Approach

Figure 4 illustrates how a cross-blockchain-based patients' data search system works. It shows how a client application enables first responders to search for a patient's emergency-relevant data, which may be recorded on one or more regional blockchain networks. The following components describe our architecture.

A Web/Mobile Application It is accessible to the first responders on their mobile device. A web service using RESTful API available on their eCPR ambulance system can be used to request the data as well.

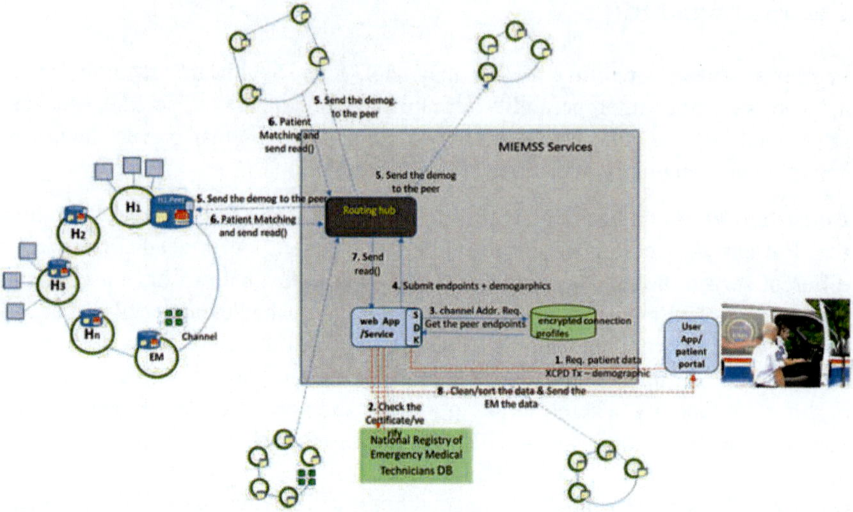

Fig. 4 Cross-blockchain health data lookup/update platform

Patient Identification and Matching This is performed on the HLF networks because a matching service is already incorporated in the chaincode/smart contract to match a patient before allowing it to be recorded on the ledger. This approach prevents any centralized patient demographic data, which meets the blockchain core value and reduces administrative task of constantly sending and updating patient's demographics on a centralized database that is time-consuming and costly. The results coming from different networks pertaining to a single patient need to be matched against the patient's demographic data provided by the first responders to ensure its validity again. Here, the matching process takes less time because the number of records gathered from different HLF networks has been significantly reduced. Then the patient's data will be sorted based on the date/time it has been updated on the ledgers. For patients' matching algorithm embedded in the chaincode, the best practice is to follow the Sequoia project's proposed rules to improve matching algorithms for cross-organizational patient identity management and matching. It indicates that organizations that use historical records for patient matching have a higher maturity rate [6].

Routing Hub To broadcast transactions to the HLF networks simultaneously and get the result back to the service provider application.

Data Availability on the Networks Since all peer nodes on a single channel have identical ledger, in case one peer node fails unexpectedly, the other peer node endpoints will be used to query the data. On the other hand, to handle the transaction scalability and performance, the requests can be broadcast by a load balancer and can be sent to different peers sitting on a same network to reduce the task burden on

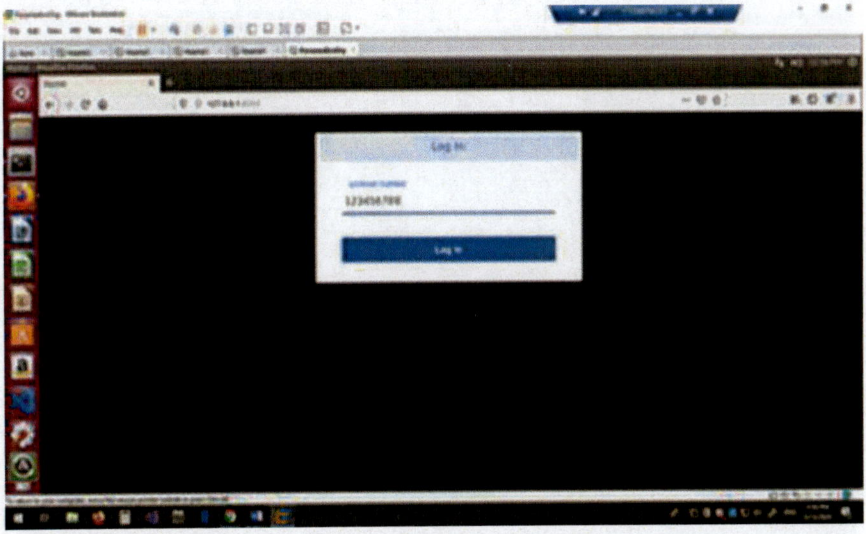

Fig. 5 Login page

one peer. This way, multiple peers on the same network can perform different tasks coming from different transactions. Thus, high-level availability will be guaranteed.

Consistent View of the Data An HLF network has a consistent view of a patient's data because all members use the same chaincode/smart contract–shared processing logic to record the data with the same data standard and format on the identical ledger. Thus, we have a consistent view of a patient's data in all regional networks. In our approach, mutually exchanging of data between HLF networks is not the case as a patient's data will be collected across networks and sorted based on date. If data obtained from one network is understandable, then the data obtained from other networks will be understandable as well. In case all networks decide to have the same view of a patient's data, then interoperability is required that looks like the same problem with EHR interoperability but in smaller scale as interoperability issue has been removed from members of a network to inter-network level. There is effort to solve this problem [19].

First-responder side: A user application (a browser or patients' portal in an ambulance existing system) will connect to the web/app server where the client application resides. The client app will provide a user interface to ask the first responder's license for authentication. Then it connects to the National Registry of Emergency Medical Technicians (NREMT) Database. The NREMT will verify the identity of the first responders and send result back to the client's application (Fig. 5).

The client application will authenticate the first responders and allow them to input the patient's demographics or whatever data they have found or discovered in the time of encounter. The system will require the first responder to input different

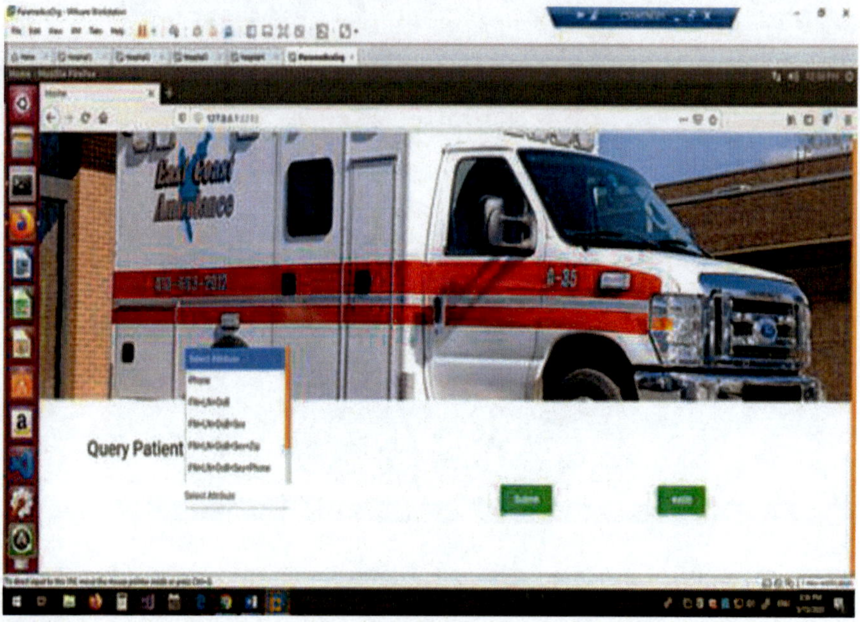

Fig. 6 Search for the patient's data

combinations of patient traits based on the identity data they have gathered from the patient at the scene (Fig. 6).

Then, the applications will use the connection profile to connect to peers on different networks. The client's application will send the request to a routing hub to broadcast message to the different HLF networks synchronously. The peers get the request, verify the emergency service provider's identity, and will call the chaincode to query the state database to perform the patient's matching process, and if it matches, it will create a read set containing the patient's data and will send it to the client application. It will get all coming data and sort it based on the date in descending format. It performs matching algorithm again to have more clean data and will send it to the first responders. The following screenshot displays the result of submitting request to the networks (Fig. 7).

By clicking on view link, paramedics can view the patient's data (Fig. 8).

The paramedics can also use Update Report link to add the patient's care report/summary and submit it to the networks to be recorded and updated there. Once clicked, a form appears and is populated with patient's data and boxes for paramedics/EMT license number so that it clears who has written the care report. The following screenshots depict these interactions (Fig. 9).

After submitting the report, a message will appear on the screen indicating the patient's report has successfully been added to the ledgers (Figs. 10, 11, 12, and 13).

If the query for a patient's data returns no record, it indicates the patient's data does not exist in any HLF networks. In this situation, the system allows paramedics to submit the care summary to all networks.

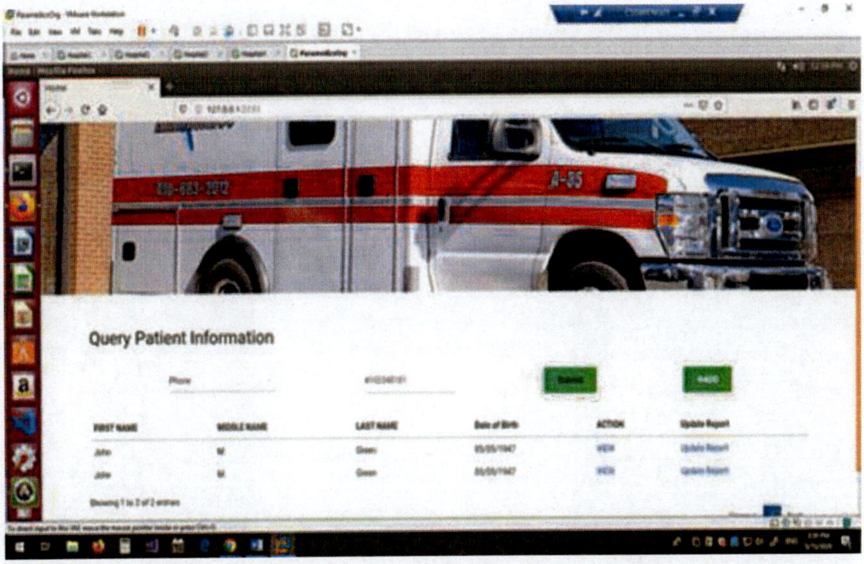

Fig. 7 The result of search obtained from both networks

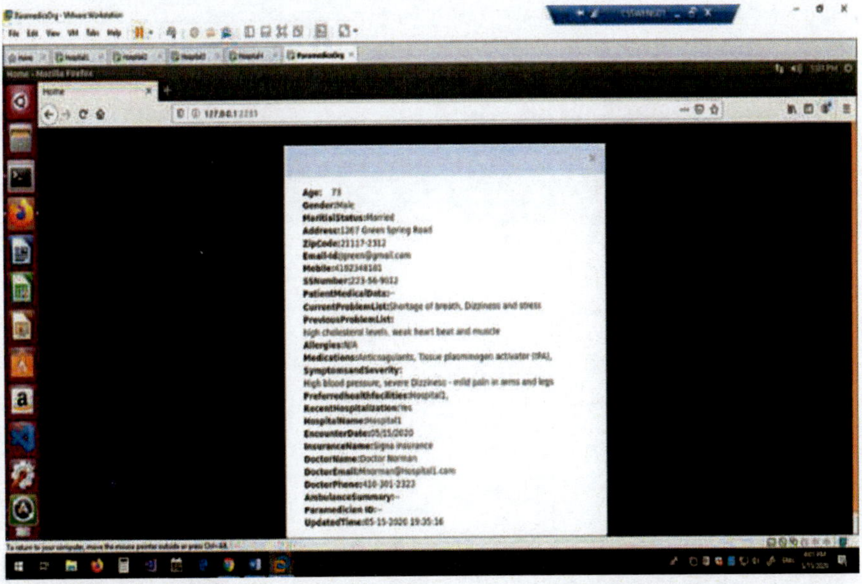

Fig. 8 Patient's data detail

By pressing ADD button, it navigates the new page allowing them to enter the patient's data and care report.

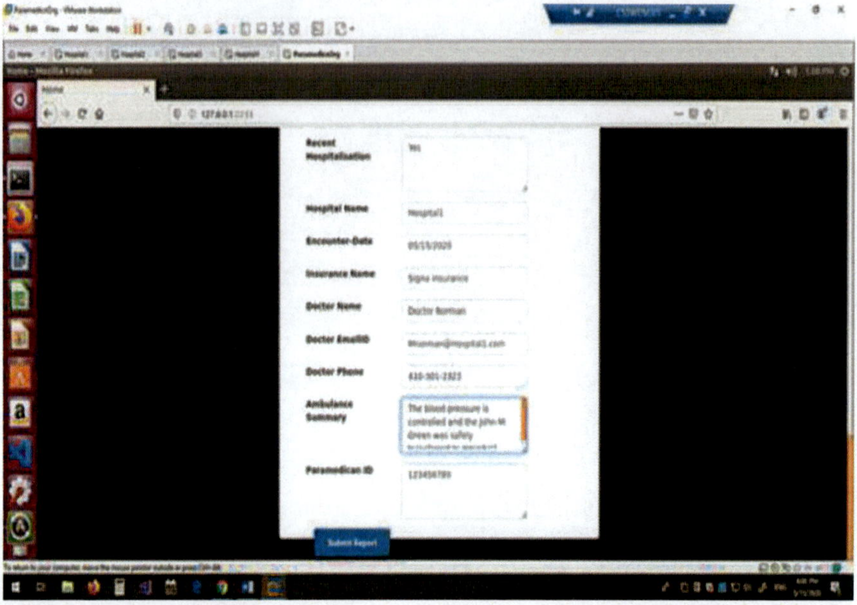

Fig. 9 Adding and submitting the patient's care report

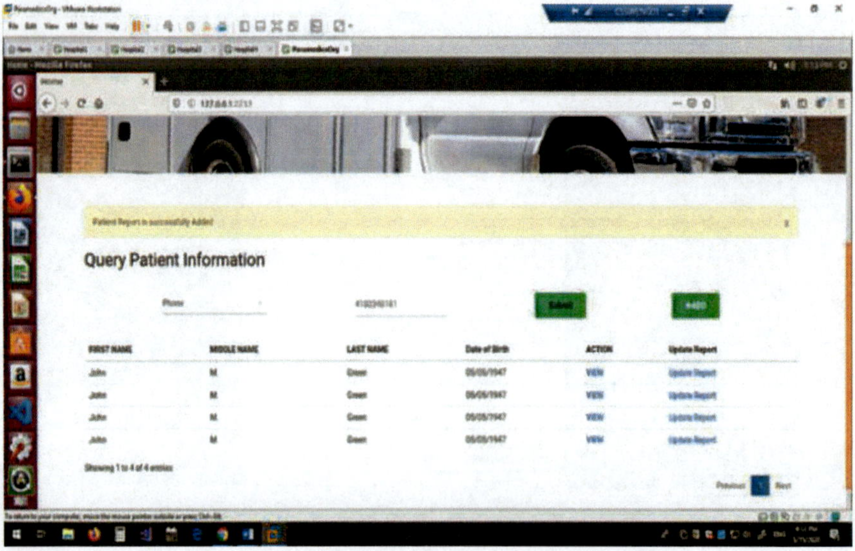

Fig. 10 The result of search for the added patient's care report

To test if the care report has successfully committed to the ledgers on both networks (Fig. 14).

To view the care summary, the user clicks the view link (Fig. 15).

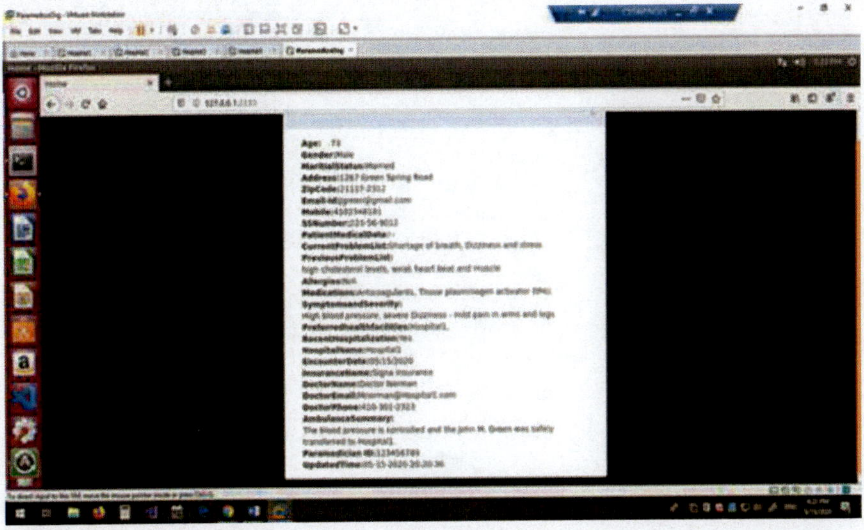

Fig. 11 Ambulance care report and the paramedic's ID

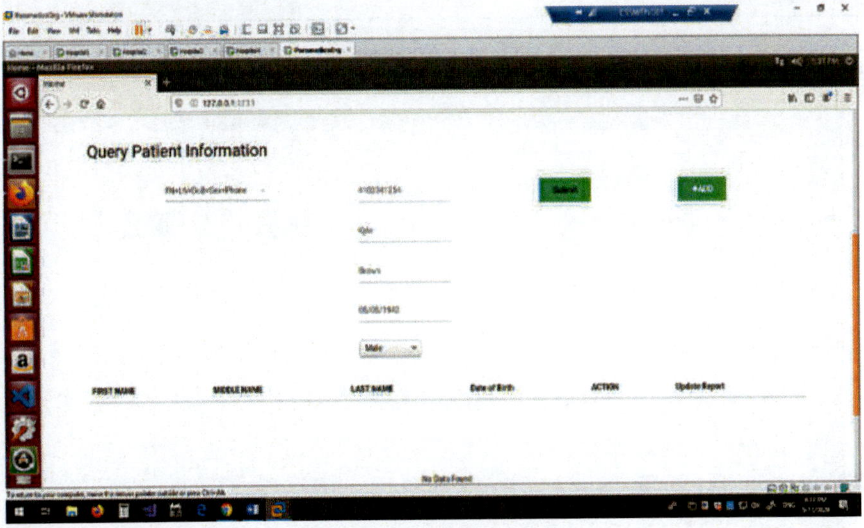

Fig. 12 The result of search when no data exist for the patient

Access Control to HLF Networks

In our use case, the organization representing first responders and providing a cross-blockchain service is not required to be a member of any HLF networks. It reduces administrative work on the organization, and it is cost-effective as well. The networks when configured can define organization' role in their configuration file to allow the organization' users (first responders) to submit transactions. For

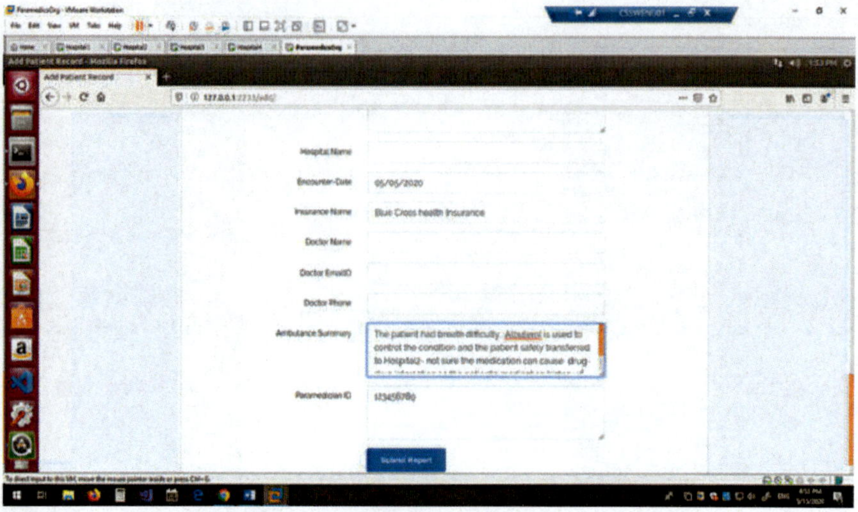

Fig. 13 Adding the patient's care report/summary

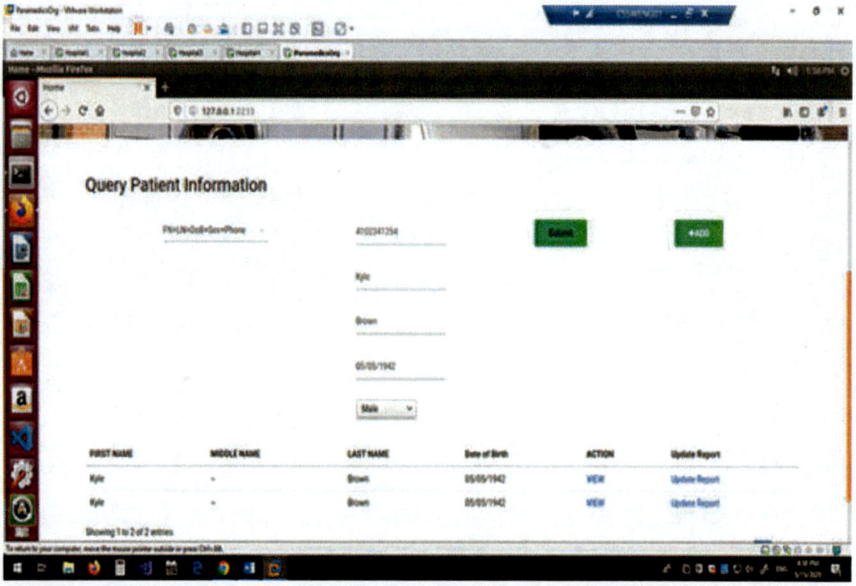

Fig. 14 Evidence of the patient's care report committed on the ledgers on both networks

secure access, each network's admin will create a TLS certificate/crypto-materials for the emergency service provider organization to connect securely to the network and sign the transaction. In this scenario, we use mutual TLS to make sure none of the clients and peers are malicious. Any network's proxy server can monitor the incoming messages to make sure they are coming from known endpoints. This is

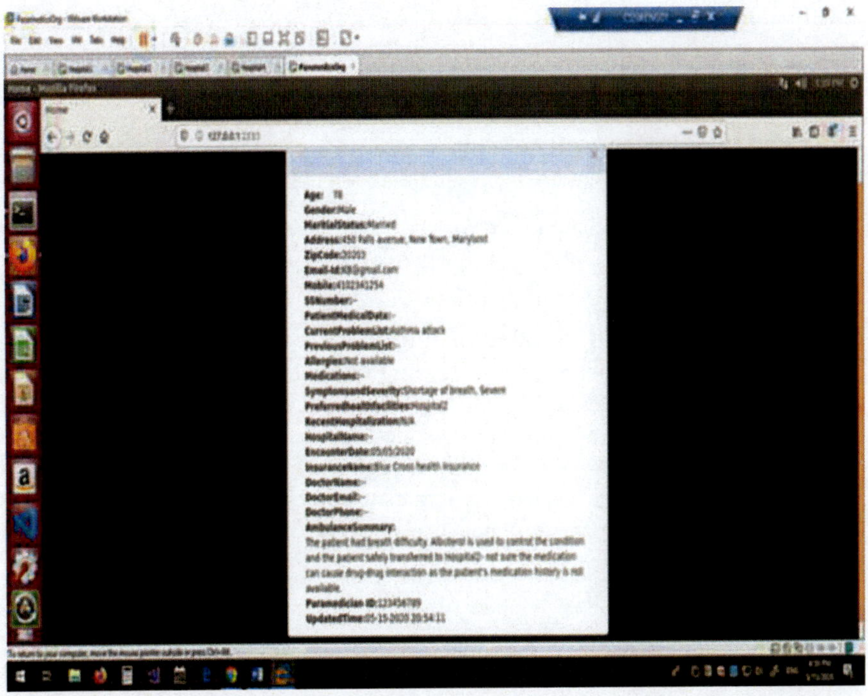

Fig. 15 The patient's care report detail on one of the networks

a mutual agreement between the cross-blockchain service provider and the HLF networks' members. In fact, the healthcare facilities like hospitals and clinics are primary sources of a patient's care so they own the ledger and need to be a member of the networks, and first responders can contribute to the data on the ledger. On the other hand, it is not practical for organizations like emergency service providers, department of health and human services, or research entities to be a member by having peer nodes on all networks as it can lead to scalability and performance issues, and maintaining such a system would be problematic.

Use Cases

For validating our system architecture and capturing the high-level requirements, we have defined the use cases shown in Figs. 5 and 6. Additionally, these use case diagrams help the reader to understand the system expected behavior. In Fig. 5, the primary actor/user that triggers the use case is first responders including paramedics/EMTs who provide their license numbers. The system needs to verify the user identity before allowing them to supply further information like a patient's demographics to query the patient's data. So the NREMT organization as a cooperative adjacent system is used to help identify and authenticate the first responder. All other steps have already been explained using screenshots. We split the system architecture into two use case diagrams. The first one depicts interaction between a human actor and a system/app, and the second use case depicts the interaction between two automated systems: client application and network peers. We have excluded exception cases from the figures. Exceptions are unwanted system behaviors that prevent the system to accomplish its goal. For example, in case the NREMT database is not available or the paramedics enter the wrong identity, then the application needs to handle it and send the correct message to the users.

The second use case diagram depicts how the mobile/web application used by first responders interacts with HLF subnetwork/channel to ask for the patient's data.

Sequence Diagram
For any system especially complex ones, interactions among components depend on the services each component provides to the other to support its functionality. This service can be a message, input/output, or calling a function. The sequence diagram in Fig. 7 illustrates the flow of the logic and the order in which these services and functions take place and how long they are active during system overall functionality. We used the sequence diagrams to combine and clarify the messages exchanged between components in both use cases and the functions each component performs using that service.

5 Our Challenges

Due to the scope of this complex system, measuring its security, scalability, and performance in a developer environment is of a challenge. It heavily depends on the security, scalability, and performance of connecting systems, especially HLF networks. Practically, a complex system performance will be evaluated ahead of time, while the number of organizations adopting the solution will be increasing. The performance of the system is a key factor for first responders, so even if this platform has been implemented in a developer environment, we will not be able to measure its performance with existing operational systems as it takes quite a bit of time to ensure its efficiency in the real-world environment.

The following use case diagrams depict the transactions among objects (Figs. 16 and 17).

The following sequence diagram describes the flow of messages, events, and actions between objects in our system.

In Fig. 18, we have not incorporated some transactions for simplicity such as submitting the patients' care report to HLF networks or when the patient is not found on any network.

Implementation Summary We have implemented two Hyperledger Fabric network; each one consists of two hospitals sitting on different virtual machines (VM). One emergency data providing service, a web/mobile application runs on the fifth VM named paramedicsOrg representing first responders and support their transactions. The host operating system is Windows 10 Enterprise, the hypervisor

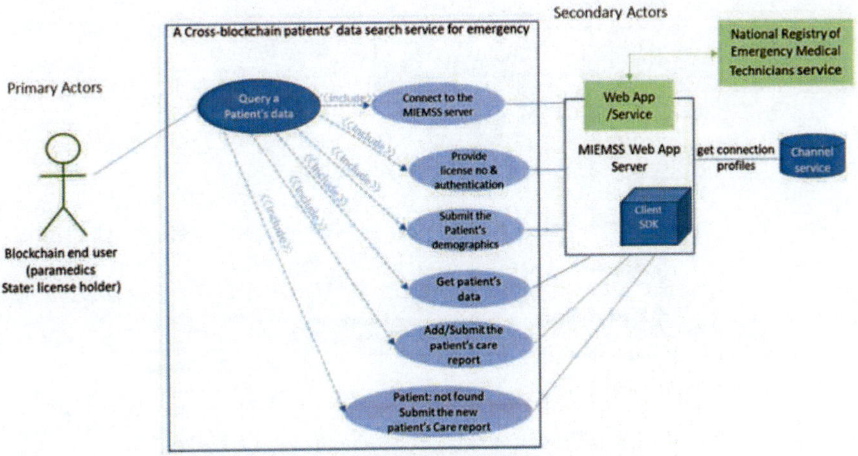

Fig. 16 Transaction between the user and the web app/service

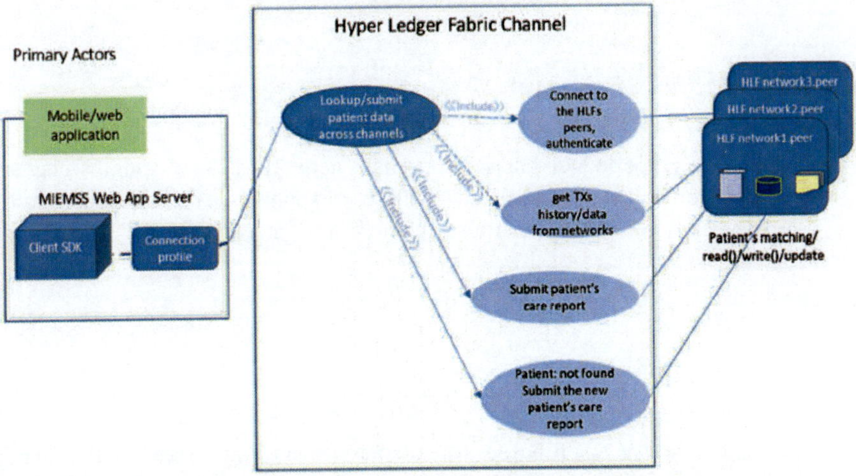

Fig. 17 Transaction between the web app/service and the Hyperledger Fabric networks

is VMware Workstation Pro, and the virtual machine's OS is Linux Ubuntu 16.04 Xenial.

We have used the Django framework to implement the client application. The application is completely developed in Python programming language, as there are four types of sd client such as Python fabric sdk, Golang sdk, Node.js sdk, and Java sdk, among which the Python is easier to implement in the developer environment. It is also flexible with any platform and is robust too. We have used the JSON connection profiles to connect to peers sitting on the networks. A connection profile describes a set of components, including peers, orderers, and certificate

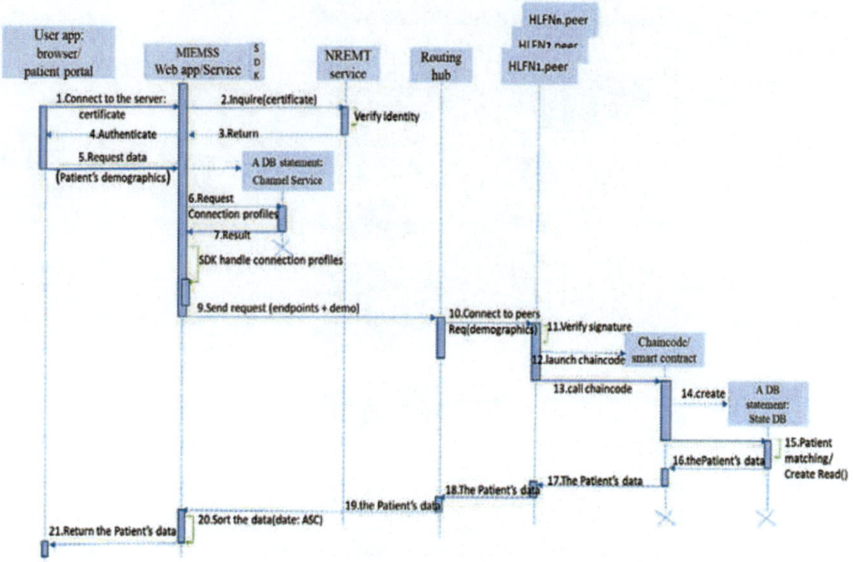

Fig. 18 Sequence diagram for message flow

authorities in a Hyperledger Fabric blockchain network. It also contains channel and organization information related to these components. A connection profile is primarily used by an application to configure a gateway handles all network interactions.

6 Conclusion

In this chapter, we have proposed a new approach on how to access a patient's emergency medical data across HLF networks. It keeps the patient's data within the healthcare facility and provides provenance to the data. The key point of our effort is that we eliminated the need of obtaining patients' demographic information from healthcare facilities to identify a patient and then provide the emergency data service to search for the patient's clinical and medical data. The identification will be performed within each HLF network. Another point is that the organization providing the emergency service does not need to have a peer node on the networks. It will have the privilege of acting like a user of those networks. We have explained the advantage of this mechanism earlier in this approach. We can increase the system's performance and data availability by distributing the transactional load to different peers sitting on the same HLF network since all peers of the same network have identical ledgers.

Any new technology or approach needs to respect the large investments/funds made to enable exchanging and sharing of patient's data across healthcare ecosystem. The blockchain is a new technology, and it will be operating in a small scale and scale up over time like any other technologies. It grows up over time while ensuring its effectiveness and efficiency.

7 Future Direction

This approach can also serve patients to search for their own data by providing their own credentials to the system. Even in an emergency case, a double check on the data accuracy can be available in place if a patient's data can be searched for by patients themselves or by first responders in certain situation using the patient's credential with the patient's consent. It increases the system availability in case NREMT is not available. Since HLF is a cross-organizational solution for sharing data, the users of healthcare facilities including patients are authenticated and authorized to access their own data by their organizational credentials. One solution might suggest using a patient's credentials on one HLF network to search across multiple networks. Since we do not know which network has the patient's credentials, a second task of patient's credential search will slow down the system significantly when thousands or millions of patients are the case.

A first-responder identity can be verified by their license issuer data source (NREMT), whereas there is no single place to refer to and identify a patient's credential to log in and search for their data. If one suggestion is going to be that the service provider application can provide patient's credentials, then maintenance and security issues might occur. The third parties' credential will also not be a secure approach to the solution in the healthcare domain. Therefore, a new research is required on how to manage patients' authentication to use this service.

References

1. H. Wu, E.M. LaRue, Linking the health data system in the U.S.: Challenges to the benefits. Int. J. Nurs. Sci **4**(4), 410–417 (2017)
2. G. Mears, et al., National EMS assessment Table of Contents (2011), pp. 1–550
3. ISO/IEC 24760:2011, "A framework for identity management," Fg-Secmgt.Gi.De (2011)
4. "Health IT Standards," HealthIT.gov, 04-Jun-2019. [Online]. Available: https://www.healthit.gov/topic/standards-technology/health-it-standards
5. N. Shen et al., Understanding the patient privacy perspective on health information exchange: A systematic review. Int. J. Med. Inform. **125**, 1–12 (2019)
6. Patient consent for electronic health information exchange and interoperability, HealthIT.gov, 18-Sep-2019. [Online]. Available: https://www.healthit.gov/topic/interoperability/patient-consent-electronic-health-information-exchange-and-interoperability
7. M. Reisman, EHRs: The challenge of making electronic data usable and interoperable. P T Peer Rev. J. Formul. Manag. **42**(9), 572–575 (2017)

8. C. Rathert, T.H. Porter, J.N. Mittler, M. Fleig-Palmer, Michelle seven years after meaningful use: Physicians' and nurses' experiences with electronic health records. Health Care Manage. Rev. **44**(1), 30–40 (2019)
9. "Hyperledger Fabric Glossary," Hyperledger fabric. [Online]. Available: https://hyperledger-fabric.readthedocs.io/en/release-1.2/glossary.html
10. On May 15, 2018, Senate Bill 17, *Health Information Exchanges – Definitions and Regulations,* was signed into law, changing the definition of an HIE
11. N. Menachemi, S. Rahurkar, C.A. Harle, J.R. Vest, The benefits of health information exchange: An updated systematic review. J. Am. Med. Inform. Assoc. **25**(9), 1259–1265 (2018)
12. Q. Ahrq, Regional Health eDecisions: A guide to connecting health information exchange in primary care
13. J. Adler-Milstein, D.W. Bates, A.K. Jha, Operational health information exchanges show substantial growth, but long-term funding remains a concern. Health Aff (Millwood) **32**(8), 1486–1492 (2013)
14. S. Jamison, "On the road to RHIO: What state CIOs need to know," (859), pp. 1–10, 2007
15. "7.9 Common Example Scenarios in FHIR," Usecases - FHIR v4.0.1. [Online]. Available: https://www.hl7.org/fhir/usecases.html
16. E. O'Dowd, "FHIR may not help healthcare orgs achieve semantic interoperability," HIT-Infrastructure, 24-Sep-2018. [Online]. Available: https://hitinfrastructure.com/news/fhir-may-not-help-healthcare-orgs-achieve-semantic-interoperability
17. D. Devine, "With FHIR in Place is There Room for Blockchain in Healthcare? - Huron," Huron Consulting Group. [Online]. Available: https://www.huronconsultinggroup.com/resources/healthcare/fhir-blockchain-healthcare
18. I.A. Qasse, M.A. Talib, Q. Nasir, Inter blockchain communication: A survey, in *International Conference Proceedings Series* (2019)
19. G.G. Dagher, C.L. Adhikari, T. Enderson, Towards secure interoperability between heterogeneous blockchains using smart contracts (November 2017)

Robotic Process Automation-Based Glaucoma Screening System: A Framework

Somying Thainimit, Panaree Chaipayom, Duangrat Gansawat, and Hirohiko Kaneko

1 Introduction

Glaucoma is an ocular disease that progressively damages the optic nerve. Generally, there are no warning signs in early-stage glaucoma. The disease develops gradually and often without noticeable sight loss. However, advanced glaucoma can lead to irreversible blindness. According to the World Health Organization (WHO), glaucoma is considered the second most common disease that causes blindness [1]. Currently, there is no cure for glaucoma. However, early detection and treatment can prevent disease progression [2]. To early detect glaucoma, annual eye examination and screening with optic nerve check is a practical recommendation.

Glaucoma diagnosis involves visual field test, examining physical history of patients, intraocular pressure (IOP), measuring structure changes of an optic nerve head such as disk diameter, CDR, etc. These tests are often performed by medical professionals. Therefore, performing mass glaucoma screening requires tremendous resources of time, cost, and medical staff. Incorporating technologies into retinopathy screening helps to improve cost-effectiveness of a screening program. Many automatic ocular detection and screening systems are developed and well validated

S. Thainimit (✉) · P. Chaipayom
Department of Electrical Engineering, Kasetsart University, Bangkok, Thailand
e-mail: fengsyt@ku.ac.th; panaree.c@ku.th

D. Gansawat
National Electronics and Computer Technology Center, Pathum Thani, Thailand
e-mail: duangrat.gansawat@nectec.or.th

H. Kaneko
Department of Information and Communications Engineering, Tokyo Institute of Technology, Yokohama, Japan
e-mail: kaneko.h.ab@m.titech.ac.jp

H. R. Arabnia et al. (eds.), *Advances in Computer Vision and Computational Biology*, Transactions on Computational Science and Computational Intelligence,
https://doi.org/10.1007/978-3-030-71051-4_44

[3–8]. However, they are still not widely used. This is because most systems are proprietary and limited in capturing and transmitting ocular images. These limitations are relaxed with the advance of sensors and communication technology [9, 10].

Recently, a new emerging technology called robotic process automation (RPA) is widely integrated into streamline business processes to enrich human interaction experience and to reduce time and cost of operations [11]. The RPA is a software tool that partially or fully replicates repetitive routine actions of an actual human such as manipulating administrative data, automatically generating response to simple customer service queries, and communicating with other digital systems. The software robot can be integrated with existing systems without disturbing the essential infrastructure of the system, making it easier to implement. The RPA is widely deployed in several industries such as banking, insurance, healthcare, and retails. M. Ratia [12] tested the effectiveness of RPA in the private healthcare sector by deploying RPA in analysis of the value-creating function. The test reported that RPA can increase efficiency in repetitive procedures and also can be used for health care. Feiqi et al. [13] proposed a framework for applying RPA in the confirmation process of the auditing service. The study reported benefits of RPA in minimizing human errors in paperwork and in increasing scale of some procedures from sampling to testing the entire population.

In health care, leveraging RPA presents opportunities and benefits that can free up clinicians' time and improve patient care delivery. The RPA does not only reduce time and improve patient engagement and care but also can address massive scale of population health screening such as remote eye screening. This can be done by assisting workflows of remote monitoring and operation management such as registration and appointment scheduling.

This chapter presents a mobile application that integrated RPA with a glaucoma screening system. The system can be further scaled up for other ocular disease screening. For the first phase, the proposed system automatically analyzes the OD shape using fundus images. Combined with basic eye pressure measurement information if it exists, the preliminary glaucoma condition is analyzed at the remote site. If the obtained preliminary analysis is found to be abnormal and further examination by experts should be performed, both eye specialists and patients can set an appointment through this application. Details of the proposed system framework are elaborated in Sect. 2. The next section also includes investigation results of two automatic optic disk measurements. The framework and investigation results are discussed in Sects. 3 and 4 is a conclusion.

2 The RPA-Based Glaucoma Screening System

The proposed embedded RPA glaucoma screening system is developed based around the mobile technology. The mobile application allows users to easily upload their own fundus eye images, views preliminary machine learning (ML)-based glaucoma analysis, and allows users to request for a further appointment if needed. Our purposed framework also gathers relevant examination history of patients such as the information of the responsible physician and medical information within the mobile application.

2.1 Design of the Screening System

Figure 1 depicts the functionality of the proposed system. With the advanced retinal acquisition and secured telecommunication, portable fundus photography coupled with tele- or web-based data transfer is available [9, 10, 14]. Users can obtain their fundus eye images at both local and remote hospitals that provided professional fundus imaging by clinicians. The application can upload, display, and transfer images to the server for automatic ML preliminary glaucoma analysis and for specialist analysis. Users can request to queue up for physician and hospital visits.

The application facilitates physician in glaucoma diagnosis by gathering patient's information, history of medical record, and the preliminary analysis result. The gathering work is performed by RPA, which helps to reduce error-prone manual

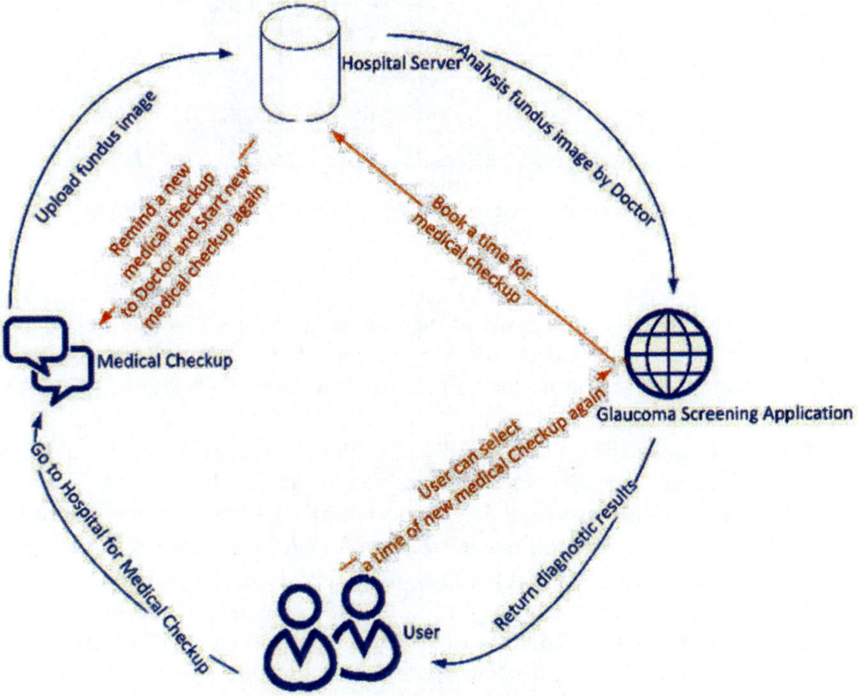

Fig. 1 Functionality of the glaucoma screening application

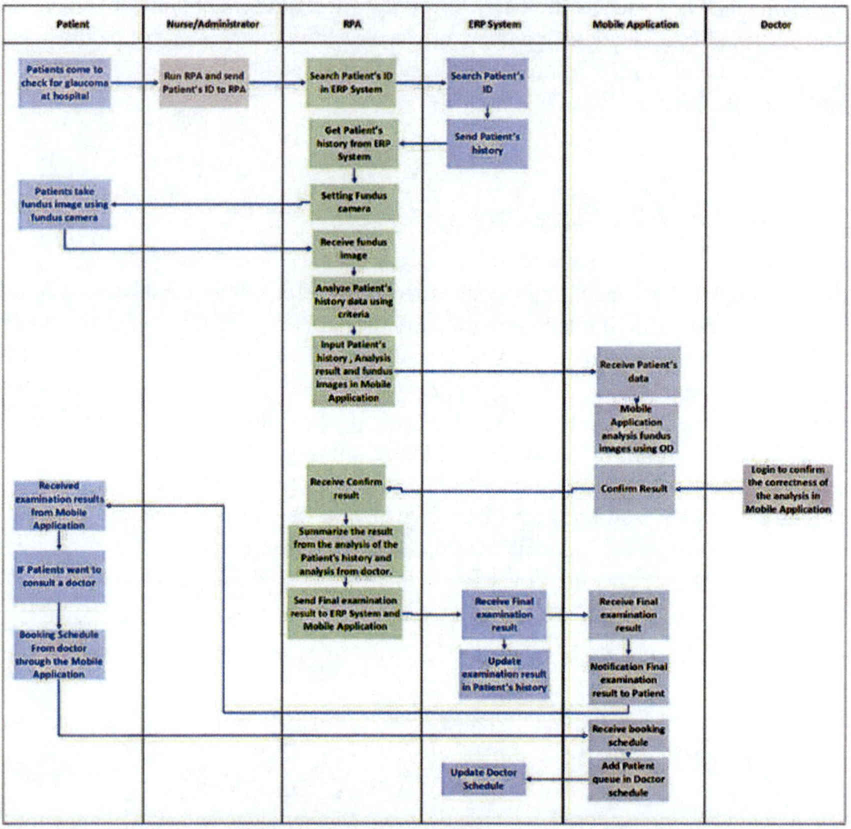

Fig. 2 Task operations of the RPA and its involved parties in the proposed glaucoma screening application

process. It also reduces work hours of medical and administrative staff, efficiently manages schedules for patients and doctors, and allows remote diagnosis. These make screening possible in isolated regions and in places with limited physicians and resources.

The task operations of the involved parties in the framework are illustrated in Fig. 2. With the use of RPA, doctor's examination queue is in the hospital enterprise resource planning (ERP) system. Doctors can maximally manage the number of patients and prioritize patient's queue based on preliminary diagnosis result. Thus, the RPA-based system increases productivity and efficiency. The application aids expert diagnosis. The physician can display fundus eye images, clinical parameters, patient's histories, and related ML-based analysis results such as OD measurement. For the final diagnosis, the physician needs to interpret, check clinical parameters, and index values. The ML-based clinical data such as OD size can be corrected by the physician before giving the final diagnosis decision. Then, the RPA process summarizes and updates the results and relevant information on the ERP and mobile application systems. The mobile application notifies the patient about the decision and makes an appointment for the next examination if needed.

2.2 *User Interface*

As for the user interface (UI) design of mobile applications, we designed a system to support the works of the medical and administrative staff by securely integrating historical records and relevant information of each patient. The data collection in the form of periodic data helps in improving accuracy of progressive glaucoma diagnosis.

Figure 3 displays example interfaces of the mobile application. User's profile and medical histories are shown in Fig. 3a. The taken fundus images can be uploaded for automatic glaucoma analysis using the ML-based optic nerve head analysis. At the first phase of the project, a measured size of the optic disk is included in the application. Other automatic measurements such as cup size or CDR can be integrated in the next phase of the project. The application allows the doctor to modify the size of the OD through the interfaces shown in Fig. 3b, c before making final diagnosis decision. The user can view both the ML and the doctor's decision. The next appointment can be requested both from the user and the doctor.

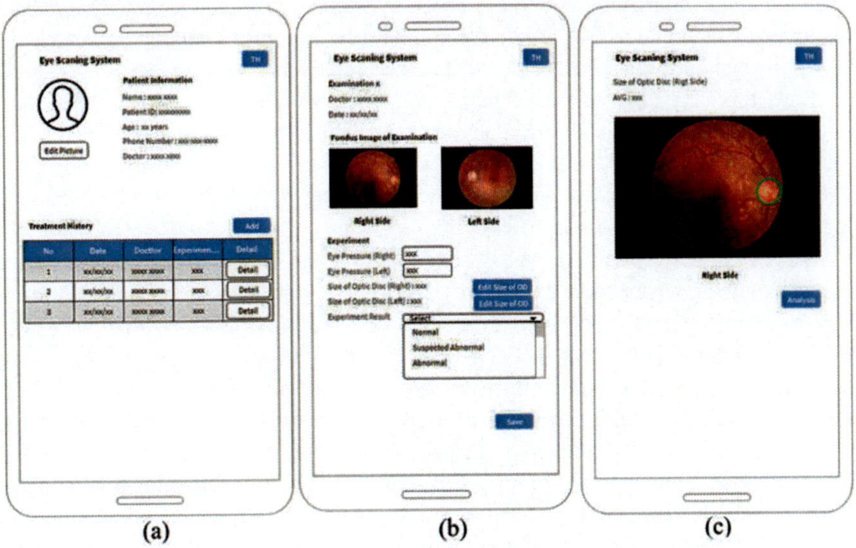

Fig. 3 User interface of the proposed system

2.3 Machine Learning-Based Analysis

For the first phase of the project, the framework integrates optic nerve head or optic disk measurement using machine learning algorithm. Assessment of the optic disk is one common measurement for glaucoma diagnosis since glaucoma causes deformation in the optic disk and causes the optic cup to enlarge. Optic disk deformation can be measured in several ways such as disk diameter, vertical cup-to-disk ratio (CDR), ISNT rule, peripapillary atrophy (PPA), and notching [15]. During the first phase of this work, the OD diameter is combined with the intra-ocular pressure for glaucoma diagnosis.

The accurate OD segmentation is needed in order to quantify the size of OD. This chapter investigated two segmentation methods: adaptive thresholding and U-net deep learning techniques. Issac et al. [16] proposed segmenting disk by adaptively thresholding the red channel of eye images. The red channel image is firstly illuminated and contrast normalized by subtracting the input image with its average intensity and standard deviation. Next, the histogram of the normalized image is smoothed using a Gaussian filter of size $W \times 1$. The threshold value is adapted to contrast the smoothed image reflected by the standard deviation of both Gaussian window and the normalized image. The threshold value to segment the optic disk is defined by

$$Th = (0.5 * W) - (2 * \sigma_G) - \sigma_R, \tag{1}$$

where Th is the threshold for optic disk segmentation, W is the size of Gaussian window (W is equal to 60), σ_G is the standard deviation of Gaussian window, and σ_R is the standard deviation of the normalized red channel eye image.

Sevastopolsky [17] proposed using a U-net deep learning for optic disk segmentation. The U-net is a fully convolutional neural network, capable of training on extremely small datasets and yielding good promising results. The U-net architecture consists of two major parts: contracting path (left side) and expansive path (right side), as shown in Fig. 4.

The contracting part of U-net is constructed using typical convolutional neural network layers, whereas the expansive path consists of transposed 2D convolutional layers. Each process block constitutes two convolutional layers with 3×3 pixel filters. A number of filters in each layer are indicated above the layer's output represented by a blue rectangle in Fig. 4. An example is the first convolutional layer that has 32 filters. Each convolution is followed by the rectified linear unit (ReLU) activation function and the dropout regularization. The 2×2 max pooling is applied for down-sampling the image. For each block in the expansive path, the resulted image is upsized by two (unsampling) using the transpose convolution. The obtained feature image is then concatenated with the corresponding image from the contracting path. At the last layer, a 1×1 convolution and a sigmoid activation are applied to obtain the designed segmentation output.

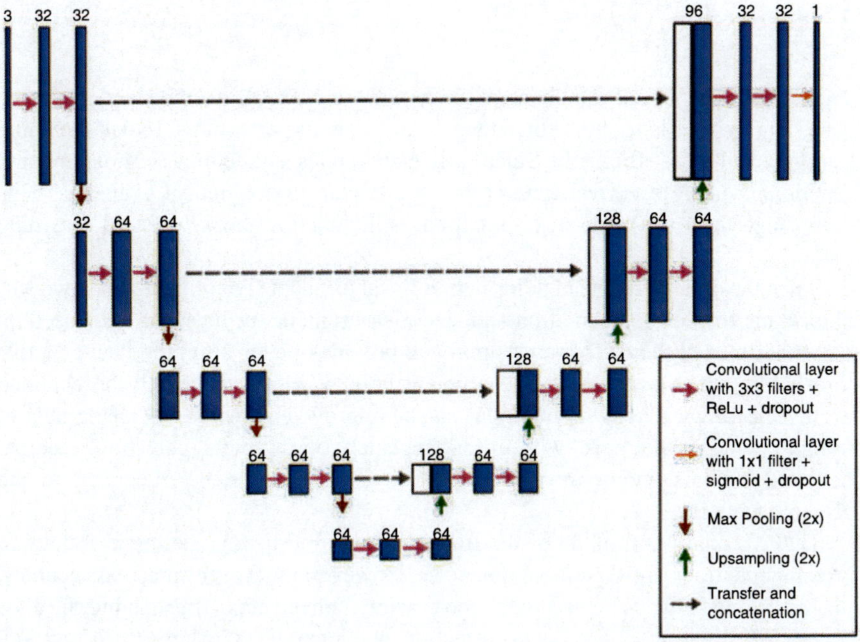

Fig. 4 The U-net architecture proposed by Sevastopolsky [17] for optic disk segmentation

Table 1 Comparisons of optic disk segmentations (Drishti-GS1)

Algorithms	IoU	Dice
Adaptive thresholding [16]	0.71613	0.82975
CNN [17]	0.76149	0.85969
Average	0.73881	0.84772

Both OD segmentation techniques are investigated using Drishti-GS1 dataset [15]. This dataset consists of a total of 101 images with 31 normal and 70 glaucomatous images. The ground truth was collected from four glaucoma experts. The obtained segmented OD is compared with the ground truth OD in terms of intersection over union (IoU) and Dice coefficients. The (IOU) score and Dice score are defined as follows:

$$\mathrm{IOU} = \left|\frac{A \cap B}{A \cup B}\right| \text{ and Dice} = \frac{2\,|A \cap B|}{|A| + |B|}, \tag{2}$$

where A is a segmented output map and B is a correct binary output map (the ground truth). These quality measures do not depend on object scale and class imbalance. The obtained results are listed in Table 1.

3 Discussions

The primary purpose of establishing the framework of the RPA-embedded glaucoma screening system is to aid clinicians and hospitals in performing ocular screening remotely and more efficiently. Since early glaucoma is asymptomatic, structural and functional vision tests over time can help clinician to distinguish glaucoma at its early stage; historical data of each patient is included in the RPA-based screening system.

Since the optic nerve head deformation is a significant sign of glaucoma, two ML algorithms for OD segmentation and size measurement are investigated. Based on our experiments, the CNN-based approach provides better accuracy than adaptive thresholding. The average Dice coefficient is 0.84772. Even though the obtained average accuracy is not very high, this can be improved by increasing the number of training data. Furthermore, with the advancement of automatic detection research, better algorithms and more ocular disease detections can be integrated to the screening system.

The ML analysis module of the framework is used as a guideline in follow-up recommendations and in remote diagnosis. However, in terms of medical accuracy, diagnosis must always be verified by professional physicians. Thus, an interface for formal investigation, clinical data correction, and approval is included in the system.

Integrating RPA- and ML-based module in the screening system offers many bene-fits for clinicians, hospitals, and patients. RPA module of the system can directly prompt the physician if the ML-based diagnosis is severe. Due to its high risk, RPA can be set to allow patients to override the regular checkup by requesting a new visit that is more recent. In addition, the physician can set to prioritize a patient's visit based on the severity level obtained from the ML-based diagnosis. Some patients may automatically refer to retaken images before directly visiting the physician. In a remote place with limited clinicians and resources, this maximizes resource utilization efficiency.

The RPA module in the screening system is also designed to help patients and clinicians in accessing retinal images, examination results, and scheduling. The software RPA improves interaction experiences among patients and clinicians. The human errors are also reduced. With deploying the RPA in the repeated tasks such as test result reporting and appointment scheduling. The working hours and waiting time are reduced.

The screening system can be extended further by applying the RPA in registration process. The new and existing registrants can be validated using the RPA robot. This makes remote screening easier to use, costless, and time efficient, and it increases feasibility of performing nationwide ocular screening.

4 Conclusion

The authors aim to develop a mobile application and RPA embedded glaucoma screening system. This work presents the framework of the system that allows collecting patient's eye data, efficiently aiding medical professionals in glaucoma diagnosis, and also facilitates patients in notifying examination results and scheduling appointments. In this system, we have images of the patient's eyes taken periodically to promote early glaucoma detection. By embedding the RPA with the screening system, cost and time operations are significantly reduced. The patient experience is also improved, and timely treatment can be achieved. Moreover, the RPA provides efficient resource management; hence, it enables the system to be more suitable for massive ocular screening. In the future, we plan to develop more efficient system by adding various analysis techniques and applying the RPA in registration and financial process.

Acknowledgments This research was supported by the Thailand Graduate Institute of Science and Technology (grant no: SCA-CO-2560-4524-TH).

References

1. R.N. Weinreb, T. Aung, F.A. Medeiros, The pathophysiology and treatment of Glaucoma: A review. JAMA (2015)
2. T.R. Einarson et al., Screening for glaucoma in Canada: A systematic review of the literature. Can. J. Ophthalmol., 709–721 (2006)
3. Z. Zhang, R. Srivastava, H. Liu, et al., A survey on computer aided diagnosis for ocular diseases. BMC Med. Inform. Decis. Mak. **14** (2014)
4. K.P. Noronha, U.R. Acharya, K.P. Nayak, et al., Automated classification of glaucoma stages using higher order cumulant features. Biomed. Signal Proc. Control, 174–183 (2014)
5. U. Raghavendra, H. Fujita, S.V. Bhandary, et al., Deep convolution neural network for accurate diagnosis of glaucoma using digital fundus images. Inf. Sci., 41–49 (2018)
6. H. Fu, J. Cheng, Y. Xu, et al., Disc-aware ensemble network for glaucoma screening from fundus image. IEEE Trans. Med. Imaging (2018)
7. U. Raghavendra, H. Fujita, S.V. Bhandary, et al., Deep convolution neural network for accurate diagnosis of glaucoma using digital fundus images. Inf. Sci. **441**, 41–49 (May 2018)
8. J.D.L. Araújo, J.C. Souza, O.P.S. Neto, et al., Glaucoma diagnosis in fundus eye images using diversity indexes. Multimed. Tools Appl., 78 (2019)
9. J. Cuadros, G. Bresnick, EyePACS: An adaptable telemedicine system for diabetic retinopathy screening. J. Diabetes Sci. Technol. **3**(3), 509–516 (2009)
10. K. Jin, H. Lu, Z. Su, et al., Telemedicine screening of retinal diseases with a handheld portable non-mydriatic fundus camera. BMC Ophthalmol., 17 (2017)
11. A. Asquith, G. Horsman, Let the robots do it! – Taking a look at robotic process automation and its potential application in digital forensics. For. Sci. Int. Rep. **1** (2019)
12. M. Ratia, J. Myllarniemi, N. Helander, Robotic process automation – Creating value by digitalizing work in the private healthcare? in *AcademicMindtrek'18*, (2018)
13. F. Huang, M.A. Vasarhelyi, Applying robotic process automation (RPA) in auditing: A framework. Int. J. Account. Inform. Syst. (2019)

14. N. Panwar et al., Fundus photography in the 21st century—A review of recent technological advances and their implications for worldwide healthcare. Telemed. J. E Health, 198–208 (2016)
15. J. Sivaswamy et al., A comprehensive retinal image dataset for the assessment of glaucoma from the optic nerve head analysis. JSM Biomed. Imag. Data Papers **2**(1), 1004 (2015)
16. A. Issac, M. Parthasarthi, M.K. Dutta, An adaptive threshold based algorithm for optic disc and cup segmentation in fundus images. Int. Con. Signal Proc. Integr. Networks, 143–147 (2015)
17. A. Sevastopolsky, Optic disc and cup segmentation methods for glaucoma detection with modification of U-net convolutional neural network. J. Pattern Recogn. Image Anal. Adva. Math. Theory Appl. (2017)

Introducing a Conceptual Framework for Architecting Healthcare 4.0 Systems

Aleksandar Novakovic, Adele H. Marshall, and Carolyn McGregor

1 Introduction

We live in the era of big data where enormous amounts of information are collected each second in both structured and unstructured formats across a number of different platforms and devices. The data underpins all modern enterprises nowadays, and the healthcare industry is no different. When presenting at the doctor's surgery with symptoms, it is the data about the patient that the doctor uses to make an informed diagnosis of their condition, and likewise, it is data that informs the treatments and medications that should be administered and the follow-up during recovery.

This data revolution is impacting significantly on the healthcare industry. The ever evolving health sector consists of a number of inter-related processes whose change not only has an impact on the overall healthcare delivery of care and services but also has an impact on clinicians, healthcare providers and, ultimately, the patient. This complexity of co-existing multiple processes can benefit from big data analytics. In fact, a health sector that fully integrates big data analytics is essential.

The past 7 years has seen the introduction, expansion and maturing of big data analytics in healthcare research and practice. In particular, it offers data tools that can collate, manage and analyse vast amounts of data, structured and unstructured

A. Novakovic (✉) · A. H. Marshall (✉)
School of Mathematics and Physics, Queen's University Belfast, Belfast, UK

C. McGregor
Faculty of Business and IT, Ontario Tech University, Oshawa, Canada

Faculty of Engineering and IT, University of Technology, Sydney, Australia
e-mail: c.mcgregor@ieee.org

H. R. Arabnia et al. (eds.), *Advances in Computer Vision and Computational Biology*, Transactions on Computational Science and Computational Intelligence,
https://doi.org/10.1007/978-3-030-71051-4_45

in nature [1]. There are many sources from which healthcare data can be generated, from clinical to genomic or pharmacological to behavioural, hence emphasizing just some of the variety in healthcare data available. The data is quite often collected and stored across multiple systems which may well be placed in a number of different physical locations and organisations such as healthcare centres, hospitals, government departments and research labs. Each one of these organisations is being overwhelmed by the continuous increase in overall data volume and speed at which it is being generated, illustrating the velocity of big data in healthcare. Data repositories are also experiencing growth in size and complexity so not only by variety, volume, and velocity but also by veracity that exists due to data inconsistency. Such characteristics are commonly known, well-versed features of big data and well-accepted concepts of any modern-day system.

The extra consideration in the healthcare domain is the sensitivity of personal data and the need for a platform that encompasses vast amounts of personal data both from patient records and from medical devices and transforms it into intelligent healthcare systems. The smart environment needs to inform, personalise and support diagnosis and treatment pathways. In this context, any Healthcare 4.0 system shall take one or both of the following two forms: (1) the real-time analysis helps to find out irregularities in the collected data and acts as fast as possible to prevent undesired consequences on the patient's health, or (2) the long-term analysis uses the massive data collected from Internet of things (IoT) devices to uncover insights and identify trends and opportunities.

Consider a hospital setting where there is a central system that records the patient information for a busy intensive care unit. Data will be recorded by the clinical staff regarding the patient condition and treatment alongside data streaming onto the system from medical devices such as a ventilator recording critical information on the ventilation being administered to the patient. It is impossible for a clinician to view all the data for a specific patient; however, real-time analysis of the data can create early alarms to alert the clinician of a change in condition, and additionally, the data can be used to identify any underlying trend or gradual change in the patient's condition. This can act as a decision support mechanism for the clinician and potentially flag up certain characteristics that would otherwise go unnoticed. Likewise, in the community, patients currently diagnosed with type 1 diabetes can have data recorded from their mobile devices such as their insulin pumps that can calculate the required dose of insulin which is monitored in real-time but also can be used in long-term analysis to consider the long-term risk of developing one of the possible multiple complications associated with the condition.

It has previously been predicted that quality of care of the patient and the overall efficiency of the system will be vastly increased with the full implementation of Electronic Health/Care Records (EHRs/ECRs) along with the systematic collection of physiological data by healthcare providers [2]. However, this is not yet the reality, despite advances in data collection and storage [3]. The key challenges are within the implementation of new approaches to inform decisions based on vast amounts of data and the ability to embed such new algorithms into the healthcare system. Even to this day, clinical decision support systems are not being used to their full potential and are being restricted to draw from just one data set or have predefined rules embedded within.

Our previous research considered real-time clinical decision support systems (CDSS) identifying the lack of current relevant metrics and clinical feedback as the biggest hindrance to the development of real-time CDSS [4, 5]. This motivated us to develop a set of new performance analytics techniques, with particular emphasis on CDSS for improving the quality of care of mechanically ventilated patients. This resulted in new suitable metrics to evaluate a CDSS working as decision support to the clinicians. But what happens when there is more than one CDSS or when there are several different algorithms performing different functions in one healthcare system? Another challenge is how the algorithms potentially share and use knowledge from one another while protecting patient data, confidentiality and intellectual property.

Although there are many studies proposing architectural solutions for various use cases, such as mechanical ventilation [5, 6] and neonatal care [7], all of these solutions lack flexibility as they are tightly coupled to existing clinical systems. Furthermore, the systems are very complex in nature, each using a different blend of technologies and cloud services which makes practical implementation of proposed systems and collaboration between research teams difficult, if not impossible. For example, the published proposal may rely on using Python programming language and cloud-based technologies and services, while employees in the IT department of the hospital are specialized in. NET technologies and may not have access to the cloud applications. This results in a system that cannot be accessed or implemented by the hospital team, and so the proposed solution and benefits of improved quality of care are not realised.

In order to reap the full benefits of new Healthcare 4.0 systems, such hurdles need to be overcome to release the users and researchers from the ongoing challenges of technology differences and dealing with sensitive personal data. To the best of our knowledge, there is no paper that proposes a solution that would enable easier access to the healthcare data and collaboration between medical practitioners and researchers. We propose a unique approach that utilizes the Apache Kafka data streaming platform as the underpinning technology to build a conceptual framework with the goal to provide a set of guidelines for overcoming such challenges.

This chapter is organised as follows. Section 2 provides a brief overview of Apache Kafka discussing the challenges related to architecting and building big data pipelines in general. Section 3 addresses these challenges by introducing a framework as a set of guidelines for building scalable, secure and fault-tolerant data pipelines particularly for the Healthcare 4.0 industry. Section 4 provides an overview of related work and describes how our architectural solution differs from anything that has been done previously, and Section 5 concludes this chapter and offers our thoughts on future research.

2 Relevant Theoretical Concepts

2.1 Apache Kafka

Apache Kafka [8] is an open-source distributed messaging platform [9] built for collecting and distributing large volumes of data, at high velocities. The entire Kafka's ecosystem is based on the producer-consumer messaging pattern [10] characterised by five key components: message, topic, producer, consumer and broker.

The *messages* are basic data units within the ecosystem, which are generated by the processes called *producers*. In order to achieve the efficiency in the performance, the producers send messages in batches to the centralised *cluster* consisting of single or multiple servers (also known as *broker/s*) where they get organised into categories called *topics*. Using the RDBMS terminology, the closest analogy to explain the concepts of messages and topics would be rows and tables in the database, respectively.

For achieving high scalability and redundancy, each topic can furthermore be segregated into multiple *partitions* and each partition replicated across multiple brokers within the cluster to obtain performance far superior to the ability of a single server. It is important to highlight that all of the messages belonging to a single batch are published to the same topic and partition in an append-only manner.

Opposite to the producers, the *consumers* are the processes that are used for reading messages from single or multiple topics, in the same order as they are being produced (i.e. first in, first out (FIFO) principle).

Customised producers and consumers in Apache Kafka can be defined either by using low-level producer-consumer API or by using the higher level Connect framework. The former approach is used in instances where researchers have full access to the underlying systems' programming logic and are able to modify the code of the application they want to connect an application to so that they can either push data into or pull data from Kafka. Alternatively, the Connect framework is used for the scalable and reliable streaming data between Apache Kafka and other externally managed data stores that are not necessarily written by the researchers for which the code cannot be modified [11].

Data streaming between Kafka and other external data stores is performed using processes called *connectors*, which can be either *source* or *sink connectors*. Source connectors are used for ingesting entire data sources (e.g. relational and non-relational databases, key-value stores, file systems, search indexes, etc.) and streaming the updates to Kafka topics when these occur, while sink connectors are used for delivering data from Kafka topics into destination data sources (e.g. warehouses, data lakes, etc.) for batch analysis [12]. A plethora of source and sink connectors that can be used for connecting Kafka with various data sources can be found on the Confluent Hub portal [13].

Features that differentiate Kafka from other similar producer-consumer messaging systems (e.g. RabbitMQ, ActiveMQ, etc.) are the way in which the messages are immediately purged upon consuming and its unique capability to persist the topics and their messages on disk for some configurable amount of time or until the designated storage space is filled. This feature enables consumers to replay the messages when needed which is crucial for the fault tolerance of the downstream systems and can facilitate longer-term analytics. All persistence settings can be tuned for each topic separately, and upon exceeding either the allowed disk's quota or the retention time, the messages are automatically deleted from the system [14].

2.2 Challenges in Building Data Integration Systems

Narkhede et al. [11] state that the most important characteristics to take into consideration when designing data pipelines with a focus on integrating multiple systems are timeliness, security, reliability and scalability. Apache Kafka meets all of these requirements as the technology for the implementation of these data integration systems:

1. *Timeliness:* Generally speaking, the timeliness characteristic refers to the capability of the data integration systems to provide support for the variable consumption needs of different consumer systems. For instance, some consumers might expect to receive their data within just a few milliseconds of its generation, while others may wish to receive it weekly in bulk. Bearing in mind that Apache Kafka is a distributed messaging platform with scalable and reliable storage capabilities, it can act as a huge buffer for received messages enabling decoupling time-sensitivity requirements between the producers and consumers. This allows producers to write to the Kafka cluster as frequently or infrequently as required and consumers to read and deliver the messages either as they arrive or to work in batches and read the messages that were accumulated in the cluster over time or all at once [11].
2. *Security:* When it comes to the data integration pipelines, the main security considerations are those related to the (i) encryption, (ii) authentication and (iii) authorisation. Kafka provides support for SSL encryption of the data as it is transferred from the data sources to Kafka topics or from the topics to sinks, which is of huge importance especially when the data cross data centre boundaries. To prevent unauthorised and unauthenticated access to the data, Kafka supports the implementation of role-based access control (RBAC) authorisation and SASL authentication mechanisms. Additionally, Kafka also provides audit logs to track access [11].
3. *Reliability:* The main reliability concern is the design of data integration pipelines that avoid single points of failure and permit fast and automatic recovery from all kinds of failure events. In Kafka, the data delivery reliability can be ensured through two different delivery mechanisms: *at-least-once* and *exactly once delivery* [11].

4. *Scalability:* The requirement for the data integration pipelines is to support very high throughputs and to be able to scale out in order to support increased messaging loads, when it is needed. By acting as a buffer between producers and consumers, Kafka does not require the coupling of consumer throughput to producer throughput, as is the case with many other messaging brokers. Instead, because of its capabilities to accumulate received messages on disk, Kafka has the ability to scale either side of the pipeline by adding consumers or producers independently and matching the changing throughput requirements [11].

3 A Conceptual Framework for Architecting Healthcare 4.0 Applications

In this section, we introduce the conceptual framework with the primary goal of bringing in the standardisation and ease that is required for the development of Healthcare 4.0 applications. Our proposal extends and enhances the current development of healthcare applications which follows a three-tiered architecture consisting of the Data Emitting Layer (DEL), the Healthcare Gateway Layer (HGL) and the Application Layer (APL).

As the name suggests, DEL includes any possible healthcare data emitting mechanism which includes, but is not limited to, devices for collecting medical images (X-rays, CAT scans, magnetic resonance, etc.), devices for collecting sensory readings such as those necessary for vital signs monitoring (e.g. pulse rate, respiration rate, blood pressure, body temperature, etc.), or data from the healthcare professionals who, having collected information about the patient, are in charge of writing the diagnosis and prescriptions or admitting and discharging patients to and from the hospital. Depending on the source and type of the collected data, using various protocols (such as TCP, HTTP, MQTT, and Bluetooth), this information is then transported to HGL where it is usually persisted in the electronic medical records (EMR), Hadoop Distributed File System (HDFS), AWS S3, or similar storage solutions for further processing and analysis. The healthcare providers are the key stakeholders so they have to maintain both DEL and HGL due to the sensitivity of the patient information. The researchers and academic collaborators outside of these organisations need to pass rigorous security checks and obtain special data access rights to be able to utilise just a small portion of the information for the purpose of developing clinical decision support systems and other advanced applications in the APL. Each healthcare organisation has its own set of internal policies, hence making the requesting of these permissions and eventual access to the data a very lengthy process which generally can take several months. If we take into account that every healthcare organisation will utilise a different combination of technologies and programming languages for running their internal IT infrastructure (.NET vs JVM vs other programming stacks, cloud vs on-premise deployment, different cloud providers if the cloud is used, relational vs non-relational databases for storing information and different vendors of these technologies, etc.), research organisations need to be prepared for a huge degree of flexibility and adaptability in order to start using the data from these systems. Cumulatively, this all causes a serious negative impact to the speed of development of Healthcare 4.0 applications, thus raising the need for creating a standardised framework for easier collaboration between the healthcare providers and research organisations.

To overcome these issues, we propose adding an additional layer to decouple communication between HGL and APL. We name this extra layer the Data Pipeline Layer (DPL), and due to the reasons previously described, we selected Apache Kafka as its underpinning technology. Figure 1 provides an overview of the proposed architecture.

To facilitate data transfer between Kafka and existing data sources in HGL and APL, we propose using Kafka Connect. The main motivation for proposing this framework is the fact that it provides out-of-the-box features like configuration management, offset storage, parallelization, error handling, and support for different data types, and most importantly, it is extremely flexible as it can be used by non-developers who would only need to configure the connectors for communication with the data sources [11].

The healthcare providers (data owners) should be in charge of maintaining the Kafka cluster and source connectors. Due to the advanced security capabilities which enable data encryption and protection of data stored in Kafka, from unauthorised and unauthenticated access, healthcare providers are able to pre-plan what datasets they are willing to share with potential research collaborators and have a fine-grain control over adequate data access rights. Research organisations with the right data access permission would be able to start using healthcare data by attaching their preferred sink connector to the Kafka cluster provided by the healthcare organisation. Similar to how data exchanges between HGL and APL, if the data sharing agreement permits, Apache Kafka could be used for establishing the connection, hence fostering the collaboration between the research organisations in the Research Collaboration Layer (Fig. 1).

4 Related Work

The Apache Kafka has been increasingly used as a distributed streaming platform in real-time processing of IoT events [15], Industry 4.0 [16] and smart cities [9].

Gokalp et al. [17] created a real-time patient monitoring system which collected patients' vital sign parameters: heart rate, blood pressure, respiration, skin temperature, and blood oxygen level SpO2 using IoT devices. Kafka was used as a message broker to distribute the data from IoT devices to Apache Storm [18] which processed the data in real time and warned clinicians if collected values crossed predefined thresholds.

There are two fundamental differences between their work and the conceptual framework proposed in this chapter. The first difference is in the way that Kafka

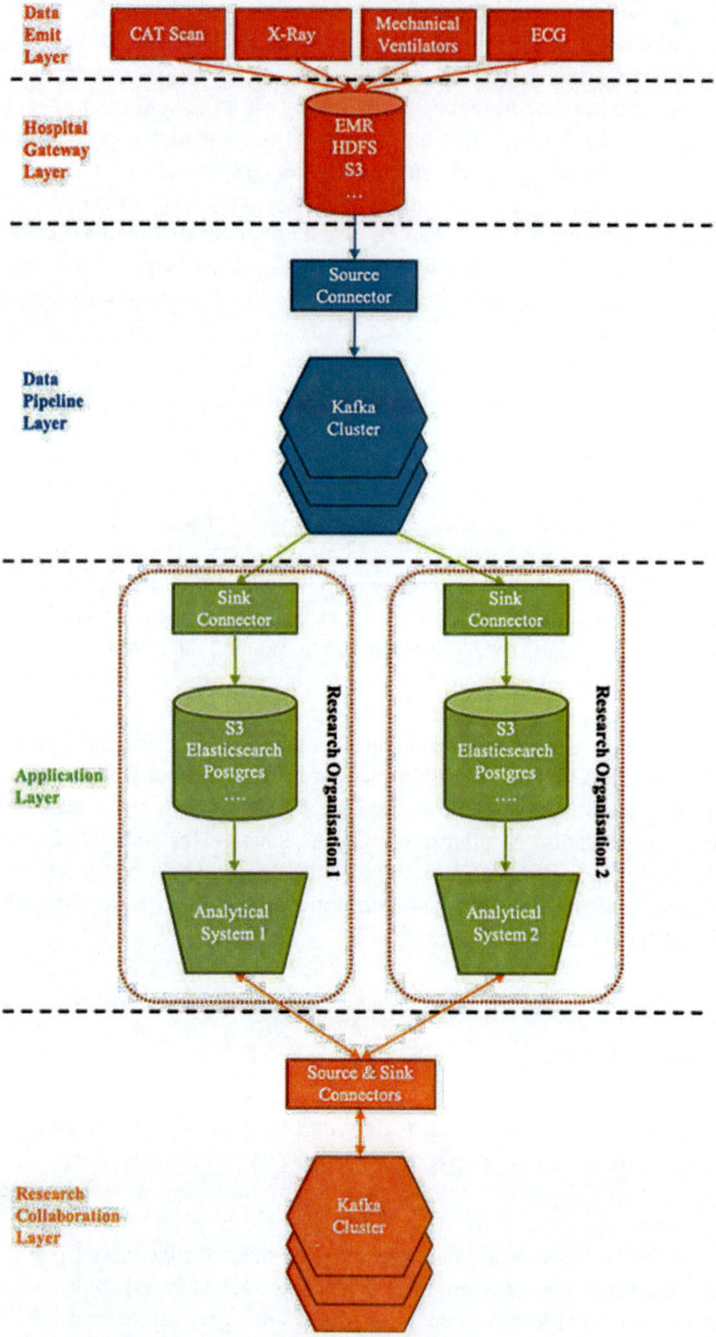

Fig. 1 A conceptual framework for architecting Healthcare 4.0 applications

communicates with the DEL. Gokalp et al. [17] have full access to the underlying systems' programming logic and are able to modify the application code they want to connect to so that they can push data into Kafka directly from the IoT devices. The majority of Healthcare 4.0 projects do not have this condition as the healthcare providers are the data owners. Hence, the Kafka Connect framework is a better alternative.

The second difference is in the transformations that the pipelines perform. Gokalp et al. [17] use the ETL (extract-transform-load) approach where the data pipeline, or in their case Apache Storm [18], makes modifications to the data as it passes through. The main disadvantage of this method is that valuable information is getting lost in the process which automatically creates restrictions on those who want to process the data further down the pipeline [11]. Hence, in our chapter, we propose using the ELT (extract-load-transform) process instead providing maximum flexibility to users of the target system, since they have access to all the data in the original format [11]. Figure 2 provides an illustration of the proposed architecture for a research organisation utilising data for their healthcare analytics applications from two different healthcare providers.

The Artemis platform makes use of the Vines device connectivity software to enable data acquisition from medical devices within neonatal ICUs [19]. Vines utilises RabbitMQ. Vines was chosen due to the proprietary messaging protocol for the output signals from many medical devices including those used within the collaborating NICUs for the Artemis deployments. Decoupling of the data collection and data acquisition components from the remaining analytics, data storage and visualisation components of Artemis was proposed in [20]. Both Vines and Python scripts were assessed for their applicability for the data acquisition function within the context of low resource settings with a case study context of the NICU within Belgaum Children's Hospital, India. The component nature of Artemis enables the Vines component to be easily replaced by the architecture proposed in this chapter.

A key challenge for different healthcare providers is ensuring that new medical device procurement procedures ensure procured support output of data streams and utilise standardised and well-documented messaging protocols rather than proprietary messaging approaches.

5 Conclusions and Further Directions

This chapter introduces a novel conceptual framework as a consistent architecture for Healthcare 4.0 applications. The framework proposes Apache Kafka as the core technology for creating data integration pipelines bringing standardisation to the healthcare systems, enabling easier communication between healthcare providers and researchers.

The architecture offers a safe and secure environment in which multiple applications and algorithms from different organisations and providers can seamlessly

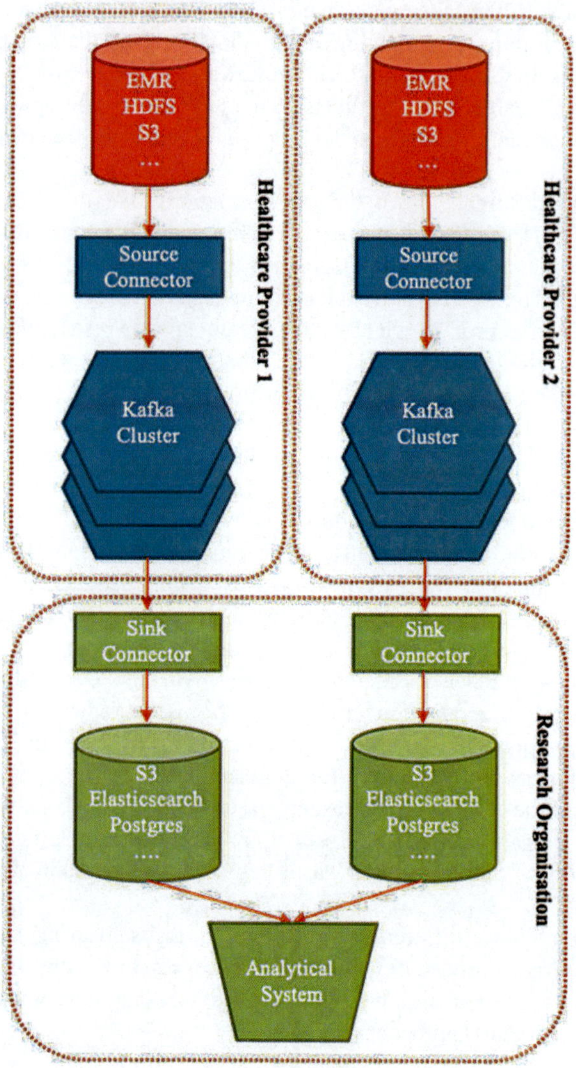

Fig. 2 A research organisation utilising data from two different healthcare providers

"plug" into the healthcare providers' Kafka "socket" to utilise sensitive data without any issue with data access, or security. Each healthcare provider has their "socket" created for each organisation, and likewise, each organisation may have multiple "sockets" in which they can "plug" into to access the relevant healthcare data set and provide their service.

Further directions of the research are to deploy previously designed healthcare analytics applications to the new architecture in a hospital setting.

Acknowledgments This work has been supported by Queen's University Belfast, United Kingdom, and Ontario Tech University, Canada.

References

1. A. Belle, R. Thiagarajan, S.M.R. Soroushmehr, F. Navidi, D.A. Beard, K. Najarian, *Big Data Analytics in Healthcare*, vol 2015 (Hindawi Publishing Corporation, 2015), pp. 1–16
2. T.D. Gunter, N.P. Terry, The Emergence of National Electronic Health Record Architectures in the United States and Australia: Models, Costs, and Questions. J. Med. Internet Res. **7**(1), e3 (2005)
3. A.S. Kellerman, What it will take to achieve the as-yet-unfulfilled promises of health information technology. Health Aff. **32**(1), 63–68 (2013)
4. A.H. Marshall, A. Novakovic, Analysing the performance of a real-time healthcare 4.0 system using shared frailty time to event models, in *2019 IEEE 32nd International Symposium on Computer-Based Medical Systems (CBMS)*, (Cordoba, Spain, 2019)
5. A. Novakovic, A.H. Marshall, Introducing the DM-P approach for analysing the performances of real-time clinical decision support systems. Knowl.-Based Syst. **198**, 105877 (2020)
6. C.J. Gillan, A. Novakovic, A.H. Marshall, M. Shyamsundar, D.S. Nikolopoulos, Expediting assessments of database performance for streams of respiratory parameters. Comput. Biol. Med. **100**, 186–195 (2018)
7. S. Balaji, M. Patil, C. McGregor, A cloud based big data based online health analytics for rural NICUs and PICUs in India: Opportunities and challenges, in *2017 IEEE 30th International Symposium on Computer-Based Medical Systems (CBMS)*, (Thessaloniki, Greece, 2017)
8. Apache Kafka, [Online]. Available: https://kafka.apache.org. Accessed 28 Feb 2020
9. J.Y. Fernandez-Rodriguez et al., Benchmarking real-time vehicle data streaming models for a smart city. Inf. Syst. **72**, 62–76 (2017)
10. C. Barba-Gonzales et al., On the design of a framework integrating an optimization engine with streaming technologies. Futur. Gener. Comput. Syst. **107**, 538–550 (2020)
11. N. Narkhede, G. Shapira, T. Palino, *Kafka: The Definitive Guide* (O'Reilly Media, Inc, 2017)
12. Kafka Connect, [Online]. Available: https://bit.ly/2SSpLEH. Accessed 28 Feb 2020
13. Confluent Hub, [Online]. Available: www.confluent.io/hub/. Accessed 28 Feb 2020
14. P. Dobbelaere, K.S. Esmaili, Kafka versus RabbitMQ: A comparative study of two industry reference publish/subscribe implementations: Industry Paper, in *DEBS '17: Proceedings of the 11th ACM International Conference on Distributed and Event-based Systems*, (Barcelona, Spain, 2017)
15. D. Plaza-Corral, I. Medina-Bulo, G. Ortiz, J. Boubeta-Puig, A stream processing architecture for heterogeneous data sources in the Internet of Things. Comp. Stand. Inter. **70**, 1–13 (2020)
16. R. Sahal, J.G. Breslin, M.I. Ali, Big data and stream processing platforms for Industry 4.0 requirements mapping for a predictive maintenance use case. J. Manuf. Syst. **54**, 138–151 (2020)
17. M.O. Gokalp, A. Kocyigit, E. Eren, A visual programming framework for distributed Internet of Things centric complex event processing. Comput. Electr. Eng. **74**, 581–604 (2019)
18. Apache Storm, [Online]. Available: https://storm.apache.org. Accessed 28 Feb 2020
19. C. McGregor, C. Inibhunu, J. Glass, I. Doyle, A. Gates, J. Madill, J.E. Pugh, Health analytics as a service with artemis cloud: Service availability, in *Proceedings of the 42nd IEEE Engineering in Medicine and Biology Conference*, (Montreal, Canada, 2020)
20. M. Bastwadkar, C. McGregor, S. Balaji, A cloud based big data health-analytics-as-a-service framework to support low resource setting neonatal intensive care unit, in *Proceedings of the 4th International Conference on Medical and Health Informatics (ICMHI 2020)*, (Kamakura City, Japan, 2020)

A Machine Learning-Driven Approach to Predict the Outcome of Prostate Biopsy: Identifying Cancer, Clinically Significant Disease, and Unfavorable Pathological Features on Prostate Biopsy

John L. Pfail, Dara J. Lundon, Parita Ratnani, Vinayak Wagaskar, Peter Wiklund, and Ashutosh K. Tewari

1 Introduction

One man out of nine will be diagnosed with prostate cancer during his lifetime, making prostate cancer the most commonly diagnosed solid organ malignancy in men. Worldwide, there were 1,276,106 new cases reported in 2018 [1]. In the United States alone, there is expected 191,930 new cases and 33,330 deaths attributable to prostate cancer for 2020 [2]. The advent of prostate-specific antigen (PSA) to aid in prostate cancer (PCa) diagnosis in the late 1980s has drastically influenced both the diagnosis of and mortality from prostate cancer [3]. Current guidelines for screening and early detection of prostate cancer recommend utilizing PSA and/or abnormal digital rectal exam (DRE) to guide the need for transrectal ultrasound (TRUS)-guided prostate biopsy [4].

Although most men with prostate cancer have elevated PSA levels, the current evidence regarding the benefit of population-based serum PSA screening for PCa remains controversial with recent reports showing that roughly 15% of men with a PSA level below 4 ng/mL are also diagnosed with prostate cancer [5–7]. Recently, clinicians have employed the use of several other pre-biopsy measures such as PSA dynamics, Prostate Health Index (PHI), 4Kscore®, and novel biomarkers to more accurately assess which patients are at an increased risk for harboring PCa [8, 9].

Overdiagnosis is a clinical and ethical challenge; in the context of PCa, it refers to a diagnosis of PCa that would not otherwise affect a patient's quality of life or cause death. It could occur because either the cancer cells are slow growing or well differentiated and that patient co-morbidity results in death from other causes before meaningful clinical progression of the PCa [10]. One potential approach to

J. L. Pfail (✉) · D. J. Lundon · P. Ratnani · V. Wagaskar · P. Wiklund · A. K. Tewari
Department of Urology, Icahn School of Medicine at Mount Sinai, New York, NY, USA
e-mail: John.Pfail@icahn.mssm.edu

H. R. Arabnia et al. (eds.), *Advances in Computer Vision and Computational Biology*, Transactions on Computational Science and Computational Intelligence,
https://doi.org/10.1007/978-3-030-71051-4_46

help reduced overdiagnosis is through the development and use of predictive tools to aid in the differentiation of clinically significant from indolent tumors.

Approximately 1.3 million prostate biopsies are performed every year in the United States [11]. Several risk tools have been described in the literature that predict the outcome of prostate biopsy [12]. However, fewer studies have aimed to predict the detection of clinically significant disease or unfavorable pathology which is associated with adverse outcomes in prostate cancer [13–15]. Existing risk tools are derived predominantly in single ethnicity groups, using data from northern European countries in the ERSPC trials [16].

There is a need for novel and accurate tools to help identify each patient's risk of PCa, clinically significant disease, and likelihood of having unfavorable pathology using prognostic parameters in patients from a multiethnic cohort, as one might experience in practice in the United States. The aim of this study is to create an easy-to-use risk calculator for the prediction of (i) prostate cancer, (ii) clinically significant disease, and (iii) unfavorable pathology in a multiethnic cohort of males presenting for consideration of prostate biopsy to a clinical practice in a large academic urology practice in the United States.

2 Methods

2.1 *Study Population*

After receiving Institutional Review Board approval, we identified 2734 patients in a prospectively maintained database who were assessed for prostate cancer and underwent prostate biopsy between 2014 and 2019.

2.2 *Outcome and Study Design*

The outcomes of interest in the present study were the presence of prostate cancer, clinically significant disease, and unfavorable pathology. The presence of prostate cancer was defined as Gleason grade $\geq$6 (Gleason grade group [GGG] $\geq$1). Clinically significant disease was defined as GGG $\geq$3. Unfavorable pathology was defined as pT3a or pT3b and GGG $\geq$3. Variables included in our model consisted of PSA, age, race, and MRI characteristics. This included the Prostate Imaging-Reporting and Data System (PI-RADS) for scoring prostate lesions.

2.3 Statistical Analysis

The sample size was based on the available data from all patients who were assessed for prostate cancer and underwent prostate biopsy between 2014 and 2019. Descriptive statistics including frequencies and proportions were reported for categorical variables, while medians and interquartile ranges (IQRs) were reported for continuous variables.

Data was divided into a training and holdout testing set using an 80%:20% ratio. The training set was used to train the classifiers, and the hold-out set was used to evaluate the predictive ability of the model.

To identify the relative importance of each feature, feature selection was performed using the least absolute shrinkage and selection operator (LASSO) regression method [17]. Prediction models were built using an ensemble model incorporating machine learning techniques such as logistic regression, decision tree, random forest, and support vector machine to predict each outcome: a diagnosis of prostate cancer, significant prostate cancer, and unfavorable pathology.

The performance of the prediction tool was assessed as previously described [18]. Briefly, discriminative ability was assessed using receiver operating characteristic (ROC) curves. Area underneath the ROC curve (AUC) was calculated for each risk calculator. Calibration plots were computed by comparing observed proportions of cancer to mean calculated risks by the respective risk calculator deciles observed in the cohort. The Hosmer–Lemeshow chi-square test was used to compare the same observed rates to predicted risks across the deciles for each calculator. For this test, a $p < 0.05$ indicates a poor agreement between predicted risks and actual observed risk. Decision curve analysis was performed to assess for the gain derived from the respective risk calculator over the corresponding net benefit curves of two alternative strategies: referring no patients or all patients to biopsy. Decision curve analysis was performed using the *rmda* package in R version 3.6.0 [19]. All other analyses were conducted in R version 3.6.0. All tests were two-sided with a significance threshold of $p < 0.05$.

3 Results

3.1 Study Population Characteristics

Our final study cohort consisted of 2734 patients who underwent systemic TRUS biopsy for evaluation of prostate cancer. Overall, 1528 (55.9%) patients had prostate cancer, 1318 (48.2%) had clinically significant prostate cancer, and 725 (26.5%) had unfavorable pathology on final biopsy report (Table 1). Additionally, 1119 (40.9%) patients underwent MRI-targeted fusion biopsy in addition to systemic TRUS biopsy. The median age of our cohort was 64 (IQR: 58–69) years old with a

Table 1 Descriptive characteristics of 2734 patients who underwent prostate biopsy at a single academic institution

	[ALL]	Cancer	CS cancer	Unfavorable pathology
Variable	$N = 2734$	$N = 1528$	$N = 1318$	$N = 725$
Median (IQR) age	64.0 [58.0;69.0]	64.0 [58.0;68.0]	64.0 [59.0;69.0]	66.0 [61.0;70.0]
Race, *n* (%)				
Other	2510 (91.8%)	1361 (89.1%)	1184 (89.8%)	659 (90.9%)
African American	224 (8.19%)	167 (10.9%)	134 (10.2%)	66 (9.10%)
Median (IQR) PSA, ng/mL	6.20 [4.30;9.98]	7.00 [4.84;11.8]	7.40 [4.98;12.2]	8.50 [5.28;14.4]
Median (IQR) PSA-d, ng/mL	0.14 [0.08;0.22]	0.18 [0.11;0.27]	0.18 [0.12;0.28]	0.20 [0.12;0.31]
DRE, *n* (%)				
Normal	1770 (64.7%)	814 (53.3%)	638 (48.4%)	276 (38.1%)
Abnormal	964 (35.3%)	714 (46.7%)	680 (51.6%)	449 (61.9%)
PI-RADS, *n* (%)				
0	1452 (53.1%)	573 (37.5%)	465 (35.3%)	236 (32.6%)
3	268 (9.80%)	150 (9.82%)	112 (8.50%)	42 (5.79%)
4	565 (20.7%)	402 (26.3%)	361 (27.4%)	182 (25.1%)
5	449 (16.4%)	403 (26.4%)	380 (28.8%)	265 (36.6%)
Systemic bx: Yes, *n* (%)	2734 (100%)	1528 (100%)	1318 (100%)	725 (100%)
Targeted bx, *n* (%)				
No	1615 (59.1%)	988 (64.7%)	833 (63.2%)	462 (63.7%)
Yes	1119 (40.9%)	540 (35.3%)	485 (36.8%)	263 (36.3%)
Gleason grade group, *n* (%)				
0	1206 (44.1%)	0 (0%)	0 (0%)	0 (0%)
1	210 (7.68%)	210 (13.7%)	0 (0%)	0 (0%)
2	593 (21.7%)	593 (38.8%)	593 (45.0%)	0 (0%)
3	315 (11.5%)	315 (20.6%)	315 (23.9%)	315 (43.4%)
4	227 (8.30%)	227 (14.9%)	227 (17.2%)	227 (31.3%)
5	183 (6.69%)	183 (12.0%)	183 (13.9%)	183 (25.2%)

median PSA of 6.20 (IQR: 4.30–9.98) ng/mL. The majority (64.7%) of our patients had a normal DRE at time of presentation.

3.2 *Prediction of Prostate Cancer, Significant Disease, and Unfavorable Pathology*

After performing internal validation, the AUCs of the models were 82% (95% CI: 80.4–83.5), 83.8% (95% CI: 82.3–85.2), and 88.1% (95% CI: 86.7–89.5) for

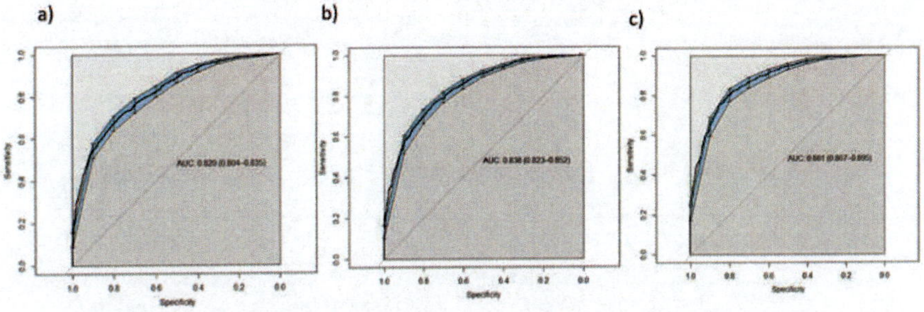

Fig. 1 Receiver operating characteristic (ROC) curves for the detection of (**a**) prostate cancer, (**b**) clinically significant prostate cancer, and (**c**) unfavorable pathology on initial prostate biopsy

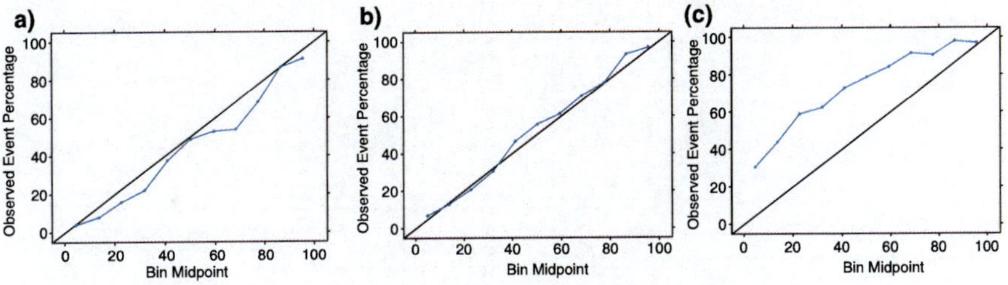

Fig. 2 Calibration plots of observed vs predicted probability of (**a**) prostate cancer, (**b**) clinically significant prostate cancer, and (**c**) unfavorable pathology on initial prostate biopsy

predicting prostate cancer, clinically significant disease, and unfavorable pathology, respectively (Fig. 1).

The calibration plots, exploring the relationship between observed and predicted values, are shown in Fig. 2. Calibration plots can be said to describe the reliability of the predicted risk. Calibration plots indicate that the derived risk tools are well calibrated; across all calculated risks, the model accurately estimates the risk of a biopsy diagnosis being positive (Fig. 2a) and having significant prostate cancer (Fig. 2b) and underestimates the risk of unfavorable pathology (Fig. 2c).

Decision curves for PCa diagnosis, clinically significant disease, and unfavorable pathology were plotted in Fig. 3. Decision curves calculate a "net benefit" so as to provide a metric of the clinical utility of using such a risk tool. Across the entire range of clinically useful threshold probabilities, there is a superior net benefit for each outcome, predicting prostate cancer (Fig. 3a) and predicting clinically significant prostate cancer (Fig. 3b) and unfavorable pathology (Fig. 3c), than if one was to have adopted a strategy of either performing a biopsy in everyone or no one.

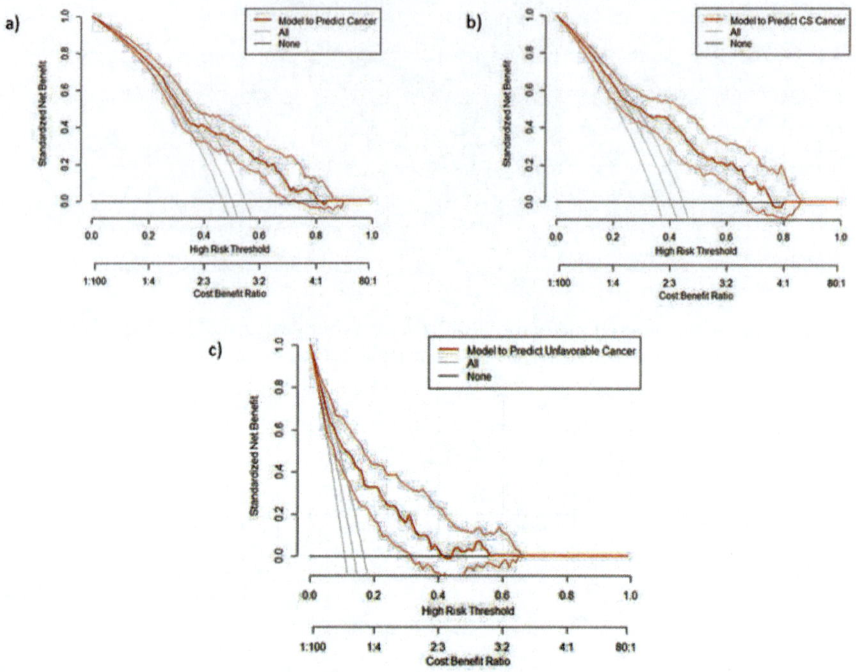

Fig. 3 Decision curve analyses showing the net benefit associated with the use of the predictive models for the prediction of (**a**) prostate cancer, (**b**) clinically significant prostate cancer, and (**c**) unfavorable pathology on initial biopsy

4 Discussion

Personalizing diagnostic guidelines for prostate cancer represents a great challenge, as it requires urologists to balance the risks of overdiagnosis vs the benefits of early cancer detection. Given this, clinicians often employ a combination of PSA levels, PSA dynamics, and novel biomarkers along with other clinical factors, such as family history, age, DRE, and MRI findings in their decision to treat patients.

The aim of the present study was to produce models for the prediction of (i) prostate cancer, (ii) clinically significant prostate cancer, and (iii) unfavorable pathology among men with no previous history of PCa who presented for consideration of biopsy. The predictors used in our models included PSA, age, race, and MRI characteristics. Our models are therefore based on readily available variables, which can easily be used in clinical practice.

In our patient cohort, the overall rate of cancer detection and clinically significant disease was 55.9% and 48.2%, respectively. A similar study, which assessed the added value of prostate cancer antigen 3 in the identification of men at risk for harboring prostate cancer, reported that 46% and 20% of patients were diagnosed with any PCa and high-grade PCa (Gleason sum >= 7) following systemic

TRUS-guided biopsy [14]. However, in our study, 40.9% of patients underwent MRI-targeted biopsies in addition to the standard systemic biopsy. The use of MRI with MRI-US fusion-targeted biopsy has been shown to detect more clinically significant prostate cancer than systemic biopsy, which may have contributed to the relatively high diagnostic rate in our cohort [20].

Among current models, Bjurlin et al. created novel pre-biopsy nomograms, which incorporated PSA density, age, and MRI findings to predict the probability of overall PCa and clinically significant PCa on MRI-targeted and combined MRI-targeted and systematic prostate biopsy. In biopsy-naive patients, the AUC for predicting any cancer was 78%, and the AUC for predicting clinically significant disease was 84% [21]. Similarly, Zaytoun et al. retrospectively reviewed 1551 men who underwent initial extended prostate biopsy and created two nomograms to predict PCa (AUC: 73%) and high-grade PCa (AUC: 71%) using age, race, PSA level, percent-free PSA, family history of PCa, and DRE findings [22]. In addition, conventional screening with PSA has repeatedly been shown to underperform in accurately detecting prostate cancer, with a recently reported AUC of 66%. Granted, there has been some diagnostic improvement with the advent of PHI and PI-RADS scoring. However, the performance of PHI is still poor, with an AUC of 77% for predicting PCa in males with a PSA of 4–10 ng/ml [23]. Additionally, the PI-RADS v2 score is not perfect as recent reports using the threshold of $\geq$4 showed an AUC of 79% for predicting clinically significant cancer [24]. Therefore, the predictive accuracy of our models for PCa (AUC: 82%) and CS-PCa (AUC: 84%) is comparable to those in previous reports, and they perform significantly better than traditional screening methods utilizing PSA, PI-RADS v2 score, or PHI alone.

In addition to stronger performance, our proposed models offer several advantages over those currently in the literature. The application of previous predictive nomograms has focused mainly on the overall cancer detection rate, with little differentiation between the presence of clinically significant or indolent tumors. With the rising concerns of over-detection and emerging active surveillance for patients with favorable low-risk disease, accurately determining an individual's risk for clinically significant PCa is of utmost importance [25]. The statistical models employed by such multivariate risk tools can improve the efficiency of prostate cancer detection and exceed that of other common approaches such as age-normalized PSA [26–28].

Despite the satisfactory performance of previous models, to the best of our knowledge, this is the only study which aims at predicting unfavorable pathology from pre-biopsy clinical characteristics, with an AUC of 88%. It is well known that there is a significant difference in patient outcomes between different grade groups [29, 30]. However, recent reports suggest a misclassification between certain histologically distinct carcinoma patterns [31]. For example, within grade group 2 ($3 + 4 = 7$), a small focus of "poorly formed glands" is assigned the same risk group designation as a small focus of "cribriform glands." It has been reported that the presence of cribriform glands is correlated with worse outcomes [32, 33]. By applying our nomogram, we believe that there is the potential to both reduce overdiagnosis and increase the accuracy of a clinician's ability to counsel patients presenting for biopsy consideration.

Our study is not without limitations. A major limitation of our study is inherent in the retrospective nature, which comes with intrinsic limitations and potentials for bias including selection bias. In addition, 40.9% of the biopsies in our cohort were targeted, which may limit the generalization of our proposed models. Lastly, the presented results were obtained from a large single academic institution serving a large and multiethnic catchment area and need to be externally validated.

5 Conclusions

Machine learning methods can be used to predict the clinically meaningful outcomes of prostate biopsies and demonstrate excellent discriminative ability and calibration and provide a superior net benefit than other commonly employed strategies over a wide range of threshold risk probabilities. Such multivariable risk prediction models can be used to further aid patient counselling for those undergoing prostate biopsy.

Acknowledgments This work would not have been possible without the consent and participation of the patients undergoing investigation for prostate cancer, and we would like to acknowledge their selfless contribution to the advancement of medical care.

References

1. F. Bray et al., Global cancer statistics 2018: GLOBOCAN estimates of incidence and mortality worldwide for 36 cancers in 185 countries. CA Cancer J. Clin. **68**, 394–424 (2018). https://doi.org/10.3322/caac.21492
2. R.L. Siegel, K.D. Miller, A. Jemal, Cancer statistics, 2020. CA Cancer J. Clin. **70**, 7–30 (2020). https://doi.org/10.3322/caac.21590
3. T. Byers et al., A midpoint assessment of the American Cancer Society challenge goal to halve the U.S. cancer mortality rates between the years 1990 and 2015. Cancer **107**, 396–405 (2006). https://doi.org/10.1002/cncr.21990
4. N. Mottet et al., EAU-ESTRO-SIOG guidelines on prostate cancer. Part 1: screening, diagnosis, and local treatment with curative intent. Eur. Urol. **71**, 618–629 (2017). https://doi.org/10.1016/j.eururo.2016.08.003
5. J.J. Fenton et al., Prostate-specific antigen-based screening for prostate cancer: Evidence report and systematic review for the US preventive services task force. JAMA **319**, 1914–1931 (2018). https://doi.org/10.1001/jama.2018.3712
6. R.M. Martin et al., Effect of a low-intensity PSA-based screening intervention on prostate cancer mortality: The CAP randomized clinical trial. JAMA **319**, 883–895 (2018). https://doi.org/10.1001/jama.2018.0154
7. G.L. Andriole et al., Mortality results from a randomized prostate-cancer screening trial. N. Engl. J. Med. **360**, 1310–1319 (2009). https://doi.org/10.1056/NEJMoa0810696
8. D. Lundon, S. Loeb, Prostate-specific antigen velocity risk count to discern significant from indolent prostate cancer. Rev. Urol. **16**, 154–156 (2014)

9. R.W. Foley et al., Improving multivariable prostate cancer risk assessment using the prostate health index. BJU Int. **116**, 31–31 (2015)
10. L. Klotz, Prostate cancer overdiagnosis and overtreatment. Curr. Opin. Endocrinol. Diabetes Obes. **20**, 204–209 (2013). https://doi.org/10.1097/MED.0b013e328360332a
11. S. Loeb, H.B. Carter, S.I. Berndt, W. Ricker, E.M. Schaeffer, Complications after prostate biopsy: Data from SEER-Medicare. J. Urol. **186**, 1830–1834 (2011). https://doi.org/10.1016/j.juro.2011.06.057
12. D.F. Osses, M.J. Roobol, I.G. Schoots, Prediction medicine: Biomarkers, risk calculators and magnetic resonance imaging as risk stratification tools in prostate cancer diagnosis. Int J Mol Sci **20**, ARTN 1637 (2019). https://doi.org/10.3390/ijms20071637
13. X.K. Niu et al., Developing a new PI-RADS v2-based nomogram for forecasting high-grade prostate cancer. Clin. Radiol. **72**, 458–464 (2017). https://doi.org/10.1016/j.crad.2016.12.005
14. J. Hansen et al., Initial prostate biopsy: Development and internal validation of a biopsy-specific nomogram based on the prostate cancer antigen 3 assay. Eur. Urol. **63**, 201–209 (2013). https://doi.org/10.1016/j.eururo.2012.07.030
15. M.W. Kattan et al., Counseling men with prostate cancer: A nomogram for predicting the presence of small, moderately differentiated, confined tumors. J. Urol. **170**, 1792–1797 (2003). https://doi.org/10.1097/01.ju.0000091806.70171.41
16. M.J. Roobol et al., Prediction of prostate cancer risk: The role of prostate volume and digital rectal examination in the ERSPC risk calculators. Eur. Urol. **61**, 577–583 (2012). https://doi.org/10.1016/j.eururo.2011.11.012
17. I. Berger et al., National variation in opioid prescription fills and long-term use in opioid naive patients after urological surgery. J. Urol. **202**, 1038–1044 (2019). https://doi.org/10.1097/Ju.0000000000000343
18. D.J. Lundon et al., Prostate cancer risk assessment tools in an unscreened population. World J. Urol. **33**, 827–832 (2015). https://doi.org/10.1007/s00345-014-1365-7
19. K.F. Kerr, M.D. Brown, K. Zhu, H. Janes, Assessing the clinical impact of risk prediction models with decision curves: Guidance for correct interpretation and appropriate use. J. Clin. Oncol. **34**, 2534–2540 (2016). https://doi.org/10.1200/JCO.2015.65.5654
20. X. Meng et al., Relationship between prebiopsy multiparametric magnetic resonance imaging (MRI), biopsy indication, and MRI-ultrasound fusion-targeted prostate biopsy outcomes. Eur. Urol. **69**, 512–517 (2016). https://doi.org/10.1016/j.eururo.2015.06.005
21. M.A. Bjurlin, A.B. Rosenkrantz, S.S. Taneja, Prediction of prostate cancer risk among men undergoing combined MRI-targeted and systematic biopsy using novel pre-biopsy nomograms that incorporate MRI findings REPLY. Urology **112**, 120–120 (2018). https://doi.org/10.1016/j.urology.2017.09.037
22. O.M. Zaytoun et al., Development of improved nomogram for prediction of outcome of initial prostate biopsy using readily available clinical information. Urology **78**, 392–398 (2011). https://doi.org/10.1016/j.urology.2011.04.042
23. N.D. Shore et al., A comparison of prostate health index, total PSA, %free PSA, and proPSA in a contemporary US population-The MiCheck-01 prospective trial. Urol. Oncol. (2020). https://doi.org/10.1016/j.urolonc.2020.03.011
24. S.Y. Park et al., Prostate cancer: PI-RADS version 2 helps preoperatively predict clinically significant cancers. Radiology **280**, 108–116 (2016). https://doi.org/10.1148/radiol.16151133
25. N. Perlis, L. Klotz, Contemporary active surveillance: Candidate selection, follow-up tools, and expected outcomes. Urol. Clin. North Am. **44**, 565–574 (2017). https://doi.org/10.1016/j.ucl.2017.07.005
26. F.K. Chun, P.I. Karakiewicz, H. Huland, M. Graefen, Role of nomograms for prostate cancer in 2007. World J. Urol. **25**, 131–142 (2007). https://doi.org/10.1007/s00345-007-0146-y
27. S.S. Salami et al., Multiparametric magnetic resonance imaging outperforms the Prostate Cancer Prevention Trial risk calculator in predicting clinically significant prostate cancer. Cancer **120**, 2876–2882 (2014). https://doi.org/10.1002/cncr.28790
28. D.G. Murphy et al., The Melbourne Consensus Statement on the early detection of prostate cancer. BJU Int. **113**, 186–188 (2014). https://doi.org/10.1111/bju.12556

29. M.S. Leapman et al., Application of a prognostic gleason grade grouping system to assess distant prostate cancer outcomes. Eur. Urol. **71**, 750–759 (2017). https://doi.org/10.1016/j.eururo.2016.11.032
30. J.I. Epstein et al., A contemporary prostate cancer grading system: A validated alternative to the gleason score. Eur. Urol. **69**, 428–435 (2016). https://doi.org/10.1016/j.eururo.2015.06.046
31. J.K. McKenney et al., Histologic grading of prostatic adenocarcinoma can be further optimized analysis of the relative prognostic strength of individual architectural patterns in 1275 patients from the canary retrospective cohort. Am. J. Surg. Pathol. **40**, 1439–1456 (2016). https://doi.org/10.1097/Pas.0000000000000736
32. C.F. Kweldam et al., Disease-specific survival of patients with invasive cribriform and intraductal prostate cancer at diagnostic biopsy. Mod. Pathol. **29**, 630–636 (2016). https://doi.org/10.1038/modpathol.2016.49
33. C.F. Kweldam et al., Cribriform growth is highly predictive for postoperative metastasis and disease-specific death in Gleason score 7 prostate cancer. Modern Pathol. **28**, 457–464 (2015). https://doi.org/10.1038/modpathol.2014.116

Using Natural Language Processing to Optimize Engagement of Those with Behavioral Health Conditions that Worsen Chronic Medical Disease

Peter Bearse, Atif Farid Mohammad, Intisar Rizwan I. Haque, Susan Kuypers, and Rachel Fournier

1 Introduction

Untreated behavioral health conditions worsen chronic medical disease, leading to poor member outcomes and low-value, high-cost medical utilization. Supporting health plan members with health coaching to address behaviors and social determinants of health leads to improved outcomes and high-value care. For this purpose, member engagement specialists (MESs) employ a skilled call center model to perform the initial outreach to members. Given the sensitive nature of the topics, MESs are highly trained. We hypothesized that MESs use words and phrases that are both positively and negatively associated with engagement and that natural language processing on call transcripts would uncover those words and phrases.

Call centers typically employ audio recordings which generate large amounts of audio data. The analysis of audio data is used to understand the conversation dynamics of call participants. Examples of such dynamics include analysis of the audio calls to objectively quantify how well the interaction between the service representative and the customer took place. This is achieved through development of metrics and key performance indicators driven primarily through data mining techniques for improving the overall quality of service. The manual analysis of audio data is time and labor intensive, thus nearly impossible to implement for drawing useful insights with large datasets. Automated approaches, on the other hand, employ either voice analytics built directly through audio analysis or are based on text analytics built upon speech-to-text transcription. A typical process flow for development of text analytics is shown in Fig. 1.

P. Bearse · A. F. Mohammad · I. R. I. Haque (✉) · S. Kuypers · R. Fournier
Catasys Inc., Santa Monica, CA, USA
e-mail: pbearse@catasys.com; amohammad@catasys.com; ihaque@catasys.com; skuypers@catasys.com; rfournier@catasys.com

H. R. Arabnia et al. (eds.), *Advances in Computer Vision and Computational Biology*, Transactions on Computational Science and Computational Intelligence,
https://doi.org/10.1007/978-3-030-71051-4_47

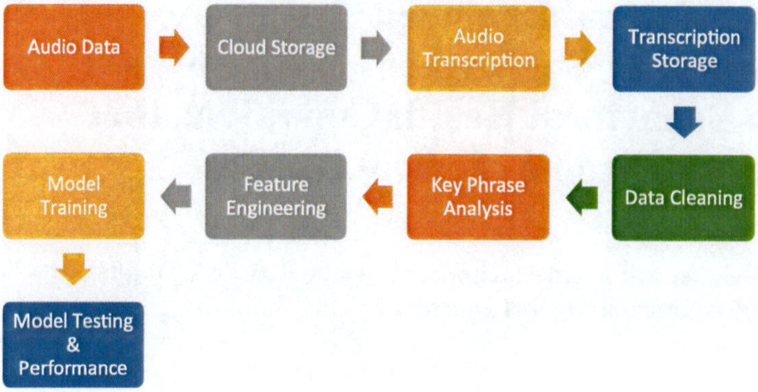

Fig. 1 Call center text analytics development based on automated speech-to-text transcription

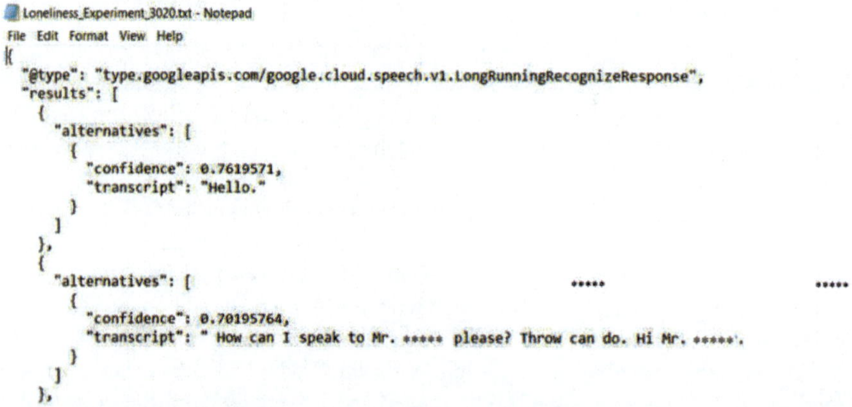
Loneliness_Experiment_3020.txt - Notepad
File Edit Format View Help


```
{
  "@type": "type.googleapis.com/google.cloud.speech.v1.LongRunningRecognizeResponse",
  "results": [
    {
      "alternatives": [                                    *****          *****
        {
          "confidence": 0.7619571,
          "transcript": "Hello."
        }
      ]
    },
    {
      "alternatives": [
        {
          "confidence": 0.70195764,
          "transcript": " How can I speak to Mr. ***** please? Throw can do. Hi Mr. *****",
        }
      ]
    },
```


Fig. 2 Sample speech-to-text transcription. Patient name has been redacted due to protected health information

As shown in Fig. 1., the process starts with the storage of audio data in the cloud environment. This is followed by generation of automatic speech-to-text transcription. A sample transcription is shown in Fig. 2.

As seen from Fig. 2, before the transcribed files can be analyzed, pre-processing is required to remove irrelevant data elements. From Fig. 2, everything is removed except the quoted text that follows the keyword "transcript." Figure 3 shows the sample transcribed file after data cleaning process.

As seen from Fig. 3, the transcribed results are not accurate which can be due to multiple reasons including noisy audio data, inaccurate results from the transcription model, misidentification of the spoken word by the transcription model and cross talk, etc. After data cleaning, keyword analysis is performed which helps in building up the preliminary data labels for further text classification using machine learning approaches. Keyword analysis is followed by feature engineering which involves the

```
               Hello                                    How can I         **********
speak to Mr ****** please? Throw can do Hi Mr ****** It's **********
your care coach calling from contract How are you? Okay how you
doing? Do you and alright thank you I just wanted to touch base
just to see if you needed anything or had any updates or anything
since we had talked last know Did you check on that Lubin issuer
for macaroni?                                  I miss look back
at my notes Here I know I had a call I don't know
So I left a voicemail That was oh my gosh when we talked last you
miss you and they never did They never reach out cuz I left and I
talked with one of the representatives after we talked at the end
of July and then they were swinging a reaching out and then did
nobody over to to the lady She couldn't talk to him
```

Fig. 3 Transcribed speech after data cleaning. Names have been redacted

extraction of suitable features to help distinguish between different classes of text. Finally, the model is trained and tested, and accuracy is determined for choosing a suitable classifier for the given problem.

In the current research, we propose an approach for determining the outcome of call center calls made to prospective members for their enrollment in a specially designed mental and behavioral therapy program. The purpose of the program is to identify and provide timely intervention to care-avoidant mental and behavioral health patients to prevent adverse medical outcomes such as hospitalization and mortality. Ultimately, the program aims to develop skills allowing patients to manage the challenges associated with their behavioral health conditions. In this way, the treatment effect of the program is durable allowing graduates to lead healthier lives and, at the same time, reducing projected costs to healthcare system.

In the next section, an overview of natural language processing (NLP) is provided. It is followed by data collection and characteristics in Sect. 3, methodology in Sect. 4, results in Sect. 5, and finally conclusion.

2 Natural Language Processing Tasks

The various natural language processing tasks can be broadly classified into two categories:

- Syntactic analysis
- Semantic analysis

These tasks belong to the "text parsing and exploratory data analysis" phase of the NLP workflow (Fig. 4).

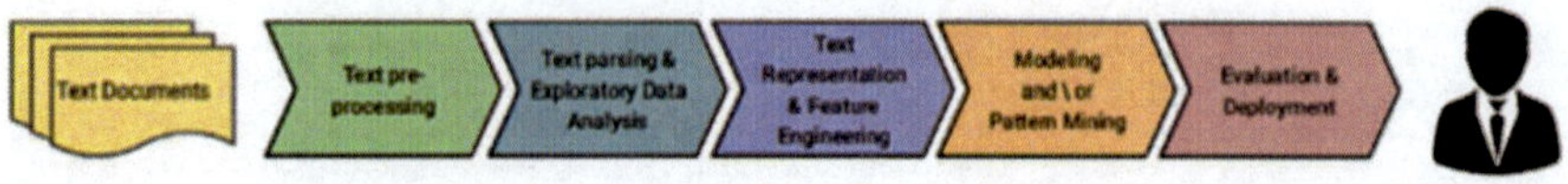

Fig. 4 Standard NLP workflow [3]

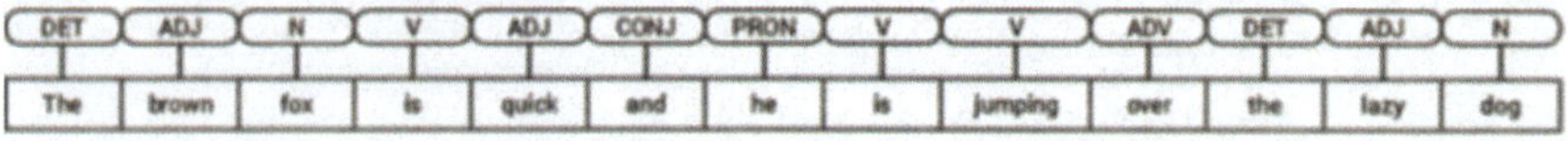

Fig. 5 POS tagging for a sentence [3]

2.1 Syntactic Analysis

The syntax is the arrangement of the words in a language that form a sentence with meaning. A syntactically correct sentence has a proper grammatical meaning. There are many tasks for syntactic analysis, the key ones of which are as follows [1].

Lemmatization/Stemming It refers to the process of reducing various inflected forms of a word into a single form for easier analysis [1]. That is, if there are many variations of a word, it is stripped to one form. Usually the variations are stripped down to the root of the word, because of which lemmatization is preferred over just stemming [2].

Stemming just strips a word of its plurality, prefixes, or suffixes and returns the root stem, e.g., removing "s" and removing "ing." Another difference is that in lemmatization, the lemma or the root word, called the lemma, is always lexicographically correct, while a root stem need not [3].

Morphological Segmentation It refers to dividing a word into many tiny bits called morphemes [1], through stemming. These morphemes cannot be divided any further. Dog, cat, dance, love, earth, etc., are morphemes. However, "unsociable" can be split into "un," "social," and "able," each of which is a morpheme.

Word, Intent, Sentence, and Topic Segmentation A string of many words in a language can be divided into individual words for better analysis. This is word segmentation. Likewise, the text of words could be divided based on the intent, motive, or idea in the text. The words can also be split sentence by sentence or topic-wise. These are some types of segmentation of texts in a language (Fig. 5).

Parts-of-Speech Tagging It involves identifying the part of speech for every word in a sentence. Parts of speech (POS) are the lexical categories in which the words in a sentence of most human languages fall into like noun, verb, adjective, and adverb. This tagging helps in specific analysis of finding the prominent words used and analysis of the grammar in a language [3].

Parsing The process of analyzing sentences by splitting the words into phrases and terms based on the grammar is called parsing. Parts-of-speech tagging, shallow

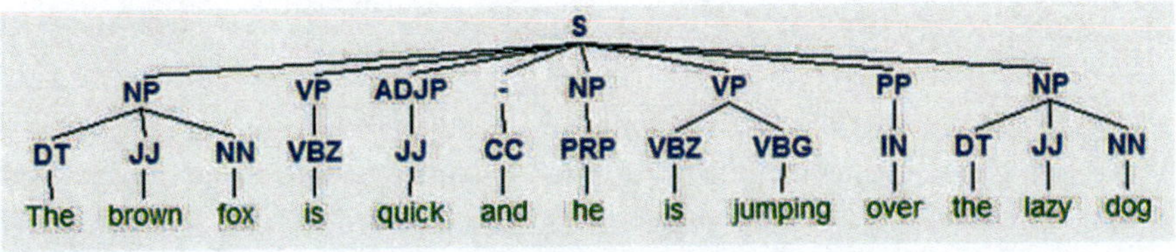

Fig. 6 An example of shallow parsing depicting higher-level phrase annotations [3]

parsing or chunking, constituency parsing, and dependency parsing are various types of parsing a given set of sentences [3].

The chunking uses phrases like the parts-of-speech tags such as noun phrase, adjective phrase, and adverb phrase as in Fig. 6. The constituency parsing uses grammar-based rules called phrase structure rules that determine what each structure in the sentence consists of and the order in which they occur. For example, S → AB is a phrase structure rule that denotes that the structure S constitutes of constituents A and B in the order A followed by B [3].

The dependency parsing uses the relationship between the various tokens in a sentence. For this purpose, it uses dependency-based grammar, and it helps to infer both the structural and semantic relationships.

2.2 *Semantic Analysis*

Semantics analysis comprises of inferring the meaning of a given sentence. This is a bit complex to achieve and needs the use of algorithms to understand the meaning of words and interpret them according to the context. This is particularly the area that is still yet to evolve more [1].

Named Entity Recognition (NER) In any text, there are usually some words that give more information about the context of the text. These words could refer to specific places, people, and organizations that could be first identified and classified. These are typically proper names, and a naive approach would be to identify the nouns in the text and segment or classify them into predefined classes [3].

Word Sense Disambiguation (WSD) It is an open problem that infers the "sense" or meaning of a word based on the usage of the word in a particular context. This classifies the words based on their possible senses and their neighbor words.

Natural Language Generation (NLG) It is the process of converting structured data into natural language. It follows a process similar to a human turning idea into written work or speech. This is the mechanism used by chatbots and text-to-speech conversion software.

3 Data Collection and Characteristics

Using claims and eligibility data provided by health insurers, clinical knowledge is combined with machine learning algorithms to identify candidates for the treatment program. Based on this list, a member engagement specialist (MES) makes a cold call to a prospective member. The call conversation dynamics are shown in Fig. 7.

As seen from Fig. 7, after the initial introduction by the MES caller, the prospective member is provided a brief overview of the program highlighting how it can be useful for managing mental health and behavioral issues. This is followed by an explanation of the process and what the member can expect to gain from participation. Finally, the member is asked if she would like to enroll in the program or, alternatively, if she would like to receive further information regarding the program or refuse altogether. When members show positive sentiments about enrollment or request further information, their calls are transferred to care coaches for potential enrollment. This transfer of call to the care coach is regarded as the successful outcome of the cold call by the member engagement specialist. And in this research study, we analyze MES calls for successful transfer to the care coach.

The audio dataset comprised of 9254 calls with size varying in between 30 MB and 50 MB. The call duration varied approximately between 30 and 50 minutes. The calls were recorded at 128 kbps using mono channel. The calls were transcribed using Google Cloud Speech to Text API. The analysis was performed using Python in Jupyter™ Notebook available with Anaconda Navigator™.

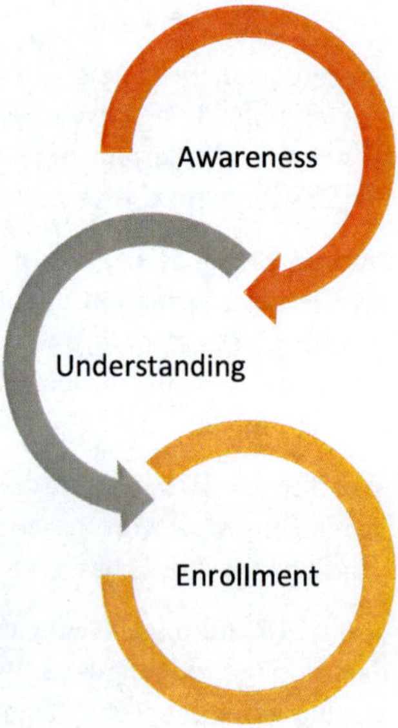

Fig. 7 Conversation dynamics of call between member engagement specialist and prospective member

4 Methodology

Initially, keyword search was applied to search for the instances of "transfer" keyword for generation of data labels to identify calls in which "transfer to care coach" event took place. Then sentence extraction was performed by extracting five words before and after the keyword "transfer." This was done to clarify the context behind the use of keyword "transfer." One of the sentences extracted from the calls is shown in Fig. 8.

Once the data labels were generated, the data was split into training and validation sets so that various classifiers can be trained and tested. This was followed by feature engineering, in which raw text was transformed into feature vectors based on count vectors; term frequency–inverse document frequency (TF-IDF) vectors at word level, N-gram level, and character level; word embedding vectors; and topic model vectors.

Count vectors are basically matrices where rows represent the individual transcription file, columns represent terms, and the corresponding value indicates the frequency. Simply stated each cell of the matrix provides the frequency count of a specific term in each transcribed file.

A TF-IDF vector is determined using the equations provided below.

$$\text{TF}(x) = \frac{\text{Number of times term}'x'\text{ occurs in a transcribed file}}{\text{Total number of terms in the transcribed file}}$$

$$\text{IDF}(x) = \ln\left(\frac{\text{Total number of transcribed files}}{\text{Number of transcribed files containing term}'x'}\right)$$

This is a useful measure of relative importance for a specific term in a transcribed file in comparison to the entire collection of transcribed files which we can refer to as corpus. TF-IDF vectors were generated for individual word level terms, a combination of words using N-grams, and a combination of characters using N-grams.

Word embeddings provide a dense vector representation of text in which the position of the word in the vector space is determined through text from the transcribed file. Finally, the topic modeling is a technique for grouping words based on different topics to generate a collection of topics vector. In other words, each transcribed file is a distribution over topics.

Additionally, words and phrases for NLP were selected using a qualitative design. Researchers used a two-pronged approach for this. First, they listened

```
'Would you like me to transfer you to that therapist now'
```

Fig. 8 Sample sentence extracted for keyword "transfer"

to calls between MESs and prospective members and coding words and phrases frequently used by the MESs. The coded words and phrases were then divided into two categories: those used by high-performing agents and those used by low- to mid-performing agents. A second researcher read through a sample of the call transcriptions for words and phrases MESs used in calls that resulted in either a transfer to a care coach or not. Words and phrases were coded into categories. Each category represented a reason that people do not seek the medical care they need, which is the target member. Some examples are denial, lack of trust in doctors and the medical profession, hopelessness, fear, and lack of access to care.

The hypothesis is that words trigger either positive or negative sentiments in relation to seeking medical care. Those that are associated with positive sentiments around how the program could help them would more likely result in a call being transferred to a care coach.

5 Results

The keyword analysis for the term "transfer" is shown in Fig. 9.

The keyword search resulted in total count of instances equal to 2300. However, for some of the calls, the keyword was used more than once as seen from Fig. 9. The unique count per call was equal to 1529.

The performance result for various classifiers in terms of their accuracy, training time (normalized), and testing time (normalized) is shown in Fig. 10.

As seen from Fig. 10, the best classifier is a linear support vector machine (SVM) which has one of the highest accuracies with minimal training and testing time. The XGBoost classifier, on the other hand, has a similar accuracy but has longer training time associated with it.

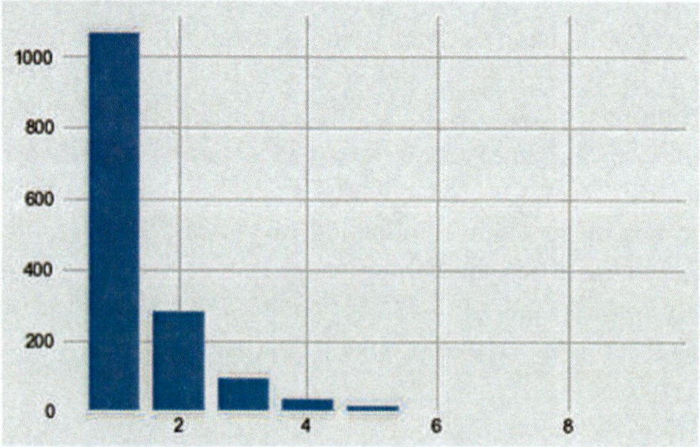

Fig. 9 Keyword "transfer" frequency per call on x-axis and count on y-axis

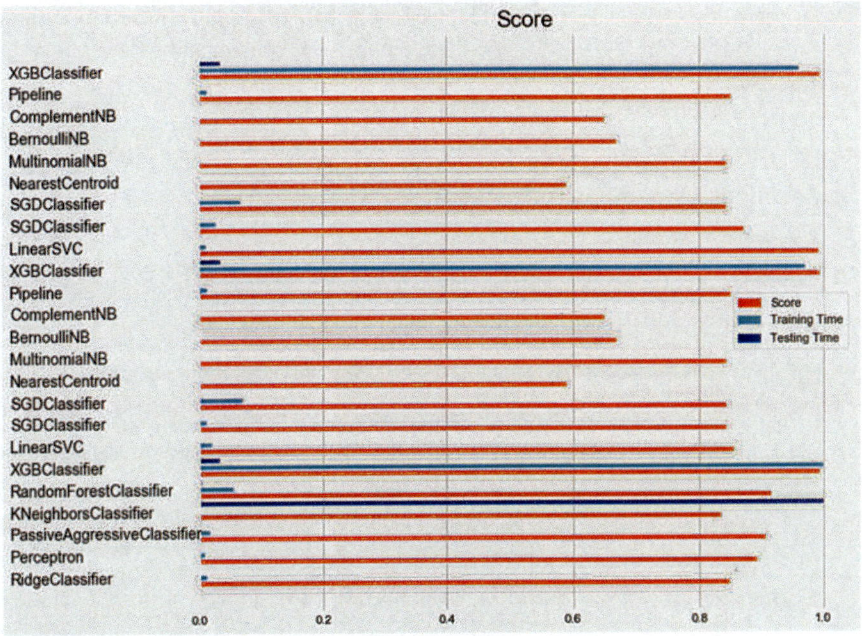

Fig. 10 Performance comparison of various classifiers

Based on the analysis of high performer and low/mid-performers, the following words and phrases were selected using the qualitative design.

High performers say:	Low/mid-performers say:	Words associated with stigma and shame:
Skill building counselor	Counselor	Psychiatrist
Personalized	Tailored	Mental health
Medical doctor	Psychiatrist	Mental health services
Medication management	Psychiatry	Addiction

6 Conclusion

The results indicate that the proposed approach for determining the outcome of call center calls made to prospective members can be used to determine various outcomes based on NLP algorithms. This is significant for identification and provision of timely intervention to care-avoidant mental and behavioral health patients. Additionally, key phrases or words that trigger positive sentiments regarding a program in relation to seeking medical care would be more likely to result in the call being transferred to a care coach. The work will be expanded in future to include keyword analysis for high performers and low/mid-performers and will be tested on a larger dataset.

References

1. M.J. Garbade, A Simple Introduction to Natural Language Processing, October 2018. [Online]. Available: https://becominghuman.ai/a-simple-introduction-to-natural-language-processing-ea66a1747b32
2. Why Natural Language Processing (NLP) is a core AI Technology, October 2018. [Online]. Available: https://witanworld.com/article/2018/10/28/naturallanguageprocessing-nlp/
3. D.D.J. Sarkar, A Practitioner's Guide to Natural Language Processing (Part I) — Processing & Understanding Text, June 2018. [Online]. Available: https://towardsdatascience.com/a-practitioners-guide-to-natural-language-processing-part-i-processing-understanding-text-9f4abfd13e72

Smart Healthcare Monitoring Apps with a Flavor of Systems Engineering

Misagh Faezipour and Miad Faezipour

1 Introduction

Smartphone devices and applications (apps) have become an integral part of the advanced technology era. Attributes such as embedded software, hardware, and connectivity have allowed for smartphones to serve as an attractive interface to collect, process, and analyze health-related data. Users, patients, and healthcare professionals can connect through the online/communication features of the smartphone to further facilitate telemedicine platforms. Such interfaces are especially useful for monitoring the health status of patients with chronic conditions and those that require immediate attention. Given the current circumstances of the ongoing COVID-19 global pandemic, where self-quarantine and physical distancing is a must, remote smartphone-based healthcare monitoring can potentially be an effective alternative. Several thousands of mobile health applications have already been developed and made available through the online stores. With the foreseeable evolution in technology and healthcare, the number is expected to grow exponentially [1–3].

To date, many smartphone-based healthcare monitoring apps have been developed [4, 5]. There is also a large number of core algorithms that have been introduced which are ready to be deployed as smartphone-based healthcare monitoring

M. Faezipour (✉)
Department of Engineering Technology, Middle Tennessee State University, Murfreesboro, TN, USA
e-mail: misagh.faezipour@mtsu.edu

M. Faezipour
Departments of Computer Science & Engineering and Biomedical Engineering, University of Bridgeport, Bridgeport, CT, USA
e-mail: mfaezipo@bridgeport.edu

H. R. Arabnia et al. (eds.), *Advances in Computer Vision and Computational Biology*, Transactions on Computational Science and Computational Intelligence,
https://doi.org/10.1007/978-3-030-71051-4_48

apps. Machine learning is the main idea behind the data analysis of the vast majority of such algorithms. Some apps/algorithms focus on the brain/cognitive functionality [6], monitor the cardiac status [1, 7, 8], or report the breathing/respiratory function [9, 10]. Other apps/algorithms deal with assessing other health-related conditions such as the skin [11], eye-vision and pressure [12], hearing aids [13], dietary assistance, etc. [1, 7]. The efficiency of healthcare monitoring apps is usually considered by the depth (level) of which it sustains patient well-being and care.

With numerous smartphone healthcare monitoring apps available, ultimately, the users would want to select the most efficient app. As the number of smart healthcare monitoring apps increases, the factors and inter-relationships would increase, resulting in a complex system. A method such as systems engineering capable of successfully dealing with such complexity is needed. Systems engineering is an "integrative and transdisciplinary approach to enable the successful realization, use, and retirement of engineered systems, using systems principles and concepts, and technological, scientific, and management methods" [14]. One of the goals of systems engineering is to better realize the behavior of a system and its problems. Systems thinking is one of the most common approaches in systems engineering and will be utilized in this paper.

Systems thinking is a systems engineering approach that can help to address complex systems. Systems thinking is referred to a world view where everything is seen holistically. In this method, the whole world would be observed as a complex system and the aim is to understand the inter-relationships and inter-connections [15]. Systems thinking assists to comprehend how various elements in the smart-based healthcare monitoring apps interact. System dynamics is an approach within systems thinking that supports understanding the dynamic feedback behavior and structure in complex systems. System dynamics was first developed by Forrester [16]. Many areas within healthcare have deployed applications of system dynamics [17–20].

2 Proposed Ideas

2.1 Causal Model

A systems thinking, and particularly, a systems engineering approach is introduced to delve into the factor and factor relationships influencing the efficiency of generic smartphone-based healthcare monitoring apps. For this, a causal model is first proposed to visualize the feedback and connections of the system factors and their inter-relationships.

Figure 1 illustrates the graphical depiction of our proposed causal model for smartphone-based healthcare monitoring systems in general. Causal models provide an underlying basis for system dynamics. The model diagram consists of the factor

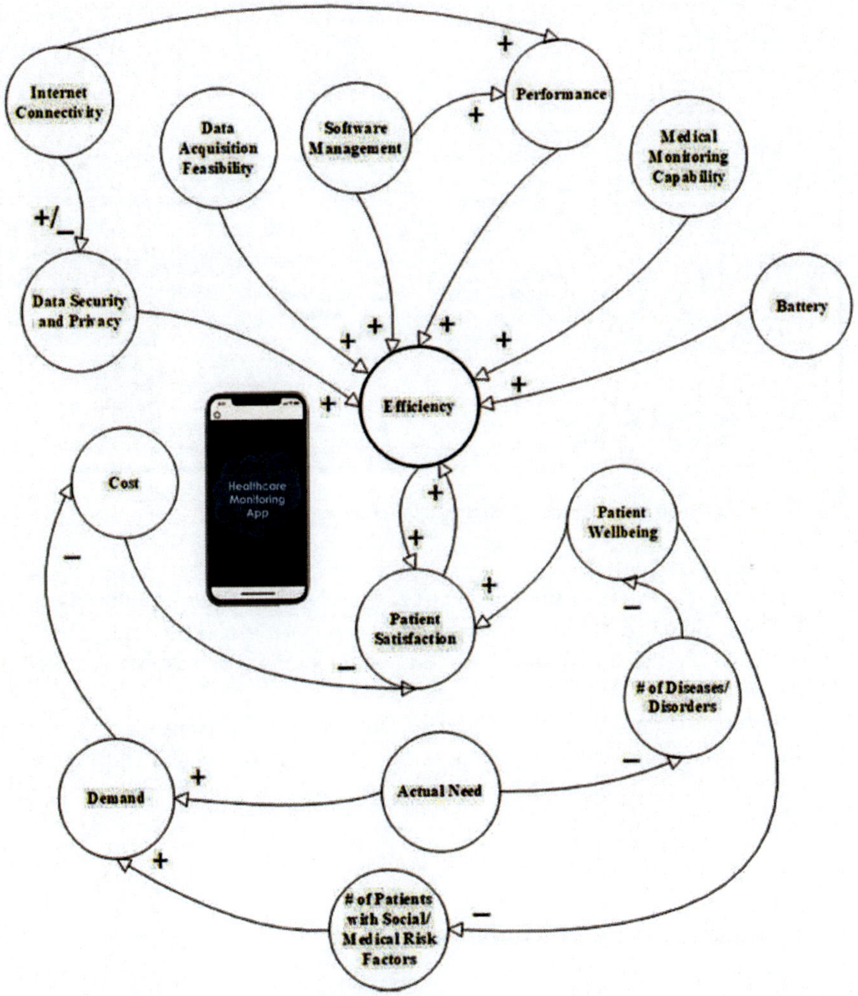

Fig. 1 Causal model of a generic smartphone-based healthcare monitoring system

elements along with their causal links (arrows). The sign of each arrow denotes an increasing (+) or decreasing (−) relationship.

A set of key factors and their inter-relations are considered for our proposed causal model. A review of the literature [18, 21, 22] suggests that factors such as patient well-being and satisfaction, cost, device's data acquisition feasibility, software/app management, and medical monitoring capability as well as the app's performance, are deemed the most influential factors determining the efficiency of the healthcare monitoring app. A more comprehensive set of factors can be viewed from our proposed causal model. Since this is a generic model, the factors of the model shall be fine-tuned according to any specific healthcare app. As an example,

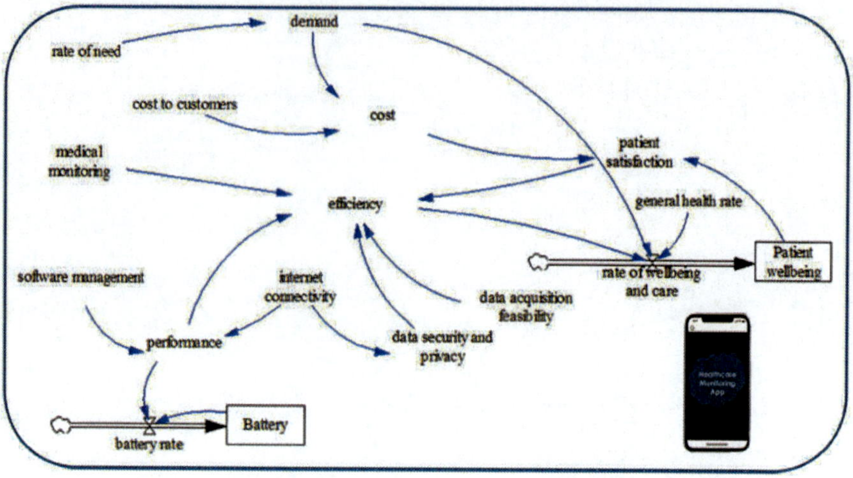

Fig. 2 System dynamics model of healthcare monitoring app

for a skin monitoring app, the number (#) of diseases/disorders would reflect the number of incidents of unhealthy (abnormal) skin lesions, and the data acquisition module could be the smartphone's camera that captures the image of skin lesions [23].

As observed from Fig. 1, the model structure involves feedback and nonlinear (complex) increasing/decreasing relationships among the factors. For example, when the performance measure factors of the app improves, the efficiency increases as well.

2.2 *System Dynamics Model*

With the base of the proposed causal model, we suggest a system dynamics model to study the behavior of the system model factors and assess the efficiency of smartphone-based healthcare monitoring apps. The structure of the proposed system dynamics model is presented in Fig. 2.

The system dynamics model is generated using the Vensim® Pro [24] software. As can be seen from Fig. 2, only a subset of the proposed causal model is considered where stocks (Patient Well-being, Battery), flows (rate of well-being and care, battery rate), and auxiliary variables (efficiency, performance, etc.) are introduced. System dynamics modeling can operate with various settings and scenarios to observe the dynamics of the model factors affecting the efficiency of the healthcare app.

3 Expected Outcome

As this research work is under progress, the simulation results and outcomes are yet to be explored and validated. Nonetheless, we expect the app's performance and medical monitoring capability factors, including software management, that mostly deal with the data analysis algorithm, to have the highest impact on the efficiency of smart healthcare monitoring apps.

To observe the precise dynamics of the model, social factors such as patient well-being, satisfaction, and care with clinical implications should be studied over the duration of months and years. We envision that such systems engineering modeling would unveil the complex dynamics of various factors and can suggest the most efficient smart-health apps.

References

1. K. Vinay, K. Vishal, Smartphone applications for medical students and professionals. Nitte Univ. J. Health Sci. **3**(1), 59 (2013)
2. C. Kratzke, C. Cox, Smartphone technology and apps: rapidly changing health promotion. Global J. Health Education Prom. **15**(1) (2012)
3. M. Faezipour, A. Abuzneid, Smartphone-based self-testing of COVID-19 using breathing sounds. Telemed. e-Health **26**, 1202–1205 (2020)
4. G. Gupta, Are medical apps the future of medicine? Medical J. Armed Forces India **69**(2), 105 (2013)
5. M. Bradway, C. Carrion, B. Vallespin, O. Saadatfard, E. Puigdomènech, M. Espallargues, A. Kotzeva, mhealth assessment: conceptualization of a global framework. JMIR mHealth uHealth **5**(5), e60 (2017)
6. K.A.I. Aboalayon, M. Faezipour, W.S. Almuhammadi, S. Moslehpour, Sleep stage classification using EEG signal analysis: a comprehensive survey and new investigation. Entropy **18**(9), 272 (2016)
7. O.A. Alsos, A. Das, D. Svanæs, Mobile health it: The effect of user interface and form factor on doctor–patient communication. Int. J. Med. Inf. **81**(1), 12–28 (2012)
8. M. Faezipour, A. Saeed, S.C. Bulusu, M. Nourani, H. Minn, L. Tamil, A patient-adaptive profiling scheme for ECG beat classification. IEEE Trans. Inf. Technol. Biomed. **14**(5), 1153–1165 (2010)
9. A. Abushakra, M. Faezipour, Augmenting breath regulation using a mobile driven virtual reality therapy framework. IEEE J. Biomed. Health Inf. **18**(3), 746–752 (2014)
10. A. Abushakra, M. Faezipour, Acoustic signal classification of breathing movements to virtually aid breath regulation. IEEE J. Biomed. Health Inf. **17**(2), 493–500 (2013)
11. O. Abuzaghleh, B.D. Barkana, M. Faezipour, Noninvasive real-time automated skin lesion analysis system for melanoma early detection and prevention. IEEE J. Translat. Eng. Health Med. **3**, 1–12 (2015)
12. M. Aloudat, M. Faezipour, El-Sayed, A., Automated vision-based high intraocular pressure detection using frontal eye images. IEEE J. Transl. Eng. Health Med. **7**, 1–13 (2019)
13. A.M. Amlani, B. Taylor, C. Levy, R. Robbins, Utility of smartphone-based hearing aid applications as a substitute to traditional hearing aids. Hearing Rev. **20**(13), 16–18 (2013)
14. D.D. Walden, G.J. Roedler, K. Forsberg, R.D. Hamelin, T.M. Shortell, *Systems Engineering Handbook: A Guide for System Life Cycle Processes and Activities* (Wiley, New York, 2015)

15. J. Sterman, System dynamics: systems thinking and modeling for a complex world. ESD Int. Symp. ESD-WP-2003 **01**(13), 1–31 (2002)
16. J.W. Forrester, System dynamics, systems thinking, and soft OR. Syst. Dyn. Rev. **10**(2–3), 245–256 (1994)
17. M. Faezipour, S. Ferreira, Applying systems thinking to assess sustainability in healthcare system of systems. Int. J. Syst. Syst. Eng. **2**(4), 290–308 (2011)
18. M. Faezipour, S. Ferreira, A system dynamics perspective of patient satisfaction in healthcare. Procedia Comput. Sci. **16**, 148–156 (2013)
19. M. Faezipour, S. Ferreira, A system dynamics approach for sustainable water management in hospitals. IEEE Syst. J. **12**(2), 1278–1285 (2018)
20. L. de Andrade, C. Lynch, E. Carvalho, C.G. Rodrigues, J.R.N. Vissoci, G.F. Passos, R. Pietrobon, O.K. Nihei, M.D. de Barros Carvalho, System dynamics modeling in the evaluation of delays of care in ST-segment elevation myocardial infarction patients within a tiered health system. PloS One **9**(7), e103577 (2014)
21. J. Ware, M. Kosinski, B. Gandek, *SF-36 Health Survey: Manual and Interpretation Guide Lincoln* (QualityMetric Incorporated, Lincoln, 2000)
22. M. Faezipour, The empowered patient wants shared decision making–how can system dynamics modeling help?, in *Proceedings of the International System Dynamics Conference* (2018)
23. O. Abuzaghleh, M. Faezipour, B.D. Barkana, SkinCure: An innovative smart phone-based application to assist in melanoma early detection and prevention (2015). Preprint arXiv:1501.01075
24. Vensim Software (2020). https://vensim.com/vensim-software/#professional-amp-dss. Accessed 29 May 2020

Using Artificial Intelligence for Medical Condition Prediction and Decision-Making for COVID-19 Patients

Mohammad Pourhomayoun and Mahdi Shakibi

1 Introduction and Background

In late 2019, a novel form of coronavirus, named SARS-CoV-2 (which stands for severe acute respiratory syndrome coronavirus 2), started spreading in the province of Hubei in China and claimed numerous human lives [1–5]. In February 2020, the WHO selected an official name, COVID-19 (which stands for coronavirus disease 2019), for the infectious disease caused by the novel coronavirus and later in March 2020 declared a COVID-19 pandemic [5, 6].

Coronavirus is a family of viruses that usually causes respiratory tract disease and infections that can be fatal in some cases such as in SARS, MERS, and COVID-19. The novel coronavirus might have jumped from an animal species into the human population and then begun spreading [7]. A recent study has shown that once the coronavirus outbreak starts, it will take less than 4 weeks to overwhelm the healthcare system. Once the hospital capacity gets overwhelmed, the death rate jumps [8].

Machine learning has been shown to be an effective tool in predicting medical conditions and adverse events and helping caregivers with medical decision-making [9–13]. In this study, we proposed a data-driven predictive analytics algorithm based on artificial intelligence (AI) and machine learning to determine the health risk and predict the mortality risk of patients with COVID-19. The developed system can help hospitals and medical facilities decide who has higher priority to be hospitalized, triage patients when the system is overwhelmed by overcrowding, and eliminate delays in providing the necessary care. The algorithm predicts

M. Pourhomayoun · M. Shakibi (✉)
Department of Computer Science, California State University, Los Angeles, CA, USA
e-mail: mpourho@calstatela.edu; mshakib@calstatela.edu

H. R. Arabnia et al. (eds.), *Advances in Computer Vision and Computational Biology*, Transactions on Computational Science and Computational Intelligence,
https://doi.org/10.1007/978-3-030-71051-4_49

the mortality risks based on patients' physiological conditions, symptoms, and demographic information.

The proposed system includes a set of algorithms for preprocessing the data to extract new features, handling missing values, eliminating redundant and useless data elements, and selecting the most informative features. After preprocessing the data, we use machine learning algorithms to develop a predictive model to classify the data, predict the medical condition, and calculate the probability and risk of mortality.

The rest of this chapter is organized as follows. In Sect. 2, we will introduce the different methods and model architecture and discuss each method by providing detailed information about the model, data preprocessing, and challenges that we encountered and the steps to mitigate these challenges, feature selection, and feature extraction. In Sect. 3, we describe the results and conclusion.

2 Data Processing and Predictive Analytics

2.1 Dataset

In this chapter, we used a dataset of more than 117,000 laboratory-confirmed COVID-19 patients from 76 countries around the world including both male and female patients with an average age of 56.6 [3]. The disease confirmed by detection of virus nucleic acid [3]. The original dataset contained 32 data elements from each patient, including demographic and physiological data. At the data cleaning stage, we removed useless and redundant data elements such as data source, admin ID, and admin name. Then, data imputation techniques were used to handle missing values.

After analyzing the data, we found out that 74% of patients had recovered from COVID-19. To have an accurate and unbiased model, we made sure that our dataset is balanced. A balanced dataset with equal observations for both recovered and deceased patients was created to train and test our model. The data observations (patients) in the training dataset have been selected randomly, and they are completely separated from the testing data. Figure 1 shows a high-level architecture of our system.

2.2 Data Processing

The outcome label contained multiple values for the patient's health status. We considered patients discharged from the hospital or patients in stable situation with no more symptoms as recovered patients.

A total of 80 features were extracted from *symptoms* and *doctors' medical notes* about the patient's health status.

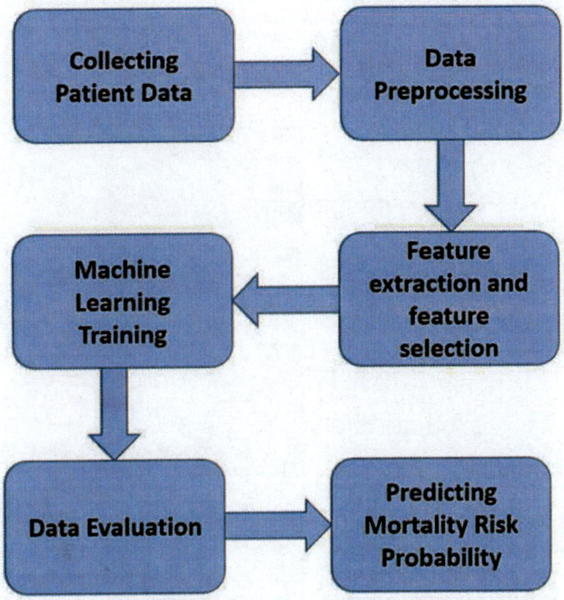

Fig. 1 High-level system architecture

We also extracted additional 32 features from patient's demographic and physiological data. Hence, there were 112 features. We consulted with a medical team to make sure that the best features are extracted and selected.

The next step is feature selection. The primary purpose of feature selection is to find the most informative features and eliminate redundant data to reduce the dimensionality and complexity of the model [11]. We used univariate and multivariate filter method and wrapper method to rank the features and select the best feature subset [11]. Filter methods are very popular (especially for large datasets) since they are usually very fast and much less computationally intensive than wrapper methods. Filter methods use a specific metric to score each individual feature (or a subset of features together). The most popular metrics used in filter methods include correlation coefficient, Fisher score, mutual information, entropy and consistency, and chi-square parameters [11].

After applying different filter and wrapper methods, we chose 42 features out of 112 features. Our final feature set includes demographic features such as age, sex, province, country, age, travel history, general medical information such as comorbidities (diabetes, cardiovascular disease, etc.), and also patient symptoms such as chest pain, chills, colds, conjunctivitis, cough, diarrhea, discomfort, dizziness, dry cough, dyspnea, emesis, expectoration, eye irritation, fatigue, gasp, headache, lesions on chest radiographs, little sputum, malaise, muscle pain, myalgia, obnubilation, pneumonia, myelofibrosis, respiratory symptoms, rhinorrhea, somnolence, sputum, transient fatigue, and weakness.

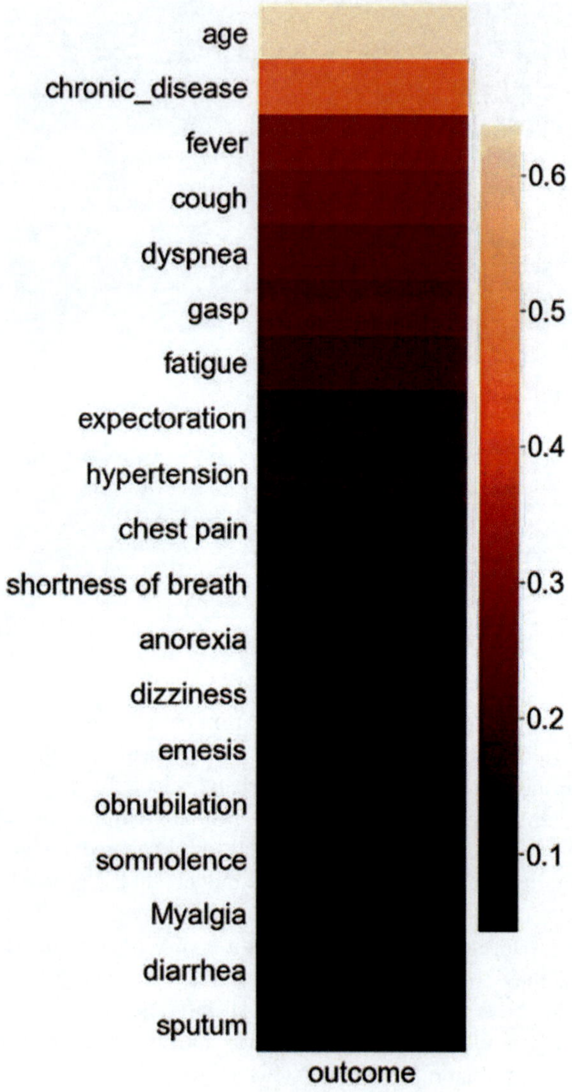

Fig. 2 Correlation heatmap for the most correlated features to the mortality risk

Fig. 2 shows the correlation between features and the outcome, i.e., mortality risk. As Fig. 2 illustrates, some features like age and chronic diseases (comorbidities) were the top features with high correlation to the patient's mortality risk.

2.3 Machine Learning and Predictive Analytics Algorithms

After selecting the best feature subset, we used various machine learning algorithms to build a predictive model. In this research, we used different algorithms including support vector machine (SVM), neural networks, and random forest [14–16].

The neural network algorithm achieved the best performance and accuracy. We used grid search to find the best hyper-parameters for the neural network. A model hyperparameter is a characteristic of a model that is external to the model, and its value cannot be estimated from data. We set the hyperparameter value before the learning process begins. Grid search will build a model on each hyperparameter combination that is possible. The grid search will go through every hyperparameter and store the model for each combination. And in the end, it will return the best hyperparameter. The best neural network results were achieved with two hidden layers with ten neurons in the first layer and three neurons in the second layer. We used sigmoid function as the hidden layer activation function and used stochastic gradient optimizer, constant learning rate, and the regularization rate of alpha = 0.01.

The SVM model was configured with linear kernel and regularization parameter $C = 1.0$.

The random forest algorithm is an ensemble learning method combined with multiple decision tree predictors that are trained based on random data samples and feature subsets [16]. We configured the random forest algorithm with 20 trees in the forest.

2.4 Evaluation

To evaluate the developed model, we first used *K-fold random cross-validation* to evaluate the overall accuracy. There are three main steps for K-fold cross-validation. In the first step, we partition the dataset randomly into k-equal, non-overlapping sections which are called fold. In the second step, we use one of the sections as testing set at a time and the combination of the other (k-1) sections as the training set; we will perform training stage and testing stage and compute the accuracy based on the split each time. Repeat this procedure k times so that each one of the K sections is used as testing set one time, and as a part of training set for (k-1) times in the last step, we calculate the average of the accuracies as the final result. In this research, we used ten-fold cross-validation (Fig. 3). Figure 4 demonstrate the K-fold architecture.

Furthermore, to evaluate the sensitivity and specificity, we split the dataset randomly with no overlap into a training set (%70) and a testing set (%30) and generated receiver operating characteristic (ROC) curves for every algorithm to measure and compare and calculated the area under the curve (AUC) and confusion matrix. Again, we made sure that there is no overlap (no common patient) between

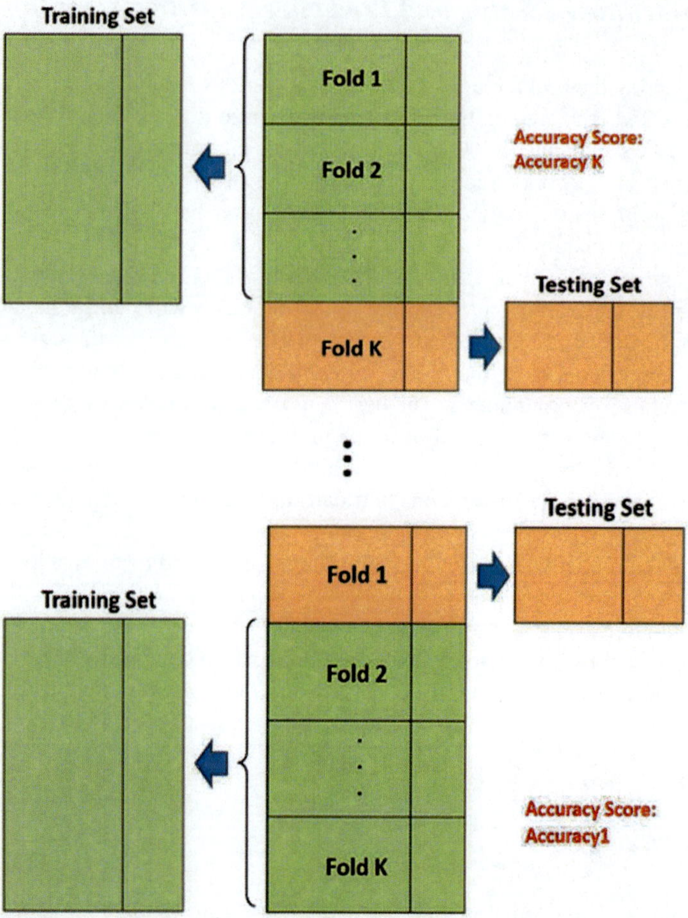

Fig. 3 Cross-validation for evaluation

training and testing datasets at any level. The next section will provide the results and performance of the developed system.

3 Results

The purpose of this study is to create a predictive algorithm to help hospitals and medical facilities maximize the number of survivors by providing an accurate and reliable tool to help medical decision-making and triage COVID-19 patients more effectively and accurately during the pandemic.

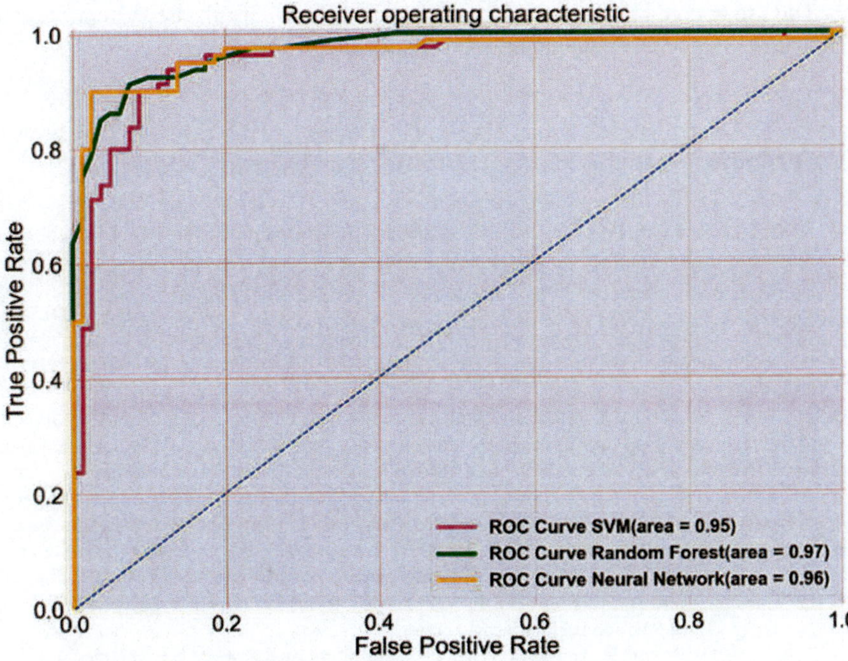

Fig. 4 ROC curve comparison for all algorithms

Table 1 The accuracy of mortality prediction in patients with COVID-19 using ten-fold cross-validation

Neural network using ten-fold cross-validation	93.75%
Random forest using ten-fold cross-validation	91.88%
SVM using ten-fold cross-validation	90.63%

As explained in Sect. 2, several metrics such as accuracy, ROC, AUC, and confusion matrix have been used to evaluate the developed model.

Table 1 demonstrates the prediction accuracy for predicting mortality in patients with COVID-19 using ten-fold cross-validation for various machine learning algorithms.

Figure 4 demonstrates and compares the ROC curves and AUC for every machine learning algorithm that was used in this research.

The results demonstrate that the developed algorithm is able to accurately predict the mortality risk in patients with COVID-19 based on the patients' physiological conditions, symptoms, and demographic information.

This system can help hospitals, medical facilities, and caregivers decide who needs to get attention first before other patients, triage patients when the system is overwhelmed by overcrowding, and also eliminate delays in providing the necessary care.

This study could expand to other diseases to help the healthcare system respond more effectively during an outbreak or a pandemic.

References

1. T. Ellerin, H. Farid, D. Krakower, H.E. LeWine, C. McCarthy, B. Memon, J. Sharp, R.H. Shmerling, J. Sperling, Harvard Health Publishing Coronavirus Resource Center Experts
2. Q. Li et al., Early transmission dynamics in Wuhan, China, of novel coronavirus–infected pneumonia. N. Engl. J. Med, NEJMoa2001316 (2020). https://doi.org/10.1056/NEJMoa2001316
3. B. Xu, B. Gutierrez, S. Mekaru, et al., Epidemiological data from the COVID-19 outbreak, real-time case information. Nature Sci Data **7**, 106 (2020). https://doi.org/10.1038/s41597-020-0448-0. In: Nature
4. I.I. Bogoch, A. Watts, A. Thomas-Bachli, C. Huber, M.U.G. Kraemer, K. Khan, Pneumonia of unknown aetiology in Wuhan, China: Potential for international spread via commercial air travel. J. Travel Med. **27**(2) (2020., taaa008). https://doi.org/10.1093/jtm/taaa008
5. Statement on the second meeting of the International Health Regulations (2005) Emergency Committee regarding the outbreak of novel coronavirus (2019-nCoV), World Health Organization (WHO). Archived from the original on 31 January 2020. Retrieved 11 February 2020
6. WHO Director-General's opening remarks at the media briefing on COVID-19, World Health Organization (WHO) (Press release). 11 March 2020. Retrieved 12 March 2020
7. L. Maragakis, M.P.H. Johns Hopkins Medicine
8. T. McConghy, B. Pon, E. Anderson, When does Hospital Capacity Get Overwhelmed in USA? Germany? A model of beds needed and available for Coronavirus patients. trent.st (2020)
9. A. Kalatzis, B. Mortazavi, M. Pourhomayoun, Interactive dimensionality reduction for improving patient adherence in remote health monitoring, in *The 2018 International Conference on Computational Science and Computational Intelligence (CSCI'18)*, (Las Vegas, 2018)
10. D.R. Chang, M. Pourhomayoun, Risk prediction of critical vital signs for ICU patients using recurrent neural network, in *The 2019 International Conference on Computational Science and Computational Intelligence*, (Las Vegas, 2019)
11. M. Pourhomayoun et al., Multiple model analytics for adverse event prediction in remote health monitoring systems, in *Proceedings of the IEEE EMBS Conference Healthcare Innovation & Point-of-Care Technologies*,
12. S. Yoo, A. Kalatzis, N. Amini, M. Pourhomayoun, Interactive predictive analytics for enhancing patient adherence in remote health monitoring, in *The 8th ACM MobiHoc2018 Workshop on Pervasive Wireless Healthcare*, (2018)
13. M. Pourhomayoun, E Martin, T Kim, V. Martin, M Kuko, M Kwon, Multi-label Classification of Single and Clustered Cervical Cells Using Deep Convolutional Networks
14. C. Cortes, V. Vapnik, *Machine Learning* (1995), pp. 273–297
15. V. Vapnik, The Nature of Statistical Learning Theory
16. L. Breiman, Random forests. Mach. Learn. (2001)

An Altmetric Study on Dental Informatics

Jessica Chen and Qiping Zhang

1 Introduction

1.1 Definition of Dental Informatics

Dental informatics (DI) is the application of computer and information science to improve dental practice, research, and program administration [8]. Similarly, Schleyer [4] defined dental informatics as the use of computers and technology to improve multiple aspects of dentistry (e.g., dental practice and management in dental healthcare).

Even with the growing number of articles released yearly, more research needs to be further done. Several studies called for a systematic review of the field, and many directions of the related research are proposed [4, 6]. In addition, given dental informatics is a comparatively new field, there's not as much analysis done. In order for more articles and publications to be completed in this field, researchers will need to know what aspects have and have not been researched, what journals are the key sources, what affiliation/organizations are key players, etc.

J. Chen
Jericho High School, Jericho, NY, USA
e-mail: Jessica.Chen@jerichoapps.org

Q. Zhang (✉)
Long Island University, Brookville, NY, USA
e-mail: Qiping.Zhang@liu.edu

H. R. Arabnia et al. (eds.), *Advances in Computer Vision and Computational Biology*, Transactions on Computational Science and Computational Intelligence,
https://doi.org/10.1007/978-3-030-71051-4_50

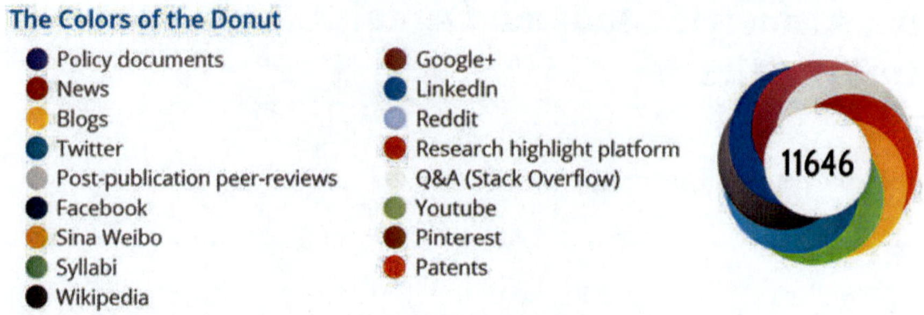

Fig. 1 An example of Altmetric attention score

1.2 Altmetric Attention Score and Altmetric Explorer

Altmetric Explorer is a platform that enables users to browse and report on all of the mentions from various online sources for research outputs, including articles, dataset, patent, and public policies. Figure 1 lists major online sources Altmetric tracks, which include citations on Wikipedia and public policy documents, discussions on research blogs, mainstream media coverage, bookmarks on reference managers like Mendeley, and mentions on social networks such as Twitter.

The Altmetric score (shown as the number inside an Altmetric "donut" in Fig. 1) is a weighted count of all the mentions Altmetric has tracked for an individual research output and is designed as an indicator of the amount and reach of the attention an item has received.

Altmetric provides citation-based information about how often journal articles and other scholarly outputs, like datasets, are discussed and used around the world. Altmetric cleans and normalizes the data from sources and then makes it available for analysis. Figure 2 is a screenshot of Altmetric Explorer. On the top of the page, you can type in search queries to find your interested research outputs. The searching results will be grouped into six categories: Highlights, Research Outputs, Timeline, Demographics, Mentions, and Journals. The dashboard of attention breakdown will display an overview of attention by social media, policy and patents, news and blogs, academic sources, and other sources. This is very helpful for scholars and practitioners to understand the impact of research outputs on the Internet. While traditional bibliometric studies focus on the scholarly communication in academic databases, Altmetric data will provide online social media communication of similar research outputs. Together we will be able to understand the research trends in both academic and practical worlds on the same research topic.

The research question of this study is: what are the research trends in dental informatics? The objective of the study is to identify the major characteristics of dental informatic research based on Altmetric data and provide implications to research and practical communities of dental informatics.

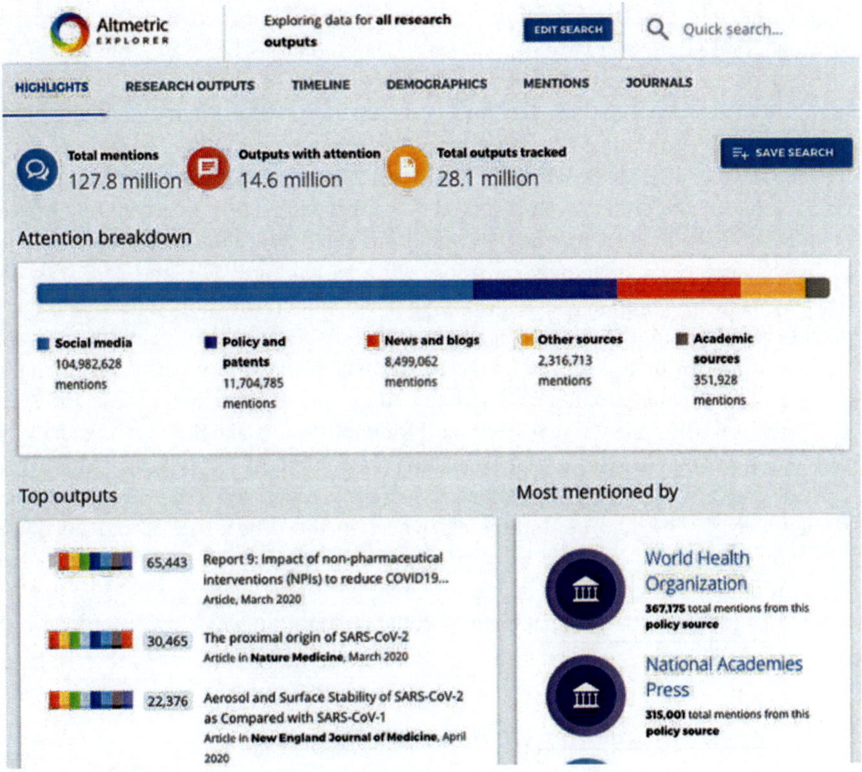

Fig. 2 A screenshot of Altmetric Explorer interface

2 Literature Review

2.1 Dental Informatics

Dental informatics is a relatively new field that incorporates computer and information science into dental practice [8]. Information science focuses on the implication, application, and support of computer technology and telecommunications. Oftentimes, information technology applications are a result of dental informatics research [6]. Currently, dental informatics applications are identified as such because there is a combination of computer technology and high-tech devices for unique dental use. Some examples are intra-oral imagery, laser handpieces, and office management systems. The data and information collected from high-tech devices are the dental informatics aspect of the system [8]. As of December 2003, there are approximately 600 papers published between 1975 and 2003 with a growth rate of about 50 papers annually [4]. Compared to other fields, dental informatics has a small number of publications, but the 10% annual growth from 1993 to 2003 means that DI is growing three times faster than other medical fields, which typically grow at a rate of 3% annually [4].

Since dental informatics is a relatively new field in the dental industry, it has not been fully developed, making the ability to transform oral medicine into a learning healthcare close to impossible. If information technology is able to be incorporated into the dental field, there would be an increase in efficiency for clinical practice. One reason for the underdeveloped field is the difficulties of implementing clinical computing. First of all, most dental offices are small and, therefore, cannot afford to spend large sums of money on information technology (IT), and 75.3% of all dentists work in a solo practice. Along with the amount of money needed for IT, dental computer applications are complex. This is because they need to maintain large amounts of data, such as images, treatment plans, and medical history of a patient, in an organized manner. There are companies that maintain these software and hardware components, making it hard for dentists to make their own form of IT sites. In a survey consisting of 39 questions, a sample of 1159 participants were sent the surveys. The results showed that 24.6% of respondents had computers at chairside, 62.3% had computers elsewhere in the office, 13.1% did not have computers, and 10.4% did not respond to the survey [5]. Informatics has contributed substantially to the growth of dental research, but more attention could be put on helping large and distant research teams collaborate through electronic tools [4].

2.2 Dental Informatics Challenges

There are multiple challenges in the field of dental informatics. In the field, there is no one system that can access the likelihood of successful outcomes for dental treatments. If such a system could be created, doctors and patients would have an easier time looking at the results of treatments and surgeries. Along with this, seeing results beforehand will ease the minds of patients, making the patients more likely to agree to the procedure that needs to take place. Besides a system that gives an estimation of outcomes for dental treatments, a decision aid for patients could be made. Currently, doctors have to speak with each patient about the procedures that might take place. This is time-consuming for the doctors, leading the patients to not have an in-depth understanding of the operation taking place. If a decision aid is created, patients will have a deeper understanding of what is going to take place, if the procedure takes place, and will be more engaged in the process as a whole. Along with a deeper understanding for the patient, doctors will not have to go through the procedures with the patient one on one, giving the doctors more time to think about procedures that have to be done and complete surgeries for patients [8].

In the last decade, there has been a rapid growth in the number of healthcare professionals and students with new technologies, such as computers. For example, 85% of dentists use computers in their offices, and the number of clinical uses for computers is growing. In the past 10 years, the clinical use of information technology in the dental field has increased substantially [2].

2.3 Support Systems

One solution to dental informatics challenges is a clinical decision support system (CDSS). CDSS are computer programs that help make expert decisions for health professionals. The programs use clinical knowledge to make educated decisions after analyzing patient data. The inference engine (IE) component of the CDSS is the main part of the system. The IE uses knowledge on the system and patients to draw conclusions regarding certain conditions. The collection of patient data, such as demographics, allergies, and medications, may be stored in the databases [2].

An alternative to the paternalistic care model is shared decision-making (SDM), which enables both patients and clinicians to reach mutual agreement on healthcare and treatment decisions. In SDM, patients are given all available pieces of evidence and information about a medical problem and the treatment choices. As SDM is a relatively new concept, there are multiple obstacles, such as task complexity, lack of time, and missing information [3].

2.4 Doctor-Patient Relationship

The strength of a doctor-patient relationship is important. The value of the relationship has been linked to important outcomes of care, including treatment compliance, clinical outcomes, malpractice, and switching physicians. Through the Internet, websites with a biography on the doctor can be found. This can give patients a sense of the doctor's values. Along with information about doctors, a website with information about a patient's personal health records can help enhance the relationship between doctor and patient. When patients have access to their own information, they find it easier to talk to their doctor, which enables them to feel more in control. This sense of control may lead to more trust in the relationship [1].

2.5 Ontology in Dental Informatics

One definition of ontology is "a formal, explicit specification of a shared conceptualization" [7]. As of 2012, there have been relatively few ontologies available for use in the dental community [9]. In order to build a comprehensive ontology for a particular domain, the relevant medical and oral terms have to be taken from the same scientific literature, such as peer-reviewed publications, government health education websites, and medical/dental textbooks. Moreover, accurate identification of relationships needs to happen in order for ontologies to be correctly evaluated [7].

2.6 *Applications of Dental Ontologies*

Ontologies can serve as a semantic backbone for linked data initiatives that want to make their data available on the Web in a form that is susceptible to machine-based processing. One benefit of making data available in an easily accessible format is that it opens up analytic opportunities. If the data is easily accessible, there are more opportunities for such data to be analyzed to reveal new relationships and contingencies. In some cases, these opportunities can lead to new insights and scientific discoveries. When data is made available on the Web, it becomes available in a form that allows for filtering, retrieval, and manipulation required for knowledge discovery. In the dental field, patient dental records are the main point of interest in Web-based platforms. Through conditions reported by patients, diagnosis made by dentists, advice given to patients, and various treatments administered, important information about predisposing health factors can be provided. There are many problems with patient dental records, such as the ethics of using patient data without consent or keeping patient confidentiality [9].

2.7 *Major Research Areas in Dental Informatics*

Training and Education

The way ontologies have been used to support training and education is indirect. Ontologies are used as a resource that supports the operation of e-learning systems. Along with being used in e-learning systems, ontologies have been used in augmented reality applications to assist students in learning about the preparation of teeth for all-ceramic restorations [9].

Compliance and Legal Issues

In some countries, the provision of dental services is regulated by the government and national agencies. One use of ontologies is to help support dental practitioners in understanding and complying with such regulations. The use of ontologies makes recording patient information easier for regulatory authorities to detect incidences of malpractice and noncompliance [9].

Evidence-Based Dentistry

Evidence-based dentistry (EBD) is a form of evidence-based medicine (EBM) that stresses the integration of scientific and clinical evidence with the expertise of individual dental practitioners to improve patient care. The actual means of integrating EBD into routine clinical practice remains unclear. EBD requires access to the latest empirical data regarding specific medical conditions and prevailing views on what constitutes best practice in certain situations [9].

3 Method

3.1 Dataset

In total, there were 11,211 articles from 2010 to 2020. In this dataset, metadata of research output includes article information (article title, journal title, subject keywords, affiliation, and publication year) and impact information (Altmetric attention score, policy mentions, Facebook mentions, news mentions, patent mentions, and Twitter mentions).

3.2 Procedure

Step 1. Determine Seed Query Keywords

To get the data used for this project, Altmetric Explorer was used. In order to determine the keywords used to collect data, the keyword "dental informatics" was initially used to search through Google Scholar. Among the search results, the author's keywords were examined. The top three keywords, "oral medicine," "dental computing," and "dental research trends," as well as "dental informatics," were chosen as our seed query keywords for this study.

Step 2. Search and Download Raw Data

After inserting seed query keywords into the search bar in Altmetric Explorer, research outputs, timeline, demographics, mentions, and journals appeared for each keyword. All of this information was allowed to be exported to Excel. When the data was separately exported, the information in the four keywords were combined together based on their subunits, such as mentions and journals, into one Excel sheet for easy manipulation.

Step 3. Data Clean-Up

In order to find the research trends in each subunit, the data had to be analyzed. Therefore, pivot tables were used in Excel to find the trends in the data. This is the main form of data manipulation used.

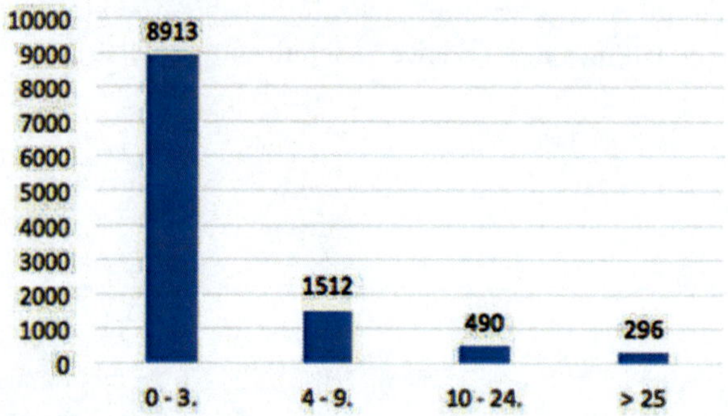

Fig. 3 Distribution of Altmetric attention score of dental informatics articles (2010–2020)

First, duplicated data had to be identified. After combining duplicates into one row, pivot tables were used for each of the subunits. Next, the simplified information was put into diagrams, such as pie charts, bar graphs, and charts. Through diagrams, the data for each subunit was easier to understand, making the research trends more distinct.

4 Results

4.1 Attention Score

The attention score for a research output provides insight into the amount of attention an output has received, with weights on specific types of sources due to the amount of attention brought by the source. Figure 3 shows the distribution of Altmetric attention score for articles on dental informatics in the past 10 years. Figure 4 shows the percentage of such distributions. In our research output data, the Altmetric attention score distribution was mainly in the range of 0–3, which composed 80% of the research output. In the attention score distribution, the highest Altmetric attention score was 1832. This explains that the majority of dental informatics research has little attention on social media.

4.2 Timeline for Mentions

Figure 5 shows a timeline of mentions in Twitter and Facebook. As shown in Fig. 5, the mentions varied on social media. For example, Twitter mentions have been rising since 2011, but Facebook mentions have stayed at a relatively low level. Therefore, if individuals wanted to find information on dental informatics on social media, Twitter would be a better source to look on rather than Facebook.

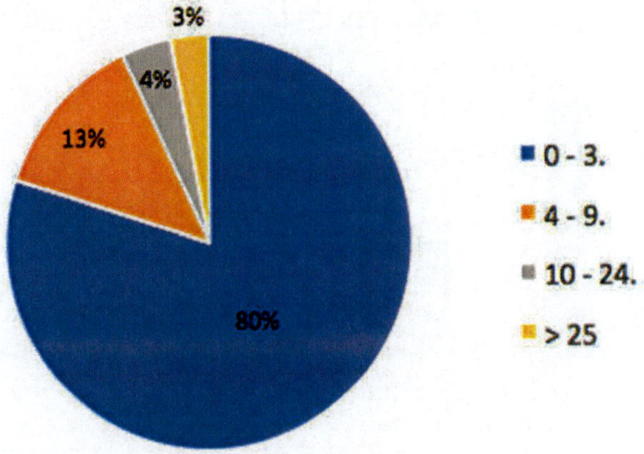

Fig. 4 Percentage of Altmetric attention score for dental informatics articles (2010–2020)

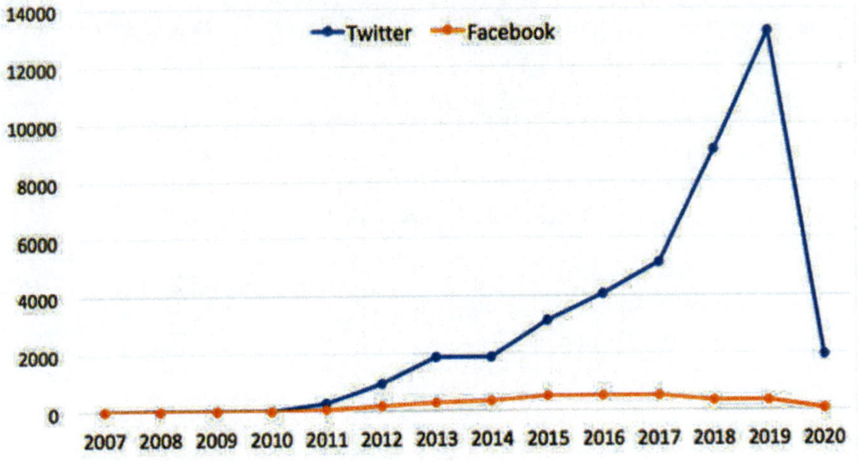

Fig. 5 Timeline for mentions on Twitter and Facebook

4.3 Twitter Demographics by Countries

For Twitter demographics, Fig. 6 shows that the top four countries of tweeters and tweets are the United States, United Kingdom, Spain, and Canada, but about 40% of tweeters or tweets do not indicate their country.

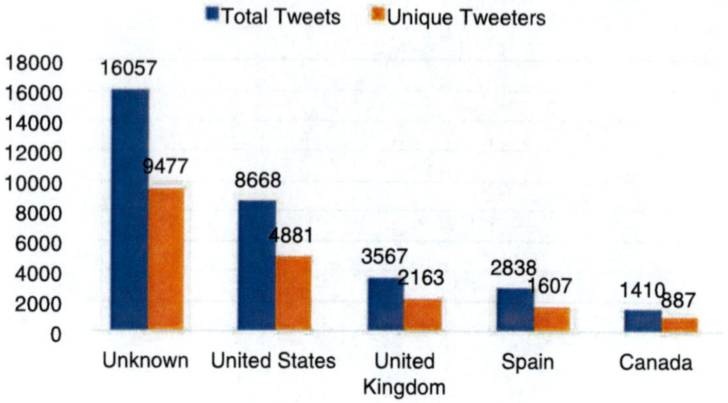

Fig. 6 Twitter demographics by top four countries

Table 1 Top ten journals for dental informatics

Rank	Journal title	Total mentions	%
1	New England Journal of Medicine	15,100	24%
2	Journal of Medicinal Chemistry	6826	11%
3	JAMA Internal Medicine	4833	8%
4	Annals of Emergency Medicine	2654	4%
5	Annals of Internal Medicine	2459	4%
6	Oral Surgery, Oral Medicine, Oral Pathology and Oral Radiology	1972	3%
7	Science Translational Medicine	1606	3%
8	Bioorganic & Medicinal Chemistry Letters	1538	2%
9	Journal of Oral Pathology & Medicine	1232	2%
10	Oral Surgery, Oral Medicine, Oral Pathology, Oral Radiology & Endodontology	1010	2%

4.4 *Top Ten Journals for Dental Informatics*

Table 1 shows the top ten journals with the most mentions. The top two journals, *New England Journal of Medicine* and *Journal of Medicinal Chemistry*, attracted more than one-third of mentions (35%). Interestingly, only two (#6 and #10) out of the top ten list are dental-specific journals.

4.5 *Frequency of Top Five Mention Categories*

There are 17 types of mention measures in Altmetric. However, many of them were practically zero in our collected data, showing that dental informatics does not receive enough publicity. Figure 7 lists top five mention categories whose

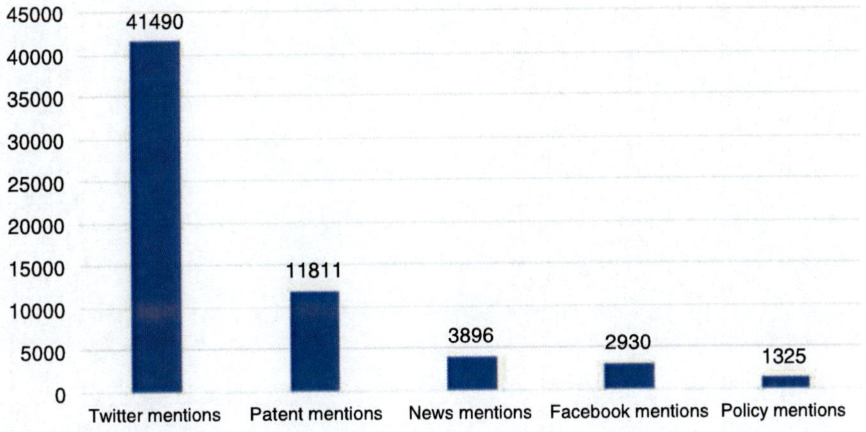

Fig. 7 Top five social media mentions

frequencies were above 1000. Twitter mentions highest (over 40,000), followed by patent mentions (11,811), news mentions (3896), Facebook mentions (2930), and policy mentions (1235).

4.6 Publications per Year

As shown in Fig. 8, in the 1900s, the number of publications annually has always been on the low side. It was not until around the 2000s did the publication rate increase. Over the past 10 years, the annual number of publications seems to be increasing at a fast rate.

4.7 Top 15 Publication Affiliations

Table 2 shows the top 15 affiliations of the first authors. The top affiliation is Merck Sharp & Dohme (MSD), an American multinational pharmaceutical company and one of the largest pharmaceutical companies in the world. Within the top 15 affiliations of the first authors, only four are outside the USA (#5, #9, #10, and #11), and seven out of nine colleges/universities are in the USA (shaded in Table 2). Thus, Altmetric data shows that US affiliations contributed majority of articles on dental informatics.

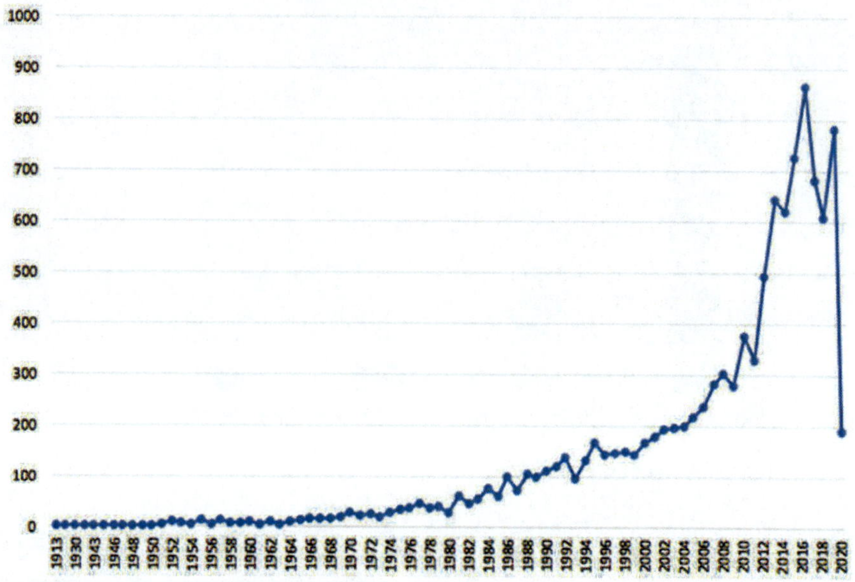

Fig. 8 Number of publications per year

Table 2 Top 15 affiliations of the first authors

Rank	Affiliation Name of First Authors	Count
1	MSD (United States)	115
2	Pfizer (United States)	90
3	University of Michigan–Ann Arbor	79
4	University of Rochester	68
5	Academic Center for Dentistry Amsterdam	65
5	University of California, San Francisco	65
7	Brigham and Women's Hospital	63
7	Harvard University	63
9	King's College London	62
10	Great Ormond Street Hospital	61
11	University of Queensland	59
12	Johns Hopkins University	54
13	Bristol-Myers Squibb (United States)	53
14	The Ohio State University	52
15	University of California, Los Angeles	50

5 Discussion and Conclusion

The findings from this study support what has been reviewed in the literature review. That is, dental informatics is a field that has a small number of publications, but it is growing at a fast rate. As shown in Fig. 7, the rate of publications since the 2000s has been increasing, regardless of the small number of publications. In addition, Fig. 5

displays how Twitter mentions have been rising since 2011. Dental informatics has recently started to gain interest from the public and will continue to do so as more individuals become aware of the challenges.

In Table 1, the top journal has 15,100 mentions, and the leading journal is *New England Journal of Medicine*. The total mentions of the leading journal have more than doubled those of the second ranked journal (*Journal of Medicinal Chemistry*). With the top two journals combined, the two attract more than one-third of mentions. Furthermore, only two out of top ten journals are dental-specific one. This implies that mentions of dental informatic articles on social media mainly went to those that were published on top journals in the field.

It is worthwhile to mention that 80% of research outputs with an attention score of 0–3 further show how little attention is put on the field of dental informatics on social media. In essence, dental informatics needs more publicity and research from researchers, scientists, and the public. There is an increase in multiple aspects, such as social media mentions and publications, but not enough to match other popular fields.

In the future, more recent data from Altmetric Explorer can be recollected and analyzed. The data analyzed was collected in March 2020, making the 2020 data incomplete. Since new journals come out daily, there may be an increase in attention scores or mentions.

References

1. M. Kirshner, The role of information technology and informatics research in the dentist-patient relationship. Adv. Dent. Res. **17**(1), 77–81 (2003)
2. E.A. Mendonça, Clinical decision support systems: Perspectives in dentistry. J. Dent. Educ. **68**(6), 589–597 (2004)
3. S.G. Park, S. Lee, M.K. Kim, H.G. Kim, Shared decision support system on dental restoration. Expert Syst. Appl. **39**(14), 11775–11781 (2012)
4. T.K. Schleyer, Dental informatics: A work in progress. Adv. Dent. Res. **17**(1), 9–15 (2003)
5. T.K. Schleyer, T.P. Thyvalikakath, H. Spallek, M.H. Torres-Urquidy, P. Hernandez, J. Yuhaniak, Clinical computing in general dentistry. J. Am. Med. Inform. Assoc. **13**(3), 344–352 (2006)
6. T. Schleyer, U. Mattsson, R. Ni Riordain, V. Brailo, M. Glick, R.B. Zain, M. Jontell, Advancing oral medicine through informatics and information technology: A proposed framework and strategy. Oral Dis. **17**, 85–94 (2011)
7. T. Shah, F. Rabhi, P. Ray, K. Taylor, A guiding framework for ontology reuse in the biomedical domain, in *Proceedings of 2014 47th Hawaii International Conference on System Sciences (HICSS)*, January 6–9, 2014,, (IEEE, Hawaii, 2014), pp. 2878–2887
8. D.F. Sittig, M. Kirshner, G. Maupome, Grand challenges in dental informatics. Adv. Dent. Res. **17**(1), 16–19 (2003)
9. P.R. Smart, M. Sadraie, Applications and uses of dental ontologies, in *e-Society*, (Berlin, Germany, 2012, 2012)

Part VI
Bioinformatics & Computational Biology – Applications and Novel Frameworks

A Novel Method for the Inverse QSAR/QSPR to Monocyclic Chemical Compounds Based on Artificial Neural Networks and Integer Programming

Ren Ito, Naveed Ahmed Azam, Chenxi Wang, Aleksandar Shurbevski, Hiroshi Nagamochi, and Tatsuya Akutsu

1 Introduction

Drug design is one of the important targets of bioinformatics and computational biology. Quantitative structure activity/property relationship (QSAR/QSPR) analysis is a major approach for computer-aided drug design. In particular, inverse QSAR/QSPR plays an important role [12, 18], which is to infer chemical structures from given chemical activities/properties. Inverse QSAR/QSPR is often formulated as an optimization problem to find a chemical structure maximizing (or minimizing) an objective function under various constraints. In this formalization, objective functions reflect certain chemical activities or properties, and are often derived from a set of training data consisting of known molecules and their activities/properties using statistical machine learning methods.

In many machine learning methods, input data are represented as vectors of real or integer numbers, which are called *feature vectors*. In QSAR/QSPR, chemical compounds are also represented as vectors of real or integer numbers, which are often called *descriptors*. Using these chemical descriptors, various heuristic and statistical methods have been developed for finding optimal or nearly optimal graph structures under given objective functions [8, 12, 16]. In many cases, inference or enumeration of graph structures from a given feature vector is a crucial subtask in these methods because it is quite difficult to directly handle chemical graphs. Var-

R. Ito · N. A. Azam (✉) · C. Wang · A. Shurbevski · H. Nagamochi
Department of Applied Mathematics and Physics, Kyoto University, Kyoto, Japan
e-mail: r.ito@amp.i.kyoto-u.ac.jp; azam@amp.i.kyoto-u.ac.jp; chenxi@amp.i.kyoto-u.ac.jp; shurbevski@amp.i.kyoto-u.ac.jp; nag@amp.i.kyoto-u.ac.jp

T. Akutsu
Institute for Chemical Research, Kyoto University, Uji, Japan
e-mail: takutsu@kuicr.kyoto-u.ac.jp

H. R. Arabnia et al. (eds.), *Advances in Computer Vision and Computational Biology*, Transactions on Computational Science and Computational Intelligence,
https://doi.org/10.1007/978-3-030-71051-4_51

ious methods have been developed for this enumeration problem [6, 9, 11, 15] and the computational complexity of the inference problem has been analyzed [2, 13]. On the other hand, enumeration in itself is a challenging task, since the number of molecules (i.e., chemical graphs) with up to 30 atoms (vertices) C, N, O, and S, may exceed 10^{60} [4].

As in many other fields, Artificial Neural Network (ANN) and deep learning technologies have recently been applied to inverse QSAR/QSPR. For example, variational autoencoders [7], recurrent neural networks [17, 20], and grammar variational autoencoders [10] have been applied. In these approaches, new chemical graphs are generated by solving a kind of inverse problems on neural networks, where neural networks are trained using known chemical compound/activity pairs. However, the optimality of the solution is not necessarily guaranteed in these approaches. In order to guarantee the optimality mathematically, a novel approach has been proposed [1] for ANNs, using mixed integer linear programming (MILP).

Recently, a new framework has been proposed [3, 5, 21] by combining two previous approaches: efficient enumeration of tree-like graphs [6], and MILP-based formulation of the inverse problem on ANNs [1]. This combined framework for inverse QSAR/QSPR mainly consists of two phases. The first phase solves (I) PREDICTION PROBLEM, where a prediction function $\psi_{\mathcal{N}}$ on a chemical property π is constructed with an ANN $\mathcal{N}$ using a data set of chemical compounds G and their values $a(G)$ of π. The second phase solves (II) INVERSE PROBLEM, where (II-a) given a target value y^* of the chemical property π, a feature vector x^* is inferred from the trained ANN $\mathcal{N}$ so that $\psi_{\mathcal{N}}(x^*)$ is close to y^* and (II-b) then a set of chemical structures G^* such that $f(G^*) = x^*$ is enumerated. In (II-b) of the abovementioned previous methods [3, 5, 21], an MILP is formulated for acyclic chemical compounds. However, their methods were applicable only to acyclic chemical graphs (i.e., tree-structured chemical graphs). This is a big limitation because the ratio of acyclic chemical graphs in a major chemical database (PubChem) is only 2.91%.

To break this limitation, we significantly extend the MILP-based approach for inverse QSAR/QSPR so that monocyclic chemical compounds can be efficiently handled. The ratio of acyclic and monocyclic chemical graphs in the database (PubChem) is 16.26%. We propose a novel MILP formulation for (II-a) along with a new set of descriptors. One big advantage of this new formulation is that an MILP instance has a solution if and only if there exists a monocyclic chemical graph satisfying given constraints, which is useful to significantly reduce redundant search in (II-b). We conducted computational experiments to infer monocyclic chemical compounds on several chemical properties.

2 Preliminary

Let $\mathbb{R}$ and $\mathbb{Z}$ denote the sets of reals and non-negative integers, respectively. For two integers a and b, let $[a, b]$ denote the set of integers i with $a \leq i \leq b$.

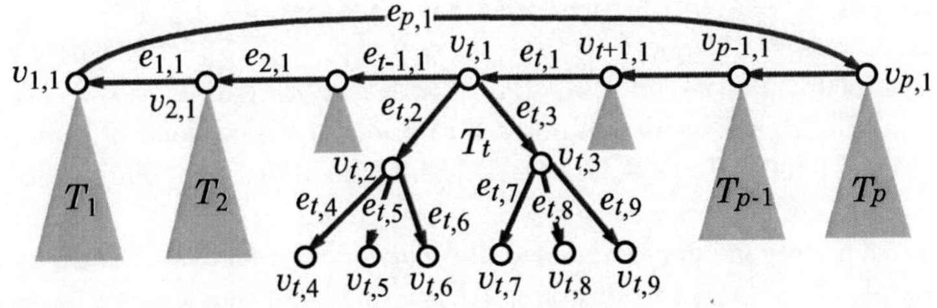

Fig. 1 An illustration of the monocyclic skeleton graph $H(2, 3, 2, p)$

Graphs Let $H = (V, E)$ be a graph with a set V of vertices and a set E of edges. For a vertex $v \in V$, the set of neighbors of v in H is denoted by $N_H(v)$, and the *degree* $\deg_H(v)$ of v is defined to be $|N_H(v)|$. Define the *1-path connectivity* $\kappa_1(H)$ of H to be $\sum_{uv\in E} 1/\sqrt{\deg_H(u)\deg_H(v)}$. We call a connected graph H with exactly one cycle of length at least 3 *monocyclic*. The *core* of a monocyclic graph H is defined to be an induced subgraph $H' = (V', E')$ such that V' is the set of vertices in a cycle of H. The *core size* $\mathrm{cs}(H)$ is defined to be $|V'|$, and the *core height* $\mathrm{ch}(H)$ is defined to be the maximum length of a path between a vertex $v \in V'$ to a leaf of H without passing through any edge in E'.

For positive integers a, b, and c with $b \geq 2$, let $T(a, b, c)$ denote the rooted tree such that the number of children of the root is a, the number of children of each non-root internal vertex is b and the distance from the root to each leaf is c. In the rooted tree $T(a, b, c)$, we denote the vertices by $v_1, v_2, \ldots, v_n$ $(n = a(b^c - 1)/(b - 1) + 1)$ with a breadth-first-search order, and denote the edge between a vertex v_i with $i \in [2, n]$ and its parent by e_i. For each vertex v_i in $T(a, b, c)$, let $\mathrm{Cld}(i)$ denote the set of indices j such that v_j is a child of v_i, and $\mathrm{prt}(i)$ denote the index j such that v_j is the parent of v_i when $i \in [2, n]$.

Given positive integers a, b, c, and p with $b \geq 2$ and $p \geq 3$, the *monocyclic skeleton graph* $H(a, b, c, p)$ is defined to be a monocyclic graph that is obtained from p disjoint copies T_t, $t = 1, 2, \ldots, p$ of tree $T(a, b, c)$ by joining the p roots of these trees with p edges to form a cycle C that consists of the p roots. In $H(a, b, c, p)$, let $v_{t,i}$ denote the vertex in the t-th copy T_t that corresponds to a vertex v_i of tree $T(a, b, c)$, and assume that the unique cycle C visits the p roots in the order $v_{p,1}, v_{p-1,1}, \ldots, v_{2,1}, v_{1,1}$ denoting the edge between $v_{t+1,1}$ and $v_{t,1}$ by $e_{t,1}$. Figure 1 illustrates an example of the monocyclic skeleton graph $H(2, 3, 2, p)$.

Chemical Graphs We represent the graph structure of a chemical compound as a graph with labels on vertices and multiplicity on edges in a hydrogen-suppressed model. Let Λ be a set of labels each of which represents a chemical element such as C (carbon), O (oxygen), N (nitrogen), and so on, where we assume that Λ does not contain H (hydrogen). Let mass(a) and val(a) denote the mass and valance of a chemical element a $\in \Lambda$, respectively. In our model, we use integers $\mathrm{mass}^*(\mathtt{a}) = \lfloor 10 \cdot \mathrm{mass}(\mathtt{a}) \rfloor$, a $\in \Lambda$. We introduce a total order $<$ over the elements in Λ according to their mass values; i.e., we write a $<$ b for chemical elements a, b $\in \Lambda$

with $\mathrm{mass}(\mathtt{a}) < \mathrm{mass}(\mathtt{b})$. Choose a set $\Gamma_<$ of tuples $\gamma = (\mathtt{a}, \mathtt{b}, k) \in \Lambda \times \Lambda \times [1, 3]$ such that $\mathtt{a} < \mathtt{b}$. For a tuple $\gamma = (\mathtt{a}, \mathtt{b}, k) \in \Lambda \times \Lambda \times [1, 3]$, let $\overline{\gamma}$ denote the tuple $(\mathtt{b}, \mathtt{a}, k)$. Set $\Gamma_> = \{\overline{\gamma} \mid \gamma \in \Gamma_<\}$, $\Gamma_= = \{(\mathtt{a}, \mathtt{a}, k) \mid \mathtt{a} \in \Lambda, k \in [1, 3]\}$ and $\Gamma = \Gamma_< \cup \Gamma_=$. A pair of two atoms a and b joined with a bond of multiplicity k is denoted by a tuple $\gamma = (\mathtt{a}, \mathtt{b}, k) \in \Gamma$, called the *adjacency-configuration* of the atom pair.

We use a hydrogen-suppressed model. A *chemical graph* over Λ and Γ is defined to be a tuple $G = (H, \alpha, \beta)$ of a graph $H = (V, E)$, a function $\alpha : V \to \Lambda$ and a function $\beta : E \to [1, 3]$ such that (1) H is connected; (2) $\sum_{uv \in E} \beta(uv) \leq \mathrm{val}(\alpha(u))$ for each vertex $u \in V$; and (3) $(\alpha(u), \alpha(v), \beta(uv)) \in \Gamma$ for each edge $uv \in E$. Let $\mathcal{G}(\Lambda, \Gamma)$ denote the set of chemical graphs over Λ and Γ. Nearly 68% of the monocyclic chemical graphs with at most 200 non-hydrogen atoms registered in chemical database PubChem have maximum degree at most 3 for all non-core vertices in the hydrogen-suppressed model.

Descriptors In our method, we use only graph-theoretical descriptors for defining a feature vector, which facilitates our designing an algorithm for constructing graphs. Given a chemical graph $G = (H, \alpha, \beta)$, we define a *feature vector* $f(G)$ that consists of the following 12 kinds of descriptors: $n(G)$: the number of vertices in G; $\mathrm{cs}(G)$: the core size of G; $\mathrm{ch}(G)$: the core height of G; $\kappa_1(G)$: the 1-path connectivity of G; $\mathrm{dg}_i(G)$ $(i \in [1, 4])$: the number of vertices of degree i in G; $\mathrm{ce}^{\mathrm{cr}}_{\mathtt{a}}(G)$ $(\mathtt{a} \in \Lambda)$: the number of core vertices with chemical element $\mathtt{a} \in \Lambda$; $\mathrm{ce}^{\mathrm{nc}}_{\mathtt{a}}(G)$ $(\mathtt{a} \in \Lambda)$: the number of core vertices with chemical element $\mathtt{a} \in \Lambda$; $\overline{\mathrm{ms}}(G)$: the average of mass* of atoms in G; $b^{\mathrm{cr}}_k(G)$ $(k \in [2, 3])$: the number of double and triple bonds in core edges; $b^{\mathrm{nc}}_k(G)$ $(k \in [2, 3])$: the number of double and triple bonds in non-core edges; $\mathrm{ac}^{\mathrm{cr}}_{\gamma}(G)$ $(\gamma = (\mathtt{a}, \mathtt{b}, k) \in \Gamma)$: the number of adjacency-configurations $(\mathtt{a}, \mathtt{b}, k)$ of core edges; $\mathrm{ac}^{\mathrm{nc}}_{\gamma}(G)$ $(\gamma = (\mathtt{a}, \mathtt{b}, k) \in \Gamma)$: the number of adjacency-configurations $(\mathtt{a}, \mathtt{b}, k)$ of non-core edges. The number k of descriptors in our feature vector $x = f(G)$ is $k = 2|\Lambda| + 2|\Gamma| + 13$.

3 A Method for Inferring Chemical Graphs

We review the framework that solves the inverse QSAR/QSPR by using MILPs [3], which is illustrated in Fig. 2. For a specified chemical property π such as boiling point, we denote by $a(G)$ the observed value of the property π for a chemical compound G. As the first phase, we solve (I) PREDICTION PROBLEM with the following three steps.

Phase 1

1. Let DB be a set of chemical graphs. For a specified chemical property π, choose a class $\mathcal{G}$ of graphs such as acyclic graphs or monocyclic graphs. Prepare a data set $D_\pi = \{G_i \mid i = 1, 2, \ldots, m\} \subseteq \mathcal{G} \cap \mathrm{DB}$ such that the value $a(G_i)$ of

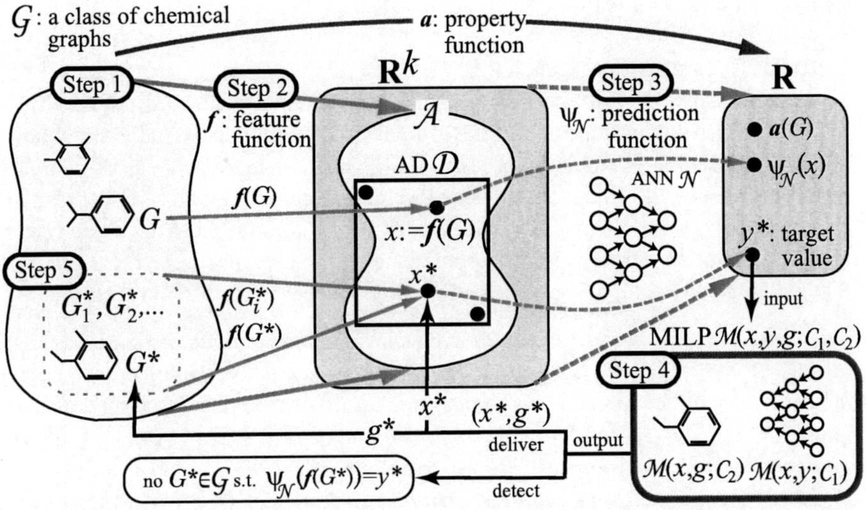

Fig. 2 A property function a, a feature function f, a prediction function $\psi_{\mathcal{N}}$, and an MILP that either delivers a vector (x^*, g^*) that forms a chemical graph $G^* \in \mathcal{G}$ such that $\psi_{\mathcal{N}}(f(G^*)) = y^*$ (or $a(G^*) = y^*$) or detects that $\mathcal{G}$ contains no such chemical graph G^*

each chemical graph G_i, $i = 1, 2, \ldots, m$ is available. Set reals $\underline{a}, \overline{a} \in \mathbb{R}$ so that $\underline{a} \leq a(G_i) \leq \overline{a}$, $i = 1, 2, \ldots, m$.

2. Introduce a feature function $f : \mathcal{G} \to \mathbb{R}^k$ for a positive integer k. We call $f(G)$ the *feature vector* of $G \in \mathcal{G}$, and call each entry of a vector $f(G)$ a *descriptor* of G.
3. Construct a prediction function $\psi_{\mathcal{N}}$ with an ANN $\mathcal{N}$ that, given a vector in $x \in \mathbb{R}^k$, returns a real $\psi_{\mathcal{N}}(x)$ with $\underline{a} \leq \psi_{\mathcal{N}}(x) \leq \overline{a}$ so that $\psi_{\mathcal{N}}(f(G))$ takes a value nearly equal to $a(G)$ for many chemical graphs in D.

A vector $x \in \mathbb{R}^k$ is called *admissible* if there is a graph $G \in \mathcal{G}$ such that $f(G) = x$ [3]. Let $\mathcal{A}$ denote the set of admissible vectors $x \in \mathbb{R}^k$. In this paper, we use the range-based method to define an applicability domain (AD) [14] to our inverse QSAR/QSPR. Set $\underline{x_j}$ and $\overline{x_j}$ to be the minimum and maximum values of the j-th descriptor x_j in $f(G_i)$ over all graphs G_i, $i = 1, 2, \ldots, m$ (where we possibly normalize some descriptors such as $\mathrm{ce}_{\mathrm{a}}^{cr}(G)$, which is normalized with $\mathrm{ce}_{\mathrm{a}}^{cr}(G)/n(G)$). Define our AD $\mathcal{D}$ to be the set of vectors $x \in \mathbb{R}^k$ such that $\underline{x_j} \leq x_j \leq \overline{x_j}$ for the variable x_j of each j-th descriptor, $j = 1, 2, \ldots, k$. See Fig. 2 for an illustration of functions a, f, and ψ and sets $\mathcal{A}$ and $\mathcal{D}$. As the second phase, we solve (II) Inverse Problem for the inverse QSAR/QSPR by treating the following inference problems.

(II-a) Inference of Vectors
Input: A real y^* with $\underline{a} \leq y^* \leq \overline{a}$.
Output: Vectors $x^* \in \mathcal{A} \cap \mathcal{D}$ and $g^* \in \mathbb{R}^h$ such that $\psi_{\mathcal{N}}(x^*) = y^*$ and g^* forms a chemical graph $G^* \in \mathcal{G}$ with $f(G^*) = x^*$.

(II-b) Inference of Graphs
Input: A vector $x^* \in \mathcal{A} \cap \mathcal{D}$.
Output: All graphs $G^* \in \mathcal{G}$ such that $f(G^*) = x^*$.

To treat Problem (II-a), we use MILPs for inferring vectors in ANNs [1]. In MILPs, we can easily impose additional linear constraints or fix some variables to specified constants. We include into the MILP a linear constraint such that $x \in \mathcal{D}$ to obtain the next result. In the previous method [5], they tried to find a vector $x^* \in \mathbb{R}^k$ such that $\psi_{\mathcal{N}}(x^*) = y^*$ in (II-a), which may not be admissible. Afterwards, Azam et al. [3] included into (II-a) another vector g that represents a chemical graph so that any inferred vector x^* becomes admissible whenever the MILP is feasible.

Theorem 1 *Let $\mathcal{N}$ be an ANN with a piecewise-linear activation function for an input vector $x \in \mathbb{R}^k$, n_A denote the number of nodes in the architecture, and n_B denote the total number of break-points over all activation functions. Then there is an MILP $\mathcal{M}(x, y; \mathcal{C}_1)$ that consists of variable vectors $x \in \mathcal{D}$ ($\subseteq \mathbb{R}^k$), $y \in \mathbb{R}$, and an auxiliary variable vector $z \in \mathbb{R}^p$ for some integer $p = O(n_A + n_B)$ and a set $\mathcal{C}_1$ of $O(n_A + n_B)$ constraints on these variables such that: $\psi_{\mathcal{N}}(x^*) = y^*$ if and only if there is a vector (x^*, y^*) feasible to $\mathcal{M}(x, y; \mathcal{C}_1)$.*

The constraints that we included in the MILP $\mathcal{M}(x, y; \mathcal{C}_1)$ in Theorem 1 to define our AD $\mathcal{D}$ are as follows.

AD constraints in $\mathcal{C}_1$:
constants:
Integers $\mathrm{cs}^* \geq 3$ and $\mathrm{ch}^* \geq 1$; An integer $d_{\max} \in \{3, 4\}$;
An integer $n^* \in [\mathrm{cs}^* + 1, \mathrm{cs}^* \cdot (d_{\max} - 1)^{\mathrm{ch}^*}]$;
variables x for descriptors:
$\mathrm{Mass} \in \mathbb{Z}$; $\kappa \in \mathbb{R}$; $\mathrm{dg}(d) \in [0, n^*]$ $(d \in [1, 4])$;
$\mathrm{ce}^{\mathrm{cr}}(\mathrm{a}), \mathrm{ce}^{\mathrm{nc}}(\mathrm{a}) \in [0, n^*]$ $(\mathrm{a} \in \Lambda)$;
$\mathrm{b}^{\mathrm{cr}}(k), \mathrm{b}^{\mathrm{nc}}(k) \in [0, n^* - 1]$ $(k \in [1, 3])$;
$\mathrm{ac}^{\mathrm{cr}}(\gamma), \mathrm{ac}^{\mathrm{nc}}(\gamma) \in [0, n^*]$ $(\gamma \in \Gamma)$;
constraints:

$$n^* \min_{G \in D} \frac{\kappa_1(G)}{n(G)} \leq \kappa \leq n^* \max_{G \in D} \frac{\kappa_1(G)}{n(G)};$$

$$n^* \min_{G \in D} \frac{\mathrm{dg}_d(G)}{n(G)} \leq \mathrm{dg}(d) \leq n^* \max_{G \in D} \frac{\mathrm{dg}_d(G)}{n(G)}, d \in [1, 4];$$

$$\min_{G \in D} \overline{\mathrm{ms}}(G) \leq \mathrm{Mass} \leq \max_{G \in D} \overline{\mathrm{ms}}(G);$$

$$n^* \min_{G \in D} \frac{\mathrm{ce}^{\mathrm{cr}}_{\mathrm{a}}(G)}{n(G)} \leq \mathrm{ce}^{\mathrm{cr}}(\mathrm{a}) \leq n^* \max_{G \in D} \frac{\mathrm{ce}^{\mathrm{cr}}_{\mathrm{a}}(G)}{n(G)}, \mathrm{a} \in \Lambda;$$

$$n^* \min_{G \in D} \frac{b^{\mathrm{cr}}_k(G)}{n(G)} \leq \mathrm{b}^{\mathrm{cr}}(k) \leq n^* \max_{G \in D} \frac{b^{\mathrm{cr}}_k(G)}{n(G)}, k \in [2, 3];$$

$$n^* \min_{G \in D} \frac{\mathrm{ac}^{\mathrm{cr}}_{\gamma}(G)}{n(G)} \leq \mathrm{ac}^{\mathrm{cr}}(\gamma) \leq n^* \max_{G \in D} \frac{\mathrm{ac}^{\mathrm{cr}}_{\gamma}(G)}{n(G)}, \gamma \in \Gamma,$$

where some constraints on $\mathrm{ce}^{\mathrm{nc}}(\mathtt{a})$, $\mathrm{b}^{\mathrm{nc}}(k)$, and $\mathrm{ac}^{\mathrm{nc}}(\gamma)$ similar to those on $\mathrm{ce}^{\mathrm{cr}}(\mathtt{a})$, $\mathrm{b}^{\mathrm{cr}}(k)$, and $\mathrm{ac}^{\mathrm{cr}}(\gamma)$ are omitted.

To attain the admissibility of inferred vector x^*, we also introduce a variable vector $g \in \mathbb{R}^q$ for some integer q and a set $\mathcal{C}_2$ of constraints on x and g such that $x^* \in \mathcal{A}$ holds in the following sense: (x^*, g^*) is feasible to the MILP $\mathcal{M}(x, g; \mathcal{C}_2)$ if and only if g^* forms a chemical graph $G^* \in \mathcal{G}$ with $f(G^*) = x^*$.

We design an algorithm to Problem (II-b) based on the branch-and-bound method (see [19] for enumerating monocyclic chemical compounds).

The second phase consists of the next two steps.

Phase 2

4. Formulate Problem (II-a) as the above MILP $\mathcal{M}(x, y, g; \mathcal{C}_1, \mathcal{C}_2)$ based on $\mathcal{G}$ and $\mathcal{N}$. Find a set F^* of vectors $x^* \in \mathcal{A} \cap \mathcal{D}$ such that $(1-\varepsilon)y^* \leq \psi_{\mathcal{N}}(x^*) \leq (1+\varepsilon)y^*$ for a tolerance ε set to be a small positive real.
5. To solve Problem (II-b), enumerate all graphs $G^* \in \mathcal{G}$ such that $f(G^*) = x^*$ for each vector $x^* \in F^*$.

See Fig. 2 for an illustration of Steps 4 and 5.

In this paper, we formulate an MILP $\mathcal{M}(x, g; \mathcal{C}_2)$ for the class $\mathcal{G}$ of monocyclic chemical graphs.

4 MILPs for Monocyclic Chemical Graphs

In this section, we present a formulation to the MILP $\mathcal{M}(x, g; \mathcal{C}_2)$ in Step 4 of the framework. For inferring an acyclic chemical graph with an MILP, the previous formulation due to Azam et al. [3] is based on an idea that a required acyclic chemical graph G^* with n vertices will be constructed as a subset of $n-1$ vertex pairs as edges over an $n \times n$ adjacency matrix (or a complete graph K_n with n vertices). Afterwards, Zhang et al. [21] introduced a new formulation so that G^* will be constructed as an induced subgraph of a larger "acyclic graph," which they called "a skeleton tree." In this paper, we extend the idea of "a skeleton tree" in such a way that a required monocyclic chemical graph will be selected as an induced subgraph of a larger monocyclic graph. For integers $d_{\max}, n^*, \mathrm{cs}^*, \mathrm{ch}^* \in \mathbb{Z}$, let $\mathcal{H}(d_{\max}, n^*, \mathrm{cs}^*, \mathrm{ch}^*)$ denote the set of monocyclic graphs H such that the degree of each core vertex is at most 4, the degree of each non-core vertex is at most $d_{\max}$, $n(H) = n^*$, $\mathrm{cs}(H) = \mathrm{cs}^*$ and $\mathrm{ch}(H) = \mathrm{ch}^*$. Let $n_{\mathrm{tree}} = 1 + 2((d_{\max}-1)^{\mathrm{ch}^*} - 1)/(d_{\max}-2)$, and $n_{\mathrm{in}} = 1+2((d_{\max}-1)^{\mathrm{ch}^*-1}-1)/(d_{\max}-2)$, where n_{tree} and n_{in} are the numbers of vertices and non-leaf vertices in the rooted tree $T(2, d_{\max}-1, \mathrm{ch}^*)$, respectively. In this paper, we obtain the following result.

Theorem 2 *Let Λ be a set of chemical elements, Γ be a set of adjacency-configurations, where $|\Lambda| \leq |\Gamma|$, and $k = 2|\Lambda| + 2|\Gamma| + 13$. Given integers $d_{\max} \in [2, 4]$, $n^* \geq 3$, $\mathrm{cs}^* \geq 3$, and $\mathrm{ch}^* \geq 0$, there is an MILP $\mathcal{M}(x, g; \mathcal{C}_2)$ that consists of variable vectors $x \in \mathbb{R}^k$, $g \in \mathbb{R}^q$ for an integer $q = O(|\Gamma| \cdot \mathrm{cs}^* \cdot n_{\mathrm{tree}})$ and a set $\mathcal{C}_2$ of $O(|\Gamma| + \mathrm{cs}^* \cdot n_{\mathrm{tree}})$ constraints on x and g such that: (x^*, g^*) is feasible to $\mathcal{M}(x, g; \mathcal{C}_2)$ if and only if g^* forms a monocyclic chemical graph $G^* = (H, \alpha, \beta) \in \mathcal{G}(\Lambda, \Gamma)$ such that $H \in \mathcal{H}(d_{\max}, n^*, \mathrm{cs}^*, \mathrm{ch}^*)$ and $f(G^*) = x^*$.*

We formulate an MILP in Theorem 2 so that such a graph H is selected as a subgraph of the monocyclic skeleton graph. For a technical reason, we introduce a dummy chemical element ϵ, and denote by Γ_0 the set of dummy tuples (ϵ, ϵ, k), $(\epsilon, \mathtt{a}, k)$, and $(\mathtt{a}, \epsilon, k)$ ($\mathtt{a} \in \Lambda$, $k \in [0, 3]$). To represent elements $\mathtt{a} \in \Lambda \cup \{\epsilon\} \cup \Gamma_< \cup \Gamma_= \cup \Gamma_>$ in an MILP, we encode these elements a into some integers denoted by $[\mathtt{a}]$, where we assume that $[\epsilon] = 0$. In the following, we show our formulation of $\mathcal{M}(x, g; \mathcal{C}_2)$ for the case $d_{\max} \in \{3, 4\}$.

MILP $\mathcal{M}(x, g; \mathcal{C}_2)$

variables g **for constructing** G**:**

$v(t, i) \in \{0, 1\}$, $\deg(t, i) \in [0, 4]$, $\widetilde{\beta}(t, i) \in [0, 3]$,
$\eta(t, i) \in [1, n_{\mathrm{tree}}]$, $\widetilde{\alpha}(t, i) \in \{[\mathtt{a}] \mid \mathtt{a} \in \Lambda \cup \{\epsilon\}\}$
$(t \in [1, \mathrm{cs}^*], i \in [1, n_{\mathrm{tree}}])$;
$\delta_{\deg}(t, i, d) \in \{0, 1\}$ $(t \in [1, \mathrm{cs}^*], i \in [1, n_{\mathrm{tree}}], d \in [0, 4])$;
$\delta_{\kappa}(t, i, d, d') \in \{0, 1\}$ $(t \in [1, \mathrm{cs}^*], i \in [1, n_{\mathrm{tree}}], d, d' \in [0, 4])$;
$\delta_{\tau}(t, i, \gamma) \in \{0, 1\}$ $(t \in [1, \mathrm{cs}^*], i \in [1, n_{\mathrm{tree}}], \gamma \in \Gamma \cup \Gamma_0)$;
$\delta_{\mathrm{dd}}(t, i, d, d') \in \{0, 1\}$, $t \in [1, \mathrm{cs}^*]$, $i \in [1, n_{\mathrm{tree}}]$, $d, d' \in [0, 4]$;

constraints in $\mathcal{C}_2$**:**

For choosing a graph $H \in \mathcal{H}(d_{\max}, n^*, \mathrm{cs}^*, \mathrm{ch}^*)$, we include in $\mathcal{C}_2$ the following constraints:

$$v(t, 1) = 1, \; t \in [1, \mathrm{cs}^*]; \qquad \sum_{t \in [1, \mathrm{cs}^*], i \in [1, n_{\mathrm{tree}}]} v(t, i) = n^*;$$

$$n^* \cdot v(t, i) \geq \sum_{j \in \mathrm{Cld}(i)} v(t, j), \quad t \in [1, \mathrm{cs}^*], i \in [2, n_{\mathrm{in}}];$$

$$\deg(t, 1) = \sum_{j \in \mathrm{Cld}(1)} v(t, j) + 2, \quad t \in [1, \mathrm{cs}^*];$$

$$\deg(t, i) = \sum_{j \in \mathrm{Cld}(i)} v(t, j) + v(t, i), \quad t \in [1, \mathrm{cs}^*], \quad i \in [2, n_{\mathrm{in}}];$$

$$\deg(t, i) = v(t, i), \quad t \in [1, \mathrm{cs}^*], \quad i \in [n_{\mathrm{in}} + 1, n_{\mathrm{tree}}];$$

$$\sum_{d \in [0,4]} \delta_{\deg}(t, i, d) = 1, \quad t \in [1, \mathrm{cs}^*], \quad i \in [1, n_{\mathrm{tree}}];$$

$$\sum_{d\in[1,4]} d\cdot\delta_{\mathrm{deg}}(t,i,d)=\mathrm{deg}(t,i),\quad t\in[1,\mathrm{cs}^*],\quad i\in[1,n_{\mathrm{tree}}];$$

$$\sum_{t\in[1,\mathrm{cs}^*],\ i\in[1,n_{\mathrm{tree}}]} \delta_{\mathrm{deg}}(t,i,d)=\mathrm{dg}(d),\quad d\in[1,4];$$

$$\sum_{t\in[1,\mathrm{cs}^*],\ i\in[n_{\mathrm{in}}+1,n_{\mathrm{tree}}]} v(t,i)\geq 1;$$

$$\sum_{t\in[1,\mathrm{cs}^*],\ i\in[2,n_{\mathrm{tree}}]} \delta_{\mathrm{deg}}(t,i,4)\geq 1\ (=0)\ \text{if}\ d_{\max}=4\ (=3).$$

For choosing functions α and β so that $(H,\alpha,\beta)\in\mathcal{G}(\Lambda,\Gamma)$, we include in $\mathcal{C}_2$ the following constraints:

$$\sum_{\substack{t\in[1,\mathrm{cs}^*],\\ \gamma=(\mathtt{a},\mathtt{b},k)\in\Gamma}} \delta_\tau(t,1,\gamma)=\mathrm{ce}^{\mathrm{cr}}(\mathtt{a}),\ \mathtt{a}\in\Lambda;\qquad \sum_{\substack{t\in[1,\mathrm{cs}^*],\\ i\in[2,n_{\mathrm{tree}}],\\ \gamma=(\mathtt{a},\mathtt{b},k)\in\Gamma}} \delta_\tau(t,i,\gamma)=\mathrm{ce}^{\mathrm{nc}}(\mathtt{b}),\ \mathtt{b}\in\Lambda;$$

$$\sum_{\mathtt{a}\in\Lambda} \mathrm{mass}^*(\mathtt{a})(\mathrm{ce}^{\mathrm{cr}}(\mathtt{a})+\mathrm{ce}^{\mathrm{nc}}(\mathtt{a}))=\mathrm{Mass};$$

$$v(t,i)\leq\widetilde{\beta}(t,i)\leq 3v(t,i),\quad t\in[1,\mathrm{cs}^*],\quad i\in[1,n_{\mathrm{tree}}];$$

$$\sum_{\gamma=(\mathtt{a},\mathtt{b},k)\in\Gamma} \mathrm{ac}^{\mathrm{cr}}(\gamma)=\mathrm{b}^{\mathrm{cr}}(k),\quad k\in[1,3];\qquad \sum_{\gamma=(\mathtt{a},\mathtt{b},k)\in\Gamma} \mathrm{ac}^{\mathrm{nc}}(\gamma)=\mathrm{b}^{\mathrm{nc}}(k),\quad k\in[1,3];$$

$$\widetilde{\beta}(t,i)+\sum_{j\in\mathrm{Cld}(i)}\widetilde{\beta}(t,j)\leq\sum_{\gamma=(\mathtt{a},\mathtt{b},k)\in\Gamma}\mathrm{val}(\mathtt{b})\cdot\delta_\tau(t,i,\gamma),\ t\in[1,\mathrm{cs}^*],\ i\in[2,n_{\mathrm{tree}}];$$

$$\widetilde{\beta}(t-1,1)+\widetilde{\beta}(t,1)+\sum_{j\in\mathrm{Cld}(1)}\widetilde{\beta}(t,j)\leq\sum_{\gamma=(\mathtt{a},\mathtt{b},k)\in\Gamma}\mathrm{val}(\mathtt{b})\cdot\delta_\tau(t,1,\gamma),\ t\in[2,\mathrm{cs}^*];$$

$$\widetilde{\beta}(\mathrm{cs}^*,1)+\widetilde{\beta}(1,1)+\sum_{j\in\mathrm{Cld}(1)}\widetilde{\beta}(1,j)\leq\sum_{\gamma=(\mathtt{a},\mathtt{b},k)\in\Gamma}\mathrm{val}(\mathtt{b})\cdot\delta_\tau(1,1,\gamma);$$

$$\sum_{(\mathtt{a},\mathtt{b},2)\in\Gamma}\delta_\tau(\mathrm{cs}^*,1,(\mathtt{a},\mathtt{b},2))+\sum_{(\mathtt{a},\mathtt{b},2)\in\Gamma}\delta_\tau(1,1,(\mathtt{a},\mathtt{b},2))\leq 1.$$

For counting edges with each adjacency-configuration from functions α and β, we include in $\mathcal{C}_2$ the following constraints:

$$\sum_{\gamma\in\Gamma\cup\Gamma_0}\delta_\tau(t,i,\gamma)=1,\quad t\in[1,\mathrm{cs}^*],\quad i\in[1,n_{\mathrm{tree}}];$$

$$\sum_{\gamma=(\mathrm{a},\mathrm{b},k)\in\Gamma\cup\Gamma_0} [\mathrm{a}]\delta_\tau(t,i,\gamma) = \widetilde{\alpha}(t,\mathrm{prt}(i)),\ \ t\in[1,\mathrm{cs}^*],\ \ i\in[2,n_{\mathrm{tree}}];$$

$$\sum_{\gamma=(\mathrm{a},\mathrm{b},k)\in\Gamma\cup\Gamma_0} [\mathrm{b}]\delta_\tau(t,i,\gamma)=\widetilde{\alpha}(t,i),\ \ t\in[1,\mathrm{cs}^*],\ \ i\in[2,n_{\mathrm{tree}}];$$

$$\sum_{\gamma=(\mathrm{a},\mathrm{b},k)\in\Gamma} [\mathrm{a}]\delta_\tau(t,1,\gamma) = \widetilde{\alpha}(t+1,1),\ \ t\in[1,\mathrm{cs}^*-1];$$

$$\sum_{\gamma=(\mathrm{a},\mathrm{b},k)\in\Gamma} [\mathrm{a}]\delta_\tau(\mathrm{cs}^*,1,\gamma) = \widetilde{\alpha}(1,1);$$

$$\sum_{\gamma=(\mathrm{a},\mathrm{b},k)\in\Gamma} [\mathrm{b}]\delta_\tau(t,1,\gamma) = \widetilde{\alpha}(t,1),\ \ t\in[1,\mathrm{cs}^*];$$

$$\sum_{\gamma=(\mathrm{a},\mathrm{b},k)\in\Gamma\cup\Gamma_0} k\delta_\tau(t,i,\gamma)=\widetilde{\beta}(t,i),\ \ t\in[1,\mathrm{cs}^*],\ \ i\in[1,n_{\mathrm{tree}}];$$

$$\sum_{t\in[1,\mathrm{cs}^*]} (\delta_\tau(t,1,\gamma)+\delta_\tau(t,1,\overline{\gamma})) = \mathrm{ac}^{\mathrm{cr}}(\gamma),\ \ \gamma\in\Gamma_<;$$

$$\sum_{t\in[1,\mathrm{cs}^*]} \delta_\tau(t,1,\gamma) = \mathrm{ac}^{\mathrm{cr}}(\gamma),\ \ \gamma\in\Gamma_=,$$

where some constraints on $\mathrm{ac}^{\mathrm{nc}}(\gamma)$ similar to those on $\mathrm{ac}^{\mathrm{cr}}(\gamma)$ are omitted. To compute the 1-path connectivity, we include in $\mathcal{C}_2$ the following constraints:

$$\sum_{d,d'\in[0,4]} \delta_{\mathrm{dd}}(t,i,d,d') = 1,\ \ t\in[1,\mathrm{cs}^*],\ \ i\in[1,n_{\mathrm{tree}}];$$

$$\sum_{d,d'\in[0,4]} d\delta_{\mathrm{dd}}(t,1,d,d') = \deg(t+1,1),\ \ t\in[1,\mathrm{cs}^*-1];$$

$$\sum_{d,d'\in[0,4]} d\delta_{\mathrm{dd}}(\mathrm{cs}^*,1,d,d') = \deg(1,1);$$

$$\sum_{d,d'\in[0,4]} d'\delta_{\mathrm{dd}}(t,1,d,d') = \deg(t,1),\ \ t\in[1,\mathrm{cs}^*];$$

$$\sum_{d,d'\in[0,4]} d\delta_{\mathrm{dd}}(t,i,d,d') = \deg(t,\mathrm{prt}(i)),\ \ t\in[1,\mathrm{cs}^*],\ \ i\in[2,n_{\mathrm{tree}}];$$

$$\sum_{d,d'\in[0,4]} d'\delta_{\mathrm{dd}}(t,i,d,d') = \deg(t,i),\ \ t\in[1,\mathrm{cs}^*],\ \ i\in[2,n_{\mathrm{tree}}];$$

$$(1-\xi)\kappa \le \sum_{\substack{t\in[1,\mathrm{cs}^*],i\in[1,n_{\mathrm{tree}}],\\ d,d'\in[1,4]}} \delta_{\mathrm{dd}}(t,i,d,d')/\sqrt{dd'} \le (1+\xi)\kappa,$$

where a tolerance ξ is set to be 0.001. To reduce the number of monocyclic chemical graphs G that are isomorphic to each other over the skeleton monocyclic graph, we include in C_2 the following constraints, where $\mathrm{dsn}(t, i) \in [1, n_{\mathrm{tree}}]$ represents the number of descendants of a vertex $i \in [1, n_{\mathrm{tree}}]$ in tree T_t, $t \in [1, \mathrm{cs}^*]$. Define $\eta(t, j) \triangleq 21|\Lambda|\mathrm{dsn}(t, j) + 20\widetilde{\alpha}(t, j) + 4\mathrm{deg}(t, j) + \widetilde{\beta}(t, j)$.

$$\mathrm{dsn}(t, i) \geq \sum_{j \in \mathrm{Cld}(i)} \mathrm{dsn}(t, j) + v(t, i), \quad t \in [1, \mathrm{cs}^*],\ i \in [1, n_{\mathrm{tree}}];$$

$$\sum_{t \in [1, \mathrm{cs}^*]} \mathrm{dsn}(t, 1) \leq n^*; \eta(t, j_1) \geq \eta(t, j_2), \quad t \in [1, \mathrm{cs}^*],\ j_1, j_2 \in \mathrm{Cld}(1),\ j_1 < j_2;$$

$$\eta(t, j_1) \geq \eta(t, j_2), \quad t \in [1, \mathrm{cs}^*],\ i \in [2, n_{\mathrm{in}}],\ j_1, j_2 \in \mathrm{Cld}(i),\ j_1 < j_2, \text{ for } d_{\max} = 3;$$

$$\eta(t, j_1) \geq \eta(t, j_2) \geq \eta(t, j_3), \quad t \in [1, \mathrm{cs}^*],\ i \in [2, n_{\mathrm{in}}],$$
$$j_1, j_2, j_3 \in \mathrm{Cld}(i),\ j_1 < j_2 < j_3, \text{ for } d_{\max} = 4;$$

$$\eta(1, 1) \geq \eta(t, 1), \quad t \in [2, \mathrm{cs}^*]; \eta(2, 1) \geq \eta(\mathrm{cs}^*, 1).$$

5 Experimental Results

We constructed a system for inferring monocyclic chemical graphs and conducted experiments on a PC with Intel Core i5 1.6 GHz CPU and 8 GB of RAM running under the Mac OS operating system version 10.14.6. We select three chemical properties: heat of combustion (Hc), octanol/water partition coefficient (K_{OW}), and boiling point (Bp).

Results on Phase 1 We collected Hc, K_{OW}, and Bp information provided by HSDB from PubChem as data set. Table 1 shows the size and range of data sets that we prepared for each chemical property, where we denote the following: π: one of the chemical properties Hc, K_{OW}, and Bp; $|D_\pi|$: the size of data set D_π for property π; $|\Lambda|$: the number of chemical elements over data set D_π (hydrogen atoms are added at the final stage); $[\underline{n}, \overline{n}]$: the minimum and maximum number $n(G)$ of non-hydrogen atoms over data set D_π; $[\underline{\mathrm{cs}}, \overline{\mathrm{cs}}]$, $[\underline{\mathrm{ch}}, \overline{\mathrm{ch}}]$: the minimum and maximum core size and core height over chemical compounds in D_π, respectively; and $[\underline{a}, \overline{a}]$: the minimum and maximum values of $a(G)$ for property π over data set D_π.

In Step 2, we set a graph class $\mathcal{G}$ to be the set of all monocyclic chemical graphs over the sets Λ and Γ in Table 1.

In Step 3, we used `scikit-learn` version 0.21.6 with Python 3.7.4 to construct ANNs $\mathcal{N}$ where the tool and activation function are set to be MLPRegressor and ReLU, respectively. We tested several different architectures of ANNs for each chemical property. To evaluate the performance of the resulting prediction function $\psi_{\mathcal{N}}$ with cross-validation, we partition a given data set D_π into five subsets $D_\pi^{(i)}$, $i \in [1, 5]$ randomly, where $D_\pi \setminus D_\pi^{(i)}$ is used for a training set and $D_\pi^{(i)}$ is used for

Table 1 Results on phase 1

	Steps 1 and 2						Step 3			
π	$\lvert D_\pi \rvert$	$\lvert \Lambda \rvert$	$[\underline{n}, \overline{n}]$	$[\underline{\text{cs}}, \overline{\text{cs}}]$	$[\underline{\text{ch}}, \overline{\text{ch}}]$	$[\underline{a}, \overline{a}]$	Act.	Arch.	L-time	R^2
Hc	87	5	[3,28]	[3,8]	[0,8]	[302.9,13749.1]	ReLU	(45,15,1)	0.499	0.908
Kow	146	4	[3,38]	[3,8]	[0,19]	[−1.98,13.45]	ReLU	(39,5,1)	0.181	0.857
Bp	117	3	[3,30]	[3,15]	[0,12]	[-32.8,413.0]	ReLU	(37,5,1)	0.576	0.874

a test set in five trials $i \in [1, 5]$. Further, Table 1 shows the results on Step 3, where Act.: denotes the choice of activation function; Arch.: $(a, b, 1)$ gives the architecture of the ANN, consisting of an input layer with a nodes, a middle layer with b nodes, and an output layer with a single node; L-time: the average time (sec.) to construct ANNs for each trial; R^2: the average of coefficient of determination over the five test sets.

For each chemical property π, we selected the ANN $\mathcal{N}$ that attained the best test R^2 score among the five ANNs to formulate an MILP $\mathcal{M}(x, y, z; \mathcal{C}_1)$ in the second phase.

Results on Phase 2 We implemented Steps 4 and 5 in Phase 2 as follows.

Step 4 In this step, we solve the MILP $\mathcal{M}(x, y, g; \mathcal{C}_1, \mathcal{C}_2)$ formulated based on the ANN $\mathcal{N}$ obtained in Phase 1. To solve an MILP in Step 4, we use `CPLEX` version 12.8.

In our experiment, we choose a target value $y^* \in [\underline{a}, \overline{a}]$ and fix or bound some descriptors in our feature vector as follows: fix n^* to be some four integers in $[\underline{n}, \overline{n}]$; choose $d_{\max} = 3$ or 4; fix cs* to be each integer in [3, 6]; and fix ch* to be each in $[\text{ch}_{\min}, \text{ch}_{\max}]$, where $\text{ch}_{\min}$ (resp., $\text{ch}_{\max}$) is the minimum (resp., maximum) possible core height of a monocyclic graph with n^* vertices, cs* core vertices, and the maximum degree $d_{\max}$ of non-core vertices. This scheme results in 13 to 19 MILP instances for each pair $(y^*, d_{\max}, n^*)$. Each of these MILP instances is either feasible or infeasible and we find one feasible vector (x^*, g^*) to each feasible MILP instance, where a monocyclic chemical graph G^* can be immediately constructed from the resulting vector g^*. We set $\varepsilon = 0.02$ in Step 4.

Table 2 shows the results on Step 4, wherein: y^*_π: a target value in $[\underline{a}, \overline{a}]$ for a property π; n^*: a specified number of vertices in $[\underline{n}, \overline{n}]$; $|F^*|$/#I: #I means the number of MILP instances in Step 4, and $|F^*|$ means the size of set F^* of vectors x^* generated from all feasible instances among the #I MILP instances in Step 4; IP-time: the time (sec.) to solve all the #I MILP instances to find a set F^* of vectors x^*.

Step 5 In this step, we modified the algorithm proposed in [19] to enumerate all monocyclic graphs $G^* \in \mathcal{G}$ such that $f(G^*) = x^*$ for each $x^* \in F^*$. We stop the execution when either the total number of graphs inferred over all vectors $x^* \in F^*$ exceeds 100 or the execution time exceeds 1 h.

Table 2 shows the results on Step 5, where we denote the following: #G^* (): the number of all (or up to 100) monocyclic chemical graphs G^* such that $f(G^*) = x^*$

Table 2 Results on phase 2, steps 4 and 5

			$d_{max} = 3$				$d_{max} = 4$			
π	y^*	n^*	$\lvert F^*\rvert/\#I$	IP-time	$\#G^*$	G-time	$\lvert F^*\rvert/\#I$	IP-time	$\#G^*$	G-time
Hc	3000	11	17/19	15.7	100 (0)	0.732	13/13	27.7	93 (0)	1.566
	8000	18	12/17	45.5	100 (0)	285.3	12/16	141.2	100 (0)	913.3152
	10,000	23	8/15	33.5	8 (0)	>1h	8/16	91.3	8 (0)	>1h
	12,000	28	4/15	19.0	4 (0)	>1h	4/15	71.3	4 (0)	>1h
Kow	2	11	17/19	16.3	100 (1)	0.785	13/13	33.0	100 (2)	1.374
	3	18	15/17	46.0	100 (0)	1163.5	15/16	166.9	100 (0)	2001.5
	6	28	11/15	78.2	11 (0)	>1h	10/15	240.3	10 (0)	>1h
	12	38	3/13	32.2	3 (0)	>1h	3/14	92.9	3 (0)	>1h
Bp	200	11	17/19	11.6	100 (1)	0.707	13/13	26.4	100 (1)	2.466
	250	18	12/17	27.7	100 (0)	692.3	11/16	97.1	100 (0)	2069.0
	300	24	8/15	29.1	14 (0)	>1h	8/16	102.5	8 (0)	>1h
	350	30	3/14	20.5	3 (0)	>1h	3/15	81.6	3 (0)	>1h

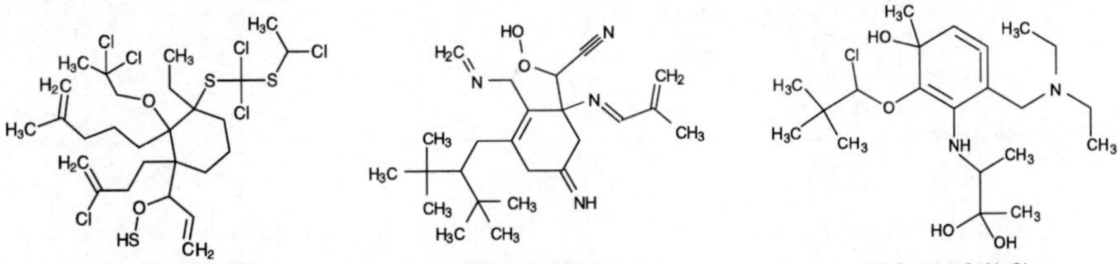

(a) $C_{27}H_{42}O_2S_3Cl_6$ (b) $C_{24}H_{38}O_2N_4$ (c) $C_{27}H_{37}O_4N_2Cl$

Fig. 3 Monocyclic chemical graphs inferred in Step 4 or 5: (**a**) Kow, $d_{max}=4$, $n^* = 38$, $y^*=12$, $cs^* = 6$, $ch^* = 5$; (**b**) Bp, $d_{max} = 4$, $n^* = 30$, $y^* = 350$, $cs^* = 6$, $ch^* = 4$; (**c**) Hc, $d_{max} = 4$, $n^* = 28$, $y^*=12{,}000$, $cs^*=6$, $ch^*=4$

for some $x^* \in F^*$ (where $|F^*|$ such graphs G^* have been found after Step 4); The number of chemical graphs already registered in the database PubChem among the generated graphs is indicated in parentheses; G-time: the running time (sec.) to execute Step 5, where "> 1h" means that the execution time exceeds the limit.

From Table 2, we observe that for all chemical properties we tested, each of the tested instances for finding a monocyclic chemical graph with specified sizes $n^* \leq 38$, $cs^* \leq 6$, and $ch^* \leq 5$ for a specified target y^* was solved within 1–10 s on average based on our novel MILP formulation. Note that our MILP formulation includes a constraint on the ranged-based applicability domain (AD), and we expect that all the inferred monocyclic chemical graphs obey some tendency on the structures of chemical compounds in the tested data set D_π. We observe that most of such inferred chemical graphs are not registered in the PubChem database.

Figure 3 illustrates some monocyclic chemical graphs inferred in the computational experiment.

6 Concluding Remarks

In this paper, we proposed a new method for the inverse QSAR/QSPR to monocyclic chemical graphs by significantly enhancing the framework due to Azam et al. [3] and the MILP formulation due to Zhang et al. [21], and implemented it for inferring monocyclic chemical graphs using a feature vector f with only graph-theoretical descriptors. This enhancement is very important because most useful chemical compounds have cycles, and it is an essential step towards building similar frameworks that can handle multi-cyclic chemical compounds [22]. From the results on some computational experiments with real data from the PubChem database, we observe that the proposed method runs efficiently for chemical compounds with up to around $n = 30$ atoms in a hydrogen-suppressed model (40–60 atoms including hydrogens). Furthermore, our method could find many novel and realistic compounds, which suggests that the proposed framework is useful for designing novel drugs. It is left as a future work to improve the efficiency of the enumeration algorithm in Step 5.

References

1. T. Akutsu, H. Nagamochi, A mixed integer linear programming formulation to artificial neural networks, in *Proceedings of the 2nd International Conference on Information Science and Systems* (ACM, New York, 2019), pp. 215–220
2. T. Akutsu, D. Fukagawa, J. Jansson, K. Sadakane, Inferring a graph from path frequency. Discret. Appl. Math. **160**(10–11), 1416–1428 (2012)
3. N.A. Azam, R. Chiewvanichakorn, F. Zhang, A. Shurbevski, H. Nagamochi, T. Akutsu, A method for the inverse QSAR/QSPR based on artificial neural networks and mixed integer linear programming, in *Proceedings of the 13th International Joint Conference on Biomedical Engineering Systems and Technologies—Volume 3: BIOINFORMATICS* (2020)
4. R.S. Bohacek, C. McMartin, W.C. Guida, The art and practice of structure-based drug design: A molecular modeling perspective. Med. Res. Rev. **16**(1), 3–50 (1996)
5. R. Chiewvanichakorn, C. Wang, Z. Zhang, A. Shurbevski, H. Nagamochi, T. Akutsu, A method for the inverse QSAR/QSPR based on artificial neural networks and mixed integer linear programming *ICBBB2020*, Paper K0013 (2020)
6. H. Fujiwara, J. Wang, L. Zhao, H. Nagamochi, T. Akutsu, Enumerating tree-like chemical graphs with given path frequency. J. Chem. Inf. Model. **48**(7), 1345–1357 (2008)
7. R. Gómez-Bombarelli, J.N. Wei, D. Duvenaud, J.M. Hernández-Lobato, B. Sánchez-Lengeling, D. Sheberla, J. Aguilera-Iparraguirre, T.D. Hirzel, R.P. Adams, A. Aspuru-Guzik, Automatic chemical design using a data-driven continuous representation of molecules. ACS Central Sci. **4**(2), 268–276 (2018)
8. H. Ikebata, K. Hongo, T. Isomura, R. Maezono, R. Yoshida, Bayesian molecular design with a chemical language model. J. Comput.-Aided Molecular Design **31**(4), 379–391 (2017)
9. A. Kerber, R. Laue, T. Grüner, M. Meringer, MOLGEN 4.0. Match Commun. Math. Comput. Chem. **37**, 205–208 (1998)
10. M.J. Kusner, B. Paige, J.M. Hernández-Lobato, Grammar variational autoencoder, in *Proceedings of the 34th International Conference on Machine Learning*, vol. 70 (2017), pp. 1945–1954
11. J. Li, H. Nagamochi, T. Akutsu, Enumerating substituted benzene isomers of tree-like chemical graphs. IEEE/ACM Trans. Comput. Biol. Bioinf. **15**(2), 633–646 (2016)

12. T. Miyao, H. Kaneko, K. Funatsu, Inverse QSPR/QSAR analysis for chemical structure generation (from y to x). J. Chem. Inf. Model. **56**(2), 286–299 (2016)
13. H. Nagamochi, A detachment algorithm for inferring a graph from path frequency. Algorithmica **53**(2), 207–224 (2009)
14. T.I. Netzeva, et al., Current status of methods for defining the applicability domain of (quantitative) structure-activity relationships: the report and recommendations of ECVAM workshop 52. Altern. Lab. Anim. **33**(2), 155–173 (2005)
15. J.L. Reymond, The chemical space project. Accounts Chem. Res. **48**(3), 722–730 (2015)
16. C. Rupakheti, A. Virshup, W. Yang, D.N. Beratan, Strategy to discover diverse optimal molecules in the small molecule universe. J. Chem. Inf. Model. **55**(3), 529–537 (2015)
17. M.H.S. Segler, T. Kogej, C. Tyrchan, M.P. Waller, Generating focused molecule libraries for drug discovery with recurrent neural networks. ACS Central Sci. **4**(1), 120–131 (2017)
18. M.I. Skvortsova, I.I. Baskin, O.L. Slovokhotova, V.A. Palyulin, N.S. Zefirov, Inverse problem in QSAR/QSPR studies for the case of topological indices characterizing molecular shape (Kier indices). J. Chem. Inf. Comput. Sci. **33**(4), 630–634 (1993)
19. M. Suzuki, H. Nagamochi, T. Akutsu, Efficient enumeration of monocyclic chemical graphs with given path frequencies. J. Cheminf. **6**(1), 31 (2014)
20. X. Yang, J. Zhang, K. Yoshizoe, K. Terayama, K. Tsuda, ChemTS: an efficient python library for de novo molecular generation. Sci. Technol. Adv. Mat. **18**(1), 972–976 (2017)
21. F. Zhang, J. Zhu, R. Chiewvanichakorn, A. Shurbevski, H. Nagamochi, T. Akutsu, A new integer linear programming formulation to the inverse QSAR/QSPR for acylic chemical compounds using skeleton trees, in *Proceedings of the 33rd International Conference on Industrial Engineering and Other Applications of Applied Intelligent Systems* (2020)
22. J. Zhu, C. Wang, A. Shurbevski, H. Nagamochi, T. Akutsu, A novel method for inference of chemical compounds of cycle index two with desired properties based on artificial neural networks and integer programming. Algorithms **13**(5), 124 (2020)

Predicting Targets for Genome Editing with Long Short Term Memory Networks

Neha Bhagwat and Natalia Khuri

1 Introduction

Since the discovery of the DNA double helix, scientists have been working towards developing techniques for breaking, building, and modifying the DNA [16]. Genome editing is an important research topic and its applications range from disease prevention and cure to the resurrection of species and the creation of new, healthy foods [3, 22, 39].

An increasingly popular genome editing tool is a CRISPR/Cas system due to its simplicity, cost-effectiveness, and the ease of engineering [16, 23]. CRISPR stands for Clustered Regularly Interspaced Short Palindromic Repeats, and Cas refers to CRISPR-associated endonucleases. The CRISPR/Cas system provides immunity in Bacteria and Archaea [15], which can be re-purposed to edit DNA sequences in genomes of other organisms, including mammals. CRISPR/Cas genome editing comprises three steps. First, a target genome is scanned by an endonuclease, to find a target DNA sequence complementary to the single guide RNA (sgRNA). Second, the endonuclease creates a break in the target DNA, which is then repaired by the host's DNA repair complexes in the third step. Target genome sequences are typically of size 20 nucleotides (nt), and they are complementary to the subsequences of the sgRNA, called crispr RNAs or crRNAs (Fig. 1). Notably, Cas endonucleases bind next to a protospacer adjacent motif (PAM). In case of the most common CRISPR-associated endonuclease, Cas9, the PAM sequence is NGG, any nucleotide (N) followed by two guanines (GG).

N. Bhagwat
Department of Computer Science, San José State University, San José, CA, USA

N. Khuri (✉)
Department of Computer Science, Wake Forest University, Winston-Salem, NC, USA
e-mail: natalia.khuri@wfu.edu

H. R. Arabnia et al. (eds.), *Advances in Computer Vision and Computational Biology*, Transactions on Computational Science and Computational Intelligence,
https://doi.org/10.1007/978-3-030-71051-4_52

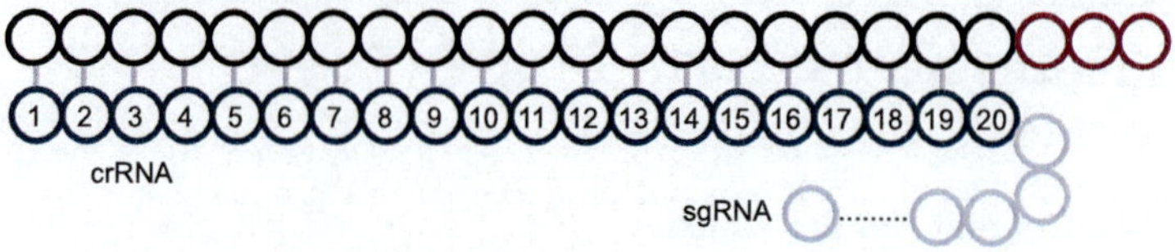

Fig. 1 Schematic diagram of the target DNA sequence (black) bound to crRNA (blue) of the sgRNA (blue and gray). PAM motif (purple) comprises three nucleotides

Designing guide RNAs is an important problem in making CRISPR/Cas systems reliable. While all 20-mer sequences adjacent to PAM can be rapidly detected in a genome, predicting which 20-mers will be active in CRISPR/Cas experiments is challenging [13, 14]. For instance, the same target sequence may be present in several loci in the genome. Thus, a sgRNA could bind at one or more of these unintended sites leading to a non-specific genome editing [31, 35]. Whether or not significant off-target effects occur in the CRISPR/Cas genome editing is still under debate; however, it is important to minimize them during the design of sgRNAs.

The accuracy and efficiency of sgRNAs depend on the properties of the sgRNA, their targets, as well as on the conditions of the experiment. For example, targeting non-coding regions of mammalian genes, such as untranslated 3′ and 5′ regions, is ineffective, and the activity of sgRNA diminishes upon binding in close proximity to a C-terminus of a coding sequence [14, 38]. Several other patterns within sgRNAs have been linked to their efficiency. For example, a subsequence of 10 to 12 nt, immediately preceding PAM, defines a seed region critical for the recognition by CAS endonucleases [35]. Other properties of high-activity sgRNAs include preferences for guanine in position 20 and adenosine in the middle of sgRNAs, as well as avoidance of cytosines in positions 3 and 20 [13, 16, 37, 38].

On the other hand, two dinucleotide patterns, `TT` and `GCC`, at the 3′ end of the sgRNA sequence may lead to a drastic reduction in efficiency [17]. Moreover, although single-base mismatches are tolerated in the 5′ end of the sgRNAs, they increase the probability of binding to unintended regions [14, 21]. Finally, structural and epigenetic factors have also been correlated with the sgRNA activity [6, 20, 36].

The availability of several large-scale CRSIPR/Cas experimental data sets [6, 13, 14] creates an opportunity for the development of regression and classification models to predict genome targets for sgRNAs. The practical applications for these two techniques differ. Regression methods attempt to select sgRNA molecules that will bind their targets most efficiently, that is given a sample of sgRNA molecules and a putative binding site, the goal is to predict a binding coefficient for each sgRNA. Therefore, regression methods are mostly used to improve the design of the genome editing systems, when the genome target is known.

Classification task involves solving a different type of problems, namely, given a large set of experimentally tested sgRNA molecules and a genome sequence, the goal is to predict which sgRNAs will bind to a given genome and where the binding will occur. Thus, the main application for the classification task is the prediction of putative targets in a long genomic sequence.

Therefore, the main objective of this work was to investigate the utility and accuracy of a deep learning classifier in the prediction of editing sites in human and mouse genomes. We developed a classifier that relies on a Long Short Term Memory (LSTM) network, a special class of Recurrent Neural Networks (RNN) [18, 19]. RNNs are networks with loops that allow the neural network to retain information. Due to the presence of these loops, RNNs are amiable for applications that involve sequences of characters, and LSTM networks have been shown to accurately learn long-term dependencies [18], including patterns of bacterial and archaeal CRISPR arrays [12]. Deep learning is computationally expensive and relies on the availability of large training data sets. Therefore, we also built two feature-based machine learning predictors and compared their performance with the LSTM model. To the best of our knowledge, this is the first application of LSTM networks in the prediction of genome editing targets.

The remainder of this work is organized as follows. We review prior computational efforts for the prediction of genome editing sites in Sect. 2. In Sect. 3, we present the workflow for the development and validation of our three classifiers. The results are discussed in Sect. 4, and we conclude the paper with some remarks and future directions in Sect. 5.

2 Prior Work

Both classical and deep machine learning have been successfully used in various bioinformatics applications and problem domains, including sequence analyses and pattern recognition in genomes [26, 27, 34]. In CRISPR-based genome editing, computational work often focuses on optimizing the design of sgRNA libraries using regression. These workflows begin with the construction of libraries of sgRNAs that target a number of genes, followed by the identification of the most and the least active sgRNAs and the derivation of their features. In the last step, regression models are fit to the experimental data [14]. In addition to predicting the efficacy of sgRNAs, such models add insights into molecular properties of efficient sgRNA molecules. For example, a gradient-boosted regression tree model, trained with approximately 4000 sgRNAs, has about 50% agreement between predicted and observed sgRNA activities [13]. As a result, optimized sgRNA libraries for human and mouse genomes can be designed for downstream experiments.

Classification models also exist to separate sgRNAs into classes based on their binding efficiency. Among these models, classifiers built with the Support Vector Machine (SVM) are widespread. For example, after experimentally determining activities of 1841 sgRNAs, top 20% and bottom 20% active sgRNAs were used to train binary classifiers [14]. SVM and logistic regression models relied on 72 sequence-based features, such as position-dependent nucleotides and dinucleotides in the (a) 20-mer target sequence, (b) four nucleotides upstream of the target site, and (c) six nucleotides downstream of the target site. Additionally, two features measuring the GC content were incorporated into the feature set. In a leave-one-gene out validation, SVM model achieved an area under the Receiver Operating Characteristic (ROC) curve (AUC) between 70 and 80% per gene. The classifier was also applied to predict activity of an independent test set and high consistency was observed between predicted and experimentally determined sgRNA activities.

Another popular SVM-based classifier, sgRNAScorer, contributed to the development of an in vivo library-on-library large-scale assay, which probed approximately 1400 genomic loci [6]. In a tenfold cross-validation experiment, the SVM model achieved the average accuracy of 73.2%, when trained with an expanded feature set. The expanded feature set included epigenetic features, such as target accessibility, in addition to features derived from the sequences. In the follow up experiments, it was confirmed that epigenetic features of the target site play an important role for the sgRNA specificity.

Likewise, WU-CRISPR uses SVM with radial kernel and it improves upon other classification models by introducing a filtering step into the predictor. The package first filters sgRNAs with empirically determined criteria, such as contiguous uracil or guanine motifs, GC content, and so on, and then classifies them. WU-CRISPR achieved an AUC of 92% in a tenfold cross-validation and 91% in a leave-one-gene-out validation [38].

While classical machine learning methods for sgRNA classification show good results, they all require feature engineering. Neural Deep learning (DL) networks can circumvent this requirement and automatically extract useful features from large data sets [28]. For example, a semi-supervised tool, DeepCRISPR, begins the training process by learning, in an unsupervised manner, the representation of sgRNAs from a large set of all 20-mers adjacent to PAM and follows by fine-tuning of the network with labeled sgRNAs [8]. More specifically, a deep convolutional denoising neural network (DCDNN) was used in the unsupervised step and a convolutional neural network (CNN) in the second step. DeepCRISPR can be executed in a classification or a regression mode; in the classification task, it achieves an average AUC of 79.6%.

Finally, another DL-based tool, DeepCas9, also uses a CNN and trains a regression model. The training proceeds by expanding short nucleotide sequences into their binary representations and then inputting the encoded vectors to a CNN. DeepCas9 model achieved a Spearman correlation of 0.23 to 0.61 between predicted and experimental sgRNA activities for various data sets [40].

Our work differs from previous approaches in two ways. First, we focus on learning patterns in experimentally screened sgRNAs to predict their putative targets in human and mouse genomes. Rather than classifying sgRNA into top and bottom activity groups, we are interested in learning how well patterns can be learned from a large data set of diverse sgRNA target sites. The main motivation for this is that sgRNAs may bind at unintended locations in the target genome and hence, it is important to identify both on-target and off-target sites.

Second, unlike prior deep learning models for the sgRNA design, which rely on a CNN, we developed an RNN model motivated by its ability to retain dependencies between the elements of a sequence [33]. Recently, an LSTM-based predictor for archaeal and bacterial CRISPR arrays has been developed and validated *in silico*, achieving 94% sensitivity and 97% specificity in classifying individual CRISPR repeats [12].

Third, we also compared the LSTM-based model with two classical feature-based algorithms, such as SVM and Random forest (RF), rather than with other DL approaches. Our rationale for this comparison is that feature-based classifiers are faster to train and do not require specialized hardware or cloud-based services, which may not be readily available to experimental laboratories. Additionally, in classical machine learning, feature importance can be estimated, providing some insights into learned patterns that explain the interaction between the sgRNAs and their targets. Thus, it is important to understand whether the LSTM network outperforms simpler models, rather than investigate if it outperforms other DL tools, such as CNN-based predictors.

3 Materials and Methods

In this work, we implemented a standard machine learning workflow (Fig. 2) comprising three steps. First, input sequences were converted to a representation suitable for training, then the models were selected with the tenfold cross-validation using the accuracy metric as an optimization criterion. Additionally, we compared the performance of the LSTM and classical machine learning models using a held-out validation data set.

In what follows, we show that our deep learning LSTM model outperformed the SVM and RF classifiers. We also demonstrate a practical application of how an LSTM network can be trained with sgRNA data from one species (mouse) and used to predict sgRNA binding in genome of another species (human).

3.1 Data Collection

We created the data sets of mouse and human sequences as follows. First, we downloaded sequences of experimentally validated sgRNAs along with the accession numbers of their target transcripts [13]. The human data set comprised 19,114 unique transcripts and 76,441 sgRNAs, and the mouse data set consisted of 19,674 unique transcripts and 78,637 sgRNAs.

Next, we used accession numbers as queries and retrieved the corresponding genomic sequences from the National Center for Biotechnology Information (NCBI) [1] with BioPython (v.1.73) [10]. Each transcript was scanned for the presence of a PAM motif on the forward and reverse complement DNA strands, and each 20-mer adjacent to a PAM motif was considered for the inclusion in the final data set. Between 8 and 9546 putative sgRNA targets were found in each human

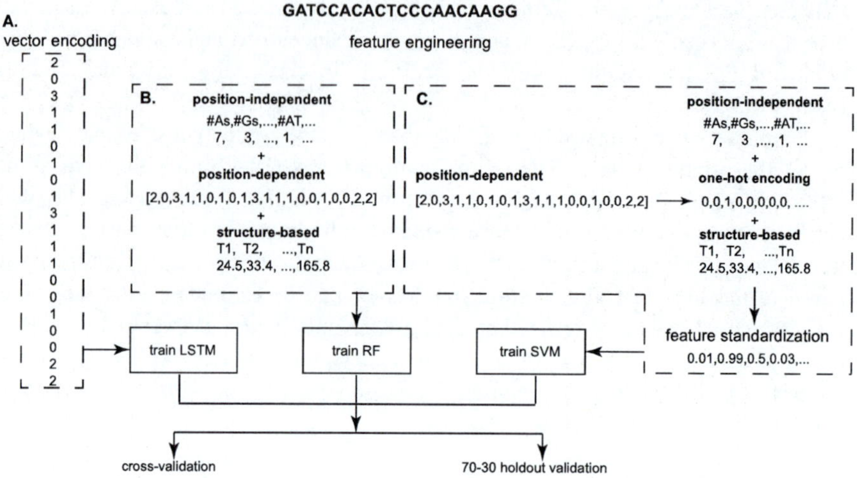

Fig. 2 Schematic diagram of the LSTM, RF, and SVM workflows. (**a**) In LSTM, sequences are encoded into numerical vectors. (**b**) In RF, features are engineered from sequence and structure-dependent properties. (**c**) In SVM, features are engineered from sequence and structure-dependent properties and standardized to between 0 and 1

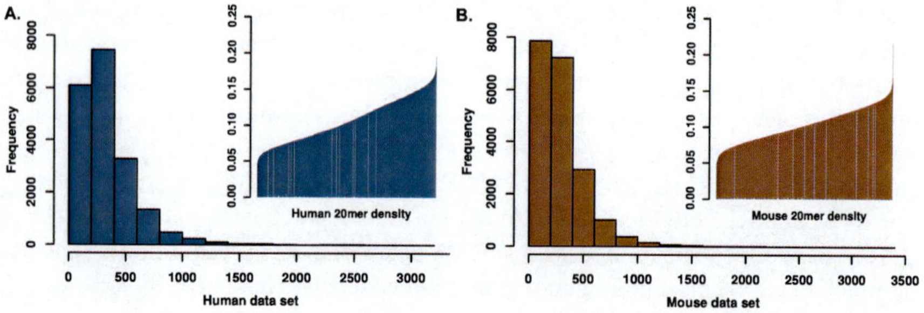

Fig. 3 Distribution of putative sgRNA targets per transcript. (**a**) Human putative targets per transcript are shown in blue (not included are three human transcripts with 1431, 4194, and 9546 putative targets). (**b**) Mouse putative sgRNA targets per transcript are shown in brown. Insets display the density of 20-mers adjacent to PAM in human and mouse transcripts, respectively

transcript. In the mouse genome, 3–3386 putative targets were found per transcript. On average, there were 339 putative targets per transcript in the human genome, and 295 putative targets per transcript in the mouse genome (Fig. 3). The density of putative sgRNA targets in human transcripts ranged between 0.04 and 0.19, and the average density was 0.11. Similarly, the density of putative sgRNA targets in the mouse genome was on average 0.11 and ranged between 0.04–0.22 (Fig. 3).

Next, each 20-mer target sequence was compared with all known sgRNAs and if a match was found, the 20-mer was added to a positive data set. Otherwise, this

Table 1 Description of the human and mouse data sets

Organism	Transcripts	Positives	Negatives	Total
Human	18,589	46,877	46,877	93,754
Mouse	19,157	48,794	48,794	97,588

20-mer was assigned to the negative class. We discarded all transcripts without experimentally validated sgRNAs.

Finally, negative data set was randomly under-sampled, such that the number of positive and negative 20-mers for each transcript was equal. For example, if only three positive 20-mers were identified for a given transcript, three negative 20-mers were randomly chosen, and the remainder of negative 20-mers was discarded.

As a result, the two data sets comprised of 93,754 positive and negative 20-mers from 19,114 human transcripts, and 97,588 positive and negative 20-mers from 19,675 mouse transcripts (Table 1).

3.2 *Sequence Encoding and Feature Engineering*

We converted the sequences of the positive and negative 20-mers into formats suitable for machine learning. For training an LSTM network, we devised a numerical vector representation (Fig. 2), and for classical machine learning, we engineered features from sequences and predicted two-dimensional structures.

More specifically, in the LSTM sequence encoding, we converted each target sequence into a numeric vector, by replacing each nucleotide with an integer (Fig. 2a). Additionally, we experimented with including PAM sequences into input vector; we denote this feature set as LSTM-23.

For the SVM and RF modeling, the engineered features were derived from the sequence and structure of the 20-mers. More specifically, we computed position-dependent, position-independent, and structure-based features as follows.

- **Position-dependent** features ($n = 39$) were represented by nucleotides and dinucleotides, which occur in each position of the 20-mers.
- **Position-independent** features ($n = 84$) consisted of the counts of occurrences of 4 nucleotides, 16 dinucleotides, and 64 trinucleotides in each 20-mer.
- **Structure-based** features ($n = 5$) of a 20-mer comprised its overall melting temperature, melting temperature of its parts, and its minimum free energy. The three parts of the 20-mer, for which melting temperatures were calculated separately were (a) 5-mers next to a PAM motif, (b) 8-mers adjacent to the 5-mer, and (c) 5-mers adjacent to the 8-mer. The melting temperatures were calculated using nearest neighbor thermodynamics-based function provided in the BioPython package [10] and the minimum free energy was calculated with the RNAfold package [29].

Position-dependent features were further processed as follows. For RF modeling, we encoded categorical values into integer representations, and used them along with the position-dependent and structure-based features ($n = 128$) (Fig. 2b).

For SVM modeling, categorical values were expanded into one-hot encoded vectors using the OneHotEncoder from the sklearn API. More specifically, categorical features were converted into a binary vector of size N, where N is the number of possible categories of each feature. All elements of the resulting vector were set to "0," except for the element denoting a specific categorical value. This element was set to "1." Finally, all three types of features ($n = 473$) were standardized prior to training an SVM classifier (Fig. 2c).

In summary, 473 features were used in the SVM model, 128 features in the RF model, and input vectors of size 20 and 23 were used in the LSTM and LSTM-23 models, respectively. All models were tuned using a tenfold cross-validation process, consisting of a repeated splitting of the training data sets into 10 subsets [25]. We used the tenfold cross-validation to get robust estimates of the models' performances with a reasonable computational cost. More specifically, in each experiment, nine subsets were used to train the models and one subset was used to estimate the performance of a model. This validation process was repeated 10 times, thus, each subset was used once as a validation set. The results of these experiments were used to compute the average performance metrics and tune the parameters for each model.

3.3 Long Short Term Memory Network

The LSTM network was built using keras [7]. It consisted of five layers, namely an embedding layer, an LSTM layer, a dense layer, a dropout layer, and finally, a second dense layer with the Adam optimizer [24]. Both dense layers used sigmoid activation functions. The best models were obtained with 25 epochs and accuracy was used as an optimization criteria to tune the parameters.

The embedding layer stores weights learned from the training data and outputs a two-dimensional vector to the LSTM layer. The LSTM layer has a chain-like structure, similar to an RNN architecture. The difference between the two layers lies in the form of the repeating module. In case of RNNs, the repeating module is in the form of a single neural network layer, whereas in LSTMs, the repeating module comprises four neural network layers arranged in a specific manner to capture dependencies. The dense layers connect every neuron in the previous layer to every neuron in the dense layer. The two dense layers are separated by a dropout layer which prevents over-fitting. The dropout layer takes as an argument a float value between 0 and 1. This argument represents the fraction of neurons that are dropped.

3.4 Classical Machine Learning Models

For comparison, we trained two feature-based machine learning models using SVM and RF algorithms. SVM tries to identify a hyperplane in an N-dimensional space, where N is the number of features used for classification, such that the hyperplane effectively divides a set of inputs into distinct classes [11]. Several hyperplanes may achieve this purpose, and the aim is to find a hyperplane that clearly distinguishes the inputs while maintaining a maximum distance between the inputs and the plane. RF classifiers identify the class of the input sequence based on votes of a set of decision trees. These decision trees are created using subsets of the training data [4].

Both algorithms were trained to predict binary labels, and we made use of the implementations of SVM and RF algorithms in the sklearn Python API. Tenfold cross-validation was used to tune the parameters, and accuracy was used as an optimization criterion. The best SVM model was found with a linear kernel. The parameters *gamma*, *coef0* and *degree* were set to auto, 0.0, and 3, respectively.

For RF model, the best model was trained with 80 trees using Gini impurity [30] as the measure of the quality of splits. The other parameters were set to the default sklearn values [5].

3.5 Validation Protocol and Performance Measurements

All classifiers were validated in a hold-out experiment as follows. Each of the two data sets was divided into two non-overlapping subsets consisting of 70 and 30% of the data. We used data stratification to partition the original subsets, thus ensuring that each subset contained the same class ratios as the original data sets.

Using validation data sets, we estimated three performance metrics for the LSTM, SVM, and RF models, namely accuracy, sensitivity, and specificity. These metrics were computed using a classification threshold score of 0.5. We note that the classification cutoff could either be raised to reduce the number of false positives or lowered to reduce the number of false negatives.

4 Results

Experiment 1: Cross-Validation Here, we estimated the performance in a tenfold cross-validation experiment. Additionally, we compared the accuracy of LSTM model with (LSTM-23) and without PAM (LSTM-20) sequences. On average, accuracy of LSTM networks was higher than the accuracy of RF and SVM models for human and mouse data sets (Fig. 4). The LSTM-23 models, which included the PAM sequence, outperformed LSTM-20.

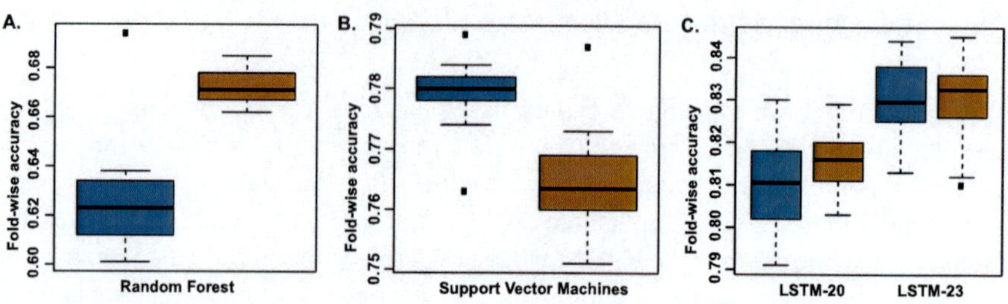

Fig. 4 Distribution of fold-wise accuracy values in tenfold cross-validation for the human (in blue) and the mouse (in brown) data sets

The RF and LSTM models had better accuracy in predicting targets in the mouse data compared to the human data, as evidenced by higher average accuracy and tighter distribution of fold-wise accuracy values. For instance, the fold-wise accuracy of RF model ranged from 66.2 to 68.5% for the mouse data set compared to 60.1–69.4% for human data set. On the other hand, the SVM model had a stronger performance with the human data set than with the mouse data set.

Experiment 2: Hold-Out Validation In the hold-out validation, the three models were trained with 70% of the data and validated with 30%. The models were tuned using accuracy as an optimization criterion. The two LSTM models showed the strongest performance followed by the SVM model with a linear kernel (Table 2). More specifically, the accuracy of the LSTM-20 model was 81.6% for the mouse and 82.5% for the human data sets, respectively. At the 0.5 classification cutoff, the LSTM-20 model achieved sensitivity of 80.1% and specificity of 83.2% for mouse data set. For the human data set, LSTM-20 model had sensitivity of 80.8% and specificity of 84.2%. Finally, we estimated area under the Receiver Operating Characteristic curve (AUC) for all classifiers. For the mouse data set, AUC values were 0.81, 0.79, and 0.69 for the LSTM-20, SVM, and RF models, respectively, and those for the human data set were 0.83, 0.77, and 0.64, respectively.

The performance of the LSTM network was further improved by including the PAM sequence in the input vector. More specifically, the accuracy for the mouse data set was 83.2% for the LSTM trained with 23-mers as compared to 81.6% for the LSTM trained with 20-mers. Similarly, the accuracy for the human data set also improved from 82.5% for 20-mers to 83.1% for 23-mers. The AUC metric was approximately 0.83 for both, the mouse and human data sets (Table 2). We examined the concordance between predictions of the four classifiers and found that about 25% of mouse and 15% of human hold-out data were similarly labeled by all four models.

Experiment 3: Cross-Species Prediction Finally, we investigated if the predictions of CRISPR/Cas9 targets in the human genome could be made by training the LSTM network with the mouse data. This experiment was carried out using the two classifiers that were observed to give the best results for the mouse and

Table 2 Performance in the hold-out validation. Best results are shown in boldface

	Mouse				Human			
Metrics	LSTM-20	LSTM-23	SVM	RF	LSTM-20	LSTM-23	SVM	RF
Accuracy	0.81	**0.83**	0.79	0.68	0.82	**0.83**	0.77	0.63
AUC	0.81	**0.83**	0.79	0.68	0.82	**0.83**	0.77	0.63
Specificity	0.80	**0.84**	0.78	0.80	0.80	**0.84**	0.85	0.77
Sensitivity	**0.83**	0.81	0.81	0.56	**0.84**	0.81	0.68	0.50

Table 3 Performance of the cross-species experiment with training on the mouse data set and testing on the human data set

Metrics	LSTM-20	LSTM-23
Accuracy	0.81	0.81
AUC	0.81	0.81
Specificity	0.81	0.81
Sensitivity	0.80	0.81

human data sets in the 70–30 hold-out experiment—LSTM-20 and LSTM-23. In this experiment, each model was trained using the complete mouse data set and tested with the complete human data set. The accuracy of LSTM-20 and LSTM-23 was 80.7 and 81.3%, respectively. The AUC and specificity was 81% for both classifiers and sensitivity was 80% for the classifier trained with 20-mers and 81% for the classifier trained with 23-mers, respectively (Table 3).

5 Conclusion

While genome editing is poised to bring positive changes in many application domains, its widespread adoption is subject to technical barriers and ethical concerns [2]. One of the technical challenges is to design efficient and specific single guide RNAs, which will direct CRISPR-associated nucleases to their intended targets in a given genome. In this work, we proposed a method for evaluating whether a sgRNA molecule will bind to its target. The proposed classifier relies on deep learning, and we compared its performance with two classical feature-based classifiers. While classical machine learning algorithms, such as Support Vector Machines and Random forest, were trained with 128 and 473 sequential and structural features, respectively, deep learning with LSTM did not require extensive feature engineering. It derived its power from large quantities of training data, albeit incurring higher training costs.

The LSTM model displayed a substantial increase in accuracy of 13 and 19% in the mouse and human data sets, respectively, compared to RF. The difference between the evaluated metrics for the LSTM model and the SVM model was not as pronounced as the difference between the same metrics for the LSTM model and the RF model. The LSTM model was observed to have an accuracy of approximately 2 and 5% over the SVM model for the mouse and human data sets, respectively. Our results also support the inclusion of PAM sequences in the encoded input vectors for the LSTM models. The LSTM-23 model showed an improvement over the LSTM-20 model in accuracy of 1.6 and 0.6% in the mouse and human data sets, respectively.

Our results demonstrated that differences exist in the predictions made by each model. Therefore, in practice, it is recommended to use multiple tools to find overlapping predictions. We note that the data set construction also influences performance estimates. We aimed to create a balanced data set of positive and negative training examples. However, it is possible that the random selection of the non-functional sgRNAs may have affected the results of our classifiers. Future work will focus on evaluating different schemes for balancing the data sets.

Although direct comparison with existing CNN-based predictors is not possible due to differences in training sets, intended task, and/or lack of detailed implementation description, our AUC values are on par or better than previously reported results [8]. Finally, given the strong performance of the LSTM network, its results could be further improved by experimenting with different RNN configurations, such as Bidirectional Recurrent Neural Networks (BRNN) [32] and/or Gated Recurrent Units (GRU) [9]. Because these models process training data and dependencies in both directions, additional dependencies could be automatically discovered, possibly leading to performance improvement.

References

1. S.F. Altschul, W. Gish, W. Miller, W.Myers, E., J.Lipman, D.: Basic local alignment search tool. Journal of Molecular Biology **215**, 403–410 (1990)
2. D. Baltimore, P. Berg, M. Botchan, D. Carroll, R.A. Charo, G. Church, J.E. Corn, G.Q. Daley, J.A. Doudna, M. Fenner, H.T. Greely, M. Jinek, G.S. Martin, E. Penhoet, J. Puck, S.H. Sternberg, J.S. Weissman, K.R. Yamamoto, A prudent path forward for genomic engineering and germline gene modification. Science **348**(6230), 36–38 (2015)
3. R. Barrangou, J.A. Doudna, Applications of CRISPR technologies in research and beyond. Nat. Biotechnol. **34**, 933–941 (2016)
4. L. Breiman, Random forests. Mach. Learn. **45**(1), 5–32 (2001)
5. L. Buitinck, G. Louppe, M. Blondel, F. Pedregosa, A. Mueller, O. Grisel, V. Niculae, P. Prettenhofer, A. Gramfort, J. Grobler, R. Layton, J. VanderPlas, A. Joly, B. Holt, G. Varoquaux, API design for machine learning software: Experiences from the scikit-learn project, in *ECML PKDD Workshop: Languages for Data Mining and Machine Learning* (2013), pp. 108–122
6. R. Chari, P. Mali, M. Moosburner, G.M. Church, Unraveling CRISPR-Cas9 genome engineering parameters via a library-on-library approach. Nat. Methods **12**, 823–826 (2015)
7. F. Chollet, et al., Keras (2015). https://keras.io
8. G. Chuai, H. Ma, J. Yan, M. Chen, N. Hong, D. Xue, C. Zhou, C. Zhu, K. Chen, B. Duan, F. Gu, S. Qu, D. Huang, J. Wei, Q. Liu, DeepCRISPR: optimized CRISPR guide RNA design by deep learning. Genome Biol. **19**(1), 80 (2018)
9. J. Chung, C. Gulcehre, K. Cho, Y. Bengio, Empirical evaluation of gated recurrent neural networks on sequence modeling (2014). Preprint arXiv:1412.3555
10. P. Cock, T. Antao, J. Chang, B. Chapman, C. Cox, A. Dalke, I. Friedberg, T. Hamelryck, F. Kauff, B. Wilczynski, M. de Hoon, Biopython: freely available python tools for computational molecular biology and bioinformatics. Bioinformatics **25**, 1422–1423 (2009)

11. C. Cortes, V. Vapnik, Support-vector networks. Mach. Learn. **20**(3), 273–297 (1995)
12. S. Deshmukh, P. Heller, N. Khuri, A long-short term memory network for detecting CRISPR arrays, in *2019 18th IEEE International Conference On Machine Learning And Applications (ICMLA)* (IEEE, Piscataway, 2019), pp. 619–624
13. J.G. Doench, N. Fusi, M. Sullender, M. Hegde, E. Vaimberg, K.F. Donovan, I. Smith, Z. Tothova, C. Wilen, R. Orchard, H.W. Virgin, J. Listgarten, D. Root, Optimized sgRNA design to maximize activity and minimize off-target effects of CRISPR-Cas9. Nat. Biotechnol. **34**, 184–191 (2016)
14. J.G. Doench, E. Hartenian, D.B. Graham, Z. Tothava, M. Hegde, I. Smith, M. Sullender, B.L. Ebert, R.J. Xavier, D.E. Root, Rational design of highly active sgRNAs for CRISPR-Cas9–mediated gene inactivation. Nat. Biotechnol. **32**, 1262–1267 (2014)
15. P. Donohoue, R. Barrangou, A. May, Advances in industrial biotechnology using CRISPR-Cas systems. Trends Biotechnol. **36**(2), 134–146 (2018)
16. J.A. Doudna, E. Charpentier, The new frontier of genome engineering with CRISPR-Cas9. Science **346**(6213), 1258,096 (2014)
17. R. Graf, X. Li, V. Chu, K. Rajewsky, sgRNA sequence motifs blocking efficient CRISPR/Cas9-mediated gene editing. Cell Reports **26**(5), 1098–1103.e3 (2019)
18. A. Graves, *Supervised Sequence Labelling with Recurrent Neural Networks* (Springer, Berlin, 2012)
19. S. Hochreiter, J. Schmidhuber, Long short-term memory. Neural Comput. **9**, 1735–1780 (1997)
20. M.A. Horlbeck, L.B. Witkowsky, B. Guglielmi, J.M. Replogle, L.A. Gilbert, J.E. Villalta, S.E. Torigoe, R. Tjian, J.S. Weissman, Nucleosomes impede Cas9 access to DNA in vivo and in vitro. eLife **5**, e12,677 (2016)
21. P. Hsu, E. Lander, F. Zhang, Development and applications of CRISPR-Cas9 for genome engineering. Cell **157**, 1262–1278 (2014)
22. P.D. Hsu, E.S. Lander, F. Zhang, Development and applications of CRISPR-Cas9 for genome engineering. Cell **157**(6), 1262–1278 (2014)
23. M. Jinek, K. Chylinski, I. Fonfara, M. Hauer, J.A. Doudna, E. Charpentier: A programmable dual RNA guided DNA endonuclease in adaptive bacterial immunity. Science **337**(6096), 816–821 (2012)
24. D.P. Kingma, J. Ba, Adam: A method for stochastic optimization (2014). Preprint arXiv:1412.6980
25. R. Kohavi, A study of cross-validation and bootstrap for accuracy estimation and model selection, in *Proceedings of the 14th International Joint Conference on Artificial Intelligence,IJCAI'95*, vol. 2 (Morgan Kaufmann Publishers Inc., San Francisco, CA, 1995), pp. 1137–1143
26. A. Lapedes, C. Barnes, C. Burks, R. Farber, K. Sirotkin, Application of neural networks and other machine learning algorithms to DNA sequence analysis. Technical Report, Los Alamos National Lab., NM (USA) (1988)
27. P. Larranaga, B. Calvo, R. Santana, C. Bielza, J. Galdiano, I. Inza, J.A. Lozano, R. Armananzas, G. Santafé, A. Pérez, et al., Machine learning in bioinformatics. Briefings Bioinf. **7**(1), 86–112 (2006)
28. G. Lo Bosco, M.A. Di Gangi, Deep learning architectures for DNA sequence classification, in *Fuzzy Logic and Soft Computing Applications*, ed. by A. Petrosino, V. Loia, W. Pedrycz (Springer International Publishing, Cham, 2017), pp. 162–171
29. R. Lorenz, S. Bernhart, C.H. zu Siederdissen, H. Tafer, C. Flamm, P. Stadler, I. Hofacker, Viennarna package 2.0. Algorithms for Molecular Biology **6**, 6–26 (2011)
30. B.H. Menze, B.M. Kelm, R. Masuch, U. Himmelreich, P. Bachert, W. Petrich, F.A. Hamprecht, A comparison of random forest and its Gini importance with standard chemometric methods for the feature selection and classification of spectral data. BMC Bioinf. **10**, 213 (2009)
31. V. Pattanayak, S. Lin, J.P. Guilinger, E. Ma, J. Doudna, D.R. Liu, High-throughput profiling of off-target DNA cleavage reveals RNA-programmed Cas9 nuclease specificity. Nat. Biotechnol. **31**, 839–843 (2013)

32. M. Schuster, K.K. Paliwal, Bidirectional recurrent neural networks. IEEE Trans. Signal Proces. **45**(11), 2673–2681 (1997)
33. S.K. Sønderby, C.K. Sønderby, H. Nielsen, O. Winther, Convolutional LSTM networks for subcellular localization of proteins, in *International Conference on Algorithms for Computational Biology* (Springer, Berlin, 2015), pp. 68–80
34. S. Sonnenburg, G. Rätsch, S. Henschel, C. Widmer, J. Behr, A. Zien, F. De Bona, A. Binder, C. Gehl, V. Franc, The shogun machine learning toolbox. J. Mach. Learn. Res. **11**(60), 1799–1802 (2010)
35. S. Tsai, Z. Zheng, N. Nguyen, M. Liebers, V. Topkar, V. Thapar, N. Wyvekens, C. Khayter, A. John Iafrate, L. Le, M.J. Aryee, J.K. Joung, GUIDE-Seq enables genome-wide profiling of off-target cleavage by CRISPR-Cas nucleases. Nat. Biotechnol. **33**, 187–197 (2014)
36. M.I.E. Uusi-Mäkelä, H.R. Barker, C.A. Bäuerlein, T. Häkkinen, M. Nykter, M. Rämet, Chromatin accessibility is associated with CRISPR-Cas9 efficiency in the zebrafish (danio rerio). PLOS ONE **13**(4), 1–15 (2018)
37. T. Wang, J.J. Wei, D.M. Sabatini, E.S. Lander, Genetic screens in human cells using the CRISPR-Cas9 system. Science **343**, 80–84 (2013)
38. N. Wong, W. Liu, X. Wang, WU-CRISPR: characteristics of functional guide RNAs for the CRISPR/Cas9 system. Genome Biol. **16**(1), 218 (2015)
39. A.V. Wright, J.K. Nuñez, J.A. Doudna, Biology and applications of CRISPR systems: Harnessing nature's toolbox for genome engineering. Cell **165**(1–2), 29–44 (2016)
40. L. Xue, B. Tang, W. Chen, J. Luo, Prediction of CRISPR sgRNA activity using a deep convolutional neural network. J. Chem. Inf. Model. **59**(1), 615–624 (2019)

MinCNE: Identifying Conserved Noncoding Elements Using Min-Wise Hashing

Sairam Behera, Jitender S. Deogun, and Etsuko N. Moriyama

1 Introduction

Noncoding regions such as introns and intergenic regions of a genome are usually more divergent and exhibit higher molecular evolutionary rates compared to exon regions. Conserved noncoding elements (CNEs) are the genomic regions that show unusually extreme conservation. These elements are mostly clustered around the genes and play important roles in regulating the transcription process [1]. These elements (or regions) are also referred as conserved noncoding sequences (CNSs), ultraconserved elements (UCEs), or ultraconserved noncoding elements (UCNEs). The identification of CNEs in animal and plant genomes poses different challenges due to their sizes. CNEs in plants are shorter (15$\sim$50 bp) compared to animal CNEs ($\geq$ 100 bp) [2, 3]. The two major approaches that have been used to identify CNEs are alignment-based and alignment-free methods. The approaches can also be classified based on pairwise or multiple sequence comparison. Pairwise methods work on exactly two input sequences. Therefore, it requires multiple pairwise operations to process more than two sequences. The use of more than two sequences at once also poses challenges for scalability and computational efficiency compared to pairwise operations. Probabilistic data structures and approximate methods are often used to address scalability challenges.

The alignment-based approaches for CNE identification employ either pairwise or multiple sequence alignment methods. The most commonly used alignment tools are BLAST [4], QUOTA-ALIGN [5], LASTZ [6], BLASTZ [7], and MULITZ [8]. In some studies, CNEs are identified by manual or automated curation of BLASTN

S. Behera (✉) · J. S. Deogun · E. N. Moriyama
University of Nebraska-Lincoln, Lincoln, NE, USA
e-mail: sbehera@cse.unl.edu; emoriyama2@unl.edu

H. R. Arabnia et al. (eds.), *Advances in Computer Vision and Computational Biology*, Transactions on Computational Science and Computational Intelligence,
https://doi.org/10.1007/978-3-030-71051-4_53

results [2, 3]. Others used global alignment with sliding window [9] or whole-genome alignment [10] to identify CNEs.

Among the first alignment-free tools that were developed for finding CNEs in plants were STAG-CNS [11] and DiCE [12]. STAG-CNS used suffix tree-based indexing and a directed acyclic graph to discover order-aware exact-matched CNEs in various grass species, where the minimum length of CNEs can be as short as 8 bp. DiCE is the extension of the STAG-CNS approach, where the exact-matched CNEs are further processed in a brute-force manner allowing a given percentage of mismatches. CNEFinder [13] identifies CNEs longer than 200 bp in animal genomes. It finds the maximal exact matches (MEMs) between two given sequences using k-mer-based methods and then extends the MEMs to produce the CNEs. CNEFinder employs a pairwise approach, whereas STAG-CNS and DiCE are designed to work with multiple sequences simultaneously. The approach used in DiCE for finding CNEs with mismatches is not computationally efficient due to its brute-force nature. This motivated us to design an efficient algorithm for the CNE identification problem.

In this study, we propose an efficient alignment-free method, called MinCNE. MinCNE identifies the CNEs conserved among more than two sequences with user-defined constraints. Instead of finding exact-matched (identical) k-mers, our method clusters the similar k-mers with a given mismatch rate using min-wise hashing (minhash) and locality-sensitive hashing (LSH). These two hashing approaches are highly efficient for clustering the elements using the Jaccard similarity measure. It ensures that the CNEs with the user-defined similarity are grouped together. MinCNE can identify CNEs as short as 100 bp. With its fast and efficient resource usage as well as the user-customizable similarity threshold, MinCNE is expected to contribute to discovery of more CNEs from a wide range of organisms.

2 Materials and Methods

Given a set of sequences, $S = \{s_1, s_2, \cdots, s_n\}$, a minimum CNE length, k, and a similarity threshold, θ, MinCNE uses minhash and LSH strategies to identify all CNEs of length $\geq k$ present in all input sequences. The algorithm used in MinCNE is given in Algorithm 1, and the flowchart summarizing the MinCNE process is shown in Fig. 1. MinCNE is written in C++ and distributed under the GNU Public License (GPL). The source codes and relevant documents are freely available at https://github.com/srbehera/MinCNE.

2.1 Minhash Signatures

The minhash is useful when the Jaccard similarity needs to be measured for large datasets. The Jaccard similarity index, which is also known as Intersection over

Algorithm 1: Identify CNEs using minhash and LSH

```
Input: Set of sequences S = {s_1, ··· , s_n},
Parameter: k-mer size, number of hash functions N, q-gram size, band size b, similarity
           threshold θ, hash functions H
Functions: minHash, edlib, LSH
Output: List of CNEs with start and end positions
Initialize cluster set C ← ϕ (empty)
Initialize list L ← ϕ (empty)
/* process all but the first sequence */
for each sequence s_i ∈ {s_2, s_3, ··· , s_n} in the S do
    extract all k-mers and put in set K_i
    for each k-mer k_j ∈ {k_1, k_2, ··· , k_{|s_i|-k+1}} in K_i do
        /* generate minhash signature of k-mer by using q-grams
           and set of hash functions H */
        min_sketch ← minhash(k_j, q, H)     // set of N 64-bit integers
        r ← N/b
        B ← LSH(min_sketch, b, r)           // set of bucket ids
        Assign sequence k_i in buckets whose ids are in B
/* process the first sequence */
extract all k-mers and put in set K_1
for each k-mer k_j ∈ {k_1, k_2, ··· , k_{|s_1|-k+1}} in K_1 do
    create a cluster C and assign k_j to it
    min_sketch ← minhash(k_j, q, H)
    r ← N/b
    B ← LSH(min_sketch, b, r)               // set of bucket ids
    for each bucket_id b_k in {b_1, b_2, ··· , b_r} in B do
        B ← Bucket with id b_k
        if B has k-mers from n − 1 sequences then
            for each k-mer k_u in B do
                per_id ← edlib(k_j, k_u)
                if per_id ≥ θ then
                    Put k_u into C
    Process the cluster C to keep the one k-mer from each sequence with highest per_id
    score with k_j
    if C has n elements then
        Add C to C
    Clusters that contain consecutive k-mers are merged and put into CNE list L
return L
```

Union, is used to represent the similarity between two sets. The similarity index between the two sets X and Y is given as

$$J(X, Y) = \frac{|X \cap Y|}{|X \cup Y|} \tag{1}$$

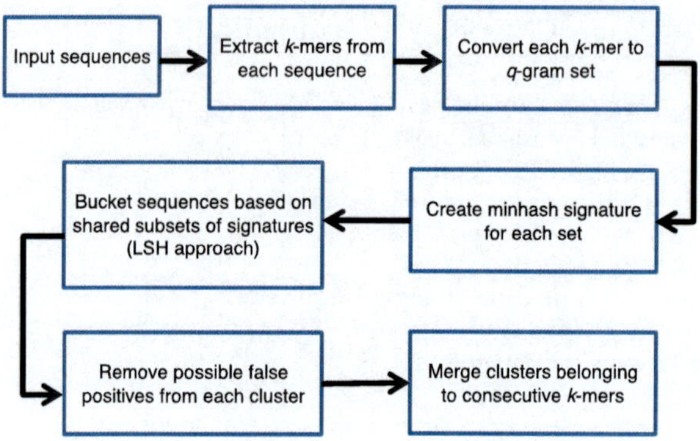

Fig. 1 Flowchart of MinCNE: k-mers extracted from each sequence are converted first to q-gram sets and next to minhash signatures. LSH creates the initial cluster. k-mers in each cluster are compared to remove potential false positives. Clusters are merged to generate the final set of CNEs

The earliest work of estimating the Jaccard similarity between sets of any sizes using minhash is found in [14]. A set of hash functions is used to convert each of the two sets into a minhash signature as follows. Each independent hash function generates a hash value for each element of the set. The minimum value among all hash values generated by the same hash function across all elements of the set is collected as an element of the minhash signature. With N independent hash functions, the minhash signature is a set of N elements corresponding to these minimum values. Therefore, the size of a minhash signature depends on the number of the independent hash functions used and independent of the size of the original set.

Let h_{min} be a minhash function and the collection of minimum hash values of the sets X and Y be $h_{min}(X)$ and $h_{min}(Y)$, respectively. It is shown that the probability of the two minimum hash value sets being equal is the Jaccard similarity of the sets X and Y [14]:

$$P(h_{min}(X) = h_{min}(Y)) = J(X, Y) \tag{2}$$

Given the minhash signatures of the two sets, both with the size N, let z be the number of minhash values that are shared, i.e., $|h_{min}(X) \cap h_{min}(Y)|$. Then, an unbiased estimate of the Jaccard similarity is obtained by dividing z by N [15].

For MinCNE, the input sequences are preprocessed by enumerating all k-mers from each sequences. Each k-mer is further tokenized by extracting all possible q-grams (q-mers, $q << k$). A hash function converts each token into a 64-bit integer, and the minimum among them is selected. This process is repeated several times with different hash functions. With N different hash functions, a 64-bit integer vector of size N is generated for each k-mer. This vector is the minhash signature for the k-mer. This process is equivalent to selecting N random q-grams from a k-mer. It is expected that if two k-mers are similar, they share many q-grams. The Jaccard similarity between two k-mers, i.e., the proportion of shared q-grams between them, can be approximated by comparing the signatures as discussed above. However, the pairwise comparison of every possible k-mers is still computationally expensive. Therefore, the LSH algorithm is used to cluster the k-mers with similarities.

2.2 LSH-Based Clustering

LSH indexing was first developed for a general approximate nearest-neighbor search problem in high-dimensional spaces [16]. A family of hash functions is chosen in such a way that the collision probabilities of those hash functions are always high for similar inputs and low for dissimilar inputs. A formal definition of LSH functions is found in [16]. The minhash function h_{min} belongs to the family of LSH functions for the Jaccard distance, as the probability of collision is equal to the Jaccard similarity.

A minhash LSH index is built as follows. Once the minhash signatures are generated from all input data (e.g., sequences each represented by a set of q-grams), all signatures are divided into b bands of a fixed size r. If the minhash signature size is N, then $N = b * r$. We define the hash function H, which generates a bucket signature B_i for the ith band by taking minhash signature values from positions $i * 1$ to $i * r$ as input:

$$B_i = H(h_{min,i*1}, h_{min,i*2}, \dots, h_{min,i*r}) \quad (3)$$

The bucket signature B_i maps a band in a signature to a bucket so that minhash signatures with the same bucket signature on the band i are mapped to the same bucket. The minhash signatures of the two sets compared are mapped to buckets using the same set of hash functions. The two sets are considered to be the candidates of a similar pair if the signatures map to at least one same bucket. The time complexity of searching the candidate pairs using the LSH algorithm depends on the number of minhash functions (the minhash signature size) and is sub-linear with respect to the total number of sets in the search space. Let j be the Jaccard similarity between the sets X and Y, i.e., $j = J(X, Y)$. The probability that X and Y are the candidate pair is calculated as

$$P(j|b, r) = 1 - (1 - j^r)^b \quad (4)$$

While the sets that meet a given Jaccard similarity threshold should have a high probability of becoming a candidate pair, those that do not meet the threshold should have low probabilities of becoming candidate pairs. The parameters such as the number of the bands b and band size r need to be adjusted to achieve these requirements.

In MinCNE, the LSH algorithm is used for clustering of k-mers as follows. The minhash signature of each k-mer is broken into a series of bands. A hash function is generated for each band and this becomes the bucket id. The index of the k-mer is put into this bucket. If the signatures of two k-mers share a band, then their indices

Table 1 Generation of minhash signatures for two k-mer sequences S_1 and S_2

S_1						S_2					
5-grams	H_1	H_2	H_3	H_4	H_5	5-grams	H_1	H_2	H_3	H_4	H_5
`caagt`	11	67	9	89	56	`cagtc`	18	12	59	97	29
`aagtc`	98	53	16	9	67	`agtct`	88	32	99	7	23
`agtct`	88	32	99	7	23	`gtcta`	2	78	52	92	50
`gtcta`	2	78	52	92	50	`tctag`	10	7	88	70	39
`tctag`	10	7	88	70	39	`ctagt`	13	14	96	89	5
`ctagt`	13	14	96	89	5	`tagta`	58	61	28	1	15
`tagta`	58	61	28	1	15	`agtag`	76	58	43	11	52
`agtag`	76	58	43	11	52	`gtaga`	92	62	14	3	6
`gtaga`	78	42	59	82	31	`tagat`	19	39	23	88	97
`tagac`	66	71	45	92	4	`agatg`	86	10	77	31	3
`agacg`	32	38	93	72	21	`gatga`	44	96	29	9	47
`gacga`	69	51	94	6	7	`atgac`	29	52	75	95	53
`acgac`	73	71	99	88	14	`tgact`	20	23	9	82	88
`cgact`	92	75	8	62	22	`gactt`	59	40	86	18	28

$H_1, \cdots, H_5$ are hash functions, and hash values shown in red are the minimum values of each column

(start positions in the sequences) will be found in the same bucket. The chances of finding the two similar k-mers in the same bucket increase with the increase in the number of bands.

How a pair of k-mers is compared using the minhash signatures and LSH-based clustering is shown in the following example. Consider the following two k–mers where $k = 18$:

S_1 : `caagtctagtagacgact`
S_2 : `cagtctagtagatgactt`

Each k-mer is first converted into a q-gram set that contains every possible q-grams of the k-mer. Setting both q and the minhash signature size N to 5, five hash functions ($H_1, \cdots, H_5$) are used to generate five hash values as illustrated in Table 1. The minhash signature of each k-mer is the vector containing the minimum value from each hash function (shown in red in Table 1). Thus, the minhash signatures of the above two k-mers will be given as

$$Sig(S_1) = < 2, 7, 8, 1, 4 >$$
$$Sig(S_2) = < 2, 7, 9, 1, 3 >$$

With the number of bands b=5 and band size r=1, we have the following clusters: C_1: $<1, 2>$, C_2: $<1, 2>$, C_3: $< 2 >$, C_4: $< 1 >$, C_7: $< 1, 2 >$, C_8: $< 1 >$, C_9: $< 1 >$

2.3 CNE Identification

Once the clusters are identified, the next task is to identify the CNEs. A CNE is required to be present in all given sequences. Therefore, we first discard the clusters that do not contain k-mers from all sequences. In the above example, clusters C_3, C_4, C_8, and C_9 will be discarded. The k-mers clustered by LSH are likely to have higher Jaccard similarity scores than those that are not clustered. To ensure that the similarity between every pair is greater than or equal to the given threshold (θ), sequences of each k-mer pairs in each cluster are compared. Edit distances are calculated using edlib, a lightweight and fast C++ library [17]. The clusters containing consecutive k-mers are merged and extended until the similarity score drops below the threshold. For example, if we have the following five clusters containing the start positions of 200-mers in the original sequence:

C_i: *<10456, 39898, 78907 >*
C_j: *<10457, 39899, 78908 >*
C_k: *<10458, 39900, 78909 >*
C_l: *<10459, 39901, 78910 >*
C_m: *<10460, 39902, 78911 >*

these clusters can be merged to generate a CNE of length 205. The start and end positions of three CNEs identified are as follows:

<10456-10660, 39898-40102, 78907-79111>

In this study, the size of the minhash signature (N) was set to 50 generated by 50 minhash functions. Other settings used include q = 13, b = 25, r = 2, and k = 200. The threshold for pairwise sequence similarity (θ) was set to 95%. These parameters were found to be optimal for the test sequences used in this study and no false positives were produced. Depending on the target CNEs, k-mer size can be set as short as 100.

2.4 Benchmark Dataset

UCNEbase [18] is a publicly available database that contains the information about UCNEs of 18 vertebrate genomes. There are currently ~4300 CNEs present in the database. Almost half of them are from intergenic regions and others are from either intron or untranslated exon regions. The non-coding regions of the human genome that exhibits more than 95% identity with chicken sequences are considered to be UCNEs. The minimum length of UCNE is 200 bp. To the best of our knowledge, this is the most recently updated database for CNEs of the human genome. We therefore chose this database to be the current benchmark. It should be noted that no independent verification has been performed for any CNEs under the definition of UCNEbase. We selected human intergenic UCNEs found in the following five gene regions: ZEB2, TSHZ3, EBF3, BCL11A, and ZFHX4. From 1 Mbp regions both upstream and downstream of the coding regions of the five genes, UCNEbase recognized 271 UCNEs in total. The genomic sequences from five vertebrate species included human (hg19), mouse (mm10), opossum (monDom5), chicken (galGal3), and zebra finch (taeGut1).

2.5 Performance Evaluation

All experiments were run on the CentOS Linux server with Intel® Xeon® CPU E5–2630 v4 at 2.20GHz. All programs were run on a single core.

An identified CNE is considered to be a true positive if sequences identified from all species used have more than 95% sequence identity with the benchmark CNE sequences. The CNE-finding performance was examined using following metrices:

- *TP* (true positives): the number of identified CNEs that are present in UCNEbase,
- *FP* (false positives): the number of identified CNEs that are not found in UCNEbase,
- *FN* (false negatives): the number of CNEs that are present in UCNEbase but are not identified by the tool,
- precision or positive predictive value: $\frac{TP}{(TP+FP)}$, and
- recall or true positive rate: $\frac{TP}{(TP+FN)}$.

Note that we did not include negative data; hence, no true negative was counted. CNEs were identified from the 1 Mbp upstream and downstream of each gene region. Some of these test regions overlapped with exon regions of neighboring genes. Since our benchmark dataset was derived from UCNEbase, which does not recognize any conserved sequences from exon regions, any CNE candidates identified in these regions were excluded from the analyses.

We compared the performance of MinCNE with CNEFinder. CNEFinder works only on a pair of sequences for CNE identification. Therefore, direct performance comparisons were performed using only human and chicken sequences. The time and space efficiency of CNEFinder for multiple sequence comparisons was estimated based on the number of operations needed to be executed.

3 Results and Discussion

3.1 CNE Identification Performance

We first compared the CNE-finding performance between MinCNE and CNEFinder. Because CNEFinder can be used only for pairwise comparisons, we limited the comparison for human and chicken sequences.

As shown in Table 2, both MinCNE and CNEFinder were able to identify most of the benchmark CNEs. Out of 271 CNEs, MinCNE and CNEFinder missed 7 and 9 CNEs in total, respectively. MinCNE was able to find all 44 CNEs for EBF3 and 80 out of 81 CNEs for TSHZ3. CNEFinder identified all CNEs for TSHZ3 but missed only one for EBF3. For ZFHX4, both MinCNE and CNEFinder failed to identify the same set of three out of 57 CNEs. The recall values were $\geq 95\%$ and $\geq 91\%$ for MinCNE and CNEFinder, respectively. About a half of the FNs were the same CNEs missed by both MinCNE and CNEFinder (4 of 7 and 4 of 9, respectively). As noted above, the 1 Mbp test regions included some exon sequences of other genes. Both MinCNE and CNEFinder found CNE candidates in these regions (shown as N/A in Table 2), with many of them from the same regions. Neither of the tools produced FPs from any gene regions. Thus, the precision values were one for all tests.

Unlike CNEFinder, MinCNE can identify CNEs among multiple sequences at once. To demonstrate this capability, we performed the CNE identification using MinCNE with the sequences from three, four, and five species. The performance was exactly the same as shown in Table 2 (the same numbers of TPs and FNs were identified). This was expected because the two species compared in Table 2 are human and chicken, which are the most divergent pair of species among those compared (human, mouse, opossum, zebra finch, and chicken). Therefore, even when more species were included, since they were more closely related to either human or chicken, it did not increase the number of CNEs identified. It should also be noted that MinCNE identified all corresponding CNEs from additional species without exception. This demonstrates that MinCNE can efficiently and accurately identify CNEs from multiple genomes.

3.2 Time and Space Usage

The time and space usage of MinCNE was examined using different numbers of sequences. For CNEFinder, usages for more than two sequences were estimated based on the number of operations required in either serial or parallel execution. For example, if there are 10 datasets used in an experiment, there will be 45 pairwise operations. For serial executions, the estimated time for CNEfinder will be 45 times of a single execution. If all the executions are done in parallel, then the estimated time for the completion of all executions will be the same as for a single execution.

Table 2 Comparision of MinCNE and CNEFinder using human and chicken dataset

Gene	UCNEbase	TP		FN		Recall		N/A[a]	
		MinCNE	CNEFinder	MinCNE	CNEFinder	MinCNE	CNEFinder	MinCNE	CNEFinder
ZEB2	63	61	61	2	2	0.97	0.97	25	21
TSHZ3	81	80	81	1	0	0.99	1	16	16
EBF3	44	44	43	0	1	1	0.98	25	24
BCL11A	32	31	29	1	3	0.97	0.91	15	15
ZFHX4	57	54	54	3	3	0.95	0.95	20	18

[a] All these sequences were found in the exon regions of other genes and not counted for the performance analysis

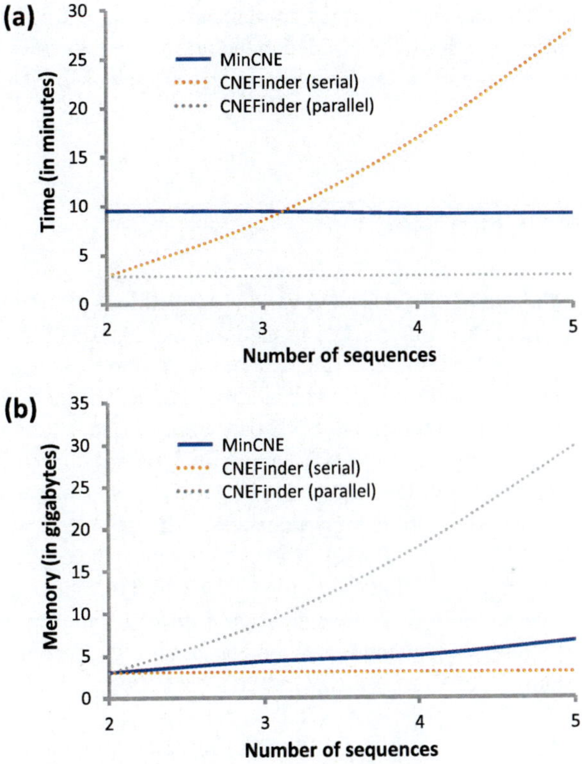

Fig. 2 Time (**a**) and space (**b**) usage of MinCNE and CNEFinder: for CNEFinder, only the time and memory amount used for the two-sequence comparison was based on the actual observation. Other data were estimates

CNEFinder was faster than MinCNE when only two sequences were used (3 min by CNEFinder and ~9 min by MinCNE; Fig. 2a). The LSH-based clustering stage of MinCNE produces many clusters including many redundant ones. The processing of those clusters is the time-consuming step of MinCNE. The minhash signature generation and initial clustering time increases sub-linearly with increase in the number of sequences. However, the time for identifying CNEs from the clusters decreases with increase in the number of sequences. This is because if a cluster does not contain a k-mer that is found in every sequence, it is eliminated. Therefore, the time usage with MinCNE did not increase with the number of sequences. In contrast, CNEFinder will require to be run ten times longer to compare five sequences. If these ten operations are executed serially, as shown in Fig. 2a, CNEFinder will take almost 30 min. CNEFinder will also require additional time for the post-processing of results from all pairwise runs.

The memory consumption of MinCNE was comparable to CNEFinder. Both tools used approximately 3 GB of RAM. As shown in Fig. 2b, the space usage increased only gradually when more sequences were used with MinCNE. Similar to computational time analysis, CNEFinder will need to be run ten times either serially or parallely for five sequences. For parallel executions, the space usage for CNEFinder will increase by ten times. Additional space is also needed for CNEFinder for post-processing of pairwise results.

Although the current implementation of MinCNE does not support multi-threading, this will be added in the future version of MinCNE. With multi-threading, the advantage of using time and space efficient MinCNE is expected to be even more significant.

4 Conclusion

Minhash has been used in various applications of bioinformatics especially for analyzing large datasets. We applied this technique in MinCNE, a new computationally efficient CNE finder. MinCNE does not require whole genome alignment or multiple pairwise alignments for generating indices for the given sequences. Unlike other CNE-finding tools, MinCNE can work on more than two sequences at once. Our previous tool STAG-CNS found only exact-matched CNEs [11]. This requirement was relaxed in DiCE [12]. However, DiCE was not computationally efficient especially with multiple long sequences. With MinCNE, we addressed these challenges. MinCNE is also flexible and the sequence identity threshold can be customized. Although CNEFinder uses the k-mer-based technique and computationally efficient, it works only on two sequences at once. It requires multiple pairwise operations if multiple sequences need to be analyzed. Currently available CNE databases such as Ancora [19], CEGA [20], cneViewer [21], CONDOR [22], UCBase [23], UCNEbase [18], and VISTA [24] are mostly static and not updated regularly. MinCNE, with its computational efficiency, high sensitivity, and the flexibility, will be useful for studies in large-scale comparative genomics. The approximation techniques used by minhash and LSH can be further improved to reduce both space and time efficiency.

Acknowledgments We thank Drs. Schnable and Voshall (UNL) for suggestions and critical comments on the earlier and current works. Some part of this work was completed utilizing the Holland Computing Center of the University of Nebraska, which receives support from the Nebraska Research Initiative. This work has been supported by NSF EPSCoR RII Track-1: Center for Root and Rhizobiome Innovation (CRRI) Award OIA-1557417 to ENM.

References

1. D. Polychronopoulos, J.W.D. King, A.J. Nash, G. Tan, B. Lenhard, Conserved non-coding elements: developmental gene regulation meets genome organization. Nucl. Acids Res. **45**(22), 12611–12624 (2017)
2. S. Stephen, M. Pheasant, I.V. Makunin, J.S. Mattick, Large-scale appearance of ultraconserved elements in tetrapod genomes and slowdown of the molecular clock. Mol. Biol. Evol. **25**(2), 402–408 (2008)
3. G. Turco, J.C. Schnable, B. Pedersen, M. Freeling, Automated conserved non-coding sequence (CNS) discovery reveals differences in gene content and promoter evolution among grasses. Front. Plant Sci. **4**, 170–170 (2013)

4. S.F. Altschul, W. Gish, W. Miller, E.W. Myers, D.J. Lipman, Basic local alignment search tool. J. Mol. Biol. **215**(3), 403–410 (1990)
5. H. Tang, E. Lyons, B. Pedersen, J.C. Schnable, A. Paterson, M. Freeling, Screening synteny blocks in pairwise genome comparisons through integer programming. BMC Bioinf. **12**, 102 (2011)
6. R.S. Harris, Improved pairwise alignment of genomic DNA. Ph.D. Thesis, The Pennsylvania State University (2007)
7. S. Schwartz, W.J. Kent, A. Smit, Z. Zhang, R. Baertsch, R. Hardison, D. Haussler, W. Miller, Human-mouse alignments with blastz. Genome Res. **13**, 103–110 (2003)
8. M. Blanchette, W.J. Kent, C. Riemer, L. Elnitski, A. Smit, K. Roskin, R. Baertsch, K. Rosenbloom, H. Clawson, E. Green, D. Haussler, W. Miller, Aligning multiple genomic sequences with the threaded blockset aligner. Genome Res. **14**, 708–722 (2004)
9. L. Baxter, A. Jironkin, R. Hickman, J. Moore, C. Barrington, P. Krusche, N.P. Dyer, V. Buchanan-Wollaston, A. Tiskin, J. Beynon, et al., Conserved noncoding sequences highlight shared components of regulatory networks in dicotyledonous plants. Plant Cell **24**(10), 3949–3965 (2012)
10. A. Haudry, A.E. Platts, E. Vello, D.R. Hoen, M. Leclercq, R.J. Williamson, E. Forczek, Z. Joly-Lopez, J.G. Steffen, K.M. Hazzouri, et al., An atlas of over 90,000 conserved noncoding sequences provides insight into crucifer regulatory regions. Nat. Genet. **45**(8), 891–898 (2013)
11. X. Lai, S. Behera, Z. Liang, Y. Lu, J.S. Deogun, J.C. Schnable, Stag-CNS: an order-aware conserved noncoding sequences discovery tool for arbitrary numbers of species. Mol. Plant **10**(7), 990–999 (2017)
12. S. Behera, X. Li, J.C. Schnable, J.S. Deogun, Dice: discovery of conserved noncoding sequences efficiently, in *2017 IEEE International Conference on Bioinformatics and Biomedicine (BIBM)* (2017), pp. 79–82
13. L.A.K. Ayad, S.P. Pissis, D. Polychronopoulos, CNEFinder: finding conserved non-coding elements in genomes. Bioinformatics **34**(17), i743–i747 (2018)
14. A.Z. Broder, M. Charikar, A.M. Frieze, M. Mitzenmacher, Min-wise independent permutations. J. Comput. Syst. Sci. **60**, 630–659 (3).
15. E. Zhu, F. Nargesian, K.Q. Pu, R.J. Miller, LSH ensemble: internet-scale domain search. Proc. VLDB Endowment **9**(12), 1185–1196 (2016)
16. P. Indyk, R. Motwani, Approximate nearest neighbors: towards removing the curse of dimensionality, in *Proceedings of the Thirtieth Annual ACM Symposium on Theory of Computing, STOC'98* (ACM, New York, 1998), pp. 604–613
17. M. Šošić, M. Šikić, Edlib: a C/C++ library for fast, exact sequence alignment using edit distance. Bioinformatics **33**(9), 1394–1395 (2017)
18. S. Dimitrieva, P. Bucher, UCNEbase–a database of ultraconserved non-coding elements and genomic regulatory blocks. Nucl. Acids Res. **41**(D1), D101–D109 (2012)
19. P.G. Engström, D. Fredman, B. Lenhard, Ancora: a web resource for exploring highly conserved noncoding elements and their association with developmental regulatory genes. Genome Biol. **9**, R34–R34 (2007)
20. A. Dousse, T. Junier, E.M. Zdobnov, CEGA - a catalog of conserved elements from genomic alignments. Nucl. Acids Res. **44**(D1), D96–D100 (2015)
21. J. Persampieri, D.I. Ritter, D. Lees, J. Lehoczky, Q. Li, S. Guo, J.H. Chuang, cneViewer: a database of conserved non-coding elements for studies of tissue-specific gene regulation. Bioinformatics **24**(20), 2418–2419 (2008)
22. A. Woolfe, D.K. Goode, J.E Cooke, H. Callaway, S.F. Smith, P.J. Snell, G. McEwen, G. Elgar, Condor: a database resource of developmentally associated conserved non-coding elements. BMC Develop. Biol. **7**, 100 (2007)
23. V. Lomonaco, R. Martoglia, F. Mandreoli, L. Anderlucci, W. Emmett, S. Bicciato, C. Taccioli, UCbase 2.0: ultraconserved sequences database (2014 update). Database 2014 (2014)
24. A. Visel, S. Minovitsky, I. Dubchak, L.A. Pennacchio, VISTA enhancer browser–a database of tissue-specific human enhancers. Nucl. Acids Res. **35**(suppl 1), D88–D92 (2006)

An Investigation in Optimal Encoding of Protein Primary Sequence for Structure Prediction by Artificial Neural Networks

Aaron Hein, Casey Cole, and Homayoun Valafar

1 Introduction

Proteins are variable length chains of amino acid residues. Anfinsen's dogma states that simply the sequence of amino acid residues is enough to determine the unique, three-dimensional shape of a given protein [2]. However, in practice determining that structure purely from the first principles of physics and thermodynamics is computationally intractable especially for challenging proteins such as those that undergo dynamics or membrane proteins. Nevertheless, determining the structure is vital in determining the function of the protein. Perturbations in the structure of a protein can lead to a misfolding of the protein, which can lead to the manifestation of diseases. Alzheimer's disease, type 2 diabetes mellitus, and Parkinson's disease [3] can be cited as examples of this phenomenon. In all of those cases, proteins fail to fold "properly" causing a disruption in the natural cellular functions. It stands to reason that the cure to these diseases would involve drugs or therapies to correct the misfolded proteins.

Although there are experimental methods to determine protein structure [5, 20], these methods are highly time and cost intensive. In contrast, computational approaches to protein structure determination have many advantages such as reduced cost, increased effectiveness, and speed. Computational approaches can also be conducted in the absence of the biological sample. Although purely physics-based simulation of protein folding is intractable at this time, the recent advances in big data and machine learning have given rise to inception of data driven strategies to protein structure determination.

A. Hein (✉) · C. Cole · H. Valafar
Department of Computer Science, University of South Carolina, Columbia, SC, USA
e-mail: ahein@email.sc.edu; coleca@email.sc.edu; homayoun@cec.sc.edu

H. R. Arabnia et al. (eds.), *Advances in Computer Vision and Computational Biology*, Transactions on Computational Science and Computational Intelligence,
https://doi.org/10.1007/978-3-030-71051-4_54

Previous works in this field have detailed the use of various machine learning techniques in order to make these predictions. These techniques have included support vector machines [17, 21] as well as a number of different neural network architectures [11–13, 18, 19, 23, 24]. Due to their obvious advantages, the most successful approaches to structure prediction of proteins have consisted of artificial neural networks (ANN). Although ANNs provide several advantages over other existing machine learning techniques, they do require optimization in numerous categories including selection of a proper model of ANN, ANN architecture, and input/output encoding. Nearly all of the previous reports [12, 13, 18, 19, 23, 24] have consisted of an investigation of different architectures and models of ANN to improve the performance. While the selection of the most appropriate model and architecture is an important aspect of an ANN-based approach, the proper selection of input and output encoding scheme has been poorly investigated despite its impact on the problem outcome.

Here we present an investigation and evaluation of multiple input encodings including schemes based off of 10 different substitution matrices and 11 different window sizes while presenting a new approach that improves ANN's predictions compared to the previous approaches when tested on a single class of proteins. More specifically, we have utilized protein CATH class 1.10.510.10 that consists of 5814 protein structures in order to develop and evaluate different input encoding schemes. We have tested general improvements of our new proposed encoding scheme on 7 models of different architectures as well as two other protein CATH classes 2.60.120.200 and 3.90.1150.10 that collectively encompassed 4505 protein structures. In general, we observed a 4°–5° improvement in the prediction of the both torsion angles across different ANN models and architectures.

2 Background and Method

2.1 Protein Structure Formation in Rotamer Space

An amino acid is an organic compound that is made up of an amine group (consisting of a nitrogen and two hydrogens) and a carboxyl group (consisting of a carbon with two oxygens and a hydrogen) connected by a carbon atom. This central carbon is known as the alpha carbon (C_α). The C_α atom also has a hydrogen bonded to it in addition to a side chain. This side chain is different for each amino acid. For example, glycine has a very simple side chain consisting of a single hydrogen atom, whereas aspartate's side chain consists of a carbon with two oxygen atoms. A protein is a series of amino acids that have bonded together in what is known as a peptide bond. During a peptide bond, the carbon from the carboxyl group of the first amino acid bonds with the nitrogen from the amine group of the second amino acid. Additionally, the oxygen and hydrogen from the carboxyl group of the first amino acid bond with a hydrogen from the amine group of the second amino acid to form water (H_2O) that is released. The resulting structure's backbone consists of N–C_α–C–N–C_α–C. When this bond occurs, the angle that describes the rotation between the two amino acid residues is known as ω (omega). It is almost always fixed at 180°. However, the other angles in the structure are much less rigid. It is these angles that define the protein's secondary and tertiary structure. The angle that describes the rotation around the bond between the nitrogen and alpha carbon is referred to as the ϕ (phi) angle, while the angle that describes the rotation around the bond between the alpha carbon and the carboxyl carbon is known as the ψ (psi) angle.

2.2 Methodology

All previous approaches to protein structure prediction using machine learning have striven to achieve more accurate predictions of the backbone dihedral angles ϕ (phi) and ψ (psi) for each amino acid. As early as 1988, Quin and Sejnowski [19] used machine learning and neural networks to predict these angles. In this earliest attempt, a window size of 13 amino acids and one-hot encoding was used to represent the data for input to the ANN. Since then, many others have used machine learning and neural networks in an attempt to achieve a more accurate prediction of these torsion angles. Reporting in chronological order: in 2005, Wood and Hirst proposed a method for predicting secondary structures and the ψ angles called DESTRUCT [23]. This method relied on the position specific scoring matrix (PSSM) from PSI-BLAST[1] as well as the ϕ angle as input data for their models. PSI-BLAST uses the BLOSUM62 scoring matrix [14] as the starting point by default, although other matrices can be used that will impact the encoding of the protein. Additional use of neural networks to predict the torsion angles was made in the ANGLOR[24], REALSPINE 2.0 [25], REALSPINE 3.0 [8], SPINE XI [9], SPINE X [10], SPIDER 2 [13], RaptorX [12], and deep learning method works[18] with all of them including the PSSM from PSI-BLAST in their input features.

2.3 The Explored Encoding Schemes

Our exploration of the new encoding schemes was motivated by three constraints. First was to avoid dependence on an encoding mechanism that is time-variant such as the use of PSSM that is continuously changing due to deposition of new proteins. Second was to develop a method that did not require a heavy pre-processing step. The final constraint was to develop an encoding mechanism that will broadly improve structure prediction across different protein classes, models, and architectures of ANN. To that end, we used a one-hot encoding as well as ten other encoding schemes based on different BLOSUM [15] and PAM [7] substitution matrices including BLOSUM62 [14] (used in PSSM creation by PSI-BLAST),

BLOSUM30, BLOSUM45, BLOSUM65, BLOSUM80, BLOSUM 100, PAM30, PAM60, PAM120 and PAM250. A 21 position array was used for the encoding with the last position being reserved for other or unknown amino acid residues. As the name implies, one hot encoding involves creating a zero-filled array where each column represents one particular value. To set that value, the column is set to one, while all other entries in the array remain zero. For example, in one-hot encoding (which has been commonly used in previous works), alanine is represented by a column in a 21 unit vector. We used the same ordering across all of the encodings, which was A R N D C Q E G H I L K M F P S T W Y V X. Therefore, ALA would be converted into [1, 0, 0, 0, 0, 0, 0, 0, 0, 0, 0, 0, 0, 0, 0, 0, 0, 0, 0, 0]. With the BLOSUM62 encoding, the row corresponding to alanine would be used resulting in the encoding [4, −1, −2, −2, 0, −1, −1, 0, −2, −1, −1, −1, −1, −2, −1, 1, 0, −3, −2, 0, 0].

Using our amino acid encoding, the complete proteins were then presented to the ANN using a sliding window of an odd number of amino acids. We explored window sizes ranging from 3 to 23 residues with the aim of predicting the torsion angles of the middle residue. After the residue was encoded, the ϕ and ψ angles of all residues were encoded using the sine and cosine functions as described in the RaptorX [12] and deep learning works [18]. For each angle, the sine and cosine were evaluated and used as the predicted outputs during the training sessions. This had the benefit of compressing the values between -1 and 1 that map directly to the output of the $tanh()$ activation function while also allowing us to unambiguously retrieve the original angle using the $arctan2()$ function.

2.4 Target Proteins

In our investigations, we used three protein classes (shown in Table 1) reported by the CATH classification mechanism as training data. CATH [6] is a method of classifying proteins by [C]lass, [A]rchitecture, [T]opology, and [H]omologous superfamily. We focused primary on the 4 Classes at the top of the CATH hierarchy. They are mainly alpha (1), mainly beta (2), alpha beta (3), and few secondary structures (4). We chose to exclude class 4 for two reasons. First it is the smallest class with only 4519 domains. Limited data makes it more difficult to train a neural network and to provide a meaningful review of the encoding and window sizes. Second, the catch-all nature of the class indicates much more diverse proteins that may be difficult or impossible for a neural network to learn during training.

In total, these three classes represented more than 10,000 proteins with structural sampling of α-helical, β-sheet, and mixed α/β proteins. In order to establish the generalization principle of our developed encoding, we used the proteins in Class 1 (1.10.510.10) to select the optimal encoding mechanism and used Classes 2 and 3 to validate the performance of our selected encoding.

Table 1 A summary of the structures and CATH classes used in this experiment

CATH class	Domains	Unique PDBs
1.10.510.10	5814	4042
2.60.120.200	2284	965
3.90.1150.10	2221	919

Table 2 A summary of ANN architectures investigated in this chapter

Model	Architecture
DNN 1	3 layer feed forward neural network
DNN 2	6 layer feed forward neural network
LSTM 1	1 LSTM layer with 2 fully connected layers before output
LSTM 2	2 LSTM layer with 2 fully connected layers before output
LSTM 3	4 LSTM layer with 2 fully connected layers before output
LSTM 4	8 LSTM layer with 2 fully connected layers before output
LSTM 5	64 LSTM layer with 2 fully connected layers before output

2.5 *Data Processing*

Prediction of the secondary or tertiary protein structure practically involves predicting the ϕ (phi) and ψ (psi) angles that are located around the C_α atom of each residue. These angles are commonly referred to as the torsion angles of the amino acid. In order to produce the ϕ and ψ angles, we made use of the online PDBMine tool [4]. The PDBMine database includes the backbone torsion angles for over 140,000 proteins and is accessible via an online web portal as well as via direct API calls. The content of PDBMine can be used for retrieval of protein torsion angles, or for data mining purposes that can assist in the folding of proteins [4]. In this work, the use of PDBMine eliminated the need to process and store large amounts of data while also improving the overall repeatability. One caveat of note is that PDBMine can have multiple models or versions of the same protein because multiple models can exist in the PDB. We were concerned that using all of them would skew the data set and give more weight to those proteins. Therefore, then there were multiple models of a protein in the PDB, and we used the first model that was returned and discarded the others.

2.6 *Artificial Neural Network Architectures*

Although the goal of this chapter is not to develop or identify the best model but rather to identify the most suitable encoding and window size, it was required to try multiple models with the above encodings and window sizes in order to compare their initial performance. We explored different particularizations of our input encoding on feed forward and LSTM neural network architectures. For each CATH data set, we explored different architectures as shown in Table 2. There is some intuition that an LSTM [16] might perform well when predicting the torsion angles due to the sequential nature of the data. However, for completeness, other model architectures were also used. We trained each data set on two "regular" feed forward neural networks and on five LSTM networks. Each neural network architecture contained a different number of layers, but the other training parameters remained constant. In between all of the dense layers, dropout regularization [22] was used with a 30% dropout rate.

All of the models were trained with an initial learning rate of 0.01 that was set to reduce if learning plateaued during training using mean squared error as the loss function. Although many of the papers cited in this work used mean absolute error as defined in Eq. (1), it can be argued that mean squared error as defined in Eq. (2) is a better metric for training in this particular instance. RMSE gives more weight to larger errors since the errors are squared prior to summation. This seemed preferable as a large error would more drastically affect the structure of the protein.

$$MAE = \frac{1}{n}\sum_{i=1}^{n}|y_i - \hat{y}_i| \tag{1}$$

$$RMSE = \sqrt{\frac{1}{n}\sum_{i=1}^{n}(y_i - \hat{y}_i)^2}. \tag{2}$$

A total of 2541 models were investigated as part of this survey. Training on a CPU led to an estimated completion time of about 9 months. In order to decrease training time, a GPU was utilized. Each model was trained for 50 epochs and with a batch size of 4096 in an attempt to maximize GPU utilization. Training with the GPU lowered the initial estimated training time from 265 days with a single CPU to only 45 days. The training process was also configured to stop once the validation loss plateaued and the models were no longer benefiting from additional training. All of the layers used the ReLU activation function with the exception of the output layers that all used the tanh activation function.

2.7 Training, Testing, and Evaluation Protocols

Three models were trained for each model architecture, window size, and encoding combination. One was trained to predict only the ϕ angle. A second was trained to predict only the ψ angle, and a third was trained to predict both angles simultaneously. The thought was that perhaps information about both angles might lead to more accurate predictions.

Rather than encoding the data and then splitting into training, testing, and validation sets, we randomly divided the list of proteins into a 70/20/10 split for training, validation, and testing. The data was then encoded after the split. This ensured that the entire protein was included in the same data set although there was a small impact to the final percentages. In other words, because protein can be of a different length, when encoded it will produce a different number of samples. A protein that is 20 residues long when encoded with a window size of 5 will produce 16 samples, whereas a protein that is 30 residues long will produce 26 samples. If the 30 residue protein was included in the training set and the 20 residue protein was included in the validation set, the training set would have a few more samples. Although the training set included 70% of the proteins, it was not exactly 70% of the total samples. The models then were trained using a training set that was made up of 70% of the data and a validation set that was 20% of the data. 10% of the data was held out as a testing set and not used for training at all.

In order to gauge the effectiveness of the encodings, the predictions were then converted back into angles in degrees and the mean absolute error was calculated based on the angles. The lower the error, the better the model. This allowed us to compare these results with those achieved in the previous works. After the error results were compared and the best model architecture, encoding, and window size were identified, additional models were trained on the additional two CATH classes. Because CATH Class 1 is made up of mostly α-helical structures, we wanted to ensure that our findings were applicable across proteins with different secondary structures, so we selected two additional CATH classes to use as additional data sets. This provided verification that the data processing has the potential to be expanded across all proteins in the future. For this additional validation, separate models were trained using CATH 2.60.120.200 and then trained again using CATH 3.90.1150.10. The only difference from the initial training was that they were trained for 150 epochs as opposed to only 50 epochs but with early stopping still applied. This was done in an attempt to improve the results and further validate that the results were good enough to pursue additional research using this data preparation. In order to make an accurate comparison, CATH 1.10.510.10 was used again to train with 150 epochs on the narrowed selection.

3 Results and Discussion

3.1 *Root Mean Squared Error Versus Mean Absolute Error*

In order to evaluate the model performance, we examined the error rate when making predictions on the previously discussed testing set. Because the root mean squared error was used for training, we looked at that first. Tables 3, 4, and 5 show the 20 lowest RMSE achieved across all 2541 models trained as well as the encoding, window size, and architecture that produced the lowest error. Specifically, Table 3 shows the 20 models with the lowest RMSE for predicting the ϕ angles. Table 4 shows the models with the lowest RMSE for predicting the ψ angles. The

Table 3 Lowest MSE for phi prediction

Score	Encoding	Window size	Model arch
0.062	one hot[0,1]	9	lstm 5
0.062	one hot[0,1]	11	lstm 5
0.063	one hot[0,1]	13	lstm 5
0.064	one hot[0,1]	15	lstm 5
0.065	one hot[0,1]	7	lstm 5
0.068	blosum30	7	lstm 5
0.068	blosum45	7	lstm 5
0.069	one hot[0,1]	5	lstm 5
0.069	one hot[0,1]	17	lstm 5
0.069	blosum62	7	lstm 5
0.069	blosum65	7	lstm 5
0.071	one hot[0,1]	19	lstm 5
0.071	blosum45	5	lstm 5
0.073	blosum62	5	lstm 5
0.073	blosum65	5	lstm 5
0.075	pam250	5	lstm 5
0.075	blosum80	7	lstm 5
0.076	pam250	7	lstm 5
0.076	blosum65	9	lstm 5
0.077	pam120	7	lstm 5

Table 4 Lowest MSE for psi prediction

Score	Encoding	Window size	Model arch
0.097	one hot[0,1]	19	lstm 5
0.098	one hot[0,1]	13	lstm 5
0.103	one hot[0,1]	11	lstm 5
0.103	one hot[0,1]	15	lstm 5
0.104	one hot[0,1]	9	lstm 5
0.107	blosum62	7	lstm 5
0.112	one hot[0,1]	7	lstm 5
0.113	blosum30	7	lstm 5
0.113	blosum30	9	lstm 5
0.113	blosum62	9	lstm 5
0.115	blosum30	11	lstm 5
0.116	blosum45	9	lstm 5
0.117	blosum45	13	lstm 5
0.119	blosum45	7	lstm 5
0.119	blosum65	11	lstm 5
0.12	pam250	7	lstm 5
0.12	blosum45	11	lstm 5
0.121	blosum45	5	lstm 5
0.123	pam250	11	lstm 5
0.124	pam250	9	lstm 5

Table 5 Lowest MSE for phi and psi prediction

Score	Encoding	Window size	Model arch
0.097	one hot[0,1]	11	lstm 5
0.103	one hot[0,1]	15	lstm 5
0.104	one hot[0,1]	17	lstm 5
0.107	one hot[0,1]	7	lstm 5
0.107	one hot[0,1]	9	lstm 5
0.111	blosum30	9	lstm 5
0.111	blosum45	7	lstm 5
0.111	blosum62	9	lstm 5
0.113	blosum62	7	lstm 5
0.113	blosum65	7	lstm 5
0.114	one hot[0,1]	13	lstm 5
0.114	blosum30	7	lstm 5
0.114	blosum65	11	lstm 5
0.115	blosum45	9	lstm 5
0.116	blosum80	9	lstm 5
0.119	pam250	7	lstm 5
0.119	blosum45	11	lstm 5
0.12	pam250	9	lstm 5
0.121	one hot[0,1]	5	lstm 5
0.122	pam250	5	lstm 5

models with the lowest RMSE for predicting both the ϕ and ψ angles at the same time are in Table 5.

Because much of the past work in this field has relied on the mean absolute error, we believed it important to look at that as well in order to make comparisons. Tables 6, 7, and 8 show the lowest MAE error rates for ϕ, ψ, and both ϕ and ψ angles, respectively. It is worth pointing out that the RMSE will always have a value greater than or equal to the MAE. Instances where a model has a low MAE but a higher RMSE respective to other models indicate that when mistakes were made in the predictions they are generally larger mistakes. Also of note is that in our case, when training we are looking at the RMSE of the prediction that is of the sine and cosine of the angles and that was what we included in the tables. When we calculate the MAE, we are calculating the MAE of the actual angles for comparison purposes. That means that the MAE will look larger because it is given in angle degrees and not the sine and the cosine.

3.2 Optimal Architecture

Although our goal was not to determine an optimal architecture, we did examine all of our explored neural network architectures to determine if any of the architectures performed better than the others. Interestingly, all of the best performing models

Table 6 Lowest angle MAE for phi prediction

Score	Encoding	Window size	Model arch
14.294	one hot[0,1]	9	lstm 5
14.313	one hot[0,1]	11	lstm 5
14.421	one hot[0,1]	13	lstm 5
14.433	one hot[0,1]	7	lstm 5
14.571	one hot[0,1]	15	lstm 5
15.087	blosum65	7	lstm 5
15.133	blosum45	7	lstm 5
15.278	one hot[0,1]	5	lstm 5
15.29	blosum62	7	lstm 5
15.591	blosum30	7	lstm 5
15.615	one hot[0,1]	17	lstm 5
15.758	one hot[0,1]	19	lstm 5
15.823	blosum62	5	lstm 5
15.883	blosum65	5	lstm 5
15.915	blosum45	5	lstm 5
16.057	pam250	5	lstm 5
16.506	blosum30	9	lstm 5
16.522	blosum30	5	lstm 5
16.553	blosum65	9	lstm 5
16.574	pam250	7	lstm 5

were the deep (64 layer) LSTM model. This indicates that our intuition about an LSTM being a good choice for these types or predictions was correct. This is most likely due to the LSTM's strengths when looking at data in a series as well as the fact that this was the deepest network trained.

3.3 *Encoding and Window Size*

When analyzing the best performing models, we were surprised to see that regardless of whether the model was trained to predict ϕ, ψ, or both, the five models with the lowest error were all trained using the one-hot encoded data. In fact, eight out of the twenty models with the lowest error when predicting only the ϕ angle used one-hot encoding as well as six out of the twenty models with the lowest error when predicting only the ψ angle. The next best encoding was BLOSUM45 that accounted for two of the twenty ϕ models and five of the twenty ψ models. This seems to indicate that one-hot encoding is a perfectly acceptable method of encoding the amino acids for use in training these types of models. This went against our intuition that one-hot encoding would serve as a baseline for comparison but would not perform as well as the encodings based off of substitution matrices because of the number of 0's in the encoding. We believed this would be the case because neural networks are basically a series of multiplication of a weight and the input value

Table 7 Lowest angle MAE for psi prediction

Score	Encoding	Window size	Model arch
23.289	one hot[0,1]	19	lstm 5
24.864	one hot[0,1]	13	lstm 5
25.227	one hot[0,1]	11	lstm 5
25.257	one hot[0,1]	15	lstm 5
25.335	one hot[0,1]	9	lstm 5
25.88	blosum62	7	lstm 5
26.313	one hot[0,1]	7	lstm 5
26.357	blosum30	9	lstm 5
26.408	blosum45	5	lstm 5
26.455	blosum62	9	lstm 5
26.465	blosum30	7	lstm 5
26.617	blosum45	9	lstm 5
26.655	blosum30	11	lstm 5
26.869	blosum45	13	lstm 5
27.056	blosum65	11	lstm 5
27.161	blosum45	7	lstm 5
27.378	pam250	7	lstm 5
27.47	blosum45	11	lstm 5
27.513	pam250	9	lstm 5
27.561	pam250	11	lstm 5

Table 8 Lowest angle MAE for phi and psi prediction

Score	Encoding	Window size	Model arch
22.616	one hot[0,1]	11	lstm 5
23.229	one hot[0,1]	9	lstm 5
23.249	one hot[0,1]	17	lstm 5
23.586	one hot[0,1]	15	lstm 5
23.994	one hot[0,1]	7	lstm 5
24.067	blosum62	9	lstm 5
24.224	blosum30	9	lstm 5
24.371	one hot[0,1]	13	lstm 5
24.483	blosum45	7	lstm 5
24.515	blosum62	7	lstm 5
24.532	blosum30	7	lstm 5
24.782	blosum65	11	lstm 5
24.924	blosum45	9	lstm 5
25.132	blosum45	5	lstm 5
25.148	blosum65	7	lstm 5
25.166	blosum45	11	lstm 5
25.173	blosum80	9	lstm 5
25.215	one hot[0,1]	5	lstm 5
25.328	pam250	9	lstm 5
25.614	pam250	5	lstm 5

Table 9 Multiple CATH class results

Size	Pred	1.10.510.10		2.60.120.200		3.90.1150.10	
		MSE	A. MAE	MSE	A. MAE	MSE	A. MAE
7	Phi	0.066	14.853	0.077	17.076	0.081	16.635
	Psi	0.105	25.646	0.101	26.061	0.132	26.66
	Phi/Psi	0.111	24.844	0.104	24.904	0.139	26.162
9	Phi	0.063	14.331	0.074	16.472	0.086	17.515
	Psi	0.106	25.324	0.093	24.535	0.16	30.05
	Phi/Psi	0.102	23.018	0.112	25.774	0.136	25.806
11	Phi	0.06	14.017	0.077	17.004	0.073	15.846
	Psi	0.096	24.418	0.119	29.377	0.148	28.6
	Phi/Psi	0.099	22.96	0.118	26.32	0.133	25.157
13	Phi	0.06	14.137	0.08	17.90	0.075	15.736
	Psi	0.098	24.879	0.105	27.427	0.129	26.443
	Phi/Psi	0.099	22.831	0.125	27.119	0.132	25.269

and anything multiplied by 0 equals 0. This can lead to difficulty training where there are a large number of 0's as is the case in one-hot encoding. Since one-hot encoding performed so well here, we have to assume that the additional relationship information we believed the substitution matrices to contain was not useful to the neural network.

The window size for the best performers was not nearly as clear as the best type of encoding was. Although the model with the lowest error when predicting ϕ used a window size of 9, only two of the twenty models with the lowest error were training on data with a window size of 9 as opposed to eight of the twenty models that were trained on data with a window size of 7. Compare this with the models that were predicting the ψ angles where five of the twenty models with the lowest error used a window size of 7, five used a window size of 9, and five used a window size of 11. The correlation seems to be that ϕ predictions did better with a window size of 5 or 7 and ψ predictions did better with larger window sizes of 7, 9, or 11. When attempting to predict both the ϕ and ψ angles simultaneously, window sizes of 7 and 9 were most consistently accurate with six models each out of the twenty models with the lowest error. Our conclusion is that 7 is the best window size overall for training models with these predictions. It is worth noting that no models with window sizes of 3, 21, or 23 were among the best performers.

3.4 Expanded CATH Selection

As previously discussed, after identifying the best model, encoding, and window sizes, new models were trained using CATH 1.10.510.10, CATH 2.60.120.200, and CATH 3.90.1150.10 to ensure that similar results were achieved with proteins from different CATH classifications. This more focused retraining used only the deep LSTM (64 layer) architecture with one-hot encoding and more limited window sizes of 7, 9, 11, and 13. Each model was trained for 150 epochs, but with the same early stopping criteria. After training, the results were very similar to the first model as shown in Table 9. The results for the model trained on CATH 1.10.510.10 changed very little with the addition of more epochs. Those differences can be attributed to the nondeterministic nature of model training. For example, dropout regularization chooses nodes to ignore at random. This could result in different nodes being ignored in a different training. The results for the model trained on CATH 2.60.120.200 performed about 2° worse for the ϕ angle prediction and almost identically for the ψ angles. Finally, the results for the model trained on CATH 3.90.1150.10 performed about 1° worse than the original model. This could be because CATH 2 is contains mostly, β-sheets and the ϕ and ψ angles for those are a little more difficult to predict than the ϕ and ψ angles for the mostly α-helical proteins or it could be due to other difference in the data sets or the test and validation sets. Regardless, the results show great promise compared to the results found in previous works.

3.5 *Overall Performance*

Spider 2 [13] achieved a MAE of 19° for ϕ angle prediction and 30° for ψ angle prediction. RaptorX [12] improved on that by 0.5° for ϕ and 1.4° for ψ. We achieved a MAE of 14°–16° for ϕ angle prediction and 23°–25° for ψ angle prediction depending on the CATH class predicted. However, our results were limited to predictions over proteins in specific CATHs, whereas the past work used proteins across a much wider spectrum. As the goal of this work was to survey encoding and window size options and to identify an encoding, window size, and neural network architecture for future work, these results seem very promising.

4 Conclusions and Future Work

One of the biggest opportunities for future work lies in attempting to tune the neural network architecture to achieve better results. We did not focus on the network architecture or attempt to fine-tune the hyperparameters. As such there are multiple potential improvements to be made to the model architecture to improve the predictions. Additionally, this work was performed on only three CATHs, but ideally the predictions work for any CATH and without the protein being classified beforehand. There are multiple ways this might be accomplished, which presents its own avenue of research.

Acknowledgments We would like to thank Chris Ott and the IFES-TOS Lab at the University of South Carolina for modifying the PDBMine interface, which was supported by NIH Grant Number P20 RR-016461 to Dr. Homayoun Valafar, to allow us to query proteins for the torsion angles required for this work.

References

1. S.F. Altschul, T.L. Madden, A.A. Schaffer, J. Zhang, Z. Zhang, W. Miller, D.J. Lipman, Gapped blast and PSI-blast: a new generation of protein database search programs. Nucleic Acids Res. **25**(17), 3389–3402 (1997)
2. C.B. Anfinsen, Principles that govern the folding of protein chains. Science **181**(4096), 223–230 (1973). https://doi.org/10.1126/science.181.4096.223, https://science.sciencemag.org/content/181/4096/223, https://science.sciencemag.org/content/181/4096/223.full.pdf
3. G. Ashraf, N. Greig, T. Khan, I. Hassan, S. Tabrez, S. Shakil, I. Sheikh, S. Zaidi, M. Akram, R.J. Nasimudeen, C.K. Firoz, A. Naeem, I. Alhazza, G. Damanhouri, M. Kamal, Protein misfolding and aggregation in Alzheimer's disease and type 2 diabetes mellitus. CNS Neurol. Disord. Drug Targets **13**, 1280–1293 (2014). https://doi.org/10.2174/1871527313666140917095514
4. C.A. Cole, C. Ott, D. Valdes, H. Valafar, PDBMine: a reformulation of the protein data bank to facilitate structural data mining (2019). arXiv: 1911.08614v1
5. C.A. Cole, N.S. Daigham, G. Liu, G.T. Montelione, H. Valafar, REDCRAFT: a computational platform using residual dipolar coupling NMR data for determining structures of perdeuterated proteins without NOEs (2020). bioRxiv https://doi.org/10.1101/2020.06.17.156638, https://www.biorxiv.org/content/early/2020/07/01/2020.06.17.156638, https://www.biorxiv.org/content/early/2020/07/01/2020.06.17.156638.full.pdf
6. N.L. Dawson, T.E. Lewis, S. Das, J.G. Lees, D. Lee, P. Ashford, C.A. Orengo, I. Sillitoe, CATH: an expanded resource to predict protein function through structure and sequence. Nucleic Acids Res. **45**(D1), D289–D295 (2017)
7. M.O. Dayhoff, R.M. Schwartz, A model of evolutionary change in proteins, in *in Atlas of Protein Sequence and Structure*, Chap. 22 (1978)
8. E. Faraggi, B. Xue, Y. Zhou, Improving the prediction accuracy of residue solvent accessibility and real-value backbone torsion angles of proteins by guided-learning through a two-layer neural network. Proteins **74**(4), 847–856 (2009)
9. E. Faraggi, Y. Yang, S. Zhang, Y. Zhou, Predicting continuous local structure and the effect of its substitution for secondary structure in fragment-free protein structure prediction. Structure **17**(11), 1515–1527 (2009). https://doi.org/10.1016/j.str.2009.09.006, http://www.sciencedirect.com/science/article/pii/S0969212609003724
10. E. Faraggi, T. Zhang, Y. Yang, L. Kurgan, Y. Zhou, Spine x: improving protein secondary structure prediction by multistep learning coupled with prediction of solvent accessible surface area and backbone torsion angles. J. Comput. Chem. **33**(3), 259–267 (2012)
11. T.M. Fawcett, S.J. Irausquin, M. Simin, H. Valafar, An artificial neural network approach to improving the correlation between protein energetics and the backbone structure. Proteomics **13**(2), 230–238 (2013)
12. Y. Gao, S. Wang, M. Deng, J. Xu, RaptorX-angle: real-value prediction of protein backbone dihedral angles through a hybrid method of clustering and deep learning. BMC Bioinformatics **19**(4), 100 (2018)
13. R. Heffernan, K. Paliwal, J. Lyons, A. Dehzangi, A. Sharma, J. Wang, A. Sattar, Y. Yang, Y. Zhou, Improving prediction of secondary structure, local backbone angles and solvent accessible surface area of proteins by iterative deep learning. Sci. Rep. **5**(1), 11476 (2015)
14. S. Henikoff, J.G. Henikoff, Amino acid substitution matrices from protein blocks. Proc. Natl. Acad. Sci. USA **89**(22), 10915–10919 (1992)

15. S. Henikoff, J.G. Henikoff, Amino acid substitution matrices from protein blocks. Proc. Natl. Acad. Sci. **89**(22), 10915–10919 (1992). https://doi.org/10.1073/pnas.89.22.10915, https://www.pnas.org/content/89/22/10915, https://www.pnas.org/content/89/22/10915.full.pdf
16. S. Hochreiter, J. Schmidhuber, Long short-term memory. Neural Comput. **9**(8), 1735–1780 (1997). https://doi.org/10.1162/neco.1997.9.8.1735
17. P. Kountouris, J.D. Hirst, Prediction of backbone dihedral angles and protein secondary structure using support vector machines. BMC Bioinformatics **10**(1), 437 (2009)
18. H. Li, J. Hou, B. Adhikari, Q. Lyu, J. Cheng, Deep learning methods for protein torsion angle prediction. BMC Bioinformatics **18**(1), 417 (2017)
19. N. Qian, T.J. Sejnowski, Predicting the secondary structure of globular proteins using neural network models. J. Mol. Biol. **202**(4), 865–884 (1988)
20. P. Shealy, M. Simin, S.H. Park, S.J. Opella, H. Valafar, Simultaneous structure and dynamics of a membrane protein using REDCRAFT: membrane-bound form of Pf1 coat protein. J. Magn. Reson. **207**(1), 8–16 (2010)
21. J. Song, H. Tan, M. Wang, G.I. Webb, T. Akutsu, Tangle: two-level support vector regression approach for protein backbone torsion angle prediction from primary sequences. PLoS ONE **7**(2), 1–16 (2012). https://doi.org/10.1371/journal.pone.0030361
22. N. Srivastava, G. Hinton, A. Krizhevsky, I. Sutskever, R. Salakhutdinov, Dropout: a simple way to prevent neural networks from overfitting. J. Mach. Learn. Res. **15**, 1929–1958 (2014)
23. M. Wood, J. Hirst, Protein secondary structure prediction with dihedral angles. Proteins **59**, 476–81 (2005). https://doi.org/10.1002/prot.20435
24. S. Wu, Y. Zhang, Anglor: a composite machine-learning algorithm for protein backbone torsion angle prediction. PLoS ONE **3**(10), 1–8 (2008). https://doi.org/10.1371/journal.pone.0003400
25. B. Xue, O. Dor, E. Faraggi, Y. Zhou, Real-value prediction of backbone torsion angles. Proteins **72**, 427–433 (2008). https://doi.org/10.1002/prot.21940

Rotation-Invariant Palm ROI Extraction for Contactless Recognition

Dinh-Trung Vu, Thi-Van Nguyen, and Shi-Jinn Horng

1 Introduction

With the tremendous growth of technology and the variety of its applications on industry and daily lives, security awareness has extended from individuals to organizations. In the early years, PIN, passwords, and smart cards were the most popular security tools. Although they are simple to use, they can be easily attacked if the code lacks complexity. Users also cannot have access to their system if they forget the code or lose the cards. However, biometrics emergence provides the alternative security solution not only for identification but also for authentication of the system. By using human's physiological or behavioral traits, biometrics allows a person to be identified and authenticated in a convenient, fast, and reliable way. Common physical traits include fingerprints, ear, hand or palm geometry, vein, retina, iris and facial characteristics. Behavioural traits include voice, signature, keystroke pattern and gait [12].

Among many biometrics, the hand-based biometrics such as hand geometry [22], fingerprint [13], finger vein [2], inner knuckle print [16], palm print, and palm vein [25] have received increasing attention. Each trait has strengths and weaknesses when it is being used typically depending on the requirement of applications.

D.-T. Vu · T.-V. Nguyen
Department of Computer Science and Information Engineering, National Taiwan University of Science and Technology, Taipei, Taiwan

Faculty of Information Technology, Vietnam Maritime University, Haiphong, Vietnam

S.-J. Horng (✉)
Department of Computer Science and Information Engineering, National Taiwan University of Science and Technology, Taipei, Taiwan

H. R. Arabnia et al. (eds.), *Advances in Computer Vision and Computational Biology*, Transactions on Computational Science and Computational Intelligence,
https://doi.org/10.1007/978-3-030-71051-4_55

Fingerprints were first introduced for person identification system over 100 years ago [10]. It was recognized that the distinctive finger ridges and minutiae points for each person become important features to identify individuals. Fingerprint system can be easily implemented at low cost, but it is unstable in the case of wet, dirty fingers or unclear prints from old people. Also, finger size becomes suitable in embedded system.

The palm region is the large inner area of a hand surrounded by the fingers, thumb, and wrist. Palm is hairless and unable to tan. The palm print and the palm vein show less distortion when capturing them, even if they contain abundant features such as principal lines, ridges, minutiae, and texture. However, the palm print is vulnerable to damage caused by working environment or accidents; then it downgrades the system performance.

The vein structure is the network of blood vessels hidden under the skin in the human body; the veins are responsible for carrying blood toward the heart. There are many kinds of veins in the hands such as finger veins, palm veins, dorsal veins, and wrist veins. Generally, veins are difficult to observe in visible light. The spectrum ranges of near infrared (NIR) between 690 nm and 900 nm provide better view of the hand veins and the palm veins [7]. Human veins are proven to be stable, unique, and robust to spoof for each person and even different between twins. Therefore, vein-based techniques are more efficient compared to other modalities for identifying a person.

The palm vein system originally was built for fixing hand positions with several pegs support. This system lacks flexibility because users are restricted to position their hand. On the other hand, there is an issue that arises when the hand is in contact with the hygienic device. Therefore, there is a need to develop contactless palm vein system. Consequently, users can freely pose their hands toward the device without having physical contact with the imaging device. There are a number of challenges to be addressed in contactless palm vein recognition such as lighting conditions, hand appearance, noisy background, rotation, and translation. This study proposes a new rotation-invariant palm ROI extraction method for the palm print and the palm vein recognition system.

2 Related Works

According to some studies about the palm print and palm vein, authors generally pay attention to the ROI detection, image enhancement, feature extraction, and recognition phase [3]. Among the processes of the recognition, the palm ROI extraction plays the most important role. An accurate and reliable extracted ROI leads to better result on the next step and impacts on final recognition performance. In this section, there are a number of palm ROI extraction methods discussed.

Basically, the palm ROI extraction composes of two main steps: first, the hand region segmentation from input image and, second, the extracted area of vein interest in the hand region. The hand segmentation is to separate the hand foreground and the background areas. This process can be categorized into one of three basic methods such as hand edge-based, region-based, or combination. Naturally, this step aims to get distinctive binarized image from the input. In the contact system, it is easier to own a binarized image because the devices are typically set up to capture one background. But it becomes harder in the contactless system due to non-uniform illumination, background, deformation, etc. Knowing how to overcome these difficulties, the techniques to binarize image can be applied on any palm database. The main difference among other studies is in the second step. Once the hand images are segmented, some conventional algorithms continue to detect key points and extract the palm ROI from these key points. Nonetheless, some others do not need these key points. They simply eliminate finger region and wrist; then the image is scaled to get the ROI. Zhang et al. [23], Wang et al. [20], and Leng et al. [9] proposed their methods using reference points to localize ROI. The flow for ROI extraction of these algorithms consists of common steps: (1) binarizing the images, (2) detecting the key points, (3) performing transformation, and (4) obtaining the ROI. Extracted ROI can be represented in rectangular, circular, or square form.

Zhang et al. [23] proposed the well-known palm print region extraction and also work on the palm vein images. First, an original input image is filtered, and a threshold is applied to convert to a binarized image. Then, authors used boundary tracking algorithm to obtain the boundaries of the gaps between fingers. This feature is considered as a reference point to determine a coordinate system. The final step is extracting a sub-image of a fixed size on a certain area of the palm. This region of interest is used next for feature extraction. From the beginning, this algorithm is designed for contacting palm print recognition systems, but later methods improved from the original to applicable version for contactless scenario.

Wang et al. [20] applied this idea on fusion image of the palm print and the palm vein. Authors emphasized the importance of a fixed and restricted hand position during the capturing process. Leng et al. [9] used hand-shape-based segmentation method. This method also finds out the valley points between index-middle fingers and ring-little fingers as in Zhang et al.'s [23] method and performs some transformation steps before getting the desired area of the palm. Leng et al.'s [9] method exposed the disadvantages in case fingers are closed or palm is rolled. Nonetheless, Han's method [5] did not use any key point as previous referred papers. This method omitted fingers and wrist parts from a hand silhouette. The centroid of the palm is kept after gradually removing horizontal and vertical columns with a threshold.

In the contactless recognition systems, the rotation solving is one of the open issues attracting much devotion. Michael et al. [11] had put forward another palm ROI extraction in contactless scenes. This paper introduced a palm print and knuckle print technique tracking to detect and capture these features from low resolution stream. However, a maximum rotation is up only to 30°. Ouyang et al. [15] and Kang and Wu [8] claimed that their approaches are possible to work well under any hand rotation. However, the benchmark databases they used for validation only have maximum hand rotations of up to 45° and 60°, respectively [7]. El-Sallam et al. [4] proposed ROI techniques modified from the previous works and possible to handle the case of orientation of a variety of fingers. The abovementioned methods did not work on a special condition in which some fingers are drawn close to one another. The valley point between middle-ring fingers is wrongly detected since these two fingers are too close to each other. Besides, the contours of fingers are affected by the presentation of fingernails, thus reducing the performance of methods.

Recently, Zhang et al. [25] introduced a palm print and palm vein recognition based on DCNN and applied their palm ROI extraction method in previous studies [24] on their large own collected dataset. Low-pass filter as Gaussian is first used to convert an input image to a binary image. Next, they got the two tangent points of the gap boundaries of the fingers with the tangent line. After defining the coordinate, a square region of side length is extracted.

Jhinn et al. [7] claimed that their approach is suitable for large hand rotation problem. However, they found that their ROI formulation was applied precisely if the hand is facing up and the angle difference between the little valleys and index valley is 250.99°. Moreover, the proposed ROI method does not fulfill the case of the middle or ring deformity.

3 Proposed Palm ROI Extraction Method

In this study, a rotation-invariant palm ROI extraction method for contactless system is proposed. The fundamental framework of the proposed approach includes six steps, illustrated in Fig. 1. The details for each step are presented in the following sections.

3.1 Hand Segmentation

The hand segmentation is a process using image thresholding algorithm to extract the hand region from the background. For most hand images acquired by the hand acquisition device, the contrast between the background and the hand region is large enough for applying Otsu's thresholding method [14] which calculates a global threshold to segment the hand region. However, there are still some areas of few hand images where the contrast between the hand region and the background is similar causing difficulties in hand segmentation. In this case, a global threshold computed using Otsu' thresholding algorithm is regularly large, and the segmented hand area is eroded. It is possible to apply a fixed threshold estimated through testing to separate the hand area more smoothly. However, in case where the fingers are closed, a fixed threshold much smaller than the global threshold is not able to separate those fingers. Alternatively, the adaptive thresholding method [21] where the threshold is calculated for each small area of the image can be applied in this case. The contour between the closed fingers is clearer but still disjointed.

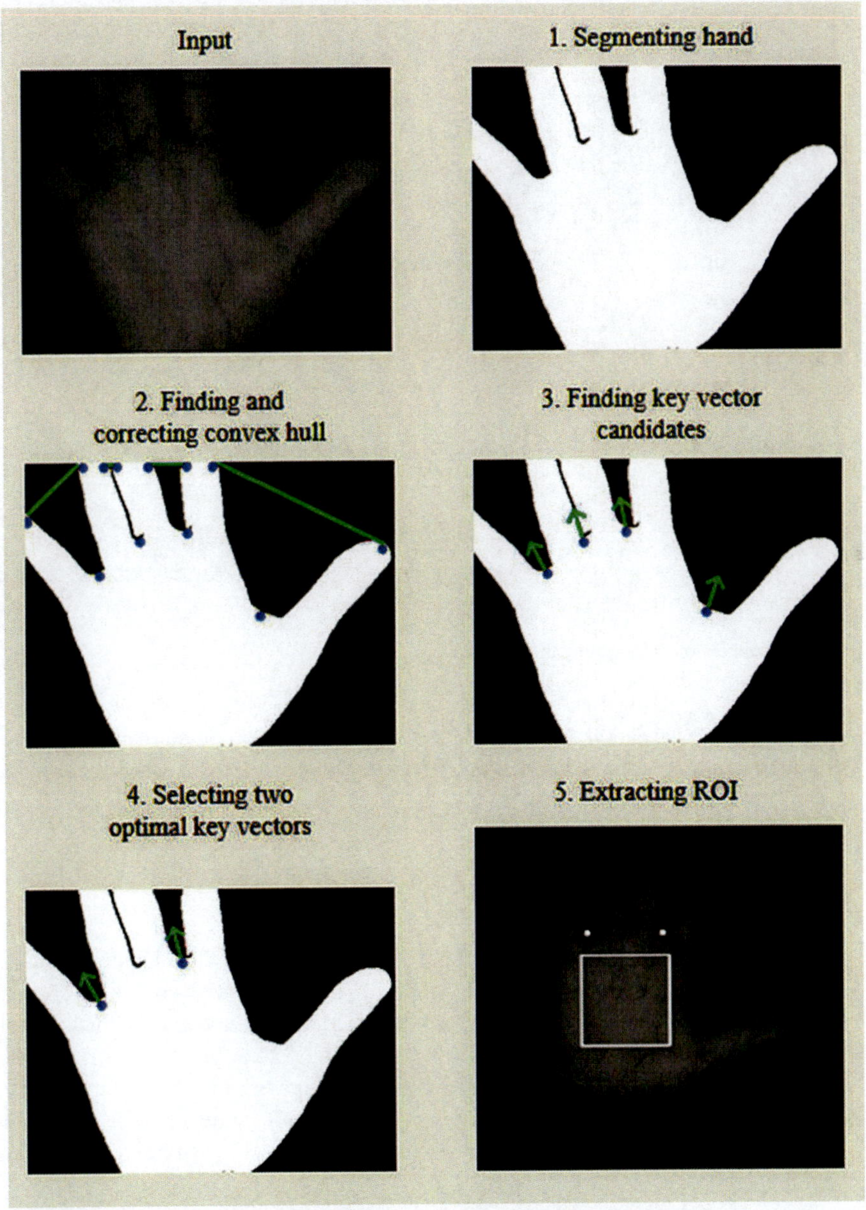

Fig. 1 Fundamental framework of the proposed approach

Our experiments indicate that the combination of thresholding methods provides better result. First, a fixed threshold is used to obtain a smooth binary mask of the hand image. Second, the adaptive thresholding method is applied on the irregular

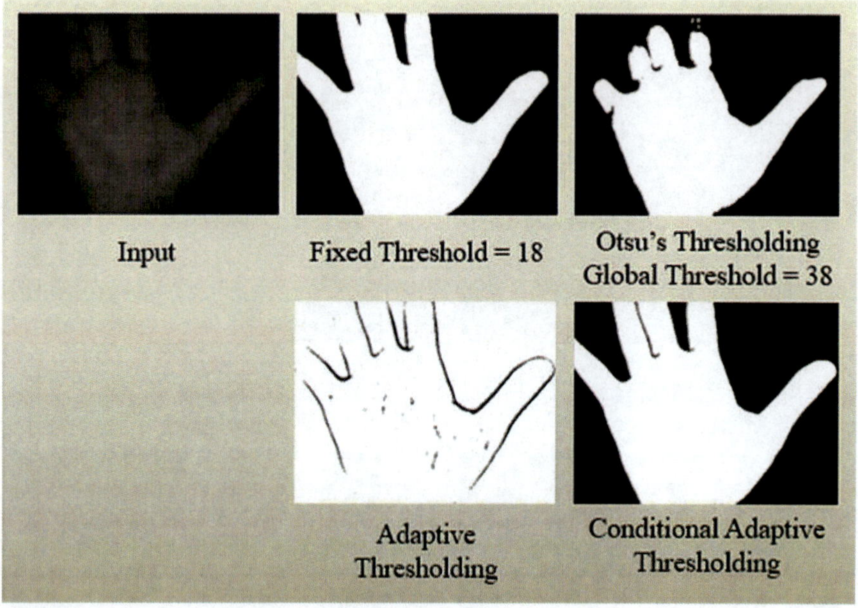

Fig. 2 Examples of thresholding methods

region of interest specified by that binary mask. This combination is known as "conditional adaptive thresholding" (CATh) [6]. This description is shown in Fig. 2.

3.2 *Finding and Correcting Convex Hull*

A binary image is received after the hand segmentation step. The hand contour is extracted from this image using the algorithm [19]. Based on this contour, a convex hull is discovered using Sklansky's algorithm [18]. Between the two convex hull points on the hand contour, a potential valley containing a key point to determine the ROI position is possible. These key points are also known as the convexity defects of the contour. However, in case where two convex hull points are located on the same specified border of the hand image, more than one convexity defect between them may exist.

The convex hull correcting method is proposed to collect all the convexity defects. This algorithm is simply based on tracking the change in the distance of the contour points between two certain convex hull points to the corresponding convex hull edge. Convex hull edge is a possible sub-convex separated with corresponding convexity defects. This process also ignores sub-convex hull edges that have the angle between two convex hull points, and convexity defect is too large. This process is represented in Fig. 3.

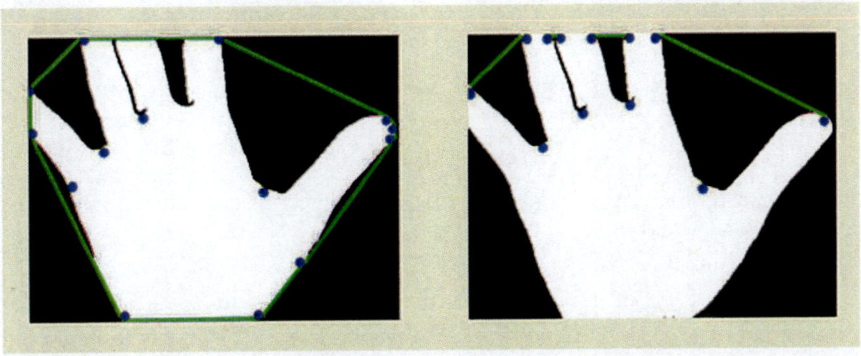

Fig. 3 Finding and correcting convex hull

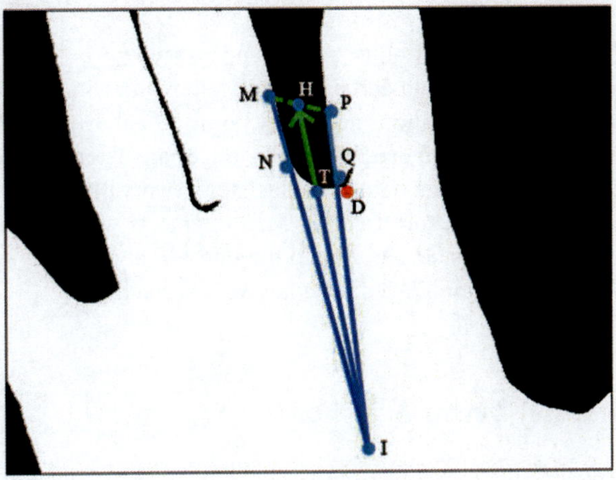

Fig. 4 Finding key vectors

3.3 Finding Key Vector Candidates

This is a preeminent step in our method. A key vector is represented by a line segment with a definite direction from its tail (key point) to its head to specify the direction of fingers. Generally, each convexity defect obtained from the previous step can be specified as a key point with the midpoint of the corresponding convex hull edge to form a key vector. However, the CATh algorithm used in step 1 may cause the not smooth hand contour and result in the position deviation of the convex defects (red point D) from the expected key points (blue point T) as illustrated in Fig. 4. To solve this problem, a key vector finding algorithm is proposed as follows.

First, for each convexity defect, this algorithm tracks the angle variation on the hand contour to find points which indicates two valley edges. Figure 5 demonstrates how to calculate the angle at a particular position on contour. The angle at point

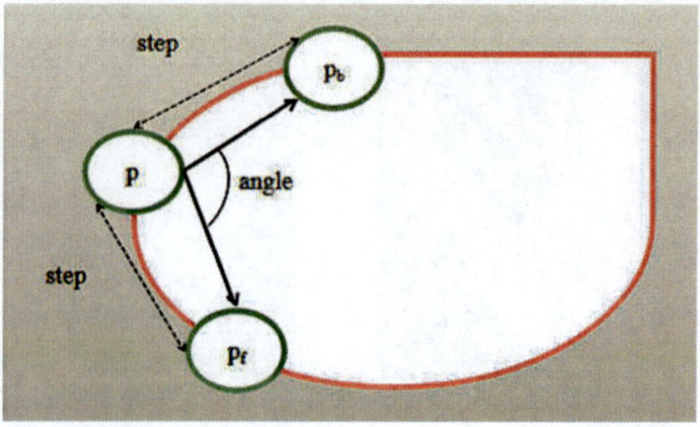

Fig. 5 Calculation of the angle of a contour point

p is the angle between three points: p_b, p, and p_f, where p_f and p_b are forward and backward points of p with a certain jumping step on contour, respectively. It is obvious that the closer the positions are to key points or valley points on the contour, the smaller the angle. Based on that, two valley edges are determined for finding key vectors. Figure 4 illustrates the details of this step. Two valley edges, *MN* and *PQ*, intersect at point *I*. The bisector of corner *MIP* intersects with the contour segment between two contour points, *M* and *P*, and the line *MP* at expected key point *T* and point *H*, respectively. Vector *TH* here is a key vector candidate.

3.4 Optimal Key Vector Selection

In this step, two optimal key vectors are selected from the candidates acquired from the previous step. They are key vectors between index-middle and ring-little fingers, and they are used to specify the rotation direction of the hand. The way to choose these vectors is as follows. If the number of candidates is two, then they are two optimal key vectors. Otherwise, three vectors are selected, confirming that the angle between their tails (key points) is largest and greater than 120°. As in Fig. 6, two optimal key points, T_1 and T_2, are formed with the tail T_3 of the key vector between middle-ring fingers at the largest angle θ. It is obvious that two selected optimal vectors are not related to the valley between index-thumb fingers, therefore our proposed method is still possible to extract the palm ROI if this valley is not found.

In addition, to determine the exact rotation direction of the hand to the vertical direction, it is necessary to indicate which key point is on the left and which is on the right. It is easy to see that the point on the left is T_1 because the vector T_1H_1 forms with the vector T_1T_2 a clockwise angle or a negative angle while the vector T_2H_2 forms with the vector T_2T_1 a counterclockwise angle or a positive angle.

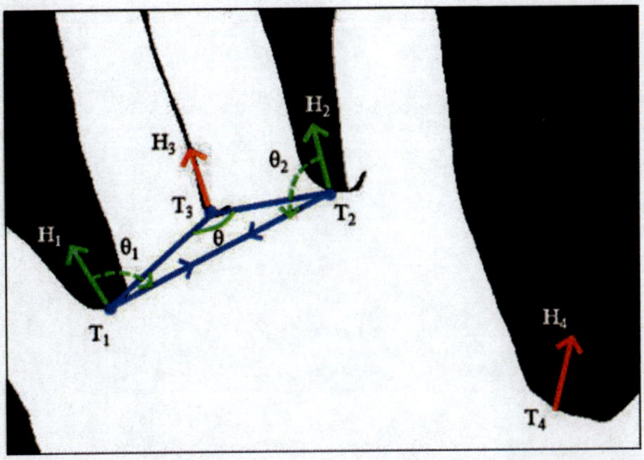

Fig. 6 Selection of two optimal key vectors

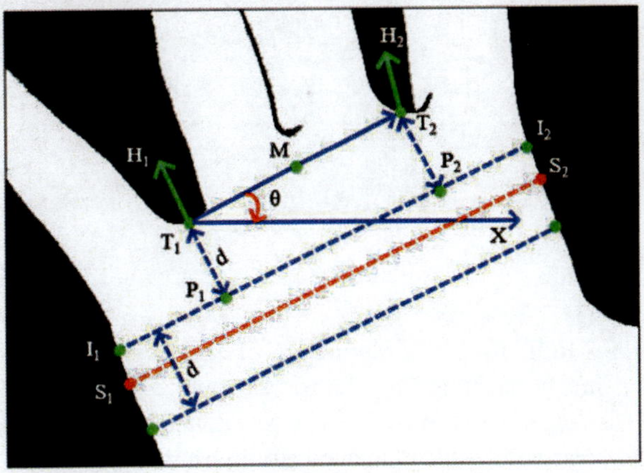

Fig. 7 Calculation of the hand rotation angle and scale

3.5 ROI Extraction

This step is similar to approaches proposed in Qin et al. [17], which involves three tasks: (i) calculating the hand rotation angle, (ii) finding the hand scale, and (iii) rotating the hand by rotation angle and extracting ROI. As shown in Fig. 7, the rotation angle θ is formed by rotating from the vector T_1T_2 to the horizontal vector T_1X. In order to find the hand scale, we locate line P_1P_2 that parallels to line T_1T_2 as well as far from it a certain distance $d = T_1T_2 \times \lambda_1$, where λ_1 is an optional positive factor smaller than 1.0. Line P_1P_2 intersects with hand contour at I_1, I_2. Then, the hand scale S_1S_2 is the longest line in lines paralleling to line I_1I_2, where the distance from line S_1S_2 to line I_1I_2 does not exceed distance d and S_1, S_2 are on hand contour also.

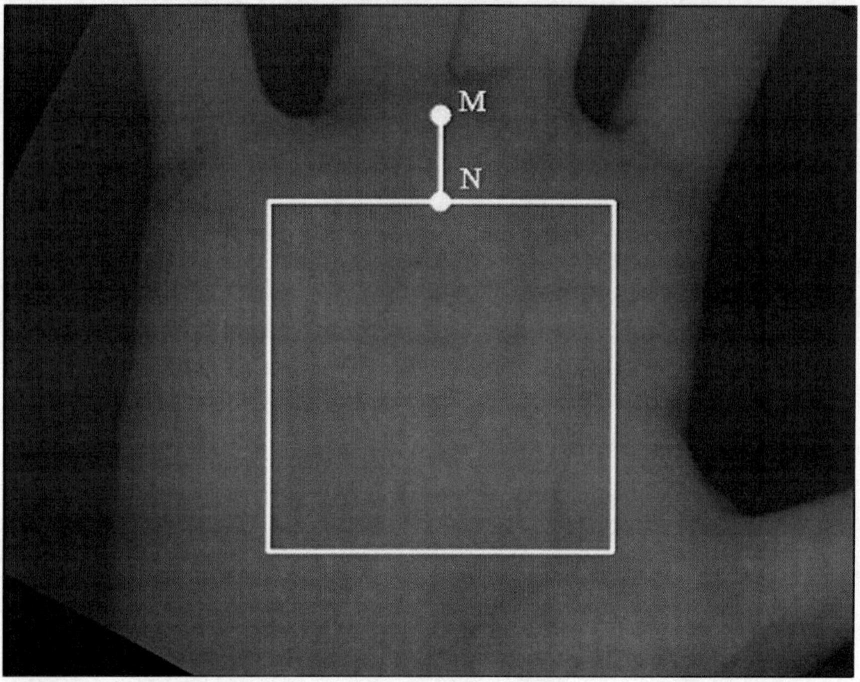

Fig. 8 Locating ROI position

For extracting ROI, first, a midpoint M of line segment T_1T_2 is calculated. Next, the hand image is rotated by the rotation angle θ, and the new coordinate of midpoint M is recalculated. Based on the coordinate of midpoint M and the hand scale S_1S_2, the position of ROI is located. In Fig. 8, the line MN is perpendicular to the horizontal axis, and distance from M to N is equal to $S_1S_2 \times \kappa_2$ where κ_2 is an optional positive factor smaller than 1.0 and N is the midpoint of the top edge of ROI. The edge size of ROI is equal to $S_1S_2 \times \kappa_3$ where κ_3 is also an optional positive factor smaller than 1.0.

4 Experiments and Discussion

The performance of our proposed method is assessed on the Tongji Contactless Palm Vein Dataset [25] in 12 different rotation angles and a self-collected palm print dataset with arbitrary rotation angles.

Table 1 The name of incorrect ROI images extracted using Zhang et al.'s method

Session	Name of incorrect ROI images
1	00529, 02499, 02504, 02509, 03130, 03650, 04173, 04177, 04307, 05169, 05441, 05442, 05596, 05762
2	03297, 03738, 04703, 05292

4.1 Performance Evaluation on Tongji Contactless Palm Vein Dataset

This dataset includes 12,000 images captured from 600 different palms in two separate sessions. However, in this dataset, all the hands are in the vertical direction meaning that there is slight change in the rotation angle of the hands. Therefore, to evaluate the performance of the proposed method in terms of the rotation invariant, each image in this dataset is rotated in 12 angles from 0° to 360° counterclockwise with a step of 30°, and there are 144,000 images in total. ROI images are compared with each other using the histogram comparison method using correlation metric as mentioned in Bradski and Kaehler [1]. This experiment is divided into two phases as follows.

In the first phase, for each original image, the ROI histogram at rotation angle 0° is compared with the remaining rotation angles. Since the ROI images matched to each other are extracted from the same image, the histogram comparison method should return a high match about over 0.98. All matchings in this experiment returned high correlation scores above 0.98 meaning that the accuracy of our proposed method is 100%. In the second phase, since Tongji University also released ROI images extracted using their method [24], each of these ROI images is compared to 12 ROI images corresponding to 12 different angles obtained by our proposed algorithm. This experiment returned 216 wrong matchings with low correlation scores. However, to verify that the wrong matchings come from the ROI extracted using Zhang et al.'s method or our proposed method, the incorrect ROI images are compared with other ROI images of the same corresponding palm. After verifying, the result indicates that all incorrect ROI images are the ones extracted using Zhang et al.'s method. The total number of incorrect images is 18, and the names are listed in Table 1, since each one is incorrectly matched with 12 corresponding ROI images extracted using our method. Some examples are listed in Fig. 9.

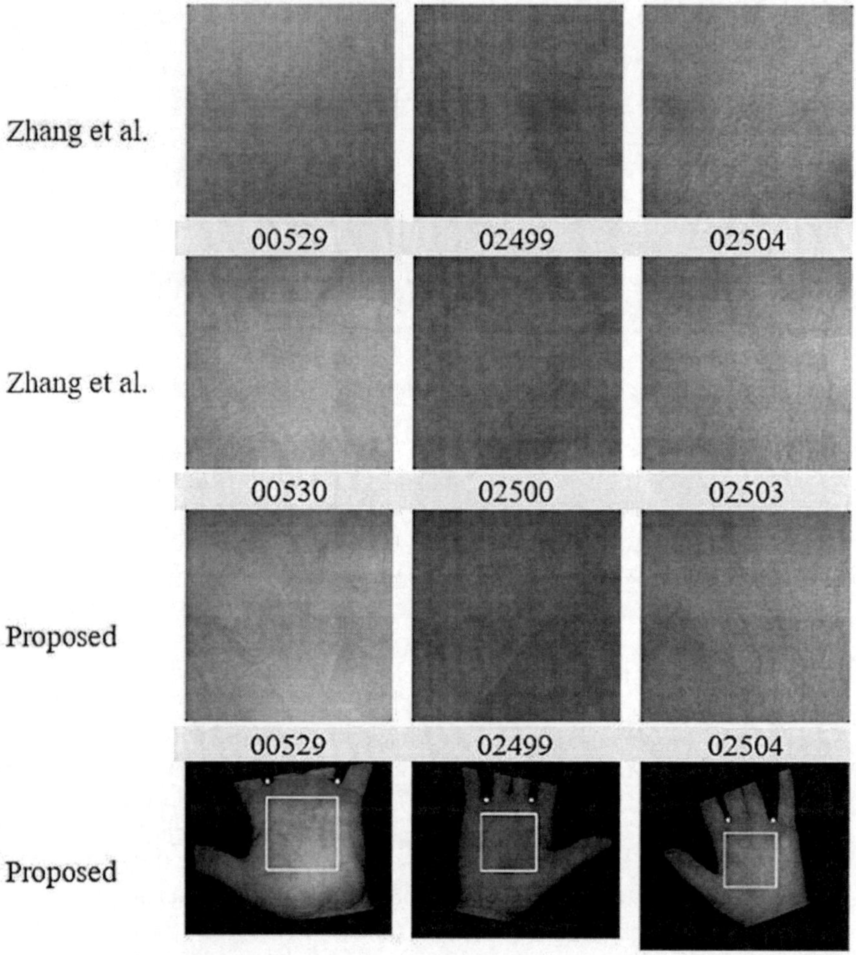

Fig. 9 Examples of extracted palm ROI images of each method, where the first row contains incorrect ROI images from Zhang et al.'s method compared to the other ones extracted using Zhang et al.'s method from the same palm and our proposed method at the second row and third row, respectively, and the fourth row contains resulting images from our method for verifying, in which the white points indicate the optimal detected key points and the white box indicates the detected palm ROI

4.2 Performance Evaluation on a Self-Collected Palm Print Dataset

A mobile application has been built using the front camera of a smartphone to collect palm print images with arbitrary hand poses. There are 50 volunteers in total. Each volunteer is captured ten images of the left hand and ten images of the right

Table 2 The distribution of rotation angles in the self-collected palm print dataset

Range (degree)	Number of correct detections
(−180, −150)	4
(−150, −120)	2
(−120, −90)	5
(−90, −60)	25
(−60, −30)	109
(−30, 0)	318
(0, +30)	294
(+30, +60)	148
(+60, +90)	69
(+90, +120)	16
(+120, +150)	3
(+150, +180)	6
All	999

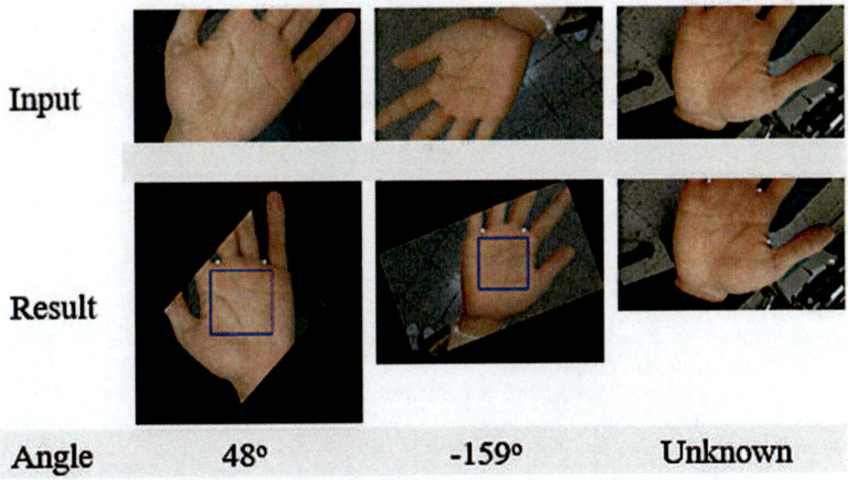

Fig. 10 Examples of extracted palm ROI images of our proposed method on the self-collected dataset, where the white-color points indicate the detected key points and the blue-color box indicates the detected palm ROI

hand; the total captured palm print images are 1000. The rotation angles calculated using our proposed method are random from $-180°$ to $180°$, but due to the limited wrist rotation of the volunteers as well as the operator, these values are to focus on the range from $-90°$ to $90°$, as shown in Table 2. The total number of correct detections is 999, which means that there is only one failed detection out of 1000 detections as shown in Fig. 10 and the correct detection rate is up to 99.99%. The failed detection here is due to the fact that the proposed algorithm cannot find the key vector between middle-ring fingers, which makes it impossible to identify the two optimal key vectors exactly described in step 4.

5 Conclusion

This study proposed a robust rotation-invariant palm ROI extraction method for palm vein and palm print recognition. The proposed method combines conditional adaptive thresholding, convex hull correction, and finding key vectors to specify the rotation angle as well as rotation direction of the hand. This combination is possible to significantly increase the palm ROI extraction success rate, especially in cases where fingers are closed or the hand is rolled in an arbitrary direction. The experimental results on the public contactless palm vein dataset and our self-collected palm print dataset have shown the high performance of our proposed method. The extracted ROI can then be an input to any recognition system using deep learning and the recognition rate can be improved.

Acknowledgments The authors thankfully acknowledge the School of Software Engineering, Tongji University, for providing contactless palm vein dataset used in this work.

This work was supported in part by the Ministry of Science and Technology under contract number 108-2218-E-011-006, and it was also partially supported by the "Center for Cyber-physical System Innovation" from The Featured Areas Research Center Program within the framework of the Higher Education Sprout Project by the Ministry of Education (MOE) in Taiwan.

References

1. G. Bradski, A. Kaehler, *Learning OpenCV: Computer Vision with the OpenCV Library* (O'Reilly Media, Inc, 2008)
2. S. Brindha, Finger vein recognition. Int. J. Renew. Energy Technol. **4**, 1298–1300 (2017)
3. W. Damak, R.B. Trabelsi, M.A. Damak, D. Sellami, Dynamic roi extraction method for hand vein images. IET Comput. Vis. **12**(5), 586–595 (2018)
4. A. El-Sallam, F. Sohel, M. Bennamoun, Robust pose invariant shape-based hand recognition, in *2011 6Th IEEE Conference on Industrial Electronics and Applications*, (IEEE, 2011), pp. 281–286
5. Y. Han, Z. Sun, F. Wang, T. Tan, Palmprint recognition under unconstrained scenes, in *Asian Conference on Computer Vision*, (Springer, 2007), pp. 1–11
6. A. Horváth, S. Spindler, M. Szalay, I. Rácz, Preprocessing endoscopic images of colorectal polyps. Acta. Technica. Jaurinensis **9**(1), 65–82 (2016)
7. W.L. Jhinn, M.G.K. Ong, L.S. Hoe, T. Connie, Contactless palm vein roi extraction using convex hull algorithm, in *Computational Science and Technology*, (Springer, 2019), pp. 25–35
8. W. Kang, Q. Wu, Contactless palm vein recognition using a mutual foreground-based local binary pattern. IEEE Trans. Inf. Forensics Sec. **9**(11), 1974–1985 (2014)
9. L. Leng, G. Liu, M. Li, M.K. Khan, A.M. Al-Khouri, Logical conjunction of triple-perpendicular-directional translation residual for contactless palmprint preprocessing, in *2014 11th International Conference on Information Technology: New Generations*, (IEEE, 2014), pp. 523–528
10. D. Maltoni, D. Maio, A.K. Jain, S. Prabhakar, *Handbook of Fingerprint Recognition* (Springer Science & Business Media, 2009)
11. G.K.O. Michael, T. Connie, A.T.B. Jin, Robust palm print and knuckle print recognition system using a contactless approach, in *2010 5Th IEEE Conference on Industrial Electronics and Applications*, (IEEE, 2010), pp. 323–329

12. S. Pal, U. Pal, M. Blumenstein, Signature-based biometric authentication, in *Computational Intelligence in Digital Forensics: Forensic Investigation and Applications*, (Springer, Cham, 2014), pp. 285–314
13. V. Mura, G. Orru, R. Casula, A. Sibiriu, G. Loi, P. Tuveri, L. Ghiani, G.L. Marcialis, Livdet 2017 fingerprint liveness detection competition 2017, in *2018 International Conference on Biometrics (ICB)*, (IEEE, 2018), pp. 297–302
14. N. Otsu, A threshold selection method from gray-level histograms. IEEE Trans. Syst. Man Cybern. **9**(1), 62–66 (1979)
15. C.-S. Ouyang, R.-C. Wu, C.-C. Wang, An improved neural network-based palm biometric system with rotation detection mechanism, in *2010 International Conference on Machine Learning and Cybernetics*, vol. 6, (IEEE, 2010), pp. 2927–2932
16. E. Perumal, S. Ramachandran, A multimodal biometric system based on palmprint and finger knuckle print recognition methods. Int. Arab J. Inf. Technol. **12**(2) (2015)
17. H. Qin, M.A. El Yacoubi, J. Lin, B. Liu, An iterative deep neural network for hand-vein verification. IEEE Access **7**, 34823–34837 (2019)
18. J. Sklansky, Finding the convex hull of a simple polygon. Pattern Recogn. Lett. **1**(2), 79–83 (1982)
19. S. Suzuki et al., Top logical structural analysis of digitized binary images by border following. Comp. Vis. Graph. Image Process. **30**(1), 32–46 (1985)
20. J.-G. Wang, W.-Y. Yau, A. Suwandy, E. Sung, Person recognition by fusing palmprint and palm vein images based on "laplacianpalm" representation. Pattern Recogn. **41**(5), 1514–1527 (2008)
21. P.D. Wellner, Adaptive thresholding for the digitaldesk, in *Xerox, EPC1993-110*, (1993), pp. 1–19
22. A.L.N. Wong, P. Shi, Peg-free hand geometry recognition using hierarchical geomrtry and shape matching, in *MVA*, (Citeseer, 2002), pp. 281–284
23. D. Zhang, W.-K. Kong, J. You, M. Wong, Online palmprint identification. IEEE Trans. Pattern Anal. Mach. Intell. **25**(9), 1041–1050 (2003)
24. L. Zhang, L. Li, A. Yang, Y. Shen, M. Yang, Towards contactless palmprint recognition: A novel device, a new benchmark, and a collaborative representation based identification approach. Pattern Recogn. **69**, 199–212 (2017)
25. L. Zhang, Z. Cheng, Y. Shen, D. Wang, Palmprint and palmvein recognition based on DCNN and a new large-scale contactless palmvein dataset. Symmetry **10**(4), 78 (2018)

Mathematical Modeling and Computer Simulations of Cancer Chemotherapy

Frank Nani and Mingxian Jin

1 Introduction

Cancer is a disease in which certain cells proliferate in disregard of the regulatory mechanisms that act to regulate the growth of normal cells. Cancerous cells bio-transform to stages of greater malignancy, characterized by oncogene activation/mutation, heterogeneity, invasiveness, and metastasis [5, 9, 11, 20]. In general, such a cellular proliferation is called neoplasia and hence cancer is sometimes referred to as a neoplastic disease. The term tumor, which denotes swelling, is commonly used to refer to a neoplasm, while cancer is a generic term for all malignant neoplasms. A malignant tumor, or cancer, is a configuration of neoplastic cells in an anatomic organ or tissue such that these (cancer) cells differ from normal (non-cancer) cells in histopathologic, morphologic, immunologic, and cytokinetic characteristics [24].

In cancer treatment today, four major modalities are commonly used in efforts to obtain long-term time durations of cancer annihilation. These four are surgery, radiotherapy, chemotherapy, and immunotherapy. For certain cancer types, debulking or destruction of localized primary cancer is performed using surgery and/or radiation therapy. However, in most instances, there is a metastatic invasion by disseminated cancer cells into one or more anatomic regions of the body, leading to secondary neoplasms. Cancer chemotherapy has demonstrated a definite capacity for eradicating disseminated metastatic cancer and is widely used [8, 15, 23].

The ultimate role of mathematical modeling in cancer chemotherapy is to provide a fundamental theoretical basis for experimental design of efficacious therapy and

F. Nani · M. Jin (✉)
Department of Mathematics and Computer Science, Fayetteville State University, Fayetteville, NC, USA
e-mail: fnani@uncfsu.edu; mjin@uncfsu.edu

H. R. Arabnia et al. (eds.), *Advances in Computer Vision and Computational Biology*, Transactions on Computational Science and Computational Intelligence,
https://doi.org/10.1007/978-3-030-71051-4_56

to make qualitative predictions in regards to the dynamic evolution or the disease based on the cytokinetic parameters of the tumor/patient and the drug parametric configuration. Models for cancer chemotherapy can be classified as deterministic or stochastic. Model sub-classifications into cell-cycle specific and cell-cycle non-specific also exist. Cell cycle specific models have been developed and analyzed in ([4, 12–14, 17, 19, 21, 25]), and many more. Some cell cycle non-specific models have also been found (e.g. [7, 26–27]).

The deterministic theory of cancer chemotherapy presupposes that the population sizes of normal and cancer cells are large enough to be described by continuous variables, which are not affected by random cellular fluctuations. Deterministic mathematical models of tumor growth by diffusion have been developed in the literature (e.g. [1]). These models use systems of partial differential equations. However, when diffusive dynamics and spatial variations are neglected or minimal, the systems of deterministic ordinary and functional differential equations can be used. A simplified version of ODE models was considered by Gatenby [10] and Panetta [22], who used Lotka-Volterra type dynamics to model cancer chemotherapy.

By constructing and analyzing mathematical models of cancer chemotherapy, the clinical doctors could use such information to discard non-efficacious treatment protocols and also to compare pre-treatment protocols and provide optimal therapies. When tumor biopsies are clinically performed at various stages of the therapy, medical oncologists and clinical researchers would be able to monitor the dynamic prognosis and progress of the chemotherapy.

The simultaneous use of multiple anti-cancer drugs may lead to additive drug toxicities and unwholesome side effects. This can be resolved by encapsulating the drug cocktails in monoclonal antibody-conjugated drug carriers, such as liposomes. The dynamics of liposomes have been modeled by Nani and Oguztoreli [19]. The monoclonal antibody guides the drug encapsulated liposomes to the cancer-bearing organ, where the drug cocktails could be delivered locally with minimal whole-body toxicities. Nevertheless, the use of an anti-neoplastic drug may create an aggressive drug-resistant phenotype that may repopulate the tumor. Liposomes, which escape capture by the reticulo-endothelial system or the mononuclear-phagocytic system, are called stealth liposomes [2, 6]. Liposomes are the most valuable nanocarriers in clinical use because of their biocompatibility, bio-degradation, and effective encapsulation of hydrophilic or hydrophobic drugs. Mastrotto et al. [16] investigated liposome coatings with respect to their stealth performances using computational molecular dynamics modeling.

This chapter utilizes a system of clinically plausible deterministic non-linear differential equations which depict the pathophysiology of malignant cancers. The cytokinetic properties of normal cells, cancer cells, and the pharmacokinetics of the chemotherapy drug are described, respectively, by biophysically measurable growth parameters, stoichiometric rate constants, and Michaelis–Menten type reaction profiles. The fundamental clinical properties of cancer chemotherapy will be analyzed using computer simulations that elucidate the therapeutic efficacy of stealth liposomes in high dose chemotherapy.

The chapter is organized as follows. Section 2 presents the model with parameter definitions. Sections 3 and 4 give theoretical analyses on two specific cases. Section 5 shows computer simulations with explanation. Section 6 summarizes the research.

2 The Cancer Chemotherapy Model

2.1 Definition of Variables, Parameters, Rate Constants, and Auxiliary Functions

$x_1(t)$: the number of normal non-cancerous cells in the anatomic organ, tissues, or physiologic region of the cancer patient at any time t.

$x_2(t)$: the number of cancerous/malignant neoplastic cells in the cancer-bearing organ, tissue, or physiologic region of the cancer patient at any time t.

$x_3(t)$: the number of moles of chemotherapy drug per unit volume of the cancer-bearing anatomic organ, tissue, or physiologic region of the cancer patient at any time t.

$G_i(x_i)$: the net proliferation defined by $G_i(x_i) = B_i(x_i) - D_i(x_i)$, represents the physiologic proliferation rate for non-cancerous cells ($i = 1$) and cancer cells ($i = 2$).

$B_i(x_i)$: the growth factor and genetically modulated cellular proliferation rate in the cancer-bearing patient. The cytokinetic rate variables of $B_i(x_i)$ are genetically controlled for normal cells ($i = 1$) but for cancer cells ($i = 2$), the growth suppressor control is subverted by the processes of angiogenesis, neo-vascularization, and metastasis.

$D_i(x_i)$: the cell-loss rate function due to necrosis, exfoliation, apoptosis, endogenous immune surveillance activity and other natural processes for normal cell ($i = 1$) and cancer cells ($i = 2$).

$Q_k(x_1, x_2)$: the rate function depicting cell-loss lethal competition between normal cells and cancerous cells for nutrients, such as oxygen, amino-acids, and minerals, and also for space for proliferation. The cancer cells (for $k = 2$) has a greater competitive advantage over normal cells ($k = 1$).

$P_k(x_i, x_3)$: the chemotherapy-induced cytotoxic activity rate function for normal cells ($k = 1$) and cancer cells ($k = 2$). Here x_3 depicts the drug molecule concentration.

$\Phi(x_1, x_2; t)$: the rate function which represents the concentration, at any time t, of the anti-neoplastic chemotherapy drug in the cancer-bearing anatomic organ of the cancer patient.

2.2 The Model Equations

The prototype mathematical model has the generic form:

$$\begin{aligned}\dot{x}_1 &= B_1(x_1) - D_1(x_1) - Q_1(x_1, x_2) - P_1(x_1, x_3)\\ \dot{x}_2 &= B_2(x_2) - D_2(x_2) - Q_2(x_1, x_2) - P_2(x_2, x_3)\\ \dot{x}_3 &= \begin{cases} 0, & 0 \le t < \tau \\ \Phi(x_1, x_2, x_3; t), & \tau \le t \end{cases}\end{aligned} \tag{1}$$

Where

$\dot{x}_1$: the rate of change of the number density of non-cancerous/normal cells in the cancer-bearing organ
$\dot{x}_2$: the rate of change of the number density of cancer cells in the cancer-bearing organ
$\dot{x}_3$: the intra-tumoral perfusion rate of the anti-cancer drug
τ*:* the time taken by the drug molecules to attain therapeutic concentrations in the cancer-bearing organ.

2.3 The Basic Cancer Chemotherapy Model for Solid Tumors

In this research, the relevant basic mathematical model consists of the following system of coupled non-linear differential equations:

$$\begin{aligned}\dot{x}_1 &= \frac{a_1 x_1}{1+s_1 x_1} - b_1 x_1 - q_1 \frac{x_1 x_2}{1+x_1} - c_1 \frac{x_1 x_3}{\mu_1 + x_3}\\ \dot{x}_2 &= a_2 x_2 \left(1 - \frac{x_2}{K_2}\right) - q_2 \frac{x_1 x_2}{1+x_2} - c_2 \frac{x_2 x_3}{\mu_2 + x_3}\\ \dot{x}_3 &= Q f(t) - c_3 x_3 - \frac{c_{11} x_1 x_3}{\mu_1 + x_3} - \frac{c_{22} x_2 x_3}{\mu_2 + x_3}\\ x_1(t_0) &= x_{10}\\ x_2(t_0) &= x_{20}\\ x_3(t_0) &= x_{30}\end{aligned} \tag{2}$$

Where:

t_0: the time when chemotherapy intervention initiated in the cancer patient
$\{a_1, s_1, b_1\}$: cytokinetic parameters for normal/non-cancerous cells
K_1: the genetically limited carrying capacity of normal cells in the cancerous-bearing organ. In particular,

$$K_1 = \frac{1}{s_1}\left(\frac{a_1}{b_1} - 1\right)$$

$\{c_1, \mu_1\}$: the cyto-reductive or cytotoxic parameters of the chemotherapy drug in normal/non-cancer cells

q_1: inter-specific competition rate constant of normal cells with respect to cancer cells. It depicts the call-loss rate coefficient during competition with cancer cells.

a_2: tumor growth rate constant, which measures the tumor-doubling potential

K_2: the carrying capacity of the cancer cells in the tumor-bearing organ. This can be limited by the availability of space in the anatomic region in the vicinity of the tumor bearing organ

q_2: inter-specific competition rate constant of cancer cells with respect to normal cells. It represents the cell-loss rate coefficient during competition with normal cells

$\{c_2, \mu_2\}$: the tumoricidal rate parameters of the chemotherapy drug in malignant neoplastic cells of the tumor.

Q: the intravenous continuous infusion dose rate

$f(t)$: the intravenous infusion function. This function has the shape of multiple Heaviside step functions with intermediary gaps during which the patient does not receive any infusion so as to reduce systemic toxicity and reduce toxic build-up of drug residue. In particular, $f(t)$ has the form: $f(t) = |$ ceil (sin nt)

$\{c_{11}, c_{22}\}$: the respective stoichiometric coefficients depicting drug absorption efficiency in normal-cells and cancer cells

c_3: the washout rate of the anti-cancer drug from the anatomic organ bearing the cancerous tumor.

$\{x_{10}, x_{20}, x_{30}\}$: the initial values, respectively, of the normal cells, cancer cells, and initial loading dose of the chemotherapy drug.

3 Theoretical Analysis of No-Treatment Case

In this section and the following section, the cancer chemotherapy model will be analyzed with respect to the concepts of existence of non-negative solutions, consequences of no pharmacological intervention, and the therapeutic efficacy of the use of stealth liposomes in cancer chemotherapy.

3.1 Existence of Non-negative Solutions

Consider the cancer chemotherapy model Eq. (2). The system equations can be reduced to the system of differential equations:

$$\dot{x}_1 \le \frac{a_1 x_1}{1 + s_1 x_1} - b_1 x_1$$

$$\dot{x}_2 \le a_2 x_2 \left(1 - \frac{x_2}{K_2}\right)$$

$$\dot{x}_3 \le Q_0 \max_{t \in R_+} f(t) - c_3 x_3$$

Let $\max_{t \in R_+} f(t) = 1$. There exists a t $\in$ R_+ such that for $t > T_{01} + \varepsilon$, $\limsup x_1(t) \le K_1$ where $K_1 = \frac{1}{s_1}\left(\frac{a_1}{b_1} - 1\right)$ and $a_1 > b_1$. Also, there exists a $T_{02} \in R_+$ such that $t > T_{02} + \varepsilon$, $\limsup x_2(t) \le K_2$. Similarly, there exists a $T_{03} \in R_+$ such that for $t > T_{03} + \varepsilon$, $\limsup x_3(t) \le K_3$ where $K_3 = \frac{Q}{c_3}$. Thus, for $t > \max\{T_{01}, T_{02}, T_{03}\}$, there is an invariant set A where

$$A = \left\{(x_1, x_2, x_3) \in R_+^3 | 0 \le x_1 \le K_1, 0 \le x_2 \le K_2, 0 \le x_3 \le K_3\right\}$$

such that all solution trajectories of (2) with initial values $(x_{10}, x_{20}, x_{30}) \in R_+^3$ will eventually enter the compact attractor set A and become ultimately bounded and entrapped in A for all $t \in R_+$.

3.2 *Model for No-Treatment Case and Analysis of Equilibrium Points*

Suppose no chemotherapy or intervention such as immunotherapy or radiotherapy is attempted for the cancer patient, the model equations reduce to the following system:

$$\begin{aligned} \dot{x}_1 &= \tfrac{a_1 x_1}{1+s_1 x_1} - b_1 x_1 - q_1 \tfrac{x_1 x_2}{1+x_1} \\ \dot{x}_2 &= a_2 x_2 \left(1 - \tfrac{x_2}{K_2}\right) - q_2 \tfrac{x_1 x_2}{1+x_2} \\ x_1(t_0) &= x_{10} \\ x_2(t_0) &= x_{20} \end{aligned} \tag{3}$$

The patho-physiological outcomes or equilibrium/rest points are $E_1 = [0,0]$, $E_2 = [K_1,0]$, $E_3 = [0, K_2]$, and $E_4 = [\overline{x}_1, \overline{x}_2]$, which are depicting, respectively, annihilation of normal cells and cancer cells in the cancer-bearing organ; tumor eradication whilst normal cells repopulate to carrying-capacity; elimination of normal cells in the tumor-bearing organ whilst cancer cells repopulate to carrying capacity; and co-existence of both normal cells and cancer cells at levels below their carrying capacity in the tumor-bearing organ. Under pathophysiological conditions, the most likely outcomes are $E_1(0,0)$, and $E_3(0, K_2)$. If the patient has a competent immune system, the outcomes $E_2(K_1,0)$ and $E_4(\overline{x}_1, \overline{x}_2)$ are possible, if the tumor is de-bulked using surgery to reduce x_{10} to sub-clinical level.

The Jacobian matrices of linearization in the neighborhood of each of the equilibrium points are listed as follows in (4).

$$\begin{aligned}
J\{E_1(0,0)\} &= \begin{bmatrix} a_1 - b_1 & 0 \\ 0 & a_2 \end{bmatrix} \\
J\{E_2(K_1,0)\} &= \begin{bmatrix} \frac{a_1}{(1+s_1K_1)^2} - b_1 & -\frac{q_1K_1}{1+K_1} \\ 0 & a_2 - q_2K_1 \end{bmatrix} \\
\{E_3(0,K_2)\} &= \begin{bmatrix} a_1 - b_1 - q_1K_2 & 0 \\ -\frac{q_2K_2}{1+K_2} & -a_2 \end{bmatrix} \\
J\{E_4(\overline{x}_1,\overline{x}_2)\} &= \begin{bmatrix} \frac{a_1}{(1+s_1\overline{x}_1)^2} - b_1 - \frac{q_2\overline{x}_2}{(1+\overline{x}_1)^2} & -\frac{q_1\overline{x}_1}{1+\overline{x}_1} \\ -\frac{q_2\overline{x}_2}{1+\overline{x}_2} & a_2 - \frac{2q_2\overline{x}_2}{K_2} - \frac{q_2\overline{x}_1}{(1+\overline{x}_2)^2} \end{bmatrix}
\end{aligned} \tag{4}$$

Theorem 1 Suppose

(i) The isoclines $\frac{a_1x_1}{1+s_1x_1} - b_1x_1 - q_1\frac{x_1x_2}{1+x_1}$ and $a_2x_2\left(1 - \frac{x_2}{K_2}\right) - q_2\frac{x_1x_2}{1+x_2}$ do not intersect
(ii) $a_1 - b_1 > 0$
(iii) $\frac{a_1}{(1+s_1K_1)^2} - b_1 > 0$ and $a_2 - q_2K_2 > 0$
(iv) $a_1 - b_1 - q_1K_2 < 0$

Then the patho-physiological outcome $E_3(0, K_2)$ is a global attractor and consequently the cancer cells will annihilate the normal cells in the cancer-bearing organ/tissue or anatomic region of the patient's body.

Proof Condition (i) of the theorem implies the non-existence of $E_4(\overline{x}_1, \overline{x}_2)$. The conditions (ii) and (iii) imply that the equilibrium points E_1(0,0) and $E_2(K_1$,0), are hyperbolic sources and unstable locally, as they repel the flow in both x_1 and x_2 directions. Using the Poincare-Bendixson theorem and condition (iv) of the theorem, it can be shown that the omega limit set of Eq. 2 is $E_3(0, K_2)$, In particular, every solution trajectory with initial point(x_{10}, x_{20}) in $R_+^2 = \{(x_1, x_2) \in R^2 | x_1 \geq 0, x_2 \geq 0\}$ will approach this equilibrium as t tends to infinity. Thus, $E_3[0, K_2]$ is a global attractor.

4 Theoretical Analysis of Continuous Intravenous Infusion Case

4.1 Model for Continuous Intravenous Infusion Case

Suppose the chemotherapy drug is infused at a constant optimal dose rate Q_0 continuously. Then $f(t) \equiv 1$, and the model equations reduce to

$$
\begin{aligned}
\dot{x}_1 &= \tfrac{a_1 x_1}{1+s_1 x_1} - b_1 x_1 - q_1 \tfrac{x_1 x_2}{1+x_1} - c_1 \tfrac{x_1 x_3}{\mu_1 + x_3} \\
\dot{x}_2 &= a_2 x_2 \left(1 - \tfrac{x_2}{K_2}\right) - q_2 \tfrac{x_1 x_2}{1+x_2} - c_2 \tfrac{x_2 x_3}{\mu_2 + x_3} \\
\dot{x}_3 &= Q_0 - c_3 x_3 - \tfrac{c_{11} x_1 x_3}{\mu_1 + x_3} - \tfrac{c_{22} x_2 x_3}{\mu_2 + x_3} \\
x_1(t_0) &= x_{10} \\
x_2(t_0) &= x_{20} \\
x_3(t_0) &= x_{30}
\end{aligned} \tag{5}
$$

The possible patho-physiological outcomes or equilibrium points are listed as follows:

$$E_1 = [0, 0, \bar{x}_3],\ E_2 = [0, \hat{x}_2, \hat{x}_3],\ E_3 = [\tilde{x}_1, 0, \tilde{x}_3],\ \text{and } E_4 = [\check{x}_1, \check{x}_2, \check{x}_3]$$

These equilibrium points depict, respectively, the annihilation of both normal and cancer cells by the cytotoxic cancer drug; the annihilation of normal cells only in tumor bearing organ; the clinically-desirable case of annihilation of cancer cells only; and co-existence between normal cells and cancer cells in the presence of anti-cancer drug residual concentration.

4.2 Analysis of $E_3 = [\tilde{x}_1, 0, \tilde{x}_3]$

The necessary condition for existence for this equilibrium is that $\tilde{x}_1$ and $\tilde{x}_3$ are solution to the equations:

$$a_1 x_1 - b_1 x_1 - c_1 \frac{x_1 x_3}{\mu_1 + x_3} = 0$$

$$Q_0 - c_3 x_3 - \frac{c_{11} x_1 x_3}{\mu_1 + x_3} = 0 \tag{6}$$

If stealth liposomes are used, then $c_1 = 0$ and c_{11} is negligible. This the Jacobian matrix of linearization of the system (5) in the neighborhood of $E_3(\tilde{x}_1, 0, \tilde{x}_3)$ is given below.

$$J\left\{E_3\left(\tilde{x}_1, 0, \tilde{x}_3\right)\right\} = \begin{bmatrix} \frac{a_1}{\left(1+s_1\tilde{x}_1\right)^2} - b_1 & -\frac{q_1 \tilde{x}_1}{1+\check{x}_1} & 0 \\ 0 & a_2 - q_2 \tilde{x}_1 & 0 \\ 0 & -\frac{c_{11} x_1 x_3}{\mu_1 + \tilde{x}_3} & -c_3 \end{bmatrix}$$

Theorem 2 Suppose

(i) $\tilde{x}_1$ and $\tilde{x}_3$ are solution to (6.0)
(ii) $\frac{a_1}{\left(1+s_1\tilde{x}_1\right)^2} - b_1 < 0$
(iii) $a_2 - q_2\tilde{x}_1 < 0$
Then the patho-physiological outcome $E_3(\tilde{x}_1, 0, \tilde{x}_3)$ is a hyperbolic sink and a local attractor and consequently, the cancer will be in clinical remission.

Proof The first condition of the theorem guarantees the local existence of $E_3(\tilde{x}_1, 0, \tilde{x}_3)$. The conditions (ii) and (iii) imply that the eigenvalue of the Jacobian matrix of linearization has negative real parts. This $E_3(\tilde{x}_1, 0, \tilde{x}_3)$ is a local asymptotically stable equilibrium point, and hence a local attractor. Thus the cancer will be in clinically observable remission [3, 18].

5 Computer Simulations

In this section, some intrinsic mathematical principles of cancer chemotherapy will be elucidated using investigative computer simulations, involving clinically plausible hypothetical cancer patient patho-physiologic parametric configurations. The parameter values used in the simulations are computer-generated estimates and are used qualitatively to elucidate the fundamental principles of cancer chemotherapy.

5.1 Simulation #1 – No-Treatment Case

As discussed in Sect. 3, the no-treatment case in cancer chemotherapy has at most four physiological outcomes, namely, E_1 = [0,0], E_2 = [K_1,0], E_3 = [0, K_2], and $E_4 = [\bar{x}_1, \bar{x}_2]$.

Consider a patient with the physiological parametric configuration in Table 1 below.

The results of the simulations are displayed in Fig. 1.

In the absence of chemotherapy, the patient with physiological parametric configuration P_1 will observe that the cancer cells have completely annihilated all

Table 1 Parametric configuration P_1

Normal cells	Cancer cells	Chemo drug
$x_{10} = 10{,}000$	$x_{20} = 1700$	$x_{30} = 0$
$a_1 = 1.98$	$a_2 = 3.5$	$Q = 0$
$b_1 = 0.05$	$K_2 = 10{,}000$	$c_3 = 0$
$S_1 = 0.0005$	$q_2 = 0.0125$	$c_{11} = 0$
$q_1 = 1.25$	$c_2 = 0.095$	$c_{22} = 0$
$c_1 = 0.07$	$\mu_2 = 1$	
$\mu_1 = 1$		

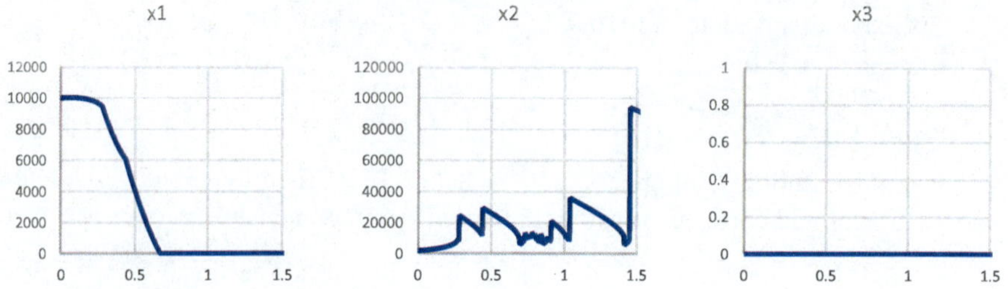

Fig. 1 Simulation results for P_1

Table 2 Parametric configuration P_2

Normal cells	Cancer cells	Chemo drug
$x_{10} = 10{,}000$	$x_{20} = 800$	$x_{30} = 1000$
$a_1 = 1.98$	$a_2 = 3.5$	$Q = 50{,}000$
$b_1 = 0.05$	$K_2 = 10{,}000$	$c_3 = 0.0035$
$S_1 = 0.0005$	$q_2 = 0.0125$	$c_{11} = 0.125$
$q_1 = 1.25$	$c_2 = 0.095$	$c_{22} = 0.9$
$c_1 = 0.07$	$\mu_2 = 1$	
$\mu_1 = 1$		

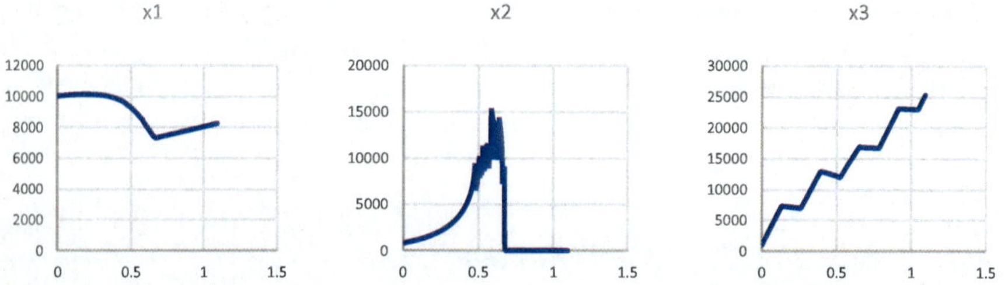

Fig. 2 Simulation results for P_2

the normal cells in the cancer-bearing anatomic tissue or organ. This could result in total incapacitation or death of the patient.

5.2 Simulation #2 – High-Dose Chemotherapy

In this simulation, the hypothetical patient was subjected to high-dose chemotherapy, using the parametric configuration displayed in Table 2.

The simulation results are exhibited in Fig. 2.

This simulation shows that aggressive chemotherapy using high dose rate of the pharmacological drug is able to annihilate the cancer cells during one cycle, so this approach is the potential systemic toxicity of the cancer patient.

Table 3 Parametric configuration P_3

Normal cells	Cancer cells	Chemo drug
$x_{10} = 20{,}000$	$x_{20} = 1000$	$x_{30} = 1000$
$a_1 = 2.45$	$a_2 = 3.5$	$Q = 50{,}000$
$b_1 = 0.05$	$K_2 = 10{,}000$	$c_3 = 0.35$
$S_1 = 0.0005$	$q_2 = 0.125$	$c_{11} = 0.125$
$q_1 = 0.9$	$c_2 = 0.095$	$c_{22} = 0.9$
$c_1 = 0.07$	$\mu_2 = 1$	
$\mu_1 = 1$		

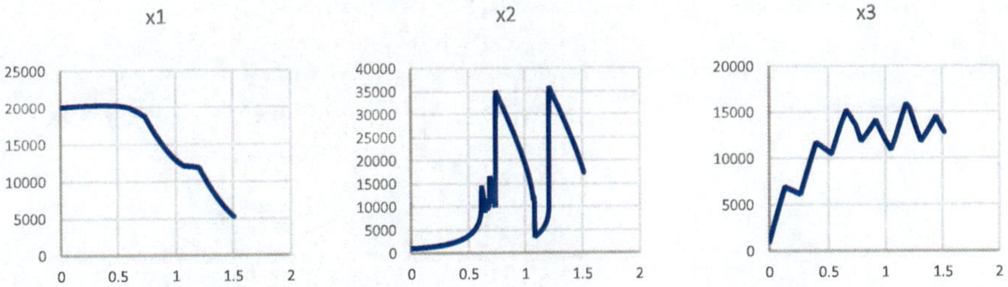

Fig. 3 Simulation results for P_3

5.3 *Simulation #3 – Therapeutic Failure*

The effect of less-aggressive chemotherapy and use of stealth-liposomes as drug carriers to target tumor-bearing organs are investigated with regards to their therapeutic efficacy. The hypothetical cancer patient has the following physiological parametric configuration (Table 3):

The simulation results are displayed in Fig. 3 as follows.

These simulation results depict a scenario of therapeutic failure in which the normal cells in the cancer-bearing organ seem to be undergoing monotonic decline just after the mid-way point of the first cycle of chemotherapy, whereas the cancer cells appear to be undergoing oscillations after the mid-way point of the first cycle of chemotherapy. The cancer dynamics seem to be constrained below a manageable threshold of 35,000 cells. However, the decline of normal cells can lead to organ failure. This problem can be resolved in the next simulation using stealth liposomes to deliver the pharmacologic drug without systemic toxicity and death of normal cells (see [2, 6]).

5.4 *Simulation #4 – Chemotherapy wth Stealth Liposome*

As discussed in Sect. 4, the hypothetical patient in this scenario is given intravenous infusion using mono-clonal antibody-conjugated stealth liposomes with pharmacokinetics as described by Nani and Oguztorelli [19].

Table 4 Parametric configuration P_4

Normal cells	Cancer cells	Chemo drug
$x_{10} = 20{,}000$	$x_{20} = 1000$	$x_{30} = 1000$
$a_1 = 2.45$	$a_2 = 3.5$	$Q = 50{,}000$
$b_1 = 0.05$	$K_2 = 10{,}000$	$c_3 = 0.35$
$S_1 = 0.0005$	$q_2 = 0.125$	$c_{11} = 0.125$
$q_1 = 0.9$	$c_2 = 0.095$	$c_{22} = 0.9$
$c_1 = 0$	$\mu_2 = 1$	
$\mu_1 = 1$		

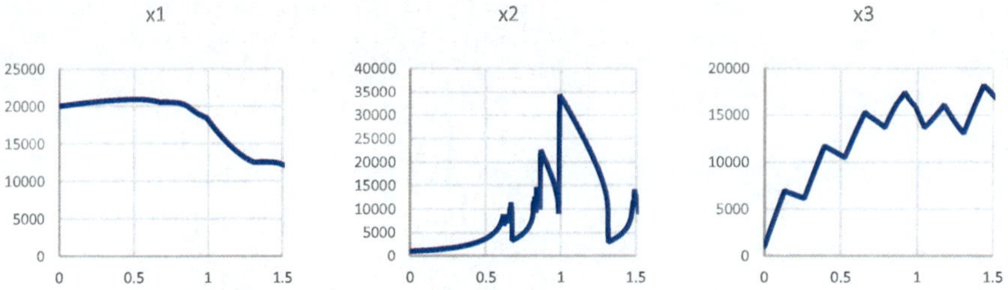

Fig. 4 Simulation results for P_4

The physiological parametric configuration P_4 is such that $c1 = 0$ as shown in Table 4.

The effect of use of stealth liposome is the minimization of toxicity of the chemotherapy drug to normal and non-cancerous cells and tissues. Thus the normal cell cytotoxicity rate constant is set to zero in the parametric configuration used for the simulations. In Fig. 3, the normal cell number without stealth liposome was 5000 as compared to Fig. 4, which showed the normal cell number as 12,500 due to the use of the stealth liposomes.

The repeat of the simulations with parametric configuration P_3 using $c_1 = 0$ to implement effect of stealth liposomes gives the results as shown in Fig. 4.

6 Summary

In this chapter, we have presented a plausible mathematical model system of deterministic non-linear differential equations, which depict the pathophysiology of malignant cancers. The cytokinetic properties of normal cells, cancer cells, and the pharmacokinetics of the chemotherapy drug are described, respectively, by biophysically measurable growth parameters, stoichiometric rate constants, and Michaelis–Menten type reaction profiles. Theoretical clinically-plausible criteria are presented depicting the scenarios of cancer remission under stealth-liposome chemotherapy and the consequences of the no-treatment case. Investigative computer simulations confirm the clinically observed reduction in cytotoxicity of anti-cancer drug when encapsulated in stealth liposomes. The simulations also show that when no intervention is done, cancer cells will eventually annihilate normal cells in the tumor-bearing organ.

References

1. J. Adams, A mathematical model of tumor growth II: Effects of geometrical and spatial non-uniformity on stability. Math. Biosci. **86**, 183–211 (1987)
2. T.A. Allen, Stealth liposomes: Five years on. J. Liposome Res. **2**(3), 289–305 (2008)
3. H. Amann, *Ordinary Differential Equations (An Introduction to Non-Linear Analysis)* (Walter de Gruyter, New York, 1990), pp. 200–265
4. O. Arino, M. Kimmel, Asymptotic analysis of cell cycle models based on unequal division. SIAM J. Appl. Math. **47**, 128–145 (1987)
5. J.L. Bos, The ras oncogene family and human carcinogenesis. Mutat. Res. **195**, 255–271 (1988)
6. B. Čeh, M. Winterhalter, P.M. Frederick, et al., Stealth Liposomes from theory to product. Adv. Drug Deliv. Rev. **24**(2–3), 165–177 (1997)
7. M. Eisen, Mathematical models in cell biology and cancer chemotherapy, in *Lecture Notes in Biomathematics*, vol. 40, (Springer, Bew Youk, 1979), pp. 122–218
8. E. Frei III, Curative cancer chemotherapy. Cancer Res. **45**, 6523–6548 (1985)
9. C. Gamkke, A. Hall, C. Moroni, Activation of an N-ras gene in acute myeloblastic leukaemia. Proc. NaH. Acad. Sci. **82**, 879–882 (1984)
10. R.A. Gatenby, Models of tumor-host interaction as competing populations: Implications for tumor biology and treatment. J. Theor. Biol. **176**, 447–455 (1995)
11. Genetech, Stages of NSCLC. (2007).. Retrieved January 17, 2008, from http://www.avastin.com/avastin/patient/lung/learn/stages/index.m
12. M. Gyllenberg, K. Woo, G.F. Webb, Age-structure in tumor populations with quiescence. Math. Biosci. **86**, 67–95 (1987)
13. M. Kim, K.B. Woo, S. Perry, Quantitative approach to the design of anti-tumor drug dosage schedule via cell cycle kinetics and systems theory. Ann. Biomed. Eng. **5**, 12 (1977)
14. H. Knolle, Cell kinetic modeling and the chemotherapy of cancer, in *Lecture Notes in Biomathematics*, vol. 75, (Springer, New York, 1988)
15. L.A. Liotta, Cancer cell invasion and metastasis. Sci. Am. **1992**, 54–63 (1992)
16. F. Mastrotto, C. Brazzale, F. Bellato, et al., In vitro and in vivo behavior of liposomes decorated with PEGs with different chemical features. Mol. Pharm. **17**(2), 472–487 (2020)
17. S. Michelson, J.T. Leith, Growth factors and growth control of heterogeneous cell populations. Bull. Math. Biol. **55**, 993–1011 (1993)
18. F.K. Nani, Models of Chemotherapy and Immunotherapy (Doctoral Thesis, University of Alberta, 1998) (1998)
19. F.K. Nani, M.N. Oguztoreli, Modeling and simulation of liposomal drug delivery to the central nervous system, in *Biomedical Modelling and Simulation*, ed. by J. Eisenfeld, D. S. Levine, M. Witten, (Elsevier Science Publishers B. V., North-Holland, London, 1992), pp. 351–367
20. A. Neri et al., Analysis of ras oncogene mutations in human lymphoid malignancies. Proc. Batl. Acad. Sci. **85**, 9268–9272 (1988)
21. M.N. Oguztoreli, C.P. Tsokos, J. Akabutu, A kinetic study of chemotherapy. Appl. Math. Comput. **12**, 255–300 (1983)
22. J.C. Panetta, A mathematical model of periodically pulsed chemotherapy: Tumor recurrence and metastasis in a competitive environment. Bull. Math. Biol. **58**, 425–447 (1996)
23. M. C. Perry (ed.), *The Chemotherapy Sourcebook* (Williams and Wilkins, Baltimore, 1992), pp. 213–220
24. H.G. Pitot, *Fundamentals of Oncology* (Marcel Dekker, New York, 1986)

25. G.E. Swan, Tumor growth models and cancer chemotherapy, in *Cancer Modelling*, ed. by F. R. Thompson, B. W. Brown, (New York, Marcel-Dekker, 1987), pp. 91–180
26. S.L. Weekes, B. Barker, S. Bober, et al., A multi-component mathematical model of cancer stem cell driven tumor growth dynamics. Bull. Math. Biol. **76**(7), 1762–1782 (2014)
27. T.E. Wheldon, *Mathematical Models in Cancer Research* (Adam Hilger, Bristol, 1988), pp. 67–82

Optimizing the Removal of Fluorescence and Shot Noise in Raman Spectra of Breast Tissue by ANFIS and Moving Averages Filter

Reinier Cabrera Cabañas, Francisco Javier Luna Rosas, Julio Cesar Martínez Romo, and Iván Castillo Zúñiga

1 Introduction

Breast cancer represents 15% of all female cancer deaths, which is exceeded only by lung cancer in the United States [1]. Early diagnosis is the key factor to increasing the survival rate for cancer patients and, therefore, it is important to develop quick, less-invasive, objective methods for diagnosing breast cancer.

Raman spectroscopy is a high-resolution photonic technique that provides in a few seconds chemical and structural information of almost any organic and/or inorganic material or compound, allowing its identification. The analysis by Raman spectroscopy is based on the analysis of the light scattered by a material by making a monochromatic light beam strike it; when this happens, a small portion of the light is inelastically scattered, undergoing slight changes in frequency that are characteristic of the material analyzed and independent of the frequency of the incident light. This technique is currently being applied in multiple scientific areas, such as physics and chemistry, but it has taken great importance in biochemistry, specifically in virus detection [2]. Numerous studies have investigated the application of Raman spectroscopy on the detection of normal, precancerous, and cancerous breast tissues [3, 4], demonstrating that it could detect the changes in molecular structure and composition that occur during tumor formation in the main biomolecules that make up the cell and tissue, such as carbohydrates, lipids, proteins, and nucleic acids. These changes are detected, when clinical symptoms occur, from the analysis and

R. C. Cabañas (✉) · F. J. L. Rosas · J. C. M. Romo
Computer Science Department, Instituto Tecnológico de Aguascalientes, Aguascalientes, Ags., Mexico

I. C. Zúñiga
Systems and computation Department Instituto Tecnológico del Llano Aguascalientes, Aguascalientes, Ags., Mexico

H. R. Arabnia et al. (eds.), *Advances in Computer Vision and Computational Biology*, Transactions on Computational Science and Computational Intelligence,
https://doi.org/10.1007/978-3-030-71051-4_57

detection of tumor medical images. Molecular spectroscopy has, in this sense, great advantages for determining an early diagnosis of the tumor [5].

However, one of the great problems of Raman spectra and specifically of biological tissue is that the Raman scattering (RS), which characterizes the composition of the sample, is accompanied by noise generated by the measuring instrument, external sources, and noise due to fluorescence. The latter may be orders of magnitude greater than the Raman signal, preventing the obtaining of information associated with its molecular composition. Therefore, it is necessary to eliminate the noise in the spectra before the analysis stage.

Noise removal is one of the most important data-processing operations. Despite its wide use in various types of signals, there is no general strategy to carry out this procedure, since it largely depends on the problem treated, the signal-to-noise ratio (*S*/*N*) and the shape of the signals. Noise elimination process must be carried out with special care to avoid loss of information, and to adapt to the signal to be analyzed. For noise elimination, two different approaches have been used: the experimental and the computational. The methods that use the experimental approach are based on adjustments or improvements to the instrumentation and these include shifted excitation and time-limited systems [6]. Experimental methods like the previous ones are a little complex because they involve long acquisition times that hinder their use for applications in biological tissue; for these reasons, the use of computational methods has increased due to their speed, easy implementation, and low cost. Some computational methods that stand out include adjustment methods, highlighting the modified multipolinomial adjustment method and the Vancouver Algorithm [7, 8], the methods based on wavelet transforms [9] and the morphological algorithms [10].

In this work, ANFIS (Adaptive Neuro-Fuzzy Inference System), an integrating system between neural networks and fuzzy-logic that has previously been applied as an artificial intelligence tool in some areas, such as architecture, the automotive industry, in biochemistry, and in medicine [11], is used to characterize the contribution of fluorescence noise that is generated in Raman signals from healthy and damaged breast tissue, the procedure consists of developing an algorithm that allows to subtract the Raman peaks from the signal until a continuous signal at intervals is obtained and that signal will act as input to the diffuse neural network; the same, through an own adjustment system using the backpropagation error, will adjust the background curve of the signal and filling in the empty spaces where the peaks were.

This obtained signal will be assumed as the fluorescence background masking the signal and will be subtracted from the original signal. To eliminate small fluctuations that occur around the average value of the signal, moving averages filters are used, which allow smoothing the signal and suppressing high-frequency noise.

This procedure ensures that the signal is clean of noise and in a position to be correctly identified for future diagnostic and prediction procedures. Furthermore, in this chapter, we demonstrate that it is possible to optimize the response time in the pre-processing of Raman signals of healthy and damaged breast tissue, when we eliminate fluorescence and shot noise in large quantities of biological samples, achieving an improvement of 59.67% in relation to the processing of data sequentially, which makes it a valuable tool in the field of medicine for future applications of diagnosis and prediction of diseases.

2 Materials and Methods

2.1 *ANFIS (Adaptative Neuro-Fuzzy Inference System)*

ANFIS (Adaptive Neuro Fuzzy Inference System) integrates Neural Networks with fuzzy logic inheriting the characteristics of both and allows you to tune or create the rule base of a fuzzy system using the backpropagation algorithm from the data collection of a process. It is an architecture functionally equivalent to a fuzzy rule system based on the Takagi and Sugeno mode [12, 13].

The Neuro-Diffuse system is a traditional diffuse system in which each stage can be represented by a layer of neurons to which neural network learning capabilities can be provided to optimize the knowledge of the system. By having trainable parameters, the delta rule algorithms and backpropagation error are applicable [14]. Some parameters allow to establish the training set of the ANFIS system, and some common rules presented by the first-order fuzzy model are necessary.

2.2 *Moving Averages*

Moving Averages is a fairly simple prediction method that has been used in commerce and has not been altered for more than half a century [15]. A window of size N is selected, and the mean or average of the variable for the N data is obtained, allowing the average to move as the new data of the variable in question are observed. This smoothens out possible strong oscillations or outliers.

The increase of any moving average depends exclusively on the shape of the function f and the size of the selected window. The mean movement of order N (MA_f) of a series f of values $Y_1, Y_2, Y_3, \ldots, Y_N$ is defined by the sequence of values corresponding to the arithmetic means:

$$\mathrm{MA}_f = \left(\frac{Y_1 + Y_2 + Y_N}{N}; \frac{Y_2 + Y_3 + Y_{N+1}}{N}; \frac{Y_3 + Y_4 + Y_{N+2}}{N}; \ldots \right) \quad (1)$$

Where $Y_1, Y_2, Y_3, \ldots, Y_N$ are the most recent observations of the closed interval; N is the size of the Interval within the function f.

2.3 Parallel Computing

Parallel computing is a form of computation in which many instructions are performed simultaneously, operating over the principle that big problems can often be divided into smaller ones, which are then solved simultaneously (in parallel).

The hardware that supports parallel computing consists of multicore computers, symmetric multiprocessors, distributed computers, such as task clusters stations, and specialized parallel processors, such as FPGA, GPU, and built in circuits of specific applications (AISC). With the development of hardware that supports parallel programming, especially the development of multicore computers, parallel programming architectures become more important than before [16].

The most common forms of parallelism, include: task parallelism, pipeline parallelism, and data parallelism [16]. In the task parallelism, also known as functional parallelism, is a development structure in which independent figures from parts of a method can be performed simultaneously in different processors. In the case of pipeline parallelism, the problem is separated in a series of tasks. Any of the tasks will be performed in a separate process or processor. Each parallel process is usually referred to as a pipeline state. The exit as a pipeline state serves as the entrance of another state, therefore, in a given time each pipeline state is working over a different dataset. The data parallelism is mainly centered over the same process that will be applied simultaneously over different parts of a dataset. Let us say, similar operating sequences or functions are carried out in parallel over a large element data structure. Moreover, if given enough parallel resources, the computing time of the data structure in parallel is usually independent from the problem size. One of the parallelism methods mentioned previously, or their combination, should be used in parallel applications.

3 Experiments

Raw Raman spectra were provided to us by the University of Guadalajara, Jalisco, Mexico, and were taken from samples of cancerous and healthy breast tissues; the samples were obtained by excisional biopsy of patients diagnosed with infiltrating ductal cancer and preserved in formalin; in order to obtain the Raman spectra, histological cuts were made on the samples. The Raman spectra were obtained using a Raman Renishaw system model 1000-B; this system uses a laser diode of $\lambda = 830$ nm and a grating of 600 lines/mm. The laser was focused on the samples with a Leica microscope model DMLM (objective of 50×), at approximately 35 mW of power. Each spectrum was collected in the region from 680 to 1780 cm^{-1}, with an exposition time of 10s. Finally, the wavenumber resolution was of 2 cm^{-1} and the Raman system was calibrated with a silicon semiconductor at the Raman peak in 520 cm^{-1}. With this experimental setup, 10,000 Raman spectra were recorded from healthy and diseased tissue zones of the biopsies.

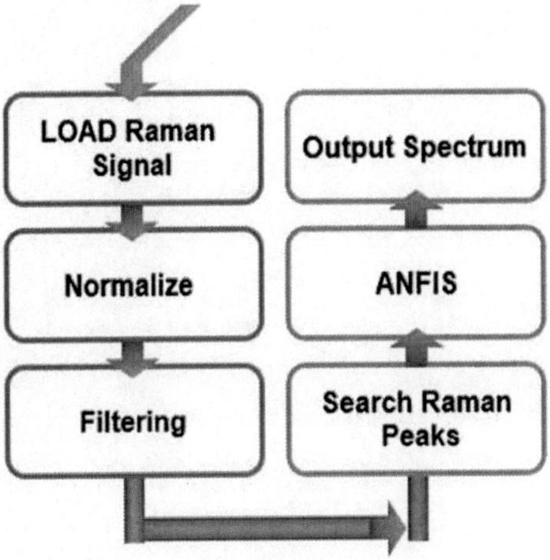

Fig. 1 Program sequence designed to eliminate noise in Raman spectra

4 Results and Discussion

4.1 Description of the Proposed Algorithm for Fluorescence and Shot Noise Reduction

As previously mentioned, the Raman signal is made up of the useful signal, (characteristic of the molecular vibrations that occur inside the excited molecule) and a noise signal inherent in the measurement process, mainly high-frequency noise and fluorescence background.

$$Y = X_{\text{true}} + b + n \tag{2}$$

Where X_{true} is the Raman spectra free of noise and fluorescence, b is the background fluorescence, n is the noise in the signal and finally Y is the raw Raman signal acquired with the spectrometer containing fluorescence and shot noise. In such a way that, to obtain a noise-free signal, it is necessary to subtract the identified background fluorescence and shot noise from the raw signal.

The strategy followed is to design a mechanism to eliminate possible peaks in the raw Raman signal by detecting their start and end points. By suppressing these peaks, we will have a continuous signal at intervals such as the one shown in Fig. 5, the objective of using ANFIS is to apply an interpolation to determine the possible shape of the fluorescence signal in the empty spaces of the signal, to finally subtract it from the measured spectrum. Figure 1 shows a diagram highlighting each of the stages involved in the fluorescence removal process.

Stage 1. Load the Raman Signal In this step, the data vector is loaded from an Excel file, it contains two columns corresponding to the intensity values of the

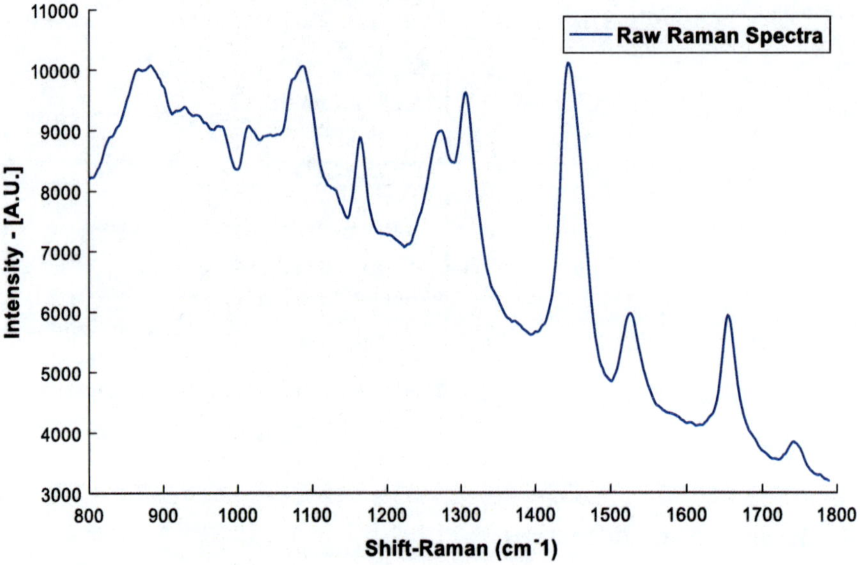

Fig. 2 Raman signal of healthy breast tissue without processing

spectrum and the shift Raman, respectively. In Fig. 2, we have an example of a raw Raman spectrum corresponding to healthy breast tissue.

Stage 2. Normalizing the Data This stage was performed in order to keep the signal under the same scale on the two coordinate axes, it was achieved through an interpolation algorithm, on the *y*-axis the maximum and minimum values of the spectrum were calculated, the minimum value is subtracted from the original spectrum and the result is divided by the maximum value, leaving the intensity values between 0 and 1, on the *x*-axis an arbitrary value of 574 values corresponding to the length of the data was taken.

This is the best way to work with the signals because the signals would be on the same scale and the slope on each Raman signal will be easily located and very similar.

Stage 3. Signal Filtering A moving averages filter is applied with the purpose of smoothening the signal as a previous step to the correction of the baseline; the procedure is performed with a vector of fixed size previously defined and the central part of the result that is equal in size is rescued to the original data. With this method, it is possible to overshadow the high frequency noise that affects the spectrum and dissolve the small peaks in the signal that can cause confusion in the interpretation of the data. Figure 4 shows the high frequency noise that was subtracted from the healthy breast tissue Raman signal (Fig. 3).

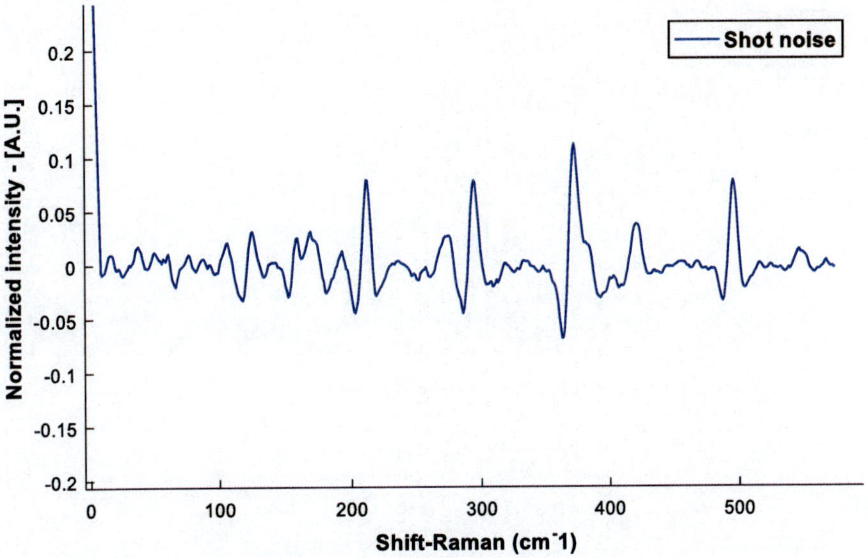

Fig. 3 Shot noise removed from the Raman signal of healthy breast tissue by moving averages Filter

Stage 4. Looking for Raman Peaks Candidates With this objective, different algorithms were implemented that allow detection of all the signal peaks and subtraction of them from the original signal, considering their starting and ending points.

The way this problem is solved is as follows:

1. Initially, all the maximum points of the signal are discovered; for this, it was necessary to implement a window algorithm with a window size equal to 15 samples, when we sampled the signal in this way the maximum values inside the window were found and assumed as possible Raman peaks if they were centered in the window; if they incline to one side they are discarded.

   Through this method, we detect the portions of the spectrum that may have a peak shape and that could later be identified as legitimate Raman peaks.
2. Once all the possible signal peaks are obtained, the maximum values are taken for evaluation, keeping the same window size and is evaluated point by point from the maximum value descending on both sides of the possible peak (to the right is increased by 1 unit and the left is decreased by one unit with respect to the x-axis), a least squares procedure is applied at each point to obtain the equation of the line that best describes the points corresponding to each window, the angle of inclination is calculated in each step with respect to the abscissa and is compared, taking as a criterion that the inclination of the peak is represented by an angle of more than 60°, since for smaller angles, they would make the appearance of the peak disappear and the structure of the signal would be affected

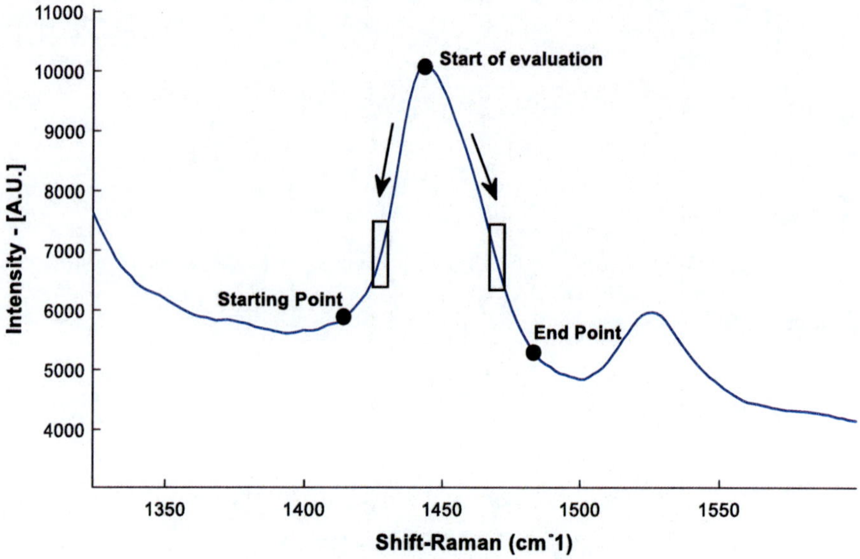

Fig. 4 Evaluation to find the start and end points of the peak

with the introduction of morphological errors. The point where the condition is not met is taken as the starting and ending point of the peak.

In Fig. 4, we can observe the procedure described above. We can see that the start and end points of the peak (points where the condition is not met) do not have the same height, and the rectangles try to represent the angle that is formed between the points with respect to the axis of the abscissa (Fig. 5).

Stage 5. ANFIS, Configuration Developed ANFIS is used at the junction of the points, where each peak detected in the previous stage begins and ends. An adaptive network is constructed functionally equivalent to the fuzzy model Sugeno type, whose scheme can be seen in Fig. 6.

The procedure to apply ANFIS will be explained step by step:

Preparation of the Data For explanatory purposes, the vector containing the signal will be known as y or output and the vector containing the abscissa data will be known as x or input. Those definitions allow us to define the training set of the ANFIS system.

Training with ANFIS To explain the training procedure, a portion of the spectrum has been selected; the values required for training are the scale in which the Raman peaks do not appear on the x-axis as input and the amplitude y as the output variable or target that presents the Raman peak. In Fig. 7, we can see a portion of the spectrum that we selected for illustrative purposes, where the representation of the training vectors is framed on the x- and y-axes. The scale we take on the x-axis goes

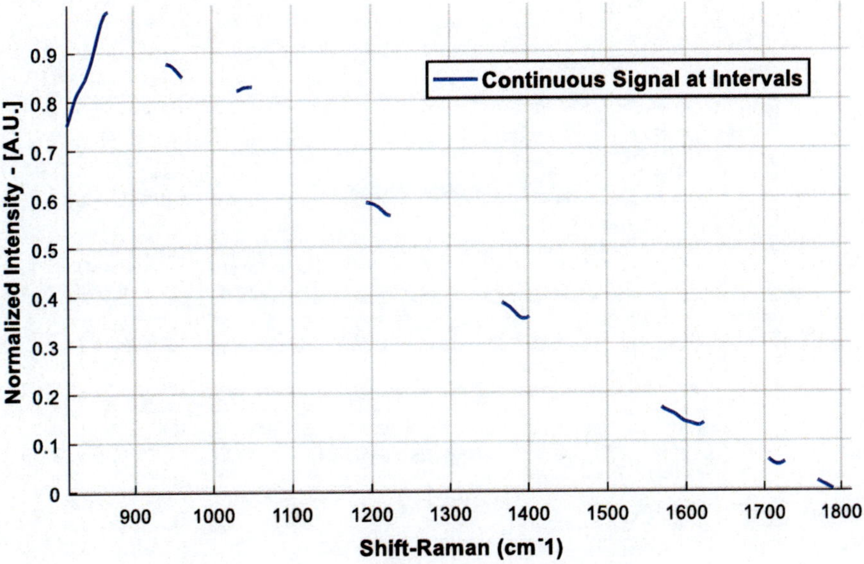

Fig. 5 Raman signal continues at intervals with the peak regions removed

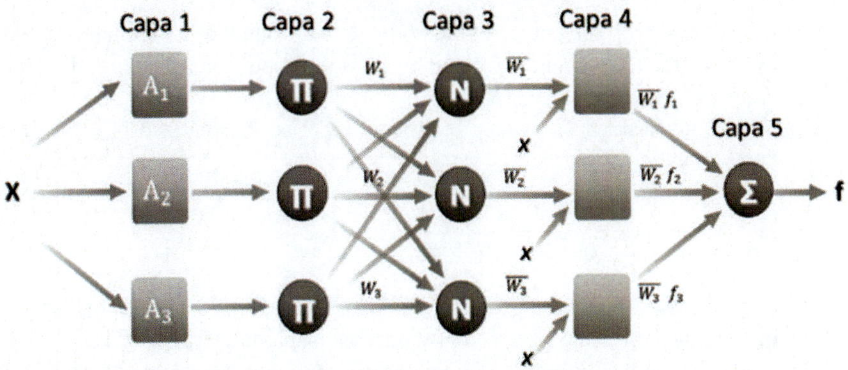

Fig. 6 ANFIS network structure. One input, three rules one output

from 941.7 cm^{-1} to 1051 cm^{-1} as the input variable and the amplitude y as the output or target variable. In the mentioned interval, there is a Raman peak in the interval between 962.4 cm^{-1} and 1032 cm^{-1}.

Forward propagation phase *Layer 1* (see Fig. 6) receives vector X and calculates the degree of membership $\mu_{Ak}(X)$ of the fuzzy set for each of the values X_i of the vector according to the membership function A_k associated with each input; in this case, a Gaussian membership functions with three trainable parameters

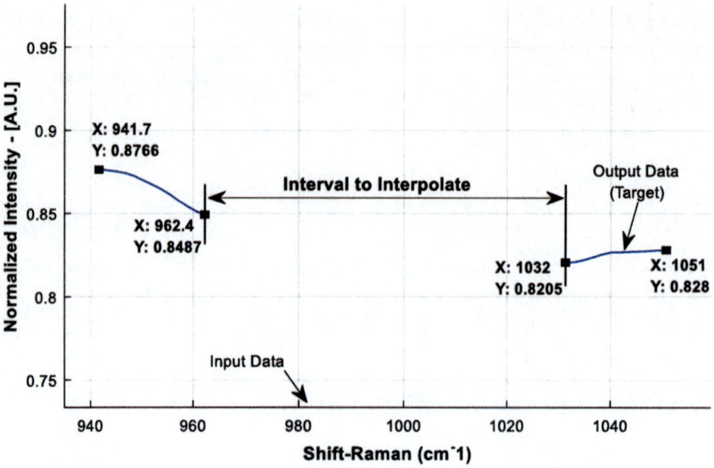

Fig. 7 Portion of the spectrum selected for training

$$A_k = \text{gauss}\ (x, \sigma, c) = e^{-\left(\frac{x-c}{\sigma}\right)^2} \quad (3)$$

In *layer 2* (layer π), the output of the nodes is the product of all the input signals, but in this case, the antecedent is formed by a unique condition (if x is ...); therefore, the output of this layer $w = \mu_{Ak}(X)$.

In *layer 3* (layer *N*), every element $w_{i,j}$ is normalized to the sum $w_{i,1} + w_{i,2} + w_{i,3}$

$$\overline{w_i} = \frac{w_i}{w_1 + w_2}\ , i = 1, 2 \quad (4)$$

In the next stage of forward propagation, *layers 4 and 5* of the presented network structure are involved. The parameters (consequent parameters) p, q, and r of the linear models that are weighted by the inputs are candidates for training in this phase and represent the inferred fuzzy output set. Every node in this layer is an adaptive node with a function:

$$\overline{w}_i f_i = \overline{w}_i \left(p_i(x) + q_i(y) + r_i\right) \quad (5)$$

In which, f_i are those described in the rules of the fuzzy system [12]. Finally, the defuzzification is carried out, the outputs are processed and integrated as a summation of all the input signals.

$$\text{output} = \sum \overline{w}_i f_i \quad (6)$$

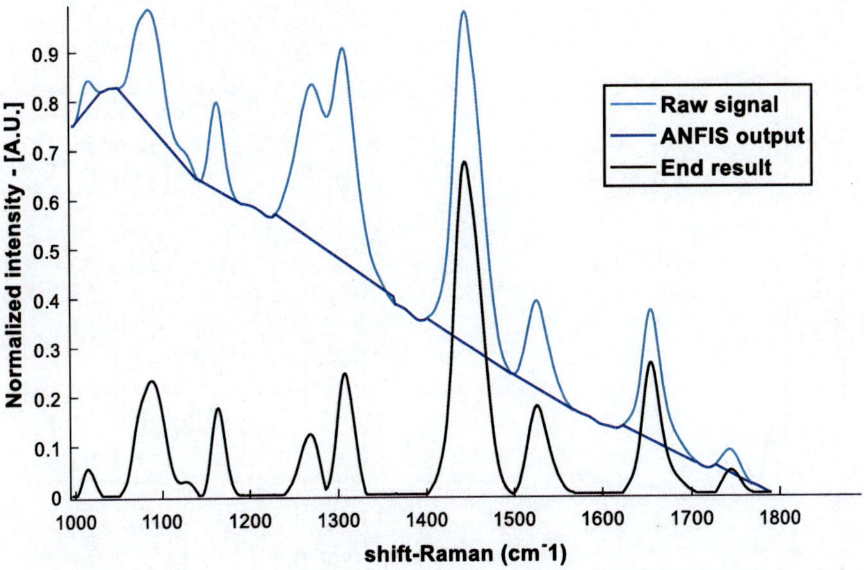

Fig. 8 Raman spectrum corresponding to healthy breast tissue. Cyan, the Raman spectrum after the application of the moving averages filtering; blue, the fluorescence background rescued by the final adjustment of ANFIS; black, the noise-free Raman spectrum

The backpropagation algorithm uses the sum of the square error between the desired output and the output of the ANFIS system to adjust all the trainable parameters of layer 1 of the system. The error is back propagated from layer m to layer m-1; thus, from layer 5 to 4 there is an error signal of 5–4, from 4 to 3 the signal is 4–3, and so on, until the error signal 2–1 is reached. The latter is the one used to adjust the nonlinear trainable elements of layer 1, which are the parameters σ and c of the fuzzy sets A_k. The described process of forward propagation and back propagation is performed iteratively up to a certain number of epochs (100 in this case) or until the error decreases to a specific value.

Figure 8 shows the final result in three graphs; the first one, of cyan color, shows the values of the Raman spectrum of healthy breast tissue after the application of moving average filters; the blue one shows the output values of ANFIS that translates as the fluorescence background of the analyzed spectrum; and finally the black one shows the graph of the output values, after applying the subtraction of the spectra mentioned above.

Figure 9 shows the final result in three graphs; the first one, in cyan color, shows the Raman spectrum values of damaged breast tissue after the application of moving averages filter; the blue one shows the output values of ANFIS which is translated as the fluorescence background of the analyzed spectrum; and finally the black one shows the graph of the output values, after applying the subtraction of the spectra mentioned above.

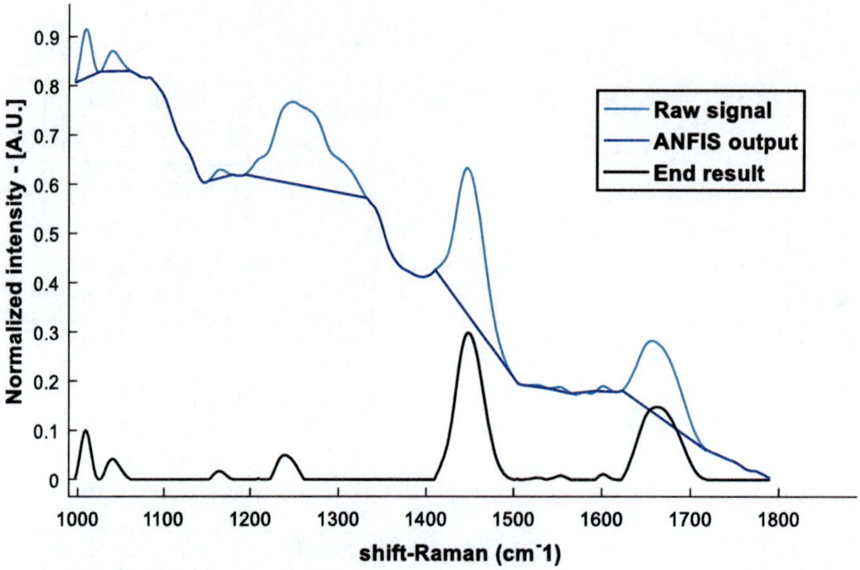

Fig. 9 Raman spectrum corresponding to damaged breast tissue. Cyan, the Raman spectrum after the application of the moving averages filtering; blue, the fluorescence background rescued by the final adjustment of ANFIS; black, the noise-free Raman spectrum

4.2 *Healthy Breast Tissue and Damaged Breast Tissue: Morphology and Chemistry*

In this section, we present the results of Raman studies on normal (non-cancerous) and damaged (cancerous) breast tissues after the application of the implemented algorithm to eliminate fluorescence and high-frequency noise that made it difficult to interpret the spectrum to extract valuable information about the morphological and chemical components present in the breast tissue.

In Fig. 8 (healthy tissue) and Fig. 9 (damaged tissue), we can see the result of applying moving averages filtering and the ANFIS algorithm to eliminate the fluorescence and the shot noise signals and get a spectrum that allows us to make a diagnosis or prediction with the minimum error rate –cyan, the Raman spectrum after the application of the moving averages filtering; blue, the fluorescence background rescued by the final adjustment of ANFIS; black, the noise-free Raman spectrum.

The breast contains two types of tissues: glandular and stromal. The glandular elements consist of lobes and ducts and the stromal elements provide the support network for the glandular units and include the extracellular matrix, the fibroblasts (responsible for producing the extracellular matrix, a support network of structural proteins and carbohydrates, mainly collagen and glycosaminoglycans), fat, and blood vessels. Fat is the only other important morphological structure present and constitutes most of the normal breast tissue.

Many of the morphological structures in benign and malignant breast lesions are like those in normal breast tissue. For example, fibrosis occurs in both benign and malignant breast lesions and involves stromal proliferation. However, some morphological characteristics of diseased breasts are different from those of normal breast tissue. For example, breast cancer most often originates from the lobes and ducts as a rapid proliferation of epithelial cells, associated with nuclear enlargement, pleomorphism (variation in size and shape), and hyperchromatism (darker staining), atypical mitosis and DNA aneuploidy (gain or loss of a chromosome). These morphological changes are not associated with a large-scale production of new chemicals, but with a change in the relative concentrations of chemicals that are already present in the breast [17]. With this basic understanding of the chemistry and architecture of the breasts, and the changes induced by the progression of the disease, it is possible to explain all the main Raman spectral characteristics of normal and damaged breast tissue.

In Fig. 11, we can see the main differences between healthy and damaged tissue from the same patient, the results showed a clear distinction between Raman spectra collected from normal and cancerous tissues in the spectroscopic region of 1000–1800 cm^{-1}, by the positions of the peaks and the proportions of the spectral peaks characteristic of the cellular components. As we can see, the signs are characterized by 9 prominent peaks at 1004, 1080, 1158, 1266, 1304, 1444, 1521, 1660, and 1750 cm^{-1} [6, 18–20].

When making assignments, the methyl balancing modes and C-C stretch modes are between 1000 and 1200 cm^{-1}; in-plane C-H curves, methyl strains (−CH3), and C = C stretch modes are between 1200 and 1600 cm^{-1}.

The Raman peak at 1660 cm^{-1} corresponds to the amide I protein due to carbonyl stretching (C = O); the peak of 1260 cm^{-1} corresponds to the amide III protein due to the stretching of the C-N single link and the bending of N-H. It was found that a lipid peak at 1750 cm^{-1} in the spectra of healthy tissues decreased considerably in the spectrum of damaged tissue. The differences in the spectra of cancerous and normal tissues in the intensity ratio of the peaks in 1444 and 1663 cm^{-1} are surprising, which implies an increase in protein concentration.

The most pronounced differences can be observed in the regions of bands 1521 and 1158 cm^{-1} assigned to carotenes and the regions of bands 1444, 1660, 1750 cm^{-1} that have been assigned to lipids. A detailed inspection in Fig. 10 shows that the Raman bands of carotenes are very strong in healthy tissues, while in damaged tissues, they are not observed. The Raman intensities of the lipid peaks (fatty regions) are significantly smaller in damaged tissue than in healthy tissue (bands 1444, 1750, 1080 cm^{-1} [21], for a deeper description we can address to [22, 23].

We now know that Raman spectra of breast tissue are mainly dominated by lipids and carotenes; through Raman spectroscopy and using a good computational method, such as that described in this work for the elimination of fluorescence and shot noise, it is possible to reliably extract particular characteristics of healthy

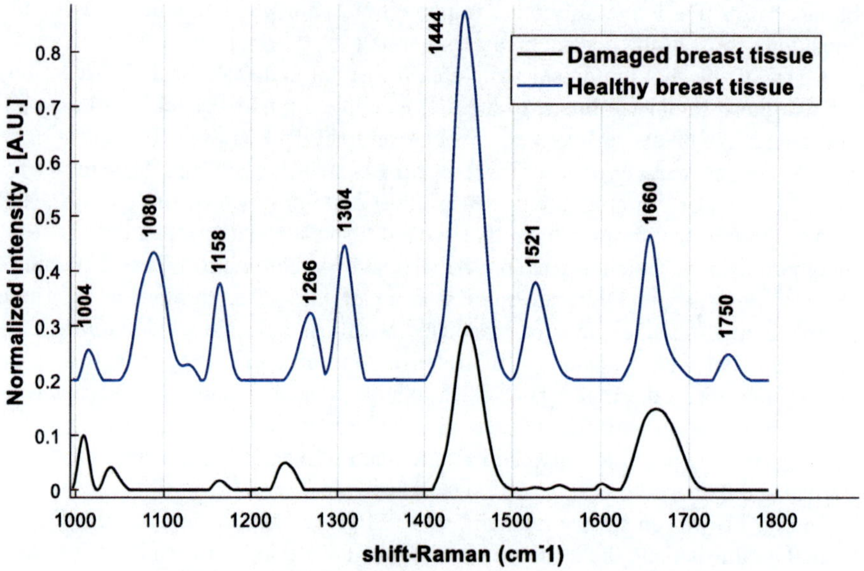

Fig. 10 Raman spectrum of normal and damaged breast tissue (invasive ductal carcinoma) of the same patient

tissue and damaged tissue that allow us to carry out the identification and even early diagnosis of the disease; however, the process of noise reduction becomes more expensive when we treat large amounts of data at the same time; we speak of computational time because the amount of computational resources required increases with the amount of data to process.

The optimization of noise elimination reported in this chapter can have an immediate application to improve the response time of spectroscopic processes that guarantees the diagnosis of diseases.

4.3 *Optimum Design in the Removal of Fluorescence and Shot Noises in Raman Spectrum of Healthy and Damaged Breast Tissues*

Today, data is in all kinds of formats – from traditional databases to hierarchical data stores created by end users, through OLAP systems, text documents, email, measurement data, signal data, video, audio, stock information, and financial transactions, among many others. According to some calculations, 80% of the data of the organizations are not numerical [24]. However, these should also be included in the analysis and decision-making process. Speed designates how quickly data is generated and how fast it must be processed to satisfy demand.

Table 1 Sequential and parallel processing times in suppression of fluorescence and shot noise in Raman spectra of breast tissue

Raman spectra	ANFIS algorithm and moving averages filter	
Biological examples (healthy breast tissue and damaged breast tissue)	Sequential process	Parallel process
1000	40.466077	16.7695
2000	84.093451	32.1250
3000	124.565025	49.9149
4000	166.294112	70.7037
5000	206.913026	81.4252
6000	247.760978	97.4377
7000	300.533240	113.1972
8000	338.862996	142.6557
9000	372.606862	151.0356
10,000	404.099370	169.9889

In this section, we show how we can optimally preprocess high-volume of Raman signals from biological examples (data parallelism) by applying MATLAB multi-core technology [25]. As we have seen, there are many sources of noise that attack the weak Raman signal. In order to achieve material identification, it is essential to have a good signal-to-noise ratio in the Raman spectrum. Currently, there are different methods implemented to combat these imperfections in Raman spectra, experimental methods, such as shifted excitation and computational methods, such as morphological filtering [26] and polynomial algorithms are used to suppress noise from high and low frequency highlighting the advantage of seconds in terms of low cost and ease of implementation; however, the implementation of these methods involves computation time especially when we preprocess large amounts of Raman signals; for this reason, we decided to use Parallel computing with multicore technology to optimize the response time of the preprocessing of large volumes of Raman spectroscopic signals in samples of healthy and damaged breast tissue.

In Table 1, we can observe the sequential and parallel processing time what takes for the suppression of fluorescence and shot noise in Raman spectra of breast tissue using the moving averages filtering to smoothen the signal as a previous step to operations of the developed ANFIS algorithm, which provides a close baseline in the regions where there are Raman bands which are subtracted from the raw Raman spectrum leaving the signal in the base band.

To eliminate the shot noise on signal f, we use a moving average filter with a window size of $N = 7$, guaranteeing smoothening of the signal without damaging the identifying characteristics of the spectrum.

The arithmetic mean in this case is calculated as:

$$\mathrm{MA} = \frac{\sum_{i=1}^{N}(f)}{N} \tag{7}$$

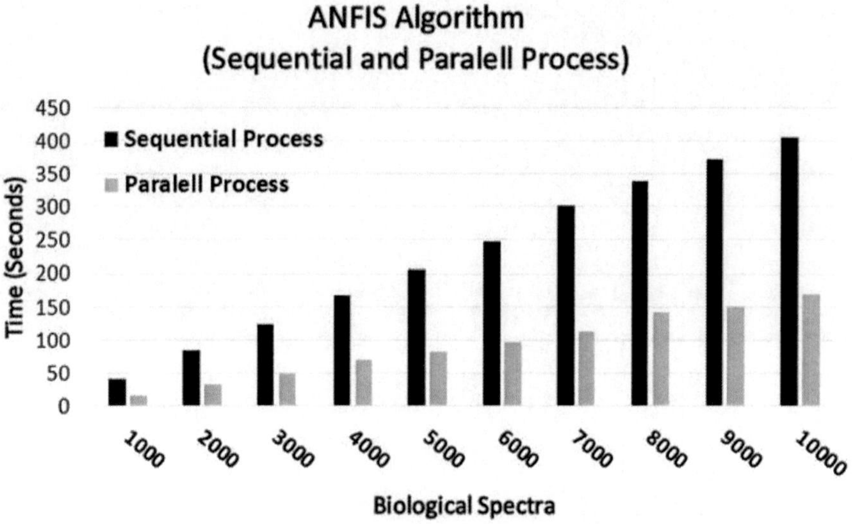

Fig. 11 Sequential and parallel processing time using the ANFIS algorithm to eliminate the fluorescence background and moving averages filtering for high frequency noise (shot noise)

In Eq. (7), N is the base of moving averages. Although there is no specific rule on how to select the bases for moving averages (N), it is recommended that N be large when the behavior of the data is stable over time. Conversely, if the variable shows changing patterns; it is recommended to use a small value of N. In practice, values for N between 2 and 10 are normal.

As we can see in Table 1, we started with 1000 spectra of samples of healthy and damaged breast tissue, we continued with increments of 1000 spectra until we achieve the suppression of fluorescence and shot noise of 10,000 Raman spectra.

In the graph in Fig. 11, we clearly observe that we obtain an improvement in the processing time of the data for the elimination of fluorescence and high frequency noise when we implement the ANFIS algorithm and the filtering of moving averages with multicore technology to the set of biological spectra (data parallelism), we can clearly observe the significant reduction in processing time with a gain of approximately 59.67%.

5 Conclusions

A Raman spectrum is a fingerprint of the material being analyzed since it is composed of (a) Raman scattering (RS), which characterizes the molecular composition of the sample through the position of the Raman peaks described by the wave number; there are also numerous disturbances that are added to the spectrum during the measurement process, such as (b) fluorescence noise and (c) shot noise;

sometimes these are several orders of magnitude greater than the useful signal so that it could be masked, making it difficult to appreciate correctly, for this reason it must be eliminated.

We used an own algorithm based on ANFIS (Adaptive Neuro Fuzzy Inference System) to reveal the fluorescence background of the spectra and the filtering of moving averages to eliminate the shooting noise; both disturbances, causing the masking of the data and the difficult appreciation of its useful content. This preprocessing takes considerable computation time when we process large amounts of Raman spectroscopic signals.

In this work, we have shown that it is possible to optimize the preprocessing time of large volumes of Raman spectroscopic signals in samples of biological materials like healthy and damaged breast tissue through parallel processing that consists of dividing the tasks to be performed in a multicore environment.

This optimized method can have specific applications in the field of medicine or industry since it guarantees to carry out diagnostic and classification applications in a considerably short time.

Acknowledgments The authors thank the Instituto Tecnológico Nacional of Mexico/Instituto Tecnológico de Aguascalientes and the Universidad Central de los Lagos of the Universidad de Guadalajara, to the Centro de Investigaciones en Óptica, Campus Aguascalientes (CIO-Ags.) for supporting this research.

References

1. R.L. Siegel, K.D. Miller, A. Jemal, Cancer statistics, 2015. CA Cancer J. Clin. **65**(1), 5–29 (2015)
2. Y.T. Yeh et al., A rapid and label-free platform for virus capture and identification from clinical samples. Proc. Natl. Acad. Sci. U. S. A. **117**(2), 895–901 (2020)
3. Q. Li, Q. Gao, G. Zhang, Classification for breast cancer diagnosis with Raman spectroscopy. Biomed. Opt. Exp. **5**(7), 2435 (2014)
4. J.C. Martínez Romo, F.J. Luna-Rosas, R. Mendoza-González, A. Padilla-Díaz, M. Mora-González, E. Martínez-Cano, Improving sensitivity and specificity in breast cancer detection using raman spectroscopy and bayesian classification. Spectrosc. Lett. **48**(1), 40–52 (2015)
5. L.A. Austin, S. Osseiran, C.L. Evans, Raman technologies in cancer diagnostics. Analyst **141**(2), 476–503 (2016)
6. M. T. Gebrekidan, C. Knipfer, F. Stelzle, J. Popp, S. Will, A. Braeuer, A shifted-excitation Raman difference spectroscopy (SERDS) evaluation strategy for the efficient isolation of Raman spectra from extreme fluorescence interference, J. Raman Spectrosc, (2016)
7. C.A. Lieber, A.M. Ahadevan-jansen, Automated method for subtraction of fluorescence from biological raman spectra. Appl. Spectrosc. **57**(11), 1363–1367 (2003)
8. J. Zhao, H. Lui, D.I. Mclean, H. Zeng, Automated autofluorescence background subtraction algorithm for biomedical raman spectroscopy. Appl. Spectrosc. **61**(11), 1225–1232 (2007)
9. M.T. Gebrekidan, C. Knipfer, A.S. Braeuer, Vector casting for noise reduction. J. Raman Spectrosc. (2020)
10. F. Javier et al., *Optimal Design in the Removal of Fluorescence and Shot Noise in Raman Spectra from Biological Samples* (2018), pp. 78–84

11. E.D. Übeyli, Adaptive neuro-fuzzy inference system employing wavelet coefficients for detection of ophthalmic arterial disorders. Expert Syst. Appl. **34**(3), 2201–2209 (2008)
12. M. Sugeno, G.T. Kang, Structure identification of fuzzy model. Fuzzy Sets Syst. **28**(1), 15–33 (1988)
13. T. Takagi, M. Sugeno, Derivation of fuzzy control rules from human operator'S control actions. IFAC Proc. Ser. **16**(13), 55–60 (1984)
14. J.-S. R. Jang, C.-T. Sun, and E. Mizutani, Neuro-Fuzzy and Soft Computing: A Computational Approach to Learning and Machine Intelligence. 1997
15. C.C. Soberón-celedón, J.R. Molina-contreras, C. Frausto-reyes, J. Carlos, Removal of fluorescence and shot noises in Raman spectra of biological samples using morphological and moving averages filters. **0869**(3), 14–19 (2016)
16. W. Gao, Q. Kemao, H. Wang, F. Lin, H.S. Seah, Parallel computing for fringe pattern processing: A multicore CPU approach in MATLAB® environment. Opt. Lasers Eng. **47**(11), 1286–1292 (2009)
17. K.E. Shafer-Peltier et al., Raman microspectroscopic model of human breast tissue: Implications for breast cancer diagnosis in vivo. J. Raman Spectrosc. **33**(7), 552–563 (2002)
18. R. Raman, "Resonance Raman and Raman Spectroscopy for Breast Cancer Detection," 2013
19. B. Brozek-Pluska, M. Kopec, J. Surmacki, H. Abramczyk, Raman microspectroscopy of noncancerous and cancerous human breast tissues. Identification and phase transitions of linoleic and oleic acids by Raman low-temperature studies. Analyst **140**(7), 2134–2143 (2015)
20. C.J. Frank, R.L. McCreary, D.C.B. Redd, Raman spectroscopy of normal and diseased human breast tissues. Anal. Chem. **67**(5), 777–783 (1995)
21. F. Javier, et al., PCA and parellel svm to optimize the diagnostic of breast cancer based on raman spectroscopy, **2025**(Who), 1–13 (2017)
22. J. Surmacki, J. Musial, R. Kordek, H. Abramczyk, Raman imaging at biological interfaces: applications in breast cancer diagnosis. Mol. Cancer, 1–12 (2013)
23. B. Brozek-pluska, J. Musial, R. Kordek, and E. Bailo, "Raman Spectroscopy and Imaging: Applications in Human Breast Cancer," 2012
24. V. Prajapati, Big Data Analytics with R and Hadoop, no. 1. 2013
25. U. P. D. E. Cartagena, A. Juan, F. Rodríguez, and E. Autor, "Programación Matlab En Paralelo Sobre Clúster Computacional: Evaluación De Prestaciones," 2010
26. R. P. P. Mª José Tosina Muñoz, Filtro Morfológico, eliminacion de fluorescencia

Re-ranking of Computational Protein–Peptide Docking Solutions with Amino Acid Profiles of Rigid-Body Docking Results

Masahito Ohue

1 Introduction

Protein–peptide interactions involving a globular protein and a flexible linear peptide are important for understanding cellular processes and regulatory pathways; hence, such interactions are common targets for drug discovery [1]. Many recent studies reported the biological functions of short open reading frames-encoded peptides or micropeptides encoded in noncoding RNAs [2–6]. However, many peptide– and protein–peptide interactions remain to be uncovered, which can drastically shift the field of traditional genome biology.

Various protein–peptide docking prediction tools have been developed recently for determination of the structures of protein–peptide complexes [7–16] and reviewed in [17]. Protein–peptide docking involves certain computation steps such as initial conformation sampling, structural refinement, and rescoring, similar to traditional protein–protein docking or protein–ligand docking techniques. Thus, these prediction tools offer broad steps that can be used for a single purpose. CABS-dock [15, 16] is one of the few tools that is capable of predicting a protein–peptide complex in a one-step process based on protein structure and peptide sequence information. Specifically, CABS-dock generates candidate complex structures with $C\alpha$-$C\beta$-side group protein model (CABS model [18])-based replica exchange Monte Carlo dynamics simulations and then performs all-atom modeling by MODELLER [19]. With the rapid increase in the generation and deposition of peptide structure information in public database such as PeptiDB [20], template-

M. Ohue (✉)
Department of Computer Science, School of Computing, Tokyo Institute of Technology, Yokohama City, Kanagawa, Japan
e-mail: ohue@c.titech.ac.jp

H. R. Arabnia et al. (eds.), *Advances in Computer Vision and Computational Biology*, Transactions on Computational Science and Computational Intelligence,
https://doi.org/10.1007/978-3-030-71051-4_58

based prediction is also a powerful tool for protein–peptide docking when the peptide template is identified [7].

Despite the wide array of methods recently developed in the field of protein–protein and ligand–peptide docking, it remains a challenge to effectively achieve protein–peptide docking. For example, the targets of Critical Assessment of PRedicted Interactions (CAPRI), T65, T66, and T67 are very difficult to predict accurately as protein–peptide complexes, resulting in frequent incorrect answers, especially for T65 and T66 [21]. Thus, further attempts at accuracy improvement for such predictions are very important. Despite apparent similarities, compared with the diverse prediction approaches available for protein–protein docking or protein–ligand docking, the field of protein–peptide docking methodology is still in an immature phase [22, 23].

The computational techniques used in protein–protein docking are arguably more important for protein–peptide docking. This is not simply because the peptide chain consists of amino acids (as in a protein), but several protein structure informatics can also be appropriated for protein–peptide docking. Protein–protein docking first developed with a fast Fourier transform-based exhaustive search technique using rigid bodies as one of the elemental technologies; MEGADOCK [24] is an example based on this approach. By considering the structure of a protein as rigid, structural sampling can be achieved over the entire space with a short calculation time. The latest tools (MEGADOCK 4.0 [25] and Hex [26]) are capable of evaluating trillions of conformations in seconds on GPU accelerators, and protein–protein docking tools are used casually. Although the conformations predicted with these tools tend to include many false-positive complexes, the so-called decoy conformations that result from a rigid-body search can be used in reevaluating the predicted conformations [27–29] or provide information for the search direction in redocking [30]. This can expand the application of these tools from predicting a single complex structure to prediction of the post-docking processes.

However, rigid-body sampling is not sufficiently efficient to be used for highly flexible proteins [31]. This is a reasonable outcome considering the basis of "rigid." Therefore, when dealing with flexible proteins, many more false-positive candidates will be generated. Accordingly, this approach has been considered to be difficult to apply to problems such as protein–peptide docking. In this study, we address this problem by incorporating the rigid-body sampling results to the re-ranking of protein–peptide docking solutions. Because sampling with a rigid-body model results in many false positives, we propose the "decoy profile" as the environment in which the binding site is favored by rigid-body samples. We then developed a new protein–peptide docking re-ranking method with the decoy profile. The method can be performed with very light computation requirements. Moreover, since only rigid-body docking sampling is used, the method does not need the training datasets of protein–peptide complex structures that are required with machine learning-based methods.

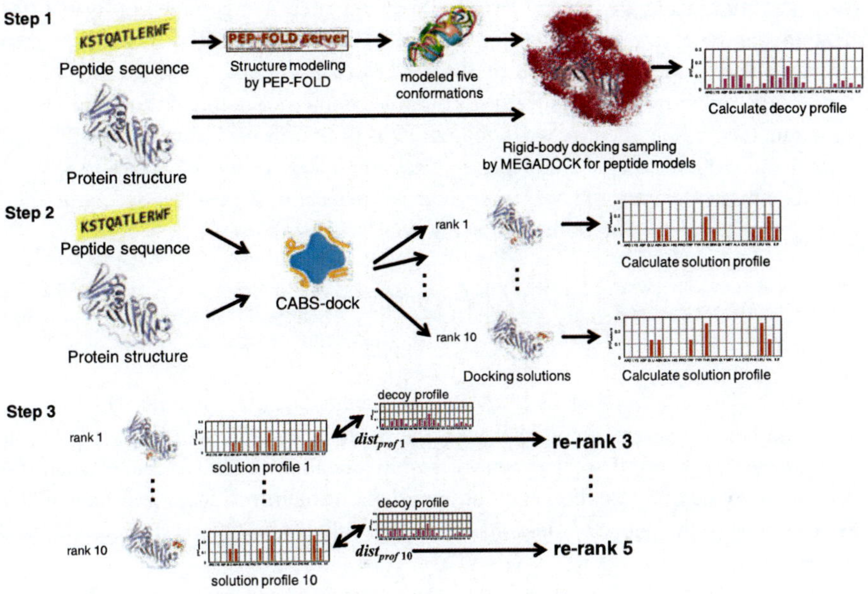

Fig. 1 Overview of the proposed method

2 Materials and Methods

2.1 *Protein–Peptide Docking Re-ranking*

An overview of the proposed method is presented in Fig. 1. The purpose of protein–peptide docking is to predict the complex structure based on an input protein tertiary structure and a peptide sequence.

In the proposed method, a vector of the relative frequencies of the number of protein residues with which the peptide makes contact (solution profile) is obtained for the generated protein–peptide complex solution. In addition, we independently obtain the residue contact profile of the decoys (decoy profile) among a large number of rigid-body docking samples to provide a clue for estimating the peptide binding preference. In other words, the decoy profile attempts to pseudo-estimate the ideal interaction surface environment for peptide binding to the target protein. Finally, the similarity between the solution profile and the decoy profile is determined by the Euclidean distance. A better solution is considered as one in which the solution profile is the closest to the decoy profile, and then the re-ranking process is performed accordingly.

The proposed method is conducted by the following three steps:

Step 1: calculate the decoy profile,
Step 2: calculate the solution profile, and
Step 3: calculate the profile–profile distance and re-rank.

Step 1: Calculating the Decoy Profile We generated five peptide conformations from the input peptide sequence using the PEP-FOLD server [32]. The input protein structure and modeled peptide structures were then docked using MEGADOCK rigid-body docking software [25] to sample numerous peptide docking poses simultaneously. Specifically, we sampled 3600 poses for each peptide model, and a total of $3600 \times 5 = 18{,}000$ poses were generated using MEGADOCK. The contact amino acid profile was then determined using these "decoy" structures (decoy profile) according to the following equation:

$$\mathbf{prof}_{decoys} = \left(\frac{\sum_{\text{decoy}} n_{con,i}}{\sum_{\text{decoy}} N_{con}} \right)_{i \in \text{aa}} \tag{1}$$

where $n_{con,i}$ is the number of residues i in contact with the peptide, N_{con} is the total number of residues in contact with the peptide, and $i \in$ aa represents the 20 standard amino acids. The judgment of residue–peptide contact is made when the distance between any of the heavy atoms of the protein residue i and any of the heavy atoms of the peptide is less than 4 Å. The values of $n_{con,i}$ and N_{con} are then incremented.

Step 2: Calculating the Solution Profile To obtain solutions of the protein–peptide complex, the following vector (solution profile) was calculated:

$$\mathbf{prof}_{solution_k} = \left(\frac{n_{con,i}}{N_{con}} \right)_{i \in \text{aa}} \tag{2}$$

where $n_{con,i}$ and N_{con} are defined as above for the decoy profile calculation.

Although some residues can more easily make contact, whereas others will be less able to make contact due to the difference in the number of amino acids in a protein, normalization by the relative frequency of amino acids in a protein was not necessary in this case because the profiles were only compared for the same protein–peptide target.

In this study, the solutions of the protein–peptide complex were generated by CABS-dock [16]. We ran CABS-dock with default settings using the target peptide sequence and protein structure and then calculated the profiles of each of the 10 solutions generated by CABS-dock.

Step 3: Calculating the Profile–Profile Distance and Re-ranking The profile–profile distance $dist_{prof}$ between the decoy profile and each solution profile was calculated as follows:

$$dist_{prof_k} = \left\| \mathbf{prof}_{solution_k} - \mathbf{prof}_{decoys} \right\| \quad (k = 1, \ldots, 10) \tag{3}$$

The solutions with smaller $dist_{prof_k}$ values were then re-ranked so that they come out on top.

Table 1 Protein–peptide complexes

PDB ID	Protein	Peptide
1PRM	c-Src tyrosine kinase SH3 domain	Proline-rich ligand PLR1
1X2R	Kelch-like ECH-associated protein 1	Nrf2/Neh2 peptide
1RXZ	DNA polymerase sliding clamp	PCNA-binding motif
2FMF	Chemotaxis protein CheY	C-terminal 15-mer helix of CheZ

Table 2 Peptide sequences

PDB ID	Peptide Sequence	# Peptide residues
1PRM	AFAPPLPRR	9
1X2R	LDEETGEFL	9
1RXZ	KSTQATLERWF	11
2FMF	QDQVDDLLDSLGF	13

2.2 *Dataset*

Protein–Peptide Complex Dataset Among the 10 protein–peptide complexes in the dataset generated by Dagliyan et al. [14], those with 9 or more residues were selected for use in this study. Tables 1 and 2 show the details of the dataset. The number of peptide residues ranged from 9 to 13; all hydrogen atoms and HETATM records in the PDB structure data were deleted. Only 1PRM was a nuclear magnetic resonance (NMR) structure. For the NMR structure, only the coordinates of the first state were used for the input structure.

Protein–Peptide Docking Solutions The holo (bound) state of the protein structure was obtained as a PDB file, and the sequence information of the peptide was input to CABS-dock to obtain the docking solutions. The peptide secondary structure information was not used, and the number of simulation cycles was set to 50, which is the default parameter for CABS-dock.

Rigid-Body Docking Decoys The sequence information of each peptide was input into PEP-FOLD, resulting in five peptide conformations for each peptide. The target protein structure and peptide conformations were then entered into MEGADOCK version 4.0.2 to obtain 3600 rigid-body docking solutions (decoys) per peptide conformation for a total of 18,000 decoys. The protein PDB file was set to `-R` and the peptide PDB file was set to `-L` using the `-N 3600` option; default parameters were used for the other settings of MEGADOCK.

2.3 *Evaluation of Prediction Performance*

Evaluation of the Predicted Structure The docking solution was evaluated using the all-heavy-atom root mean square deviation (RMSD) between the native peptide structure and the docking solution peptide when the protein structure was superimposed. We defined a near-native solution (correct answer) when the RMSD was less than 10 Å. The RMSD was calculated using ProDy library [33].

Solution Ranking Evaluation The rankings of the 10 predicted structures output by CABS-dock with those obtained after re-ranking were compared using the proposed method. The area under the receiver operating characteristics curve (AUC), calculated from the rank position of the near-native solution (Eq. (4)), was also used to compare the rankings as follows:

$$\mathrm{AUC} = 1 - \frac{\sum_{i=1}^{n} r_i}{n(N-n)} + \frac{n+1}{2(N-n)} \tag{4}$$

where n is the number of near-native solutions, N is the number of all solutions (= 10), and r_i is the rank of each near-native solution. For example, if the 2nd- and 4th-ranked docking solutions were found to be near-native among the 10 solutions, then $n = 2$, $N = 10$, $r_1 = 2$, and $r_2 = 4$; thus, $\mathrm{AUC} = 1 - \frac{2+4}{2\cdot(10-2)} + \frac{2+1}{2\cdot(10-2)} = 0.8125$. Note that in this study, the focus was on the top 10 solutions of CABS-dock, and the AUC value for 10 solutions will be different from the measure used for common docking results such as those dealing with thousands of candidates. For example, a result of $n = 1, N = 10$, and $r_1 = 8$ that yields a low value of AUC = 0.222 is considered to be a generally good result for protein–peptide docking. In this study, the AUC value was simply used as an indicator to check whether the ranking had been improved by our method.

3 Results and Discussion

3.1 CABS-Dock and Re-ranking Results

Table 3 shows the RMSD, rank, and ranking change based on the proposed method, along with the AUC values of the docking solutions for CABS-dock. Protein–peptide docking with CABS-dock generated near-native solutions in the top rank with the exception of 1PRM.

In addition, when considering the best near-native solution rankings for re-ranks, 1RXZ moved down a rank from first to second but otherwise did not deteriorate. Overall, 1PRM, which had no near-native solution at #1, had the best near-native solution rank improvement by moving up from position 8 to position 6.

With respect to the ranking of near-native solutions based on AUC values, 1RXZ and 2FMF showed a slight deterioration in ranking, whereas 1PRM and 1X2R showed good improvement. In particular, the enrichment of near-native solutions for 1X2R improved significantly. The improved peptides were all 9-mer, suggesting that the effect of re-ranking may be higher when the number of residues is less than 10. However, this may also be related to the performance of the PEP-FOLD

Table 3 Results of CABS-dock solutions and re-ranking by the proposed method. Bold values represent near-native solutions

	1PRM		1X2R		1RXZ		2FMF	
Rank	RMSD (Å)	Re-rank	RMSD (Å)	Re-rank	RMSD (Å)	Re-rank	RMSD (Å)	Re-rank
1	24.40	8	**9.83**	6	**5.38**	3	**7.80**	3
2	19.79	7	**8.21**	5	**5.86**	2	**7.74**	2
3	17.70	2	31.97	10	25.53	6	**8.55**	1
4	14.68	10	39.26	3	26.95	8	**8.30**	4
5	19.31	3	20.35	7	24.75	4	20.91	7
6	16.71	9	37.43	9	33.30	7	12.91	5
7	16.06	1	**7.22**	1	24.83	1	33.18	10
8	**6.54**	6	**9.00**	2	25.58	9	**8.93**	9
9	18.15	4	**8.81**	4	25.75	10	33.38	6
10	23.76	5	**8.45**	8	35.09	5	28.21	8
AUC	0.222	0.444	0.333	0.792	1.000	0.875	0.880	0.840

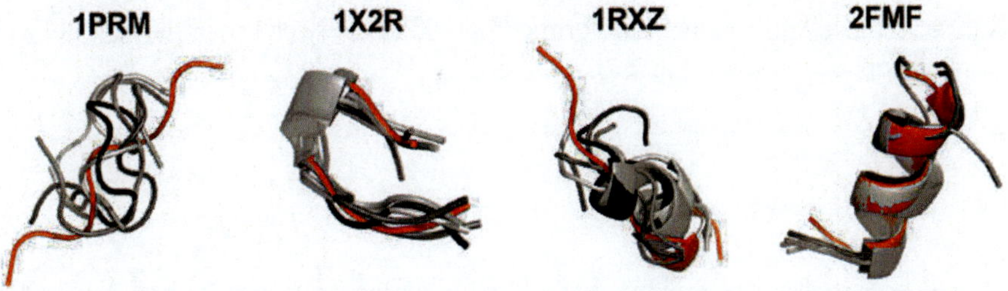

Fig. 2 PEP-FOLD conformation sampling results. Red peptides represent the binding form obtained from the PDB complex, and gray peptides represent the results from PEP-FOLD sampling

conformation sampling. Figure 2 shows the sampling results of PEP-FOLD. For the most successful case (1X2R), the conformation sampling of peptides by PEP-FOLD yielded a structure close to that of the native form. Conversely, no peptide conformation similar to the native form was obtained for 1PRM. Thus, it is likely that the performance of conformation sampling affects the re-ranking according to the decoy profile.

3.2 *Example of Predicted Structures*

The native structure and some solutions for 1X2R are shown in Fig. 3. As shown in Fig. 3a, we can confirm that the solutions located around the correct binding site have RMSDs less than 10 Å. Similarly, solutions with RMSDs greater than 10 Å bound at completely different sites than the correct site. The green-colored peptide in Fig. 3, which ranked at the top after re-ranking, was at a position and orientation

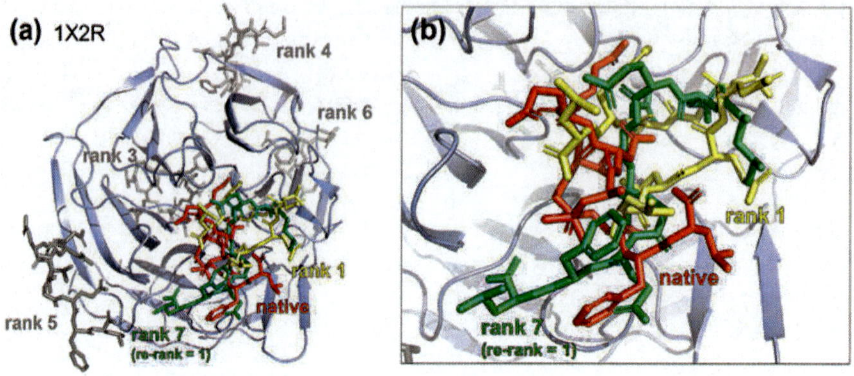

Fig. 3 Results of 1X2R peptide docking and re-ranking. (**a**) Overall image of the protein, and (**b**) enlarged image of the area around the native binding site

closer to those of the native-like form compared to the structure of the original top-ranked peptide (yellow) (Fig. 3b).

4 Conclusion

We have proposed a re-ranking method using amino acid residue contact information from rigid-body docking results to improve protein–peptide docking calculations. Application of the proposed method to four protein–peptide docking solution sets showed general improvement in the ranking of near-native solutions with our re-ranking approach. As the number of peptide residues increased, the degrees of freedom increased and improvement became generally more difficult; however, the re-ranking prevented worsening predictions.

Peptides have received particular attention in recent years as an important drug discovery modality. Therefore, accurate prediction of the modes of peptide binding to their target proteins will lead to accelerated peptide drug discovery. Although some difficulties remain that need to be overcome owing to the low number of peptide complexes in the PDB at present, development of a dataset for protein–peptide docking is also currently underway [34]. Although archive sets of docking solutions (Dockground [35] and ZLAB decoy set [36]) are available in the field of protein–protein docking, no such equivalent resource is available in the field of protein–peptide docking. The construction of a large-scale archive set of protein–peptide docking solutions and the development and exhaustive evaluation of methods based on these solutions are needed to accelerate peptide drug discovery as an important challenge to undertake.

Acknowledgments This work was supported in part by KAKENHI (grant nos. 15K16081, 18K18149, and 20H04280) from the Japan Society for the Promotion of Science (JSPS) and the Mizuho Foundation for the Promotion of Sciences.

References

1. M. Rubinstein, M.Y. Niv, Peptidic modulators of protein-protein interactions: progress and challenges in computational design. Biopolymers **91**(7), 505–513 (2009). https://doi.org/10.1002/bip.21164
2. S.A. Slavoff, A.J. Mitchell, A.G. Schwaid, et al., Peptidomic discovery of short open reading frame-encoded peptides in human cells. Nat. Chem. Biol. **9**(1), 59–64 (2013). https://doi.org/10.1038/nchembio.1120
3. S.J. Andrews, J.A. Rothnagel, Emerging evidence for functional peptides encoded by short open reading frames. Nat. Rev. Genet. **15**(3), 193–204 (2014). https://doi.org/10.1038/nrg3520
4. J. Ma, C.C. Ward, I. Jungreis, et al., Discovery of human sORF-encoded polypeptides (SEPs) in cell lines and tissue. J. Proteome Res. **13**(3), 1757–1765 (2014). https://doi.org/10.1021/pr401280w
5. S.A. Slavoff, J. Heo, B.A. Budnik, et al., Human short open reading frame (sORF)-encoded polypeptide that stimulates DNA end joining. J. Biol. Chem. **289**(16), 10950–10957 (2014). https://doi.org/10.1074/jbc.C113.533968
6. D.M. Anderson, K.M. Anderson, C.-L. Chang, et al., A micropeptide encoded by a putative long noncoding RNA regulates muscle performance. Cell **160**(4), 595–606 (2015). https://doi.org/10.1016/j.cell.2015.01.009
7. H. Lee, L. Heo, M.S. Lee, et al., GalaxyPepDock: a protein–peptide docking tool based on interaction similarity and energy optimization. Nucl. Acids Res. **43**(W1), W431–W435 (2015). https://doi.org/10.1093/nar/gkv495
8. N. London, B. Raveh, E. Cohen, et al., Rosetta FlexPepDock web server-high resolution modeling of peptide-protein interactions. Nucl. Acids Res. **39**(suppl), W249–W253 (2011). https://doi.org/10.1093/nar/gkr431
9. I. Antes, DynaDock: a new molecular dynamics-based algorithm for protein–peptide docking including receptor flexibility. Proteins Struct. Funct. Bioinform. **78**(5), 1084–1104 (2010). https://doi.org/10.1002/prot.22629
10. G.M. Morris, R. Huey, W. Lindstrom, et al., AutoDock4 and AutoDockTools4: automated docking with selective receptor flexibility. J. Comput. Chem. **30**(16):2785–2791 (2009). https://doi.org/10.1002/jcc.21256
11. O. Trott, A.J. Olson, AutoDock Vina: improving the speed and accuracy of docking with a new scoring function, efficient optimization, and multithreading. J. Comput. Chem. **31**(2), 455–461 (2010). https://doi.org/10.1002/jcc.21334
12. M. Trellet, A.S.J. Melquiond, A.M.J.J. Bonvin, A unified conformational selection and induced fit approach to protein–peptide docking. PLoS One **8**(3), e58769 (2013). https://doi.org/10.1371/journal.pone.0058769
13. M. Trellet, A.S.J. Melquiond, A.M.J.J. Bonvin, Information-driven modeling of protein–peptide complexes. Methods Mol. Biol. **1268**, 221–239 (2015). https://doi.org/10.1007/978-1-4939-2285-7_10
14. O. Dagliyan, E.A. Proctor, K.M. D'Auria, et al., Structural and dynamic determinants of protein–peptide recognition. Structure **19**(12), 1837–1845 (2011). https://doi.org/10.1016/j.str.2011.09.014
15. M. Blaszczyk, M. Kurcinski, M. Kouza, et al., Modeling of protein–peptide interactions using the CABS-Dock web server for binding site search and flexible docking. Methods **93**, 72–83 (2016). https://doi.org/10.1016/j.ymeth.2015.07.004

16. M. Kurcinski, M. Jamroz, M. Blaszczyk, et al., CABS-Dock web server for the flexible docking of peptides to proteins without prior knowledge of the binding site. Nucl. Acids Res. **43**(W1), W419–W424 (2015). https://doi.org/10.1093/nar/gkv456
17. M. Ciemny, M. Kurcinski, K. Kamel, et al., Protein–peptide docking: opportunities and challenges. Drug Discov. Today **23**(8), 1530–1537 (2018). https://doi.org/10.1016/j.drudis.2018.05.006
18. A. Kolinski, Protein modeling and structure prediction with a reduced representation. Acta Biochim. Pol. **51**(2), 349–371 (2004).
19. N. Eswar, B. Webb, M.A. Marti-Renom, et al., Comparative protein structure modeling using MODELLER, in *Current Protocols in Protein Science* (Wiley, Hoboken, 2007)
20. N. London, D. Movshovitz-Attias, O. Schueler-Furman, The structural basis of peptide-protein binding strategies. Structure **18**(2), 188–199 (2010). https://doi.org/10.1016/j.str.2009.11.012
21. CAPRI ROUND 29 (2020). http://www.ebi.ac.uk/msd-srv/capri/round29/round29.html. Last accessed 9 May 2020
22. S.-Y. Huang, Search strategies and evaluation in protein–protein docking: principles, advances and challenges. Drug Discov. Today **19**(8), 1081–1096 (2014). https://doi.org/10.1016/j.drudis.2014.02.005
23. M.A. Khamis, W. Gomaa, W.F. Ahmed, Machine learning in computational docking. Artif. Intell. Med. **63**(3), 135–152 (2015). https://doi.org/10.1016/j.artmed.2015.02.002
24. M. Ohue, Y. Matsuzaki, N. Uchikoga, et al., MEGADOCK: an all-to-all protein-protein interaction prediction system using tertiary structure data. Protein Pept. Lett. **21**(8), 766–778 (2014). https://doi.org/10.2174/09298665113209990050
25. M. Ohue, T. Shimoda, S. Suzuki, et al., MEGADOCK 4.0: an ultra-high-performance protein-protein docking software for heterogeneous supercomputers. Bioinformatics **30**(22), 3281–3283 (2014). https://doi.org/10.1093/bioinformatics/btu532
26. D.W. Ritchie, V. Venkatraman, Ultra-fast FFT protein docking on graphics processors. Bioinformatics **26**(19), 2398–2405 (2010). https://doi.org/10.1093/bioinformatics/btq444
27. G.-Y. Chuang, D. Kozakov, R. Brenke, et al., DARS (decoys as the reference state) potentials for protein-protein docking. Biophys. J. **95**(9), 4217–4227 (2018). https://doi.org/10.1529/biophysj.108.135814
28. E. Chermak, A. Petta, L. Serra, et al., CONSRANK: a server for the analysis, comparison and ranking of docking models based on inter-residue contacts. Bioinformatics **31**(9), 1481–1483 (2015). https://doi.org/10.1093/bioinformatics/btu837
29. G. Launay, M. Ohue, J.P. Santero, et al., Rescoring ensembles of protein-protein docking poses using consensus approaches. bioRxiv 2020.04.24.059469 (2020). https://doi.org/10.1101/2020.04.24.059469
30. N. Uchikoga, Y. Matsuzaki, M. Ohue, et al., Re-docking scheme for generating near-native protein complexes by assembling residue interaction fingerprints. PLoS ONE **8**(7), e69365 (2013). https://doi.org/10.1371/journal.pone.0069365
31. J. Janin, Protein–protein docking tested in blind predictions: the CAPRI experiment. Mol. Biosyst. **6**(12), 2351 (2010). https://doi.org/10.1039/c005060c
32. Y. Shen, J. Maupetit, P. Derreumaux, et al., Improved PEP-FOLD approach for peptide and miniprotein structure prediction. J. Chem. Theory Comput. **10**, 4745–4758 (2014). https://doi.org/10.1021/ct500592m
33. A., Bakan, L.M. Meireles, I. Bahar, ProDy: protein dynamics inferred from theory and experiments. Bioinformatics **27**(11), 1575–1577 (2011). https://doi.org/10.1093/bioinformatics/btr168
34. A.S. Hauser, B. Windshügel, LEADS-PEP: a benchmark data set for assessment of peptide docking performance. J. Chem. Inf. Model. **56**(1), 188–200 (2016). https://doi.org/10.1021/acs.jcim.5b00234
35. S. Liu, Y. Gao, I.A. Vakser, Dockground protein-protein docking decoy set. Bioinformatics **24**, 2634–2635 (2008). https://doi.org/10.1093/bioinformatics/btn497
36. ZLAB decoy sets (2020). https://zlab.umassmed.edu/zdock/decoys.shtml. Accessed 9 May 2020

Structural Exploration of Rift Valley Fever Virus L Protein Domain in Implicit and Explicit Solvents by Molecular Dynamics

Gideon K. Gogovi

1 Introduction

The Rift valley fever virus (RVFV) is an arbovirus in the Bunyavirales order, Phenuiviridae family, and Phlebovirus genus. It was first discovered in 1931 in the Great Rift Valley of Kenya, East Africa [1]. Since that time, it has caused periodic outbreaks in human and livestock populations throughout Africa and has even spread into the Arabian Peninsula. The virus is vectored by mosquitoes, and, as such, outbreaks tend to follow periods of heavy rainfall that increase significantly mosquito populations [1]. The virus infects ruminants and pseudoruminants leading to abortions in pregnant animals and high mortality among young animals. It is a negative-sense RNA virus that contains three segments of viral RNA, the S, M, and L segments and can also be transmitted to humans causing febrile illness with the possibility for severe disease [2]. The structure of the RVFV L protein, which is made up of a sequence of 2092 amino acids, has a flexible termini of about 200 amino acids each and a high proportion of helical regions [3]. The structure of the C-terminal 117 amino acid-long domain of the RVFV L protein as modeled using X-ray crystallography shows high similarity to the influenza virus PB2 cap-binding domain and the putative non-functional cap-binding domain of reptarenaviruses [4].

The interest of investigating the behavior of peptides, polypeptides, or proteins in solvent environments has grown rapidly in recent years and now constitutes a wide literature composed of thousands of research articles. Notably, Guo and Mei [5] studied the solvation effect on the structure and folding dynamics of a small peptide, nonstructural protein 4B (NS4B) H2 in both pure water and water/2,2,2-Trifluoroethanol (TFE) cosolvent in both explicit and implicit solvents. In this study,

G. K. Gogovi (✉)
Department of Computational and Data Sciences, George Mason University, Fairfax, VA, USA
e-mail: ggogovi@gmu.edu

H. R. Arabnia et al. (eds.), *Advances in Computer Vision and Computational Biology*, Transactions on Computational Science and Computational Intelligence,
https://doi.org/10.1007/978-3-030-71051-4_59

the force field parameters for water are taken from the TIP3P water model, and those for TFE generated from the general AMBER force field (GAFF).

The distribution of solvent molecules around the peptide indicated that folding is triggered by the aggregation of TFE on the peptide surface, but in pure water it undergoes a large structural deformation. Exploration of the effects of different pHs on the structural characteristics of α-syn12 dimer using temperature replica exchange molecular dynamics (T-REMD) simulations in explicit solvent shows that the free energy surfaces contain ten highly populated regions at physiological pH, while there are only three highly populated regions contained at acidic pH [5].

A study of free energy of peptide unfolding in vacuum using the end-to-end distance of reaction coordinate [6] by simulating deca-alanine (Ala_{10}) were also performed using the 104-atom compact helical model used by Park et al. [7]. Although sufficient in vacuum, the study showed that end-to-end distance is incapable of capturing the full complexity of deca-alanine folding in water. Instead, the a-helical content was used as a second reaction coordinate, and this led to the deduction of a more descriptive free energy landscape.

The amphiphilic peptide of the triacylglycerol lipase, which plays a critical role in guarding the gate for ligand access, was also studied by Nellas et al. [8] by comparing the conformations of this peptide at several water–oil interfaces and in protein environments using atomistic simulations with explicit solvents. In the oil-containing solvents, this peptide was found to able to retain a folded structure. However, when the peptide is immersed in a low-polarity solvent environment, it exhibits a "coalesced" helix structure, which has both α-helix and 3_{10}-helix components.

The structural stability and preference of a protein are highly sensitive to the its accommodating environment. Solution pH is one of the most important environmental factors that affects the structure and dynamics of proteins [9, 10]. This work seeks to study the behavior of the functional cap-binding domain in RVFV in the presence of different water models. Solvents influence protein structure to a great extent.

In this work, extensive molecular dynamics simulation studies of RVFV L protein domain in five different water models are conducted to understand the solvent effect on the protein structure and dynamics. The well-known AMBER 18 [11] package with the ff14SB force field [12] is used for the simulations. Even with several perspectives and results from laboratory experiments on different proteins, it is important to have a visual understanding of the dynamics of protein structure and changes in different solvent environments. This requires understanding of the dynamics at a molecular level, which can be achieved with molecular dynamics simulation.

Effect of solvents on the protein structure due to protein–solvent interaction has been widely studied with experimental and computational techniques (Fig. 1). However, molecular-level understanding of protein structural behaviors in the presence of some simple solvents is still not fully understood. This work focuses on detailed molecular dynamics simulations of solvent effect on a functional cap-binding domain of Rift valley fever virus (RVFV) L protein in different water

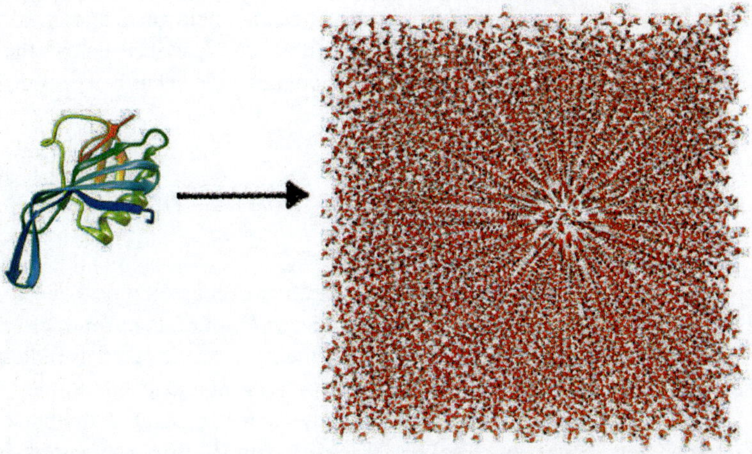

Fig. 1 Initial conformation of system. RVFV L protein domain placed in a cubic periodic box

models and also in implicit solvent in order to well understand the structural and dynamical behaviors of the L protein domain. In order to achieve this, several structural and dynamic properties are presented and conclusions drawn.

The chapter is organized as follows. Section 2 describes the methods used including the computational setups and details of the simulations including the force fields used. Section 3 contains our results and discussions from the simulation process. The conclusions of this chapter are presented in Sect. 4.

2 Methods

2.1 Details of the Simulations

Molecular dynamics (MD) simulations of a functional cap-binding domain in Rift valley fever virus L protein in implicit and explicit solvents were carried out using the AMBER 18 package with the ff14SB force field [12]. Five different water models, namely, TIP3P, TIP4P, OPC, SPC/E, and SPCE/Fw [14–17] were adopted as the aqueous media for the simulations with 10521 molecules for the explicit solvent. Before solvating the peptide in the different water models, an NVT MD simulation for 1 ns was performed to thermalize the solvents in periodic boxes of size 72.5 Å per side with a cutoff distance of 12 Å and a time step of 1 fs after an energy minimization. This was followed by an equilibration with NPT simulation for 40 ns with a time step of 2 fs using velocity rescale thermostat [18] and a pressure of 1 bar with the Berendsen barostat [19] for the pressure correction. Another 1 ns NVT was performed after the NPT. The densities of the solvents were obtained from the NPT simulations (see Sect. 3). Finally, production runs along 20 ns for each solvent box at the respective equilibrium densities that maintained a temperature of $T = 298\_2$ K was perform with NVE ensemble. As described below, the NVE simulations are used for calculation of the solvent energies and their self-diffusion coefficients computed from

$$D = \frac{1}{6t}\frac{1}{m}\sum_{k=1}^{m}\frac{1}{N}\sum_{i=1}^{N}(\mathbf{r}_i(t) - \mathbf{r}_i(t_{0k}))^2 + D_{PBC} \tag{1}$$

where $\mathbf{r}_i$ is the position of the ith molecule's center of mass at time t and N is the number of molecules in the solvent. Each NVE run is split into m time series, each starting from a reference position $\mathbf{r}_i(t_{0k})$, and their average is taken as indicated in Eq. 1. The last term is the correction due to the periodic boundary conditions (PBCs) [20], $D_{PBC} = \frac{2{:}837297 k_B T}{6\pi\eta L}$, with k_B being Boltzmann's constant, T temperature, L computational box length, and η solvent viscosity. The viscosity value is taken from experiment at 298 K: $\eta = 0.8937$ mPa s [21].

The next step is the preparation of systems with the RVFV L protein peptide, solvated in each of the different water models. The starting coordinates of the peptide were taken from the X-ray crystallographic structure (PDB ID: 6QHG) [4]. This peptide is made up of 117 amino acids making up a total of 1849 atoms including the hydrogen atoms. For the explicit solvent simulations, the visualization and analysis package, chimera [13], was used to place the RVFV L protein peptide in a cubic periodic box of size 72.5 Å per side. Energy minimization was performed using the steepest descent method followed by conjugate gradient to remove possible clashes between atoms that may be too close. The cutoff distance was increased to 16 Å after the introduction of the peptide. Position restraints were used on heavy atoms during annealing, when the system was gradually heated from $T = 0$ K to $T = 293.15$ K in 50 ps with periodic boundary conditions.

The systems were thermalized again for 100 ns at a constant volume and a temperature of $T = 293.15$ K before equilibration with NVT ensemble for another 100 ns at the same temperature via the Langevin thermostat with a collision frequency of 5 ps^{-1} and a time step of 1 fs. Ewald sums are used in all calculations for the long-range electrostatics within the particle mesh implementation (PME) [22]. Finally, using the generated ff14SB force field parameters and the AMBER package, another simulation of 300 ns NVT molecular dynamics was performed for the peptide using the generalized Born model for implicit solvent model [23] at $T = 293.15$ K with a dielectric constant, $\varepsilon = 78.5$. Energy minimization was performed using the steepest descent method followed by conjugate gradient to relax the system. Position restraints were again used on heavy atoms during annealing, when the system was gradually heated from $T = 0$ K to $T = 293.15$ K in 50 ps.

Along the MD simulations, the energetics and several structural properties of the peptide such as the end-to-end distance R_{ee}, radius of gyration

$$R_g^2 = \sum_{i=1}^{N} (\mathbf{r}_i - \mathbf{r}_{cm})^2 / N \tag{2}$$

and the hydrodynamic radius

$$\frac{1}{R_{hyd}} = \frac{1}{N^2} \sum_{i=1}^{N-1} \sum_{j>i}^{N} \frac{1}{r_{ij}} \tag{3}$$

are examined, where $\mathbf{r}_i$ are atomic position vectors referred to the peptide center of mass, $\mathbf{r}_{cm}$ is the center of mass position vector, r_{ij} are distances between atoms i and j, and N is the number of atoms in the peptide. Other properties examined are the root-mean-square deviation, $RMSD$ with reference to the starting structure coordinates, and the solvent-accessible surface area ($SASA$).

The $SASA$ is one measure of protein behavior that is governed by the interactions or non-interactions of hydrophobic and hydrophilic amino acids with water [24]. The solvent molecules create a surface tension near the protein–solvent interface which affects protein dynamics and structure. Because of this, a good solvent model is expected to reproduce the SASA. This is used as a metric of comparison between the different water models used in the study. The Linear Combinations of Pairwise Overlaps (LCPO) method [25] is used for approximating the SASA.

LCPO calculates the SASA of each atom by estimating the overlap between the atom and neighboring atoms. The more a protein atom is overlapped by other protein atoms, the less the atom is exposed to the solvent. LCPO defines the SASA of an atom with four terms:

$$\begin{aligned} A_i = {} & P_1 S_i + P_2 \sum_{j \in N(i)} A_{ij} + P_3 \sum_{\substack{j,k \in N(i) \\ k \in N(j) \\ k \neq j}} A_{jk} \\ & + P_4 \sum_{j \in N(i)} A_{ij} \sum_{\substack{k \in N(i) \\ k \in N(j) \\ k \neq j}} A_{jk} \end{aligned} \tag{4}$$

where the overlap between spheres i and j is

$$A_{ij} = \pi R_i [2R_i - r_{ij} - (1/r_{ij})(R_i^2 - R_j^2)]$$

The parameters $P1$, $P2$, $P3$, and $P4$ are parameterized for different atom types. The first term involves the surface area of the atom before overlap, $S_i = 4\pi R_i^2$, where R is the atomic radius (i.e., vdW radius plus probe radius of 1.4 Å). The second term estimates the total overlaps of all neighboring ($j \in N(i)$ means any atom j for which $r_{ij} < R_i + R_j$) atoms with atom i. The third term is the sum of overlaps of i's neighbors with each other. The more i's neighbors overlap each other, the more they over subtracted surface area in the second term. The fourth term is a further correction for multiple overlaps. Each overlap of j with i is weighted by how much j is overlapped with all mutual neighbors k.

Along with the potential energy of the peptide calculated, the interaction energy between the solvent and the solute molecule is calculated with the formula

$$E_{\text{Int}} = E_{\text{Sys}} - (E_{\text{solvent}} + E_{\text{peptide}}) \tag{5}$$

where E_{Sys} is the energy of the whole system, E_{solvent} is the energy of the solvent component of the system, and E_{peptide} is the energy of the peptide. The results of these simulations are given in Sect. 3.

3 Results and Discussion

For the RVFV L protein peptide, we investigated the behavior of sequence of 117 amino acids in the C-terminal explicitly in five water models and also in an implicit solvent environment using the generalized Born (GB) model by setting the dielectric constant to match experimental values. All methods used in the simulations are described in detail in Sect. 2, while the results obtained from each of the various steps in this workflow are presented below.

3.1 Properties of All-Atom MD-Simulated Solvents

Table 1 presents comparison of some properties calculated from the MD simulations to experiment and other simulations. It can be seen that the results are in good agreement with other simulations and also with experiment. This tells how good the model potential used in this work is representing experiment.

3.2 Analysis of Dictionary of Secondary Structures of Proteins (DSSP)

α-helices, β-sheets, and turns are the common secondary structures in proteins with the common element of most of these structures being the presence of characteristic hydrogen bonds. Because their backbone ϕ and ψ angles repeat, helices are classified as repetitive secondary structure. Conversely, if the backbone dihedral angle pairs are the same for each residue, the resulting conformation will assume a helical conformation about some axis in space. Helices were often designated by the number of residues per helical turn and the number of atoms in

Table 1 Solvent properties compared to experiment and other simulations: potential energy (PE), density (ρ), self-diffusion coefficient (D), and temperature (T)

Property	TIP3P	TIP4P	SPC/E	SPC/Fw	OPC
This work: PE kJ/mol	−40.08 ± 0.03	−31.09 ± 0.03	−46.78 ± 0.03	−45.32 ± 0.03	−38.57 ± 0.03
Other works: PE* kJ/mol	−39.8 ± 0.08 [26]	−41.8 [27]	−45.4 ± 0.03 [26]	–	–
This work: ρ g/cm^3	0.985 ± 0.004	0.993 ± 0.004	0.998 ± 0.004	0.992 ± 0.003	0.996 ± 0.004
Other works: ρ* g/cm^3	0.998 [26]	1.001 [28]	0.998 [26]	1.012± 0.016 [17]	0.997 ± 0.001 [15]
This work: D ($\times 10^{-5}$cm^2/s)	5.8798 ± 0.0009	3.7466 ± 0.0007	2.7159 ± 0.0006	3.2230 ± 0.0004	2.3527 ± 0.0004
Other works: D* ($\times 10^{-5}$cm^2/s)	5.9 [26] ± 0.09	3.9 [28]	2.8 ± 0.06 [26]	2.32 ± 0.05 [17]	2.3 ± 0.02 [15]
This work: T K	298.16 ± 2	298.04 ± 1	298.13 ± 2	298.02 ± 1	298.51 ± 1
Other works: T* K	299.2 ± 1 [26]	298.15 [27]	298.2 ± 1 [26]	301 ± 1 [17]	298.16 [15]

Expt. [14, 29, 30]: PE=−41.5 kJ/mol, ρ = 0.997 g/cm^3, D = 2.3$\times 10^{-5}$cm^2/s, 298.15 K one hydrogen-bonded ring[31]. Helices are the most abundant form of secondary structure containing approximately 32–38% of the residues in globular proteins [32].

The α-helix is the most abundant helical conformation found in globular proteins accounting for 32–38% of all residues [32, 33]. The 3_{10}-helix is not a common secondary structural element in proteins. Only 3.4% of the residues are involved in 3_{10}-helices in the Kabsch and Sander database [32], and nearly all those in helical segments contain 1–3 hydrogen bonds. α-helices sometimes begin or end with a single turn of a 3_{10}-helix. The π-helix is an extremely rare secondary structural element in proteins. Hydrogen bonds within a π-helix display a repeating pattern in which the backbone C=O of residue i hydrogen bonds to the backbone HN of residue $i + 5$. One turn of π-helix is also sometimes found at the ends of regular α-helices

The β-sheets are another major structural element in globular proteins containing 20–28% of all residues [32, 33]. β-sheets are found in two forms designated as parallel or antiparallel based on the relative directions of two interacting β strands. The basic unit of a β-sheet is a β strand with approximate backbone dihedral angles $\phi = -120$ and $\psi = +120$ producing a translation of 3.2–3.4 Å/residue for residues in antiparallel and parallel strands, respectively. Antiparallel β-sheets are thought to be intrinsically more stable than parallel sheets due to the more optimal orientation of the interstrand hydrogen bonds. The hydrogen bonds in a parallel β-sheet are not perpendicular to the individual strands resulting in component parallel to the strand [34].

Turns are another classical secondary structures with approximately one-third of all residues in globular proteins. Turns are located primarily on the protein surface and accordingly contain polar and charged residues. The behavior of these secondary structures in the RVFV L protein domain is investigated. The disappearance, reappearance or the movement of the helices and sheets from a residue to another within protein domain in the final structures from the simulations are analyzed. The results of this analysis are presented in Fig. 2. These results also show how the SPC/E and the implicit solvent simulations produced structures that are not too different from the initial structure. Even though the other water models look like they also try to maintain the structure of the peptide, there is enough evidence from Fig. 2 that to some extent they destabilize the protein.

3.3 Structural Properties and Energetics of the Peptide from MD Simulations

Table 2 presents the average values of some structural properties of the peptide over the 100 ns of the NVT simulations. It is observed from the SASA calculated from the different solvent models that, in simulations where TIP3P, OPC, and SPCE/Fw water models were used, the protein surface area increased drastically by 23.75,

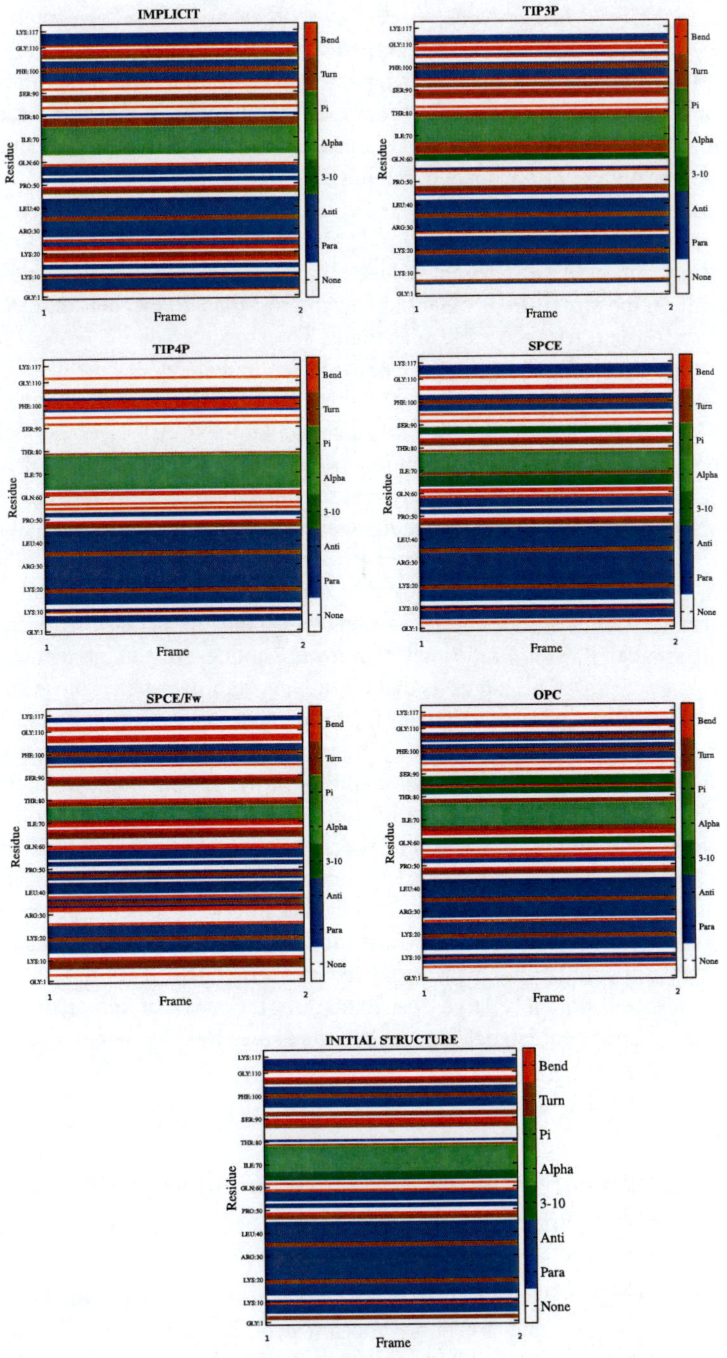

Fig. 2 DSSP Analysis of the RVFV L protein domain

25.23, and 21.74%, respectively, whereas the SPC/E and TIP4P presented a much smaller percentage increase of 3.98, and 10.92%, respectively (see Table 2), for the SASA. This signifies that these water models do not allow the protein to clench tight but rather make the protein bigger/lager than its size in the stable state. The implicit solvent simulation however produces an average SASA value that showed a decrease of 4.96% with respect to the initial structure.

A possible measure of protein size is radius of gyration, R_g, calculated with Eq. (2). An approximation of the Stokes radius measurable from size-exclusion chromatography is hydrodynamic radius, R_{hyd}, Eq. (3). While R_g is slightly more dependent on the structure of the protein of interest than R_{hyd}, their ratio R_g/R_{hyd} provides information on the molecular shape. The characteristic R_g/R_{hyd} value of a globular protein is ≈ 0.77 or $(3/5)^{1/2}$ [35]. When molecules deviate from globular to nonspherical or elongated structures, then R_g/R_{hyd} tends toward values away from 0.77. The R_g/R_{hyd} values in Table 2 show that the RVFV L protein domain is strongly not spherical, with a ratio ranging from 0.491 to 0.522. Correlation between the R_{hyd} of folded or unfolded proteins and the number of residues indicates that the structure of the domain in the different water models are consistent with denatured proteins through the empirical equation $R_{hyd} = (2.21 \pm 1.07)117^{0.5\pm0.02}$ [36].

Also, worth mentioning is that, a plot of the ratio of the radius of gyration to the hydrodynamic radius of the peptide in water against the interaction energy shows the relatively smaller R_g/R_{hyd} ratios having a lower peptide–solvent interaction energy than the larger ratios. This suggests that the solvent stabilizes better those structures leading to smaller ratios. Another useful property is the end-to-end distance R_{ee} defined as the distance between the centers of mass of the two end residues of the peptide chain. This describes the flexibility of the protein domain. Table 2 also shows the RMSD between the starting structure (6QHG), which also corresponds to the structure with the lowest potential energy, and the other structures from the different simulations. These RMSDs are of considerable importance, indicating that the models have significant structural differences between each structure and the initial structure across the different water models. The structures obtained from the implicit solvent simulation however showed an average RMSD of 0.33 ± 0.02 nm, which is also considerably large even though is the smallest across the different solvent environments studied. This was expected since initial structure is considered to be the most stable.

3.4 *Cluster Analysis of the MD Trajectory of the RVFV L Protein Peptide*

One of the popular clustering techniques in Machine Learning is the hierarchical clustering algorithms that are either top-down or bottom-up strategic ordering. Bottom-up algorithms treat each "information" as a singleton cluster at the outset and then successively merge or agglomerate pairs of clusters until all clusters

Table 2 Property and energetics evaluation of RVFV peptide in the solvents at $T = 293.15$ K: root-mean-square deviation ($RMSD$), radius of gyration (Rg), hydrodynamics radius (R_{hyd}), end-to-end distance (R_{ee}), solvent-accessible surface area ($SASA$), potential energy (PE), and interaction energy (E_{int})

Model	$RMSD$ (nm)	R_g (nm)	R_{hyd} (nm)	R_g/R_{hyd}	R_{ee} (nm)	$SASA$ (nm^2)	PE (kJ/mol)	E_{int} (kJ/mol)
TIP3P	0.63 ± 0.04	1.64 ± 0.02	3.14 ± 0.02	0.522	2.54 ± 0.38	833.7 ± 26.1	−5415 ± 259	−428885 ± 703
TIP4P	0.37 ± 0.02	1.51 ± 0.02	3.02 ± 0.02	0.500	2.90 ± 0.39	747.3 ± 21.6	−5787 ± 345	−443791 ± 815
SPC/E	0.33 ± 0.01	1.45 ± 0.01	2.94 ± 0.01	0.493	2.45 ± 0.09	700.5 ± 15.2	−6400 ± 262	−498772 ± 790
SPC/Fw	0.82 ± 0.03	1.65 ± 0.02	3.19 ± 0.02	0.517	2.39 ± 0.19	820.2 ± 20.0	−5396 ± 246	−484335 ± 760
OPC	0.62 ± 0.03	1.65 ± 0.02	3.18 ± 0.02	0.519	2.36 ± 0.32	843.7 ± 18.7	−5278 ± 297	−549610 ± 738
Implicit solvent	0.33 ± 0.02	1.43 ± 0.02	2.91 ± 0.02	0.491	2.46 ± 0.26	640.3 ± 20.9	−6753 ± 297	
6QHG	0.00	1.51	2.91	0.519	2.28	673.71	−8227.469	

have been merged into a single cluster that contains all information. Bottom-up hierarchical clustering is therefore called hierarchical agglomerative clustering (HAC) and does not require a prespecified number of clusters. Top-down clustering requires a method for splitting a cluster and proceeds by splitting clusters recursively until individual documents (trajectories) are reached. The monotonicity of the merge operation in HAC is one fundamental assumption. In this chapter, the bottom-up hierarchical clustering approach was employed to cluster the MD trajectories of the RVFV L protein domain. Hierarchical agglomerative clustering on the backbone atoms of the peptide using average linkage and stopping when either 5 clusters are reached or the minimum Euclidean distance between clusters is 3.0 Å was used. The results from the clustering analysis are presented in an RMSD time series plot in Fig. 3. Under the stopping criteria used, it was found that across all the explicit solvent and the implicit solvent simulations, a cluster of 5 was produced. The fractional cluster proportion within each solvent environment however varies. Figure 3 again shows how the peptide atomic position changes along the 100 ns run with respect to the position.

4 Conclusions

Using an all-atom molecular dynamics, we studied the structural and dynamical behavior of RVFV L protein C-terminal domain in both implicit and explicit solvents. Hierarchical agglomerative clustering analysis was also performed on the atomic trajectories obtained from the MD simulation. It was found that under the clustering criteria used, 5 clusters were obtained in all the water models and the implicit solvent environment. The structures obtained from the simulations are far from being globular as evidenced by ratio R_g/R_{hyd} in the range [0.491 0.522]. Nonetheless, in the SPC/E water model and the implicit solvent, the protein domain likes to remain compact with the α-helices and β-sheets somewhat in place like the initial structure (see Figs. 2 and 4).

Based on energetics, the more stable structures were those obtained from the implicit solvent simulation with the next more stable being structures from the SPC/E water model simulation. The RVFV L protein domain structures produced from the OPC water models turn to have the lowest interaction energy showing a strong attraction between the peptide and water molecules. The interaction energy also shows how the models obtained from TIP3P water model simulation demonstrate the most repulsiveness as compared to the other models. Structural characterization of the atomic trajectories enabled a better understanding of the structural and dynamical behavior of the domain under the conditions of the water models studied along time.

Considering the fact that information on RVFV L protein or its domains being sparse, the findings presented in this chapter on structural behavior of the domain will facilitate protein–solvent and protein–protein interaction studies as well as the journey toward drug discovery. In an ongoing research on this and other RVFV L

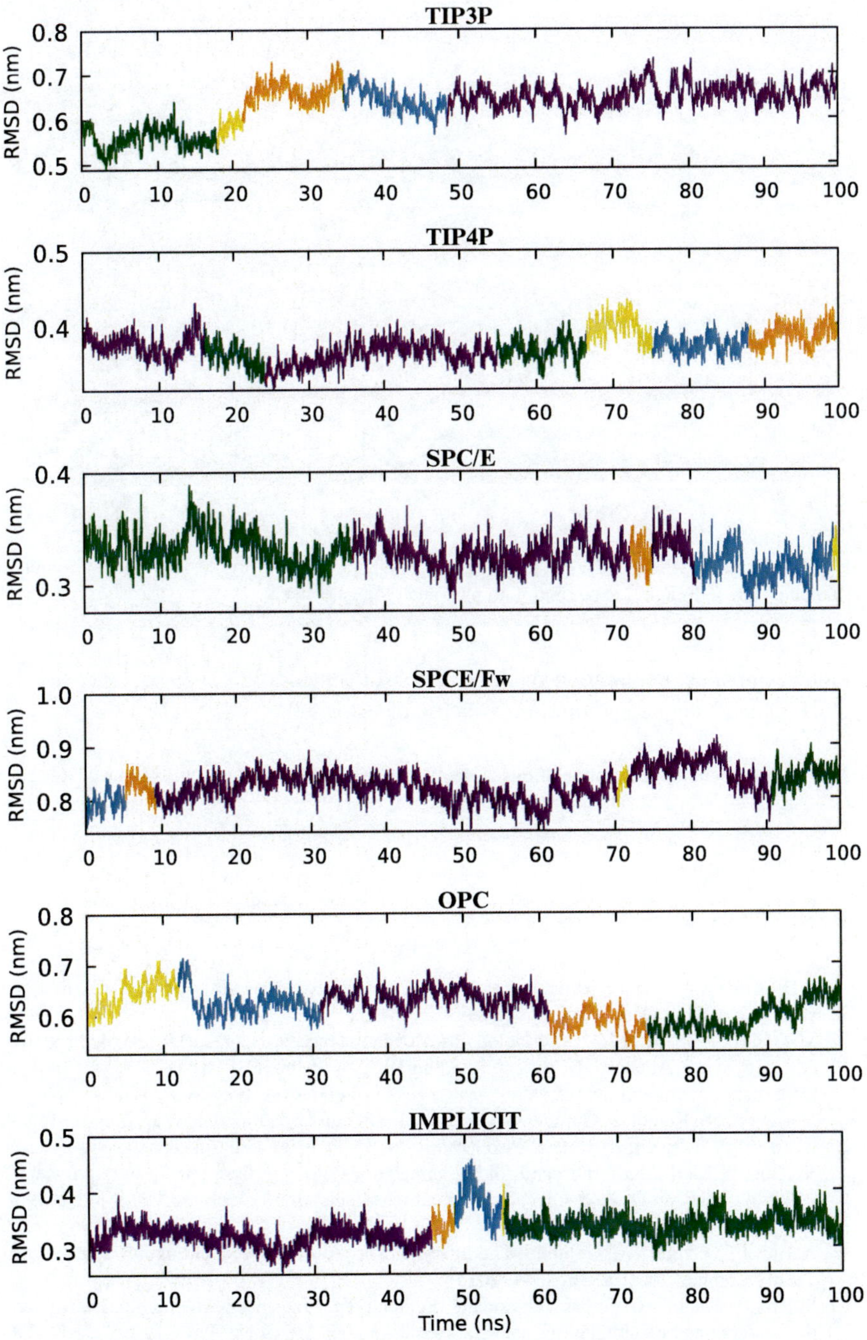

Fig. 3 Cluster distribution along the MD trajectory of the RVFV domain from the hierarchical agglomerative clustering. RMSD values as a function of time over the trajectory which are colored based on their cluster memberships along the 100 ns MD NVT runs at 293.15 K

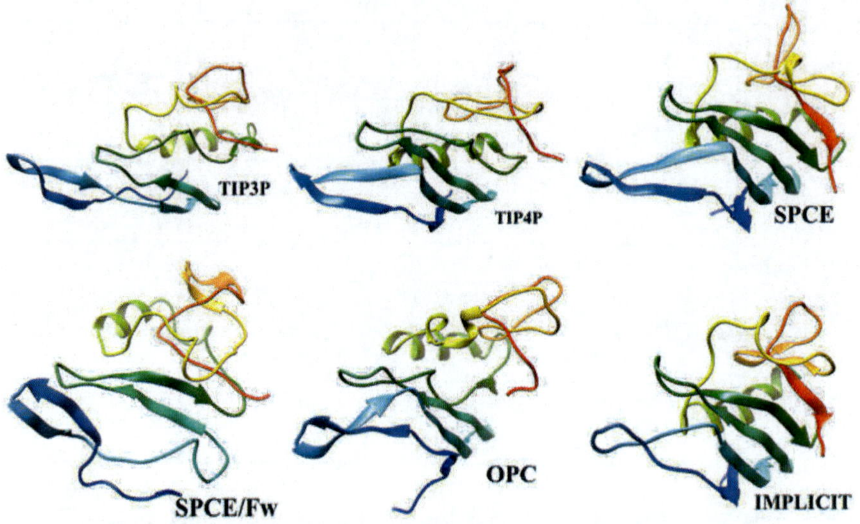

Fig. 4 Atomic structure of RVFV L protein C-terminal domain from the various environments studied. N and C-termini are colored with blue and red respectively

protein domains, exploration of the structural behaviors in dense solvents such as glycerol and its aqueous solutions is being investigated.

Acknowledgments All the simulations were done in the ARGO cluster of the Office of Research Computing at George Mason University, Fairfax VA.

References

1. B.H. Bird, S.T. Nichol, Breaking the chain: rift valley fever virus control via livestock vaccination. Curr. Opin. Virol. **2**(3), 315–323 (2012).
2. M. Bouloy, F. Weber, Molecular biology of rift valley fever virus. Open Virol. J. **4**, 8 (2010).
3. G.K. Gogovi, F. Almsned, N. Bracci, K. Kehn-Hall, A. Shehu, E. Blaisten-Barojas, Modeling the tertiary structure of the rift valley fever virus l protein. Molecules **24**(9), 1768 (2019)
4. N. Gogrefe, S. Reindl, S. Günther, M. Rosenthal, Structure of a functional cap-binding domain in rift valley fever virus l protein. PLoS Pathogens **15**(5), e1007829 (2019)
5. M. Guo, Y. Mei, Equilibrium and folding simulations of ns4b h2 in pure water and water/2, 2, 2-trifluoroethanol mixed solvent: examination of solvation models. J. Mol. Model. **19**(9), 3931–3939 (2013)
6. A. Hazel, C. Chipot, J.C. Gumbart, Thermodynamics of deca-alanine folding in water. J. Chem. Theory Comput. **10**(7), 2836–2844 (2014)
7. S. Park, F. Khalili-Araghi, E. Tajkhorshid, K. Schulten, Free energy calculation from steered molecular dynamics simulations using jarzynski's equality. J. Chem. Phys. **119**(6), 3559–3566 (2003)
8. R.B. Nellas, Q.R. Johnson, T. Shen, Solvent-induced α-to 3_{10}-helix transition of an amphiphilic peptide. Biochemistry **52**(40), 7137–7144 (2013)

9. M. Perutz, Electrostatic effects in proteins. Science **201**(4362), 1187–1191 (1978)
10. B. Garcia-Moreno, Adaptations of proteins to cellular and subcellular pH. J. Biol. **8**(11), 98 (2009)
11. D. Case, I. Ben-Shalom, S. Brozell, D. Cerutti, T. Cheatham III, V. Cruzeiro, T. Darden, R. Duke, D. Ghoreishi, M. Gilson, et al., Amber 2018. University of California, San Francisco (2018)
12. J.A. Maier, C. Martinez, K. Kasavajhala, L. Wickstrom, K.E. Hauser, C. Simmerling, ff14sb: improving the accuracy of protein side chain and backbone parameters from ff99sb. J. Chem. Theory Comput. **11**(8), 3696–3713 (2015)
13. E.F. Pettersen, T.D. Goddard, C.C. Huang, G.S. Couch, D.M. Greenblatt, E.C. Meng, T.E. Ferrin, UCSF chimera–a visualization system for exploratory research and analysis. J. Comput. Chem. **25**(13), 1605–1612 (2004)
14. W.L. Jorgensen, J. Chandrasekhar, J.D. Madura, R.W. Impey, M.L. Klein, Comparison of simple potential functions for simulating liquid water. J. Chem. Phys. **79**(2), 926–935 (1983)
15. S. Izadi, R. Anandakrishnan, A.V. Onufriev, Building water models: a different approach. J. Phys. Chem. Lett. **5**(21), 3863–3871 (2014)
16. H. Berendsen, J. Grigera, T. Straatsma, The missing term in effective pair potentials. J. Phys. Chem. **91**(24), 6269–6271 (1987)
17. Y. Wu, H.L. Tepper, G.A. Voth, Flexible simple point-charge water model with improved liquid-state properties. J. Chem. Phys. **124**(2), 024503 (2006)
18. G. Bussi, D. Donadio, M. Parrinello, Canonical sampling through velocity rescaling. J. Chem. Phys. **126**(1), 014101 (2007)
19. H.J. Berendsen, J.V. Postma, W.F. van Gunsteren, A. DiNola, J.R. Haak, Molecular dynamics with coupling to an external bath. J. Chem. Phys. **81**(8), 3684–3690 (1984)
20. I.-C. Yeh, G. Hummer, System-size dependence of diffusion coefficients and viscosities from molecular dynamics simulations with periodic boundary conditions. J. Phys. Chem. B **108**(40), 15873–15879 (2004)
21. J.R. Rumble, D.R. Lide, T.J. Bruno, *CRC Handbook of Chemistry Physics* (CRC Press, Boca Raton, 2017)
22. U. Essmann, L. Perera, M.L. Berkowitz, T. Darden, H. Lee, L.G. Pedersen, A smooth particle mesh ewald method. J. Chem. Phys. **103**(19), 8577–8593 (1995)
23. V. Tsui, D.A. Case, Theory and applications of the generalized born solvation model in macromolecular simulations. Biopolymers Original Res. Biomol. **56**(4), 275–291 (2000)
24. S.Y. Mashayak, D.E. Tanner, Comparing solvent models for molecular dynamics of protein. University of Illinois at Urbana-Champaign, Champaign (2011)
25. J. Weiser, P.S. Shenkin, W.C. Still, Approximate atomic surfaces from linear combinations of pairwise overlaps (LCPO). J. Comput. Chem. **20**(2), 217–230 (1999)
26. P. Mark, L. Nilsson, Structure and dynamics of the tip3p, spc, and spc/e water models at 298 k. J. Phys. Chem. A **105**(43), 9954–9960 (2001)
27. M.W. Mahoney, W.L. Jorgensen, A five-site model for liquid water and the reproduction of the density anomaly by rigid, nonpolarizable potential functions. J. Chem. Phys. **112**(20), 8910–8922 (2000)
28. J.L. Abascal, C. Vega, A general purpose model for the condensed phases of water: Tip4p/2005. J. Chem. Phys. **123**(23), 234505 (2005)
29. R. Mills, Self-diffusion in normal and heavy water in the range 1–45. deg. J. Phys. Chem. **77**(5), 685–688 (1973)
30. W.S. Price, H. Ide, Y. Arata, Self-diffusion of supercooled water to 238 k using pgse nmr diffusion measurements. J. Phys. Chem. A **103**(4), 448–450 (1999)
31. W.L. Bragg, J.C. Kendrew, M.F. Perutz, Polypeptide chain configurations in crystalline proteins, in *Proceedings of the Royal Society of London. Series A. Mathematical and Physical Sciences*, vol. 203, no. 1074 (1950), pp. 321–357
32. W. Kabsch, C. Sander, Dictionary of protein secondary structure: pattern recognition of hydrogen-bonded and geometrical features. Biopolymers Original Res. Biomol. **22**(12), 2577–2637 (1983)

33. T.E. Creighton, *Proteins: Structures and Molecular Properties* (Macmillan, London, 1993).
34. E. Baker, R. Hubbard, Hydrogen bonding in globular proteins. Progr. Biophys. Mol. Biol. **44**(2), 97–179 (1984)
35. W. Burchard, M. Schmidt, W. Stockmayer, Information on polydispersity and branching from combined quasi-elastic and intergrated scattering. Macromolecules **13**(5), 1265–1272 (1980).
36. D.K. Wilkins, S.B. Grimshaw, V. Receveur, C.M. Dobson, J.A. Jones, L.J. Smith, Hydrodynamic radii of native and denatured proteins measured by pulse field gradient NMR techniques. Biochemistry **38**(50), 16424–16431 (1999)

Common Motifs in KEGG Cancer Pathways

Bini Elsa Paul, Olaa Kasem, Haitao Zhao, and Zhong-Hui Duan

1 Introduction

Cancer is a leading cause of death worldwide and it consists of a group of diseases involving abnormal cell growth with the potential to invade or spread to other parts of the body [1, 2]. There are more than 100 types of cancer, including breast cancer, skin cancer, lung cancer, colon cancer, prostate cancer, and lymphoma [3]. In the last decade, many important genes responsible for the genesis of various cancers have been discovered, their mutations identified, and the pathways through which they act characterized [2, 4]. A gene is the basic physical and functional unit of heredity. Genes and gene products interact in an integrated and coordinated way to support normal functions of a living cell. Signaling pathway describes a group of genes and their products in a cell that work together to control one or more cell functions, such as cell division or cell death. After the first molecule in a pathway receives a signal, it activates another molecule. This process is repeated until the last molecule is activated and the cell function is carried out. Abnormal activation of signaling pathways can lead to cancer, and drugs are being developed to block these pathways. These drugs may help block cancer cell growth and kill cancer cells [5].

KEGG (Kyoto Encyclopedia of Genes and Genomes) is a collection of databases dealing with genomes, biological pathways, diseases, drugs, and chemical sub-

Short Research Paper.

B. E. Paul · O. Kasem · H. Zhao · Z.-H. Duan (✉)
Department of Computer Science, University of Akron, Akron, OH, USA
e-mail: be23@zips.uakron.edu; ok22@zips.uakron.edu; hz28@zips.uakron.edu; duan@uakron.edu

H. R. Arabnia et al. (eds.), *Advances in Computer Vision and Computational Biology*, Transactions on Computational Science and Computational Intelligence,
https://doi.org/10.1007/978-3-030-71051-4_60

stances. KEGG is utilized for bioinformatics research and education, including data analysis in genomics, metagenomics, metabolomics, and other omics studies, modeling and simulation in systems biology, and translational research in drug development [6].

In this research, we studied gene-gene interactions in 17 different types of cancers that are presented in KEGG pathway maps and identified common network motifs, utilizing the open-source visualization platform Gephi [7].

2 Materials and Methods

The KEGG pathway maps characterizing gene-to-gene relationship in the 17 different cancers were extracted from the xml datasets in KEGG repository. The xml files can be downloaded using KEGG IDs [8]. Table 1 shows each cancer type with its corresponding identifier. The xml files were preprocessed using python scripts to obtain a graph of gene-gene interactions. Since our focus is on gene interaction, we extract only the nodes that are genes from the data and discard all other nodes. Each node in the graph has an ID that refers to the gene ID, as 1956 refers to gene EGFR and a name that refers to the name of the gene as EGFR. While each edge connecting two nodes has a name that represents the cancer pathway in which it's presented.

The graph that integrates 17 cancer pathways is a weighted graph. The edge weight, an integer representing the strength of the interaction of two genes, is equal to the sum of the number of pathways the gene-gene interaction appears in and the

Table 1 KEGG pathway identifiers and cancer types

KEGG ID	Cancer types
05210	Colorectal cancer
05212	Pancreatic cancer
05225	Hepatocellular cancer
05226	Gastric cancer
05214	Glioma
05216	Thyroid cancer
05221	Acute myeloid leukemia
05220	Chronic myeloid leukemia
05217	Basal cell carcinoma
05218	Melanoma
05211	Renal cell carcinoma
05219	Bladder cancer
05215	Prostate cancer
05213	Endometrial cancer
05224	Breast cancer
05222	Small cell lung cancer
05223	Non-small cell lung cancer

number of times the interaction appears in the same pathway, as the interaction could occur several times in the pathway through other molecules that are not genes. We assumed a threshold of 5 and extracted the edges with weights that are greater than or equal to the threshold value. Other graph attributes we considered include giant component (largest connected component), k-core, degree range, average degree, average weighted degree, network diameter, graph density, modularity, average clustering coefficient, and average path length [7].

After extracting the nodes and edges which are the genes and gene-to-gene relations from KEGG pathway, the information is saved as a .gml file. The file has 488 nodes and 3441 edges. Gephi was then used to analyze the graph with the option 'edges merge strategy' to be sum of the edges. The resulting graph contains 488 nodes and 1489 edges.

3 Results and Discussions

Figure 1 shows the initial graph with 488 nodes and 1489 edges. All edges are bidirectional and the thickness represents the weight of the edge. It is clear that the graph contains different subnetworks. The overall statistics of the graph is listed in Table 2.

We further conducted a sequence of investigations, (1) the giant component with k-core ($k = 10$). The result is a graph shown in Fig. 2 that contains two distinct components colored red and green. A total of 10 cancer pathways are implicated in the graph, including basal cell carcinoma (hsa5217), breast cancer (hsa5224), melanoma (hsa5218), chronic myeloid leukemia (hsa5220), prostate cancer (hsa5215), non-small cell lung cancer (hsa5223), gastric cancer (hsa5226), glioma (hsa5214), acute myeloid leukemia (hsa5221), and pancreatic cancer (hsa5212); (2) considering the subgraph in which the weight of each edge is greater than or equal to 5 and nodes are connected with at least one other node. The resulting graph (Fig. 3) has 63 nodes and 125 edges in 5 clusters. Only 4 types of cancer pathways are present in this subgraph, including non-small cell lung cancer (hsa05223), breast cancer (hsa05224), melanoma (hsa05218), and prostate cancer (hsa05215); (3) with the same criteria, but including edges with weights between 3 and 5. The resulting graph has 95 nodes and 205 edges as shown in Fig. 4; (4) identifying k-core with $k = 6$ of the integrated graph, resulting in a subgraph of 15 nodes and 54 edges (Fig. 5). The subgraph involves 3 cancer pathways, non-small cell lung cancer (hsa05223), breast cancer (hsa05224), and melanoma (hsa05218).

As we can observe, the integrated cancer network is sparse with graph density 0.006 and, on average, each gene is connected to 3 other genes. The average weighted degree of over 7 indicates the commonality of the genes in different cancer networks. Network diameter 16 shows the linear size of the network is 16 and the shortest path between farthest nodes are 16. The integrated cancer network consists of a total of 91 connected components, but only two strongly connected k-cores are observed. We note that although two *k*-cores ($k = 10$) are observed in Fig. 2, it

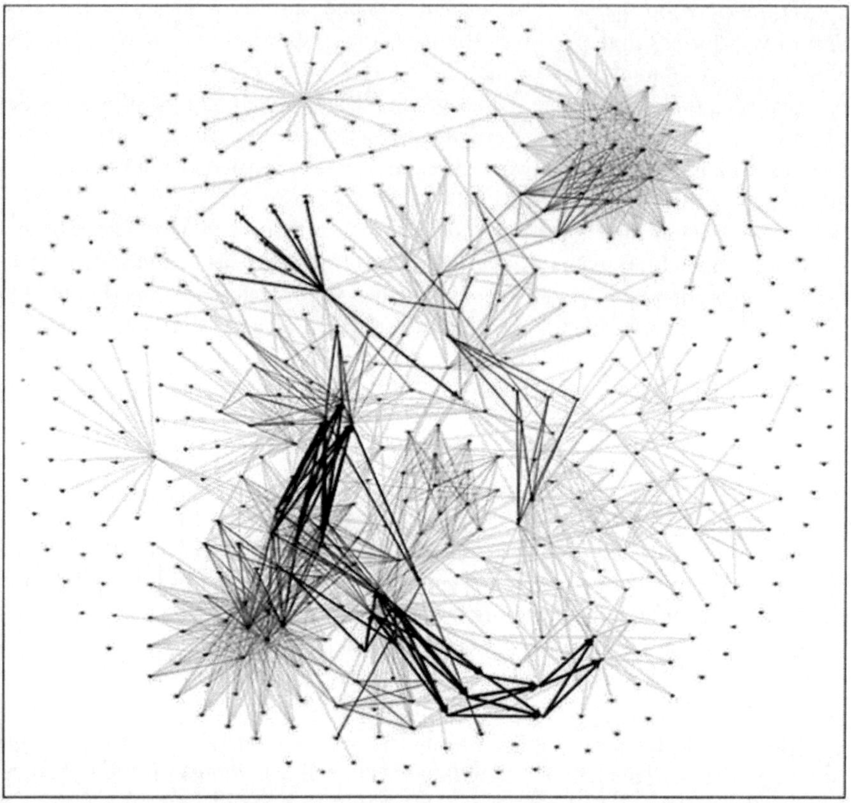

Fig. 1 Integrated graph from 17 KEGG cancer pathways with Fruchterman Reingold layout

Table 2 Statistic measures of graph attributes

Graph attributes	Values
Average degree	3.051
Average weighted degree	7.051
Network diameter	16
Graph density	0.006
Modularity	0.667
Connected components	91
Girvan-Newman clustering	114
Average clustering coefficient	0.031
Average path length	6.265

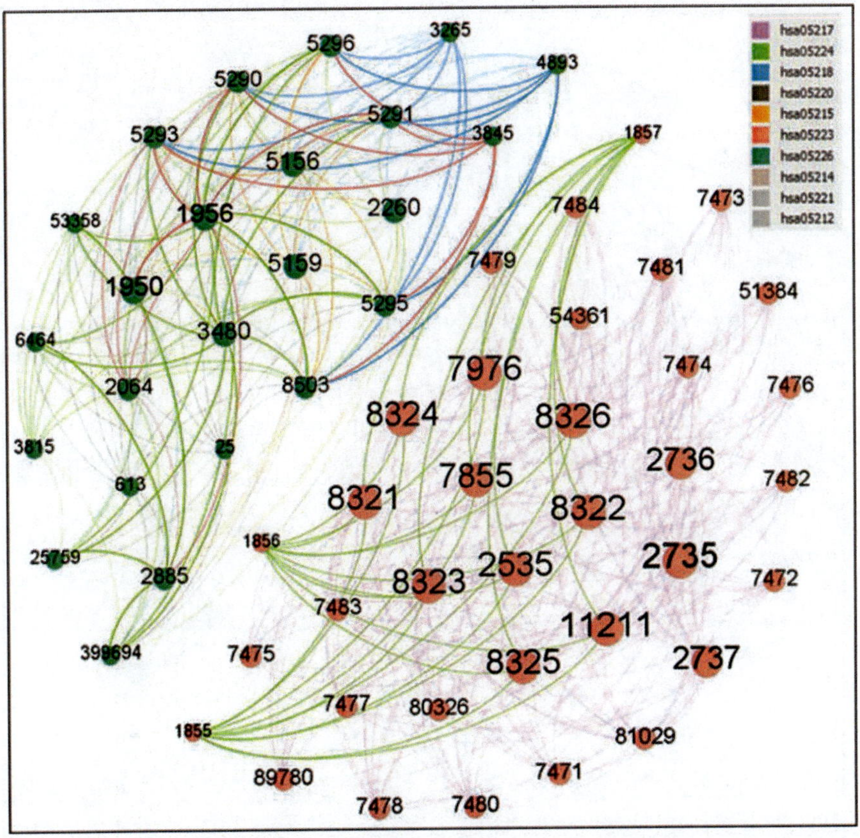

Fig. 2 Two highly connected subgraphs in the giant component with k-core ($k = 10$). The nodes are colored based on the component they belong to. The size of the node represents the degree of the node. The edges are colored based on the corresponding cancer networks

does not indicate gene-gene interactions in cancers can be divided into two different independent communities. There are many lower degree interconnections between the genes in the two components.

We observed 57.74% of edges belongs to the pathway of the basal cell carcinoma cancer type (hsa05217). It means many genes involved in basal cell carcinoma might be related to other cancer types. It's been reported that frequent skin cancers due to mutations in genes responsible for repairing DNA are linked to a threefold risk of unrelated cancers [9]. On the other hand, our analysis shows only 0.23% of edges belongs to pancreatic cancer. Medical studies show that, less commonly, cancer in other parts of the body can spread to the pancreas. However, there are reported cases that cancer found in the pancreas was metastasized from another part of the body, although this is relatively rare [10].

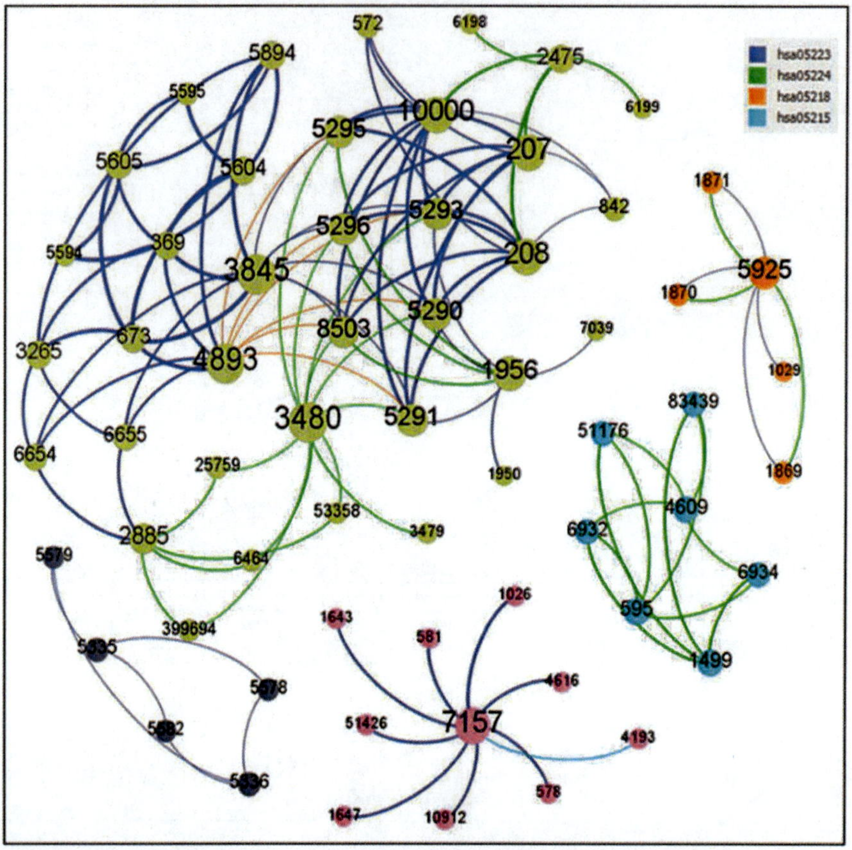

Fig. 3 Subgraph of the integrated graph, in which the weight of each edge is greater than or equal to 5

Figure 3 shows the graph is split into 5 components. We colored the nodes in 5 corresponding colors. Component 0 with light green color is the largest component with 57% of the nodes. It shows the presence of breast cancer, non-small cell lung cancer, and melanoma. The node 4893 (NRAS proto-oncogene) has the highest degree, indicating this gene is quite active in cancer. NRAS (neuroblastoma RAS viral (v-ras) oncogene homolog) encodes for the GTPase NRas protein, one of three human RAS proteins. RAS proteins are small GTPases that are central mediators downstream of growth factor receptor signaling and, therefore, critical for cell proliferation, survival, and differentiation. NRAS is implicated in the pathogenesis of several cancers. It's been reported that NRAS is altered in 2.90% of all cancers, with melanoma, colorectal adenocarcinoma, leukemia, thyroid gland neoplasm, and non-small cell lung carcinoma having the greatest prevalence of alterations [11].

Component 1 consists of nodes colored blue. All the nodes in this component have comparatively same size, which shows the degree of each node is around the

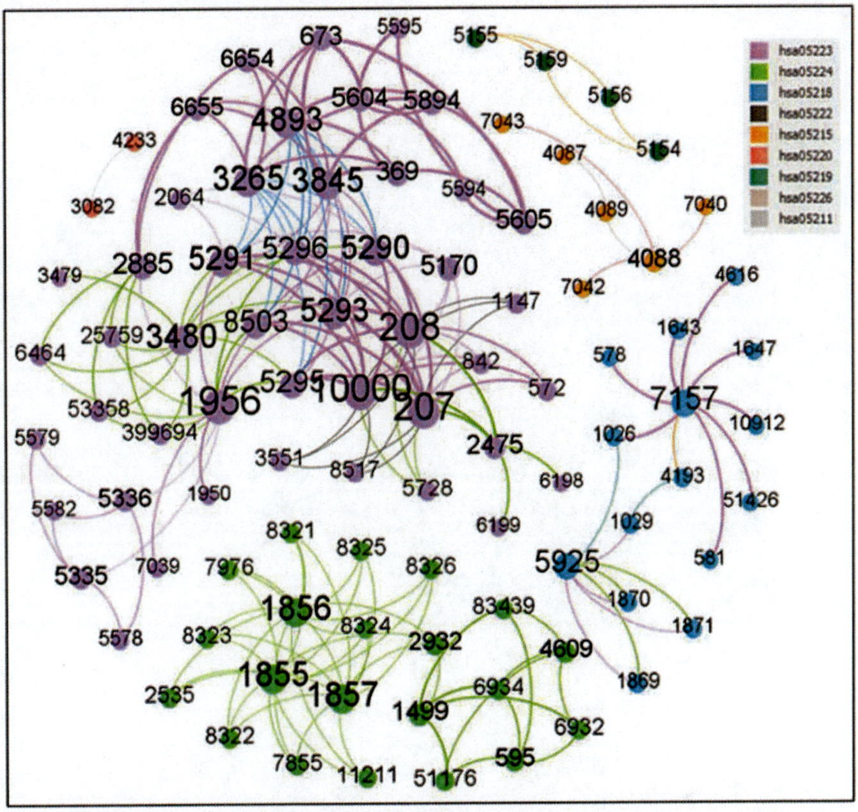

Fig. 4 Subgraph of the integrated graph in which the weight of each edge is greater than or equal to 3 and nodes are connected with at least one other node

same value, 3 or 4. All the edges are from breast cancer. We note breast cancer is also present in other components.

Genes in Component 2 are colored pink. As we see, node 7157 (tumor protein 53) is the highest degree gene and most of the edges are related to non-small cell lung cancer (NSCLC). And also there is a presence of prostate cancer. In a large number of types of human cancers, the tumor protein 53 (TP53) gene is the most frequently mutated gene. Among genetic abnormalities, the TP53 tumor suppressor gene appears to be the most frequent target, and abnormality of TP53 plays an important role in the tumorigenesis of lung epithelial cells. Indeed, mutations of the TP53 gene occur in about 50% of NSCLC. As TP53 mutants are present in almost half of NSCLC whose incidence rate is increasing every year, the possibility of abolishing their oncogenic effects is undoubtedly important for a successful treatment of NSCLC [12, 13].

Component 3 with node color orange are associated with breast cancer and non-small cell lung cancer. It's been reported annually that 1.4 million women

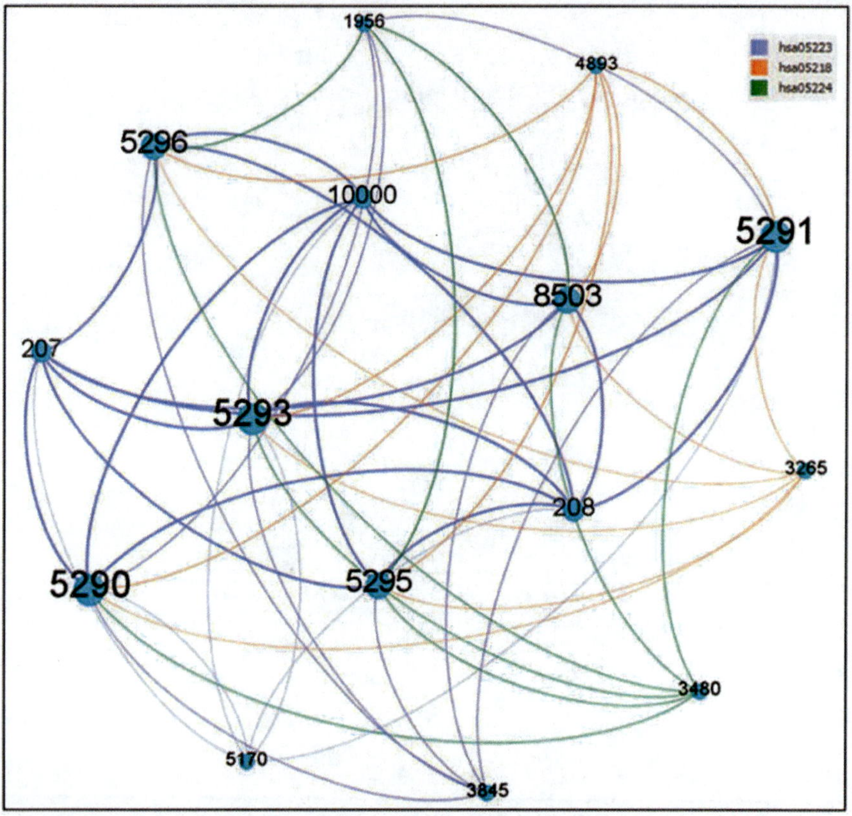

Fig. 5 K-core 6 of the integrated graph, including 15 nodes and 54 edges

worldwide are diagnosed with breast cancer and are at risk for another common malignancy: non-small-cell lung cancer (NSCLC) [14].

Component 4 with purple nodes includes interactions in non-small-cell lung cancer only.

The nodes with high weights indicate the high implication of the gene in cancers. Three nodes with high degrees include KRAS (3845), NRAS (4893), and IGF1R (3480). KRAS gene provides instructions for making a protein called K-Ras, part of the RAS/MAPK pathway. The NRAS (N-ras proto-oncogene) is a member of the Ras gene family too. All human cells contain KRAS that serves as a key regulator of signaling pathways responsible for cell proliferation, differentiation, and survival. If a mutation occurs in a KRAS gene, it may allow cells to multiply out of control, which can cause cancer. KRAS mutations play a role in some of the most common and deadly carcinomas, including lung, colorectal, and pancreatic cancers [15]. Ras pathway is a key intracellular signaling pathway. Dysregulation of this pathway is a common event in cancer as RAS family, small GTPases, is often the most frequently mutated oncogenes in human cancer [16].

KRAS G12C is particularly prevalent in non-small cell lung cancer (NSCLC), which makes up about 85% of all lung cancer cases in the U.S. Approximately 13% of Americans with NSCLC have the KRAS G12C mutation, and there are about 23,000 new cases of KRAS G12C NSCLC diagnosed every year in the U.S. alone. KRAS G12C is also found in 1–3% of colorectal and pancreatic cancer patients [17].

The NRAS gene provides instructions for making a protein called N-Ras that is involved primarily in regulating cell division. The NRAS gene belongs to a class of genes known as oncogenes. When mutated, oncogenes have the potential to cause normal cells to become cancerous. The NRAS gene is in the Ras family of oncogenes, which also includes two other genes: HRAS and KRAS. The proteins produced from these three genes are GTPases. These proteins play important roles in cell division, cell differentiation, and the self-destruction of cells [18].

IGF1R gene is linked to breast cancer. From the studies, one important pathway for breast cancer pathogenesis may be the insulin-like growth factor (IGF) signaling pathway, which regulates both cellular proliferation and apoptosis. BRCA1 has been shown to directly interact with IGF signaling such that variants in this pathway may modify risk of cancer in women carrying BRCA mutations [19].

To observe additional interactions, we reduced the degree threshold to include nodes with degree greater than or equal to 3. The results are presented in Fig. 4, showing more connections within the components observed in Fig. 3 and interactions between genes in different components.

We further identified a strongly connected k-core ($k = 6$) as showing in Fig. 5. This k-core includes genes in a very important family PI3Ks, PIK3CA (5290), PIK3CB (5291) PIK3CD (5293), PIK3R1 (5295) and PIK3R2 (5296). These genes are involved in PI3K (phosphoinositide 3-kinases) pathway which is an intracellular signaling pathway that plays key roles in regulating cell cycle and is linked to many essential cellular processes, such as cell proliferation, survival, growth, and motility. The signaling cascade is mediated through serine and/or threonine phosphorylation of a range of downstream molecules. It has been widely reported that the PI3K pathway is overactive in many cancers, thus reducing apoptosis and allowing proliferation and uncontrolled cell growth [20–24]. In addition, the alterations of PI3Ks in cancer were detailed along with the therapeutic efficacy of PI3K inhibitors in the cancer treatment [24].

4 Conclusion

In this paper, we presented the findings of our analysis of 17 KEGG cancer pathway maps. We have extracted the 17 cancer pathways from KEGG repository and integrated them to obtain a graph that consists all the involved genes. We then utilized different techniques and filtering criteria to extract and shed lights on the gene-gene interaction patterns.

As shown in Figs. 1, 2, 3, 4, and 5, the genetic pathways are sparse graphs. Typically, a gene is communicating with a handful of other genes, although a few genes serve as hubs. It has been reported that these hub genes play important roles in many different types of cancers. In addition, we identified k-cores ranging from 3 to 6, illustrating strong connections of the involved genes.

We conclude that the identified hub genes, the common gene-gene interactions, and the graph motifs in the cancer pathways enhance our understanding of gene interactions in cancers. They provide insights for cancer biologists to connect dots and generate strong hypotheses, so further biological investigations into cancer initiation, progression, and treatment can be conducted effectively.

References

1. C.P. Wild, E. Weiderpass, B.W. Stewart (eds.), World Cancer Report: Cancer Research for Cancer Prevention, World Cancer Reports, ISBN-13: 978-92-832-0448-0
2. L.A. Garraway, E.S. Lander, Lessons from the cancer genome. Cell **153**(1), 17–37 (2013). https://doi.org/10.1016/j.cell.2013.03.002
3. Cancer Types, *National Cancer Institute.* [Online]. Available: https://www.cancer.gov/types [Accessed: 5/24/2020]
4. A.L. Barabási, Z.N. Oltvai, Network biology: Understanding the cell's functional organization. Nat. Rev. Genet. **5**(2), 101–113 (2004). https://doi.org/10.1038/nrg1272
5. NCI Dictionary of Cancer Terms. *National Cancer Institute*, 2011. [Online]. Available: https://www.cancer.gov/publications/dictionaries/cancer-terms [Accessed: 24-Nov-2019]
6. KEGG: Kyoto Encyclopedia of Genes and Genomes – GenomeNet. [Online]. Available: http://www.genome.jp/kegg/ [Accessed: 24-Nov-2019]
7. M. Bastian, S. Heymann, M. Jacomy, Gephi: An open source software for exploring and manipulating networks. Int. AAAI Conf. Weblogs Soc. Media (2009)
8. XML description of colorectal cancer pathway. [Online]. Available: http://rest.kegg.jp/get/hsa05210/kgml [Accessed: 24-Nov-2019]
9. H.G. Cho, K.Y. Kuo, S. Li, et al., Frequent basal cell cancer development is a clinical marker for inherited cancer susceptibility. JCI Insight **3**(15), e122744. Published 2018 Aug 9 (2018). https://doi.org/10.1172/jci.insight.122744
10. Other associated cancers, Pancreatic Cancer UK. [Online]. Available: https://www.pancreaticcancer.org.uk/information-and-support/facts-about-pancreatic-cancer/types-of-pancreatic-cancer/other-cancers-linked-with-the-pancreas/. [Accessed: 24-Nov-2019]
11. AACR Project GENIE Consortium, AACR project GENIE: Powering precision medicine through an international consortium. Cancer Discov. **7**(8), 818–831 (2017). https://doi.org/10.1158/2159-8290.CD-17-0151
12. A. Mogi, H. Kuwano, TP53 mutations in nonsmall cell lung cancer. J. Biomed. Biotechnol. **2011**, 583929 (2011). https://doi.org/10.1155/2011/583929
13. T.H. Ecke, H.H. Schlechte, K. Schiemenz, et al., TP53 gene mutations in prostate cancer progression. Anticancer Res. **30**(5), 1579–1586 (2010)
14. M.T. Milano, R.L. Strawderman, S. Venigalla, K. Ng, L.B. Travis, Non-small-cell lung cancer after breast cancer: A population-based study of clinicopathologic characteristics and survival outcomes in 3529 women. J. Thorac. Oncol. **9**(8), 1081–1090 (2014). https://doi.org/10.1097/JTO.0000000000000213

15. O. Kranenburg, The KRAS oncogene: Past, present, and future. Biochim. Biophys. Acta **1756**(2), 81–82 (2005). https://doi.org/10.1016/j.bbcan.2005.10.001
16. Y. Pylayeva-Gupta, E. Grabocka, D. Bar-Sagi, RAS oncogenes: weaving a tumorigenic web. Nat. Rev. Cancer **11(11)**, 761–774. Published 2011 Oct 13 (2011). https://doi.org/10.1038/nrc3106
17. S. Seton-Rogers, KRAS-G12C in the crosshairs. Nat. Rev. Cancer **20**(1), 3 (2020). https://doi.org/10.1038/s41568-019-0228-3
18. K. Ohashi, L.V. Sequist, M.E. Arcila, et al., Characteristics of lung cancers harboring NRAS mutations. Clin. Cancer Res. **19**(9), 2584–2591 (2013). https://doi.org/10.1158/1078-0432.CCR-12-3173
19. D.H. Fagan, D. Yee, Crosstalk between IGF1R and estrogen receptor signaling in breast cancer. J. Mammary Gland Biol. Neoplasia **13**(4), 423–429 (2008). https://doi.org/10.1007/s10911-008-9098-0
20. J. Luo, B.D. Manning, L.C. Cantley, Targeting the PI3K-Akt pathway in human cancer: Rationale and promise. Cancer Cell **4**(4), 257–262 (2003)
21. P. Liu, H. Cheng, T.M. Roberts, J.J. Zhao, Targeting the phosphoinositide 3-kinase (PI3K) pathway in cancer. Nat. Rev. Drug Discov. **8**(8), 627–644 (2009). https://doi.org/10.1038/nrd2926
22. F. Janku, T.A. Yap, F. Meric-Bernstam, Targeting the PI3K pathway in cancer: Are we making headway? Nat. Rev. Clin. Oncol. **15**(5), 273–291 (2018). https://doi.org/10.1038/nrclinonc.2018.28
23. Y. Samuels, Z. Wang, A. Bardelli, N. Silliman, J. Ptak, S. Szabo, et al., High frequency of mutations of the PIK3CA gene in human cancers. Science **304**(5670), 554 (2004). https://doi.org/10.1126/science.1096502
24. L.M. Thorpe, H. Yuzugullu, J.J. Zhao, PI3K in cancer: Divergent roles of isoforms, modes of activation, and therapeutic targeting. Nat. Rev. Cancer **15**(1), 7–24 (2015). https://doi.org/10.1038/nrc3860

Phenome to Genome – Application of GWAS to Asthmatic Lung Biomarker Gene Variants

Adam Cankaya and Ravi Shankar

1 Introduction

Prior to doing any analysis, we utilize a medical textbook to gather a set of genes related to the metabolic biomarkers found expressed in subjects with asthma and other chronic lung conditions [1]. The relationship between variations of these genes and the asthmatic biomarkers have been previously identified by traditional candidate gene studies. We extend our knowledge of these genes into the whole genome by identifying SNPs found through GWAS methodology [2]. For our purposes, we focus on common SNPs (MAF > 1%) with an odds ratio value indicating an individual having an increased risk for developing asthma. By curating a representative set of SNPs and odds ratios, we can estimate their individual contribution towards the genetic risk of developing asthma. Once a patient knows which SNP variants are present in their genome, the individual risks of each SNP can be multiplied to determine the individual patient's overall risk of developing asthma.

1.1 Recent Literature Review

The idea of using GWAS results to help predict the risk of pathology development has been explored recently for most complex diseases. For example, an attempt has been made to use GWAS data to predict the risk of developing coronary heart disease

A. Cankaya (✉) · R. Shankar
Department of Computer & Electrical Engineering and Computer Science, Florida Atlantic University, Boca Raton, FL, USA
e-mail: acankaya2017@fau.edu

H. R. Arabnia et al. (eds.), *Advances in Computer Vision and Computational Biology*, Transactions on Computational Science and Computational Intelligence,
https://doi.org/10.1007/978-3-030-71051-4_61

[3]. The 2016 study used almost 50,000 SNPs (r^2 limit = 0.7) to create a Genomic Risk Score (GRS) that they then used to predict the risk of having a major coronary incident.

By using such a large number of SNPs, the authors attempt to capture some of the small contributions made by non-coding regions of the genome. They compared the genomic predictive capabilities to the known clinical standard Framingham risk score (FRS) on five population cohorts. The authors used the GRS and FRS individually to calculate a hazard ratio (HR) score based on the FINRISK method – the risk of acute myocardial infarction or acute disorder of the cerebral circulation within the next 10 years.

Using the traditional Framingham method, the authors calculate an average FINKRISK HR score of 1.28 compared to the genomic method score of 1.74. The difference in score is a result of the genomic method capturing "substantially different trajectories of lifetime risk not captured by traditional clinical risk scores". These different risk trajectories are expressed in the top and bottom quintiles. A meta-analysis that combined the GRS and FRS methods found an improvement on the FRS method alone for predicting the time until a major coronary event – an average improved accuracy of 1.7% compared to FRS alone. For individuals over 60 years old, the combined GRS and FRS method showed an improved accuracy of 5.1%.

Perhaps, even more importantly, the authors found that the predicted age for male patients to experience a coronary event in between the top and bottom quartiles for the genomic method is 18 years compared to the standard FRS method of 12 years. This indicates that the combined GRS and FRS method could predict an event 6 years earlier than the FRS method alone, giving patients an earlier opportunity to address risk factors.

Considering asthma, a 2017 review of 25 GWA studies of asthmatics found 39 coding genetic variants with a p-value $>5\text{x}10^{-8}$. After performing analysis to remove false-positives and limiting their results to SNPs found in European populations, the authors calculate that the remaining 28 associations collectively contribute to only 2.5% of the genetic risk for asthma. Equation 1 below shows how to calculate the variance of the risk distribution and Eq. 2 uses the variance to calculate an overall value called the "SNP Heritability" [4].

Later, we calculate an SNP Heritability of ~1.5% using ten SNPs associated with asthma. Note that Eq. 1 scales linearly with the number of variants – if we double the number of variants, assuming a similar magnitude of odds ratios and frequencies, then we will also double their collective variation.

The total variation for a sum of k SNPs with individual frequency p_k and odds ratio OR_k.

$$\text{var} = 2\sum p_k\,(1 - p_k)\,(\log \text{OR}_k)^2 \tag{1}$$

The SNP Heritability h^2 for random genetic effect g distributed as $N(0, var(g))$.

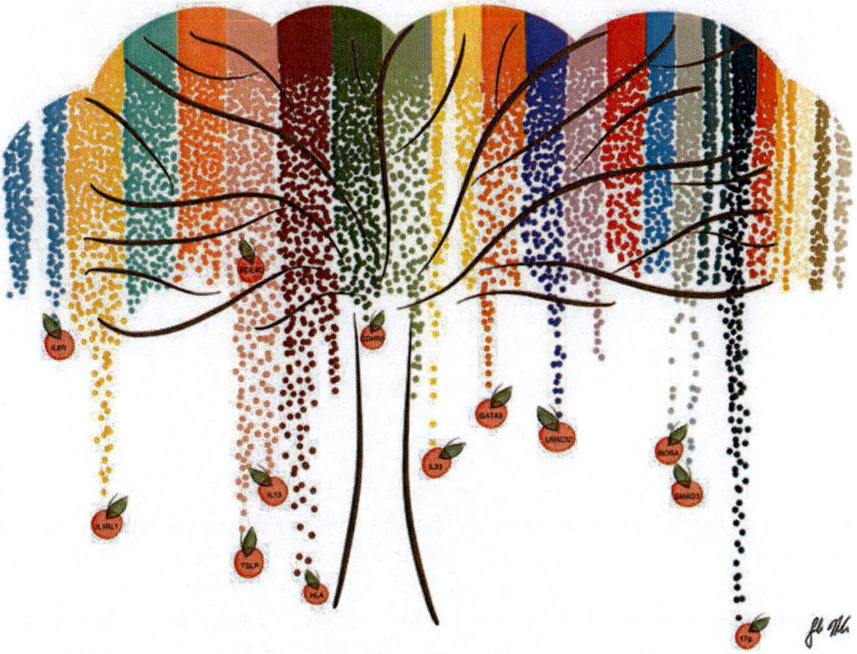

Fig. 1 The genomic variations of the asthmatic genotype illustrated as an apple tree with the "low hanging fruit" being the SNPs with the highest odds ratio. (Figure drawn by S. Mozaffari [5])

$$h^2 = \frac{\mathrm{var}(g)}{\mathrm{var}(g) + \pi^2/3} \tag{2}$$

The authors cite twin studies that show a heritability of asthma between 55% and 74% in adults – vastly larger than the previously calculated 2.5%. The authors hypothesize that the thousands of less common SNPs, each with less individual significance than 5×10^{-8}, collectively compose the majority of the inherited risk of asthma.

Using a method called linkage disequilibrium regression, the authors estimate that 1.2 million uncommon variants (MAF < 1%) contribute 13–15% of the inherited risk. This concept of the asthmatic genome is illustrated as an apple tree in Fig. 1 – each colored column is a chromosome composed of dots that represent SNPs. The observer immediately notices the "low hanging fruit" on the tree that represent the SNPs with the highest odds ratio values, while ignoring the thousands of other dots that also compose the tree [5].

This SNP-based solution to the missing/hidden heritability issue represents a step in the right direction. However, there are other factors, both experimental and genomic, that may contribute to the over/under estimation, such as poor study design, epistasis (gene-gene interactions), epigenetics factors, and the complex nature of asthmatic diseases – genetic influence could vary depending on the severity of asthma, the age of onset, or types of asthma triggered by exposure to environmental factors.

In this paper, we use a context-aware process to identify a set of genes (from a study of biomarkers [1] and other resources) and a set of tag SNPs (from the GWAS Catalog [2]) that are the most relevant to evolve our set of risk alleles. We believe this is better than a purely mechanistic process of analyzing GWAS data (that represent a potential, not experimentally validated, list). A full elucidation of this method requires one to understand all the key physiological and biological processes involved and include all the validated GWAS data (which represent potential new pathways yet to be explored).

2 Methods

The methodology we implement starts with the results of GWAS (SNPs & odds ratios) and uses them to analyze an individual patient's genome for prediction of disease phenotype development. The concept has been explored in detail by Dudley & Karczewski [6]. We expand their method by combining a priori known (experimentally verified) risk alleles with the GWAS-identified (potential) risk alleles, and using odds ratios for all these alleles from the GWAS catalog studies.

Beyond the genes we found directly corresponding to biomarkers, we also consider genes that are believed to have a role in the asthmatic metabolic process. For example, the Interleukin 7 gene, IL7, has been identified as a gene with a substantial influence on asthma biomarkers, but we go beyond IL7 to include IL7R, the Interleukin 7 Receptor gene. Although both are required for the body's metabolism of Interleukin 7, the two genes are not spatially close on the genome; IL7 is on chromosome 8, but IL7R is on chromosome 5.

We utilize the online GWAS catalog [2] to search for each of our identified genes and to gather SNPs associated with them. Each SNP entry in the GWAS catalog has information on the study it came from, including the population ethnicity statistics and a linkage disequilibrium (LD) tool (Fig. 2). We collect all SNPs related to our biomarker genes and we use the LD tool to find other SNPs that are genetically linked. When using the LD tool, we only consider SNPs that have been identified through GWAS methods and which have an r-squared value of at least 0.8. We expand the plot width to 500 kb so we can gather information on SNPs' part of other genes adjacent to the chromosome.

The LD tool requires us to select an ethnicity population before presenting a chart of the linked SNPs. By default, the ethnicity is British in England and Scotland (GBR). We try to use the LD tool to find SNPs found in similar ethnic populations as the original GWA study, but data is limited in certain ethnic groups and so our search for linked SNPs often goes beyond the original study's ethnic population. Once we have collected a set of SNPs with a high LD value, we can identify the genes each SNP represents to gather a list of additional genes in LD with our original biomarker genes.

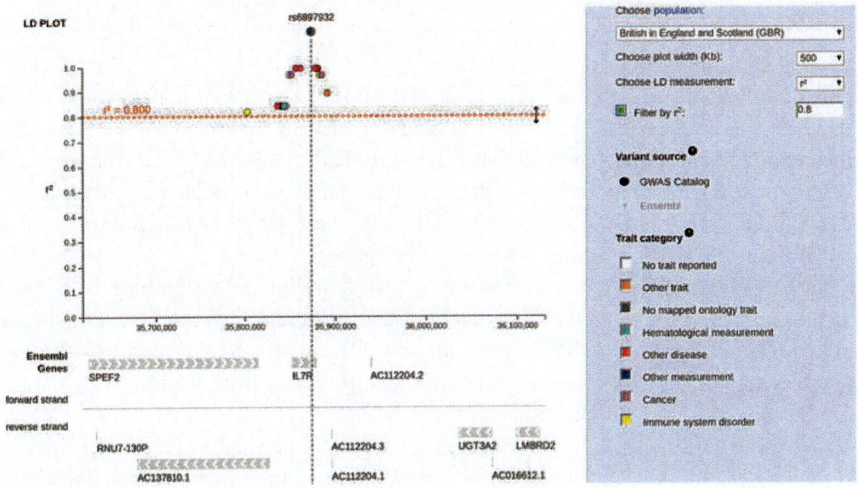

Fig. 2 The linkage disequilibrium tool provided by the GWAS catalog

Variant and risk allele	P-value	P-value annotation	RAF	OR	Beta	CI	Mapped gene	Reported trait	Trait(s)	Study accessi
rs6694672-G	9×10^{-6}	(Latino)	0.05	2.13	-	[1.52 - 2.97]	AL139418.1, CFHR5	Asthma	asthma	GCST005212
rs114647118-C	3×10^{-7}		0.99	2.08	-	[1.59 - 2.70]	TATDN1	Adult asthma	asthma	GCST007266
rs10197862-?	2×10^{-6}		NR	1.99	-	[NR]	IL1RL1, IL18R1	Asthma	asthma	GCST003176
rs10142119-G	2×10^{-7}		0.516	1.96	-	[1.52 - 2.56]	LINC01550, AL163932.1	IgE levels in asthmatics (D.f. specific)	serum IgE measurement, asthma	GCST002125
rs6563898-G	8×10^{-6}		0.523	1.82	-	[1.39 - 2.38]	CDH13	IgE levels in asthmatics (D.f. specific)	serum IgE measurement, asthma	GCST002125

Showing 191 to 195 of 1266 rows 5 rows per page ‹ 1 ... 38 39 40 ... 254 ›

Fig. 3 A selection of the GWAS catalog showing SNPs related to asthma. The entries are sorted by Odds Ratio to find the SNPs with the largest impact

To find other genes beyond those directly related to asthmatic biomarkers, we additionally search the whole GWAS catalog by filtering on the trait of asthma (Fig. 3). This provides us with hundreds of GWAS entries associated with numerous asthmatic and lung disease pathologies. We sort this list descending by Odds Ratio (OR), as we only want the most impactful SNPs with an OR greater than one (indicating an increased risk of phenotype development). We exclude entries for pathologies that are triggered by exposure to specific environmental substances – for example, we do not consider hundreds of entries related to asthma induced by toluene diisocyanate.

3 Results

Our complete set of asthma SNPs with odds ratios above one is presented below in Table 1. The first section consists of SNPs related to Interleukin 7 receptors and the second section consists of SNPs related to Th2 cytokines. These two sections represent the genes curated through biomarker studies of asthmatic patients. We expand our search beyond known biomarkers in the third section of Table 1 with a collection of SNPs from other non-biomarker genes.

The SNPs in Table 1 represent only a set of the largest magnitude odds ratio asthmatic SNPs in the GWAS catalog. They represent our attempt at a broad collection of significant SNPs with high odds ratios related to the asthmatic phenotype. With this in mind, we collect SNPs produced from studies using people of all ethnicities and who have all subtypes of asthma.

We further refine this set of SNPs into a representative smaller subset of 10 SNPs, shown below in Table 2. We have chosen to focus on ten increased risk SNPs that can be utilized to calculate a composite risk score for an individual patient. Each SNP has been identified by at least two GWA studies that have produced similar odds ratio scores. We average the odds ratio across these studies and provide it in Table 2.

We note that the distribution in ethnicity and type of asthma of Table 2 is reflective of the population of Table 1. Table 2 shows a total of ten SNPs, with nine of them being from studies focused on European patients. Further, eight of the ten SNPs are from studies on adult or non-specific age and only two of the SNPs are from child specific asthma. When making our selection of representative SNPs for Table 2, we did not consider the ethnicity or asthmatic type – the results being dominated by European and adult asthma is simply reflective of the general GWAS catalog studies being more commonly being focused on European adult patients.

Most of the ten SNPs in Table 2 come from the tag SNPs in Table 1, but some were also identified through linkage disequilibrium association [6, Sec. 6.4.5.1]. To find SNPs in low LD and to ensure none of the SNPs are in substantial LD, we make use of the online LDpair Tool [7]. It lets the user enter two SNPs and get back a detailed LD analysis. The highest r-square value we found is only 0.3157 between rs2299012 and rs1986009.

4 Discussion

We can now show how the genetic risk of a subject that expresses any of the ten SNPs from Table 2 can be adjusted based on our knowledge about the prevalence of asthma and each SNP's odds ratio/likelihood ratio. For our purposes, we are assuming that the odds ratio is approximately equal to the likelihood ratio (LR), so we use the terms interchangeably. We have conducted mathematical analysis to gain insight on the calculation of LR, given OR, MAF, and the sample size.

Table 1 Set of high odds ratio SNPs for genes associated with the asthmatic phenotype

IL-7 stimulated dendritic cell receptors					
Phenotype	**Gene**	**Tag SNP**	**SNPs in LD**	**Genes in LD**	**OR**
Eczema, allergic rhinitis, asthma	IL7R	rs6881270-C	rs11567694 rs7717955 rs11742240	AC112204.3	1.09
Asthma		rs11742240-G	rs1156769 rs7717955 rs6881270		1.057
		rs4594881-G	rs7717955 rs11567694 rs6881270 rs11742240		1.025
Th2 cytokines					
Phenotype	**Gene**	**Tag SNPs**	**SNPs in LD**	**Genes in LD**	**OR**
Asthma	IL4R	rs145986476-C			1.309
		rs3024655-G			1.139
Asthma (childhood onset)		rs3785356-T	rs4787951		1.122
Asthma	IL5	rs1986009-A	rs2244012 rs6871536 rs2040704 rs3091307 rs2706362	AC116366.3, RAD50, TH2LCRR	1.17
Asthma (childhood onset)	IL13	rs1295686-T	rs848 rs20541	TH2LCRR	1.31, 1.15
Asthma		rs1295685-A	rs848 rs20541	TH2LCRR	1.163, 1.065
Allergic disease (asthma, hay fever or eczema)		rs20541-A	rs1295685	TH2LCRR	1.234
Other genes					
Phenotype	**Gene**	**Tag SNPs**	**SNPs in LD**	**Genes in LD**	**OR**
Asthma	RNU1-21P, OR6M1	rs17744026-T			4
	AC009646.2	rs1425902-G			2.14
	CCDC195, CUL3	rs1843834-A			2.14
Asthma	AL139418.1, CFHR5	rs6694672-G	rs6003		2.13
	IL 1RL1, IL 18R1	rs10197862-A	rs3771175 rs13408661 rs3771180 rs59185885 rs950881 rs202011557	F13B, FAM183DP	1.99

(continued)

Table 1 (continued)

Phenotype	Gene	Tag SNPs	SNPs in LD	Genes in LD	OR
	AL163932.1, LINC01550	rs10142119			1.96
	CDH13	rs6563898-G			1.82
	AL355862.1, U3	rs1348135-C			1.754
	AL355862.1, U3	rs1348135-C			1.754
	TMEM132D, NLRP9P1	rs10773588-G			1.694
	RFC3P1, STAC	rs9870718-C			1.235
	THRB	rs12634582-C			1.26
	AC104837.1, ADGRL4	rs2352521-T			1.66
	AC116366.3,	rs2244012-C	rs1986009 rs3091307 rs2040704 rs6871536	IL5,	1.64
	ORMDL3, GSDMB	rs7216389-T	rs11655198 rs9901146 rs2290400 rs2305479 rs7216389	ZPBP2	1.45
Asthma & COPD	MSRA	rs117733692-?			3.332
	TAF4B	rs35614679-?			2.996
	RNF144A	rs3772010-?			2.89
	LINC01543, TAF4B	rs1677005-?			2.618
	MIR4527HG	rs11665213-?			2.232
Asthma (childhood onset)	SEMA3E	rs17446324-A			2.439
	FLG-AS1, FLG	rs61816761-A			1.97
	INSR	rs67731058-C			1.88
	CHCHD2P9, LNCARSR	rs2378383-?			1.64
Adult asthma	TATDN1	rs114647118-C			2.08
	AC246817.2	rs13277810-T			1.26
	IKZF3	rs907092-G	rs2941522 rs4795397 rs11655198 rs12939457 rs8069176 rs2305480 rs62067034	GRB7, ZPBP2, GSDMB	1.32
	RORA	rs10519067-G	rs34986765 rs110 71559 rs10519068		1.18
	STAT6	rs3122929-T	rs703816 rs167769		1.17

Table 2 A subset of 10 SNPs representing the genetics of the asthmatic response biological pathway

Gene	SNP	OR	Ethnicity	Phenotype	Biological role [8]
CDH13	rs6563898-G	1.82	East Asian	Asthma	Implicated in regulation of cell growth; expressed in endothelial cells
FLG	rs61816761-A	1.27	European	Asthma, (childhood onset)	Pro-filaggrin (filament-aggregating protein), binds to keratin fibers in epithelial cells
IL 13	rs1295686-T	1.25	European, East Asian	Asthma, (childhood onset)	Interleukin-13 induces IgG4 and IgE synthesis by human B cells; induces tissue repair program in macrophages
GSDMB	rs2305480-G	1.25	European	Asthma, (adult)	Implicated in the regulation of apoptosis in epithelial cells
IL1RL1	rs10197862-A	1.24	European	Asthma	Interleukin-1 receptor, selectively expressed on Th2 and mast cells, mediates effects of Interleukins, drives production of Th2-associated cytokines
IL5	rs1986009-A	1.17	European	Asthma	Interleukin-5, a selective eosinophil-activating growth hormone; mediates activation of white blood cell eosinophils
RORA	rs10519067-G	1.13	European, Hispanic, Afro-American/Afro-Caribbean	Asthma, (adult)	Plays an essential role in the development of type 2 innate lymphoid cells (ILC2)
IL7R	rs6881270-C	1.10	European	Asthma	Encodes receptor for Interleukin-7, a glycoprotein involved in regulation of lymphopoiesis and essential for normal development of white blood cell lymphocytes
STAT6	rs3122929-T	1.07	European, Hispanic, Afro-American/Afro-Caribbean	Asthma, (adult)	Mediates immune signaling in response to cytokines at the plasma membrane; major site of expression is the bronchial epithelium
RAD50	rs2299012-C	1.05	European	Asthma	Encodes a protein that is essential for double-stranded DNA break repair by nonhomologous DNA end joining and chromosomal integration

For typical GWAS ORs of 1.5 or less, LR can be assumed to be the same value as OR. We do have an SNP with odds ratios above 1.5 (rs6563898-G has OR = 1.82), but we assume the difference with LR to be minimal. We focus on a patient's asthmatic history (childhood vs. adult onset), along with their ethnicity and age. We primarily consider European patients because nine of the ten SNPs we are looking at were identified at least partially using a population of Europeans. We also do not consider the impact of environmental pollutants, nutrition, pharmaceuticals, or the gender of the patient.

As an example, we choose a hypothetical patient of European ethnicity, a middle-aged adult, who has had asthma their entire life – it started as a child and continues now into adulthood. Before considering their medical history or being genetically tested, their pre-test probability of having asthma can be estimated as the prevalence of asthma for their given ethnicity and age. A survey of European households found 4.72% had at least one asthmatic patient [9]. The National Surveillance of Asthma: United States, 2001–2010 identified 7.8% of white Americans having asthma in 2010, further breaking it down to 9.5% of children and 7.7% in adults [10]. For our hypothetical European adult patient, we make a rough average of these numbers and say they have a 6.0% pre-test probability of having asthma before adjusting for specific genetic variation risk.

We note that this value likely varies greatly across different environments and demographics and also does not consider the specificity of asthma diagnosis – it is possible that a percentage of the people with asthma are incorrectly diagnosed. This is especially true for complex diseases like asthma, which are not defined by a single binary diagnostic test. Asthma can be short term or long term, episodic or stable, as a symptom of a larger pulmonary syndrome or present on its own, and can be inherent in an individual or triggered intermittently by external factors.

Now that we have an estimate of the prevalence for the hypothetical patient, we can calculate the genetic risk contribution of each SNP. If a patient is found to have an SNP, we can calculate their post-test probability by multiplying the pre-test odds by the likelihood ratio of the SNP. For example, the SNP with the highest likelihood ratio for a European patient is rs61816761-A with an LR of 1.27. For a patient with an assumed 6% pre-test probability of asthma that is found to have this SNP, we can say their post-test risk of having asthma is equal to (0.06/1–0.06) $\times$ 1.27 = 0.1162 or a 8.11% probability – more than a 33% increase in the chance of having asthma.

For comparison, say instead the patient is found to have our lowest likelihood ratio SNP, rs2299012-C, with an LR of 1.05. For a patient with a 6% pre-test probability of asthma that is found to have this SNP we can say their post-test risk of having asthma is equal to (0.06/1–0.06) $\times$ 1.05 = 0.0670 or a 6.70% probability – less than a 10% increase in risk, but still a noticeable contribution. We show each SNP's individual contribution to risk in Table 3 below.

As an extreme example, let us say we have a European adult patient who expresses nine out of ten of these variants (we do not consider the impact of rs6563898-G, which was identified using only non-European populations). A person with nine of these SNPs would have an extremely rare genome – if we multiply the nine frequencies, we get a probability of having all nine SNPs present of only

Table 3 The risk allele frequency (RAF) and adjusted risk probability of asthma for each individual SNP assuming a 6% pre-test prevalence

SNP	OR	Risk allele frequency (RAF)	Post-test probability
rs6563898-G	1.82	0.523	(0.06/1–0.06) × 1.82 = 11.62%
rs61816761-A	1.27	0.0024	(0.06/1–0.06) × 1.27 = 8.11%
rs1295686-T	1.25	0.25	(0.06/1–0.06) × 2.25 = 14.35%
rs2305480-G	1.25	0.575	(0.06/1–0.06) × 1.25 = 7.98%
rs10197862-A	1.24	0.85	(0.06/1–0.06) × 1.24 = 7.92%
rs1986009-A	1.17	0.1871	(0.06/1–0.06) × 1.17 = 7.47%
rs10519067-G	1.13	0.78	(0.06/1–0.06) × 1.13 = 7.21%
rs6881270-C	1.10	0.7254	(0.06/1–0.06) × 1.10 = 7.02%
rs3122929-T	1.07	0.404	(0.06/1–0.06) × 1.07 = 6.83%
rs2299012-C	1.05	0.19	(0.06/1–0.06) × 1.05 = 6.70%

0.0000043417 or < 0.0005%. The patient would start off with a pre-test asthma probability of 6.0%, but with so many genetic contributions, their post-test risk of asthma would be 0.06 × 1.27 × 1.25 × ... 1.05 = 0.2412 or a 24.12% lifetime probability of developing asthma – more than a four-time increase compared to the general European population.

However, we cannot immediately tell the patient their lifetime risk of asthma is four times higher than normal. This statement is not necessarily the case because we are only considering the collective impact of these SNPs alone. We are also not considering the impact of the patient's environment or other cofounding factors (obesity, smoking, etc.). Additionally, we are treating all the SNPs from Table 2 as equally contributing towards the asthmatic phenotype despite some SNPs being associated with child onset and some being adult onset. Finally, we are assuming "that the allelic risk is multiplicative, such that the odds ratio for homozygous risk allele genotype is the squared odds ratio of the allelic odds ratio" [6].

Before using such risk estimates as part of a patient's medical care, we must make note that these calculations involve a single SNP or group of SNPs considered in isolation from the rest of a patient's genome. We are not considering the impact of less significant (p-value $>5 \times 10^{-8}$). As we discussed earlier, the less significant SNPs may represent the vast majority of the asthmatic heritability, with more significant SNPs composing only 2.6% of the heritability. Utilizing Eqs. 1 and 2, we estimate the total SNP heritability of ~1.5% for all ten of our most significant SNPs (Table 4).

When looking at an individual SNP's risk contribution towards a patient developing asthma, all we can actually say is that the expression of a single SNP or group of SNPs contributes a specific amount of risk to the patient. To say that the patient has a "better than average" chance of developing asthma we must consider the role of other SNPs, common and rare. We must also keep in mind that the prevalence of asthma, which we assumed to be 6%, is not at all independent of genetic factors. The prevalence is the final result of a complex disease that has ethnicity, demographic, environmental, genetic, and other risk factors.

Table 4 Calculating ~1.5% as the total genetic contribution (SNP heritability) of ten SNPs associated with asthma

SNP	OR	Risk allele frequency (RAF)	SNP heritability (h^2)
rs6563898-G	1.82	0.523	0.01016390182
rs61816761-A	1.27	0.0024	0.001194602754
rs1295686-T	1.25	0.25	0.001070447548
rs2305480-G	1.25	0.575	0.001394697109
rs10197862-A	1.24	0.85	0.0006767114757
rs1986009-A	1.17	0.1871	0.0004301349055
rs10519067-G	1.13	0.78	0.0002941154534
rs6881270-C	1.10	0.7254	0.0002078354297
rs3122929-T	1.07	0.404	0.0001264969044
rs2299012-C	1.05	0.19	0.00004204801456

5 Conclusion

Asthma is a complex disease that is known to have multiple contributing factors, including genetic and environmental components. Starting from a list of asthmatic biomarker genes and utilizing the results from genome-wide association studies, we have curated dozens of SNPs associated with asthma. We filter these SNPs to find a subset of those with high magnitude odds ratio values that are in low linkage disequilibrium with each other. We are then able to reduce this to a list of ten high risk common.

Using each SNP's odds ratio, we estimate how each SNP can impact an individual person's risk of developing asthma. Each SNP or group of SNPs that are expressed in a patient can contribute an increased risk beyond the general population prevalence. SNPs representing multiple biomarkers associated with asthma. Due to the nature of studies that compose the GWAS catalog, our list of ten SNPs is primarily sourced from European patients with an unspecific asthmatic age of onset.

Future work should also consider the role of protective SNPs present on a patient – if they do not have the pathogenic SNP associated with asthma, we could assume they instead have a protective factor that must be considered. A patient may express many polymorphisms that increase the risk of developing asthma, while simultaneously expressing many polymorphisms that lower the risk of asthma. A total "net probability" combines the odds ratios from both protective and risk factor polymorphisms. Further, biological processes might endow different additive/multiplicative weights to their effect on the overall risk. There is also an opportunity to create SNP risk profiles based on other population demographics (ethnicity, age), patient lifestyle, and environmental influences – our results are primarily related to European patients that already experience asthma. More useful for patients would be a predictive tool that could give lifetime risk predictions for younger people that have yet to develop asthma.

References

1. V. S. Vaidya, J. V. Bonventre (eds.), *Biomarkers in Medicine, Drug Discovery, and Environmental Health* (Wiley, 2010)
2. A. Buniello, J.A.L. MacArthur, M. Cerezo, L.W. Harris, J. Hayhurst, C. Malangone, A. McMahon, J. Morales, E. Mountjoy, E. Sollis, D. Suveges, O. Vrousgou, P.L. Whetzel, R. Amode, J.A. Guillen, H.S. Riat, S.J. Trevanion, P. Hall, H. Junkins, P. Flicek, T. Burdett, L.A. Hindorff, F. Cunningham, H. Parkinson, The NHGRI-EBI GWAS Catalog of published genome-wide association studies, targeted arrays and summary statistics 2019. Nucleic Acids Res. **47**(Database issue), D1005–D1012 (2019) https://www.ebi.ac.uk/gwas/
3. G. Abraham, A.S. Havulinna, O.G. Bhalala, S.G. Byars, A.M. De Livera, L. Yetukuri, E. Tikkanen, M. Perola, H. Schunkert, E.J. Sijbrands, A. Palotie, N.J. Samani, V. Salomaa, S. Ripatti, M. Inouye, Genomic prediction of coronary heart disease. Eur. Heart J. **37**(43), 3267–3278 (2016). https://doi.org/10.1093/eurheartj/ehw450
4. C.T. Vicente, J.A. Revez, M.A.R. Ferreira, Lessons from ten years of genome-wide association studies of asthma. Clin. Transl. Immunol. **6**, e165 (2017). https://doi.org/10.1038/cti.2017.54
5. C. Ober, Asthma Genetics in the post-GWAS era. Ann. Am. Thorac. Soc. **13**(Supplement 1) (2015)
6. J.T. Dudley, K.J. Karczewski, Ch.6 ‘Genetic Trait Associations’, in *Exploring Personal Genomics*, (2013)
7. M.J. Machiela, S.J. Chanock, LDlink: A web-based application for exploring population-specific haplotype structure and linking correlated alleles of possible functional variants. Bioinformatics **31**(21), 3555–3557 (Nov. 2015) https://ldlink.nci.nih.gov/?tab=ldpair
8. Online Mendelian Inheritance in Man, OMIM. McKusick-Nathans Institute of Genetic Medicine, Johns Hopkins University (Baltimore, MD). https://omim.org/. Accessed 6 July 2020
9. P. Bergquist, G.K. Crompton, Clinical management of asthma in 1999: The Asthma Insights and Reality in Europe (AIRE) study. Eur. Respir. J. **18**(1), 248 (2001)
10. J.E. Moorman et al., National surveillance of asthma: United States, 2001–2010. Vital Health Stat. **3**(35), 1–58 (Nov. 2012)

Cancer Gene Diagnosis of 84 Microarrays Using Rank of 100-Fold Cross-Validation

Shuichi Shinmura

1 Introduction

Following our completion of a new theory of discriminant analysis [17], we used Revised IP-Optimal Linear Discriminant Function (Revised IP-OLDF, RIP) [12–16] to discriminate against the Alon microarray [1]. We find that the minimum number of misclassifications (minimum NM, MNM) was zero. MNM decreases monotonously ($MNM_k \geq MNM_{(k+1)}$). If $MNM_k = 0$, all MNMs of models, including these k-variables, are zero. This indicates that the data are linearly separable data (LSD). Two classes (comprising 22 non-cancerous or "normal" patients and 40 cancer patients, respectively) are entirely separable in the 2000 gene space. We found that LSD is the crucial signal for cancer gene diagnosis. We classify the linearly separable space and subspaces as Matryoshka. We found that LSD has two special structures. First, LSD has a Matryoshka structure. The microarray (data) includes many smaller Matryoshkas up to the minimum Matryoshka (a Basic Gene Set, BGS). Because MNM of BGS is zero, all MNMs of Matryoshkas that include BGS are zero. Thus, the Matryoshka structure matches the monotonic decrease of MNM. The second structure is as follows: LINGO: Program3 can decompose data into the exclusive Small Matryoshkas (SMs) and another gene subspace (MNM > 0) using the Matryoshka Feature Selection Method (Method2). Program3 is a Method2 program. LINGO [11] is a high-quality mathematical programming (MP) solver developed by LINDO Systems Inc. When RIP discriminates microarray (n cases << p genes), we found the number of non-zero coefficients is less than equal n. LINGO: Program4 can decompose LSD into the exclusive BGSs and other gene subspace, using the same procedure used to find Yamanaka 4 genes from 24 genes. If we

S. Shinmura (✉)
Seikei University, Sakasai Kasiwa City, Chiba, Japan

H. R. Arabnia et al. (eds.), *Advances in Computer Vision and Computational Biology*, Transactions on Computational Science and Computational Intelligence,
https://doi.org/10.1007/978-3-030-71051-4_62

remove one gene from a BGS using the same method as discovering Yamanaka four genes, its MNM is not zero. SM includes nearly more than two BGSs in it. The second structure releases us from the curse of high-dimensional data [19]. We can analyze all 193 signals using the statistical software JMP [10] and propose the cancer gene diagnosis [18]. Although we have successfully found all the signals, we need to rank the importance of all signals for physicians to use for diagnosis. Thus, we evaluate all signals via the 100-fold cross-validation (Method1). We discriminate against the original data (Internal Samples, IS) using RIP and find that data is LSD (via an Internal Check, IC). If Alon et al. offer the external samples (ES) not used for analysis, we can validate the reliability of the IC by determining whether the MNM of ES is zero. However, because we cannot obtain the ES, we validate MNM (or Error Rate (ER) = MNM/n) =0 using Method1. This validation is the alternative to an External Check (EC). Machine Learning (ML) researchers use k-fold Cross Validation (k-fold CV) and focus only on test sample correct classification rate (1 – ER). They do not analyze the original data in detail and do not understand that the actual data result, such as misclassified cases, is vital for medical diagnosis. In this paper, we validate all signals via Method1 and show the critical rank of those for gene diagnosis is useful for medical research.

2 Material

2.1 Alon et al. Microarray (Alon Data)

Alon et al. studied the broad patterns of gene expression revealed by cluster analysis using 40 samples of cancerous colon tissue and 22 samples of normal colon tissue. Using an Affymetrix Hum6000 array (the first generation equipment), they analyzed over 6500 human genes from 62 samples. Although the discriminant analysis is the best method for two-class data (supervised learning data), Alon et al. analyzed both the 6500 genes and 62 tissues via cluster analysis in addition to correlation analysis based on medical knowledge. They examined the probability histogram of correlation coefficients between pairs of genes and, of the 6500 genes, specified all pairs within the 2000 genes with the highest minimal intensity across the tissues. They analyzed 2000 genes via two-way clustering based on the deterministic-annealing algorithm to organize the data in a binary tree. Lastly, they carefully examined gene clusters and tissue clusters using detailed medical knowledge.

2.2 *Gene Diagnosis by Alon Data*

Two Universal Data Structure of LSD

We downloaded six data, including the Alon data from Jeffery et al. [7], on October 28, 2015. We analyzed the six data within 54 days and found the two vital LSD data structures. (1) The six data are LSD, and two classes are utterly separable in high-dimensional gene space. We classify the linearly separable space and sub-spaces as Matryoshka. LSD has the Matryoshka structure that includes smaller Matryoshka in it up to BGS, similar to the Yamanaka four genes in a set of 24 genes. (2) LSD consists of the exclusive SMs or BGSs and another gene set (MNM > 0). Thus, we can decompose the data into all signal subspaces (MNM = 0) and noise subspace. By the second data structure, we are free from the curse of high-dimensional data and can analyze all signals using JMP. We propose a standard approach for cancer gene diagnosis. With our methods, physicians' diagnoses treat cancer in human patients.

Difficulty of SM Analysis

In 2015, we could decompose Alon data into 64 SMs using LINGO: Program3, a program of Method2. Later, we developed LINGO: Program4, which decomposes data into 129 BGSs. Each SM often includes over two BGSs. We can find 193 vital signals. In other gene sets found by Program3 and Program4, two MNMs are not zero. So, we considered those two subspaces' noise. Both programs terminate after finding the first noise subspace. If we can consider the useful meaning of other noise subspace, both programs can completely decompose data into the many exclusive SMs and several noise subspaces. Program4 can divide data into exclusive signals and noises of MNM. This shows the universal data structure of MNM. All RIP coefficients of these sub-spaces are not zero. Because SMs and BGSs are small samples, we can analyze those with six MP-based Linear Discriminate Functions (LDFs), logistic regression, Fisher's LDF, QDF, one-way ANOVA, t-test, correlation analysis, hierarchical Ward analysis, and Principal Component Analysis (PCA). However, we cannot obtain the linearly separable signals except for logistic regression, in addition to RIP and H-SVM. The logistic regression uses the algorithm of the maximum-likelihood method developed by Fisher. It is free from the assumption of the normal distribution so that it can correctly discriminate all SMs and BGSs of the six data based on the real data distribution. However, it cannot correctly discriminate against the cases on the discriminant hyperplane.

Figure 1 shows the two-way clustering of the eighth SM (SM8) via Ward's hierarchical cluster analysis. The case dendrogram on the right shows five color clusters. The 22 normal subjects (those case numbers highlighted on the left) are sorted into nine small clusters. Of the non-cancerous clusters, two are red, three are green, two are blue, and two are pale green. None of the normal subject clusters

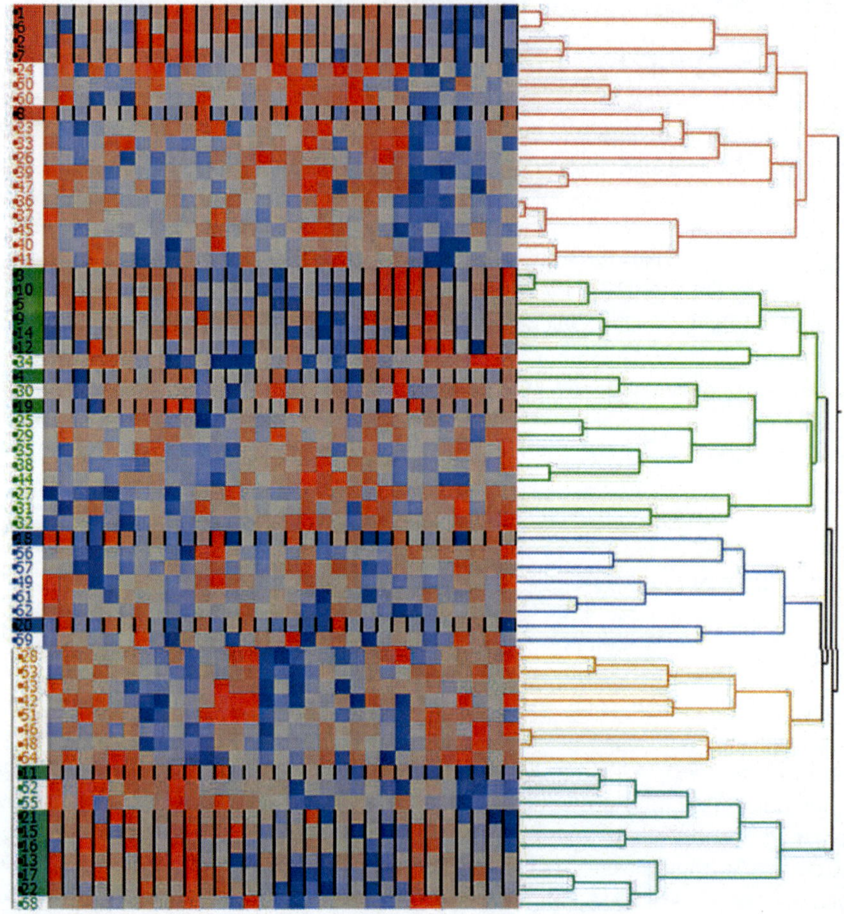

Fig. 1 Ward cluster of SM8

are orange. The 40 cancerous subjects are sorted into 10 small clusters (those case numbers on the left between highlighted numbers). The 19 small clusters on the left make up the five large clusters on the right. Four of the large clusters include both cancer and normal subjects (red, green, blue, and pale green), and a fifth cluster comprises exclusively cancerous subjects (orange). Excluding the large orange cluster, each large cluster comprises an equal number of cancerous and non-cancerous small clusters (e.g., three highlighted green clusters and three non-highlighted green clusters). This result suggests to us the following important information: (1) RIP separates non-cancerous and cancerous subjects, but those become a cluster of nine small pairs of normal and cancer clusters. Although the distance between two small clusters is small, the discriminant hyperplane separates two clusters. This fact shows the difficulties of gene data. (2) Since other SMs have the same results, however, the linear discriminant hyperplane is steady and reliable. We hypothesize that when normal patients become cancerous, they move in a specific direction that is clearly defined in the genetic space. However, since the distance is small, only RIP and H-SVM can discriminate those theoretically. There are pairs of cancer and normal subjects in the same large cluster, probably because of similar values in many other genes except several gene combinations related to cancer.

Therefore, the distance is small. The cases in orange are exclusively cancerous, including that those cancerous subjects are far from healthy in additional ways.

PCA's scatter plot show that two classes overlap. Thus, large variation cannot detect LSD signs and may show the sub-groups of cancer subjects and healthy subjects. On the other hand, small variation represented by the specific higher principal components catch the LSD. This is why statistical analysis with SM does not succeed. We introduced other similar results in Shinmura [18].

Most *t*-tests consist of three types of values: positive values, almost zero values, and negative values. Most error rates of Fisher's LDF, QDF, and Regularized Discriminant Analysis (RDA) are not zero. Thus, these discriminant functions based on the variance-covariance matrices are useless [17]. While some statisticians expect LASSO to be useful in high-dimensional genetic data analysis, the problem is that it cannot correctly identify LSD before that.

Breakthrough of RIP Discriminant Scores and Signal Data

RIP discriminated 64 SMs and made 64 RIP discriminant scores (RipDSs). We consider the 64 RipDSs of 64 SMs the cancer malignancy indexes because those can separate two classes. However, physicians must validate our claim. Because statistical methods cannot show the linearly separable signs, we make signal data that consists of 62 cases and 64 RipDSs instead of all 2000 genes.

Figure 2 shows the Ward output using the signal data. We choose five clusters, the same as we did in Fig. 1. The upper red cluster comprises the 22 normal subjects. The lower four-color clusters are the 40 cancer subjects. The two classes are entirely separable in two clusters. This result is useful because the hierarchical cluster methods use the Euclidean distance without the complex transformations. The 64 columns show the 64 RipDSs. The colormap of normal subjects (22 subjects and 64 RipDSs) is almost blue, indicating low expression levels. The colormap of the 40 cancer subjects (40 patients and 64 RipDSs) is mostly red, indicating high expression levels. The black-filled variable at the bottom is the 64th RipDS (RipDS64). Many cancer subjects of this variable are blue, indicating a low expression and showing this variable as a useless indicator of malignancy. Our result is clearer than the results of the six aforementioned medical projects. Besides, we do not need to use the self-organizing map (SOM) used by Golub et al. [6]. That tends to show untrue clustering results and is a complicated algorithm. They selected about 50 genes using a weighted voting method, not a multivariate approach. Even if the MNM of these genes is not zero, the SOM will choose the settings for classifying

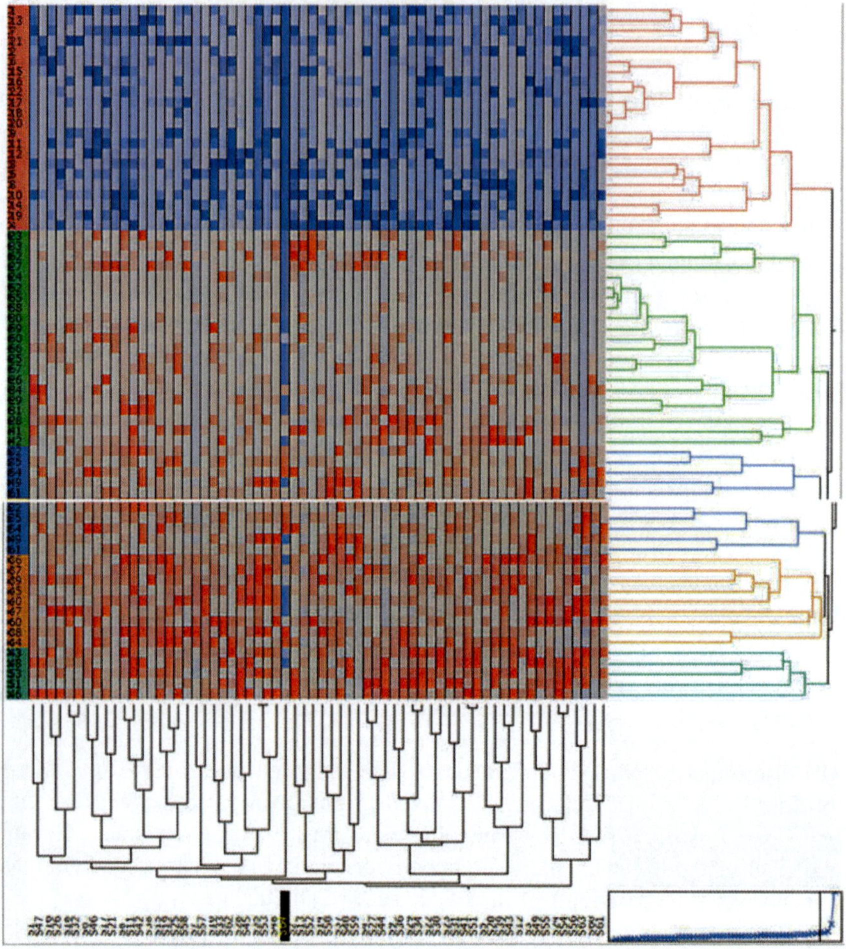

Fig. 2 Ward cluster of the signal data

data into the best two clusters, possibly resulting in false classification. Since this is a complex transformation, the result cannot be reflected in PCA. Because the positional relationship of cases is unknown, doctors cannot study cases using the combination of cluster analysis and PCA. The deterministic-annealing algorithm used by Alon et al. has the same defect.

Figure 3 shows the PCA results revealing the spatial location relationship of subjects belongs to the five clusters. The central scatter plot shows that the 22 normal cases (in red) are on the Prin1 axis at approximately −5 or less. In the same plot, the 40 cancer cases spread from the origin in a fan shape toward the positive side of Prin1. In the first quadrant, the malignancy is considered higher in order of green, blue, and orange cancer patients. In the fourth quadrant, the malignancy is higher in

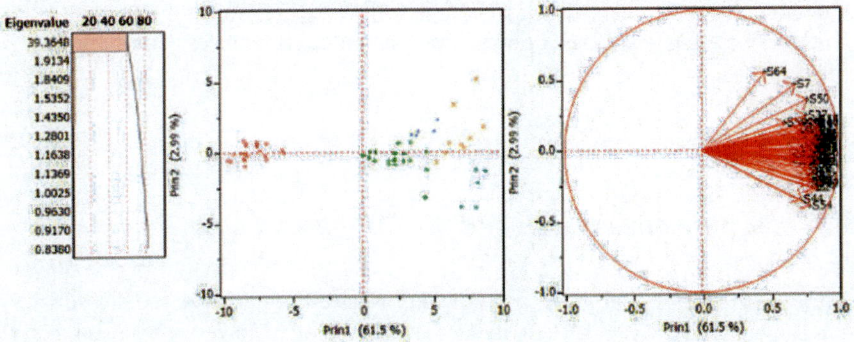

Fig. 3 PCA of the signal data

the order of green and light green cancer patients. This is useful in finding cancer subclasses. Golub et al. split the data into two clusters with SOM to find subclasses but ran into SOM's incorrect clustering disadvantage that ignores the misclassified cases.

Another problem is that we cannot examine SOM results with PCA. The plot on the left shows the first eigenvalue is 39.3, and its contribution rate is 61.5% shown in the central plot. This indicates that the two classes are on the opposite side of the origin of Prin1. This result is similar to the high-dimensional PCA result of Aoshima and Yata [2]. They found that the 6 eigenvalues of Prin1 were very large. This is because the two classes are LSD and are respectively separated on the positive and negative side of Prin1's axis. We forecast the first eigenvalue is large if two classes have almost the same number of cases. It shows a sign of LSD.

2.3 Materials in This Research

The six data had nearly the same gene diagnosis results, regardless of the different cancer types. Because of this, we expect other data to show the same results. We evaluated all signals using the RatioSV (= the distance of two SVs/ the range of RipDS×100). Because RatioSVs of 64 SMs were over 2% and those of 129 BGSs were less than 1%, we concluded not all BGSs are useful for cancer gene diagnosis. However, because RatioSV depends on only two values of the maximum and minimum valued of RipDSs, we re-evaluate all signals using Method1 in this study.

The materials of this research are 64 SMs and 129 BGSs. RIP calculates 100 NMs and 100 ERs (=NM/*n*) of 100 training samples. 100 RIPs discriminate against the test sample and calculate the 100 ERs. We obtain the minimum, maximum, and average values of 100 ERs for the training and test samples. The average ER in the training and test samples are called M1 and M2, respectively. Because M1 has the monotonic decrease like MNM, M1 of the full model is always a minimum value. Notably, we focus on M2 as it ranks important values for cancer gene diagnosis.

3 Theory

3.1 Purpose of Research and Six MP-based LDFs

If the high-dimensional gene data is LSD, we need not analyze the data directly. We can analyze SMs and BGSs by statistical methods. However, we need to rank the importance of those signals and decide the more valuable SMs and BGS for gene diagnosis. For this purpose, we validate all signals using Method1, resulting in M2s producing the gene diagnosis ranking. In this Section, we introduce six MP-based LDFs and validation methods, such as k-fold CV and Method1. We develop RIP to find the interior point of true Optimal Convex Polyhedron (OCP) defined by n-constraints ($y_i \times ({}^t\mathbf{x}_i \times \mathbf{b} + b_0) \geq 1$) in (1). We found four problems with discriminant analysis [16]. The first problem (Problem 1) involves the defects of NM. Thus, we proposed MNM instead of NM. Moreover, non-RIP LDFs must count the number of cases on the discriminant hyperplane ($f(\mathbf{x}_i) = ({}^t\mathbf{x}_i \times \mathbf{b} + 1) = 0$) to avoid Problem 1.

$$\mathrm{MIN} = \Sigma\, e_i;\, y_i \times \left({}^t\mathbf{x}_i \times \mathbf{b} + b_0\right) \geq 1\text{–}M \times e_i;\, i = 1, \ldots, n \tag{1}$$

e_i: 0/1 binary integer
$\mathbf{x}_i$: i^{th} case values
$\mathbf{b}$: p-coefficients.
b_0: the constant and free variable
M: Big M constant (10,000).

For correctly classified cases, e_i are zero. Thus, the constraints become OCP. For the misclassified cases ($e_i = 1$), it changes to ($y_i \times ({}^t\mathbf{x}_i \times \mathbf{b} + b_0) \geq -9999$). The 0/1 binary integer variables choose the two alternatives, such as SV = 1 for classified cases and SV = −9999 for misclassified cases. Our MP-based LDFs have special features as follows: (1) The $\mathbf{x}_i$ and e_i are called the decision variables. Only e_i defines the objective function (MIN = Σe_i;). However, all $\mathbf{x}_i$ are not in the objective function. (2) These LDFs choose the optimal coefficient corresponding to the interior point of OCP. All MNMs of OCP are 0 and become the optimal solution. If we change the 0/1 integer variable e_i to non-negative real values, Eq. (1) becomes the linear programming (LP) LDF called Revised LP-OLDF. Because RIP took more computational time than Revised LP-OLDF, we developed Revised IPLP-OLDF, a mixture of both models. However, because the LINGO IP solver has increasingly sped up, we need not use Revised IPLP-OLDF instead of RIP anymore.

Vapnik [24] defined a hard-margin Support Vector Machine (H-SVM) to maximize the distance of two Support Vectors (SVs) in (2). All patients in class1 are included in SV ≤ -1; other cases in class2 are included in SV ≥ 1. There are no cases between $-1 < \text{SV} < 1$. We can understand LSD-discrimination clearly. Only H-SVM and RIP can discriminate LSD theoretically. However, there is no further research on LSD-discrimination beyond us.

$$\text{MIN} = ||\mathbf{b}||^2/2;\ y_i \times ({}^t\mathbf{x}_i \times \mathbf{b} + b_0) \geq 1; \quad (2)$$

$$\text{MIN} = ||\mathbf{b}||^2/2 + c \times \Sigma e_i;\ y_i \times ({}^t\mathbf{x}_i \times \mathbf{b} + b_0) \geq 1 - e_i; \quad (3)$$

e_i: non-negative real value.
c: Penalty c that combines two objects.

After introducing H-SVM, he defined a soft-margin SVM (S-SVM) for the overlap data in (3). Because H-SVM cannot solve the overlap data, many users of SVM use S-SVM or kernel-SVM. Although users must choose the proper penalty c for S-SVM, they often use the penalty $c = 1$ without serious examination. After we examined eight choices of c such as $c = 10^6$, 10^5, 10^4, 10^3, 10^2, 10, 1, and 0.1 with six different data, we judged S-SVM with penalty $c = 10^6$ (SVM6) the best. Thus, we compared six MP-based LDFs, logistic regression, and Fisher's LDF by six different datasets using Method1. The Six MP-based LDFs are RIP, Revised LP-OLDF, Revised IPLP-OLDF, H-SVM, SVM6, and SVM1 (S-SVM with penalty $c = 1$). The six different types of ordinary datasets are: Fisher's iris data, Swiss banknote data, Student data, Cephalo-pelvic disproportion data, Japanese car data, and exam scores pass/fail determination datasets [17]. We ranked eight discriminant functions via M2. The M2 ranking is as follows: (1) RIP is the best, (2) SVM6, Revised LP-OLDF, Revised IPLP-OLDF, and logistic regression are in a group of "second best" options, and (3) Fisher's LDF and SVM1 are the worst.

3.2 *Internal and External Checks, LOO and k-fold CV LDFs*

In traditional discriminant analysis terminology, we call the original medical data the Internal Sample (IS). To evaluate NM and ER of IS is called an Internal Check (IC). We can do the IC using released IS. However, we cannot often validate IC's result by the new patients (External Sample, ES). If the medical projects collect ES after the IC, we can evaluate the ER of ES with the discriminant functions calculated by IS. We call this validation an External Check (EC). Even if we can obtain ES, we take a disadvantage of research time loss. Thus, Lachenbruch [8] promoted the Leave-One-Out (LOO) method using the training samples and validation samples generated from IS. At his time, because there was no computer, it was a good and useful validation method. The worse the ERs of EC, the less reliable the ERs of IC. Thus, the comparison of the IC and the EC is necessary. Miyake and Shinmura [9] studied the relationship between the sample ER (IC) and the population's ER (EC), assuming Fisher's assumption. Because this assumption expects the two classes to have the same normal distributions, this study is useless for cancer diagnosis because gene data do not satisfy Fisher's assumption.

Based on LOO, engineering researchers developed the *k*-fold CV. LOO is an *n*-fold CV. It divides the IS into *n* pairs. Then, it uses the divided (*n*-1) sets as a training sample (IS) and the remaining one set as a test sample (ES). We discriminate this training sample *n* times and obtain *n* ERs of test samples for final evaluation. This method was convenient for engineering researchers. They can validate quickly without obtaining new patients (ES), such as when the computer environment is poor. However, there are four complications:

1. The number of test samples is less than the training sample. Moreover, *n* sets of test samples are different.
2. For example, it is not generally possible to decide which CV is better, the.
3. Fivefold CV or the tenfold CV. It depends on the data case by case.
4. For small samples where *n* is 100 or less, there are often no differences between the variance-covariance matrices with 100 cases and 99 cases. That is, there is a tendency to affirm the current result by LDF.
5. Most problematically, many studies forget that the evaluation of the original data (the IC) is essential for medical diagnosis. Many researchers considered test sample results are crucial and do not evaluate the original data by other statistical methods.

3.3 100-Fold Cross-Validation (Method2)

Discriminant analysis is descriptive statistics, not inferential statistics. So, Fisher never formulated the standard error of LDF coefficients and ERs. Lachenbruch and Mickey proposed the LOO method for the validation technique of discriminant analysis. Golub et al. and other medical projects validate their results with LOO. However, LOO is developed (used in the era before modern computing power) and has more defects than those above. Based on the statistical framework, we proposed the following Method1. Copy the original data 100 times and consider it a test sample and pseudo-population. We assigned a uniform random number to each case and sorted it in descending order. Then, we divide it into 100 sets of training samples. We discriminate the 100 training samples and apply those functions to the test sample to obtain 100 NMs and ERs. In addition to the minimum and maximum values, we focus on the M2 calculated from 100 ERs. When comparing the models of different variables, we select the model with the minimum M2 as the best one. If we compare the best models of six MP-based LDFs, we can rank those LDFs.

4 Result

We verify 64 SMs and 129 BGSs by M2.

4.1 *Validation of 64 SMs by M2*

Method1 evaluates 64 SMs using RIP, LP, and H-SVM via M2. Table 1 shows three M2s of 64 SMs. The SN column indicates the sequential number, sorted in ascending order by H-SVM value. The SM column indicates the 64 SMs (32 SMs are omitted from the table). The RIP, LP, and H-SVM columns contain the averages of 100 test samples' ERs (M2). The last three rows are the minimum, average, and maximum values of the 64 SM's M2. The ranges of M2 via RIP, LP, H-SVM are [7.4%, 18.73%], [7.56%, 17.79%] and [4.50%, 17.34%], respectively. We can determine H-SVM is better than RIP and Revised LP-OLDF. We think the maximization of the distance of two SVs may work better than RIP and Revised LP-OLDF. The 21 M2s of SMs are $\leq$8% in the left H-SVM column. Cilia et al. [4] analyzed six data, including [1, 6]. Their results show 8.06% as the best results of their six data, so we consider 8% one threshold for gene diagnosis. In future research, we will collaborate with physicians to clarify the relationships of genes included in the 21 SMs by EC if possible. We consider SMs or BGSs that include over 100 oncogenes important cancer gene sets. This validation is straightforward for physicians.

4.2 *Evaluation of the Worst SM64 by 100-Fold Cross-Validation*

Method1 evaluates 64 SMs and finds SM64 is the worst SM among 64 SMs same as Fig.2. We evaluate the worst SM64 with eight LDFs. Those LDFs are RIP, Revised LP-OLDF (LP), H-SVM, and five S-SVMs (the penalty $c = 0, 1, 2, 3, 4$). Table 2 shows the minimum, maximum, and average values of M2 in SM64. The eight rows on the left and eight rows on the right correspond to the M1 and M2 of training samples and test samples, respectively. In the training samples, all M1s of the seven LDFs, except for SVM3, are zero. Thus, seven LDFs reveal the 100 training samples as LSD, just like Alon's original data (SM64 itself). However, SVM3 cannot discriminate against several training data. Its M1 of SM64's training data is 0.339%. However, the M2 of SM64's test data via RIP is 18.371%. M2 via RIP is worse than M2 via SVM3. This fact indicates Method1 severely evaluates M2 via RIP. Moreover, we judge SM64 is useless for cancer diagnosis because eight M2 are higher than 17.339%. The other 21 SMs from SM1 to SM21 show good results.

Table 1 Validation of 64 SMs and three LDFs by Method1

SN	SM	RIP	LP	HSVM	SN	SM	RIP	LP	HSVM
1	8	8.24	7.85	**4.50**	22	39	10.89	10.61	8.02
2	17	7.53	7.81	**5.29**	23	36	10.10	9.15	8.21
3	25	7.40	7.56	**5.66**	24	23	10.55	10.23	8.24
4	27	9.06	8.90	**5.76**	25	43	10.95	10.89	8.24
5	15	9.10	9.27	**5.84**	26	20	11.68	11.02	8.31
6	11	9.21	9.10	**6.13**	27	2	11.74	10.73	8.35
7	13	9.37	9.11	**6.26**	28	26	11.87	11.44	8.45
8	33	9.74	8.73	**6.31**	29	4	11.55	10.18	8.50
9	19	9.52	9.18	**6.58**	30	22	11.23	11.26	8.74
10	18	9.05	9.06	**6.66**	31	28	9.48	9.21	8.74
11	34	9.58	9.76	**6.98**	32	31	11.63	10.85	8.87
12	9	9.97	9.27	**7.11**	33	48	10.94	10.68	8.94
13	41	9.13	8.66	**7.11**	34	30	12.60	11.45	9.05
14	16	9.24	9.10	**7.18**	35	38	10.87	10.45	9.13
15	32	9.42	9.03	**7.18**	60	59	15.50	15.82	14.37
16	10	9.85	10.18	**7.21**	61	62	15.66	15.85	14.79
17	6	10.03	8.21	**7.27**	62	61	15.31	15.32	14.85
18	35	10.11	9.84	**7.29**	63	63	16.13	16.65	16.08
19	1	9.63	10.03	**7.31**	64	64	18.37	17.79	17.34
20	21	11.56	10.68	**7.37**		MIN	7.40	7.56	4.50
21	14	8.52	7.87	**7.56**		Mean	11.46	11.21	9.21
						MAX	18.37	17.79	17.34

Table 2 The error rate of training and test samples of SM64

	Training samples (M1)			Test samples (M2)		
	MIN	MAX	MEAN	MIN	MAX	MEAN
RIP	0	0	0	8.0645	29.032	**18.371**
LP	0	0	0	9.6774	25.807	17.790
HSVM	0	0	0	9.6774	25.807	**17.339**
SVM4	0	0	0	9.6774	25.807	**17.339**
SVM0	0	0	0	9.6774	25.807	**17.339**
SVM1	0	0	0	9.6774	25.807	**17.339**
SVM2	0	0	0	9.6774	25.807	**17.339**
SVM3	0	**4.839**	**0.339**	11.29	27.419	17.532

4.3 Validation of 129 BGSs by Method1

We used only SMs for cancer gene diagnosis because all RatioSVs of the 129 BGSs were 0.1% and were too small when compared with SMs [18]. The validation of 129 BGSs with Method1 confirms our decision based on RatioSV was right.

Table 3 Verification of BGS3 by Method1

	1	…37	…100	MIN	MAX	MEAN
Training samples	0	0	0	0	0	0
Test samples	4000	900	2200	14.52	64.52	45.44

Table 3 is the Method1 results for the third BGS (BGS3) of the 129 BGSs. The first three columns are the first, 37th, and 100th NMs, and the right three columns are the minimum, maximum, and average of 100 ERs. In the training samples, 100 NMs and 100 ERs values are zero. In the test samples, NMs show three patterns with 4000, 900, and 2200 misclassified subjects, respectively. The 4000 mean all cancer patients of the 4000 subjects are misclassified. The 2200 means all normal subjects are misclassified, and we do not understand the results from 900 subjects. At present, we cannot explain the reason for this regularity. The other 128 BGSs produce nearly the same results. Thus, Method1 concludes that BGSs are useless for cancer gene diagnosis – the same conclusion reached with RatioSVs. Presently, Program4 decomposes data into BGSs directly, regardless of SM. However, in future research, we plan to decompose each SM into the BGSs. We study the relationship between the genes contained in the pairs of SMs and BGSs. We decide to investigate which SM and BGS pairs contain over 100 oncogenes, found by medical research.

5 Discussion

Here, we focus on two points about two universal data structures of LSD and compare three types of research by medical, statistical, and ML researchers.

5.1 Two Universal Data Structures of LSD

We found two universal data structures of LSD using RIP. At first, we found the monotonic decrease of MNM in Swiss banknote data that consists of 200 bills and six variables [5]. When RIP discriminates two classes (100 genuine vs. 100 counterfeit bills), the MNM of two variables (X4, X6) is zero. All 16 models, including (X4, X6), are LSD, and the other 47 models are not LSD. This first data structure is the Matryoshka structure of LSD. Japanese automobile data (regular cars vs. compact cars) and exam data (pass students vs. fail students) were also LSD. In 2015, when we discriminated against six microarrays, we found those were LSD, also. Moreover, RIP could decompose the six data into the exclusive SMs and BGSs. In 2019, we focused on the Curated Microarray Database (CuMiDa) developed by Bruno et al. [3]. It offers 78 data of 13 carcinomas registered on GSE from 2007 to 2017. Five data have one class, 57 data have two classes (healthy vs.

cancer), and 16 data have more than three clusters (healthy vs. more than two types of cancers). We confirmed 73 new data (healthy vs. cancers) have two universal data structures. Thus, we confirmed two universal data structures of 79 microarrays in addition to three ordinary data. Moreover, we find 185 M2s of BGSs among 1666 BGSs included in 73 data become zero [20]. This indicates that 100 test samples and training samples of 185 BGSs are LSD in addition to the 185 BGS themselves. Thus, we can recommend to physicians 185 BGSs for cancer diagnosis. Presently, we cannot explain why we get the opposite evaluation of BGS as the Alon data and 73 data.

Because two data structures are confirmed by 6 old data and 73 new data stored in the US gene database after 1999, we claim that most of the high-dimensional gene data such as RNA-seq. Have the same structures. Thus, if physicians discriminate their research data using RIP and find it is LSD, they can use our theory for screening research and establish the new frontier of cancer gene diagnosis. Many researchers have studied high-dimensional gene data analysis since 1995 and could not succeed. Today, physicians can access over 50,000 genes; thus, cancer gene research has become increasingly complicated. We hope our theory will contribute to the diagnosis of cancer genes. Furthermore, we think that our results are useful for big data analysis. However, our results need validation by medical specialists before being deployed.

5.2 *Comparison of Three Types of Research*

Our research reveals that two classes (healthy vs. cancerous) are separable in SMs and BGSs. However, other researches fail by not understanding that LSD is an essential signal for cancer diagnosis. We propose that our screening methods be used at the beginning of a cancer diagnosis and expect to open a new frontier.

Medical Research

Alon et al. chose 2000 genes from 6500 genes using correlation analysis and their medical knowledge. Next, they chose several gene sets for the genetic diagnosis of cancer using cluster analysis and examined those with medical knowledge. They finally conclude that a set of 29 genes is a better gene set for cancer gene diagnosis. We have the following questions for the six medical research whose data we use: (1) Why did they ignore the discrimination of two classes? If they discriminate data by H-SVM, they can find a crucial signal (LSD). (2) Why did they not decompose the data into other gene sets using their methods similarly to Method1? Perhaps the second gene set found will likely have the same result of the first gene set. (3) Why did they not use PCA after cluster analysis? The right procedure for data analysis is discrimination, cluster analysis, and PCA in this order for the two classes decided by physicians. It is very strange for physicians to ignore misclassified patients. Misclassified cases provide much information for medical diagnosis. (4) Why did they trust the feature selection based on one-variable information, such as t-test, correlation and other methods? Only the multivariate approach, such as iPS research, can find useful gene sets for cancer diagnosis.

Statistical Approach

Many statisticians approached the high-dimensional gene data analysis as a new frontier of statistics. Their main interest was high-dimensional LDF via the singular value decomposition (SVD) that can build the high-dimensional variance-covariance matrices ($n < <p$). This extends the high-dimensional regression analysis and PCA in addition to discriminant analysis. In 2015, Sall [10], one of the founders of SAS and the developer of JMP, announced high dimensional Fisher's LDF using SVD in Tokyo. We discriminated against six data by this new LDF. For the data of Alon, Golub, Shipp [21], Singh [22], Tien [23] and Chiaretti; the six NMs (ERs) are 5 (8%), 8 (11%), 10 (10%), 3 (4%), 29 (17%) and 3 (2%) [17], respectively. These results show the fatal defect of discriminant analysis based on the variance-covariance matrices. Some statisticians expect that LASSO may be useful for gene analysis as it makes several coefficients zero. However, discriminant functions based on the variance-covariance matrices cannot discriminate LSD correctly.

Machine Learning

ML researchers are the most successful in gene data analysis when compared to statistics and other engineering research methods. Bruno et al. offer 73 benchmarks of the classification accuracies (1 – ERs) via nine classifiers and discuss the rank of nine classifiers by (mean ± SD) and medians of 73 classification accuracies. Their median rank is as follows: (1) SVM (0.94), (2) Random Forest (RF) (0.9), (3) Naïve Bayes (NB) and multilayer perceptron (MLP) (0.89), (5) k-nearest neighbors (0.86), (6) decision tree (0.81), (7) k-means (0.72), (8) Hierarchical clustering (0.55), (9) ZeroR (0.51). They conclude that SVM and RF displayed an overall higher accuracy. Their benchmarks are successful in evaluating nine classifiers using 73 supervised learning data, more than two classes that are classified by medical researches. However, their benchmarks are useless for real cancer gene diagnosis for the following reasons:

1. Each classifier can be ranked according to the number of data whose accuracy is one: (1) SVM (16), (2) MLP (14), (3) RF (10), (4) NB (8), (5) DT(1). We omit the other four classifies because those are unsupervised learning methods. This evaluation is clearer than the above evaluation because 73 data are LSD. Moreover, they use kernel-SVM. Most researchers incorrectly believe the complex kernel-SVM algorithm is superior to the simple linear discriminant hyperplane using H-SVM and S-SVM. Because H-SVM can discriminate 73 data

correctly, we claim LDFs, such as H-SVM and S-SVM, are better than kernel-SVM for LSD.

2. ML researchers need to understand the following three hierarchical reliabilities of ERs of discriminant functions: (1) Only H-SVM and RIP can discriminate LSD theoretically. (2) Other LDFs take the different ERs by the different discriminant hyperplanes. (3) QDF and kernel-SVM are the non-linear discriminant functions. Those use more variables and complex discriminant hyperplane than LDFs. However, these three categories are the discriminant functions that are the best methods for supervised learning data. ML researchers incorrectly assume discrimination and classifications are at the same levels.

6 Conclusion

In 2015, we completed the new theory of discriminant analysis and solved four problems of discriminant analysis. For the applied problem, we discriminated against six high-dimensional gene data. We found two universal data structures of six microarrays, in addition to ordinary data. We can decompose the six data into exclusive SMs and BGSs, which are crucial signals for cancer diagnosis. We analyzed those signals and proposed a formal gene data analysis for cancer diagnosis in 2017. In 2019, we discriminated against 73 data of 13 carcinomas and confirmed two universal data structures of LSD. Therefore, we confirmed that 79 data collected from 1999 to 2017 have two universal data structures that physicians can analyze for gene diagnosis. Our successful process is as follows:

1. RIP, Revised LP-OLDF, and H-SVM can discriminate data correctly. Discriminant functions based on the variance-covariance matrices cannot discriminate LSD correctly. Because of this fact, researchers fail to find proper signals. Because they cannot find the right signals, we can judge their results are wrong.
2. RIP can decompose data into many SMs and BGSs. Revised LP-OLDF can find several SMs, but it cannot see all SMs correctly [18] because of the defect of NM (Problem1). H-SVM finds one optimal solution on the whole region and cannot find one of the optimal gene subspaces, such as SM or BGS, because of the QP algorithm. However, if physicians find the right signal using H-SVM, they may find one of the SMs or BGSs using the same Program4 algorithm. If they use a high-spec PC, it is not a difficult problem.
3. Because SM and BGS are small samples having less than equal n genes, we analyzed all SMs and BGSs with ANOVA, t-test, correlation analysis, cluster analysis, PCA, Fisher's LDF, QDF, and logistic regression [18]. However, only logistic regression discriminates all SMs and BGSs of the six data correctly because the maximum likelihood obtained the logistic regression coefficients based on the real distribution. These facts indicate to us that the large variation cannot catch the LSD.

4. After many trials, we realize that RIP Discriminant Scores (RipDSs) are useful malignancy indexes. RipDSs can show the linearly separable signal correctly. Thus, we make a signal data with 62 cases and 64 RipDSs instead of 2000 genes. The five clusters of hierarchical Ward cluster separate two classes. Normal subjects become one cluster, and cancer subjects become four clusters. Next, PCA shows two classes separate on positive (cancer) and negative (normal) parts of the Prin1 in the shape of a fan. Moreover, we think that four clusters correspond to the cancer sub-classes pointed by Golub et al. Normal patients nearly locate on the Prin1 less than −5. By the breakthrough of signal data, we found that RipDSs become the malignancy indexes. The analysis of signal data from the combined Ward and PCA is precious for gene analysis. Although cancers are a heterogeneous disease, all essential results of the six data nearly reach the same conclusions. Based on these results, we proposed a formal data analysis for cancer gene diagnosis based on useful LSD information to forecast and identify cancer if physicians strictly control two classes. If RIP misclassifies several patients, physicians can treat those patients as validation samples. After we obtain the RIP using the omitted data, we examine the cases misclassified by the RIP as another external check.
5. We are successful in obtaining all signals. However, we find that 193 signals are too many. Thus, we rank the importance of the 193 signals using Method1. Three ranges of 64 M2 shows that H-SVM is better than RIP and Revised LP-OLDF. Although our two OLDFs are inferior to H-SVM, only RIP can decompose data into all signals. The 129 M2s of BGSs are over 45.43% in Table 3. Method2 and RatioSV confirm the Alon BGSs should not be used for cancer gene diagnosis.
6. In future research, we will cooperate with the medical specialists and consider the meaning of genes combination, including the pair of SM and BGSs. This research may offer the new cancer gene set for cancer gene diagnosis instead of oncogenes discovered with microscopic biology.
7. Although many microarrays provided useful information for cancer gene diagnosis, no one could solve it because the analysis technology of statistics and ML was immature. The biggest problem is the lack of LSD research. Researchers must not give up their research style, but they need to be flexible. At least, in the case of LSD, they must recognize that previous research approaches are wrong.
8. We think our research method is useful for other genes, such as RNA. By merely examining whether the data is LSD first, it is possible to avoid wrong statistical and engineering approaches in cancer research.

Acknowledgments Our research depends on the powerful LINGO solver and JMP for real data analysis of gene data supported by CuMiDa.

References

1. U. Alon et al., Broad patterns of gene expression revealed by clustering analysis of cancer and normal colon tissues probed by oligonucleotide arrays. Proc. Natl. Acad. Sci. U. S. A. **96**, 6745–6750 (1999)
2. M. Aoshima, K. Yata, Distance-based classifier by data transformation for high-dimension, strongly spiked eigenvalue models. Ann. Inst. Stat. Math. **71**, 473–503 (2019)
3. C.F. Bruno, B.C. Eduardo, I.G. Bruno, D. Marcio, CuMiDa: An extensively curated microarray database for benchmarking and testing of machine learning approaches in cancer research. J. Comput. Biol. **26-0**, 1–11 (2019)
4. N.D. Cilia et al., An experimental comparison of feature-selection and classification methods for microarray datasets. Information **10**(109), 1–13 (2019)
5. B. Flury, H. Riedwyl, *Multivariate Statistics: A Practical Approach* (Cambridge University Press, New York, 1988)
6. T.R. Golub et al., Molecular classification of cancer: class discovery and class prediction by gene expression monitoring. Science **286/5439**, 531–537 (1999)
7. I.B. Jeffery, D.G. Higgins, C. Culhane, Comparison and evaluation of methods for generating differentially expressed gene lists from microarray data. BMC Bioinformatics, 1–16 (2006)
8. P.A. Lachenbruch, M.R. Mickey, Estimation of error rates in the discriminant analysis. Technometrics **10**(1), 11 (1968)
9. A. Miyake, S. Shinmura, in *Error Rate of Linear Discriminant Function*, ed. by F. T. de Dombel, F. Gremy, (North-Holland Publishing Company, 1976), pp. 435–445
10. J.P. Sall, L. Creighton, A. Lehman, *JMP Start Statistics*, 3rd edn. (SAS Institute Inc. (Shinmura, supervise Japanese version), 2004)
11. L. Schrage, *Optimization Modeling with LINGO* (LINDO Systems Inc., 2006)
12. S. Shinmura, A new algorithm of the linear discriminant function using integer programming. New Trends Prob Stat. **5**, 133–142 (2000)
13. S. Shinmura, *The Optimal Linear Discriminant Function* (Union of Japanese Scientist and Engineer Publishing, Japan, 2010) (ISBN 978-4-8171-9364-3)
14. S. Shinmura, Problems of discriminant analysis by mark sense test data. Japanese Soc Appl Stat **4012**, 157–172 (2011)
15. S. Shinmura, End of discriminant functions based on variance-covariance matrices. ICORE2014, 5–16 (2014)
16. S. Shinmura, Four serious problems and new facts of the discriminant analysis, in *Operations Research and Enterprise Systems*, ed. by E. Pinson et al., (Springer, Berlin, 2015), pp. 15–30
17. S. Shinmura, *New Theory of Discriminant Analysis after R. Fisher* (Springer, 2016)
18. S. Shinmura, *High-dimensional Microarray Data Analysis* (Springer, 2019)
19. S. Shinmura, Release from the curse of high dimensional data analysis. Big Data, Cloud Computing, and Data Science Engineering (Stud. Comput. Intell.) **844**, 173–196 (2019)
20. S. Shinmura, *Cancer Diagnosis of 78 Microarrays Registered on GSE from 2007 to 2017. Transactions on Computational Science & Computational Intelligence* (Springer Nature, 2020b) (in Press)
21. M.A. Shipp et al., Diffuse large B-cell lymphoma outcome prediction by gene-expression profiling and supervised machine learning. Nat. Med. **8**, 68–74 (2002)
22. D. Singh et al., Gene expression correlates of clinical prostate cancer behavior. Cancer Cell **1**, 203–209 (2002)
23. E. Tian et al., The role of the Wnt-signaling antagonist DKK1 in the development of osteolytic lesions in multiple myeloma. N. Engl. J. Med. **349**(26), 2483–2494 (2003)
24. V. Vapnik, *The Nature of Statistical Learning Theory* (Springer, 1999)

A New Literature-Based Discovery (LBD) Application Using the PubMed Database

Matthew Schofield, Gabriela Hristescu, and Aurelian Radu

1 Introduction

One of the most advanced goals of studying the biomedical literature is to generate new scientific hypotheses, which can be subsequently verified experimentally, leading to new scientific Literature Based Discovery (LBD). The hypothesis is that the vast mass of biomedical knowledge may contain valuable connections between facts in seemingly unrelated areas, which have been missed by investigators whose expertise is highly focused on narrow areas. In many cases, the hypotheses are generated by connecting two distinct unrelated studies. In a very general sense, if a study describes an association between two concepts or notions A and B, and another study describes an association between B and C, the hypothesis can be advanced that, because of transitivity, an association may exist between A and C. This paradigm is known as "ABC" and it has been shown to have medical value by Don Swanson [4]. It is only natural for computer applications to employ this strategy in order to generate novel hypotheses. Many research groups have tried to introduce such applications, mostly with limited success [1–3, for recent reviews]. The main shortcoming of such an approach is that the valuable hypotheses generated automatically are included in a much larger set of hypotheses that are either obvious, already known, or do not make sense and are unlikely to be true. As a result, LBD

M. Schofield (✉) · G. Hristescu
Rowan University, Computer Science Department, Glassboro, NJ, USA
e-mail: schofielm0@students.rowan.edu; hristescu@rowan.edu

A. Radu
Department of Cell, Developmental and Regenerative Biology, Icahn School of Medicine at Mount Sinai, One Gustave L. Levy Place, New York, NY, USA
e-mail: aurelian.radu@mssm.edu

H. R. Arabnia et al. (eds.), *Advances in Computer Vision and Computational Biology*, Transactions on Computational Science and Computational Intelligence,
https://doi.org/10.1007/978-3-030-71051-4_63

packages did not yet get widespread use by the intended beneficiaries – the large number of biomedical researchers who work in various clinical and basic science areas.

2 Implementation

1. User input: The user enters a query through the interface, which is similar to the standard PubMed interface in which terms and target fields are defined.
   (a) Search terms can be defined with a target field and a word or phrase, for example (Abstract), Alzheimer's.
   (b) Search terms can be connected by Boolean operators (AND, OR, NOT) to form a Boolean expression.
   (c) A date range can be defined to only retrieve abstracts from a specific time period.
   (d) A proximity filter can be set, to only accept abstracts where certain phrases appear within a specified number of words of each other.
2. The National Center for Biotechnology Information (NCBI) PubMed Central API is used to gather PubMed IDs (PMIDs) for papers that fit the given query.
3. NCBI's PubMed Central API is used again to gather the abstracts for papers based on the previously retrieved PMIDs.
4. The application extracts triplets consisting of Subject-Predicate-Object (SPOs) from each abstract, by performing the following steps in succession (Fig. 1):
   (a) The English Core Part-of-Speech Tagging model from the natural language processing Python package spaCy is used to tokenize the abstract's text and to create a relational tree of each sentence. SpaCy (https://spacy.io/) is a top-of-the-line natural language processing package. It utilizes deep learning and various standard machine learning algorithms to perform natural language processing tasks. We primarily use its Part-Of-Speech tagging functionality in its pre-trained English-based tokenizer model.
   (b) Auxiliary and common words ("stop words") that frequently appear in PubMed abstracts are removed, such as "is," "a," "the." The most frequent words in a sample of 100,000 abstracts are extracted, considered general terms and removed.
   (c) The text is searched to locate any verbs within a pre-defined set of verbs that are involved in cause-effect relations, such as "increases," "activates," "induces," "triggers," "upregulates," etc., as well as antonyms, such as "decreases." Some of these words are frequently used in the biomedical literature, but rarely encountered in other fields.
   (d) For each verb found in step c, a search is performed for tokens that are tagged as nouns, pronouns, subjects, or objects in the sub-tree of the sentence tree where the actionable verb is the root. In addition to searching for tokens tagged as such, the system also searches for tokens that are in the list of

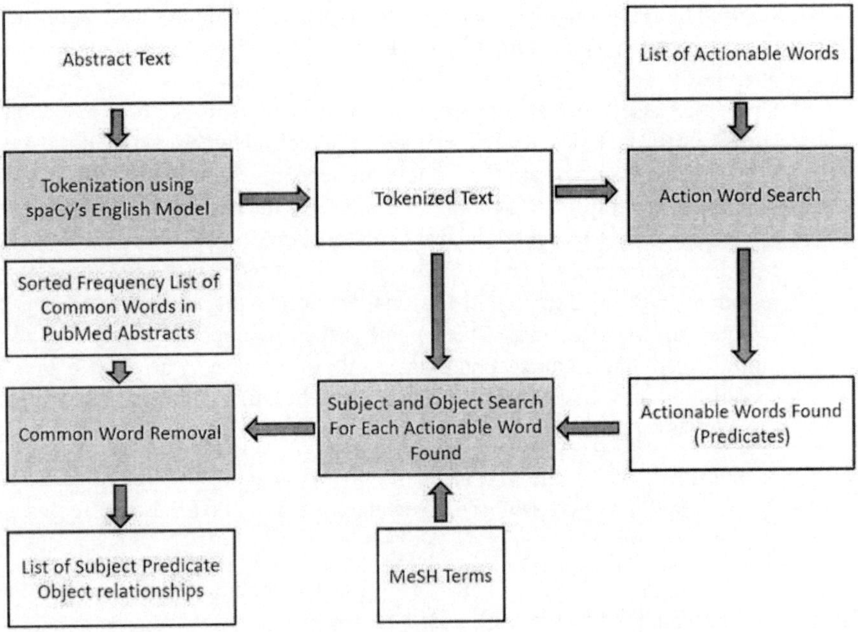

Fig. 1 An overview of our approach to extracting Subject-Predicate-Object relationships from an abstract's text

Medical Subject Heading (MeSH) terms, which are common medical terms like dyslexia, mites, and anesthesia.

(e) After this search, the system provides Subject Predicate Object (SPO) triplets, where the subject and the object represent A to B relationships, 'pronoun/noun/subject | verb | pronoun/noun/object'. Example: "sanguinarine increased intracellular free calcium concentration" (PMID 32404582).

(f) The abstract and its extracted SPOs are added to a database. This allows for future queries to search for relationships in previous queries. This database also acts as a cache, avoiding repeated searches for SPOs in already searched abstracts.

5. Steps 1–4 are repeated for a second set of abstracts. Selection of the second set is flexible and depends on the user's goal. The following options are available:

(a) Option 1: the second set is identical with set 1, in which case the database containing the SPOs and the abstracts is already available. This option can be selected if the users want to check if they missed hypotheses supported by facts in their field of expertise. This approach is suitable for fields in which extensive research was performed and large numbers of papers span a long period of time, e.g. Alzheimer's disease. Using this option in these fields may reveal meaningful connections between recent studies and much older papers, which didn't seem very relevant at the time, and which are never

referred to in the newer publications. Such papers could have been published even before the users started their career and therefore never came to their attention.
    (b) Option 2: a second set of abstracts can be used to look for connections between distinct fields, e.g. Alzheimer's disease and hypertension, if the user is an expert in the first area, but not in the second, it is unlikely that the user will be able to formulate hypotheses that bridge the two fields.
    (c) Option 3: uses as a second database the full PubMed set, or a large subset, e.g. the last 10 or 20 years. This requires much more powerful computing resources, but we estimated, using smaller subsets, that it would be feasible for our current resources. A key point is that, as opposed to the first two options, generating the second database does not have to be done for each search, but only once for each revision of the application. It is therefore acceptable for this step to take several hours or even days.

6. For each abstract within the first database, the extracted SPOs are compared to the abstracts in the second database, to create a chain of two SPOs that represent an ABC relationship.

Output: The generated ABC chains are presented to the user along with the abstracts from which they were extracted.

Example 1
Input $_1$: Dietary fish oil lowers blood viscosity, reduces platelet aggregation, and inhibits vasoconstriction;

Output $_1$: [fish oil | lowers | blood viscosity];

Input $_2$: Lower blood viscosity, reduced platelet aggregation, and inhibition of vasoconstriction prevent Raynaud syndrome;

Output $_2$: [lower blood viscosity | prevents | Raynaud syndrome];

(This is the original ABC hypothesis derived by Swanson [4]. The ability to generate this hypothesis is frequently used as a test for systems aimed at computer-assisted hypothesis generation. The hypothesis is generated by our system, too.)

Example 2
Input $_1$: ..sevoflurane treatment significantly increased the Ca(2+) concentration;

Output $_1$: [sevoflurane | increased | Ca(2+)];

Input $_2$: ..mitochondrial Ca2+ overload can damage mitochondrial recycling via mitophagy;

Output $_2$: [Ca(2+) | damage | mitochondrial recycling];

Example 3
Input $_1$: ..PGE1 will produce a depolarization of renal arterial smooth muscle;

Output $_1$: [PGE1 | will produce | depolarization];

Input $_2$: Electrical field depolarization of the brain slices stimulated the synthesis and release of serotonin;

Output $_2$: [depolarization | stimulated | release of serotonin];

3 Conclusions

We have developed a cloud-based web application for the purpose of Literature Based Discovery in medical literature using the PubMed database and natural language processing.

Future work could include the creation of Natural Language Processing models that will specifically target medical literature and a system to autonomously rate the value of the suggested hypotheses. A Part-of-Speech Tagging model that specifically targets medical literature would improve the systems performance in this specific domain as we hypothesize that medical literature has a different sentence structure than popular English. Additionally, a form of reinforcement machine learning could be used to autonomously supply a rating for each generated SPO extraction or ABC chain possible hypothesis. These generated ratings could be used by an investigator to more efficiently filter recommendations and these ratings could be used to further tune the extraction process.

References

1. V. Gopalakrishnan, K. Jha, W. Jin, A. Zhang, A survey on literature based discovery approaches in biomedical domain. J. Biomed. Inform. **93**, 103141 (2019)
2. S. Henry, B.T. McInnes, Literature based discovery: Models, methods, and trends. J. Biomed. Inform. **74**, 20–32 (2017)
3. N.R. Smalheiser, Rediscovering Don Swanson: The past, present and future of literature-based discovery. J. Data Inf. Sci. **2**(4), 43–64 (2017)
4. D.R. Swanson, Undiscovered public knowledge. Libr. Q. **56**(2), 103–118 (1986)

An Agile Pipeline for RNA-Seq Data Analysis

Scott Wolf, Dan Li, William Yang, Yifan Zhang, and Mary Qu Yang

1 Introduction

Next-generation transcriptome sequencing has experienced significant growth among biomedical researchers attempting to quantify, discover, and profile RNA's, including in their attempts at identification and examination of disease-related biomarkers and potential targets for disease treatment. The analysis of RNA-seq is to examine the cellular transcriptome through quality assessment, transcript assembly and mapping, differential expression analysis, and variant calling, including raw and filtered variants, SNPs, indels, etc. However, in the use of these structures, major issues arise among contemporary researchers: (i) implementing software solutions to these problems requires an intimate knowledge of the tools; (ii) many solutions require specific hardware to run; (iii) without a consistent, standardized pipeline, comparison of results is very difficult [1].

Particularly when working in large groups with varying protocols and expertise, disparate solutions can introduce problems. If researchers intend to collaborate seamlessly, it is necessary that each collaborator knows the analysis methods being used by others in enough specificity to replicate the analysis exactly: parameters, packages, etc. Although, in the software community, there any many ways to

S. Wolf
Princeton University, Princeton, NJ, USA

D. Li · Y. Zhang · M. Q. Yang (✉)
MidSouth Bioinformatics Center and Joint Bioinformatics Program of University of Arkansas at Little Rock and University of Arkansas fors Medical Sciences, Little Rock, AR, USA
e-mail: mqyang@ualr.edu

W. Yang
Department of Computer Science, Carnegie Mellon University School of Computer Science, Pittsburgh, PA, USA

H. R. Arabnia et al. (eds.), *Advances in Computer Vision and Computational Biology*, Transactions on Computational Science and Computational Intelligence,
https://doi.org/10.1007/978-3-030-71051-4_64

implement this: by way of assuring versioning of each piece of software along with exact parameter matching. To implement manual methods in a lab requires intense attention to detail, a high level of technical knowledge among collaborators, as well as a way to communicate changes in versioning and parameters.

Although current literature covers RNAseq pipelines and more general workflows, very few publications introduce the use of complete pipelines for full automation of analysis. Furthermore, the overarching majority of literature focuses on individual pieces of a workflow rather than establishing a collaborative structure for analysis along with piecewise integration.

For building these collaborative environments, some local and cloud-based software suites exist including publicly available ones such as Galaxy (https://galaxyproject.org/) [2, 3], Taverna [4], and Arvados (https://curoverse.com/), along with commercial workbenches such as SevenBridges (http://sbgenomics.com) and Illumina's BaseSpace (http://basespace.illumina.com/) [6]. Galaxy stands as one of the most popular open-source workbenches designed to rely on centralized resources for computing. Along with the use of centralized resources and versioning, Galaxy boasts an extensive API and a user-friendly web-based interface for the development of workflows quickly. Other than Galaxy and the other open-source suites listed above, SevenBridges, BaseSpace, and other similar workbenches offer proprietary software and support at a major cost to researcher groups, and the solutions cannot be self-hosted. Even with these resources, there is still a major gap where a self-hostable, cross-platform, self-contained pipeline structure. We fill in this gap with the introduction of our RNAseq pipeline.

In our implementation, we took on the task of establishing an end-to-end, isolated pipeline in an environment that can be identically produced, from the version level all the way to operating system and kernel, for the use of every collaborator involved in a given project. By utilizing this mirroring method for environments, we can easily ensure standardized analysis sequence within a group and bypass the need for individual-level familiarity with the analysis sequence. The group only needs to modify the platform once before dispersing a standardized Docker image curated to a given project. The software is available at https://systemsgenomics.net/html/software.html

2 Methods

2.1 Overview of RNAseq Pipeline

The RNAseq pipeline consists of a Docker (https://www.docker.com/) container, utilizing CentOS Linux 7 (Core) as a base operating system, along with tools and mapping necessary to facilitate complete analyses. Selected from a priori knowledge and various best practice reviews, the software, along with its organization and configurations, provides the workhorse element of our pipeline [6]. The exact software list can be found easily in the associated supplemental materials.

As discussed previously, the major advantage of this structure is its uniformity among collaborators and dynamic, cross-platform deployment capability. After deploying the container, users can enter the uniform environment. After entering the environment, end users can quickly change configurations in their environment and determine whether their modifications persist or reset upon an eventual restart. If a user changes the initial configuration and establishes a new baseline configuration, they can easily pass on their container to their collaborators as the updated standard form.

2.2 *Benefits of Uniform Environments*

Establishing uniform analysis environments bypasses one of the major hindrances involved in collaborative proteomics research. The containerized analysis pipelines – though being identical for every collaborator – ensure that results are consistent. Beyond this, adjusting parameters and persisting changes among collaborators is easy: just update configs and pass the new container to the group. Even beyond the ease of collaboration, the containerization of the pipeline allows for manipulation and use with technical ease through automation and a singular installation procedure.

2.3 *Challenges of Docker and Containerization*

Although the containerization approach introduces many advantages, the practice also introduces a few challenges with regards to distribution of changes, updates, and tool swaps. In order to introduce updates that are relatively simple for manual sequential analysis, one must update a variety of launch and configuration scripts, update the container, and verify the change before pushing it to collaborators. These modifications require not only an intimate knowledge of the software you are looking to change and the pipeline but also knowledge of Docker development. Beyond the technical development, Docker introduces more bulk and complication where it may not be necessary. Docker also requires users to define an absolute maximum for resources on the machine (CPU, memory, disk space, etc.) which can introduce unforeseen problems in optimization.

2.4 Hardware Configuration

In order for the pipeline to be used effectively on larger datasets, it is necessary to have hardware configurations that can take full advantage of the pipeline. Both memory and disk space commonly arise as bottlenecks in the pipeline. Running the pipeline on a shared server with many cores, lots of storage, and sufficient memory allows for optimum throughput.

2.5 Software Configuration

For the Dockerized container to function, users need to install Docker (https://www.docker.com) on the machine. After installing Docker using the associated documentation found on the website, one can import the RNAseq pipeline quickly from Docker by typing "docker pull ualrngs/rna-seq-pipeline:2.0". To help with installation and end-user usage, we included examples of pipeline usage in the following text.

In our example usage, we utilized data from the Sequencing Quality Control (SEQC) project from the Gene Expression Omnibus (GEO) database (From Dan's SEQC_testing_data document). Our data consisted of 12 paired-end transcriptome sequence samples from this study's data. To initially assess our data, we ran the pipeline's quality control command.

1. Run quality control before initializing pipeline

```
docker run --rm -v /home/yourAccount/Project1/inputRNA:/input -v
/home/yourAccount/RNA_results:/working
ualrngs/rna-seq-pipeline:2.0 quality
```

2. Run full pipeline

```
docker run --rm -v /home/yourAccount/Project1/inputRNA:/input -v
/home/yourAccount/Project1/refGenome/ refFile:/indexDir -v
/home/yourAccount/Project1/RNA-results:/working ualrngs/rna-seq-pipeline:2.0 assemble full
-k -r
```

Acknowledgments This research was supported by the NIH/R15 funding NIH/R15 (R15GM114739) and NIH/P20 GM103429.

References

1. J. Costa-Silva, D. Domingues, F.M. Lopes, RNA-Seq differential expression analysis: An extended review and a software tool. PLOS ONE **12**, e0190152 (2017). 1. PLOS ONE 12, e0190152 (2017)
2. B. Giardine et al., Galaxy: A platform for interactive large-scale genome analysis. Genome Res. **15**, 1451–1455 (2005)
3. E. Afgan et al., The Galaxy platform for accessible, reproducible and collaborative biomedical analyses: 2016 update. Nucleic Acids Res. **44**, W3–W10 (2016)
4. K. Wolstencroft et al., The Taverna workflow suite: Designing and executing workflows of Web Services on the desktop, web or in the cloud. Nucleic Acids Res. **41**, W557–W561 (2013)
5. B. Fjukstad, L.A. Bongo, A review of scalable bioinformatics pipelines. Data Sci. Eng. **2**, 245–251 (2017)
6. A. Conesa et al., A survey of best practices for RNA-seq data analysis. Genome Biol. **17**, 13 (2016)

Part VII
Biomedical Engineering and Applications

Stage Classification of Neuropsychological Tests Based on Decision Fusion

Gonzalo Safont, Addisson Salazar, and Luis Vergara

1 Introduction

Typically, most fusion approaches can be split into early fusion (i.e., feature-based), late fusion (i.e., decision-based), and hybrid fusion [1, 2]. Early fusion integrates the extracted features from several sources or modes (e.g., by concatenation of their values). Conversely, late fusion integrates the decisions obtained by multiple single classifiers. There are several advantages to the fusion of multiple classifiers, such as improved classification performance, increased confidence, or enhanced reliability [3]. Finally, hybrid fusion considers both early and late fusion.

There have been some previous works on late fusion on biomedical applications, including automatic sleep staging [4], colonic polyp detection in CT colonography [5], and the identification of auditory and visual perception processes from multimodal data [6]. Most applications have used classic decision fusion methods (e.g., majority voting and score averaging) because of their simplicity of use and robustness. However, these results could potentially be improved even further by the application of more sophisticated and powerful fusion methods.

This work compares the relative performance of several state-of-the-art late fusion methods on a challenging biomedical application: automated staging of brain signals (electroencephalograms) from epileptic patients performing learning and memory tasks. In this work, the following state-of-the-art methods for late fusion have been considered: Dempster-Shafer combination [7]; alpha integration [8]; copulas [9]; independent component analysis mixture models [10, 11]; and behavior knowledge space [12]. Besides, two classic fusion methods were implemented for

G. Safont · A. Salazar (✉) · L. Vergara
Institute of Telecommunications and Multimedia Applications, Universitat Politècnica de València, Valencia, Spain
e-mail: asalazar@dcom.upv.es

H. R. Arabnia et al. (eds.), *Advances in Computer Vision and Computational Biology*, Transactions on Computational Science and Computational Intelligence,
https://doi.org/10.1007/978-3-030-71051-4_65

comparison: score averaging (mean) and majority vote. The performance of the methods was estimated on the proposed neuropsychological test stage classification demonstrating their relative strengths and weaknesses for a real implementation.

The rest of the paper is organized as follows. Section 2 includes a review of the implemented decision fusion methods. Section 3 describes the experimental deployment. Section 4 shows and discusses the results obtained. Finally, the conclusions of this work are included in Sect. 5.

2 Late Fusion Methods

This section includes a summary of the fusion methods implemented for the proposed application of stage classification of neuropsychological tests.

2.1 *Dempster-Shafer Combination*

Evidence theory or Dempster-Shafer (DS) theory is a general framework for dealing with uncertainty and belief [7]. It has been used in applications, such as fault diagnosis [13]. To perform late fusion, we interpreted the scores produced by each classifier as probability masses, and then applied Dempster's rule of combination:

$$(m_1 \oplus m_2)(A) = \frac{1}{1-M} \sum_{B \cap C = A \neq \varnothing} m_1(B) m_2(C) \tag{1}$$

where $M = \sum_{B \cap C = \varnothing} m_1(B) m_2(C)$ and A, B and C are subsets of the whole universe, with $\varnothing$ being the empty set.

2.2 *Alpha Integration*

Alpha integration was first proposed for the binary classification (detection) problem [8, 14]. Let us assume that we have a group of D binary classifiers (detectors) working on the detection problem. Each detector will produce a score s_i, $i = 1 \ldots D$, where higher values of s_i indicate that the positive class is more likely than the negative class. In this context, alpha integration performs the optimal integration of these scores $\mathbf{s} = [s_1 \ldots s_D]^T$ into a single score s_α such that

$$s_\alpha(\mathbf{s}) = \begin{cases} \left[\sum_{i=1}^{D} w_i (s_i)^{(1-\alpha)/2} \right]^{2/(1-\alpha)}, & \alpha \neq 1 \\ \exp\left[\sum_{i=1}^{D} w_i \log(s_i) \right], & \alpha = 1 \end{cases} \tag{2}$$

where α and the coefficients $\mathbf{w} = [w_1 \ldots w_D]^T$ are the parameters to be optimized, subject to $w_i \geq 0$, $\sum_{i=1}^{D} w_i = 1$. Due to these constraints, s_α is bound between 0 and 1. It can be shown that many classical late soft fusion techniques are particular cases of alpha integration, such as the average ($\alpha = -1$ and $w_i = 1/D$, $\forall D$), the minimum ($\alpha = \infty$), and the maximum ($\alpha = -\infty$). In practice, there are many applications where the parameters of alpha integration are unknown beforehand and have to be estimated from some training data. Previous works have presented the derivations required to optimize alpha integration with respect to the least mean squares (LMSE) and the minimum probability of error (MPE) criteria [14, 15].

Alpha integration was recently generalized to multiclass classification in two methods called vector score alpha integration (VSI) [16] and separated score integration (SSI) [17]. This later method was used in this work. Essentially, SSI performs alpha integration separately on the scores corresponding to each class.

Given K classes, indexed by $k = 1 \ldots K$, and D classifiers, the i-th classifier will produce a vector of scores $\mathbf{s} = [s_{1i} \ldots s_{Ki}]^T$, $i = 1 \ldots D$. We will assume the scores are normalized to unit sum, $\sum_{k=1}^{K} s_{ki} = 1$. The true class identifier vector is defined as $\mathbf{y} = [y_1 \ldots y_K]^T$, where

$$y_k = \begin{cases} 1 \text{ if the true class is } k \\ 0 \text{ otherwise} \end{cases} \tag{3}$$

Let us define α_k and w_{ki}, $i = 1 \ldots D$, as the parameters to integrate the scores corresponding to class k. Given a set of scores $\mathbf{S} = [\mathbf{s}_1 \ldots \mathbf{s}_D]$, we can directly apply the integration function (2) to every class

$$s_{\alpha_k}(\mathbf{r}_k) = \begin{cases} \left[\sum_{i=1}^{D} w_{ki} (s_{ki})^{(1-\alpha_k)/2} \right]^{2/(1-\alpha_k)}, & \alpha_k \neq 1 \\ \exp\left[\sum_{i=1}^{D} w_{ki} \log(s_{ki}) \right], & \alpha_k = 1 \end{cases} \tag{4}$$

where $k = 1 \ldots K$ and $\mathbf{r}_k^T$ is the k-th row of matrix $\mathbf{S}$. This way, the multi class problem with K classes is converted in K separate two-class problems. The scores are then normalized so that they add up to one:

$$s_{\alpha_k}^{norm} = \frac{s_{\alpha_k}}{\sum_{k=1}^{K} s_{\alpha_k}} \tag{5}$$

Once we have fused the scores for all classes, classification is performed by selecting the class with the highest score, $\hat{k} = \arg\max_k s_{\alpha_k}^{norm} = \arg\max_k s_{\alpha_k}$. SSI is an extension of alpha integration of experts in [18] but shares its optimality under alpha risk.

As with alpha integration, the parameters of SSI usually have to be estimated from training data. Derivations to optimize the parameters of SSI with respect to the LMSE and MPE criteria were presented in [17].

2.3 Copulas

Estimating multivariate probability density functions (pdfs) is much more complex than estimating univariate pdfs, especially in cases for large dimensionality. One way to bridge this gap is the usage of copulas [9], where any multivariate pdf can be expressed as the product of a copula function and the product of univariate pdfs for each variable. This design has been extended to probabilistic graphical models called copula Bayesian networks [19]. Copulas have been applied successfully in many applications, such as financial model dependence [20].

In this work, copulas were used to build a generative classifier using the scores of the single classifiers. Briefly, copulas are used to estimate the multivariate pdf of the scores of all the classifiers for each true class. Then, for every input sample, the posterior probability of each class for that sample is computed using the Bayes theorem, and the sample is assigned to its most likely class (maximum a posteriori). We implemented the t family of copulas and the univariate pdfs were estimated using non-parametric kernel density estimation.

2.4 Independent Component Analysis Mixture Model

Independent component analysis (ICA) is a blind source separation technique that transforms the input data into a linear combination of independent components. This property allows multivariate pdfs to be expressed as a product of univariate pdfs, due to the independence of the transformed components. In addition, ICA has recently been introduced to graphical models [21–23]. Thus, ICA can be a robust alternative to copulas for multivariate pdf modeling. In this work, we considered ICA mixture models (ICAMM), which maintain the modeling capabilities of ICA with increased flexibility [10, 11]. ICAMM has been used in many different applications [24–28], including biosignal processing [29–32]. The estimation of the ICAMM parameters was performed using MIXCA [10, 11].

2.5 *Behavior Knowledge Space*

A behavior knowledge space (BKS) is a D dimensional space where each dimension corresponds to the decision of one classifier $\mathbf{k} = [k_1 \ldots k_D]^T$ [12]. In BKS fusion, this translates into the estimation of the posterior probability of the true class for every possible set of classifier decisions $\mathbf{k}$. In practice, this estimation is done by counting frequencies on a training set. BKS has been used in many applications, e.g., detecting copy-move forgery in images [33]. Unlike the previously-presented methods, BKS fuses hard decisions (classes) rather than soft decisions (scores).

3 Experiments

In a clinical setting, evaluating the learning and memory function of a patient is a fundamental aspect of their neuropsychological examination. Such evaluations are used, for instance, in testing the condition of epileptic patients before and after neurological surgery. In this work, we consider electroencephalographic (EEG) data from six epileptic subjects that were performing neuropsychological tests as part of their clinical evaluation prior to surgery. For each subject, the EEG electrodes were set according to the 10–20 system and 18 bipolar EEG channels were captured. The signals were sampled at 500 Hz, band-pass filtered between 0.5 and 50 Hz, and filtered with a notch filter at 50 Hz to remove line noise. An example of the captured EEG signals is shown in Fig. 1.

Four different neuropsychological tests were implemented: (i) the visual memory subtest of the Barcelona test (TB, [34]); (ii) the figural memory subtest of the revised Wechsler Memory Scale (WMS-R, [35]); (iii) the visual reproduction subtest of the Wechsler Adult Intelligence Scale (WAIS-III, [35]); and (iv) Sternberg's memory task [36]. The four tests consider visual stimuli and study of the learning and memory capabilities of the subject. The tests were split into three stages (classes): stimulus display (SD), retention interval (RI), and subject response (SR). An example of the sequence of stages during an actual test is shown in Fig. 2.

Briefly, during each trial of TB, the subject is shown a probe item for 3 seconds and, after a 2-second retention interval, the subject must be able to pick the probe item from a set of four similar items. There are ten trials in the test, with scoring depending on the number of correct items. WMS-R is an immediate recognition test of abstract designs. The participant is shown three abstract figures for 10 seconds. After a 2-second retention interval, the subject is shown a set of nine similar figures from which they have to select the three figures they were shown before. There are three trials of increasing difficulty, and scoring is calculated from the

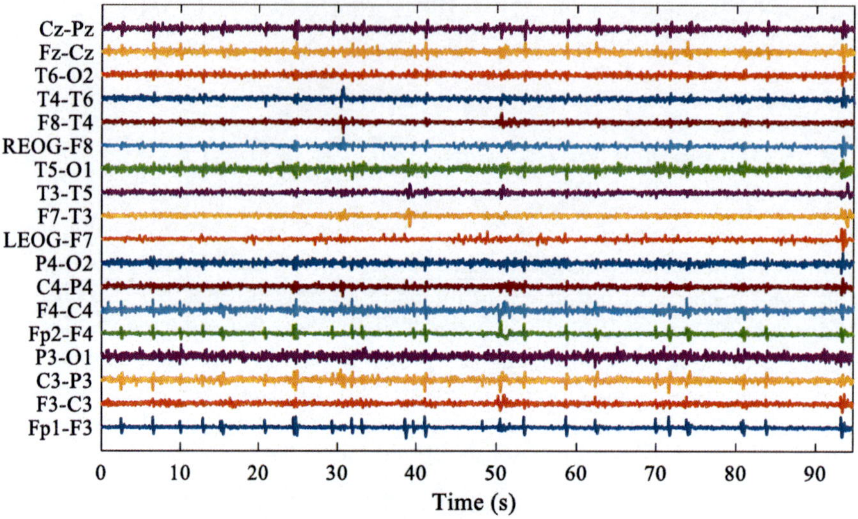

Fig. 1 Example of the captured data for one of the subjects

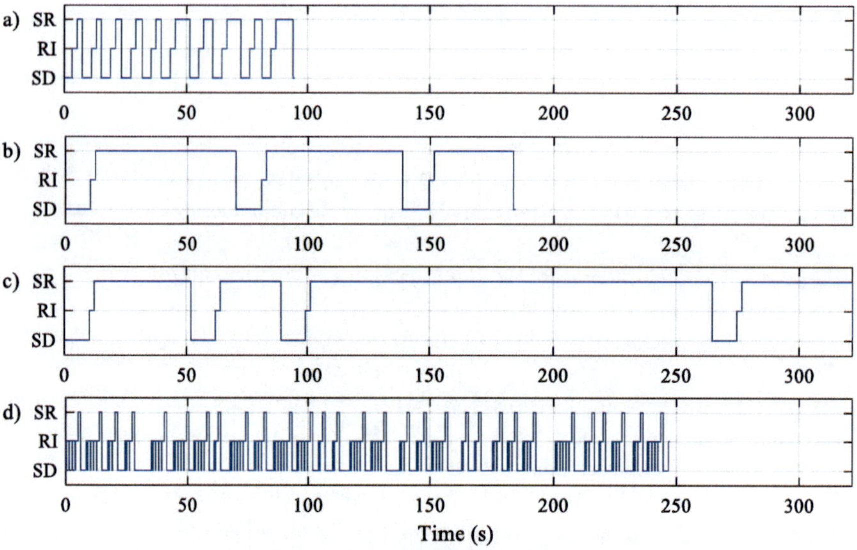

Fig. 2 Labels of the four neuropsychological tests for one of the subjects: (**a**) visual memory, TB; (**b**) figural memory, WMS-R; (**c**) visual reproduction, WAIS-III; (**d**) Sternberg's task

number of correctly-selected figures. During WAIS-III test, the subject is shown an abstract line figure during 10 seconds. The figure is then removed and, after a 10-second retention interval, the subject must draw the figure from memory. There are three trials of increasing difficulty. Scoring depends on the similarities between the original figure and the reproduction. During each trial of the Sternberg's memory task, the subject is shown 2–5 probe items (numbers). Each symbol is shown on screen for 0.2 seconds, with a 1-second blank between symbols. Then, after a 1-second retention interval, the subject is shown a test item and asked to determine whether it was one of the probe items. There are 30 trials in the test, with scoring determined by the number of correct responses.

To test the proposed fusion methods, we first performed automatic classification of the stages of the test based on features extracted from the EEG. The chosen features are commonly used in EEG signal processing [37]: average amplitude; centroid frequency; average power in the delta (0–4 Hz), theta (5–7 Hz), alpha (8–12 Hz), sigma (13–15 Hz) and beta (16–30 Hz) frequency bands; average power across all bands; and Hjorth's activity, mobility, and complexity [38]. The features were extracted in 1-second epochs with no overlap between epochs, separately for each channel. This resulted in 198 available features per epoch. Given the high dimensionality of the data with respect to the number of available samples, dimensionality reduction was performed. In this work, feature ranking was chosen [39].

The score of each feature was estimated as its average informedness (where informedness = recall + specificity – 1 [40]) using a simple classifier that only used that feature. The informedness was estimated using tenfold cross-validation. Then, the features were ranked in descending order of performance, the 10 best-ranked features were chosen, and the rest were discarded. The features were classified using four single classifiers: linear discriminant analysis (LDA); naïve Bayes (NB) with non-parametric kernel density estimation of the marginal distributions; random forests (RDF) using 50 trees; and support vector machines with a linear kernel (SVM). These classifiers were chosen for their success across many different applications. The single classifiers were applied in isolation and then fused using two classic fusion methods (mean, majority voting) and each of the fusion methods described in Sect. 2: Dempster-Shafer combination; SSI optimized with respect to the LMSE (SSI-LMSE) and MPE (SSI-MPE) criteria; copulas; ICAMM; and BKS.

Performance was estimated through a series of Monte Carlo experiments on the real EEG data. Given the limited number of epochs per subject and the need to train the classifiers and some of the fusion methods, each iteration of the experiment was split in two steps. In the first step, tenfold cross-validation was used to train and test the single classifiers, obtaining scores for each epoch from each classifier. Then, a different tenfold cross-validation was used to obtain the fused scores using the different fusion methods, in particular those that required training (alpha integration, BKS, copulas, and ICAMM). This way, all methods were trained using 90% of the samples and then tested on the remaining 10%, keeping as many values as possible for training. Performance was estimated by the classification accuracy, averaged over 100 iterations of the experiments.

4 Results and Discussion

The results obtained by the different methods for each of the tests are shown in Fig. 3. The experiments were difficult for the single classifiers, as shown by the relatively low accuracies (39.77–74.29%). RDF was the best single classifier overall, yielding the best result in three of the tests and the second best result for the figural memory subtest (Fig. 3b), where the best-performing single classifier was NB. Classic fusion methods were unable to improve over the single classifiers, with accuracies in the range of 51.14–73.60%. Conversely, in all cases, at least one of the late fusion methods was able to optimally combine the classifiers to obtain improved performance, resulting in better accuracies overall (52.30–91.44%).

The behavior of the late fusion methods was dependent on the neuropsychological test with two groups. In the first group, composed by the Barcelona test and Sternberg's task (Fig. 3a and Fig. 3d, respectively), only alpha integration was able to improve over the results of the best single classifier. In contrast, the other methods were unable to improve over the best-performing single classifier (RDF in both tests). In the second group, composed by the figural memory and visual reproduction subtests, the state-of-the-art late fusion methods were able to improve over the single classifiers, and the best result was yielded by ICAMM, with alpha integration and BKS in second place. Thus, alpha integration was shown to be more robust than the other state-of-the-art late fusion methods.

The differences in behavior of ICAMM and copulas might have owed to the number of samples available to model the multivariate pdf of the scores. In fact, there was a relation between the number of samples available to model class SR, as seen by the comparison between Figs. 2 and 3. This was confirmed by examining the scores used for training, as shown in Fig. 4. It can be seen that the class boundaries are complex, but the amount of samples of class SR available for some of the tests was not enough to estimate a robust enough model to classify new data. In contrast, alpha integration does not model the pdf of the data and instead estimates a discriminative model to the scores. The results in Fig. 3 suggest that alpha integration might be more suitable for cases where one or more of the classes have a small number of samples. Conversely, in cases with plenty of samples for all classes, a more complex pdf modeling method, such as copulas or ICAMM, might yield more complex and powerful class boundaries.

There are many possible sources of noise in EEG signals, such as line noise and artifacts (eye blinks, muscle activity . . .) [37]. This noise can make it difficult to find common patterns for the same class, reducing classification performance. Furthermore, the contribution of these sources of noise may not be uniform throughout the tests, with longer and more difficult tests leading to more eye blinks, subject fidgeting that leads to muscle noise, and so on. Noise has not been considered in this work. However, one of the advantages of decision fusion is a reduction of the effect of the noise [3]. Since multiple classifiers are considered, each with its own decision boundary, it is likely that noise will not affect all of them

Fig. 3 Average classification results obtained for each method for the four neuropsychological tests: (**a**) visual memory, TB; (**b**) figural memory, WMS-R; (**c**) visual reproduction, WAIS-III; (**d**) Sternberg's task. From left to right, the three first bars correspond to the single classifiers results, the next two bars show the results from classic fusion methods, and the last six bars correspond to the advanced fusion methods. Besides the classification accuracy, standard deviation of the results is also shown

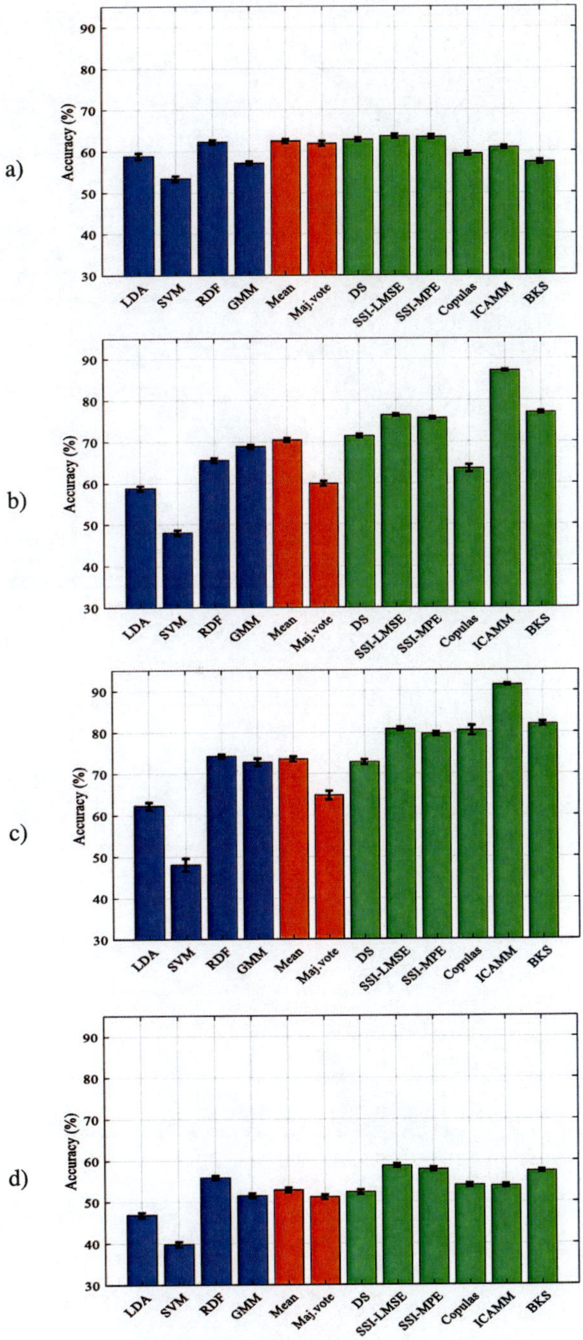

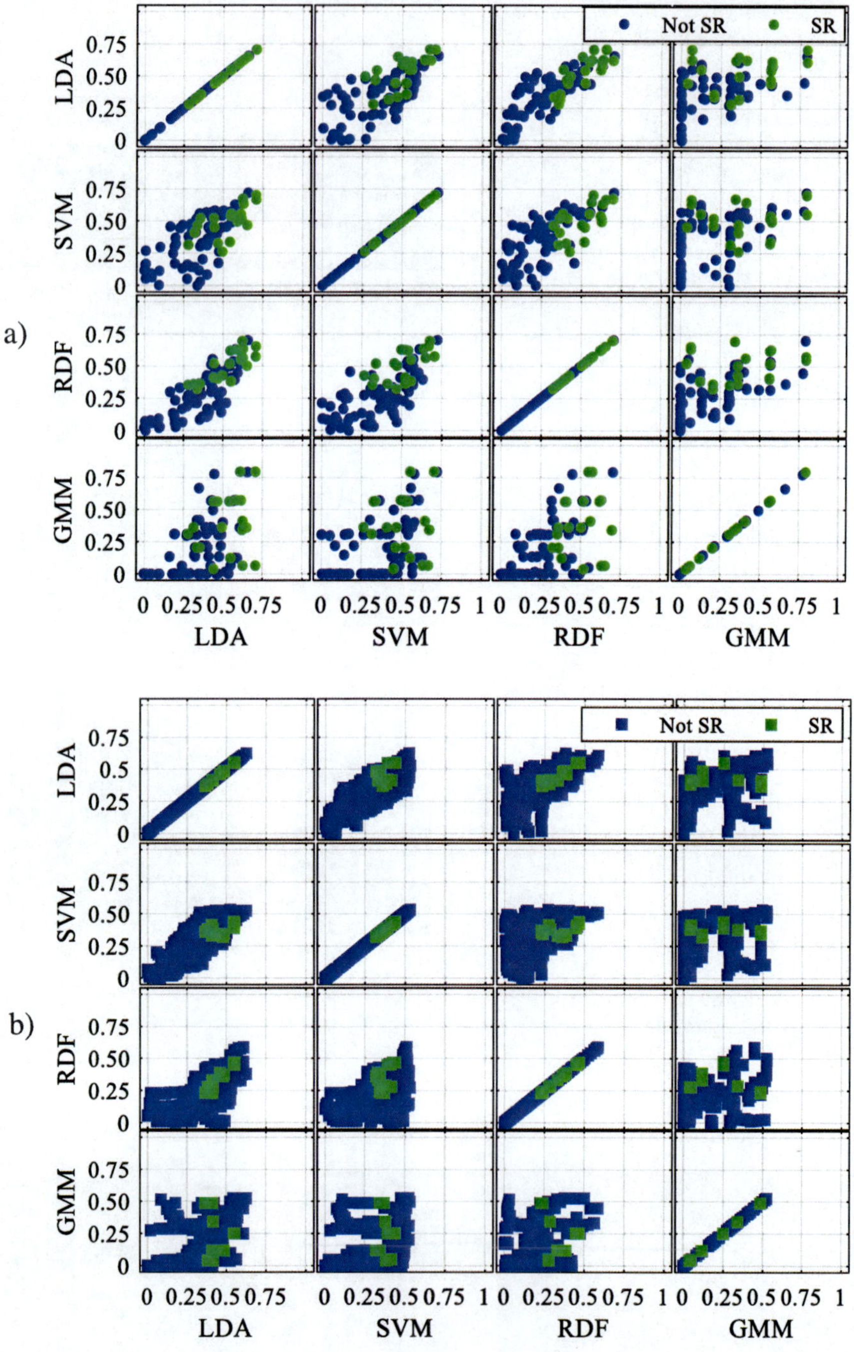

Fig. 4 Comparison of the scores of the different single classifiers produced for class SR (subject response) versus any other class (not SR) for the following neuropsychological tests: (a) visual memory, TB and (b) visual reproduction, WAIS-III

equally and thus their combination will be less affected by said noise. However, more work would be needed to confirm this possibility.

5 Conclusions

This work has tested the relative performance of several state-of-the-art late fusion methods for the automated staging of neuropsychological tests (visual and memory learning cognitive tasks) using electroencephalographic data. The considered late fusion methods were: alpha integration extended to the multiclass case (SSI); copulas; Dempster-Shafer combination (DS); independent component analysis mixture models (ICAMM); behavior knowledge space (BKS)N and two classic methods (the mean and majority vote). Those fusion methods were employed to combine the scores from four single classifiers: linear discriminant analysis; naïve Bayes; random forests; and support vector machine.

Four different neuropsychological tests were implemented. The tests were automatically staged into three classes: stimulus display, retention interval, and subject response. Late fusion methods were able to improve the performance for the automatic staging task over that of the single classifiers. In particular, ICAMM and BKs yielded the best maximum performances, but had mixed results. Conversely, alpha integration yielded a more stable result that always improved over the single classifiers. It was shown that this behavior owed to the reduced number of samples for some classes in some tests, which might hamper the estimation of complex multivariate pdfs. Several lines of research could be derived from this work, including real-time implementation for medical diagnosis and evaluation.

Acknowledgments This work was supported by Spanish Administration and European Union grant TEC2017-84743-P.

References

1. S. Yuksel, J. Wilson, P. Gader, Twenty years of mixture of experts. IEEE Trans. Neural Netw. Learn. Sys. **23**, 1177–1193 (2012)
2. B. Khaleghi, A. Khamis, F. Karray, S. Razavi, Multisensor data fusion: A review of the state-of-the-art. Inform. Fusion **14**, 28–44 (2013)
3. M. Mohandes, M. Deriche, S. Aliyu, Classifiers combination techniques: A comprehensive review. IEEE Access **6**, 19626–19639 (2018)
4. J. Zhang, Y. Wu, J. Bai, F. Chen, Automatic sleep stage classification based on sparse deep belief net and combination of multiple classifiers. Trans. Inst. Meas. Control. **38**(4), 435–451 (2015)
5. S. Wang, V. Anugu, T. Nguyen, N. Rose, et al., Fusion of machine intelligence and human intelligence for colonic polyp detection in CT colonography, in International Symposium on Biomedical Imaging: From Nano to Macro, pp. 160–164, Chicago, 2011

6. F. Putze, S. Hesslinger, C.Y. Tse, Y. Huang, C. Herff, C. Guan, T. Schultz, Hybrid fNIRS-EEG based classification of auditory and visual perception processes. Front. Neurosci. **8**, 373 (2014)
7. G. Shafer, *A Mathematical Theory of Evidence* (Princeton University Press, 1976)
8. S. Amari, Integration of stochastic models by minimizing α-divergence. Neural Comput. **19**, 2796–2780 (2007)
9. R.B. Nelsen, *An Introduction to Copulas* (Springer, 1999)
10. A. Salazar, L. Vergara, *Independent Component Analysis (ICA): Algorithms, Applications and Ambiguities* (Nova Science Publishers, New York, 2018)
11. A. Salazar, *On Statistical Pattern Recognition in Independent Component Analysis Mixture Modelling* (Springer, Berlin, Heidelberg, 2013)
12. Y.S. Huang, C.Y. Suen, A method of combining multiple experts for the recognition of unconstrained handwritten numerals. IEEE Trans. Pattern Anal. Mach. Intell. **17**(1), 90–94 (1995)
13. K.H. Hui, M.H. Lim, M.S. Leong, S.M. Al-Obaidi, Dempster-Shafer evidence theory for multi-bearing faults diagnosis. Eng. Appl. Artif. Intell. **57**, 160–170 (2017)
14. A. Soriano, L. Vergara, A. Bouziane, A. Salazar, Fusion of scores in a detection context based on alpha-integration. Neural Comput. **27**, 1983–2010 (2015)
15. A. Salazar, G. Safont, L. Vergara, E. Vidal, Pattern recognition techniques for provenance classification of archaeological ceramics using ultrasounds. Pattern Recogn. Lett. **135**, 441–450 (2020)
16. G. Safont, A. Salazar, L. Vergara, Vector score alpha integration for classifier late fusion. Pattern Recogn. Lett. (2020). https://doi.org/10.1016/j.patrec.2020.05.014
17. G. Safont, A. Salazar, L. Vergara, Multiclass alpha integration of scores from multiple classifiers. Neural Comput. **31**(4), 806–825 (2019)
18. S. Amari, *Information Geometry and its Applications* (Springer, 2016)
19. K. Karra, L. Mili, Hybrid copula Bayesian networks, in Eighth Conference on Probabilistic Graphical Models, PGM 2016, pp. 240–251, Lugano, 2016
20. D.H. Oh, A.J. Patton, Modeling dependence in high dimensions with factor copulas. J. Bus. Econ. Stat. **35**(1), 139–154 (2017)
21. J. Belda, L. Vergara, G. Safont, A. Salazar, Computing the partial correlation of ICA models for non-Gaussian graph signal processing. Entropy **21**(1), 22 (2019)
22. J. Belda, L. Vergara, A. Salazar, G. Safont, Estimating the Laplacian matrix of Gaussian mixtures for signal processing on graphs. Signal Process. **148**, 241–249 (2018)
23. J. Belda, L. Vergara, G. Safont, A. Salazar, Z. Parcheta, A new surrogating algorithm by the complex graph Fourier transform (CGFT). Entropy **21**(8), 759 (2019)
24. A. Salazar, G. Safont, L. Vergara, Semi-supervised learning for imbalanced classification of credit card transaction, in 2018 International Joint Conference on Neural Networks, IJCNN 2018, art. no. 8489755, pp. 4976–4982, Rio de Janeiro, 2018
25. A. Salazar, G. Safont, L. Vergara, Surrogate techniques for testing fraud detection algorithms in credit card operations, in 48th Annual IEEE International Carnahan Conference on Security Technology, ICCST 2014, art. no. 6986987, pp. 124–129, Rome, 2014
26. G. Safont, A. Salazar, A. Rodriguez, L. Vergara, On recovering missing ground penetrating radar traces by statistical interpolation methods. Remote Sens. **6**(8), 7546–7565 (2014)
27. A. Salazar, L. Vergara, ICA mixtures applied to ultrasonic nondestructive classification of archaeological ceramics. Eurasip J. Adv. Signal Process, 1–11 (2010)., art. no. 125201
28. A. Salazar, L. Vergara, I. Igual, J. Gosalbez, Blind source separation for classification and detection of flaws in impact-echo testing. Mech. Syst. Signal Process. **19**(6), 1312–1325 (2005)
29. G. Safont, A. Salazar, L. Vergara, A. Rodriguez, Nonlinear estimators from ICA mixture models. Signal Process. **155**, 281–286 (2019)
30. G. Safont, A. Salazar, L. Vergara, E. Gomez, V. Villanueva, Multichannel dynamic modeling of non-Gaussian mixtures. Pattern Recogn. **93**, 312–323 (2019)

31. G. Safont, A. Salazar, L. Vergara, E. Gomez, V. Villanueva, Probabilistic distance for mixtures of independent component analyzers. IEEE Trans. Neural Netw. Learn. Syst. **29**(4), 1161–1173 (2018)
32. A. Salazar, L. Vergara, R. Miralles, On including sequential dependence in ICA mixture models. Signal Process. **90**(7), 2314–2318 (2010)
33. A. Ferreira, S.C. Felipussi, C. Alfaro, P. Fonseca, J.E. Vargas-Muñoz, J.A. dos Santos, A. Rocha, Behavior knowledge space-based fusion for copy–move forgery detection. IEEE Trans. Image Process. **25**(10), 4729–4742 (2016)
34. M. Quintana, J. Pena-Casanova, G. Sánchez-Benavides, K. Langohr, R. Manero, M. Aguilar, D. Badenes, J. Molinuevo, A. Robles, M. Barquero, C. Antúnez, Spanish multicenter normative studies (Neuronorma project): Norms for the abbreviated Barcelona Test. Arch. Clin. Neuropsychol. **26**(2), 144–157 (2010)
35. E. Strauss, *A Compendium of Neuropsychological Tests* (Oxford University Press, 2006)
36. S. Sternberg, High-speed scanning in human memory. Science **153**(3736), 652–654 (1966)
37. S. Sanei, J.A. Chambers, *EEG Signal Processing* (Wiley, 2013)
38. J. Hjorth, The physical significance of time domain descriptors in EEG analysis. Electroencephalogr. Clin. Neurophysiol. **34**(3), 321–325 (1973)
39. U. Stańczyk, L.C. Jain, *Feature Selection for Data and Pattern Recognition* (Springer, Berlin, 2011)
40. D.M.W. Powers, Evaluation: From precision, recall and F-measure to ROC, informedness, markedness & correlation. J. Mach. Learn. Technol. **2**(1), 37–63 (2011)

An Investigation of Texture Features Based on Polyp Size for Computer-Aided Diagnosis of Colonic Polyps

Yeseul Choi, Alice Wei, David Wang, David Liang, Shu Zhang, and Marc Pomeroy

1 Introduction

According to recent statistics published by the American Cancer Association, colorectal cancer is the second leading cause of deaths of men and women combined, with an estimated 101,420 new cases in 2019 (American Cancer [1, 9]). Early detection and removal of polyps significantly reduces the risk of death and screenings are recommended for those 50 or older. However, using clinical optical

Y. Choi
Department of Radiology, Stony Brook University, Stony Brook, NY, USA

Stuyvesant High School, New York, NY, USA

A. Wei
Department of Radiology, Stony Brook University, Stony Brook, NY, USA

Staten Island Technical High School, Staten Island, NY, USA
e-mail: alice.wei22@sitechhs.com

D. Wang (✉)
Department of Radiology, Stony Brook University, Stony Brook, NY, USA

Syosset High School, Syosset, NY, USA

D. Liang
Department of Radiology, Stony Brook University, Stony Brook, NY, USA

Ward Melville High School, East Setauket, NY, USA

S. Zhang
Department of Radiology, Stony Brook University, Stony Brook, NY, USA

M. Pomeroy
Department of Radiology, Stony Brook University, Stony Brook, NY, USA

Department of Biomedical Engineering, Stony Brook University, Stony Brook, NY, USA

H. R. Arabnia et al. (eds.), *Advances in Computer Vision and Computational Biology*, Transactions on Computational Science and Computational Intelligence,
https://doi.org/10.1007/978-3-030-71051-4_66

colonoscopy (OC), to screen the growing population of those over 50 is severely limited by our current resources. Alternatively, computed tomography colonography (CTC) has been a rising noninvasive solution to detect possible cancers [3, 5, 6, 11, 12], decreasing the amount of people being screened under OC. Furthermore, the majority of polyps are found to be nonneoplastic, named hyperplastic, which are abnormal growths with no risk, only taking up valuable resources when removed. Therefore, being able to distinguish between hyperplastic and adenomatous polyps through CTC screenings has become crucial.

In our previous research work, texture feature extraction techniques have been established and modified to improve the accuracy of diagnoses of polyps found through CTC screenings [4, 10]. Those texture features include intensity, gradient, and curvature. Pickhardt et al. suggests that the malignancy rates of polyps increase in correlation to their size [8]. Besides polyp's malignancy rates, general kernel approach for gradient and curvature texture extraction may also get influenced by the polyp size [7]. Thus, in this study, we design experiments to investigate the effect of separating polyps based on size on the performance of machine learning.

The remainder of this chapter is organized as follows. Section 2 depicts our method for conducting feature analysis in computer-aided diagnosis of colorectal polyps. In Sect. 3, experimental design and results are reported. Finally, discussion of our work and conclusions are given in Sect. 4.

2 Materials and Methods

The aim of this study is to investigate the performance of machine learning on texture features based on different polyp sizes. Figure 1 shows a 6-mm small-sized polyp and a 22-mm medium-sized polyp visualized via two-dimensional (2D) axial image.

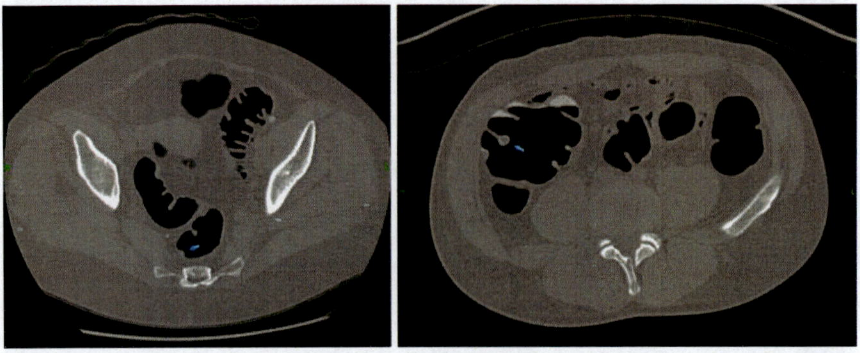

Fig. 1 A 6-mm polyp (left) and a 20-mm polyp (right) on 2D axial image

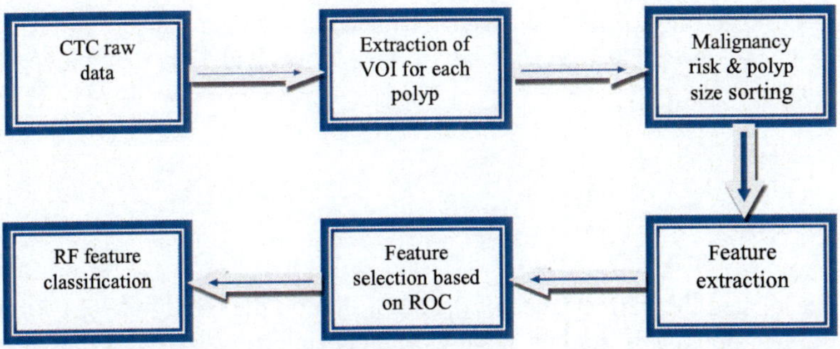

Fig. 2 Flowchart of our method for texture analysis

2.1 *Flowchart of Our Method*

The flowchart of our methods can be summarized in Fig. 2. First, from the original CT image, the volume of interest (VOI) of each polyp was extracted and further confirmed by the radiologists. Second, we applied an extended traditional Haralick model [2] with a total of 30 texture features [4], which were obtained from the VOIs of each polyp. In our study, the texture features of polyps consist of intensity, gradient, and curvature. Third, we performed a receiver operating characteristics (ROC)-based analysis to select the best feature sets. Finally, we employed a machine learning method, the Random Forest (RF) classifier, for feature classification.

2.2 *Malignancy Risk of the Polyps*

According to histopathology, polyps can be divided into two categories: nonneoplastic and neoplastic. Nonneoplastic polyps are benign polyps, including the subtypes of hyperplasic, mucosal polyp, and inflammatory, etc. On the other hand, neoplastic are malignancy risky, including serrated adenoma, tubular adenoma, tubulovillous adenoma, adenocarcinoma, etc. In this study, we labeled the nonneoplastic polyp as 0 and neoplastic polyps as 1, indicating their benign or malignancy risk accordingly.

2.3 *Data Preparation*

The dataset used in this study consists of a total number of 228 polyp masses found through a CTC database. Those polyp masses were confirmed by OC. The spatial resolution of the CT image is 0.7 by 0.7 by 1.0 mm^3. All the polyp masses have a diameter size ranging from 6 to 30 mm. Polyps were grouped into three groups based on their sizes: 6–9 mm, 10–30 mm, and a combined group of 6–30 mm. For a fair performance comparison, we have a balanced polyp pool of 114 polyps in each size group. Within each size group, all of the datasets had 57 benign polyps and 57 malignant polyps.

3 Results

We investigated the performance of the algorithm on the 6–9 mm, 10–30 mm, and 6–30 mm groups. The studied features include intensity, gradient, curvature, all combined features. We generated a measure of area under the curve (AUC) values of ROC curve. The performance was determined by assessing the sensitivity and specificity values. The averaged AUC information is illustrated in Table 1. Figure 3 shows the averaged ROC curve for the intensity feature. Figure 4 shows the averaged

Table 1 Averaged AUC information

Group	AUC information		
	6–9 mm	10–30 mm	6–30 mm
Intensity	0.7437	0.6942	0.7559
Gradient	0.6768	0.7226	0.6803
Curvature	0.5747	0.6493	0.6004
All features	0.7327	0.7915	0.7678

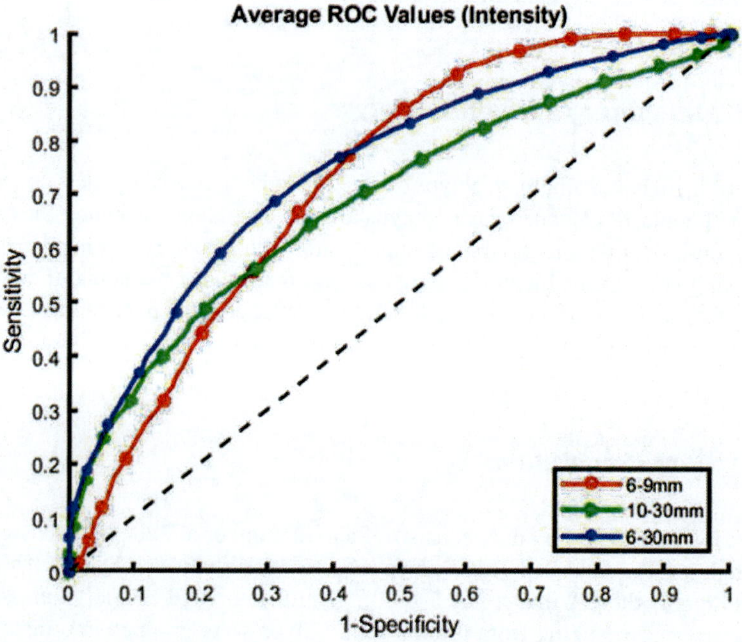

Fig. 3 The averaged ROC curves for the intensity feature

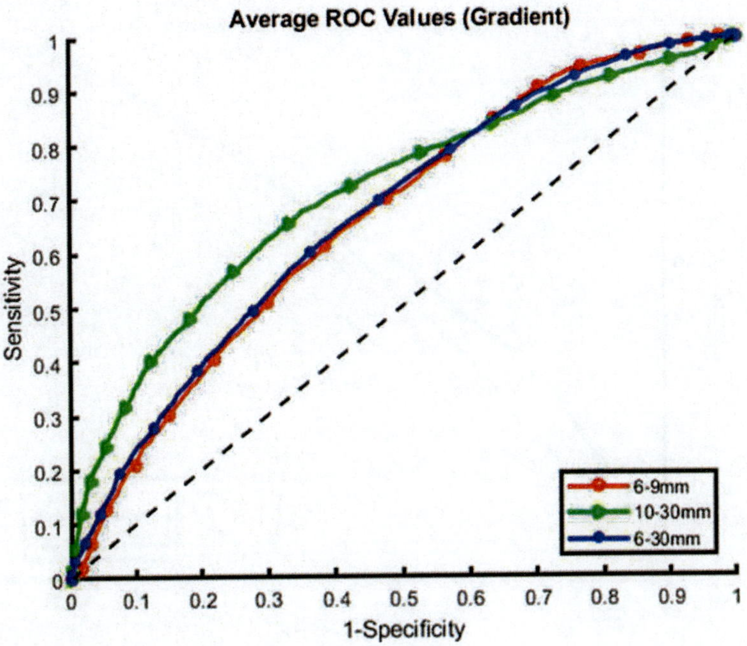

Fig. 4 The averaged ROC curves for the gradient feature

ROC curve for the gradient feature. Figure 5 shows the averaged ROC curve for the curvature feature. And Fig. 6 shows the averaged ROC curve for all combined features.

4 Discussion and Conclusions

Experimental results demonstrated that gradient and curvature were ideal distinguishing features for medium-sized polyps, whereas intensity was better for smaller-sized polyps. Due to their negligible proportions, the curvature and gradient features were flawed for the 6–9 mm polyps during the experiment. The opposite is true for the medium-sized polyp group.

When examining all features, the AUC value of the 10–30 mm polyps was greater than the AUC value of the 6–30 mm polyps, suggesting that separating the small- and medium-sized polyps would be beneficial in identifying medium-sized polyps. However, the AUC value of the 6–9 mm polyps was lower than that of the 6–30 mm polyps, suggesting that this separation may not be ideal for identifying smaller polyps. The AUC value for all polyps is greater than that of the individual group of smaller polyps because it is averaged out by the higher performance of the identification of the 10–30 mm polyps. Furthermore, the smaller polyps have less identifiable features. This study shall facilitate computer-aided diagnosis of polyps

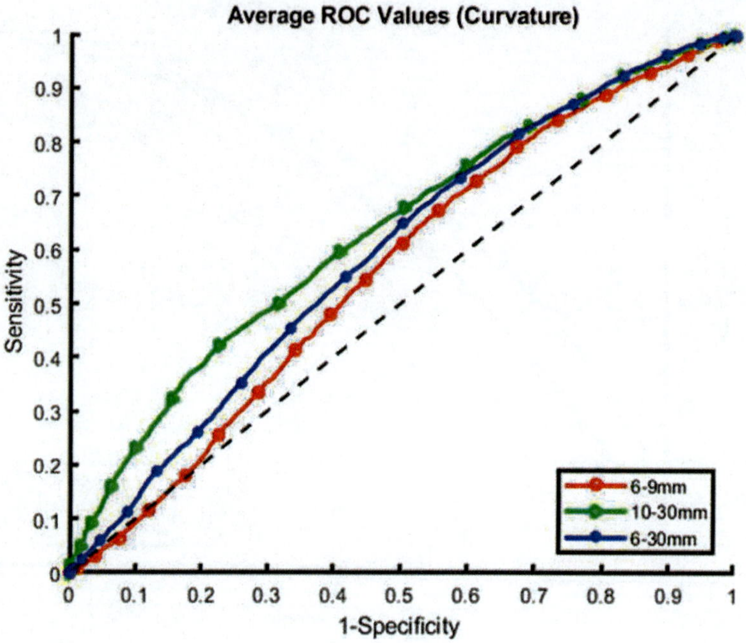

Fig. 5 The averaged ROC curves for the curvature feature

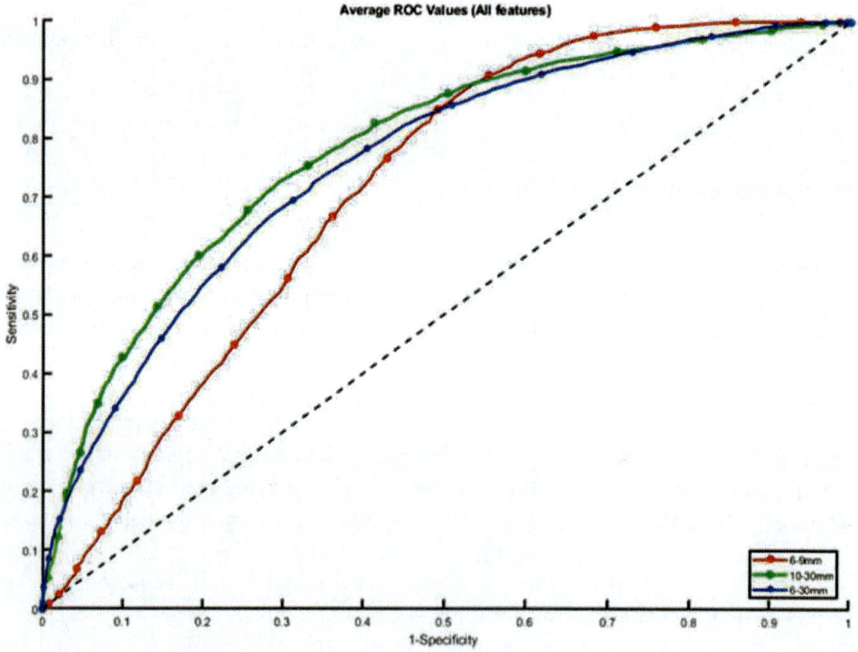

Fig. 6 The averaged ROC curves for all combined features

to achieve high performance by taking into account the contributions of different features among different polyp sizes.

Acknowledgments This work was partially supported by NIH grant #CA206171 of the National Cancer Institute and the Computer Science and Informatics Research Experience Program at Stony Brook University.

References

1. American Cancer Society, Cancer facts & figures 2019. Atlanta (2019)
2. R.M. Haralick, K. Shanmugam, I. Dinstein, Textural features for image classification. IEEE Trans. Syst. Man Cybern. **3**(6), 610–621 (1973)
3. L. Hong, A. Kaufman, Y. Wei, et al., *3D virtual colonoscopy. IEEE Biomedical Visualization Symposium* (IEEE CS Press, Los Alamitos, 1995), pp. 26–32
4. Y. Hu, Z. Liang, B. Song, et al., Texture feature extraction and analysis for polyp differentiation via computed tomography colonography. IEEE Trans. Med. Imaging **35**(6), 1522–1531 (2016)
5. Z. Liang, VC: An alternative approach to examination of the entire colon. INNERVISION **16**, 40–44 (2001)
6. Z. Liang, R. Richards, Virtual colonoscopy v.s. optical colonoscopy. Expert Opin. Med. Diagn J **4**(2), 149–158 (2010)
7. J. Liu, S. Kabadi, R.V. Uitert, et al., Improved computer-aided detection of small polyps in CT colonography using interpolation for curvature estimation. Med. Phys. **38**(7), 4276–4284 (2011)
8. P.J. Pickhardt, K.S. Hain, D.H. Kim, et al., Low rates of cancer or high-grade dysplasia in colorectal polyps collected from computed tomography colonography screening. Clin. Gastroenterol. Hepatol. **8**, 610–615 (2010)
9. R.L. Siegel, K.D. Miller, A. Jemal, Cancer statistics, 2019. CA Cancer J. Clin. **69**(1), 7–34 (2019)
10. B. Song, G. Zhang, H. Lu, et al., Volumetric texture features from higher-order images for diagnosis of colon lesions via CTC. Int. J. Comput. Assist. Radiol. Surg. **9**(6), 1021–1032 (2014)
11. D. Vining, D. Gelfand, R. Bechtold et al., Technical feasibility of colon imaging with helical CT and virtual reality. Annual Meeting of American Roentgen Ray Society, New Orleans, pp. 104 (1994)
12. H. Zhu, Y. Fan, H. Lu, et al., Improved curvature estimation for computer-aided detection of colonic polyps in CT colonography. Acad. Radiol. **18**(8), 1024–1034 (2011)

Electrocardiogram Classification Using Long Short-Term Memory Networks

Shijun Tang and Jenny Tang

1 Introduction

An electrocardiogram (ECG) is comprehensive information reflecting the electrical signal activity of the human heart. ECGs record the electrical activity of a person's heart over a period of time. Information from ECG is very helpful for physicians to detect visually if a patient's heartbeat is normal or irregular. For instance, arrhythmia is caused by improper intracardiac conduction or pulse formation, which can affect heart shape or disrupt the heart rate [1, 2].

Many methods for automatic classification of ECGs have been proposed. The arrhythmia or abnormal heartbeat from ECG can be distinguished by the time-domain [3], wavelet transform [4], support vector machine (SVM) [5], or other methods. However, these methods are highly dependent on manual design, which may increase computational complexity throughout the process as well as processing time and costs. In recent years, deep learning has been successfully used in many fields, such as image classification [6], target detection [7], and disease prediction [8]. It is also effectively used to analyze bioinformatics signals [9, 10].

Deep learning establishes the mainstream of machine learning and pattern recognition. It provides a structure in which feature extraction and classification are performed together [11]. Long short-term memory (LSTM) network is a special type of recurrent neural network (RNN) that is widely used for time series analysis.

There are 719 abnormal ECG files and 4942 normal ECG files in this research. Imbalanced ECG beat data affects the LSTM performance and results. We have

S. Tang (✉)
Department of Science and Mathematics, Alvernia University, Reading, PA, USA
e-mail: shijun.tang@alvernia.edu

J. Tang
Wilson High School, Reading, PA, USA

H. R. Arabnia et al. (eds.), *Advances in Computer Vision and Computational Biology*, Transactions on Computational Science and Computational Intelligence,
https://doi.org/10.1007/978-3-030-71051-4_67

overcome the weakness in ECG data through padding the existing abnormal ECG data and changing the performing order of the existing abnormal ECG data.

In this paper, we present a fully automatic and fast ECG classifier using a deep learning approach. This classification is based on feature processing and ECG signals. We also address imbalances in the ECG data when training LSTM network. The experimental results show that the proposed model achieved good performance on imbalanced ECG beat data.

2 Methodology

ECG classification using deep learning generally includes two basic stages: feature extraction and classification using LSTM. The details and theoretical background of ECG classification LSTM are discussed in the following sections.

2.1 *Feature Extraction of ECG Signals*

In order to accomplish ECG classification, we proposed feature extraction of ECG signals as the following steps:

1. Heartbeat detection: we take the R peak position first, then determine the position of the heartbeats.
2. RR calculation: The RR interval is defined as the time interval between successive heartbeats. The RR interval associated to a heartbeat i, RR(i), corresponds to the time difference between the heartbeat i and the previous heartbeat $(i-1)$.
3. Heartbeat normalization: Each segmented heartbeat is normalized between $[-1, 1]$. This scaling operation results in a signal that is independent of the original ECG recording position.

After processing the ECG recordings, heartbeats are represented by a set of features. One of the main goals related to the feature selection in our model is to avoid complicated features with a high computational cost.

2.2 *Method*

The softmax regression model is used as the last layer of the LSTM network structure. For the input training set, $\{(x^{(1)}, y^{(1)}), (x^{(2)}, y^{(2)}), \ldots (x^{(n)}, y^{(n)})\}$. n is the number of ECG signals. $x^{(i)}$ is an ECG signal. $y^{(i)} \in \{0, 1\}$ is the category label of the $x^{(i)}$. 0, 1 are the representations of Abnormal and Normal, respectively. If $y = 0$, $x^{(i)}$ is an abnormal signal; otherwise, $x^{(i)}$ is one of the normal types.

2.3 LSTM Recurrent Network

Long short-term memory (LSTM) is a time-recurrent neural network [12]. LSTM network includes an input gate, forget gate, and output gate. The forget gate f_t in the LSTM memory determines which information must be retained or discarded. The input gate i_t is a section where it is activated to determine whether to update the historical information to the LSTM block. c_{in} is calculated by a *tanh* function. c_t is calculated from the current candidate cell c_{in}, the previous time state c_{t-1}, the input gate information i_t, and the forget gate information f_t. o_t of the LSTM block at the current time is generated at the output gate. Finally, it determines the amount of information about the current cell state that will be output. The activation of each gate and the update of the current cell state can be calculated as follows:

$$\begin{aligned} f_t &= \text{sigmoid}\left(W_f \cdot [a_{t-1}, x_t] + b_f\right) \\ i_t &= \text{sigmoid}\left(W_i \cdot [a_{t-1}, x_t] + b_i\right). \\ c_{in} &= \tanh\left(W_c \cdot [a_{t-1}, x_t] + b_c\right) \\ c_t &= f_t \cdot c_{t-1} + i_t \cdot c_{\text{in}} \\ o_t &= \text{sigmoid}\left(W_o \cdot [a_{t-1}, x_t] + b_o\right) \\ a_t &= o_t \cdot \tanh\left(c_t\right) \end{aligned} \tag{1}$$

We calculated and obtained the feature vector from ECG signal. An output value from the output layer is used to classify the ECG signal as N, or A. In this paper, we use the three-layer LSTM architecture, including an input layer, an LSTM layer, and an output layer. The structure of the proposed LSTM network for ECG signal classification tasks is shown in Fig. 1.

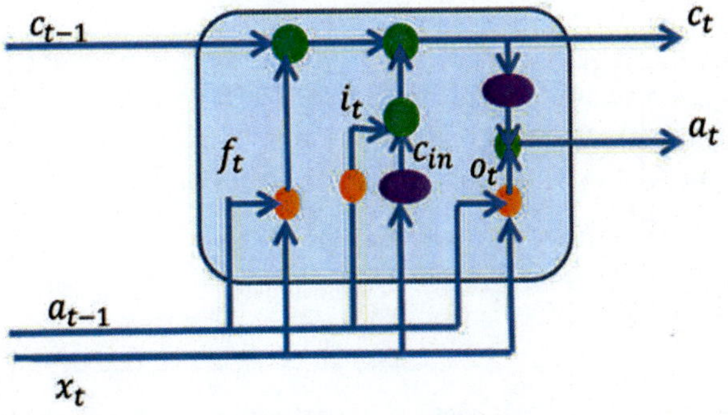

Fig. 1 Diagram of long short-term memory

3 Experimental Results

3.1 Experiment Setup

The proposed LSTM with feature extraction in this paper ran on the deep learning framework in the Microsoft Windows 10 64-bit Operating System. Computer was configured with a 16-GB Intel (R) Core (TM) i7-7700 processor.

3.2 Materials

We used the MIT-BIH arrhythmia database provided by the Massachusetts Institute of Technology [13]. Each group is approximately 30 minutes long and is sampled at a rate of 360 Hz by a 0.1–100 Hz band pass filter, for a total of approximately 650,000 sample points.

The normal category has the most data volume, and the abnormal categories include different ECG beat types. So, there is a heavy imbalance between normal and abnormal ECG beats. Because of imbalanced ECG beat data, the network model tends to learn the distribution of major ECG beat data, while there is insufficient learning of minority ECG beat data.

The dataset had a total of 5661 ECG signal files. We used 10% of all ECG data as the testing set. In the remaining ECG data, 90% of the data were used as the training set and 10% as the validation set. The training and validation sets were used to adjust the parameters and determine the optimal number of elements of the designed model. The model performance was evaluated using a testing set that was not previously used. Figures 2 and 3 show Normal ECG Signal and abnormal ECG Signal.

In Fig. 4, we can get the training progress using LSTM when performing our program. Figure 5 shows classification results. The green stars are the classified categories from LSTM; the red circles are real categories from test ECG data. 0 represents Abnormal ECG signal; 1 represents Normal ECG signal.

3.3 Evaluation

We used four metrics to evaluate the performance of the proposed network: accuracy, recall, precision, specificity. Accuracy is the proportion of correctly classified ECG signals in all ECG signals, which reflects the consistency between test results and real results. However, recall, precision, and specificity are less biased in evaluating the performance of the classifier on the imbalanced dataset. Four evaluation metrics can be calculated as follows:

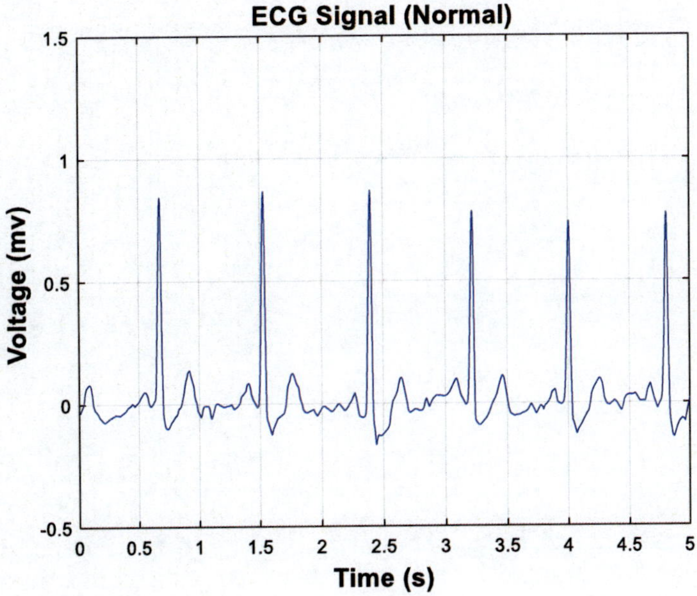

Fig. 2 Normal ECG signal

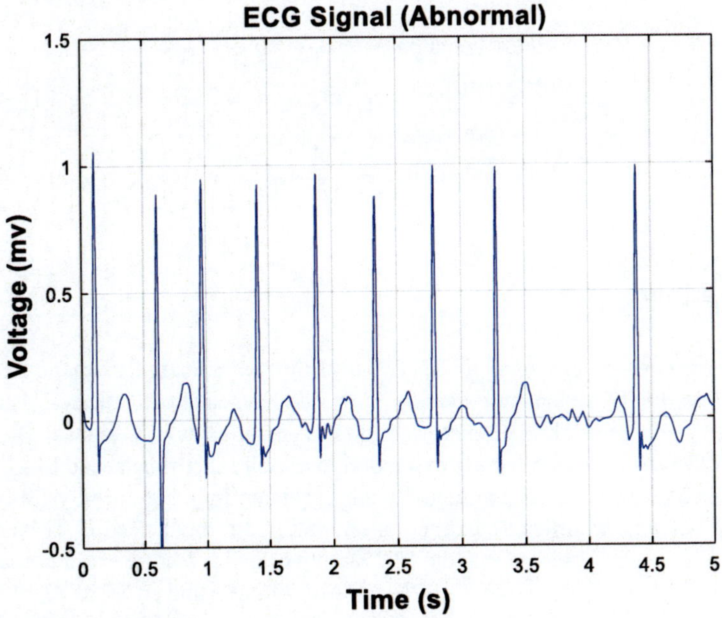

Fig. 3 Abnormal ECG signal

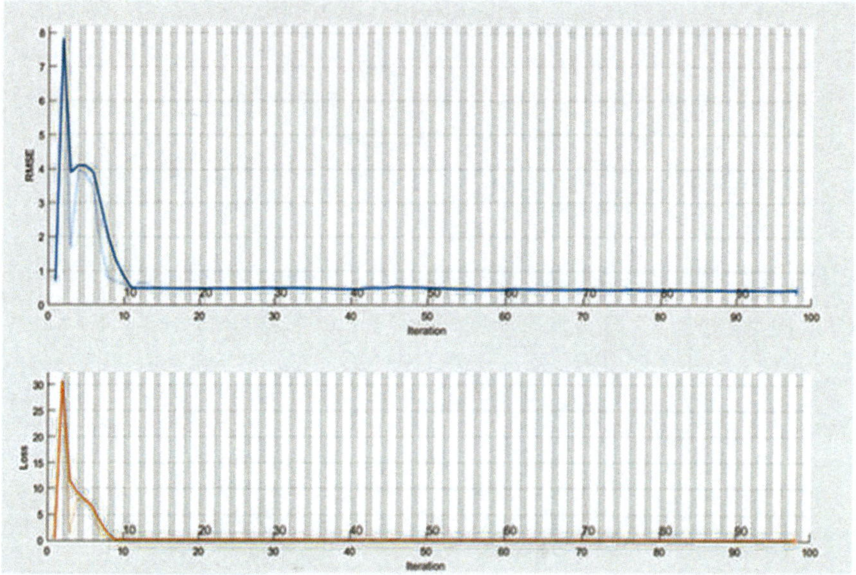

Fig. 4 Training progress using LSTM

$$
\begin{aligned}
&\text{ACC (accuracy)} = \frac{\text{TP+TN}}{\text{TP+TN+FP+FN}}\\
&\text{RE (recall)} = \frac{\text{TP}}{\text{TP+FN}}\\
&\text{PR (precision)} = \frac{\text{TP}}{\text{TP+FP}}\\
&\text{SP (specificity)} = \frac{\text{TN}}{\text{TN+FP}}
\end{aligned} \tag{2}
$$

3.4 Results

In this paper, we proposed an LSTM network with feature extraction to make imbalanced ECG signal classification. First, we have taken RR interval, half width of QRS peak, as well as their distribution as the features of ECG signals. We trained the LSTM network with feature extraction to classify the imbalanced ECG signals. Performance measures of the model were evaluated in Table 1, the validity of the LSTM network with feature extraction is verified on imbalanced ECG data. From Table 1, it can be observed that the LSTM network with feature extraction achieves an ACC of 82.14%, an RE of 87.14%, a PR of 79.22%, and an SP of 77.14%.

In this paper, we proposed an LSTM network structure to achieve the goal of imbalanced ECG signal classification. We have classified category-imbalanced ECG data through combining an LSTM network with feature extraction. From Table 1, it is evident that our proposed LSTM with feature extraction achieved

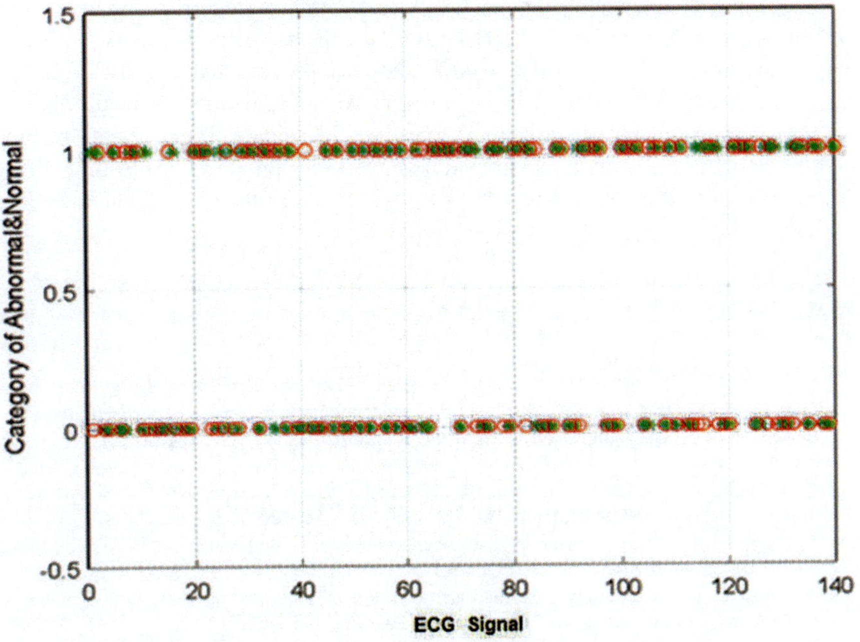

Fig. 5 Classification results. The green stars are the classified categories using LSTM; the red circles are real categories from test ECG data. 0, abnormal ECG signal; 1, normal ECG signal

Table 1 LSTM network classification results on the testing set

ACC(%)	RE(%)	SP(%)	PR(%)
82.14	87.14	79.22	77.14

good performance. This proposed method avoids the problem of undersampling or oversampling method. There are several advantages in this proposed method: (i) Feature extraction is direct and effective. Also, selection techniques are needed; (ii) the proposed method can make normal and abnormal classifications very well; (iii) our proposed method works good without denoised ECG recordings.

4 Conclusions

In this paper, we proposed a novel ECG classification algorithm based on LSTM and feature extraction to classify normal and abnormal ECG signals. The results show that the LSTM network with feature extraction achieved an accuracy, recall, precision, and specificity score of 82.14%, 87.14%, 79.22%, and 77.14%, respectively.

Experimental results of the MIT-BIH arrhythmia database demonstrate the effectiveness of the proposed LSTM network. The feature combination of both half width of QRS peak and RR interval allows us to train and classify ECG data with remarkable speeds. The proposed method can be applied to assist cardiologists in more accurately and objectively diagnosing ECG signals. The proposed method will be helpful in an online classification and will be applied in health-monitoring wireless devices and wearables.

References

1. National Heart, Lung, and Blood Institute, Arrhythmia, National Heart, Lung, and Blood Institute, Bethesda, MA, USA, (2019), https://www.nhlbi.nih.gov/health-topics/arrhythmia
2. S. Min, B. Lee, S. Yoon, Deep learning in bioinformatics. Brief. Bioinform. **18**, 851–869 (2017)
3. D. Katircioglu-Öztürk, H.A. Güvenir, U. Ravens, N. Baykal, A window-based time series feature extraction method. Comput. Biol. Med. **89**, 466–486 (2017)
4. Y. Jung, H. Kim, Detection of PVC by using a wavelet based statistical ECG monitoring procedure. Biomed. Signal Process. Control **36**, 176–182 (2017)
5. S. Raj, K.C. Ray, O. Shankar, Cardiac arrhythmia beat classification using DOST and PSO tuned SVM. Comput. Methods Prog. Biomed. **136**, 163–177 (2016)
6. E. Maggiori, Y. Tarabalka, G. Charpiat, P. Alliez, Convolutional neural networks for large-scale remote sensing image classification. IEEE Trans. Geosci. Remote Sens. **55**(2), 645–657 (2017)
7. O. Russakovsky, J. Deng, H. Su, et al., ImageNet large scale visual recognition challenge. Int. J. Comput. Vis. **115**(3), 211–252 (2015)
8. P. Lu, S. Guo, H. Zhang, et al., Research on improved depth belief network-based prediction of cardiovascular diseases. J Healthc Eng **2018**, 8954878, 9 pages (2018)
9. U.R. Acharya, S.L. Oh, Y. Hagiwara, et al., A deep convolutional neural network model to classify heartbeats. Comput. Biol. Med. **89**, 389–396 (2017)
10. W. Li, J. Li, Local deep field for electrocardiogram beat classification. IEEE Sensors J. **18**(4), 1656–1664 (2018)
11. Y. Bengio, Learning deep architectures for AI. Found. Trends Mach. Learn. **2**(1), 1–127 (2009)
12. H. Sak, A. Senior, F. Beaufays, Long short-term memory recurrent neural network architectures for large scale acoustic modeling, in Proceedings of the Fifteenth Annual Conference of the International Speech Communication Association, pp. 338–342, Singapore, Sept 2014
13. A.L. Goldberger, L.A.N. Amaral, L. Glass, et al., PhysioBank, PhysioToolkit, and PhysioNet: Components of a new research resource for complex physiologic signals. Circulation **101**(23), E215–E220 (2000)

Cancer Gene Diagnosis of 78 Microarrays Registered on GSE from 2007 to 2017

Shuichi Shinmura

1 Introduction

From 1999 to 2004, six medical projects published papers and uploaded their microarrays publicly on the Internet. The purpose of these medical studies is to identify a set of cancer genes useful for gene diagnosis of cancer, using two classes, such as healthy patients and cancer patients or patients with two types of cancer, respectively. To find multivariate oncogenes from microarray is different from traditional biological research to find one oncogene using microscopic research. A multivariate discriminant analysis is the best for this research. A multivariate approach is the best for this research. The author downloaded these six data ("six old data") in 2015 [1, 4, 5, 19, 20, 22]. We discriminated against these data using Revised IP-OLDF (RIP) and found their minimum number of misclassifications (minimum NM, MNMs) are zero [15]. This shows that two classes are linearly separable in high-dimensional gene space, and the six data are linearly separable data (LSD). LSD is a crucial signal and has two vital structures:

1. We classify the linearly separable space and subspaces as Matryoshka. LSD has the Matryoshka structure that includes smaller Matryoshkas (SM) up to the minimum SM (Basic Gene Set, BGS) in it. More importantly, finding BGS or Yamanaka four genes using the iPS study is similar to the backward stepwise of multiple regression analysis. We found success with multivariate approaches. Other researchers use a one-variable approach, like that used in traditional biological methods for finding oncogenes. This approach is useless for finding several gene sets that are important for cancer diagnosis. Ours and theirs are quite different.

S. Shinmura (✉)
Seikei University, Sakasai Kashiwa City, Chiba Pref., Japan

H. R. Arabnia et al. (eds.), *Advances in Computer Vision and Computational Biology*, Transactions on Computational Science and Computational Intelligence,
https://doi.org/10.1007/978-3-030-71051-4_68

2. LSD consists of the exclusive SMs or BGSs. This truth indicates that we are free from the curse of the high-dimensional data [17]. Thus, we can analyze all SMs and BGSs using statistical methods and propose the cancer gene diagnosis for the six data [16].

To confirm the above two truths, we discriminate 78 microarrays of 13 carcinoma types in the CuMiDa database collected from 2007 to 2017 [2]. Because the six old data and the 78 new data are LSD, we can open new frontiers for using high-dimensional genetic analysis, such as microarrays and RNA-seq., for cancer gene diagnosis. Our theory is very simple for physicians to use. If they confirm their gene data is LSD, they can analyze all SMs and BGSs using statistical methods for gene diagnosis. Using our standard procedure, we believe physicians can treat cancer using gene data.

2 Material

Table 1 shows the 78 data contained in CuMiDa. We added suffixes to instances of the same cancer types. We can get more research details by clicking the GSE number. The range of the number of cases in column N is [12, 357]. The range of the number of genes (column Gene) is [12621, 54676]. The class (or group) number is 1–7. Five data consist of 1 class, 57 data consist of 2 classes, and 16 data consist of 3 or more classes. The thirteen carcinomas are as follows: one pancreatic, thirteen breast, ten liver, four throat, nine leukemia, ten prostate, four ovary, two brain, two bladder, six lung, four renal, three gastric, ten colorectal. There are four correct classified rates (1-error rate [ER]) of nine classifiers determined by threefold cross-validation, an extension of the leave-one-out (LOO) method [6]. We omit five classifiers (Naive Bayes [NB], k-nearest neighbor [k-NN], k-means [K-M], hierarchical cluster [HC], and ZeroR) from the table. Nine classifiers can calculate the ERs using the 73 supervised learning data classified by medical researches.

Table 1 Summary of 78 microarrays on GSE DB after 2007

Type	GSE	N	Gene	Class	SVM	MLP	DT	RF
Max		357	54676	7	1	1	1	1
Min		12	12621	1	0.26	0.29	0.25	0.34
Pancreatic	GSE16515	51	54676	2	0.86	0.78	0.78	0.82
Breast5	GSE22820	139	33580	2	1	1	0.96	0.99
Breast8	GSE70947	289	35982	2	0.93	0.7	0.8	0.86
Liver2	GSE50579	76	36548	2	0.99	0.92	0.97	0.87

3 Method

When RIP discriminates against the 73 data, we find the 73 MNMs are zero and LSD. Because it takes time to find all SMs, Program3 modeled by LINGO [12] decomposes the restricted data of the first 12,621 genes into the first ten sets of SMs. LINGO: Program4 decomposes the first 10 SMs into 1666 BGSs. We analyze all SMs and BGSs of Breast5 (GSE22820) [7] via the hierarchical cluster Ward method and PCA using JMP software [11]. Other studies fail to find correct combinations of genes included in SMs and BGSs, which, given then are LSD, are the proven signal for cancer gene diagnosis. If physicians use our method as a primary screening method, they can reduce their research time and obtain useful results for diagnosis.

3.1 Revised IP-OLDF and Hard-Margin SVM

RIP in (1) directly finds the interior point of true Optimal Convex Polyhedron (OCP) [13, 14]. OCP is the feasible region of RIP defined by n constraints ($y_i \times ({}^t\mathbf{x}_i \times \mathbf{b} + b_0) \geq 1$). If data are LSD, all e_i are zero, and MNM becomes zero. The restriction by n cases releases us from the curse of high-dimensional data. Because the less than equal n coefficients of RIP are not zero and other more than (p-n) coefficients become zero naturally, RIP can select cancer genes quickly. The Branch & Bound (B&B) algorithm and OCP are the keys.

$$\text{MIN} = \Sigma e_i;\ y_i \times \left({}^t\mathbf{x}_i \times \mathbf{b} + b_0\right) \geq 1\text{–}M \times e_i;\quad i = 1, \ldots, n \tag{1}$$

$$\text{MIN} = \|b\|^2/2;\ y_i \times \left({}^t\mathbf{x}_i \times \mathbf{b} + b_0\right) \geq 1; \tag{2}$$

$\mathbf{b}$: RIP or H-SVM p-dimensional discriminant coefficients.
b_0: the constant and free variable. $\mathbf{x}_i$: p genes values of ith cases.
e_i: 0/1 binary integers corresponding to $\mathbf{x}_i$. M: Big M constant (10,000).
y_i: For the healthy class, $y_i = -1$ (class 1). For the cancer class, $y_i = 1$ (class 2).

Vapnik defined a hard-margin Support Vector Machine (H-SVM) [23] to maximize the distance of two Support Vectors (SVs) in (2). Only H-SVM and RIP can discriminate LSD theoretically. While technical researchers are responsible for separating the two classes correctly, they falsely believe that distinguishing LSD is straightforward and unworthy of research. Strangely, many researchers ignore the LSD-discrimination with H-SVM or RIP, missing an opportunity to find a crucial signal (LSD). For this reason, although they have studied gene data analysis since circa 1995, their results are useless for real gene diagnosis. However, because the quadratic programming (QP) defines H-SVM, it finds only one optimal solution in the whole region and cannot find one optimal solution of many SMs. Thus, the feature selection by H-SVM is NP-hard, like other discriminant functions.

Furthermore, they need to understand the variance-covariance matrix restricts all variables. The discriminant functions based on the variance-covariance matrix, such as Fisher's LDF, quadratic discriminant function, regularized discriminant analysis (RDA), and LASSO, never solve the curse of high-dimensional data because the variance-covariance matrix itself is the cause of the curse.

3.2 Small Matryoshka and Basic Gene Set Decomposition

At first, we developed the Matryoshka Feature Selection Method (Method2) using LINGO: Program3 explained in Section 10.5 of Shinmura [16]. It decomposes microarray into the exclusive SMs and another gene set (MNM $\geq$ 1). LINGO: Program4 decomposes high-dimensional gene data into the many exclusive BGSs and another gene set, also. BGS uses the same ideas as Yamanaka's four genes of iPS research. Dr. Takahashi found four genes from 24 genes in a similar fashion as the backward stepwise method of multiple regression and discriminant function. Cell cultures were performed with 24 combinations of 23 genes from 24 genes. If the cell culture omitting one gene generates iPS cells, it is omitted. Otherwise, it is not omitted from the 24 genes. If there are k genes omitted from 24 genes, we can omit these k genes at once and try a cell culture with 24-k genes in the second step.

In the case of 10,000 genes, Program4 evaluates 10,000 discriminations of 9999 genes in the first step. If we drop one gene from 10,000 genes and its MNM of 9999 genes is zero, we can drop this gene because this set is LSD. If its MNM is greater than zero, this gene is necessary for LSD. If k MNMs among 10,000 discriminations are zero, we can immediately drop these k genes from 10,000 genes. In the second step, Progam4 evaluates 10,000-k discriminations of 9999-k genes. In the last step, Program4 finds the first BGS. Using a Lenovo IdeaPad 320, it is difficult to repeat these iterations and build a list of all BGSs. Medical research is amply funded. Therefore, researchers can use a high-spec PC, for which the computational load is not significant. We do not know why Golub et al. [5] chose feature selection methods with one variable approach, such as the t-test, signal-noise ratio, and weighted voting. Finding a correct combination of several genes for gene diagnosis requires a multivariate approach, as used in the iPS cell research and the backward stepwise method. However, all feature selection methods used by statisticians and Machine Learning (ML) researchers lack a multivariate viewpoint, making them useless for correctly selecting genes combination.

3.3 The 100-Fold Cross-Validation for Small Sample

Starting with a statistical framework, we developed the following 100-fold Cross-Validation (Method1) [15]. We copy the original data 100 times and consider it a test sample and pseudo population. The test sample must be unique, like the population.

We assigned a uniform random number to each case and sorted it in descending order. Then, we divide it into 100 sets of training samples. We discriminate the 100 training samples and apply 100 RIPs to the test sample to obtain 100 NMs and 100 ERs. Method1 calculates an average of 100 test sample ERs as M2. M2 evaluates the vital rank of SMs and BGSs for cancer diagnosis [18]. Because the 100 training samples are samplings from the test sample and do not include several cases of the test sample, 100 RIPs misclassify several cases of the test sample. Thus, M2 can separate all BGSs into the correct signals and false signals if we can set the valid threshold. Because our test sample has the same structure as the original research data, we understand the characteristic of it.

On the other hand, the test samples of LOO and k-fold CV are not unique, and the number of cases is usually fewer than the training samples. Moreover, there were no analyses of the test samples. We cannot understand why many researchers use such flawed validation.

4 Result

4.1 Summary of Our Research (Three Studies)

In this research, we plan the following three studies:

1. In Study 1, RIP discriminates 73 data except for 5 data (with one class) and finds that the 73 MNMs are zero. Because we confirm two universal data structures of the 73 data in addition to the six older data, we expect most gene data have the same data structures.
2. In Study 2, LINGO: Program3 decomposes 57 data (with two classes) of the 73 data into 570 SMs. Program4 decomposes 570 SMs into 1666 BGSs. Method1 evaluates 1666 BGSs using their M2 values. Physicians can choose the critical BGSs for cancer gene diagnosis and ignore useless BGSs with high values of M2. The future goal is to examine the additional 16 data (those with three or more classes).
3. In Study 3, we examine several SMs and BGSs of 13 Breast cancers using JMP software. In future research studies, we will examine all of the data. After considering the results, we propose a standard gene data analysis procedure for physicians.

4.2 Confirmation of LSD and Decomposition of Ten SMs: (Study1)

We omit five microarrays (those with one class). There are 57 data (with two classes: healthy subjects and patients with cancer) and 16 data (with more than three classes:

healthy subjects and patients with more than two types of cancer). We modify the latter data into two classes (healthy subjects vs. all cancer patients). Because Brain1 (GSE50161) has five classes (one healthy class and four cancer classes), we create four new data with two classes (one class of healthy subjects vs. one class of four cancerous subjects). Thus, we make 77 new data and confirm two universal data structures of these data.

Program3 decomposes these 77 data into the first ten SMs. Table 2 shows the first ten SMs of 13 Breast cancers. Max and Min rows show the maximum and minimum values of 13 data. We omit seven SMs (SM3 through SM9) from the table. The SM1 of Breast1 consists of seven genes. The Gene column shows the number of genes included in ten SMs. The Ratio1 column shows the ratio defined by (Gene/12,621 × 100%). Ten SMs of Breast1 are 0.8% of 12,671 genes used for the SM decomposition. This value tells us that Bteast1 may have about 124 SMs in 12,621 genes. Because it contains 36,623 genes, it may have 359 SMs in 36,623 genes. Thus, we lost many useful gene sets because of the first 10 SMs' limitation. These ratios are different within the same carcinomas and between the other carcinomas. We think it shows the heterogeneity of cancer. Although cancers are heterogeneous diseases, LSD is the only signal to separate cancer and healthy patients.

Table 2 SM decompositions of 13 breast cancer

	Type	Class	SM1	SM2...	SM10	Gene	Ratio1
	Max	7	217	217	202	2070	16.4
ID	Min	2	6	3	5	52	0.4
2	Breast1	2	7	11	11	**102**	**0.8**
3	Breast2	2	65	56	57	573	4.5
4	Breast3	2	9	10	8	97	0.8
5	Breast4	2	19	16	10	153	1.2
6	**Breast5**	2	15	23	18	256	2
7	Breast6	2	15	23	18	357	2.8
8	Breast7	5	36	45	40	370	2.9
9	Breast8	2	217	210	189	2013	15.9
10	Breast9	3	17	19	24	186	1.5
11	Breast10	2	26	24	25	244	1.9
12	Breast11	6	62	69	33	512	4.1
13	Breast12	3	30	43	41	326	2.6
14	Breast13	3	31	25	30	291	2.3

Table 3 Ten SMs and BGSs included in Breast5 by Method1

	n	max	mean	MIN	MAX	MEAN
SM4	25	0	0	0	3.6	0.40
BGS41	6	0	0	0	4.32	0.45
BGS42	3	0	0	0	1.44	**0.07**
BGS43	11	0	0	1.44	7.91	**3.55**
Other4	5	6.47	4.48	5.04	12.23	6.66
SM7	22	0	0	0	5.04	0.91
BGS71	**3**	**0**	**0**	**0**	**0**	**0**
BGS72	3	0	0	0	0.72	0.02
BGS73	11	0	0	0.72	6.47	3.19
Other7	5	2.16	0.9	1.44	7.19	3.32

4.3 *Validations of SMs and BGSs of Breast5 by Method1: (Study 2)*

Program4 decomposes the first ten sets of Breast5's SMs into BGSs, and Method1 validates those by finding the M2 (the averages of 100 ERs of the test samples). Table 3 shows the fourth SM (SM4) and the seventh SM (SM7) among the 10 SMs and the BGSs included in both SMs. The last two rows of each of the SMs (Other4 and Other7, respectively) are noise (MNM > 0). The first max and mean columns show the maximum of 100 ERs of the training samples and an average of 100 ERs of the training sample (M1 value), respectively. All ERs are zero except for the ten "Others" included in ten SMs of Breast5 (Other4 and Other5). These facts tell us that 100 training samples, in addition to ten SMs and BGSs, are LSD. The second MAX and MEAN columns show the maximum of 100 ERs of the test samples and an average of 100 ERs of the test samples (M2 value), respectively. In BGS71 of SM7, we remarkably observe all ERs are zero. We believe that small M2 are useful indicators for cancer gene diagnosis. These results show that many BGSs included in the first ten SMs are helpful for diagnosis. In Alon data, RatioSVs (=200/Range of Rip Discriminant Scores) of 64 SMs were 2% or more, and the RatioSVs of 129 BGSs were 1% or less, so we judged BGSs are useless for cancer gene diagnosis [16]. This decision seems wrong for Breast5 because M2s of BGS42, BGS71, and BGS72 are less than M2s of SM4 and SM7. We evaluate the M1 and M2 compared with the ER of the original microarray (SM and BGS themselves). ML researchers, conversely, focus on the ER in the test sample, and their evaluations are useful for benchmarking the nine classifiers for unsupervised learning data. However, the first critical examination is to discriminate against the supervised learning data categorized by physicians, not using nine classifiers.

4.4 Validations of the Best BGS71 of Breast5: Study3

Program4 breaks down SM7 (22 genes) into three BGSs and Other7. BGS71 consists of 3 genes, and its M2 is zero. This shows that 100 ERs of the test sample are zero, and two classes are LSD in 100 test samples with 13,900 cases. Also, the original BGS71 and 100 training samples with 139 subjects are LSD. Researchers need to compare the original BGS71 results with the training samples and test sample validations. The M2s of SM7, BGS71, BGS72, BGS73, and Other7 are 0.91%, 0%, 0.02%, 3.19%, and 3.32%, respectively. M2 of SM7 is worse than BGS71 and BGS72. Although BGS73 is LSD, its M2 is almost the same as Other7. Thus, we do not recommend BGS73 for cancer gene diagnosis. However, if BGS73 includes several oncogenes, the reliability of M2 ranking becomes uncertain. We think that essential signals (oncogenes) found by medical research are more important than the results of data analysis.

Figure 1 shows a Ward cluster output of BGS71. The Rows of color maps are 139 individual cases, and the three columns are the BGS71 genes. The right dendrogram shows 139 subjects having two color clusters. The 129 cancer patients fall into the upper red clusters. Although the ten healthy subjects have blue colors, one of those is separate from the other nine healthy subjects. The lower dendrogram shows three variables. Because all the 100 training samples and 100 test samples of Table 3 are LSD, the healthy classes and cancer classes are well separated. However, the ten healthy cases form two groups. It may be a characteristic of breast cancer that gene data classifies clearly in this way.

Figure 2 shows the PCA three plots of BGS71. The central scatter plot shows the ten healthy subjects as blue dots and 129 cancer subjects as red dots. The one blue healthy subject in the cluster analysis corresponds to the blue case within the range of (Prin1 ≤ 3 and Prin2 ≤ 1). We can specify the location of each case via PCA after the clustering because the Ward analyzes the measurements in Euclidean space. Thus, physicians can survey the specified subjects for patient study. This is one of the reasons why we recommend hierarchical clustering instead of a Self-Organizing Map (SOP). Ward method and PCA did not show as same precise results as Figs. 1 and 2 for the six old data. Thus, we made signal data by RIP discriminant scores instead of genes. Using the signal data instead of the original data, Ward and PCA could separate two classes, just like in Figs. 1 and 2. In this study, Figs. 1 and 2 show the results of raw data, not signal data. We get a significant improvement by selecting a crucial signal ($M2 = 0$).

We test three genes using a t-test. For G71X11665, two ranges of the healthy class ($y_i = -1$) and cancer class ($y_i = 1$) are [7.06, 8.63], and [5.02, 8.09]. The *t*-value is -7.73 (*). For X11670, those are [4.9, 6.19] and [4.3, 7.029]. The *t*-value is -3.68 (*). For X11716, those are [6.32, 8.87] and [4.36, 8.16]. The *t*-value is -7.42 (*). All three *t*-values are negative and rejected by a 5% significant level. These results show that the feature selection method, based on single variable information, like the t-test, is incorrect and meaningless because these results can not mean a vital signal.

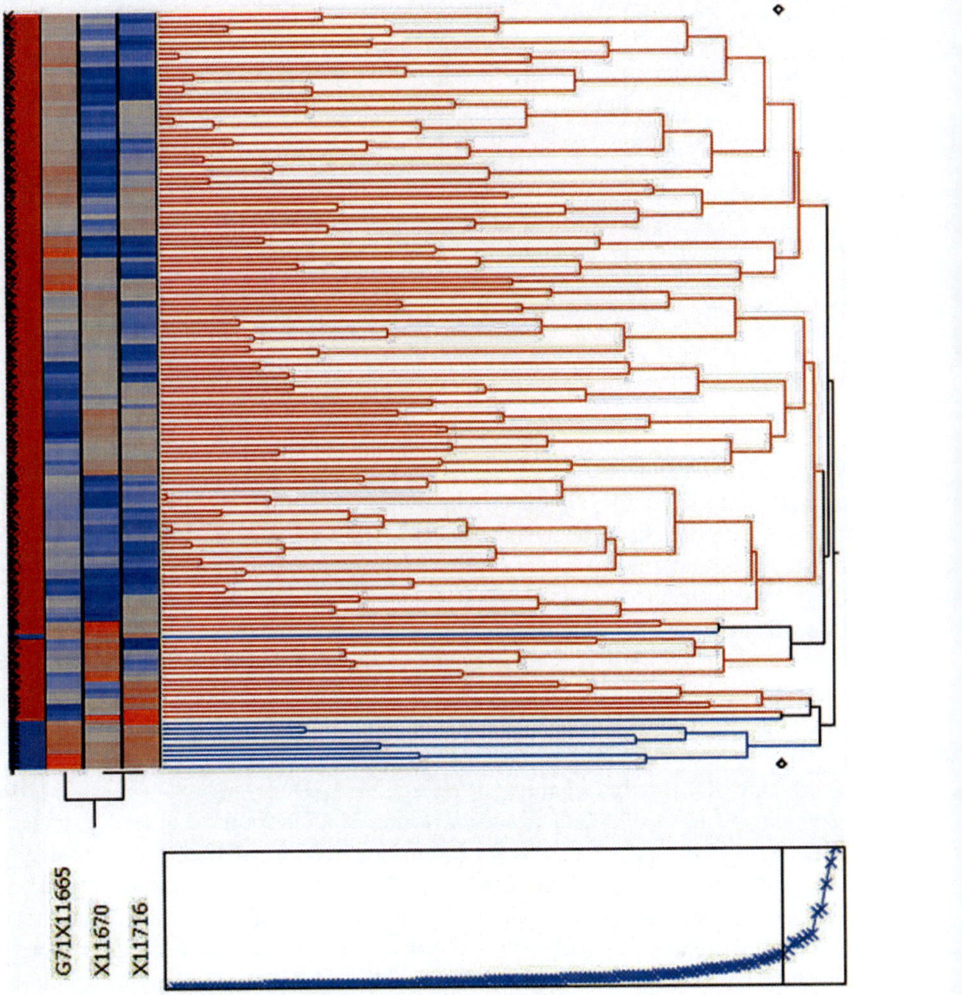

Fig. 1 Ward hierarchical cluster of BGS71 of SM7

4.5 *Validations of the Worst BGS43 of Breast5: Study3*

BGS43 (11 genes) is the worst BGS because its M2 value is the most massive 3.55% among the ten SMs and all BGSs in Breast5. The t-tests of BGS43 produce the following conclusions as same as BGS71's results: (1) Four *t*-values are negative and rejected at 5% significant level. (2) Two *t*-values are positive and rejected at 5% significant level. (3) Five *t*-values are positive and not rejected at 5% significant level. Ordinary feature selection methods never choose the last five genes and cannot find the critical signal of LSD because the last ones are necessary for LSD.

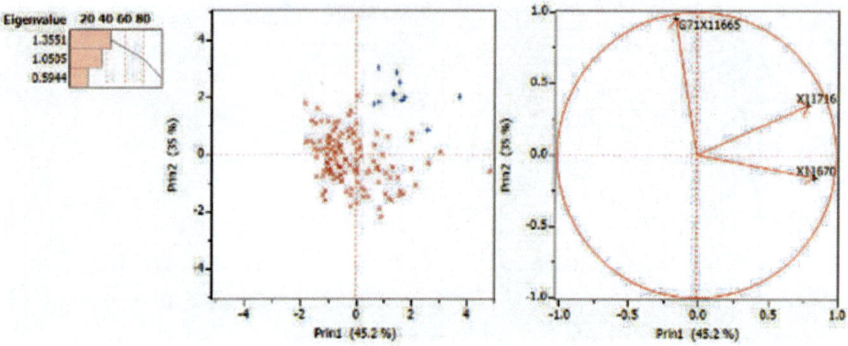

Fig. 2 PCA of BGS71 (left: eigenvalue; middle: scatter plot; right: factor loading plot)

These results again indicate that several tests calculating the difference between two averages are useless for LSD-discrimination.

Figure 3 is the cluster analysis of BGS43. Ten healthy blue cases are divided into three groups, and 129 red cancer cases are divided into four groups. The comparison of the two clusters from BGS71 and BGS43, respectively, indicates M2 is useful for evaluating the vital ranking for cancer diagnosis. If two classes from an SM or BGS become two clear clusters, we can conclude that SM or BGS is the best gene sets for cancer diagnosis. However, we expect these seven clusters may be sub-groups of cancer and healthy subjects surveyed by Golub et al.

Figure 4 shows the PCA results of BGS43. Although BGS43 (which contains 11 genes) and 100 training samples of BGS43 are LSD, several samples among 100 test samples are not LSD. The central scatter plot shows the ten healthy subjects overlapping the cancer patients. In future research, we will consider the quality check of data using the Ward method and PCA. In case the two classes of cancer subjects and healthy subjects become plural clusters, it may be a sign of the cancer sub-classes pointed by Golub et al. If physicians examine the nearest cancer subjects and healthy subjects, they may find the clue to improve the quality of data. In this study, we cannot offer the proper threshold of M2 for cancer diagnosis. Physicians may need to validate our results and determine this threshold.

5 Discussion

5.1 SM and BGS Decomposition of High-Dimensional Gene Data

We propose the high-dimensional gene data analysis of the six old data and confirm two universal data structures incorporating 77 new data collected after 2007. It is a simple approach: (1) RIP discriminates the 77 data, and all MNMs are zero. (2)

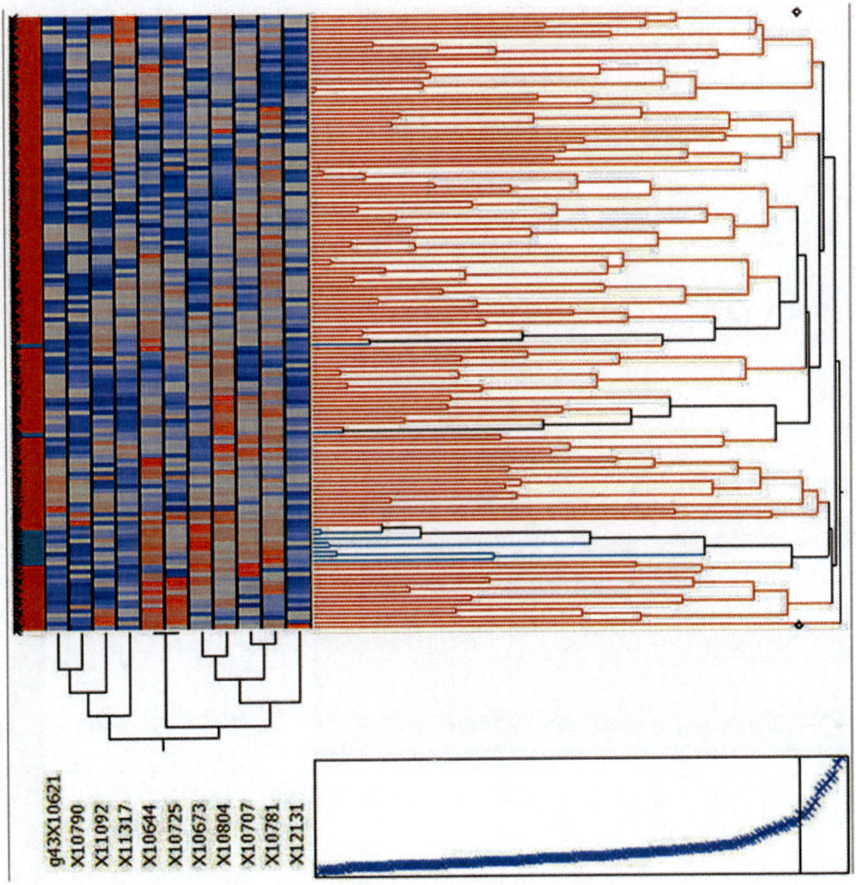

Fig. 3 Ward hierarchical cluster of BGS43

Thus, LINGO: Program3 and Program4 can break down the 77 data into 770 SMs and many BGSs. We can quickly analyze all SMs and BGSs using JMP. The analysis by LINGO and JMP are critical for cancer diagnosis.

We break down the first ten SMs of Breast5 into BGSs using Program4. Moreover, Method1 validates ten SMs and 43 BGSs of Breast5. We consider that M2 is useful for the cancer gene diagnosis ranking. Physicians can use the M2 as a reference to determine whether the selected gene sets are helpful for medical diagnosis. If the quality of healthy subjects and cancer subjects are well, we can analyze data to examine many hypotheses before medical studies.

We believe our approach is also useful for other genetic data, such as RNA-seq. If RNA-seq is not LSD, it indicates that it is less useful for cancer diagnosis than microarrays. Physicians should first check whether their research data are LSD. If it is LSD, their medical diagnosis is straightforward using the above method. If their

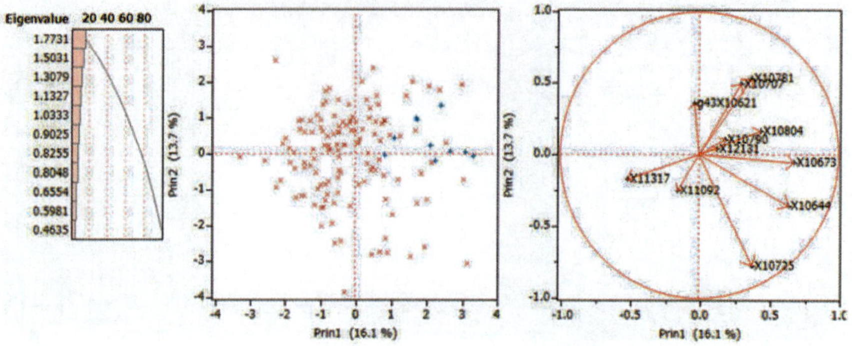

Fig. 4 PCA of BGS43

data have a few misclassified patients, they treat those cases as verification cases. After performing the above analysis with the remaining data, they can evaluate the misclassified cases carefully. This approach saves research time drastically because screening with our data analysis approach will be more efficient than traditional medical methods.

5.2 Successful Feature Selection Methods by iPS Research

iPS research is similar to our study and suggests the problems of the feature selection methods.

1. Correct Feature Selection: iPS research's first key element is to set the correct target and multivariate approach. An example of this is Professor Yamanaka, who used the gene database to identify 24 genes from over 20,000 human genes. This was the specific goal of his research. He looked for a set of genes that produced universal cells, like LSD. To that end, he specified only 24 genes activated in mouse ES cells. Dr. Takahashi, in turn, found four genes, similar to BGS, using the multivariate approach. Because Dr. Takahashi had an engineering background, he was unfamiliar with common biological logic. He confirmed a mass of universal cells generated by conducting cell experiments with 24 genes. This finding is akin to the discovery of BGS.
2. Conversely, all ordinary feature selection methods could not find the correct signal. Although many researchers pointed out the difficulties in separating signals from the noise in high-dimensional microarrays, they ignored LSD-discrimination via H-SVM or RIP. This is a crucial reason why no researchers succeeded in cancer gene diagnosis from 1995.
3. Dr. Takahashi found Yamanaka's four genes from 24 genes using an algorithm like the backward stepwise method of regression analysis. His idea is similar

to how we find BGS using Program4. He left out one of the 24 genes and experimented with 24 sets of 23 genes. Moreover, if some set of 23 genes makes a universal cell, the omitted gene is not related to the generation of the universal cell. If there were k sets, he performs the same experiment with (24-k) genes, and he finds iPS' four factors. Many studies select several independent genes with a feature selection method based on one variable. Their ways could not be used to find both Yamanaka four genes and BGS because of no consideration for multivariate aspects. Maybe it is challenging to find a set of genes, so they find one set and finish without reason. After finding one set, omitting them and repeating the analysis will find many sets like Method2. Perhaps they can't judge those superiorities or inferiorities by their threefold CV.

We believe statisticians and ML researchers ignoring LSD-researchers is the cause of the confusion in gene diagnosis. Therefore, since 1995 (when microarray technology was commercialized), they have failed to solve this high-dimensional data analysis.

5.3 *Hierarchical Structure of Number of Misclassification*

The NMs by RIP, H-SVM, Logistic Regression, Fisher's LDF, and QDF

Although the discrimination of two classes is vital knowledge for science, technologies, and applications of human society, most researchers do not understand the many defects of discriminant theory [15]. Discriminant functions, except for H-SVM and RIP, cannot discriminate LSD theoretically, and those NM and ER (=NM/n) have many defects [14]. Moreover, they do not understand the hierarchical structure of reliable NM and ER. Only RIP and H-SVM can discriminate LSD. MNM via RIP and NM via H-SVM are unique for data. "MNM = 0" is the clear definition of LSD. Other discriminant functions cannot discriminate LSD correctly, and those NMs are different by the different discriminant hyperplanes that are decided by the prior probability, discriminant threshold, and options, such as penalty c of soft-margin SVM (S-SVM). Only if two classes satisfy Fisher's assumption, NM decreases up to MNM and is equivalent to MNM. However, there is no good test for multivariate normal distribution.

Table 4 shows that SM1 and SM2 include two BGSs. The two M2s of the two Others are large values. M2 of BGS21 is zero. This means that BGS21, 100 training samples, and 100 test samples are LSD. Thus, "M2 = 0" shows a strong signal and is the most important for cancer diagnosis. Shinmura [18] shows that all M2s of 129 BGSs are larger than all M2 of 64 SMs using Alon data [1]. This fact may show the difference between the six old data in the first generation and 77 new data in the second generation. M2 of BGS22 is higher than M2 of SM2. Three M2s of other BGSs are less than the M2 of corresponding SM. Because we observe the same latter relations in other data, we consider many BGSs more useful than SMs in 77 new

Table 4 The discriminant results by RIP, Logistic Regression, LDF, and QDF

		RIP	Logistic		LDF		QDF	
SM/bgs	M2	MNM	FP	FN	FP	FN	FP	FN
SM1	0.9784	0	0	0	0	**2**	0	0
bgs11	0.8345	0	0	0	**1**	**8**	0	**1**
bgs12	0.0432	0	0	0	**1**	**8**	0	**1**
bgs13	6.8273	**7**	**0**	**13**	**0**	**34**	**0**	**4**
SM2	0.5827	0	0	0	0	**1**	0	0
bgs21	**0**	0	0	0	0	**7**	0	0
bgs22	1.3669	0	0	0	0	**10**	0	**1**
bgs23	8.3381	**9**	**1**	**46**	**3**	**35**	**0**	**16**

data. The RIP column shows MNM. "NM = 0" of H-SVM is equivalent to MNM because H-SVM can separate two classes correctly. Thus, we omit the NM of H-SVM. The sum of the False Positive (FP) and False Negative (FN) is equal to NM. Breast5 consists of ten healthy subjects and 129 cancer patients. The sample sizes of the two classes are unbalanced, which causes a harmful effect on discrimination. Many misclassified subjects are healthy subjects. Six NMs of logistic regression are zero for two SMs and four BGSs, respectively. Six NMs of Fisher's LDF are not zero. QDF discriminates two SMs and BGS21 correctly. Three NMs of BGSs are one. We confirmed that RIP and logistic regression could correctly discriminate ten SMs and 39 BGSs included in Breast5. Because the last ten Others in each SM are not LSD, ten MNMs found by RIP and ten NMs found by logistic regression are not zero. Ten NMs from logistic regression are larger than ten MNMs. Next, we check the NMs using Fisher's LDF. Although seven NMs of ten SMs are zero, three NMs of SMs and 49 NMs of all BGSs are not zero. This is the reason why ordinary discriminant functions are useless in these themes.

Hierarchical Reliability Categories of NM by Discriminant Functions

We had already pointed out the four problems of discriminant functions based on the variance-covariance matrix using six ordinary data [14, 15]. Also, we confirmed that six ERs of old data using Fisher's LDF were very high, and the ER of Tien [22] is over 17%. Failure to correctly identify LSD is the main reason for high-dimensional gene research confusion. Medical researches adopted the wrong approach of using cluster analysis without discriminant analysis. They are not interested in misclassified patients for cancer diagnosis. In 2015, we discriminated against the six old data and decomposed the six data into many SMs and BGSs within 54 days because RIP can discriminate LSD theoretically and release us from the curse of high-dimensional data. QDF separates two classes using the quadratic discriminant hyperplane and can be categorized as a non-linear discriminant function, so the four SMs and 13 BGSs are zero. These results are better than other LDFs. However, QDF needs more $p \times (p - 1)/2$ variables than LDFs. There is no research to focus on the defect of the many variables model. Table 4 suggests we categorize discriminant functions and the reliability of their discovered NMs into four categories. Only RIP, H-SVM, and logistic regression can discriminate SM and BGs correctly.

1. NM via RIP and H-SVM.
2. NM via logistic regression.
3. NM via other LDFs, such as Fisher's LDF, S-SVM, Lasso, and RDA.
4. NM via QDF and kernel-SVM that belong to the non-linear discriminant function and have the complex discriminant hyperplanes with many variables.

ML researchers must more precisely study the reliability of NMs found by the nine classifiers. Those are quite different among the categories of DT and RF, k-means, k-NN, cluster analysis, Naïve Bayes, and multilayer perceptron (or Deep Learning). Moreover, those NMs are different by data and analysts. They misunderstand that the complex algorithm classifiers, such as kernel-SVM are superior to simple linear hyperplane by RIP and H-SVM. They must stop using overlapped data because the evaluation is unclear. For methods that require setting options, they must evaluate several patters of options and choose the best option using much data. If they evaluate nine classifiers by many SMs in detail, they can understand my claim soon. They falsely believe that the reliability of discriminant functions and classifiers are the same. If the two classes have not the same values, the decision tree by the specialist, instead of the program, can always classify two classes by "NM = 0". The author developed the diagnostic logic of electrocardiogram (ECG) data using LDF and QDF at the Osaka International Cancer Institute (formerly the Center for Adult Diseases) in 1971–1975. The far superior DT developed by doctors for discriminant functions was the motivation for starting the study of discriminant theory. However, doctors updated the logic of the developed DT using new patients over one-year. That is the real validation (External Check, EC) using external samples (ES). Engineering researchers without our experience misunderstand that both DT and SVM are the same classifiers. They forget they must update their decision rule using ES and build the real system of a DT for cancer diagnosis. H-SVM and S-SVM are easier than Kernel-SVM for modifying the decision rule using ES and building a real system. However, Kernel-SVM is far easier than other classifiers, although we must choose the Kernel-SVM and S-SVM options.

6 Conclusion

Because of the diagnostic logic failure for ECG data using Fisher's LDF and QDF, we started to develop a new theory for discriminant analysis in 1975 and established it in 2015. RIP, based on the MNM criterion, discriminated six data as the applied problems of choice for the new discriminant theory. We found that the six data are LSD and could decompose data into many SMs. Because all SMs and BGSs are small samples, we could analyze those with statistical methods and propose gene diagnosis using microarrays. Although we are not physicians, the vital signal of LSD helps us to develop the correct gene diagnosis of old data as a screening method for physicians. However, we could not ask for validation by the researchers of the six projects. After many considerations, we found two universal data structures of LSD. We can decompose every data into the SMs and BGSs if data are LSD. Moreover, RIP discriminates against the 73 new microarrays of 13 different carcinomas. Because all microarrays over two classes are LSD, we decompose 73 microarrays into the first ten SMs. In this paper, we examine several vital points by ten SMs and 49 BGSs of Breast5, an instance of breast cancer [7].

Because we confirm that all microarrays collected until 2017 are LSD, we expect to obtain the same results of other gene data, such as RNA-seq and microarrays. Although cancers are heterogeneous diseases, the expression data of genes have remarkable signals, such as LSD. Thus, we can conclude the correct results. If every physician chooses the correct approach, the first step of cancer gene diagnosis is relatively straightforward. We sincerely expect physicians to treat cancer in human patients more efficiently. ML researchers misinterpret the importance of validation by test samples. Medical studies must examine our engineering results. There are the following validations:

1. Physicians found over 100 genes, such as oncogenes, tumor suppressor genes, and other genes. If some SMs and BGSs include these genes, the number of genes tell us the right signals for cancer gene diagnosis.
2. Two studies by NIH, such as Liver3 (GSE14520) and Liver10 (GSE14520), prepared the genome cohort [3, 8–10, 21, 24, 25]. Distinguished Professor Honjo promoted the validation via the genome cohort in Japan. Professor Matsuda, of Kyoto Univ.'s Graduate School of Medicine, organized the Nagahama Genome Cohort project for epidemiology. We expect NIH researchers will validate our results with their genome cohort. For this purpose, we can offer detailed information to them.
3. The authors seriously expect ML researchers to participate in a new study of indicators that show the importance of many SMs and BGSs. We hope that they develop better indicators than M2 of Method 1 if they wish to contribute to the real cancer diagnosis.

Acknowledgments Our research depends on the powerful LINGO solver and JMP for real data examinations to achieve our studies supported by CuMiDa.

References

1. U. Alon et al., Broad patterns of gene expression revealed by clustering analysis of cancer and normal colon tissues probed by oligonucleotide arrays. Proc. Natl. Acad. Sci. U. S. A. **96**, 6745–6750 (1999)
2. C.F. Bruno, B.C. Eduardo, I.G. Bruno, D. Marcio, CuMiDa: An extensively curated microarray database for benchmarking and testing of machine learning approaches in cancer research. J. Comput. Biol. **26-0**, 1–11 (2019)

3. S. Chen, H. Fang, J. Li, J. Shi, et al., Microarray analysis for expression profiles of lncRNAs and circRNAs in rat liver after brain-dead donor liver transplantation. Biomed Res Int **2019**, 5604843 (2019). PMID: 31828106
4. S. Chiaretti et al., Gene expression profile of adult T-cell acute lymphocytic leukemia identifies distinct subsets of patients with different response to therapy and survival. Blood **103/7**, 2771–2778 (2004)
5. T.R. Golub et al., Molecular classification of cancer: Class discovery and class prediction by gene expression monitoring. Science **286/5439**, 531–537 (1999)
6. P.A. Lachenbruch, M.R. Mickey, Estimation of error rates in the discriminant analysis. Technometrics **10**(1), 11 (1968)
7. R.G. Liu et al., Association of FABP5 expression with poor survival in triple-negative breast cancer implication for retinoic acid therapy. Am. J. Pathol. **178**(3), 997–1008 (2011). https://doi.org/10.1016/j.ajpath.2010.11.075
8. Y. Lu, W. Xu, J. Ji, D. Feng, et al., Alternative splicing of the cell fate determinant Numb in hepatocellular carcinoma. Hepatology **62**(4), 1122–1131 (2015). PMID: 26058814
9. S. Roessler, H.L. Jia, A. Budhu, M. Forgues, et al., A unique metastasis gene signature enables prediction of tumor relapse in early-stage hepatocellular carcinoma patients. Cancer Res. **70**(24), 10202–10212 (2010). PMID: 21159642
10. S. Roessler, E.L. Long, A. Budhu, Y. Chen, et al., Integrative genomic identification of genes on 8p associated with hepatocellular carcinoma progression and patient survival. Gastroenterology **142**(4), 957–966.e12 (2012). PMID: 22202459
11. J.P. Sall, L. Creighton, A. Lehman, *JMP Start Statistics, Third Edition* (SAS Institute Inc, 2004). (Shinmura S, supervise Japanese version)
12. L. Schrage, *Optimization Modeling with LINGO* (LINDO Systems Inc., 2006)
13. S. Shinmura, A new algorithm of the linear discriminant function using integer programming, in *New Trends in Probability and Statistics*, vol. 5, (2000), pp. 133–142
14. S. Shinmura, Four serious problems and new facts of the discriminant analysis, in *Operations Research and Enterprise Systems*, ed. by E. Pinson et al., (Springer, Berlin, 2015), pp. 15–30
15. S. Shinmura, *New Theory of Discriminant Analysis After R. Fisher* (Springer, 2016)
16. S. Shinmura, *High-Dimensional Microarray Data Analysis* (Springer, 2019)
17. S. Shinmura, Release from the curse of high dimensional data analysis, in *Big Data, Cloud Computing, and Data Science Engineering*, Studies in Computational Intelligence 844, (2019), pp. 173–196
18. S. Shinmura, Cancer gene diagnosis of 84 microarrays using rank of 100-fold cross-validation, in *Transactions on Computational Science & Computational Intelligence, Advances in Computer Vision and Computational Biology, Proceedings from IPCV'20, HIMS'20, BIOCOMP'20, and BIOENG'20*, ed. by H.R. Arabnia, (Springer Nature, Cham, 2021), pp. 805-822
19. M.A. Shipp et al., Diffuse large B-cell lymphoma outcome prediction by gene-expression profiling and supervised machine learning. Nat. Med. **8**, 68–74 (2002)
20. D. Singh et al., Gene expression correlates of clinical prostate cancer behavior. Cancer Cell **1**, 203–209 (2002)
21. Y. Sun, F. Ji, M.R. Kumar, X. Zheng, et al., Transcriptome integration analysis in hepatocellular carcinoma reveals discordant intronic miRNA-host gene pairs in expression. Int J Biol Sci **13**(11), 1438–1449 (2017). PMID: 29209147
22. E. Tian et al., The role of the Wnt-signaling antagonist DKK1 in the development of osteolytic lesions in multiple myeloma. N. Engl. J. Med. **349**(26), 2483–2494 (2003)
23. V. Vapnik, *The Nature of Statistical Learning Theory* (Springer, 1999)
24. Y. Wang, B. Gao, P.Y. Tan, Y.A. Handoko, et al., Genome-wide CRISPR knockout screens identify NCAPG as an essential oncogene for hepatocellular carcinoma tumor growth. FASEB J. **33**(8), 8759–8770 (2019). PMID: 31022357
25. X. Zhao, S. Parpart, A. Takai, S. Roessler, et al., Integrative genomics identifies YY1AP1 as an oncogenic driver in EpCAM(+) AFP(+) hepatocellular carcinoma. Oncogene **34**(39), 5095–5104 (2015). PMID: 25597408

Index

H. R. Arabnia et al. (eds.), *Advances in Computer Vision and Computational Biology*, Transactions on Computational Science and Computational Intelligence,
https://doi.org/10.1007/978-3-030-71051-4

D

E

I

M

N

Q

R

T